RAD - Aide

**OrangeBooks Publication**

1st Floor, Rajhans Arcade, Mall Road, Kohka, Bhilai, Chhattisgarh 490020

**Website**: **www.orangebooks.in**

---



**First Edition, 2025**

**ISBN:** 978-93-7426-873-5

**Price:** Rs. 2999.00



Printed in India

# RAD-AIDE

## YOUR ESSENTIAL GUIDE TO RADIATION RELATED TERMINOLOGY

A Pocket glossary for Radiation Professionals
VOLUME - I

**RAJIV KR SINGH | SUBRATA ROY**

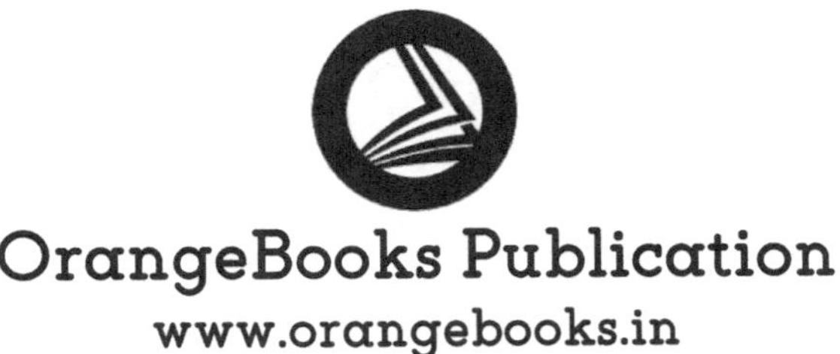

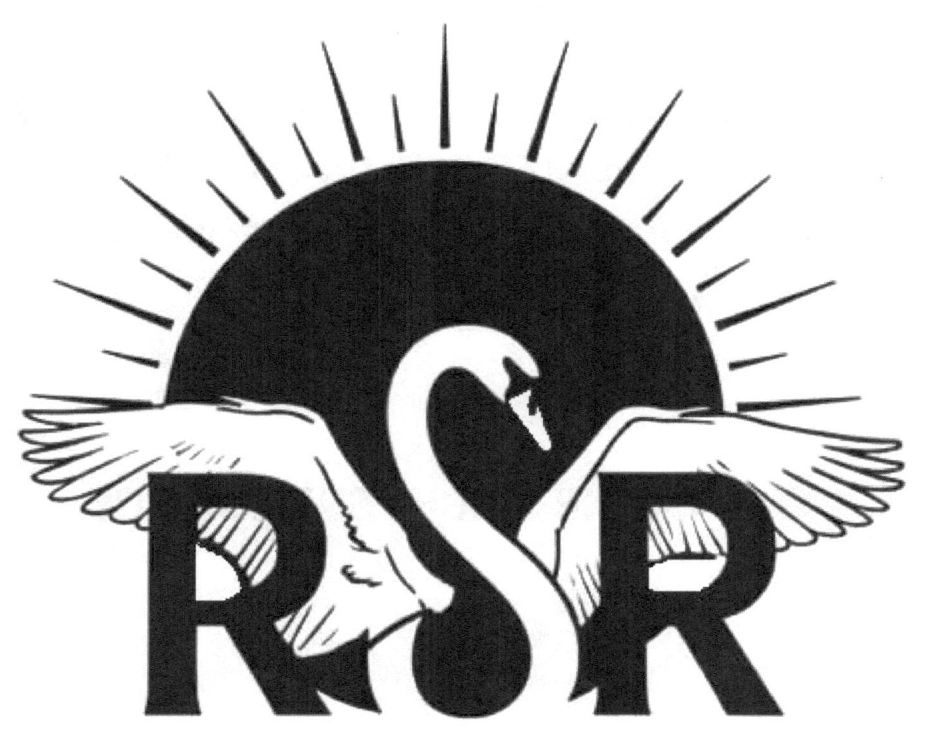
RSR

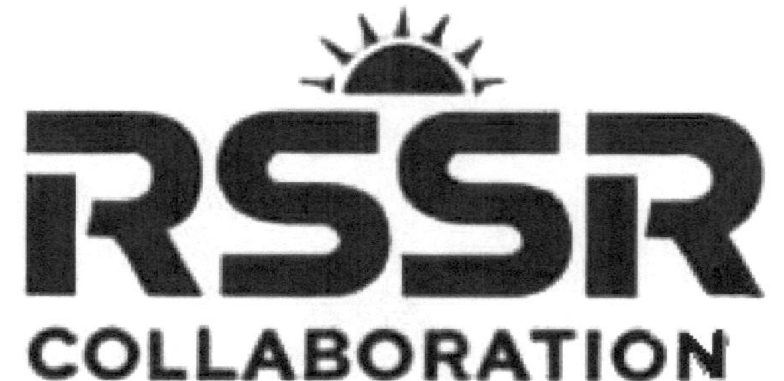
RSSR
COLLABORATION

# About the Author

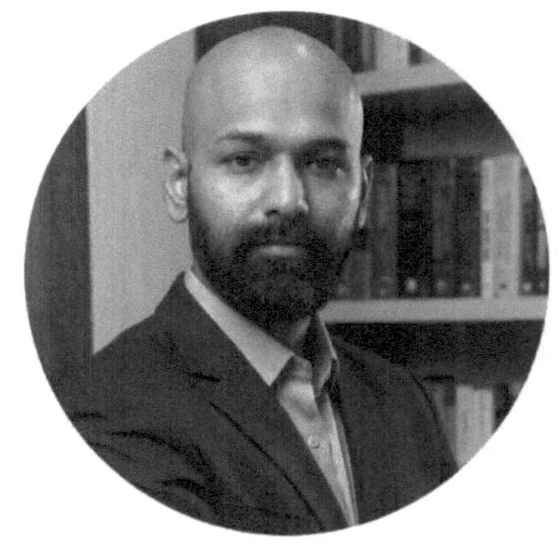

**Dr. Rajiv Kr Singh & Subrata Roy**

*Dr. Rajiv Kumar Singh (HonD) is a seasoned Senior Radiation Therapy Professional with over 18 years of dedicated clinical experience in radiation oncology. Currently serving as the Senior Chief Radiotherapist Officer at APEX Superspeciality Hospital, Varanasi, he plays a key leadership role in delivering precision-based radiotherapy, guiding clinical teams, and ensuring safe, efficient, and evidence-informed treatment workflows. Throughout his career, he has demonstrated unwavering commitment to compassionate patient care, high clinical standards, and ethical practice.*

*Dr. Singh's professional journey spans several respected cancer centres across India, including Dharamshila Narayana Superspeciality Hospital (Delhi), Shri Mata Vaishno Devi Narayana Superspeciality Hospital (J&K), Narayana Health (Bengaluru), AMRI Hospital (Kolkata) and Bhagwan Mahavir Cancer Institutes (Patna & Jaipur). Across these institutions, he gained extensive experience in advanced radiotherapy techniques including IMRT, VMAT, IGRT, SRS/SBRT, and adaptive radiotherapy workflows, contributing to treatment accuracy, patient safety, and technology-enhanced care.*

*Academically grounded, he holds a Diploma in Radio therapeutic Technology, a Bachelor's and Master's degree in Physics, and additional certifications in nutrition, therapeutic health, clinical computing, MOSAIQ documentation systems, and advanced life support. His multidisciplinary expertise strengthens his holistic understanding of cancer care and enhances his ability to integrate technology, safety protocols, and individualized treatment planning.*

*Dr. Singh is also an active academic contributor and speaker. He has delivered presentations at national seminars, CME programs, and workshops on topics such as motion management, digital documentation systems, immobilization techniques, and radiation therapy safety protocols. He has participated in major professional gatherings including ECAMPICON, ARTTI CON, and master classes on precision radiotherapy.*

***As a research contributor, he has authored scientific work, including "Role of Copper in Radiation," and written the book Radiation**: A Blessing in Disguise, reflecting his commitment to knowledge-sharing and patient education. His contributions have earned multiple recognitions, including an Honorary Doctorate from WCEPC and institutional awards for excellence, innovation, and service.*

*A professional member of ESTRO and ARTTI, Dr. Singh remains aligned with global standards of radiotherapy practice. His professional philosophy centers on precision, patient dignity, collaborative teamwork, and continuous learning. Through his leadership, clinical expertise, and academic engagement, he continues to play a meaningful role in advancing radiation therapy practice and improving the experience and outcomes of patients undergoing cancer treatment.*

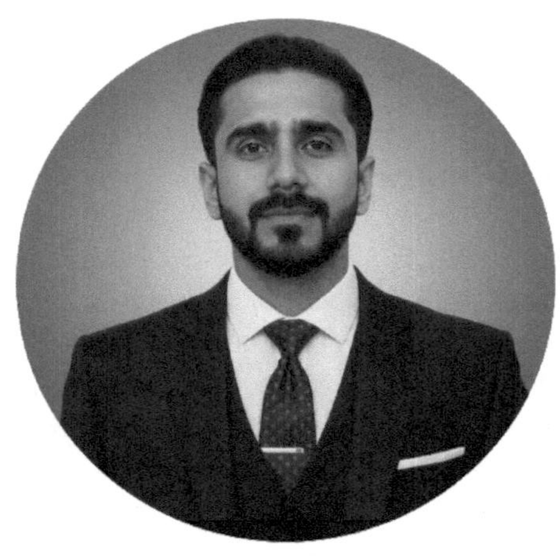

***Mr. Subrata Roy** is a distinguished Senior Radiation Therapist from India, with more than a decade of specialised experience in high precision radiation oncology, certified under the Atomic Energy Regulatory Board (AERB) through the e-LORA (e-Licensing of Radiation Applications) system. His professional journey is marked by clinical excellence, strong academic engagement, and demonstrated leadership in contemporary radiation oncology practice. A **Gold Medalist in the Bachelor of Radiation Therapy Technology** from the esteemed Tripura Institute of Paramedical Sciences, affiliated with Tripura University, Agartala, India, he has consistently demonstrated a strong commitment to delivering high-quality patient care through evidence-based practice and continuous professional development.*

*Mr. Roy currently serves as a Senior Radiation Therapist at Nanavati Max Super Speciality Hospital, Mumbai, one of India's leading tertiary cancer centres. In this role, he contributes extensively to the safe and precise delivery of advanced radiotherapy techniques, including stereotactic treatments, image-guided radiotherapy, and high-precision stereotactic radiosurgery (SRS) and stereotactic body radiotherapy (SBRT) workflows. His clinical practice is grounded in meticulous technical expertise, patient-centred care, and unwavering adherence to ethical and professional standards. His distinguished professional affiliations reflect a strong commitment to excellence and global engagement. He is associated with several esteemed regulatory and professional bodies, including the Health and Care Professions Council (HCPC, UK), the European Society for Radiotherapy and Oncology (ESTRO, EU), the American Society of Clinical Oncology (ASCO, USA), the Association of Radiation Therapy Technologists of India (ARTTI), the Indian Society of Radiographers and Technologists (ISRT), and the Asia and Middle East Society of Therapeutic Radiation and Oncology (AMSTRO, UAE). These affiliations underscore his dedication to maintaining international standards of clinical practice, safety, and professional integrity. In parallel with his clinical responsibilities, Mr. Roy is actively involved in academic and research initiatives. His areas of interest include motion management strategies, surface-guided radiation therapy, cone-beam computed tomography (CBCT) image verification, workflow optimisation, and radiation safety. He has contributed to scholarly publications, practice-improvement projects, and scientific discourse within the radiotherapy community. His growing body of work reflects a strong focus on bridging the gap between clinical application and research-driven innovation.*

*As a Radiation Therapist educator, he has served as a faculty member and invited speaker at several workshops, including those organised under the Asia-Pacific Radiation Oncology Network (IAEA ASPRONET), as well as in multiple training programmes for radiation therapists across India. His teaching philosophy centres on empowering Radiation Therapists (RTTs) through practical skill-building, technological literacy, and a strong understanding of quality and safety frameworks. His efforts have contributed to the development of a confident, research-aware, and practice-ready radiation therapy workforce.*

*Mr. Roy also contributes to the global radiotherapy academic community through his role as a peer reviewer for several national and international journals. In this capacity, he critically evaluates research manuscripts and supports the maintenance of high scientific standards, methodological rigour, and ethical publication practices. His professional philosophy emphasises precision, patient safety, interprofessional collaboration, and lifelong learning. Whether working with cutting-edge technologies, refining complex treatment workflows, or mentoring colleagues, he consistently demonstrates a balanced blend of clinical acumen and academic insight. Through his multifaceted contributions, he remains dedicated to strengthening clinical practice, advancing research, and fostering the growth and recognition of the radiation therapy profession.*

***Current Affiliation :***

***Mr. Subrata Roy***

***HCPC (UK), ESTRO (EU), ASCO (US), AERB (IN), ARTTI (IN), ISRT (IN), AMSTRO (UAE)***

***Senior Radiation Therapist (Assistant Manager)***

***Radiation Oncology Department, Nanavati Max Super Speciality Hospital, Mumbai, India***

# Preface to the First Edition

The intertwined fields of Radiation Oncology, Nuclear Medicine, and Diagnostic Radiology represent the frontline in modern cancer diagnosis and treatment. The rapid advancement in these disciplines—from molecular imaging and targeted radiopharmaceuticals to sophisticated radiation delivery—necessitates a comprehensive, up-to-date, and accessible resource for all practicing professionals.

This First Edition of Rad Aide is specifically crafted for Radiation Professionals, including residents, medical physicists, dosimetrist, radiation therapists, and practicing oncologists. Our goal is to synthesize the essential knowledge required to master the complex workflow of high-quality radiation therapy.

A Comprehensive Look at the Radiation Workflow

This book is organized to systematically follow the patient journey through the treatment process, from initial staging to final delivery and quality assurance.

**Diagnostic Foundations:** We begin with a high-yield review of Diagnostic Radiology and Nuclear Medicine principles, emphasizing their role in staging and target delineation. This includes PET, SPECT, and functional MRI, which are critical for modern treatment planning.

**Treatment Planning System (TPS) & Planning:** Detailed sections are devoted to the art and science of treatment Planning, focusing on the core functions and advanced capabilities of the TPS. Topics include contouring, dose optimization, biological modeling, and plan evaluation.

**Radiation Delivery (LINAC Machine):** Comprehensive coverage of the workhorse of radiation therapy: the LINAC Machine. This includes the principles of machine operation, beam modifiers, various delivery techniques (e.g., IMRT, VMAT, SBRT), and the safe execution of treatment.

**Quality Assurance (QA):** A dedicated, critical section covers QA protocols for all aspects of the process—from daily machine checks and patient-specific QA to chart checks and regulatory compliance.

**Why Rad Aide?**

**The demands on today's radiation professional require an intimate understanding of Radiation physics, biology, and clinical application. This volume serves as the missing link that connects the theoretical principles learned in textbooks with the practical, multi-disciplinary requirements of clinical practice. It is designed to be a quick, reliable reference for**:

Mastering the Physics and Biology underlying all modern techniques.

Standardizing technical approaches to TPS operation and treatment delivery.

Preparing for board certification and technical competency exams.

We sincerely believe that by focusing on the entire continuum of care—from imaging to dose delivery and quality control—Rad Aide will be an indispensable tool for every member of the radiation team.

**The Editors**<br>
**Dr. Rajiv Kumar Singh & Subrata Roy**<br>
*January, 2026*

# ✦ By Dr. Rajiv Kumar Singh and Subrata Roy

**RAD-Aide** presents up-to-date and accessible information on the core vocabulary of modern radiation therapy and allied sciences. It focuses on clear explanations of technical and clinical terminology frequently encountered in radiotherapy practice. This **1st Edition** has been created to support radiation therapists, educators, researchers, and students in understanding complex concepts with simplicity, precision, and clinical relevance. This reference is the result of more than a year of extensive research, academic review, and technical compilation. It comprises **over 13,000 carefully selected and defined terms** to meet the needs of professionals engaged in both clinical and academic radiotherapy environments. Each entry provides a concise meaning, relevant related terminology, and contextual examples—reflecting the language and evolution of contemporary radiation oncology.

The content of **RAD-Aide** draws from global radiotherapy literature, professional practice guidelines, and the latest research released by internationally recognized organizations. The authors have referenced peer-reviewed journals, standard oncology textbooks, institutional protocols, and leading radiotherapy publications to maintain the highest standards of accuracy, clarity, and practical value.This collective effort captures the terminology used across 21st-century radiotherapy departments and research institutions worldwide.

For this first edition, more than **1,000 new technical entries** have been incorporated, covering rapidly advancing domains such as adaptive radiotherapy, artificial intelligence in treatment planning, motion management, proton therapy, MR-guided radiotherapy, image guidance, and stereotactic body radiotherapy (SBRT). Many established concepts have also been updated with s aligned to current technological innovations and clinical practices. Consulting this resource offers a reliable and efficient way to access essential radiotherapy terminology—serving not only as a quick reference but also as a tool for continuous professional development. It is designed for use in clinical departments, academic institutions, and research environments, supporting learners and experienced professionals alike.

We envision that **RAD-Aide** will become a standard reference for radiation therapists, educators, and investigators, helping bridge the gap between theoretical knowledge and real-world application. It stands as a tribute to the ever-advancing field of radiation therapy, where innovation and compassion work together for the benefit of patients.

**With highest regard and gratitude**
To all radiation therapy professionals, educators, and researchers whose pursuit of excellence continues to inspire and improve patient care.

**Dr. Rajiv Kumar Singh**
**Subrata Roy**
*Editors and Compilers*
*First Edition — 2026*

## RAD-Aide

**Guide to Using RAD-Aide**
**RAD-Aide** is designed to provide concise and standardized s of technical, clinical, anatomical, and physics-related terminology used in radiotherapy.
It serves as a practical and authoritative reference for radiation therapists, medical physicists, dosimetrists, and allied professionals, supporting clinical practice, education, and research.
This guide explains how to use the reference efficiently.

**Format of Entries**

**Each term in** RAD-Aide **follows a unified structure to ensure clarity and rapid understanding:**

## WORD (noun):

*A clear, precise of the term.*
**Related Terms:** Associated or synonymous words
**Example in Radiotherapy:** A short clinical example (≤ 40 words)

## Explanation of Each Section

1. **WORD (noun)**
   - The term appears in bold, followed by its part of speech.
   - **The is concise, accurate, and focused on radiotherapy application.**
     Example:
     ***Collimator angle (noun):*** *The rotational position of the beam-defining jaws around the beam axis.*

2. **Related Terms**
   - **Synonyms or associated terminology supporting conceptual linkage.**
     Example:
     ***Related Terms:*** *Gantry angle, couch angle*

3. **Example in Radiotherapy**
   - **A short clinical scenario demonstrating real-world usage.**
     Example:
     ***Example in Radiotherapy:*** *Adjusted to match field shape with patient anatomy.*

## Using RAD-Aide in Daily Practice

1. **Clinical Use**
   - Clarify anatomy, OARs, treatment techniques, and procedural vocabulary.

2. **Technical Use**
   - Understand machine terminology, imaging parameters, and QA processes.

3. **Educational Use**
   - Support structured learning for students and junior clinicians.

4. **Research Use**
   - Standardize terminology across publications and multidisciplinary communication.

## Tips for Efficient Use

- Terms are organized alphabetically for quick lookup.
- Use *Related Terms* for conceptual linking.
- Refer to clinical examples for contextual clarity.
- Use alongside manuals and TPS guides for optimal understanding.

## Sample Entry

**Couch shift (noun):** Translational or rotational adjustment of the treatment couch to align the patient with the planned isocenter.

**Related Terms:** Image-guided correction, registration error

**Example in Radiotherapy:** Applied after CBCT match to correct patient position during daily treatment.

**RAD-Aide** serves as a unified reference to standardize radiotherapy terminology, enhance communication among oncology teams, and support precise, safe, and effective patient care.

# Acknowledgments

*The completion of this book would not have been possible without the support and expertise of many individualsI wish to express my profound appreciation to my editorial team, whose meticulous attention to detail and unwavering commitment to excellence greatly enhanced the final manuscript. I am equally indebted to my research collaborators and subject-matter experts, whose thoughtful perspectives informed and enriched the content presented here. I extend particular thanks to my family and close colleagues for their encouragement, patience, and belief in this work. Their support sustained me throughout the writing process. To all who contributed—directly or indirectly—to the realization of this book, I offer my deepest gratitude.*

***Dr. Ankita Patel*** *(Director) Apex Superspeciality Hospital, Varanasi, Uttar Pradesh*

***Dr. Neha Gupta*** *(HOD) Radiation Oncology Dept. Apex Superspeciality Hospital, Varanasi, Uttar Pradesh*

***Dr. Gaurav Goswami*** *(Consultant) Radiation Oncology Dept. Apex Superspeciality Hospital, Varanasi, Uttar Pradesh*

***Dr. Upendra Giri (CRSO)*** *Medical Physicists Radiation Oncology Dept. Apex Superspeciality Hospital, Varanasi, Uttar Pradesh*

***Sathi Sarkar*** *(Scientific Assistant –B) Radiation Oncology, ACTREC, TMC, Navi Mumbai*

# Contents

# A

1. **Absolute dose (noun):** The total amount of radiation energy absorbed in a given mass of tissue, measured in Gray (Gy).
 **Related Terms:** Absorbed dose, Dose measurement, and Dose calibration.
 **Example in Radiotherapy:** Absolute dose verification was performed before patient treatment to confirm machine output accuracy.
2. **Absorbed dose (noun):** The amount of radiation energy deposited per unit mass of tissue, expressed in Gray (Gy).
 **Related Terms:** Absolute dose, Equivalent dose, Dose distribution.
 **Example in Radiotherapy:** "The absorbed dose to the spinal cord was kept within tolerance limits.
3. **Accuracy (noun):** The degree to which a measured value matches the true value.
 **Related Terms:** Precision, QA, and Calibration.
 **Example in Radiotherapy:** Daily image guidance improves the accuracy of patient positioning.
4. **Accelerator (noun):** A machine that produces high-energy beams of photons or particles for medical use.
 **Related Terms:** Linear accelerator, Cyclotron, Beam delivery system.
 **Example in Radiotherapy:** "The hospital's new accelerator supports advanced stereotactic treatments."
5. **Acetabulum (noun):** The cup-shaped cavity in the pelvis that forms the hip joint.
 **Related Terms:** Pelvic anatomy, femoral head, Ilium.
 **Example in Radiotherapy:** "Pelvic fields were designed to spare the acetabulum in hip-sparing protocols."
6. **Acquisition (noun):** The process of collecting imaging or data for planning or verification.
 **Related Terms:** Image capture, Data collection, Acquisition protocol.
 **Example in Radiotherapy:** "CBCT acquisition was completed before each fraction."
7. **Action level (noun):** A predefined threshold that triggers corrective action in quality control.
 **Related Terms:** Tolerance level, QA protocol, Safety limit.
 **Example in Radiotherapy:** "An action level of ±2 mm was set for patient setup errors."
8. **Active breathing control (noun):** A technique to manage respiratory motion by controlling breath-holds during imaging or treatment.
 **Related Terms:** Respiratory gating, DIBH, Motion management.
 **Example in Radiotherapy:** "Active breathing control minimized tumor motion in left breast irradiation."
9. **Adaptive planning (noun):** Modifying the treatment plan during the course of therapy to account for anatomical or biological changes.
 **Related Terms:** Adaptive radiotherapy, Plan modification, Image-guided radiotherapy.
 **Example in Radiotherapy:** "Adaptive planning was required due to tumor shrinkage after week two."
10. **Adaptive radiotherapy (noun):** A treatment approach that uses updated imaging and planning to adapt to changes in patient anatomy or tumor response.
 **Related Terms:** Adaptive planning, IGRT, Replanning.
 **Example in Radiotherapy:** "Adaptive radiotherapy improved dose coverage for shrinking lung tumors."

11. **Add-on filter (noun):** An external device attached to the treatment head to modify beam quality or shape.
**Related Terms:** Beam modifier, Compensator, Wedge filter.
**Example in Radiotherapy:** "An add-on filter was used to reduce skin dose."

12. **Adenocarcinoma (noun):** A malignant tumor originating from glandular epithelial cells.
**Related Terms:** Carcinoma, Histopathology, Tumor type.
**Example in Radiotherapy:** "The patient was treated for adenocarcinoma of the prostate with IMRT."

13. **Administration route (noun):** The path by which a drug or agent is given to a patient.
**Related Terms:** Intravenous, Oral, Intramuscular.
**Example in Radiotherapy:** "The chemotherapy drug was administered via an intravenous route."

14. **Adverse effect (noun):** An unintended and harmful outcome resulting from treatment.
**Related Terms:** Side effect, Complication, Toxicity.
**Example in Radiotherapy:** "Skin erythema was recorded as an adverse effect after week three."

15. **Afterloader (noun):** A device used in brachytherapy to remotely position radioactive sources in applicators.
**Related Terms:** HDR brachytherapy, Source loader, Applicator.
**Example in Radiotherapy:** "The afterloader automatically retracted the source after the dwell time."

16. **Alignment (noun):** Positioning of the patient or equipment to ensure correct beam targeting.
**Related Terms:** Positioning, Setup, Isocenter.
**Example in Radiotherapy:** "Laser alignment was checked before beam delivery."

17. **Alpha particle (noun):** A positively charged particle consisting of two protons and two neutrons, emitted in radioactive decay.
**Related Terms:** Alpha radiation, Beta particle, Radioisotope.
**Example in Radiotherapy:** "Alpha particles have high LET, making them highly damaging over short distances."

18. **Alpha-beta ratio (noun):** A radiobiological parameter describing tissue sensitivity to fractionation.
**Related Terms:** Fractionation sensitivity, BED, Radiobiology.
**Example in Radiotherapy:** "Prostate cancer typically has a low alpha-beta ratio."

19. **Alternative fractionation (noun):** Any fractionation schedule differing from conventional 2 Gy per fraction.
**Related Terms:** Hypofractionation, Hyperfractionation, Accelerated treatment.
**Example in Radiotherapy:** "Alternative fractionation reduced overall treatment time to two weeks."

20. **Aluminium filter (noun):** A filter made of aluminum used to shape or harden the radiation beam.
**Related Terms:** Beam filtration, Attenuator, Wedge filter.
**Example in Radiotherapy:** "An aluminium filter was inserted to remove low-energy photons."

21. **Anatomical landmark (noun):** A recognizable structure used for patient positioning or contouring.
**Related Terms:** Fiducial marker, Bony landmark, Positioning reference.
**Example in Radiotherapy:** "The iliac crest was used as an anatomical landmark during simulation."

22. **Anatomical positioning (noun):** The arrangement of the body or its parts for imaging or treatment.
**Related Terms:** Patient setup, Immobilization, Positioning protocol.
**Example in Radiotherapy:** "Supine anatomical positioning was chosen for breast irradiation."

23. **Anatomy (noun):** The study or description of body structures.
**Related Terms:** Physiology, Structure, Morphology.
**Example in Radiotherapy:** "Knowledge of pelvic anatomy is critical in contouring."

24. **Angiogenesis (noun):** The formation of new blood vessels from existing vasculature.
**Related Terms:** Tumor growth, Vascularization, Antiangiogenic therapy.
**Example in Radiotherapy:** "Radiotherapy can indirectly inhibit tumor growth by affecting angiogenesis."

25. **Anisotropy (noun):** Variation in a property when measured in different directions.
**Related Terms:** Isotropy, Scatter pattern, Source anisotropy.
**Example in Radiotherapy:** "Source anisotropy was corrected for in brachytherapy dose calculations."

26. **Anode (noun):** Positively charged electrode in X-ray tubes where electrons strike to produce X-rays.
**Related Terms:** Cathode, X-ray tube, Target.
**Example in Radiotherapy:** "The rotating anode allowed higher tube currents for imaging."

27. **Anterior (noun):** Front surface of the body or organ.
**Related Terms:** Posterior, Superior, Inferior.
**Example in Radiotherapy:** "Markers were placed on the anterior chest wall for setup."

28. **Anterior-posterior field (noun):** Radiation beam entering from front to back of patient.
**Related Terms:** AP/PA field, Beam arrangement.
**Example in Radiotherapy:** "An anterior-posterior field was used for spine irradiation."

29. **Anthropomorphic phantom (noun):** Human-shaped model used for dosimetry or QA.
**Related Terms:** QA phantom, Dose measurement, Calibration.
**Example in Radiotherapy:** "An anthropomorphic phantom verified treatment planning accuracy."

30. **Aperture (noun):** Opening through which radiation passes, shaped by collimators or blocks.
**Related Terms:** Collimation, Field shaping, MLC.
**Example in Radiotherapy:** "A custom aperture was designed to spare the spinal cord."

31. **Application setup (noun):** Preparation and positioning of applicators or devices for treatment.
**Related Terms:** Brachytherapy setup, Immobilization, QA.
**Example in Radiotherapy:** "Application setup was verified before HDR brachytherapy."

32. **Applicator (noun):** Device delivering radiation directly to or near a tumor.
**Related Terms:** Brachytherapy, Catheter, Mold.
**Example in Radiotherapy:** "The vaginal applicator ensured accurate dose placement."

33. **Arc therapy (noun):** Technique delivering radiation continuously as the gantry rotates.
**Related Terms:** VMAT, RapidArc, Conformal therapy.
**Example in Radiotherapy:** "Arc therapy shortened treatment time significantly."

34. **Area monitoring (noun):** Measurement of radiation levels in treatment or work areas.
**Related Terms:** Radiation survey, Dosimetry, Safety monitoring.
**Example in Radiotherapy:** "Area monitoring confirmed radiation leakage was negligible."

35. **Area under curve (noun):** Mathematical integral representing cumulative dose or distribution.
**Related Terms:** Dose-volume histogram, Statistics, Treatment evaluation.
**Example in Radiotherapy:** "The area under the DVH curve indicated adequate target coverage."

36. **Artifact (noun):** Image distortion unrelated to patient anatomy.
**Related Terms:** Image quality, CT scan error, Correction.
**Example in Radiotherapy:** "Dental fillings caused CT artifacts during planning."

37. **Artificial intelligence (noun):** Computer algorithms performing tasks requiring human-like reasoning.
**Related Terms:** Machine learning, Automation, Auto-segmentation.
**Example in Radiotherapy:** "Artificial intelligence improved contouring efficiency."

38. **Assignment of isocentre (noun):** Defining the fixed treatment beam intersection point in planning.
**Related Terms:** Isocenter, Beam geometry, Target localization.
**Example in Radiotherapy:** "Isocentre assignment aligned with tumor centroid."

39. **Asymmetry (noun):** Unequal beam output or field distribution.
**Related Terms:** Beam flatness, QA, Calibration.
**Example in Radiotherapy:** "QA detected asymmetry in the photon beam profile."

40. **Attenuation (noun):** Reduction of radiation intensity as it passes through matter.
**Related Terms:** Absorption, Scatter, Shielding.
**Example in Radiotherapy:** "Beam attenuation was corrected in treatment planning."

41. **Attenuation coefficient (noun):** Measure describing how strongly a material reduces radiation per unit thickness.
**Related Terms:** Linear attenuation, Density, Tissue composition.
**Example in Radiotherapy:** "Bone's high attenuation coefficient was considered in dose calculation."

42. **Attenuator (noun):** Device reducing beam intensity before it reaches patient.
**Related Terms:** Filter, Compensator, Shield.
**Example in Radiotherapy:** "A wedge attenuator modified beam profile."

43. **Audit (noun):** Systematic review of processes or data for compliance and accuracy.
**Related Terms:** QA, Peer review, Verification.
**Example in Radiotherapy:** "An audit confirmed adherence to treatment protocols."

44. **Auto-matching (noun):** Automatic image registration aligning patient setup images with reference images.
**Related Terms:** IGRT, Image fusion, CBCT.
**Example in Radiotherapy:** "Auto-matching reduced setup time in daily CBCT."

45. **Auto-segmentation (noun):** Software-based automatic contouring of anatomical structures or targets.
**Related Terms:** Artificial intelligence, Planning efficiency, Contouring.
**Example in Radiotherapy:** "Auto-segmentation quickly outlined OARs for planning."

46. **Automatic exposure control (noun):** Imaging feature adjusting X-ray output to maintain image quality with minimal dose.
**Related Terms:** Image optimization, Patient safety, Dose reduction.
**Example in Radiotherapy:** "Automatic exposure control minimized imaging dose during setup."

47. **Automation (noun):** Use of technology to perform tasks with minimal human input.
**Related Terms:** Workflow efficiency, AI, Robotics.
**Example in Radiotherapy:** "Automation streamlined patient-specific QA checks."

48. **Axial plane (noun):** Horizontal body plane dividing superior and inferior sections.
**Related Terms:** CT slice, Transverse plane, Imaging orientation.
**Example in Radiotherapy:** "The tumor was contoured in axial CT slices."

49. **Axilla (noun):** Underarm region containing lymph nodes, often treated in breast cancer.
**Related Terms:** Nodal basin, Lymphatic drainage, Target volume.
**Example in Radiotherapy:** "The axilla was included in nodal irradiation fields."

50. **Azimuth (noun):** Angular direction in a horizontal plane, relevant for beam orientation.
**Related Terms:** Gantry angle, Beam geometry, Coordinates.
**Example in Radiotherapy:** "The azimuth angle defined non-coplanar arc entry."

51. **Absorption coefficient (noun):** Quantifies radiation energy absorbed per unit material thickness.
**Related Terms:** Attenuation, Dose calculation, Material density.
**Example in Radiotherapy:** "Soft tissue's absorption coefficient affected planning CT numbers."

52. **Abstractor (noun):** Person summarizing or indexing information for reference or research.
**Related Terms:** Indexing, Research, Documentation.
**Example in Radiotherapy:** "The abstractor compiled study data for journal submission."

53. **Accelerated aging (noun):** Artificially speeding material aging using heat or radiation to predict lifespan.
**Related Terms:** Material testing, QA, Reliability.
**Example in Radiotherapy:** "Accelerated aging tested immobilization mask durability."

54. **Accelerated partial breast irradiation (noun):** Focused breast irradiation over shorter schedules for selected patients.
**Related Terms:** APBI, Hypofractionation, Brachytherapy.
**Example in Radiotherapy:** "APBI treated early-stage breast cancer in one week."

55. **Accelerator beam shaping (noun):** Modifying treatment beams to conform to target geometry.
**Related Terms:** MLC, Collimation, Conformal therapy.
**Example in Radiotherapy:** "MLCs provide precise accelerator beam shaping."

56. **Accelerator control system (noun):** Electronic interface managing beam delivery and safety.
**Related Terms:** LINAC, QA, Beam control.
**Example in Radiotherapy:** "The accelerator control system halted the beam during a fault."

57. **Access protocol (noun):** Authorized steps to use systems or patient data securely.
**Related Terms:** Security, Workflow, Compliance.
**Example in Radiotherapy:** "Staff followed an access protocol for treatment records."

58. **Accumulated dose (noun):** Total radiation absorbed over multiple sessions.
**Related Terms:** Cumulative dose, Dose summation, BED.
**Example in Radiotherapy:** "The accumulated dose to the lung was reviewed weekly."

59. **Accumulated error (noun):** Total deviation arising from repeated setup or delivery inaccuracies.
**Related Terms:** Systematic error, QA, Positioning.
**Example in Radiotherapy:** "Image guidance reduced accumulated error during SBRT."

60. **Acoustic impedance (noun):** Property of tissue affecting ultrasound reflection and transmission.
**Related Terms:** Ultrasound imaging, Echogenicity, Sound propagation.
**Example in Radiotherapy:** "Liver lesions were localized using acoustic impedance differences."

61. **Acoustic window (noun):** An Anatomical region permitting optimal ultrasound imaging.
**Related Terms:** Imaging access, Ultrasound guidance, Anatomy.
**Example in Radiotherapy:** "The rib space served as an acoustic window for scanning."

62. **Acquired image (noun):** Diagnostic or verification image captured during planning or treatment.
**Related Terms:** CBCT, kV imaging, and Data acquisition.
**Example in Radiotherapy:** "The acquired image verified patient positioning."

63. **Acquiring sequence (noun):** Ordered steps for capturing diagnostic or planning images.
**Related Terms:** Imaging protocol, MRI, CT scanning.
**Example in Radiotherapy:** "The MRI acquiring sequence minimized motion artifacts."

64. **Acquisition matrix (noun):** Pixel grid defining image resolution during scan.
**Related Terms:** Image quality, CT, MRI parameters.
**Example in Radiotherapy:** "A 512×512 acquisition matrix improved spatial resolution."

65. **Acquisition protocol (noun):** Standardized instructions for image or data capture.
**Related Terms:** Imaging protocol, QA, Workflow.
**Example in Radiotherapy:** "A CBCT acquisition protocol ensured consistency."

66. **Activation analysis (noun):** Identifying materials via radiation-induced radioactivity.
**Related Terms:** Neutron activation, Isotopes, Material testing.
**Example in Radiotherapy:** "Activation analysis detected contaminants in shielding."

67. **Activation dose (noun):** Radiation amount required to induce measurable radioactivity.
**Related Terms:** Neutron activation, Threshold dose, Nuclear physics.
**Example in Radiotherapy:** "The activation dose was determined for component testing."

68. **Activation product (noun):** Radioactive nuclide formed by irradiating materials.
**Related Terms:** Induced activity, Neutron flux, Isotopes.
**Example in Radiotherapy:** "Activation products were monitored after beam delivery."

69. **Active detector (noun):** A Radiation detector that generates an immediate electronic signal.
**Related Terms:** Ion chamber, Real-time dosimetry, QA.
**Example in Radiotherapy:** "The active detector measured beam output instantly."

70. **Active dosimeter (noun):** A Device giving real-time radiation dose readings.
**Related Terms:** Electronic dosimeter, QA, Personal monitoring.
**Example in Radiotherapy:** "Active dosimeters ensured staff radiation safety."

71. **Active matrix display (noun):** High-resolution screen using individual transistor-controlled pixels.
**Related Terms:** Flat-panel display, Digital imaging, QA.
**Example in Radiotherapy:** "An active matrix display improved CBCT review clarity."

72. **Active source (noun):** Radioactive material emitting radiation for treatment.
**Related Terms:** Brachytherapy source, Isotope, Dwell time.
**Example in Radiotherapy:** "The active source was loaded in the applicator."

73. **Activity concentration (noun):** Radioactivity per unit volume or mass.
**Related Terms:** Bq/ml, Radiopharmaceuticals, Source strength.
**Example in Radiotherapy:** "Activity concentration guided radiotracer dosing."

74. **Acute toxicity (noun):** Early adverse effects occurring during or shortly after treatment.
**Related Terms:** Side effects, Early toxicity, Radiobiology.
**Example in Radiotherapy:** "Skin erythema was an acute toxicity of breast RT."

75. **Additive noise (noun):** Random imaging interference added to true signal.
**Related Terms:** Image quality, SNR, Artifacts.
**Example in Radiotherapy:** "Filters reduced additive noise in portal images."

76. **Adaptive planning (noun):** Updating treatment plan during therapy to reflect anatomical or biological changes.
**Related Terms:** Adaptive radiotherapy, IGRT, Replanning.
**Example in Radiotherapy:** "Adaptive planning corrected for tumor shrinkage."

77. **Adaptive dose (noun):** Adjusted radiation dose based on real-time response or anatomy.
**Related Terms:** Dose adaptation, Replanning, Response-based therapy.
**Example in Radiotherapy:** "An adaptive dose strategy improved tumor control."

78. **Add-on device (noun):** Accessory attached to equipment for beam modification or positioning.
**Related Terms:** Beam modifier, Filter, Compensator.
**Example in Radiotherapy:** "A bolus was used as an add-on device."

79. **Adenoma (noun):** Benign tumor arising from glandular tissue.
**Related Terms:** Benign tumor, Histopathology, Non-malignant.
**Example in Radiotherapy:** "The pituitary adenoma was treated using stereotactic RT."

80. **Adenopathy (noun):** Enlargement of lymph nodes, often indicating disease.
**Related Terms:** Lymphadenopathy, Metastasis, Nodal involvement.
**Example in Radiotherapy:** "Cervical adenopathy required nodal irradiation."

81. **Adenosine triphosphate (ATP) (noun):** Cellular energy carrier molecule critical for metabolism.
**Related Terms:** Biochemistry, Energy metabolism, Radiobiology.
**Example in Radiotherapy:** "ATP depletion can enhance radiosensitivity."

82. **Adjusted dose (noun):** Modified radiation dose accounting for clinical factors or uncertainties.
**Related Terms:** Dose correction, Replanning, Adaptive dose.
**Example in Radiotherapy:** "An adjusted dose was prescribed due to organ motion."

83. **Adjustment factor (noun):** Value used to correct measurements or calculations.
**Related Terms:** Calibration, Correction factor, QA.
**Example in Radiotherapy:** "A temperature adjustment factor was applied to chamber readings."

84. **Administered activity (noun):** Amount of radioactive material delivered to a patient.
**Related Terms:** Radiopharmaceutical, Bq, Dosimetry.
**Example in Radiotherapy:** "The administered activity for I-131 therapy was 3.7 GBq."

85. **Administration schedule (noun):** Planned timing for drug or radioisotope delivery.
**Related Terms:** Fractionation, Treatment schedule, Timing.
**Example in Radiotherapy:** "The chemotherapy administration schedule aligned with radiation fractions."

86. **Administrative control (noun):** Non-technical measures ensuring safe practices.
**Related Terms:** Policies, QA, Protocols.
**Example in Radiotherapy:** "Administrative controls minimized unauthorized LINAC access."

87. **Admittance criteria (noun):** Conditions required to allow patient entry to a service or trial.
**Related Terms:** Eligibility, Protocol inclusion, Screening.
**Example in Radiotherapy:** "Only patients meeting admittance criteria were enrolled in SBRT."

88. **Advanced dose modulation (noun):** Sophisticated beam intensity shaping for precise target coverage.
**Related Terms:** IMRT, VMAT, Modulation.
**Example in Radiotherapy:** "Advanced dose modulation reduced OAR exposure."

89. **Advanced localization (noun):** High-precision tumor or target positioning using modern imaging.
**Related Terms:** IGRT, Fiducial markers, CBCT.
**Example in Radiotherapy:** "Advanced localization improved prostate alignment."

90. **Advanced radiotherapy (noun):** State-of-the-art treatment using modern imaging, planning, or delivery.
**Related Terms:** IGRT, IMRT, Proton therapy.
**Example in Radiotherapy:** "Advanced radiotherapy minimized toxicity for head-and-neck cases."

91. **Advanced treatment planning (noun):** Planning using sophisticated imaging and optimization techniques.
**Related Terms:** 3D-CRT, IMRT, Monte Carlo.
**Example in Radiotherapy:** "Advanced treatment planning improved PTV coverage."

92. **Adverse dose (noun):** Dose amount causing unintended harm to tissue.
**Related Terms:** Toxicity, OAR dose, Complication.
**Example in Radiotherapy:** "An adverse dose caused spinal cord myelopathy."

93. **Affected volume (noun):** Tissue region impacted by radiation or disease.
**Related Terms:** Target volume, OAR, Dose distribution.
**Example in Radiotherapy:** "The affected volume was minimized using conformal planning."

94. **After-treatment imaging (noun):** Imaging done post-therapy to verify effects or assess toxicity.
**Related Terms:** Follow-up scan, QA, Verification.
**Example in Radiotherapy:** "After-treatment imaging confirmed tumor response."

95. **Age-specific dose (noun):** Radiation dose adapted to patient's age to reduce risk.
**Related Terms:** Pediatric dose, ALARA, Dose adjustment.
**Example in Radiotherapy:** "CT protocols used an age-specific dose for children."

96. **Aggregate activity (noun):** Total radioactive activity from all sources combined.
**Related Terms:** Summed activity, Bq, QA.
**Example in Radiotherapy:** "Aggregate activity in waste containers was monitored."

97. **Algorithmic modeling (noun):** Using mathematical algorithms to simulate or optimize therapy.
**Related Terms:** Monte Carlo, Dose calculation, Software.
**Example in Radiotherapy:** "Algorithmic modeling refined lung dose estimates."

98. **Algorithmic QA (noun):** Automated quality checks performed using programmed algorithms.
**Related Terms:** Software QA, Workflow automation, Error detection.
**Example in Radiotherapy:** "Algorithmic QA flagged planning errors automatically."

99. **Alias artifact (noun):** Imaging distortion caused by insufficient sampling resolution.
**Related Terms:** Aliasing, Imaging error, Reconstruction artifact.
**Example in Radiotherapy:** "MRI alias artifacts distorted target contouring."

100. **Aliasing (noun):** False signal representation due to undersampling.
**Related Terms:** Sampling error, Nyquist limit, Artifacts.
**Example in Radiotherapy:** "Aliasing reduced CT image quality."

101. **Alignment error (noun):** Positional deviation between planned and actual patient setup.
**Related Terms:** Setup error, Isocenter shift, QA.
**Example in Radiotherapy:** "CBCT corrected alignment errors before treatment."

102. **Alignment light (noun):** Laser system ensuring accurate patient positioning.
**Related Terms:** Isocenter, Setup, Immobilization.
**Example in Radiotherapy:** "Alignment lights verified isocenter daily."

103. **Alkaline phosphatase (noun):** Enzyme marker elevated in bone or liver disease.
**Related Terms:** Biochemical marker, Metastasis, Labs.
**Example in Radiotherapy:** "Raised alkaline phosphatase indicated bone metastases."

104. **All-body scan (noun):** Whole-body imaging for staging or follow-up.
**Related Terms:** Bone scan, PET/CT, Survey imaging.
**Example in Radiotherapy:** "An all-body scan ruled out distant metastasis."

105. **Allelic loss (noun):** Loss of one gene copy, often in cancer development.
**Related Terms:** Genetic alteration, LOH, Tumor biology.
**Example in Radiotherapy:** "Allelic loss guided personalized radiotherapy research."

106. **Allocation bias (noun):** Non-random subject assignment affecting trial validity.
**Related Terms:** Randomization error, Research bias, Protocol.
**Example in Radiotherapy:** "Proper randomization prevented allocation bias."

107. **Allowable dose (noun):** Maximum permissible radiation level to avoid harm.
**Related Terms:** Dose limit, Tolerance, OAR constraint.
**Example in Radiotherapy:** "Liver allowable dose was capped at 30 Gy."

108. **Alpha emission (noun):** Release of alpha particles from radioactive decay.
**Related Terms:** Alpha radiation, High LET, Isotopes.
**Example in Radiotherapy:** "Alpha emission is used in targeted radiotherapy."

109. **Alpha irradiator (noun):** Device emitting alpha particles for experimental or therapeutic use.
**Related Terms:** Alpha source, Laboratory device, Radiobiology.
**Example in Radiotherapy:** "An alpha irradiator studied DNA damage."

110. **Alpha radiation (noun):** High-LET radiation of short range, causing dense ionization.
**Related Terms:** Alpha particle, Heavy radiation, Radiobiology.
**Example in Radiotherapy:** "Alpha radiation selectively kills cancer cells."

111. **Alpha repair (noun):** Cellular repair of radiation-induced DNA damage caused by alpha particles.
**Related Terms:** DNA repair, Radiobiology, LET.
**Example in Radiotherapy:** "Alpha repair mechanisms affect tissue response."

112. **Alpha/beta estimation (noun):** Calculating tissue fractionation sensitivity using radiobiological data.
**Related Terms:** BED, Radiobiology, Fractionation.
**Example in Radiotherapy:** "Prostate RT used alpha/beta estimation to select dose."

113. **Alternative energy source (noun):** Non-conventional power or beam type for treatment delivery.
**Related Terms:** Proton therapy, Carbon ions, Particle beams.
**Example in Radiotherapy:** "An alternative energy source reduced neutron contamination."

114. **Alternative imaging plane (noun):** Non-standard orientation for imaging anatomy or tumor.
**Related Terms:** Sagittal, Coronal, Oblique plane.
**Example in Radiotherapy:** "Alternative imaging planes improved tumor visualization."

115. **Alternative isocenter (noun):** Additional beam reference point differing from primary isocenter.
**Related Terms:** Multiple isocenters, Planning, Non-coplanar beams.
**Example in Radiotherapy:** "An alternative isocenter optimized cranial dose."

116. **Aluminium attenuation (noun):** Reduction of beam intensity using aluminum filters.
**Related Terms:** Filtration, Beam hardening, QA.
**Example in Radiotherapy:** "Aluminium attenuation removed low-energy X-rays."

117. **Aluminium window (noun):** Thin aluminum barrier allowing controlled X-ray emission.
**Related Terms:** X-ray tube, Beam port, Filtration.
**Example in Radiotherapy:** "The tube's aluminium window shaped the output beam."

118. **Ambient background (noun):** Naturally present radiation in an environment.
**Related Terms:** Background radiation, Dose equivalent, Safety.
**Example in Radiotherapy:** "Ambient background levels were recorded during calibration."

119. **Ambient dose equivalent (noun):** Dose metric representing radiation in a given location.
**Related Terms:** Radiation protection, Monitoring, Dosimetry.
**Example in Radiotherapy:** "Ambient dose equivalent met safety standards."

120. **Ambient exposure (noun):** Radiation exposure from surrounding environment, not treatment beam.
**Related Terms:** Leakage radiation, Background dose, Survey.
**Example in Radiotherapy:** "Ambient exposure was negligible in the control room."

121. **Ambient light correction (noun):** Adjusting imaging displays to compensate for room light.
**Related Terms:** Display QA, Image quality, Calibration.
**Example in Radiotherapy:** "Ambient light correction improved CBCT contrast."

122. **Ambient radiation (noun):** Radiation naturally present or from stray sources.
**Related Terms:** Background dose, Monitoring, Survey meter.
**Example in Radiotherapy:** "Ambient radiation was measured outside the vault."

123. **Amplified beam (noun):** Radiation beam with increased energy or intensity.
**Related Terms:** LINAC, Beam gain, QA.
**Example in Radiotherapy:** "An amplified beam improved penetration for deep tumors."

124. **Amplified signal (noun):** Enhanced detector signal for clearer imaging or measurements.
**Related Terms:** Electronics, Gain, Image processing.
**Example in Radiotherapy:** "Amplified signals improved portal imaging resolution."

125. **Amplifier gain (noun):** Ratio describing signal amplification by an electronic device.
**Related Terms:** Electronics, Detector signal, QA.
**Example in Radiotherapy:** "Amplifier gain was calibrated for accurate readings."

126. **Amplitude monitor (noun):** Device measuring oscillation magnitude in respiratory or beam motion.
**Related Terms:** Motion management, RPM, Gating.
**Example in Radiotherapy:** "An amplitude monitor tracked patient breathing during DIBH."

127. **Amplitude tracking (noun):** Continuous recording of motion amplitude for gating or beam control.
**Related Terms:** Motion management, Respiratory gating, RPM.
**Example in Radiotherapy:** "Amplitude tracking ensured accurate gated delivery."

128. **Amyloidosis (noun):** Disease with abnormal protein deposits affecting organs.
**Related Terms:** Systemic disease, Imaging, Radiosensitivity.
**Example in Radiotherapy:** "Amyloidosis was incidentally detected on CT planning scans."

129. **Anal canal contouring (noun):** Outlining anal canal as an organ at risk or target.
**Related Terms:** Contouring, OAR, Planning.
**Example in Radiotherapy:** "Anal canal contouring followed RTOG guidelines."

130. **Anal cancer protocol (noun):** Standardized treatment guidelines for anal carcinoma.
**Related Terms:** Protocol, IMRT, Chemoradiation.
**Example in Radiotherapy:** "The anal cancer protocol prescribed 54 Gy with concurrent chemotherapy."

131. **Analog output (noun):** Continuous electrical signal from a device.
**Related Terms:** Signal processing, QA, Electronics.
**Example in Radiotherapy:** "Analog output from detectors was digitized for analysis."

132. **Analytical algorithm (noun):** Mathematical formula solving dose or imaging problems directly.
**Related Terms:** Pencil-beam, Analytical planning, Monte Carlo.
**Example in Radiotherapy:** "An analytical algorithm accelerated dose computation."

133. **Analytical calculation (noun):** Manual or formula-based calculation rather than simulation.
**Related Terms:** Hand calculation, QA, Verification.
**Example in Radiotherapy:** "Analytical calculations verified plan accuracy."

134. **Analytical phantom (noun):** Simple geometric model used for calculation validation.
**Related Terms:** QA phantom, Dose verification, Modeling.
**Example in Radiotherapy:** "An analytical phantom checked beam modeling."

135. **Anatomical atlas (noun):** Reference of labeled body structures for contouring or study.
**Related Terms:** Anatomy reference, Imaging atlas, Education.
**Example in Radiotherapy:** "An anatomical atlas guided OAR delineation."

136. **Anatomical data (noun):** Patient-specific structural information from imaging.
**Related Terms:** Imaging data, Contours, Modeling.
**Example in Radiotherapy:** "Anatomical data was imported for plan generation."

137. **Anatomical (noun):** Clear specification of structures or regions of interest.
**Related Terms:** Contouring, Target , Anatomy.
**Example in Radiotherapy:** "Precise anatomical improved treatment accuracy."

138. **Anatomical deformation (noun):** Shape change of tissue during treatment due to motion or response.
**Related Terms:** Deformable registration, Adaptive planning, IGRT.
**Example in Radiotherapy:** "Anatomical deformation required adaptive replanning."

139. **Anatomical model (noun):** Physical or digital representation of patient anatomy used for planning, education, or QA.
**Related Terms:** phantom, atlas.
**Example in Radiotherapy:** A 3D liver model is used to practice SBRT contouring.

140. **Anatomical plane (noun):** Standard body division (axial, sagittal, coronal) for imaging and planning.
**Related Terms:** cross-section, slice orientation.
**Example in Radiotherapy:** Dose distribution evaluated on sagittal planes for spinal tumors.

141. **Anatomical shift (noun):** Movement of organs or structures relative to baseline position.
**Related Terms:** setup error, motion.
**Example in Radiotherapy:** CBCT detects liver anatomical shift before SBRT.

142. **Ancillary software (noun):** Supporting application aiding planning, QA, or imaging analysis.
**Related Terms:** third-party tool, plugin.
**Example in Radiotherapy:** Auto-segmentation software reduces contouring time.

143. **Angular correction (noun):** Adjustment to patient/couch rotation to correct misalignment.
**Related Terms:** pitch, roll, yaw.
**Example in Radiotherapy:** 6D couch performs angular correction before beam delivery.

144. **Angular displacement (noun):** Change in rotational position measured in degrees.
**Related Terms:** rotation error, couch tilt.
**Example in Radiotherapy:** A 2° yaw displacement corrected during IGRT.

145. **Angular momentum (noun):** Physics property of rotating mass, rarely clinical but used in modeling.
**Related Terms:** rotational dynamics.
**Example in Radiotherapy:** Beamline components modeled for angular momentum in gantry design.

146. **Angular resolution (noun):** Ability to detect small rotational changes in imaging or tracking.
**Related Terms:** spatial resolution.
**Example in Radiotherapy:** Optical tracking has 0.1° angular resolution for head motion.

147. **Angular scanning (noun):** Beam or detector movement in rotational steps to cover an arc.
**Related Terms:** arc therapy, gantry rotation.
**Example in Radiotherapy:** Proton therapy uses angular scanning to shape dose.

148. **Angular spread (noun):** Divergence of beam angles or scatter.
**Related Terms:** penumbra, beam divergence.
**Example in Radiotherapy:** Collimator reduces angular spread in electron beams.

149. **Angular verification (noun):** Confirmation of correct gantry/couch angle during treatment setup.
**Related Terms:** QA, isocenter check.
**Example in Radiotherapy:** EPID images verify angular positions before arc therapy.

150. **Angular width (noun):** Angular extent of a radiation field or arc segment.
**Related Terms:** arc length, beam aperture.
**Example in Radiotherapy:** VMAT plan delivers 200° angular width arc.

151. **Animal model (noun):** Experimental animal used to study radiobiology or device safety.
**Related Terms:** preclinical study, in-vivo testing.
**Example in Radiotherapy:** Mice used to test normal-tissue radiation toxicity.

152. **Anisotropic motion (noun):** Unequal movement in different directions.
**Related Terms:** motion vector, non-uniform shift.
**Example in Radiotherapy:** Tumor exhibits anisotropic motion in SI vs. AP directions.

153. **Anisotropic resolution (noun):** Varying image clarity across different axes.
**Related Terms:** voxel size, image quality.
**Example in Radiotherapy:** CBCT shows anisotropic resolution in longitudinal axis.

154. **Annotated data (noun):** Imaging or planning datasets labeled with clinical notes.
**Related Terms:** contour dataset, structured data.
**Example in Radiotherapy:** Annotated MRI used to train auto-contouring AI.

155. **Annotated dose volume (noun):** DVH or 3D dose map marked with clinical findings.
**Related Terms:** dose metrics, labeled dataset.
**Example in Radiotherapy:** Annotated DVH highlights organs exceeding tolerance.

156. **Annotated image (noun):** Radiotherapy image marked with ROIs or comments.
**Related Terms:** tagged image, contour map.
**Example in Radiotherapy:** Portal image annotated to show misaligned fields.

157. **Anodic radiation (noun):** X-ray emission from anode interactions in tube.
**Related Terms:** bremsstrahlung, tube current.
**Example in Radiotherapy:** Diagnostic kV imaging uses anodic radiation source.

158. **Anodized filter (noun):** Metal filter with anodized coating altering beam quality.
**Related Terms:** beam hardening, filtration.
**Example in Radiotherapy:** Anodized filters optimize CT beam spectrum.

159. **Anomalous result (noun):** Unexpected finding outside predicted range.
**Related Terms:** outlier, error.
**Example in Radiotherapy:** QA detects anomalous MLC leaf position.

160. **Anomaly detection (noun):** Identifying irregular patterns automatically or manually.
**Related Terms:** outlier detection, AI.
**Example in Radiotherapy:** Machine log data scanned for anomaly detection.

161. **Anterior correction (noun):** Couch shift toward patient's front to align anatomy.
**Related Terms:** setup correction.
**Example in Radiotherapy:** CBCT indicates 2 mm anterior correction before beam.

162. **Anterior margin (noun):** PTV extension in front direction to account for motion.
**Related Terms:** setup margin.
**Example in Radiotherapy:** 5 mm anterior margin added for prostate PTV.

163. **Anterior oblique (noun):** Beam angled from front-side direction.
**Related Terms:** tangential beam.
**Example in Radiotherapy:** Breast fields planned with anterior oblique beams.

164. **Anterior shift (noun):** Patient moved forward along AP axis.
**Related Terms:** couch translation.
**Example in Radiotherapy:** CBCT requires 3 mm anterior shift in SBRT liver.

165. **Anterior structure (noun):** Organ/tissue located at front of body.
**Related Terms:** anatomy.
**Example in Radiotherapy:** Heart is anterior structure in chest imaging.

166. **Anterior tilt (noun):** Forward rotation of couch or patient.
**Related Terms:** pitch error.
**Example in Radiotherapy:** Masked patient corrected for anterior tilt.

167. **Anticoagulant protocol (noun):** Guidelines for patients on blood-thinning therapy.
**Related Terms:** medication management.
**Example in Radiotherapy:** Anticoagulant protocol checked before brachytherapy.

168. **Antigen exposure (noun):** Contact of immune system with tumor antigens.
**Related Terms:** immune recognition.
**Example in Radiotherapy:** Radiation increases antigen exposure to T-cells.

169. **Antigen presentation (noun):** Display of antigens on cell surface for immune activation.
**Related Terms:** immune response.
**Example in Radiotherapy:** Dendritic cells enhance antigen presentation post-RT.

170. **Antimetabolite (noun):** Drug disrupting DNA synthesis.
**Related Terms:** chemotherapy.
**Example in Radiotherapy:** 5-FU used as antimetabolite in chemoradiation.

171. **Antineoplastic protocol (noun):** Regimen using drugs to suppress tumor growth.
**Related Terms:** cancer therapy.
**Example in Radiotherapy:** Concurrent RT with cisplatin antineoplastic protocol.

172. **Antiproliferative effect (noun):** Inhibition of cell growth.
**Related Terms:** cytostatic.
**Example in Radiotherapy:** Radiation causes antiproliferative effect on tumor cells.

173. **Antiradiation drug (noun):** Medication protecting tissues from radiation damage.
**Related Terms:** radioprotector.
**Example in Radiotherapy:** Amifostine acts as antiradiation drug in head-neck RT.

174. **Antiradiation response (noun):** Biological defense against radiation injury.
**Related Terms:** radiotolerance.
**Example in Radiotherapy:** Hypoxic cells show natural antiradiation response.

175. **Antiscatter effect (noun):** Reduction of scattered radiation improving image quality.
**Related Terms:** grid, collimation.
**Example in Radiotherapy:** Antiscatter grid used during kV imaging.

176. **Antitumor immune response (noun):** Body's immune reaction against tumor.
**Related Terms:** immunotherapy synergy.
**Example in Radiotherapy:** RT enhances antitumor immune response via abscopal effect.

177. **Aperture correction (noun):** Adjustment of beam opening to match target.
**Related Terms:** collimation, MLC.
**Example in Radiotherapy:** Aperture correction applied to tighten VMAT fields.

178. **Aperture matching (noun):** Aligning multiple beam openings for composite dose.
**Related Terms:** field matching.
**Example in Radiotherapy:** Electron and photon fields require aperture matching.

179. **Aperture modulation (noun):** Dynamic change in beam aperture during delivery.
**Related Terms:** IMRT, VMAT.
**Example in Radiotherapy:** VMAT uses aperture modulation for dose shaping.

180. **Aperture setting (noun):** Fixed beam opening chosen for treatment.
**Related Terms:** collimator setting.
**Example in Radiotherapy:** Manual aperture setting used in 2D RT.

181. **Aperture-specific dose (noun):** Dose contribution from a single beam opening.
**Related Terms:** segment dose.
**Example in Radiotherapy:** QA checks aperture-specific dose in IMRT segments.

182. **Application dwell time (noun):** Time a brachytherapy source stays at one position.
**Related Terms:** HDR planning.
**Example in Radiotherapy:** Dwell time adjusted for uniform cervical dose.

183. **Application guide (noun):** Reference manual for device/procedure use.
**Related Terms:** protocol document.
**Example in Radiotherapy:** Vendor application guide used during TPS commissioning.

184. **Application parameter (noun):** Numerical input defining technique or protocol.
**Related Terms:** setting, variable.
**Example in Radiotherapy:** MU is a key application parameter for dose delivery.

185. **Application protocol (noun):** Standardized instructions for specific treatment method.
**Related Terms:** clinical guideline.
**Example in Radiotherapy:** Brachytherapy application protocol defines catheter loading.

186. **Application technique (noun):** Specific method to deliver treatment.
**Related Terms:** treatment approach.
**Example in Radiotherapy:** DIBH is an application technique for breast RT.

187. **Applicator angle (noun):** Orientation of brachytherapy applicator.
**Related Terms:** applicator geometry.
**Example in Radiotherapy:** Tandem applicator angle optimized for uterus alignment.

188. **Applicator configuration (noun):** Arrangement of brachytherapy components.
**Related Terms:** source path.
**Example in Radiotherapy:** Applicator configuration affects HDR dwell patterns.

189. **Applicator dose (noun):** Dose measured near or at brachytherapy applicator.
**Related Terms:** surface dose.
**Example in Radiotherapy:** QA measures applicator dose to ensure safety.

190. **Applicator geometry (noun):** Physical dimensions/shape of brachytherapy applicator.
**Related Terms:** design specs.
**Example in Radiotherapy:** Applicator geometry verified during simulation.

191. **Applicator plan (noun):** Brachytherapy plan specific to applicator placement.
**Related Terms:** loading plan.
**Example in Radiotherapy:** TPS generates applicator plan after CT simulation.

192. **Applicator shielding (noun):** Material in applicator reducing radiation to OARs.
 **Related Terms:** protective insert.
 **Example in Radiotherapy:** Tandem uses applicator shielding to protect bladder.

193. **Applicator simulation (noun):** Imaging session verifying applicator position.
 **Related Terms:** pre-planning CT.
 **Example in Radiotherapy:** Applicator simulation ensures correct intracavitary placement.

194. **Applicator spacing (noun):** Distance between brachytherapy applicators.
 **Related Terms:** catheter geometry.
 **Example in Radiotherapy:** Applicator spacing adjusted to optimize coverage.

195. **Applicator-specific QA (noun):** Quality assurance targeted to applicator devices.
 **Related Terms:** device QA.
 **Example in Radiotherapy:** HDR team performs applicator-specific QA each case.

196. **Applied dose (noun):** Actual radiation delivered to patient.
 **Related Terms:** delivered dose.
 **Example in Radiotherapy:** Applied dose verified with in-vivo dosimetry.

197. **Applied energy (noun):** Beam energy selected for treatment.
 **Related Terms:** photon energy.
 **Example in Radiotherapy:** 6 MV applied energy used for prostate IMRT.

198. **Applied field (noun):** Radiation field actually used during therapy.
 **Related Terms:** treatment field.
 **Example in Radiotherapy:** Applied field matched to PTV contour.

199. **Applied force (noun):** Physical pressure or movement during positioning.
 **Related Terms:** setup manipulation.
 **Example in Radiotherapy:** Applied force from mask secures patient head.

200. **Applied physics (noun):** Practical use of physics in clinical RT.
 **Related Terms:** medical physics.
 **Example in Radiotherapy:** Applied physics governs beam modeling in TPS.

201. **Appraisal method (noun):** Technique to evaluate quality, performance, or outcome.
 **Related Terms:** audit, assessment.
 **Example in Radiotherapy:** Peer appraisal method reviews plan quality.

202. **Approximation model (noun):** Simplified representation to estimate dose or motion.
 **Related Terms:** predictive model.
 **Example in Radiotherapy:** Approximation model estimates respiratory motion.

203. **Arbitrary unit (noun):** Non-standard scale for relative measurement.
 **Related Terms:** normalized unit.
 **Example in Radiotherapy:** EPID signal measured in arbitrary units.

204. **Arc angle (noun):** Extent of gantry rotation in arc therapy.
 **Related Terms:** arc length.
 **Example in Radiotherapy:** VMAT uses 180° arc angle around patient.

205. **Arc energy (noun):** Total beam energy delivered over arc rotation.
 **Related Terms:** MU per arc.
 **Example in Radiotherapy:** TPS calculates arc energy to meet PTV coverage.

206. **Arc fractionation (noun):** Delivering arcs in divided fractions.
**Related Terms:** hypofractionation.
**Example in Radiotherapy:** SBRT liver uses arc fractionation over 5 sessions.

207. **Arc generator (noun):** Device producing rotational treatment beams.
**Related Terms:** gantry system.
**Example in Radiotherapy:** Linac acts as arc generator for VMAT delivery.

208. **Arc initiation (noun):** Starting point of radiation arc delivery in rotational therapy.
**Related Terms:** beam-on time, gantry start angle
**Example in Radiotherapy:** In VMAT, arc initiation occurs at the preset gantry angle before dose modulation begins.

209. **Arc optimization (noun):** Process of refining arc parameters for maximal target coverage with minimal dose to organs at risk.
**Related Terms:** inverse planning, VMAT planning
**Example in Radiotherapy:** Planners use optimization algorithms to shape dose while maintaining arc efficiency.

210. **Arc rotation (noun):** Continuous gantry movement delivering radiation around a patient.
**Related Terms:** VMAT, rotational therapy
**Example in Radiotherapy:** A single 360° arc rotation delivers dose uniformly to a prostate target.

211. **Arc sequence (noun):** Ordered arrangement of multiple arcs to achieve planned dose distribution.
**Related Terms:** multi-arc plan, sequential arcs
**Example in Radiotherapy:** Head-and-neck plans may require dual arc sequences for conformity.

212. **Arc shape (noun):** The geometric path and beam aperture profile during arc delivery.
**Related Terms:** dynamic MLC, conformal arc
**Example in Radiotherapy:** Arc shape adapts to tumor contour using leaf motion.

213. **Arc smoothing (noun):** Technique minimizing abrupt dose or leaf-motion changes during arc delivery.
**Related Terms:** dose modulation, leaf sequencing
**Example in Radiotherapy:** Arc smoothing improves machine efficiency and reduces delivery error.

214. **Arc symmetry (noun):** Uniformity of beam parameters and dose around the arc path.
**Related Terms:** QA tolerance, gantry calibration
**Example in Radiotherapy:** QA checks ensure arc symmetry to avoid hotspot formation.

215. **Arc-based calculation (noun):** Dose computation method accounting for continuous gantry movement.
**Related Terms:** dynamic delivery, control points
**Example in Radiotherapy:** TPS uses arc-based calculation to predict dose in VMAT plans.

216. **Area averaging (noun):** Process of computing mean value over an irradiated region.
**Related Terms:** detector response, field uniformity
**Example in Radiotherapy:** Ion chamber readings provide area-averaged dose across a small field.

217. **Area correction (noun):** Adjustment for non-uniform detector or field response across area.
**Related Terms:** calibration factor, detector sensitivity
**Example in Radiotherapy:** Flat-panel calibration applies area correction to pixel outputs.

218. **Area (noun):** Precise specification of irradiated or imaged field boundaries.
**Related Terms:** ROI, beam aperture
**Example in Radiotherapy:** Collimator jaws define treatment area in conformal fields.

219. **Area dose (noun):** Radiation amount delivered per unit surface region.
**Related Terms:** surface dose, output factor
**Example in Radiotherapy:** Skin dose is assessed using TLDs measuring area dose.

220. **Area filter (noun):** Device modifying radiation field intensity or shape over a region.
**Related Terms:** compensator, wedge filter
**Example in Radiotherapy:** A physical wedge acts as an area filter to modulate beam.

221. **Area integration (noun):** Summation of dose or signal across a defined planar region.
**Related Terms:** dosimetry, cumulative response
**Example in Radiotherapy:** Film analysis uses area integration to calculate total exposure.

222. **Area irradiation (noun):** Exposing a predefined region to therapeutic radiation.
**Related Terms:** local treatment, field targeting
**Example in Radiotherapy:** Boost fields deliver area irradiation to tumor bed.

223. **Area of interest (noun):** Specific region selected for analysis or treatment.
**Related Terms:** ROI, target delineation
**Example in Radiotherapy:** The tumor GTV is the area of interest in contouring.

224. **Area projection (noun):** Mapping a 3D structure onto a 2D imaging plane.
**Related Terms:** DRR, imaging geometry
**Example in Radiotherapy:** DRRs are generated using area projections of CT data.

225. **Area segmentation (noun):** Process of subdividing an image or field into distinct regions.
**Related Terms:** auto-contouring, image analysis
**Example in Radiotherapy:** AI tools perform area segmentation for OAR identification.

226. **Area-specific margin (noun):** Custom expansion added around a region to account for uncertainties.
**Related Terms:** PTV margin, setup error
**Example in Radiotherapy:** Liver SBRT plans use area-specific margins to protect bowel loops.

227. **Areal correction (noun):** Adjustment compensating for area-dependent detector sensitivity.
**Related Terms:** pixel gain calibration, flat-fielding
**Example in Radiotherapy:** EPID dosimetry applies areal correction for accurate dose maps.

228. **Areal (noun):** Establishing boundaries or size of a measured planar region.
**Related Terms:** field size, ROI contour
**Example in Radiotherapy:** Collimator-defined light fields provide areal .

229. **Areal detector (noun):** Radiation sensor measuring dose over a 2D region.
**Related Terms:** EPID, film, array detector
**Example in Radiotherapy:** Flat-panel imagers serve as areal detectors during QA.

230. **Areal exposure (noun):** Radiation received per unit surface region of a detector.
**Related Terms:** entrance dose, kerma
**Example in Radiotherapy:** Gafchromic film measures areal exposure in patient-specific QA.

231. **Areal resolution (noun):** Detector ability to distinguish fine spatial details across a plane.
**Related Terms:** pixel size, imaging quality
**Example in Radiotherapy:** High areal resolution in EPIDs improves portal imaging.

232. **Argument list (noun):** Collection of input parameters for computational procedures.
**Related Terms:** programming input, algorithm settings
**Example in Radiotherapy:** TPS scripts use an argument list to automate planning tasks.

233. **Arm board (noun):** Positioning accessory supporting the patient's arm during treatment.
**Related Terms:** immobilization device, patient setup
**Example in Radiotherapy:** Breast irradiation uses an arm board to elevate the ipsilateral arm.

234. **Arm immobilizer (noun):** Device securing patient's arm to prevent movement.
**Related Terms:** positioning aid, thermoplastic mold
**Example in Radiotherapy:** SBRT spine cases use an arm immobilizer to maintain accuracy.

235. **Arteriovenous malformation (noun):** Abnormal vascular connection requiring stereotactic treatment.
**Related Terms:** AVM, radiosurgery target
**Example in Radiotherapy:** AVMs are managed using high-dose focused beams in SRS.

236. **Artifact correction (noun):** Method to reduce imaging artifacts for clearer visualization.
**Related Terms:** image reconstruction, noise reduction
**Example in Radiotherapy:** CBCT scans undergo artifact correction to improve registration.

237. **Artifact filtering (noun):** Removing unwanted image patterns or streaks via algorithms.
**Related Terms:** preprocessing, denoising
**Example in Radiotherapy:** CT artifact filtering improves HU accuracy for dose calculation.

238. **Artifact map (noun):** Spatial display showing areas affected by imaging artifacts.
**Related Terms:** quality map, reconstruction output
**Example in Radiotherapy:** TPS software generates artifact maps to highlight CT inconsistencies.

239. **Artificial contrast (noun):** Enhancement of image differences using external or computational means.
**Related Terms:** contrast agent, image enhancement
**Example in Radiotherapy:** Artificial contrast improves tumor delineation on MRI.

240. **Artificial neural network (noun):** Computational model mimicking brain neurons for prediction tasks.
**Related Terms:** AI, deep learning
**Example in Radiotherapy:** ANN models predict optimal beam arrangements automatically.

241. **Artificial radioisotope (noun):** Man-made radioactive isotope used for treatment or imaging.
**Related Terms:** radionuclide, isotope production
**Example in Radiotherapy:** Co-60 is an artificial radioisotope used in teletherapy.

242. **Artificial respiration (noun):** Mechanical ventilation to maintain breathing during procedures.
**Related Terms:** life support, ventilation
**Example in Radiotherapy:** Artificial respiration stabilizes motion during thoracic irradiation.

243. **Assignment model (noun):** Framework allocating resources or variables for optimization.
**Related Terms:** mathematical model, planning
**Example in Radiotherapy:** Beam assignment models distribute monitor units efficiently.

244. **Assignment plan (noun):** Detailed allocation of tasks, resources, or beams for a procedure.
**Related Terms:** workflow plan, scheduling
**Example in Radiotherapy:** A QA assignment plan specifies tasks for each physicist.

245. **Associated beam (noun):** Radiation beam linked to a defined target or treatment phase.
**Related Terms:** beam set, treatment field
**Example in Radiotherapy:** Each arc in VMAT is an associated beam with unique weight.

246. **Associated image (noun):** Image linked to specific reference or planning data.
**Related Terms:** fused image, registration dataset
**Example in Radiotherapy:** CBCT is an associated image aligned with planning CT.

247. **Associated risk (noun):** Probability of harm linked to a treatment or exposure.
**Related Terms:** radiation risk, complication probability
**Example in Radiotherapy:** Lung SBRT carries associated risk of radiation pneumonitis.

248. **Association bias (noun):** Systematic error due to incorrect variable correlations.
**Related Terms:** confounding, data bias
**Example in Radiotherapy:** Retrospective studies may show association bias in toxicity prediction.

249. **Assumed density (noun):** Estimated tissue density used when direct measurement is unavailable.
**Related Terms:** HU override, bulk density
**Example in Radiotherapy:** Bolus regions may use assumed density in dose calculation.

250. **Asymmetry correction (noun):** Adjustment compensating for non-uniform radiation fields.
**Related Terms:** beam calibration, off-axis correction
**Example in Radiotherapy:** Linac output factors include asymmetry correction for angled beams.

251. **Atomic time standard (noun):** Precise timekeeping reference using atomic transitions.
**Related Terms:** frequency standard, clock calibration
**Example in Radiotherapy:** Synchronizing linac systems relies on an atomic time standard.

252. **Atomic absorption (noun):** The process by which atoms absorb photons or other forms of electromagnetic energy, causing electrons to transition to higher energy levels.
**Related Terms:** Absorption spectrum, Photon interaction, Attenuation.
**Example in Radiotherapy:** Used in radiation detector calibration to measure specific energy levels absorbed by target materials.

253. **Atomic cross section (noun):** A quantitative measure of the probability that an atomic nucleus or electron will interact with a photon or particle.
**Related Terms:** Interaction probability, Scattering, Attenuation coefficient.
**Example in Radiotherapy:** Determines how likely X-rays are to interact with tissues, influencing dose distribution and treatment planning.

254. **Atomic displacement (noun):** The movement of atoms from their lattice positions due to radiation-induced collisions or energy transfer.
**Related Terms:** Radiation damage, Lattice defect, Ionization.
**Example in Radiotherapy:** Observed in radiation shielding materials exposed to high-energy beams over time.

255. **Atomic excitation (noun):** A process in which an atom absorbs energy, elevating one or more electrons to a higher energy state without ionization.
**Related Terms:** Photon absorption, De-excitation, Emission spectrum.
**Example in Radiotherapy:** Leads to secondary photon emission within detector crystals used for dosimetry.

256. **Attenuation map (noun):** An image or dataset representing the spatial distribution of attenuation coefficients within a body or object.
**Related Terms:** CT imaging, Attenuation correction, Hounsfield unit.
**Example in Radiotherapy:** Used in PET-CT to correct for tissue density differences during dose calculation.

257. **Auger electron (noun):** A low-energy electron emitted when an inner-shell vacancy in an atom is filled by another electron, releasing energy.
**Related Terms:** Auger effect, Electron emission, Inner-shell ionization.
**Example in Radiotherapy:** Exploited in Auger therapy for delivering localized energy to cancer cell DNA.

258. **Auto-contouring (noun):** The automated delineation of anatomical structures or target volumes using AI or image processing algorithms.
**Related Terms:** Auto-segmentation, AI contouring, Structure set.
**Example in Radiotherapy:** Used in adaptive radiotherapy to reduce contouring time and interobserver variability.

259. **Auto-plan generation (noun):** The automatic creation of treatment plans using predefined algorithms that optimize beam angles, doses, and constraints.
**Related Terms:** Auto-planning, Inverse planning, Optimization.
**Example in Radiotherapy:** Helps generate multiple VMAT plans quickly for clinician review.

260. **Auxiliary field (noun):** An additional radiation field used to supplement dose coverage or compensate for under dosed regions.
**Related Terms:** Boost field, Field matching, Composite field.
**Example in Radiotherapy:** Added in breast tangential planning to cover supraclavicular nodes.

261. **Axial plane (noun):** A horizontal imaging plane that divides the body into superior and inferior sections, used for image acquisition and treatment planning.
**Related Terms:** Coronal plane, Sagittal plane, Axial slice.
**Example in Radiotherapy:** CT images are reconstructed in the axial plane for contouring target volumes.

262. **Axial alignment (noun):** The precise positioning of anatomical structures or equipment along the patient's longitudinal axis.
**Related Terms:** Isocentre alignment, Setup verification, Image registration.
**Example in Radiotherapy:** Ensures the spine or target lesion is correctly centered during CBCT verification.

263. **Axial displacement (noun):** The shift or movement of a structure or beam along the patient's longitudinal (z) axis.
**Related Terms:** Longitudinal shift, Couch translation, Setup error.
**Example in Radiotherapy:** Corrected during patient setup if a tumor moves due to respiration or couch positioning errors.

264. **Axial gradient (noun):** A rate of change in a parameter such as magnetic field or dose along the axial direction.
**Related Terms:** Magnetic field gradient, Dose gradient, Spatial resolution.
**Example in Radiotherapy:** In MRI-guided systems, axial gradients help produce slice-selective imaging.

265. **Axial image reconstruction (noun):** The computational process of generating cross-sectional images from raw projection data along the axial plane.
**Related Terms:** Image reconstruction, CT acquisition, Tomographic processing.
**Example in Radiotherapy:** Used in CT simulation for accurate delineation of target volumes.

266. **Axial intensity (noun):** The magnitude of beam intensity measured along the central axis of radiation delivery.
**Related Terms:** Central axis dose, Beam profile, Flatness.
**Example in Radiotherapy:** Measured during linear accelerator QA to verify uniform beam output.

267. **Axial modulation (noun):** Adjustment of beam intensity or dose along the longitudinal axis to achieve dose conformity.
**Related Terms:** Intensity modulation, VMAT, Dose shaping.
**Example in Radiotherapy:** Used in IMRT and VMAT plans for head-and-neck tumors to improve dose homogeneity.

268. **Axial offset (noun):** A positional deviation from the planned central axis alignment.
**Related Terms:** Setup error, Couch offset, Geometric correction.
**Example in Radiotherapy:** Corrected during CBCT registration before treatment beam delivery.

269. **Axial rotation (noun):** The rotation of the patient or imaging plane around the longitudinal axis.
**Related Terms:** Rotational error, Gantry rotation, Couch angle.
**Example in Radiotherapy:** Monitored during IGRT to avoid rotational misalignments in liver SBRT cases.

270. **Axial symmetry (noun):** A condition in which dose or geometry remains uniform around the central axis.
**Related Terms:** Beam flatness, Symmetry tolerance, Calibration.
**Example in Radiotherapy:** Evaluated during monthly linac QA to ensure consistent beam performance.

271. **Axial translation (noun):** Linear movement along the z-axis used for fine patient positioning or image alignment.
**Related Terms:** Couch shift, 6D movement, Positioning correction.
**Example in Radiotherapy:** Applied to align pelvic structures with the treatment isocentre.

272. **Axillary contour (noun):** The delineation of axillary lymph node regions on planning CT or MR images.
**Related Terms:** Nodal contouring, Level I–III nodes, Target delineation.
**Example in Radiotherapy:** Required in breast cancer planning for post-mastectomy regional nodal irradiation.

273. **Axillary dissection (noun):** A surgical procedure removing axillary lymph nodes for staging or disease control.
**Related Terms:** Sentinel node biopsy, Nodal metastasis, Lymphadenectomy.
**Example in Radiotherapy:** Impacts field design and dose prescription to axillary regions.

274. **Axillary field (noun):** A radiation field specifically aimed to cover axillary lymphatic areas.
**Related Terms:** Tangential fields, Regional nodal irradiation, Supraclavicular field.
**Example in Radiotherapy:** Used as a separate or matched field in breast cancer treatments.

275. **Axillary node (noun):** Lymph node located in the axilla, commonly involved in breast and upper thoracic malignancies.
**Related Terms:** Level I–III nodes, Lymphatic drainage, Target volume.
**Example in Radiotherapy:** Included in the clinical target volume for node-positive breast cancer.

276. **Azimuthal angle (noun):** The angle between a reference direction and the projection of a vector onto a horizontal plane.
**Related Terms:** Polar coordinates, Gantry rotation, Beam geometry.
**Example in Radiotherapy:** Describes gantry orientation during arc delivery in VMAT treatments.

277. **Azimuthal asymmetry (noun):** A non-uniform distribution of dose or intensity around the azimuthal direction.
**Related Terms:** Beam asymmetry, Angular spread, Flatness deviation.
**Example in Radiotherapy:** Detected in QA tests when beam steering is misaligned.

278. **Azimuthal correction (noun):** Adjustment applied to compensate for azimuthal misalignment or asymmetry.
**Related Terms:** Beam steering, Gantry calibration, Symmetry correction.
**Example in Radiotherapy:** Performed during machine QA to ensure symmetric beam profiles.

279. **Azimuthal displacement (noun):** Rotational deviation around the central vertical axis, often affecting beam targeting accuracy.
**Related Terms:** Rotational error, Couch yaw, 6D correction.
**Example in Radiotherapy:** Corrected during patient setup in frameless stereotactic treatments.

280. **Azimuthal projection (noun):** A planar representation of data or geometry around an azimuthal coordinate system.
**Related Terms:** Cylindrical mapping, Angular reconstruction, Dose projection.
**Example in Radiotherapy:** Used in imaging algorithms for scatter correction.

281. **Azimuthal rotation (noun):** The rotation of the beam or imaging system about the vertical axis.
**Related Terms:** Couch yaw, Gantry rotation, Arc therapy.
**Example in Radiotherapy:** Defines gantry trajectory in arc-based dose delivery.

282. **Absorber material (noun):** A substance used to reduce or attenuate radiation intensity through absorption.
**Related Terms:** Shielding, Filter, Attenuator.
**Example in Radiotherapy:** Lead or tungsten used in beam shaping devices to protect normal tissue.

283. **Absorber plate (noun):** A flat material inserted to absorb scattered or primary radiation for dose control.
**Related Terms:** Filter plate, Beam modulator, Attenuation sheet.
**Example in Radiotherapy:** Utilized in dosimetry phantoms to measure absorbed dose profiles.

284. **Absorption edge (noun):** A sharp increase in attenuation coefficient when photon energy matches electron binding energy.
**Related Terms:** K-edge, Photoelectric effect, Attenuation spectrum.
**Example in Radiotherapy:** Important in kilovoltage X-ray beam filtration and detector design.

285. **Absorption peak (noun):** The energy value at which maximum radiation absorption occurs in a material.
**Related Terms:** Absorption spectrum, Resonance energy, Photon interaction.
**Example in Radiotherapy:** Determines optimal beam filtration for diagnostic kilovoltage imaging.

286. **Absorption ratio (noun):** The ratio of absorbed dose to incident energy or exposure.
**Related Terms:** Absorbed fraction, Energy transfer, Dose efficiency.
**Example in Radiotherapy:** Used to compare different phantom materials' absorption characteristics.

287. **Accelerated dose delivery (noun):** A technique delivering total prescribed dose in a shorter period using higher dose per fraction or multiple sessions per day.
**Related Terms:** Accelerated fractionation, Hypofractionation, Dose rate.
**Example in Radiotherapy:** Used in head and neck cancers to reduce tumor repopulation.

288. **Accelerated repair (noun):** An increase in cellular repair rate due to repeated sublethal radiation exposure.
**Related Terms:** Sublethal damage, Fractionation effect, DNA repair.
**Example in Radiotherapy:** Considered when adjusting overall treatment time to prevent tumor regrowth.

289. **Accelerator alignment (noun):** The geometric calibration ensuring the radiation beam is aligned with mechanical and optical isocentres.
**Related Terms:** Mechanical isocentre, Beam coincidence, QA calibration.
**Example in Radiotherapy:** Verified using Winston–Lutz tests during machine commissioning.

290. **Accelerator magnet (noun):** An electromagnet used in a linear accelerator to steer or focus charged particles.
**Related Terms:** Bending magnet, Steering coil, Beam optics.
**Example in Radiotherapy:** Guides high-energy electrons toward the target for X-ray production.

291. **Accelerator shielding (noun):** Protective structures designed to contain scattered or leakage radiation from the accelerator.
**Related Terms:** Bunker shielding, Lead barrier, Radiation protection.
**Example in Radiotherapy:** Concrete and lead walls are engineered according to workload and beam energy.

292. **Accelerator output (noun):** The measurable radiation dose rate or output from a linear accelerator under defined conditions.
**Related Terms:** Output factor, Calibration, Dose rate.
**Example in Radiotherapy:** Verified daily using a calibrated ionization chamber before treatment.

293. **Accelerator QA (noun):** A set of quality assurance tests performed to ensure the linear accelerator delivers accurate and consistent radiation doses.
**Related Terms:** Machine QA, Output constancy, Mechanical alignment.
**Example in Radiotherapy:** Includes daily, monthly, and annual checks as per AAPM TG-142 guidelines.

294. **Accelerator simulation (noun):** A virtual or computational model used to study and predict accelerator beam characteristics.
**Related Terms:** Monte Carlo simulation, Beam modeling, Commissioning.
**Example in Radiotherapy:** Used during beam modeling for treatment planning system commissioning.

295. **Accelerator upgrade (noun):** The enhancement or modification of an existing linear accelerator system to improve performance or extend service life.
**Related Terms:** Commissioning, Beam tuning, System calibration.
**Example in Radiotherapy:** May include software updates or addition of flattening filter-free (FFF) capability.

296. **Active matrix sensor (noun):** A type of digital detector with a grid of transistors that individually process imaging signals.
**Related Terms:** Flat-panel detector, Digital radiography, Image acquisition.
**Example in Radiotherapy:** Used in EPID systems for portal imaging and dosimetric verification.

297. **Active pixel detector (noun):** A sensor that records radiation intensity at individual pixels with on-chip amplification and processing.
**Related Terms:** CMOS detector, Imaging array, Active sensor.
**Example in Radiotherapy:** Employed in image-guided radiotherapy systems for high-resolution imaging.

298. **Active shielding (noun):** A system using magnetic or electric fields to reduce stray radiation or secondary particles.
**Related Terms:** Passive shielding, Electromagnetic shielding, Radiation protection.
**Example in Radiotherapy:** Implemented in proton therapy gantries to minimize neutron scatter.

299. **Activity correction (noun):** Adjustment of measured radioactivity to account for decay or detector efficiency.
**Related Terms:** Decay correction, Calibration, Half-life.
**Example in Radiotherapy:** Used in brachytherapy dose calculations for accurate source strength.

**300. Activity decay (noun):** The decrease in radioisotope activity over time as unstable atoms transform into stable ones.
**Related Terms:** Half-life, Decay constant, Radioactive decay law.
**Example in Radiotherapy:** Considered when planning I-125 seed implantations for prostate brachytherapy.

**301. Activity distribution (noun):** The spatial arrangement of radioactivity within a target or phantom.
**Related Terms:** Dose distribution, Source mapping, Heterogeneity.
**Example in Radiotherapy:** Mapped in SPECT-CT to evaluate therapeutic radionuclide localization.

**302. Activity quantification (noun):** The process of measuring and expressing the total radioactivity within a given region.
**Related Terms:** Dosimetry, Calibration factor, Quantitative imaging.
**Example in Radiotherapy:** Used to verify the delivered dose in radioisotope therapy.

**303. Adaptive gating (noun):** A respiratory management technique that adjusts beam delivery timing based on patient's real-time breathing pattern.
**Related Terms:** Respiratory gating, Motion management, 4D radiotherapy.
**Example in Radiotherapy:** Applied in lung SBRT to minimize tumor motion during treatment.

**304. Adaptive immobilization (noun):** Custom modification of immobilization devices to accommodate anatomical or positional changes over treatment sessions.
**Related Terms:** Reproducibility, Adaptive radiotherapy, Positioning device.
**Example in Radiotherapy:** Used in head-and-neck cases where patient anatomy changes due to weight loss.

**305. Adaptive modulation (noun):** Dynamic alteration of beam intensity or shape in response to anatomical or biological variations.
**Related Terms:** Intensity modulation, Adaptive planning, Dose compensation.
**Example in Radiotherapy:** Used in adaptive IMRT to compensate for tumor regression during therapy.

**306. Adaptive workflow (noun):** A clinical process integrating periodic imaging, plan adaptation, and re-optimization during a treatment course.
**Related Terms:** Online adaptation, Replanning, IGRT workflow.
**Example in Radiotherapy:** Implemented in MR-Linac systems for daily adaptive treatments.

**307. Add-on collimator (noun):** A removable beam-shaping accessory attached to the primary collimation system.
**Related Terms:** Custom block, MLC extension, Shielding device.
**Example in Radiotherapy:** Used in electron therapy to shape the beam for irregular treatment areas.

**308. Add-on wedge (noun):** An external wedge filter used to modify the beam intensity profile.
**Related Terms:** Wedge angle, Beam modifier, Isodose shaping.
**Example in Radiotherapy:** Used to achieve dose uniformity in tangential breast fields.

**309. Add-on bolus (noun):** A tissue-equivalent material placed over the skin surface to modify the dose build-up region.
**Related Terms:** Bolus material, Surface dose, Skin sparing.
**Example in Radiotherapy:** Applied over chest wall scars to increase surface dose after mastectomy.

**310. Algorithmic modeling (noun):** The use of computational algorithms to simulate physical or biological phenomena in radiotherapy.
**Related Terms:** Monte Carlo simulation, Dose calculation, Predictive modeling.
**Example in Radiotherapy:** Used in treatment planning systems to calculate dose in heterogeneous tissues.

311. **Algorithmic QA (noun):** Quality assurance process verifying the accuracy and consistency of software-based dose calculations and algorithms.
**Related Terms:** Commissioning QA, Model validation, Software verification.
**Example in Radiotherapy:** Performed when updating the treatment planning system's dose engine.

312. **Alias artifact (noun):** A distortion in digital images caused by undersampling or limited spatial resolution.
**Related Terms:** Sampling frequency, Moiré pattern, Image noise.
**Example in Radiotherapy:** Seen in CT simulation images when scan pitch is too high.

313. **Aliasing (noun):** The misrepresentation of a signal when sampling frequency is insufficient to capture its variations accurately.
**Related Terms:** Nyquist limit, Digital imaging, Signal distortion.
**Example in Radiotherapy:** Can affect MRI-based contouring if imaging resolution is inadequate.

314. **Alignment error (noun):** The deviation between planned and actual positioning of patient or equipment.
**Related Terms:** Setup error, Isocentre shift, Registration discrepancy.
**Example in Radiotherapy:** Corrected by image-guided verification before each fraction.

315. **Alignment light (noun):** Visible laser beams used to aid patient positioning and isocentre localization.
**Related Terms:** Room lasers, Setup marks, Optical alignment.
**Example in Radiotherapy:** Crosshair lasers guide patient alignment during CT simulation and treatment setup.

316. **Allowable dose (noun):** The maximum dose permitted to an organ or tissue based on safety or clinical guidelines.
**Related Terms:** Dose constraint, Tolerance dose, QUANTEC limit.
**Example in Radiotherapy:** Spinal cord allowable dose is typically limited to ≤45 Gy for conventional fractionation.

317. **Alpha emission (noun):** The release of an alpha particle (helium nucleus) from a radioactive atom during decay.
**Related Terms:** Radioactive decay, Alpha radiation, Heavy particle.
**Example in Radiotherapy:** Used in targeted alpha therapy for localized high-LET dose delivery to tumors.

318. **Alpha irradiator (noun):** A device designed to deliver controlled alpha radiation for calibration or research.
**Related Terms:** Sealed source, Alpha chamber, Radioisotope calibration.
**Example in Radiotherapy:** Utilized in laboratory settings to test radiation response of detectors.

319. **Alpha radiation (noun):** Ionizing radiation consisting of helium nuclei with high linear energy transfer and short range.
**Related Terms:** Alpha particle, LET, Ionization density.
**Example in Radiotherapy:** Forms the basis of high-LET targeted alpha radionuclide therapies.

320. **Alpha repair (noun):** The process of DNA repair following high-LET alpha particle-induced damage.
**Related Terms:** Double-strand break, DNA repair mechanism, Cell survival curve.
**Example in Radiotherapy:** Modeled in radiobiological studies assessing alpha-particle RBE.

321. **Alpha/beta estimation (noun):** Calculation of the tissue-specific alpha/beta ratio describing fractionation sensitivity in the linear-quadratic model.
**Related Terms:** Radiobiological modeling, BED, Fractionation sensitivity.
**Example in Radiotherapy:** Prostate cancer typically has a low alpha/beta ratio (~1.5 Gy), supporting hypofractionation.

322. **Alternative energy source (noun):** Non-traditional or supplementary energy used for particle acceleration or imaging systems.
**Related Terms:** Microwave power, RF source, Klystron.
**Example in Radiotherapy:** Some compact linacs use solid-state RF sources instead of magnetrons.

323. **Alternative imaging plane (noun):** A non-standard imaging orientation chosen for improved visualization or planning accuracy.
**Related Terms:** Oblique plane, Custom reconstruction, Anatomical alignment.
**Example in Radiotherapy:** Used in MRI fusion for visualizing the prostate apex more clearly.

324. **Alternative isocentre (noun):** A secondary or shifted reference point used for beam setup or verification.
**Related Terms:** Multiple isocentre, Couch translation, Setup reference.
**Example in Radiotherapy:** Applied in craniospinal irradiation to treat long target volumes.

325. **Aluminium attenuation (noun):** Reduction of X-ray beam intensity caused by passage through an aluminium filter.
**Related Terms:** Filtration, Beam hardening, Attenuator.
**Example in Radiotherapy:** Used during CT calibration to simulate tissue-equivalent attenuation.

326. **Aluminium window (noun):** A thin aluminium barrier that permits radiation transmission while sealing a detector or tube.
**Related Terms:** Detector interface, Beam port, X-ray window.
**Example in Radiotherapy:** Found in ion chambers to allow low-energy photon entry without contamination.

327. **Ambient background (noun):** The natural level of environmental radiation present in a given location.
**Related Terms:** Background dose, Natural radioactivity, Radiation survey.
**Example in Radiotherapy:** Measured during bunker QA to ensure no excess radiation leakage.

328. **Ambient dose equivalent (noun):** A quantity expressing the effective dose received from ambient radiation fields.
**Related Terms:** Equivalent dose, Dose monitoring, Hp(10).
**Example in Radiotherapy:** Used in area monitoring to assess occupational exposure levels.

329. **Ambient exposure (noun):** The amount of ionizing radiation incident on a location from environmental sources.
**Related Terms:** Exposure rate, Background radiation, Environmental monitoring.
**Example in Radiotherapy:** Measured using survey meters near treatment rooms.

330. **Amplified beam (noun):** A radiation beam whose intensity has been increased through electronic or physical means.
**Related Terms:** Beam gain, RF amplification, Signal boost.
**Example in Radiotherapy:** Achieved in linacs using RF amplifiers to accelerate electrons to therapeutic energies.

331. **Amplified signal (noun):** An electrical signal enhanced to increase its strength for detection or processing.
**Related Terms:** Electronic gain, Noise ratio, Detector output.
**Example in Radiotherapy:** Used in ion chamber electrometers to detect small current signals from low-dose beams.

332. **Amplifier gain (noun):** The ratio of output signal amplitude to input signal amplitude in an electronic amplifier.
**Related Terms:** Signal processing, Amplification factor, Sensitivity.
**Example in Radiotherapy:** Calibrated during EPID system QA to ensure consistent image brightness.

333. **Amplitude monitor (noun):** A device that tracks the intensity or variation of a signal or waveform over time.
**Related Terms:** Beam monitor, Dose monitor, Oscilloscope.
**Example in Radiotherapy:** Monitors beam pulse amplitude to maintain consistent output in electron mode.

334. **Amplitude tracking (noun):** The process of following the variations in signal or patient motion amplitude during treatment.
**Related Terms:** Motion monitoring, Gating, Respiratory tracking.
**Example in Radiotherapy:** Used in respiratory gating systems to track tumor movement in real-time.

335. **Anatomical atlas (noun):** A digital reference map of anatomical structures used for segmentation or registration.
**Related Terms:** Atlas-based segmentation, Contour library, Template model.
**Example in Radiotherapy:** Used to automatically contour organs-at-risk during treatment planning.

336. **Anatomical deformation (noun):** Change in the shape or position of anatomy over time due to motion, swelling, or weight loss.
**Related Terms:** Deformable registration, Organ motion, Adaptive planning.
**Example in Radiotherapy:** Managed in adaptive workflows for pelvic and thoracic tumors.

337. **Anatomical drift (noun):** Gradual shift in patient anatomy or organ position between imaging and treatment sessions.
**Related Terms:** Interfraction motion, Setup variation, Reproducibility.
**Example in Radiotherapy:** Detected using daily CBCT to adjust patient setup.

338. **Anatomical model (noun):** A 3D representation of human anatomy for simulation, planning, or education.
**Related Terms:** Phantom, Computational model, Atlas.
**Example in Radiotherapy:** Used in TPS to calculate dose distribution based on tissue densities.

339. **Anatomical shift (noun):** Displacement of anatomical structures relative to the treatment plan reference.
**Related Terms:** Setup error, Organ motion, Deformable registration.
**Example in Radiotherapy:** Detected by IGRT and corrected before dose delivery.

340. **Ancillary software (noun):** Supporting software tools integrated with primary systems for additional analysis or automation.
**Related Terms:** QA software, Workflow tools, Data management.
**Example in Radiotherapy:** Used to automate patient data export and plan verification.

341. **Angular verification (noun):** The process of checking the accuracy of gantry, couch, or collimator rotational angles.
**Related Terms:** Mechanical QA, Isocentre verification, Gantry calibration.
**Example in Radiotherapy:** Conducted during monthly QA using digital inclinometers or laser trackers.

342. **Attenuation coefficient (noun):** A measure of how easily a material reduces the intensity of a radiation beam.
**Related Terms:** Linear attenuation, half-value layer
**Example in Radiotherapy:** Used to calculate beam penetration through tissues during dose planning.

343. **Attenuation correction (noun):** The process of compensating for photon absorption and scatter in imaging.
**Related Terms:** PET-CT correction, image reconstruction
**Example in Radiotherapy:** Improves accuracy of PET-based target volume delineation.

344. **Audio-visual monitoring (noun):** Real-time observation of patients during treatment for safety and comfort.
**Related Terms:** Patient intercom, camera surveillance
**Example in Radiotherapy:** Therapists monitor the patient through an in-room camera during beam delivery.

345. **Automatic exposure control (noun):** Imaging system function that adjusts exposure to maintain consistent image quality.
**Related Terms:** Tube current modulation, dose optimization
**Example in Radiotherapy:** Used in CT simulators to reduce patient dose while preserving image quality.

346. **Automatic laser alignment (noun):** Self-calibrating laser system ensuring accurate patient positioning.
**Related Terms:** Simulation laser, optical alignment
**Example in Radiotherapy:** Aligns patient isocenter to CT reference marks automatically.

347. **Auto-segmentation (noun):** Software-based contouring of anatomical structures using AI or threshold algorithms.
**Related Terms:** Contour automation, structure detection
**Example in Radiotherapy:** Used to speed up OAR delineation in adaptive planning.

348. **Auxiliary beam modifier (noun):** A secondary device used to alter beam shape or intensity.
**Related Terms:** Compensator, filter
**Example in Radiotherapy:** Added to customize electron field uniformity.

349. **Axial slice thickness (noun):** The thickness of a CT image slice in the axial plane.
**Related Terms:** Image resolution, reconstruction interval
**Example in Radiotherapy:** Determines contour precision for treatment planning.

350. **Axillary node (noun):** Lymph node group in the underarm area.
**Related Terms:** Nodal region, lymphatic drainage
**Example in Radiotherapy:** Commonly included in breast cancer treatment fields.

351. **Azimuthal angle (noun):** The angular measurement around a circular plane.
**Related Terms:** Polar coordinate, gantry rotation
**Example in Radiotherapy:** Defines rotational orientation of beam geometry in TPS.

352. **Adaptive dose accumulation (noun):** The summation of dose from multiple adaptive fractions.
**Related Terms:** Re-planning, cumulative dose
**Example in Radiotherapy:** Used in adaptive SBRT to assess total delivered dose.

353. **Add-on filter (noun):** A removable device that modifies beam quality or intensity.
**Related Terms:** Wedge filter, beam hardening
**Example in Radiotherapy:** Used in orthovoltage therapy to shape the energy spectrum.

354. **Adjacent field junction (noun):** The interface between two neighboring radiation fields.
**Related Terms:** Field matching, hot spot
**Example in Radiotherapy:** Monitored to prevent dose overlap in craniospinal irradiation.

355. **Aerated lung (noun):** Lung tissue filled with air, affecting dose absorption.
**Related Terms:** Tissue density, heterogeneity correction
**Example in Radiotherapy:** Accounted for in lung IMRT dose calculation.

356. **Afterloader (noun):** A device used in brachytherapy to position and retrieve radioactive sources.
**Related Terms:** Remote afterloading, HDR system
**Example in Radiotherapy:** Delivers Ir-192 sources remotely to minimize radiation exposure.

357. **Air kerma (noun):** Kinetic energy released per unit mass of air by ionizing radiation.
**Related Terms:** Exposure, dose calibration
**Example in Radiotherapy:** Used as a primary dosimetric quantity in beam calibration.

358. **Air gap technique (noun):** Method of reducing scatter by increasing distance between patient and detector.
**Related Terms:** Scatter reduction, imaging geometry
**Example in Radiotherapy:** Used in portal imaging to improve edge .

359. **Air-cavity correction (noun):** Adjustment applied to dose calculation to account for air gaps in tissues.
**Related Terms:** Tissue inhomogeneity, electron disequilibrium
**Example in Radiotherapy:** Essential in head-and-neck IMRT near nasal cavities.

360. **Algorithm-based planning (noun):** Automated treatment optimization using mathematical models.
**Related Terms:** Dose calculation algorithm, AI planning
**Example in Radiotherapy:** Used in knowledge-based IMRT plan generation.

361. **Alignment laser (noun):** Light source indicating reference planes for patient positioning.
**Related Terms:** Isocenter alignment, simulation
**Example in Radiotherapy:** Aligns tattoos or markers during setup.

362. **Alpha-beta ratio (noun):** Radiobiological parameter describing tissue response to fractionation.
**Related Terms:** Linear-quadratic model, radiosensitivity
**Example in Radiotherapy:** Determines optimal fractionation for tumor control vs normal tissue sparing.

363. **Anatomical landmark (noun):** Recognizable structure used for patient setup and image registration.
**Related Terms:** Bony landmark, alignment point
**Example in Radiotherapy:** Used in pelvis setup via iliac crest matching.

364. **Angular velocity (noun):** The rate of rotational movement around an axis.
**Related Terms:** Gantry speed, dynamic delivery
**Example in Radiotherapy:** Controlled in VMAT for precise dose modulation.

365. **Anisotropic voxel (noun):** CT or MRI image voxel with unequal dimensions.
**Related Terms:** Image resolution, isotropic voxel
**Example in Radiotherapy:** Can cause geometric distortion during 3D reconstruction.

366. **Anterior oblique field (noun):** Treatment beam angled from the front of the patient.
**Related Terms:** Beam orientation, tangential field
**Example in Radiotherapy:** Commonly used in breast or chest wall planning.

367. **Aperture-based planning (noun):** Dose optimization using fixed field shapes instead of fluence maps.
**Related Terms:** Segmental IMRT, direct aperture optimization
**Example in Radiotherapy:** Used in simple IMRT to improve efficiency.

368. **Application catheter (noun):** Tube inserted into body cavities for brachytherapy source delivery.
**Related Terms:** Tandem, ovoid
**Example in Radiotherapy:** Used in intracavitary cervical brachytherapy.

369. **Arc modulation (noun):** Variation of beam intensity during gantry rotation.
**Related Terms:** VMAT, dynamic arc
**Example in Radiotherapy:** Optimizes dose conformity around complex targets.

370. **Areolar tissue (noun):** Loose connective tissue beneath the skin.
**Related Terms:** Subcutaneous layer, skin structure
**Example in Radiotherapy:** Affected during superficial dose delivery.

371. **Artifact correction (noun):** Image processing to reduce reconstruction errors.
**Related Terms:** Metal artifact reduction, CT correction
**Example in Radiotherapy:** Improves contouring accuracy in head-and-neck CTs.

372. **Asymmetric collimation (noun):** Independent movement of upper and lower jaws to create off-axis fields.
**Related Terms:** Half-beam block, jaw asymmetry
**Example in Radiotherapy:** Used for matching fields in breast tangents.

373. **Attenuator plate (noun):** Material used to absorb or reduce beam intensity.
**Related Terms:** Filter, beam shaper
**Example in Radiotherapy:** Used to balance dose in irregularly shaped fields.

374. **Audit phantom (noun):** Standardized phantom used in national or institutional QA audits.
**Related Terms:** End-to-end test, dosimetric verification
**Example in Radiotherapy:** Used by IAEA for inter-laboratory comparisons.

375. **Autotransformer (noun):** Electrical device that varies voltage within x-ray generators.
**Related Terms:** Power regulation, exposure control
**Example in Radiotherapy:** Used in simulator x-ray circuits.

376. **Axial plane (noun):** Horizontal plane dividing the body into upper and lower sections.
**Related Terms:** Transverse plane, CT slice
**Example in Radiotherapy:** Defines standard imaging orientation for contouring.

377. **Azimuthal modulation (noun):** Intensity variation around a circular beam delivery path.
**Related Terms:** Arc therapy, rotational modulation
**Example in Radiotherapy:** Used in proton arc therapy for dose conformity.

378. **Absolute calibration (noun):** Dosimetric calibration traceable to a national standard.
**Related Terms:** Reference calibration, chamber correction factor
**Example in Radiotherapy:** Performed using a standard ion chamber per IAEA TRS-398.

379. **Absolute dose (noun):** The measured or calculated total energy absorbed per unit mass.
**Related Terms:** Absorbed dose, dose calibration
**Example in Radiotherapy:** Verified during machine output calibration.

380. **Absorbed dose (noun):** The amount of radiation energy absorbed by tissue.
**Related Terms:** Gray (Gy), energy deposition
**Example in Radiotherapy:** Determines biological effect on tumor and normal tissues.

381. **Absorption edge (noun):** The photon energy where there is a sharp increase in absorption by a material.
**Related Terms:** K-edge, beam filtration
**Example in Radiotherapy:** Considered in shielding material design.

382. **Accessory mount (noun):** Device used to hold beam-modifying accessories on a linear accelerator.
**Related Terms:** Wedge tray, block holder
**Example in Radiotherapy:** Holds compensators or bolus material during delivery.

383. **Active breathing control (noun):** Technique for immobilizing respiratory motion during imaging or treatment.
**Related Terms:** DIBH, respiratory gating
**Example in Radiotherapy:** Used to reduce heart dose in left breast irradiation.

384. **Adaptive planning (noun):** Replanning process that adjusts for anatomical or tumor changes.
**Related Terms:** Re-optimization, adaptive radiotherapy
**Example in Radiotherapy:** Applied in head-and-neck cases to account for weight loss.

385. **Add-on block (noun):** Secondary shielding block used to define irregular field shapes.
**Related Terms:** Cerrobend block, field shaping
**Example in Radiotherapy:** Used for electron therapy of small lesions.

386. **Adenocarcinoma (noun):** A cancer originating from glandular epithelial tissue.
**Related Terms:** Carcinoma, histopathology
**Example in Radiotherapy:** Common histology in prostate and lung cancers.

387. **Administrative control (noun):** Policy-based measure ensuring radiation safety compliance.
**Related Terms:** Regulatory procedure, SOP
**Example in Radiotherapy:** Includes time, distance, and shielding guidelines.

388. **Air scatter (noun):** Scattering of radiation due to interaction with air molecules.
**Related Terms:** Photon scatter, dose fall-off
**Example in Radiotherapy:** Considered in superficial and electron treatments.

389. **Algorithm validation (noun):** Verification process ensuring dose calculation accuracy.
**Related Terms:** Benchmarking, QA validation
**Example in Radiotherapy:** Performed before clinical implementation of new TPS versions.

390. **Alignment correction (noun):** Adjustment applied to compensate for setup deviation.
**Related Terms:** Couch shift, registration correction
**Example in Radiotherapy:** Based on daily CBCT match results.

391. **Anatomic segmentation (noun):** Division of organs and structures in imaging data.
**Related Terms:** Contouring, auto-segmentation
**Example in Radiotherapy:** Used in AI-based structure detection systems.

392. **Anode heel effect (noun):** Variation in x-ray beam intensity across the field due to anode geometry.
**Related Terms:** X-ray tube, beam uniformity
**Example in Radiotherapy:** Corrected during simulator imaging calibration.

393. **Aperture block (noun):** Shield used to define custom field shape.
**Related Terms:** Cerrobend insert, beam collimation
**Example in Radiotherapy:** Used in electron cone cutouts for skin treatments.

394. **Arc therapy (noun):** Technique delivering radiation through continuous gantry rotation.
**Related Terms:** VMAT, dynamic arc
**Example in Radiotherapy:** Used in cranial and pelvic treatments for dose conformity.

395. **Area monitor (noun):** Device that continuously measures radiation levels in a treatment area.
**Related Terms:** Radiation detector, safety monitor
**Example in Radiotherapy:** Installed to ensure controlled room dose levels.

396. **Artefact (noun):** Distortion or error in imaging due to equipment or patient factors.
**Related Terms:** CT artifact, metal streak
**Example in Radiotherapy:** Can affect contouring and dose calculation accuracy.

397. **Asymmetric field (noun):** Radiation field displaced from the beam's central axis.
**Related Terms:** Half-beam block, collimator asymmetry
**Example in Radiotherapy:** Used in craniospinal junction matching.

398. **Attenuation map (noun):** Image displaying tissue attenuation properties.
**Related Terms:** CT density map, PET correction
**Example in Radiotherapy:** Used to correct photon attenuation in PET-CT fusion.

399. **Automatic positioning system (noun):** Mechanized patient setup system using pre-set coordinates.
**Related Terms:** Robotic couch, 6D alignment
**Example in Radiotherapy:** Used in stereotactic radiosurgery for submillimeter precision.

400. **Autoplanning (noun):** Software-assisted optimization generating treatment plans automatically.
**Related Terms:** AI-based planning, template planning
**Example in Radiotherapy:** Reduces planning time while maintaining clinical quality.

401. **Axial reconstruction (noun):** Image reformation process creating slices in the transverse plane.
**Related Terms:** CT reconstruction, image resampling
**Example in Radiotherapy:** Used to build planning datasets for contouring.

402. **Axillary boost (noun):** Additional dose directed to axillary lymph nodes after main breast irradiation.
**Related Terms:** Nodal boost, regional irradiation
**Example in Radiotherapy:** Delivered to control microscopic disease in high-risk axillary nodes.

403. **Axillary tail (noun):** Extension of breast tissue into the axilla.
**Related Terms:** Tail of Spence, breast anatomy
**Example in Radiotherapy:** Included in tangential fields for comprehensive breast coverage.

404. **Axon (noun):** Long projection of a neuron transmitting electrical impulses.
**Related Terms:** Neuron, myelin sheath
**Example in Radiotherapy:** Radiation-induced axonal damage may cause peripheral neuropathy.

405. **Attenuator plate (noun):** A device made of absorbing material used to reduce radiation beam intensity.
**Related Terms:** Filter, wedge, compensator
**Example in Radiotherapy:** Used in beam calibration to achieve desired dose uniformity.

406. **Attenuation coefficient (noun):** A measure describing how easily a material can attenuate radiation.
**Related Terms:** Linear attenuation, half-value layer
**Example in Radiotherapy:** Determines shielding requirements and tissue dose estimation.

407. **Audio-visual monitoring (noun):** System allowing therapists to observe and communicate with patients during treatment.
**Related Terms:** Patient surveillance, intercom
**Example in Radiotherapy:** Used to ensure patient safety and comfort during head and neck treatments.

408. **Auger electron (noun):** A low-energy electron emitted following internal conversion or photoelectric interactions.
**Related Terms:** Inner shell ionization, radiobiology
**Example in Radiotherapy:** Plays a role in localized DNA damage during radionuclide therapy.

409. **Automated contouring (noun):** Software-driven delineation of anatomical or target structures.
**Related Terms:** AI segmentation, structure set
**Example in Radiotherapy:** Reduces contouring time in adaptive radiotherapy workflows.

410. **Automated treatment delivery (noun):** Execution of radiotherapy plans via computerized control systems.
**Related Terms:** Record and verify system, linac automation
**Example in Radiotherapy:** Ensures precision and reproducibility in IMRT or VMAT delivery.

411. **Auxiliary beam modifier (noun):** Any secondary device used to shape or alter beam characteristics.
**Related Terms:** Bolus, wedge, compensator
**Example in Radiotherapy:** Used to adjust surface dose or compensate for irregular patient contours.

412. **Axial image (noun):** Cross-sectional slice perpendicular to the patient's long axis in CT or MRI.
**Related Terms:** Sagittal, coronal plane
**Example in Radiotherapy:** Used for target delineation and dose planning.

413. **Axial slice thickness (noun):** The depth of a single CT or MRI image section.
**Related Terms:** Slice interval, resolution
**Example in Radiotherapy:** Influences accuracy of contouring and dose calculation.

414. **Axillary node (noun):** Lymph node located in the armpit region.
**Related Terms:** Lymphatic drainage, breast radiotherapy
**Example in Radiotherapy:** Common target in post-mastectomy radiation fields.

415. **Azo dye marker (noun):** Tissue marker visible under imaging modalities for setup verification.
**Related Terms:** Fiducial marker, skin tattoo
**Example in Radiotherapy:** Used for permanent alignment reference in breast radiotherapy.

416. **Azimuthal angle (noun):** The angular position of a beam or object in a circular coordinate system.
**Related Terms:** Polar coordinates, gantry rotation
**Example in Radiotherapy:** Defines gantry orientation during arc-based treatments.

417. **Air cavity correction (noun):** Adjustment made in dose calculations to account for air-filled spaces.
**Related Terms:** Heterogeneity correction, dose perturbation
**Example in Radiotherapy:** Important for head and neck or lung cases with sinuses or bronchi.

418. **Air-kerma strength (noun):** Standardized measure of brachytherapy source output.
**Related Terms:** Reference air kerma rate, source calibration
**Example in Radiotherapy:** Used to specify dose rate for HDR Ir-192 sources.

419. **Air-tissue interface (noun):** Boundary between air and body tissue affecting dose distribution.
**Related Terms:** Build-up effect, backscatter
**Example in Radiotherapy:** Causes underdosing near lung or sinus interfaces.

420. **Albedo effect (noun):** The reflection of scattered photons from surfaces surrounding a radiation field.
**Related Terms:** Backscatter, dose contamination
**Example in Radiotherapy:** Considered during shielding design and phantom measurements.

421. **Algorithm accuracy (noun):** The degree of precision in dose calculation by a planning system.
**Related Terms:** Monte Carlo, collapsed cone
**Example in Radiotherapy:** Directly affects treatment plan quality in IMRT or SBRT.

422. **Alignment tolerance (noun):** The allowable deviation from the intended setup position.
**Related Terms:** Setup margin, QA
**Example in Radiotherapy:** Typically within ±2 mm for head and neck IMRT.

423. **Alloy shielding block (noun):** Custom cast metal block used to shape radiation fields.
**Related Terms:** Cerrobend, beam shaping
**Example in Radiotherapy:** Used in conventional radiotherapy before MLC era.

424. **Alpha track detector (noun):** Device used to record and measure alpha particle exposure.
**Related Terms:** Dosimeter, radiobiological assay
**Example in Radiotherapy:** Applied in environmental radon monitoring near treatment areas.

425. **Anatomical coordinate system (noun):** A standardized spatial reference used to locate body structures.
**Related Terms:** Axial, sagittal, coronal
**Example in Radiotherapy:** Assists in defining patient setup and isocenter coordinates.

426. **Anatomical landmark (noun):** Recognizable physical point used for alignment or positioning.
**Related Terms:** Bony landmark, reference point
**Example in Radiotherapy:** Used during setup verification using lasers or CBCT.

427. **Anatomical shielding (noun):** Protection of healthy organs by natural body structures.
**Related Terms:** Tissue sparing, beam arrangement
**Example in Radiotherapy:** Ribs and lungs provide partial shielding for liver fields.

428. **Anisotropy correction (noun):** Adjustment in brachytherapy dose due to directional source emission.
**Related Terms:** TG-43 formalism, anisotropy factor
**Example in Radiotherapy:** Applied for precise dose around Ir-192 sources.

429. **Annealing (noun):** Process of heating dosimeters to remove radiation history.
**Related Terms:** TLD, calibration
**Example in Radiotherapy:** Used to reset TLDs before new dose measurement cycles.

430. **Anode cooling curve (noun):** Chart showing heat dissipation rate of an X-ray tube anode.
**Related Terms:** Tube rating, heat capacity
**Example in Radiotherapy:** Ensures safe operation of diagnostic simulators.

431. **Antiscatter grid (noun):** Device that reduces scatter radiation reaching the detector.
**Related Terms:** Scatter rejection, image contrast
**Example in Radiotherapy:** Improves portal image clarity in kV imaging.

432. **Aperture block (noun):** Physical barrier defining the treatment field shape.
**Related Terms:** Collimator, MLC
**Example in Radiotherapy:** Used in electron therapy to confine the field.

433. **Apparent activity (noun):** Measured radioactivity differing from true due to geometry or attenuation.
**Related Terms:** Source calibration, decay correction
**Example in Radiotherapy:** Adjusted in brachytherapy source calibration reports.

434. **Application setup (noun):** The arrangement of equipment and patient for treatment delivery.
**Related Terms:** Positioning, immobilization
**Example in Radiotherapy:** Verified through imaging before beam-on.

435. **Arc modulation (noun):** Dynamic adjustment of dose rate and MLC position during gantry rotation.
**Related Terms:** VMAT, dynamic delivery
**Example in Radiotherapy:** Provides optimal conformity in complex dose distributions.

436. **Area monitor (noun):** Device that measures ambient radiation levels in treatment rooms.
**Related Terms:** Radiation survey, safety monitoring
**Example in Radiotherapy:** Installed near doors to detect stray leakage.

437. **Artifact reduction (noun):** Process of minimizing image distortions.
**Related Terms:** CT reconstruction, metal artifact correction
**Example in Radiotherapy:** Applied to improve contouring accuracy near dental fillings.

438. **Asymmetric collimation (noun):** Independent movement of collimator jaws to produce non-symmetric fields.
**Related Terms:** Field shaping, jaw tracking
**Example in Radiotherapy:** Useful in cranial or tangential field treatments.

439. **Atmospheric correction (noun):** Adjustment made to dosimeter readings for pressure and temperature variations.
**Related Terms:** Ion chamber correction, calibration factor
**Example in Radiotherapy:** Ensures accurate reference dose measurements.

440. **Attenuation correction map (noun):** CT-based matrix used for PET dose correction.
**Related Terms:** SUV, image fusion
**Example in Radiotherapy:** Required for PET-CT-based tumor delineation.

441. **Automatic gating (noun):** Synchronization of beam delivery with patient respiration.
**Related Terms:** Respiratory motion management, 4D-RT
**Example in Radiotherapy:** Applied in liver and lung SBRT.

442. **Autotransformer (noun):** Single-winding electrical transformer used for voltage regulation.
**Related Terms:** X-ray generator, power supply
**Example in Radiotherapy:** Stabilizes power supply for simulator imaging systems.

443. **Auxiliary dataset (noun):** Additional imaging or planning dataset supplementing the main plan.
**Related Terms:** Fusion imaging, secondary plan
**Example in Radiotherapy:** Used for adaptive planning with new CBCT scans.

444. **Average glandular dose (noun):** The average absorbed dose in glandular breast tissue during imaging.
**Related Terms:** Mammography, dose optimization
**Example in Radiotherapy:** Important for breast imaging dose audits.

445. **Axial plane correction (noun):** Adjustment made to ensure patient orientation alignment with imaging planes.
**Related Terms:** Gantry tilt, setup correction
**Example in Radiotherapy:** Ensures reproducibility during image-guided treatments.

446. **Absolute humidity (noun):** The amount of water vapor in air affecting dosimetry and equipment performance.
**Related Terms:** Environmental control, QA calibration
**Example in Radiotherapy:** Monitored in dosimetry labs for ion chamber accuracy.

447. **Anterior field border (noun):** The defined front limit of a treatment field.
**Related Terms:** Isocenter, beam arrangement
**Example in Radiotherapy:** Marked on skin for tangential breast setup.

448. **Axial rotation (noun):** Rotation around the body's long axis.
**Related Terms:** Pitch, roll
**Example in Radiotherapy:** Evaluated during setup corrections on 6D couch.

449. **Aperture optimization (noun):** Algorithm adjusting MLC shapes to improve plan quality.
**Related Terms:** IMRT planning, fluence map
**Example in Radiotherapy:** Used in inverse planning optimization.

450. **Air scatter factor (noun):** Correction for dose changes due to scatter from air to phantom interface.
**Related Terms:** Output factor, calibration
**Example in Radiotherapy:** Considered in reference dosimetry setups.

451. **Analytical anisotropic algorithm (AAA) (noun):** Dose calculation method modeling 3D radiation transport.
**Related Terms:** Monte Carlo, pencil beam
**Example in Radiotherapy:** Used in Eclipse TPS for photon dose computation.

452. **Aperture efficiency (noun):** The proportion of the beam area effectively used for treatment within the collimated field.
**Related Terms:** Beam shaping, field uniformity
**Example in Radiotherapy:** Optimized in IMRT to maintain dose conformity and reduce leakage.

453. **Apparent field size (noun):** The visible or projected treatment field as defined by light field or imaging.
**Related Terms:** Light field, radiation field
**Example in Radiotherapy:** Checked during daily QA to confirm collimator accuracy.

454. **Apposition (noun):** The contact or alignment of anatomical structures during positioning.
**Related Terms:** Alignment, immobilization
**Example in Radiotherapy:** Ensures consistent chest wall contact during breast treatments.

455. **Arc field verification (noun):** The process of checking rotational beam accuracy using imaging.
**Related Terms:** VMAT QA, gantry angle validation
**Example in Radiotherapy:** Performed in rotational dosimetry checks.

456. **Arc length (noun):** The distance covered by a rotating gantry during arc therapy.
**Related Terms:** VMAT, gantry rotation
**Example in Radiotherapy:** Determines the extent of modulation in a single arc plan.

457. **Area under curve (AUC) (noun):** A measure of cumulative response or effect derived from a plotted curve.
**Related Terms:** DVH analysis, biological modeling
**Example in Radiotherapy:** Used in TCP/NTCP modeling for outcome prediction.

458. **Artifact correction algorithm (noun):** Software process to remove noise or artifacts from images.
**Related Terms:** CT reconstruction, imaging QA
**Example in Radiotherapy:** Enhances target visibility in CBCT scans.

459. **Artificial intelligence contouring (noun):** Automated structure segmentation using AI tools.
**Related Terms:** Auto-segmentation, machine learning
**Example in Radiotherapy:** Reduces planning time for organs-at-risk in head and neck cases.

460. **Asymmetric field junction (noun):** Overlapping fields with unequal borders to ensure dose uniformity.
**Related Terms:** Field matching, craniospinal junction
**Example in Radiotherapy:** Used in craniospinal irradiation (CSI).

461. **Asymptotic dose region (noun):** Region where dose approaches a maximum steady value with increasing depth.
**Related Terms:** Depth-dose curve, dmax
**Example in Radiotherapy:** Represents build-up region stabilization in photon beams.

462. **Attenuation map (noun):** A spatial representation of attenuation coefficients for dose calculation.
**Related Terms:** CT number, electron density map
**Example in Radiotherapy:** Essential in PET-CT image fusion for planning.

463. **Automated image fusion (noun):** Computer-based registration of multimodal images.
**Related Terms:** Rigid registration, deformable registration
**Example in Radiotherapy:** Aligns MRI with CT for soft tissue .

464. **Automated patient setup (noun):** Robotic or software-controlled positioning system ensuring reproducibility.
**Related Terms:** 6D couch, image-guided setup
**Example in Radiotherapy:** Used in stereotactic treatments for submillimeter precision.

465. **Automatic beam interruption (noun):** Safety feature that halts beam output upon detecting errors.
**Related Terms:** Interlock, emergency stop
**Example in Radiotherapy:** Activated if patient moves during treatment delivery.

466. **Automatic exposure control (noun):** System regulating radiation output to achieve optimal image quality.
**Related Terms:** kVp, mAs control
**Example in Radiotherapy:** Used in kV imaging systems for portal verification.

467. **Automatic field verification (noun):** Image-based confirmation of correct field alignment before treatment.
**Related Terms:** EPID, image registration
**Example in Radiotherapy:** Ensures accuracy before daily IMRT fraction delivery.

468. **Axial coordinate (noun):** Numerical value defining position along the patient's longitudinal axis.
**Related Terms:** Spatial coordinate, DICOM reference
**Example in Radiotherapy:** Used in contouring to specify tumor extent.

469. **Axial dose distribution (noun):** The variation of dose along the longitudinal body axis.
**Related Terms:** 3D dose map, DVH
**Example in Radiotherapy:** Reviewed during plan QA to confirm homogeneity.

470. **Axial misalignment (noun):** Deviation of patient or couch along the head-foot axis.
**Related Terms:** Translational error, setup correction
**Example in Radiotherapy:** Corrected through CBCT verification.

471. **Axillary boost (noun):** Supplemental radiation dose directed to axillary lymph nodes.
**Related Terms:** Nodal irradiation, breast radiotherapy
**Example in Radiotherapy:** Applied for node-positive breast carcinoma.

472. **Axillary region (noun):** The area of the armpit containing lymphatic structures.
**Related Terms:** Axillary dissection, nodal target
**Example in Radiotherapy:** Contoured as a clinical target volume (CTV).

473. **Axonopathy (noun):** Damage to axons due to radiation exposure.
**Related Terms:** Neuropathy, late effect
**Example in Radiotherapy:** Observed in high-dose cranial or spinal treatments.

474. **Air pressure correction (noun):** Adjustment in dosimetry for barometric pressure variation.
**Related Terms:** Chamber calibration, environmental correction
**Example in Radiotherapy:** Applied during ion chamber dose measurement.

475. **Acoustic marker (noun):** Ultrasound-visible marker for non-ionizing localization.
**Related Terms:** Fiducial marker, motion tracking
**Example in Radiotherapy:** Used in prostate IGRT ultrasound guidance.

476. **Adaptive dose painting (noun):** Technique of altering dose distribution based on biological imaging.
**Related Terms:** PET-based planning, dose escalation
**Example in Radiotherapy:** Increases dose to hypoxic tumor subvolumes.

477. **Adaptive fractionation (noun):** Adjustment of dose per fraction during treatment based on response.
**Related Terms:** Biological adaptation, ART
**Example in Radiotherapy:** Implemented in adaptive head and neck protocols.

478. **Adaptive imaging protocol (noun):** Imaging strategy that modifies frequency or modality based on anatomy change.
**Related Terms:** ART imaging, CBCT scheduling
**Example in Radiotherapy:** Reduces unnecessary imaging dose in long treatment courses.

479. **Adaptive replan (noun):** Revised treatment plan to account for anatomical or tumor changes.
**Related Terms:** ART, deformation registration
**Example in Radiotherapy:** Triggered when body contour changes beyond tolerance.

480. **Adaptive workflow (noun):** Systematic process of evaluating, recontouring, and replanning adaptively.
**Related Terms:** Adaptive planning, QA protocol
**Example in Radiotherapy:** Standard in MR-Linac-guided adaptive treatments.

481. **Add-on collimator (noun):** Removable device mounted to the head of the linac to shape the beam.
**Related Terms:** Electron cone, custom collimator
**Example in Radiotherapy:** Used in small field electron treatments.

482. **Add-on filter (noun):** External filter inserted into beam path to modify intensity or spectrum.
**Related Terms:** Flattening filter, compensator
**Example in Radiotherapy:** Used for dose equalization in oblique breast fields.

483. **Adjacent field match (noun):** Alignment of two or more radiation fields to ensure dose uniformity at junctions.
**Related Terms:** Junction dose, field matching
**Example in Radiotherapy:** Important in craniospinal and spine field planning.

484. **Administration route (noun):** The method of introducing a radiopharmaceutical into the body.
**Related Terms:** Intravenous, oral route
**Example in Radiotherapy:** Determines biodistribution in therapeutic radioisotopes.

485. **Adsorbed dose (noun):** Dose deposited in a material due to adsorption rather than absorption.
**Related Terms:** Surface interaction, scatter
**Example in Radiotherapy:** Considered in dosimeter film calibration.

486. **Air gap technique (noun):** Method using space between patient and detector to reduce scatter.
**Related Terms:** Scatter reduction, geometric magnification
**Example in Radiotherapy:** Used in electron therapy to improve penumbra.

487. **Air-void correction (noun):** Adjusting dose for air pockets in immobilization or anatomy.
**Related Terms:** Heterogeneity correction, build-up loss
**Example in Radiotherapy:** Applied in head and neck thermoplastic masks.

488. **Alignment lasers (noun):** Laser system used to project reference lines on the patient for setup.
**Related Terms:** Simulation lasers, positioning
**Example in Radiotherapy:** Ensures daily reproducibility of isocenter alignment.

489. **Alloy block (noun):** Shielding block composed of lead alloy for field shaping.
**Related Terms:** Cerrobend, custom block
**Example in Radiotherapy:** Used in conventional field shaping before MLCs.

490. **Ambient dose equivalent (noun):** Dose quantity that approximates effective dose from environmental radiation.
**Related Terms:** Survey meter, radiation safety
**Example in Radiotherapy:** Measured during room leakage surveys.

491. **Analog-to-digital converter (noun):** Device that converts analog signals to digital form.
**Related Terms:** Signal processing, EPID system
**Example in Radiotherapy:** Converts detector signals into digital imaging data.

492. **Anatomical reference point (noun):** Specific landmark used to define positional reference.
**Related Terms:** Setup mark, isocenter reference
**Example in Radiotherapy:** Nasal bridge or tragus used in head setup alignment.

493. **Anode heel effect (noun):** Variation in X-ray intensity across the field due to anode geometry.
**Related Terms:** Beam uniformity, X-ray imaging
**Example in Radiotherapy:** Considered in simulator exposure balancing.

494. **Anterior oblique field (noun):** Beam incident from an oblique anterior direction.
**Related Terms:** Tangential beam, 3D conformal
**Example in Radiotherapy:** Used in cervical and thoracic spine cases.

495. **Aperture-based optimization (noun):** IMRT optimization using defined field apertures instead of fluence maps.
**Related Terms:** Segment-based planning, VMAT
**Example in Radiotherapy:** Simplifies optimization for faster plan generation.

496. **Applicator cone (noun):** Device used to guide electron beams onto the patient's surface.
**Related Terms:** Electron applicator, SSD
**Example in Radiotherapy:** Ensures correct beam collimation in electron therapy.

497. **Approximation algorithm (noun):** Simplified computation technique used for dose estimation.
**Related Terms:** Pencil beam, algorithm accuracy
**Example in Radiotherapy:** Used in early planning systems for efficiency.

**498. As-built documentation (noun):** Final technical record showing the installed configuration of a treatment system.
**Related Terms:** Commissioning report, QA records
**Example in Radiotherapy:** Maintained for equipment validation audits.

**499. Aspect ratio (noun):** Ratio of image width to height.
**Related Terms:** Image geometry, pixel size
**Example in Radiotherapy:** Important for ensuring undistorted DRR and portal images.

**500. Assisted setup (noun):** Positioning process aided by immobilization and imaging devices.
**Related Terms:** Image-guided setup, couch correction
**Example in Radiotherapy:** Used in head and neck positioning with thermoplastic mask guidance.

# B

1. **Backscatter (noun):** Radiation deflected from its original path back toward the source after interaction with matter.
   **Related Terms:** Scatter radiation, dose perturbation.
   **Example in Radiotherapy:** Considered when shielding sensitive organs behind the target.
2. **Backprojection (noun):** Image reconstruction method projecting measured data back along paths to form an image.
   **Related Terms:** Computed tomography (CT), reconstruction algorithm.
   **Example in Radiotherapy:** Used in CT simulation for treatment planning.
3. **Backpointer (noun):** Laser or device showing beam entry and exit points on the patient surface.
   **Related Terms:** Room lasers, patient positioning.
   **Example in Radiotherapy:** Helps confirm isocenter alignment in treatment setup.
4. **Backprojection algorithm (noun):** A mathematical approach to reconstructing CT images by summing backprojected rays.
   **Related Terms:** Filtered backprojection, tomography.
   **Example in Radiotherapy:** Basis for planning system image reconstruction.
5. **Backup timer (noun):** A secondary timer preventing overexposure if the primary timer fails.
   **Related Terms:** Interlocks, radiation safety.
   **Example in Radiotherapy:** Ensures treatment beam automatically stops in machine malfunction.
6. **Baffling (beam collimation) (noun):** Physical structures to block stray radiation or reduce leakage.
   **Related Terms:** Collimators, shielding.
   **Example in Radiotherapy:** Used in treatment heads to improve beam quality.
7. **Bag mask ventilation (noun):** Manual device delivering positive pressure ventilation during emergencies.
   **Related Terms:** Airway management, CPR.
   **Example in Radiotherapy:** Kept ready in case a patient loses consciousness during setup.
8. **Barium contrast (noun):** Radiopaque substance enhancing GI tract visibility on imaging.
   **Related Terms:** Contrast agents, simulation imaging.
   **Example in Radiotherapy:** Used in CT simulation to outline stomach or bowel.
9. **Barium enema (noun):** X-ray or CT study using rectal administration of barium contrast.
   **Related Terms:** Colon imaging, GI contrast.
   **Example in Radiotherapy:** Helps delineate rectum for pelvic radiotherapy planning.
10. **Barium swallow (noun):** Fluoroscopic study of the esophagus and stomach using barium.
   **Related Terms:** Esophageal imaging, contrast studies.
   **Example in Radiotherapy:** Identifies tumor extent in esophageal cancer cases.
11. **Beam attenuation (noun):** Reduction in beam intensity as it passes through material.
   **Related Terms:** Attenuation coefficient, beam quality.
   **Example in Radiotherapy:** Considered in tissue heterogeneity correction in planning.
12. **Beam axis (noun):** The central path of the radiation beam emitted from the treatment unit.
   **Related Terms:** Central axis (CAX), isocenter.
   **Example in Radiotherapy:** Used to align fields in multi-beam arrangements.

13. **Beam block (noun):** Shielding device to block unwanted parts of the treatment field.
**Related Terms:** Cerrobend block, custom shielding.
**Example in Radiotherapy:** Protects healthy tissues adjacent to tumor.

14. **Beam central axis (noun):** Line passing through the geometric center of the treatment beam.
**Related Terms:** Beam axis, isocenter.
**Example in Radiotherapy:** Reference for dose profiles and calibration.

15. **Beam collimation (noun):** Shaping of the radiation beam using collimators or jaws.
**Related Terms:** Multileaf collimator (MLC), field shaping.
**Example in Radiotherapy:** Optimizes target coverage and spares normal tissue.

16. **Beam compensator (noun):** Physical device modifying beam intensity to correct for patient contour irregularities.
**Related Terms:** Bolus, intensity modulation.
**Example in Radiotherapy:** Used in 3D-CRT to produce uniform dose distribution.

17. **Beam data acquisition (noun):** Measurement of beam characteristics for treatment planning system commissioning.
**Related Terms:** Dosimetry, commissioning.
**Example in Radiotherapy:** Involves measuring PDD, TMR, and profiles.

18. **Beam divergence (noun):** Natural spreading of the radiation beam from its source.
**Related Terms:** Source-to-axis distance (SAD), field size.
**Example in Radiotherapy:** Affects geometric penumbra and field matching.

19. **Beam flatness (noun):** Measure of uniformity of dose distribution across the beam profile.
**Related Terms:** Symmetry, beam quality.
**Example in Radiotherapy:** Evaluated during linear accelerator QA.

20. **Beam hardening (noun):** Increase in average photon energy as low-energy photons are filtered out.
**Related Terms:** Filtration, CT artifacts.
**Example in Radiotherapy:** Corrected in CT planning to improve dose calculation.

21. **Beam homogenizer (noun):** Device to make beam intensity uniform.
**Related Terms:** Flattening filter, beam shaping.
**Example in Radiotherapy:** Used in electron therapy to achieve uniform dose.

22. **Beam intensity profile (noun):** Dose distribution across a radiation beam at a specified depth.
**Related Terms:** Beam profile, dosimetry.
**Example in Radiotherapy:** Used to evaluate machine calibration and TPS modeling.

23. **Beam junction (noun):** Area where two radiation fields meet or overlap.
**Related Terms:** Field matching, dose homogeneity.
**Example in Radiotherapy:** Monitored to avoid hot or cold spots.

24. **Beam limiting device (noun):** Any device restricting the size of the treatment beam.
**Related Terms:** Jaws, MLCs.
**Example in Radiotherapy:** Defines maximum field size on a linac.

25. **Beam matching (noun):** Process of calibrating multiple treatment machines to deliver identical beams.
**Related Terms:** Cross-calibration, QA.
**Example in Radiotherapy:** Ensures consistent treatment if patient switches linacs.

26. **Beam modifier (noun):** Any device altering the shape, energy, or intensity of the beam.
**Related Terms:** Compensator, bolus.
**Example in Radiotherapy:** Used to optimize tumor coverage in 3D-CRT.

27. **Beam monitor chamber (noun):** Ion chamber in the treatment head that measures output dose.
**Related Terms:** Output calibration, QA.
**Example in Radiotherapy:** Ensures accurate MU delivery during treatment.

28. **Beam penumbra (noun):** Region at beam edge where dose rapidly falls off.
**Related Terms:** Geometric penumbra, collimator.
**Example in Radiotherapy:** Minimized to sharpen field edges.

29. **Beam quality (noun):** Energy spectrum or penetrating ability of a radiation beam.
**Related Terms:** HVL (half-value layer), beam energy.
**Example in Radiotherapy:** Determines depth dose characteristics.

30. **Beam shaping (noun):** Adjusting beam outline to match target contour.
**Related Terms:** MLC, custom blocks.
**Example in Radiotherapy:** Essential in conformal therapy techniques.

31. **Beam splitter (noun):** Optical device dividing light or radiation into two paths.
**Related Terms:** Imaging, optical systems.
**Example in Radiotherapy:** Used in some alignment or QA tools.

32. **Beam spoiler (noun):** Device introducing scatter to increase surface dose.
**Related Terms:** Bolus, buildup region.
**Example in Radiotherapy:** Used in TBI (total body irradiation).

33. **Beam stop (noun):** Shield to absorb the beam when not treating.
**Related Terms:** Beam stopper, shielding.
**Example in Radiotherapy:** Protects staff in some treatment rooms.

34. **Beam symmetry (noun):** Uniformity of dose distribution on either side of the beam central axis.
**Related Terms:** Flatness, QA.
**Example in Radiotherapy:** Monitored during linac quality checks.

35. **Beam weighting (noun):** Distribution of dose contribution among multiple beams.
**Related Terms:** Treatment planning, optimization.
**Example in Radiotherapy:** Adjusted to spare organs at risk.

36. **Beam's eye view (BEV) (noun):** Visualization of patient anatomy from beam source perspective.
**Related Terms:** Planning, imaging.
**Example in Radiotherapy:** Used to optimize MLC shape in IMRT.

37. **Bending magnet (noun):** Magnet in linac that bends electron beam path toward target.
**Related Terms:** Linac head, waveguide.
**Example in Radiotherapy:** Determines beam direction in treatment unit.

38. **Beryllium window (X-ray tubes) (noun):** Thin beryllium barrier allowing X-ray exit while minimizing absorption.
**Related Terms:** Diagnostic imaging, tube design.
**Example in Radiotherapy:** Present in kilovoltage imaging systems.

39. **Beta decay (noun):** Radioactive process where a nucleus emits a beta particle.
**Related Terms:** Beta radiation, radionuclide.
**Example in Radiotherapy:** Basis of some internal emitters.

40. **Beta particles (noun):** High-energy electrons or positrons emitted in beta decay.
**Related Terms:** Beta radiation, isotope therapy.
**Example in Radiotherapy:** Used in targeted radionuclide therapy.

41. **Beta-plus decay (noun):** A type of radioactive decay in which a proton is converted into a neutron, emitting a positron and a neutrino.
**Related Terms:** Positron emission, PET imaging.
**Example in Radiotherapy:** Used in PET scanners to visualize tumor metabolism with positron-emitting isotopes.

42. **Beta-minus decay (noun):** A radioactive decay process in which a neutron is converted into a proton, emitting an electron and an antineutrino.
**Related Terms:** Beta particles, radionuclides.
**Example in Radiotherapy:** Seen in isotopes like Strontium-90 used for palliative treatment.

43. **Beta radiation (noun):** Ionizing radiation composed of high-energy electrons or positrons emitted during beta decay.
**Related Terms:** Electron therapy, shielding.
**Example in Radiotherapy:** Requires thin shielding; relevant in brachytherapy sources.

44. **BGO scintillator (noun):** Bismuth Germanate crystal used in detectors to convert gamma photons to light.
**Related Terms:** PET detectors, scintillation.
**Example in Radiotherapy:** Used in PET/CT scanners for high-resolution imaging.

45. **Bilateral field arrangement (noun):** A treatment technique using opposed beams from both sides of the patient.
**Related Terms:** Isocenter, parallel-opposed fields.
**Example in Radiotherapy:** Applied in head-and-neck cancer treatments to balance dose distribution.

46. **Bilinear interpolation (noun):** An image reconstruction method estimating new pixel values using linear interpolation in two directions.
**Related Terms:** Image resampling, CT reconstruction.
**Example in Radiotherapy:** Used in image registration to refine CBCT alignment.

47. **Bilious contrast medium (noun):** A type of contrast used for imaging biliary tract structures.
**Related Terms:** Cholangiography, contrast studies.
**Example in Radiotherapy:** Helpful in delineating hepatobiliary structures for SBRT planning.

48. **Binary multileaf collimator (noun):** A collimator where leaves are either fully open or closed, shaping the radiation beam.
**Related Terms:** TomoTherapy, beam modulation.
**Example in Radiotherapy:** Used in helical TomoTherapy for intensity modulation.

49. **Binding energy (noun):** The energy required to disassemble a nucleus or remove an electron from an atom.
**Related Terms:** Atomic structure, photon interactions.
**Example in Radiotherapy:** Determines the energy levels of photoelectric absorption.

50. **Binning (noun):** Grouping of detector pixels to reduce image noise or data size.
**Related Terms:** Image processing, signal-to-noise ratio.
**Example in Radiotherapy:** Used in EPID imaging to enhance visualization of portal images.

51. **Biological damage (noun):** Cellular or tissue injury caused by ionizing radiation.
**Related Terms:** DNA double-strand breaks, radiobiology.
**Example in Radiotherapy:** Directly related to treatment toxicity and tumor control.

53. **Biological dose (noun):** A dose that accounts for biological effectiveness rather than physical energy deposited.
**Related Terms:** RBE (Relative Biological Effectiveness).
**Example in Radiotherapy:** Used in proton therapy to adjust for higher effectiveness per Gy.

54. **Biological equivalent dose (noun):** A dose metric considering fractionation and tissue response, often called BED.
**Related Terms:** LQ model, fractionation.
**Example in Radiotherapy:** BED calculations guide hypofractionated schedules.

55. **Biological half-life (noun):** Time taken for half of a substance to be biologically eliminated from the body.
**Related Terms:** Effective half-life, clearance.
**Example in Radiotherapy:** Important in radionuclide therapy dosimetry.

56. **Biological response modifiers (noun):** Agents that alter cellular response to radiation.
**Related Terms:** Radiosensitizers, radioprotectors.
**Example in Radiotherapy:** Amifostine reduces normal tissue toxicity during RT.

57. **Biologic target volume (noun):** Volume of tissue defined by functional or biological imaging rather than anatomy alone.
**Related Terms:** PET-based planning, GTV.
**Example in Radiotherapy:** Identifying hypoxic tumor subregions with FMISO PET.

58. **Bioluminescence imaging (noun):** Technique detecting light emitted by biochemical reactions in living cells.
**Related Terms:** Optical imaging, molecular imaging.
**Example in Radiotherapy:** Used in preclinical studies to track tumor growth or response.

59. **Biomarkers of radiation response (noun):** Biological indicators predicting or monitoring tissue response to radiation.
**Related Terms:** Genetic markers, radiosensitivity.
**Example in Radiotherapy:** $\gamma$-H2AX foci indicate DNA damage after RT.

60. **Biomodelling (noun):** Computational simulation of biological systems under radiation exposure.
**Related Terms:** Radiobiological models, LQ model.
**Example in Radiotherapy:** Used to predict tumor control probability (TCP).

61. **Biophysics of ionizing radiation (noun):** Study of physical mechanisms by which radiation interacts with living matter.
**Related Terms:** Radiation transport, energy deposition.
**Example in Radiotherapy:** Explains LET effects in particle therapy.

62. **Biosensor dosimetry (noun):** Using biological sensors to measure radiation dose.
**Related Terms:** Bioassays, microdosimetry.
**Example in Radiotherapy:** Experimental skin patches that fluoresce with radiation exposure.

63. **Biostatic equilibrium (noun):** State in which intake and elimination of a radionuclide are balanced.
**Related Terms:** Radiopharmacokinetics, clearance.
**Example in Radiotherapy:** Important in internal dosimetry for therapeutic isotopes.

64. **Biotransformation (noun):** Metabolic conversion of radiosensitizers or radioprotectors within the body.
**Related Terms:** Pharmacokinetics, radiosensitization.
**Example in Radiotherapy:** Activation of nitroimidazole compounds in hypoxic cells.

65. **Bivariate analysis (noun):** Statistical method to assess relationship between two variables.
**Related Terms:** Dose–response correlation, regression.
**Example in Radiotherapy:** Used to analyze tumor control probability vs. BED.

66. **Bladder dose constraint (noun):** Maximum permissible radiation dose to the bladder to prevent toxicity.
**Related Terms:** OAR constraints, DVH analysis.
**Example in Radiotherapy:** Prostate IMRT plans limit bladder Dmax to $<70$ Gy.

67. **Blood–brain barrier radiosensitivity (noun):** The vulnerability of the BBB to radiation damage.
**Related Terms:** Neurotoxicity, CNS protection.
**Example in Radiotherapy:** Important for dose planning in pediatric brain tumors.

68. **Blood pool imaging (noun):** A nuclear medicine scan showing blood distribution in vessels and organs.
**Related Terms:** radionuclide angiography, SPECT
**Example in Radiotherapy:** Assesses cardiac function before mediastinal RT.

69. **Blood volume changes in RT (noun):** Alterations in circulating blood due to irradiation.
**Related Terms:** hematologic toxicity, marrow dose
**Example in Radiotherapy:** Monitored during pelvic RT to prevent anemia.

70. **Bone marrow suppression (noun):** Decreased marrow activity from radiation or chemotherapy.
**Related Terms:** myelosuppression, leukopenia
**Example in Radiotherapy:** Limits dose in pelvic RT to protect hematopoiesis.

71. **Bone dose calculation (noun):** Estimating absorbed dose in osseous tissue.
**Related Terms:** heterogeneity correction, Monte Carlo
**Example in Radiotherapy:** Ensures accuracy in spine SBRT planning.

72. **Bone scintigraphy (noun):** Nuclear scan detecting bone metastases or lesions.
**Related Terms:** skeletal survey, Tc-99m MDP
**Example in Radiotherapy:** Identifies targets for palliative bone RT.

73. **Boost dose (noun):** Additional radiation after initial course to tumor bed.
**Related Terms:** sequential boost, SIB
**Example in Radiotherapy:** Breast tumor bed boost after whole-breast RT.

74. **Boost field (noun):** Radiation field delivering the boost dose.
**Related Terms:** electron boost, conformal boost
**Example in Radiotherapy:** Tangential photon fields for breast boost.

75. **Brachial plexus tolerance dose (noun):** Maximum safe radiation to avoid neuropathy.
**Related Terms:** dose constraints, QUANTEC
**Example in Radiotherapy:** Limited to $\leq 66$ Gy in head-neck RT plans.

76. **Brachytherapy afterloading (noun):** Loading radioactive sources into applicators post-placement.
**Related Terms:** HDR, LDR
**Example in Radiotherapy:** Ir-192 HDR afterloading in cervical cancer.

77. **Brachytherapy applicator (noun):** Device positioning sources at treatment site.
**Related Terms:** tandem & ovoid, vaginal cylinder
**Example in Radiotherapy:** Used in gynecologic intracavitary RT.

78. **Brachytherapy dose rate (noun):** Activity level of source delivery (LDR, HDR, PDR).
**Related Terms:** source strength, dwell time
**Example in Radiotherapy:** HDR: $>12$ Gy/hr, LDR: 0.4–2 Gy/hr.

79. **Brachytherapy dosimetry (noun):** Calculation and verification of brachytherapy dose.
**Related Terms:** TG-43, source calibration
**Example in Radiotherapy:** Used to confirm Ir-192 source strength.

80. **Brachytherapy fractionation (noun):** Division of brachytherapy dose into sessions.
**Related Terms:** HDR schedule, pulse-dose
**Example in Radiotherapy:** 7 Gy × 3 fractions for endometrial cancer.

81. **Brachytherapy seeds (noun):** Small encapsulated radioactive sources.
**Related Terms:** prostate implants, I-125
**Example in Radiotherapy:** Permanent seed implant for prostate cancer.

82. **Brachytherapy source calibration (noun):** Standardizing source activity before clinical use.
**Related Terms:** dosimetry lab, TG-43
**Example in Radiotherapy:** Ensures accurate dwell time in HDR treatments.

83. **Bragg peak (proton therapy) (noun):** Sharp proton dose maximum at specific depth.
**Related Terms:** spread-out Bragg peak, proton therapy
**Example in Radiotherapy:** Used to spare distal normal tissue in pediatric tumors.

84. **Breathing motion management (noun):** Techniques controlling tumor motion during respiration.
**Related Terms:** DIBH, gating
**Example in Radiotherapy:** RPM-guided gating for left breast RT.

85. **Bremsstrahlung radiation (noun):** X-ray emission from electron deceleration.
**Related Terms:** photon contamination, linac target
**Example in Radiotherapy:** Generated in high-energy electron beams.

86. **Brightness (image quality metric) (noun):** Degree of luminance in images.
**Related Terms:** contrast, HU levels
**Example in Radiotherapy:** Adjusted during CBCT verification.

87. **Bronchial tree contouring (noun):** Delineation of airway structures on CT.
**Related Terms:** OAR contouring, lung RT
**Example in Radiotherapy:** Avoids excessive dose during thoracic RT.

88. **Bronchogenic carcinoma (RT planning) (noun):** Lung cancer originating from bronchi.
**Related Terms:** NSCLC, tumor contouring
**Example in Radiotherapy:** Planned with 4D-CT to account for motion.

89. **Bronchoscopy-guided marker placement (noun):** Fiducial placement via bronchoscope for tumor localization.
**Related Terms:** image guidance, lung SBRT
**Example in Radiotherapy:** Improves targeting accuracy in peripheral lung lesions.

90. **Buildup cap (dosimetry) (noun):** Material covering detectors to achieve electronic equilibrium.
**Related Terms:** ion chamber, dose calibration
**Example in Radiotherapy:** Used in linac output checks.

91. **Buildup dose region (noun):** Depth where surface dose increases to maximum.
**Related Terms:** Dmax, skin sparing
**Example in Radiotherapy:** Photon beams spare superficial skin by buildup effect.

92. **Biceps brachii (noun):** Upper-arm muscle relevant to positioning.
**Related Terms:** immobilization, arm support
**Example in Radiotherapy:** Raised arm to avoid beam path in breast RT.

93. **Biceps femoris (noun):** Thigh muscle, part of hamstring group.
**Related Terms:** patient comfort, prone setup
**Example in Radiotherapy:** Cushions used to reduce strain during pelvic RT.

94. **Bifurcation of carotid artery (noun):** Division of common carotid into internal/external branches.
**Related Terms:** neck contouring, vascular dose
**Example in Radiotherapy:** Avoid hot spots in head-neck RT plans.

95. **Bifurcation of trachea (carina) (noun):** Split of trachea into left/right bronchi.
**Related Terms:** mediastinal landmark, 4D-CT
**Example in Radiotherapy:** Used for target localization in lung RT.

96. **Bilateral symmetry (patient setup) (noun):** Equal positioning of body sides during RT setup.
**Related Terms:** lasers, tattoo alignment
**Example in Radiotherapy:** Ensures reproducibility in pelvic treatments.

97. **Bile ducts (extrahepatic) (noun):** Channels carrying bile outside the liver.
**Related Terms:** hepatobiliary contouring, GI OAR
**Example in Radiotherapy:** Delineated in upper GI RT plans.

98. **Biliary tract anatomy (noun):** Structure of intrahepatic and extrahepatic bile ducts.
**Related Terms:** liver contouring, GI OAR
**Example in Radiotherapy:** Avoid high dose in cholangiocarcinoma RT.

99. **Bilobed liver segments (noun):** Anatomical division of liver into right and left lobes.
**Related Terms:** Couinaud segments, liver contouring
**Example in Radiotherapy:** Guides SBRT target localization.

100. **Bilobed lung fissures (noun):** Fissural division creating lung lobes.
**Related Terms:** bronchopulmonary anatomy, lung SBRT
**Example in Radiotherapy:** Identified to assess tumor location.

101. **Binocular vision (positioning) (noun):** Depth perception aiding setup accuracy.
**Related Terms:** visual alignment, manual matching
**Example in Radiotherapy:** RTTs use binocular cues during patient alignment.

102. **Bacteremia (noun):** Presence of bacteria in the bloodstream that may occur after invasive procedures or infections.
**Related Terms:** Sepsis, Infection control
**Example in Radiotherapy:** Care is taken during central line insertion in head and neck RT patients to avoid bacteremia.

103. **Backscatter factor (noun):** Ratio of dose including backscattered radiation to dose without backscatter at a given depth.
**Related Terms:** Scatter radiation, Dose calibration
**Example in Radiotherapy:** Used in photon beam calibration for surface dose estimation.

104. **Backscatter shield (noun):** A device or layer that prevents scattered radiation from re-entering the treatment field.
**Related Terms:** Beam modifiers, Shielding
**Example in Radiotherapy:** Lead shields are used to minimize backscatter in superficial treatments.

105. **Back-projection reconstruction (noun):** Image reconstruction method that projects measured data back into the image plane.
**Related Terms:** Filtered back projection, CT reconstruction
**Example in Radiotherapy:** Used in CT imaging to create cross-sectional slices for treatment planning.

106. **Balanced field (noun):** Radiation field arrangement ensuring equal dose distribution across the target.
**Related Terms:** Beam weighting, Isodose distribution
**Example in Radiotherapy:** Balanced fields are used in opposed lateral head-and-neck treatments.

107. **Bandwidth (noun):** The range of frequencies a system can process or transmit.
**Related Terms:** Signal-to-noise ratio, Imaging resolution
**Example in Radiotherapy:** MRI systems use wide bandwidth to reduce geometric distortion.

108. **Barometric correction (noun):** Adjustment made to ion chamber readings to compensate for atmospheric pressure variations.
**Related Terms:** Temperature-pressure correction, Dosimetry QA
**Example in Radiotherapy:** Daily output checks apply barometric correction for accurate dose readings.

109. **Base dose plan (noun):** The primary dose distribution plan on which boost or adaptive plans are built.
**Related Terms:** Composite plan, Boost dose
**Example in Radiotherapy:** The base plan covers elective nodal regions before adding a boost to the tumor.

110. **Baseline drift (noun):** Gradual change in detector or monitor readings over time.
**Related Terms:** Reproducibility, QA calibration
**Example in Radiotherapy:** Ion chamber baseline drift is checked during monthly QA.

111. **Beam attenuation coefficient (noun):** Measure of how easily a material reduces beam intensity.
**Related Terms:** Linear attenuation, Transmission
**Example in Radiotherapy:** Used to calculate shielding thickness for walls.

112. **Beam calibration protocol (noun):** Standardized procedure to measure absolute dose output of a linac.
**Related Terms:** TRS-398, AAPM TG-51
**Example in Radiotherapy:** Beam output calibration is performed according to TRS-398 protocol.

113. **Beam cutoff (noun):** The point where radiation intensity drops to zero outside the treatment field.
**Related Terms:** Penumbra, Collimation
**Example in Radiotherapy:** Beam cutoff defines field edge in MLC-shaped fields.

114. **Beam delivery verification (noun):** Confirmation that the planned beam is delivered accurately.
**Related Terms:** Portal dosimetry, Pre-treatment QA
**Example in Radiotherapy:** Performed before patient treatment using electronic portal imaging device.

115. **Beam energy constancy (noun):** The stability of radiation beam energy output over time.
**Related Terms:** Beam quality, QA checks
**Example in Radiotherapy:** Verified monthly using depth-dose measurements.

116. **Beam exit dose (noun):** The residual dose exiting the patient after beam passes through tissue.
**Related Terms:** Transmission dose, Exit fluence
**Example in Radiotherapy:** Exit dose helps verify treatment delivery using portal imaging.

117. **Beam geometry (noun):** Spatial configuration of beam angles and isocenters.
**Related Terms:** Beam arrangement, Treatment plan optimization
**Example in Radiotherapy:** Beam geometry is optimized to minimize dose to organs at risk.

118. **Beam hardening correction (noun):** Algorithmic adjustment to compensate for differential absorption in CT imaging.
**Related Terms:** Artifact correction, Image reconstruction
**Example in Radiotherapy:** Applied during CT simulation to improve HU accuracy.

119. **Beam model (noun):** Mathematical representation of linac beam characteristics in TPS.
**Related Terms:** Commissioning, Monte Carlo model
**Example in Radiotherapy:** Accurate beam model ensures precise dose calculation.

120. **Beam output drift (noun):** Variation in linac dose output with time.
**Related Terms:** QA tolerance, Calibration
**Example in Radiotherapy:** Daily constancy checks monitor output drift within 2%.

121. **Beam pattern recognition (noun):** Use of AI to identify and analyze beam delivery data.
**Related Terms:** Machine learning QA, Automation
**Example in Radiotherapy:** AI detects anomalies in beam pattern to prevent delivery errors.

122. **Beam perturbation (noun):** Alteration in beam fluence due to inhomogeneity or device interaction.
**Related Terms:** Scatter, Heterogeneity correction
**Example in Radiotherapy:** Occurs near air cavities or metal implants.

123. **Beam profile symmetry (noun):** Degree of uniformity of beam intensity on both sides of central axis.
**Related Terms:** Flatness, QA tolerance
**Example in Radiotherapy:** Checked during monthly linac QA.

124. **Beam reproducibility (noun):** Consistency of dose output under identical settings.
**Related Terms:** QA performance, Output stability
**Example in Radiotherapy:** Ensures consistent patient dose delivery daily.

125. **Beam steering (noun):** Adjustment of magnetic fields to center the electron beam in the waveguide.
**Related Terms:** Steering coils, Linac tuning
**Example in Radiotherapy:** QA engineers perform beam steering to correct asymmetry.

126. **Beam transmission factor (noun):** Fraction of primary beam transmitted through an attenuator.
**Related Terms:** Tray factor, Wedge factor
**Example in Radiotherapy:** Used to account for MLC transmission dose in IMRT plans.

127. **Beam uniformity correction (noun):** Adjustment applied to equalize dose across the field.
**Related Terms:** Flatness, Beam modulation
**Example in Radiotherapy:** Ensures homogeneous dose in TBI fields.

128. **Benchmark dose (noun):** Dose level associated with a defined biological response.
**Related Terms:** Dose–response curve, Radiobiology
**Example in Radiotherapy:** Used in risk assessment of radiation-induced effects.

129. **Beryllium target (noun):** Thin metal target used in photon production or x-ray tubes.
**Related Terms:** X-ray tube design, Target material
**Example in Radiotherapy:** Beryllium targets produce low-energy bremsstrahlung photons.

130. **Beta shielding (noun):** Material barrier used to stop beta particles while minimizing bremsstrahlung.
**Related Terms:** Plexiglass shield, Electron safety
**Example in Radiotherapy:** Acrylic barriers are used for beta-emitting source handling.

131. **Bi-exponential decay (noun):** Radioactive decay with two distinct half-lives or components.
**Related Terms:** Dual-phase kinetics, Radiopharmaceutical
**Example in Radiotherapy:** Observed in clearance of some PET tracers.

132. **Bifurcation angle (noun):** Angle formed at a branching structure like tracheal or vascular division.
**Related Terms:** Carina, Vascular anatomy
**Example in Radiotherapy:** Important for delineating mediastinal structures in thoracic RT.

133. **Biochemical recurrence (noun):** Return of disease detected by rising tumor markers after treatment.
**Related Terms:** PSA relapse, Disease monitoring
**Example in Radiotherapy:** Used to assess recurrence in prostate cancer post-RT.

134. **Bioimaging probe (noun):** Radiolabeled or fluorescent molecule used to visualize biological processes.
**Related Terms:** Tracer, Molecular imaging
**Example in Radiotherapy:** Used for tumor hypoxia mapping in planning adaptive therapy.

135. **Biological optimization (noun):** Dose optimization based on biological response models.
**Related Terms:** TCP, NTCP models
**Example in Radiotherapy:** Employed in IMRT planning to achieve desired tumor control probability.

136. **Biological weighting factor (noun):** Factor expressing radiation type effectiveness in causing damage.
**Related Terms:** RBE, Equivalent dose
**Example in Radiotherapy:** Used in calculating dose equivalent in radiation protection.

137. **Biomarker imaging (noun):** Imaging technique to visualize molecular or genetic tumor markers.
**Related Terms:** PET, Radiogenomics
**Example in Radiotherapy:** Helps personalize treatment based on tumor biology.

138. **Biodistribution study (noun):** Evaluation of tracer or radionuclide distribution in tissues.
**Related Terms:** Pharmacokinetics, Nuclear medicine
**Example in Radiotherapy:** Conducted before radionuclide therapy to predict dose deposition.

139. **Biologic effect modeling (noun):** Mathematical prediction of tissue response to radiation.
**Related Terms:** LQ model, BED
**Example in Radiotherapy:** Used to compare hypofractionation schedules.

140. **Biophysical dose model (noun):** Model combining physical dose and biological response.
**Related Terms:** Microdosimetry, Radiobiology modeling
**Example in Radiotherapy:** Employed in proton therapy RBE calculations.

141. **Biplanar field (noun):** Two-plane beam arrangement for improved conformity.
**Related Terms:** Beam geometry, Conformal RT
**Example in Radiotherapy:** Used in craniospinal irradiation.

142. **Bipolar cautery (noun):** Surgical tool using current between two tips for coagulation.
**Related Terms:** Electrocautery, Surgical RT preparation
**Example in Radiotherapy:** Used during biopsy of irradiated tissue to control bleeding.

143. **Bispectral index (noun):** EEG-derived parameter for depth of anesthesia monitoring.
**Related Terms:** Sedation control, Patient monitoring
**Example in Radiotherapy:** Monitored during pediatric anesthesia for RT simulation.

144. **Bite verification (noun):** Checking the accuracy of dental bite block position.
**Related Terms:** Immobilization, IGRT setup
**Example in Radiotherapy:** Ensures reproducibility in head-and-neck patient positioning.

145. **Bladder motion tracking (noun):** Monitoring bladder volume change during RT.
**Related Terms:** Organ motion, Adaptive planning
**Example in Radiotherapy:** Achieved via CBCT imaging for prostate RT accuracy.

146. **Bladder volume protocol (noun):** Prescribed bladder filling level for reproducible setup.
**Related Terms:** Patient preparation, Organ displacement
**Example in Radiotherapy:** Full bladder protocol minimizes bowel dose in pelvic RT.

147. **Bleomycin toxicity (noun):** Lung damage caused by chemotherapeutic agent bleomycin.
**Related Terms:** Pulmonary fibrosis, Radiosensitizer effect
**Example in Radiotherapy:** Lung dose constraints are reduced for patients on bleomycin.

148. **Block transmission factor (noun):** Fraction of radiation passing through shielding block.
**Related Terms:** Tray factor, Attenuation
**Example in Radiotherapy:** Used in manual calculations for customized blocks.

149. **Blood perfusion imaging (noun):** Technique to assess tissue blood flow using tracers.
**Related Terms:** Dynamic PET, Perfusion CT
**Example in Radiotherapy:** Evaluates tumor hypoxia regions before RT.

150. **Bolus air gap (noun):** Space between bolus and skin reducing intended surface dose.
**Related Terms:** Surface dose, Setup error
**Example in Radiotherapy:** Avoided by ensuring full bolus contact with patient skin.

151. **Bolus buildup effect (noun):** Increase in surface dose caused by tissue-equivalent material.
**Related Terms:** Skin dose, Electron therapy
**Example in Radiotherapy:** Used to treat superficial lesions with photon beams.

152. **Bone equivalent phantom (noun):** Phantom material simulating bone density for dosimetry.
**Related Terms:** Tissue equivalence, QA phantom
**Example in Radiotherapy:** Used for heterogeneity correction validation.

153. **Boundary condition (noun):** Constraint applied to model interfaces in dose calculations.
**Related Terms:** Finite element model, Monte Carlo
**Example in Radiotherapy:** Used in computational modeling of dose distribution.

154. **Brachytherapy applicator reconstruction (noun):** Process of defining applicator geometry in TPS.
**Related Terms:** Image fusion, Source localization
**Example in Radiotherapy:** Required for accurate HDR dose calculation.

155. **Brachytherapy catheter displacement (noun):** Shift of applicator from planned position.
**Related Terms:** Interfraction variation, QA verification
**Example in Radiotherapy:** Detected through post-implant CT scan before dose delivery.

156. **Brachytherapy dwell time (noun):** Time for which source remains at a specific dwell position.
**Related Terms:** Dwell position, Source path
**Example in Radiotherapy:** Optimized to achieve uniform dose to target volume.

157. **Brachytherapy needle loading pattern (noun):** Distribution of sources in interstitial implants.
**Related Terms:** Source geometry, Dosimetry
**Example in Radiotherapy:** Determines dose homogeneity in prostate seed implants.

158. **Bragg curve (noun):** Graph showing energy loss of charged particles as they penetrate matter.
**Related Terms:** Bragg peak, Proton therapy
**Example in Radiotherapy:** Basis for depth-modulated proton treatment design.

159. **Breast edema (noun):** Swelling of breast tissue after irradiation.
**Related Terms:** Skin toxicity, Late effects
**Example in Radiotherapy:** Managed through patient follow-up and physiotherapy.

160. **Breath synchronization (noun):** Coordination of beam delivery with respiratory cycle.
**Related Terms:** Gating, Motion management
**Example in Radiotherapy:** Implemented using RPM system in DIBH breast RT.

161. **Breathing phase binning (noun):** Grouping images according to respiratory phase.
**Related Terms:** 4D-CT, Motion correction
**Example in Radiotherapy:** Used to generate average CT for moving tumors.

162. **Bremsstrahlung yield (noun):** Fraction of electron energy converted into x-rays.
**Related Terms:** Photon production, Target interaction
**Example in Radiotherapy:** Increases with electron energy and target atomic number.

163. **Bronchial dose mapping (noun):** Calculation of dose delivered to bronchial structures.
**Related Terms:** Dose–volume histogram, Lung toxicity
**Example in Radiotherapy:** Evaluated in SBRT planning for central lung tumors.

164. **Bronchial wall contouring (noun):** Delineation of airway walls in thoracic RT.
**Related Terms:** OAR contouring, Lung planning
**Example in Radiotherapy:** Required for accurate toxicity prediction.

165. **Brownian motion dosimetry (noun):** Concept of nanoscale stochastic dose distribution modeling.
**Related Terms:** Microdosimetry, Nanodosimetry
**Example in Radiotherapy:** Used in advanced research for particle track simulation.

166. **Buffer gas (noun):** Inert gas used to stabilize discharge in ionization chambers.
**Related Terms:** Argon, Chamber design
**Example in Radiotherapy:** Argon-based buffer gas enhances chamber sensitivity.

167. **Build-up region modeling (noun):** Computational representation of dose increase near surface.
**Related Terms:** Skin dose, Electron contamination
**Example in Radiotherapy:** Modeled during TPS commissioning for accuracy.

168. **Burnout dose (noun):** Radiation dose beyond which no further biological repair occurs.
**Related Terms:** Cell survival curve, LQ model
**Example in Radiotherapy:** Used in radiosensitivity threshold analysis.

169. **Bypass capacitor (noun):** Electronic component stabilizing voltage in linac circuits.
**Related Terms:** RF amplifier, Power supply
**Example in Radiotherapy:** Maintains stable RF signal during beam generation.

170. **Bacterial endotoxin (noun):** Toxic component of bacterial cell walls that can cause systemic inflammation.
**Related Terms:** Pyrogen, Infection control
**Example in Radiotherapy:** Monitored in sterile preparations used for brachytherapy procedures.

171. **Backscatter electron (noun):** Electron deflected backward after interacting with matter.
**Related Terms:** Scattered radiation, Surface dose
**Example in Radiotherapy:** Increases skin dose near high-Z interfaces.

172. **Balanced modulation (noun):** Technique to regulate beam output by equalizing intensity patterns.
**Related Terms:** Intensity modulation, Dose homogeneity
**Example in Radiotherapy:** Used in IMRT to avoid hot and cold spots in dose distribution.

173. **Bandpass filter (noun):** Device that transmits frequencies within a specific range.
**Related Terms:** Image processing, Noise reduction
**Example in Radiotherapy:** Applied in imaging systems to enhance CT signal clarity.

174. **Barium sulphate suspension (noun):** Radiopaque liquid used to visualize GI tract.
**Related Terms:** Contrast medium, Simulation imaging
**Example in Radiotherapy:** Administered before pelvic CT simulation to outline rectum.

175. **Baseline alignment (noun):** Reference alignment between imaging and treatment coordinates.
**Related Terms:** Image registration, Isocenter matching
**Example in Radiotherapy:** Used in IGRT to verify pre-treatment setup.

176. **Baseline data set (noun):** Initial reference dataset used for adaptive comparison.
**Related Terms:** Deformable registration, Follow-up imaging
**Example in Radiotherapy:** Used to track anatomical changes during treatment.

177. **Basivertebral vein (noun):** Vein located within vertebral bodies that drains the spine.
**Related Terms:** Venous plexus, Spinal anatomy
**Example in Radiotherapy:** Avoided during stereotactic spinal target delineation.

178. **Beam access port (noun):** Opening in treatment head for beam exit.
**Related Terms:** Collimator assembly, Gantry head
**Example in Radiotherapy:** Inspected during linac maintenance for beam path integrity.

179. **Beam axis correction (noun):** Adjustment applied to align beam center with mechanical isocenter.
**Related Terms:** QA alignment, Laser check
**Example in Radiotherapy:** Verified during monthly mechanical QA.

180. **Beam build-up cap (noun):** Removable cap ensuring charged particle equilibrium for measurement.
**Related Terms:** Ionization chamber, Surface dose
**Example in Radiotherapy:** Used during output calibration with reference chambers.

181. **Beam centering tolerance (noun):** Allowable deviation of beam center from defined reference.
**Related Terms:** QA limits, ISO standard
**Example in Radiotherapy:** Typically maintained within ±1 mm in QA.

182. **Beam characterization (noun):** Measurement of beam parameters such as energy, profile, and symmetry.
**Related Terms:** Commissioning, Beam modeling
**Example in Radiotherapy:** Performed during acceptance testing of new linacs.

183. **Beam coherence (noun):** Measure of phase uniformity across the beam wavefront.
**Related Terms:** Coherent scattering, Beam quality
**Example in Radiotherapy:** Important in optical or laser-based dosimetry systems.

184. **Beam collimator leaf (noun):** Metal leaf used to shape beam in MLC systems.
**Related Terms:** Multileaf collimator, Beam shaping
**Example in Radiotherapy:** Each leaf is calibrated for accurate dose conformity.

185. **Beam cross-plane profile (noun):** Dose distribution measured perpendicular to the beam axis.
**Related Terms:** In-plane profile, Flatness
**Example in Radiotherapy:** Used to check beam uniformity across the treatment field.

186. **Beam current modulation (noun):** Adjustment of electron current to vary dose output.
**Related Terms:** Dose rate control, Linac operation
**Example in Radiotherapy:** Applied in dynamic arc therapy for dose modulation.

187. **Beam efficiency (noun):** Ratio of delivered dose energy to total input power.
**Related Terms:** Energy conversion, Machine performance
**Example in Radiotherapy:** Used to evaluate linac performance efficiency.

188. **Beam fluence modulation (noun):** Controlled variation in photon fluence across field.
**Related Terms:** IMRT, Fluence map optimization
**Example in Radiotherapy:** Enables conformal dose sculpting to target volume.

189. **Beam homogeneity index (noun):** Quantitative measure of uniformity within target dose.
**Related Terms:** Dose distribution, PTV coverage
**Example in Radiotherapy:** Calculated to evaluate IMRT plan quality.

190. **Beam incident angle (noun):** Angle at which beam enters patient or phantom.
**Related Terms:** Gantry angle, Beam geometry
**Example in Radiotherapy:** Optimized to minimize OAR exposure.

191. **Beam input surface (noun):** Surface point where beam first enters patient body.
**Related Terms:** SSD setup, Surface localization
**Example in Radiotherapy:** Defined precisely during simulation for reproducibility.

192. **Beam integral dose (noun):** Total energy deposited in tissue by entire beam.
**Related Terms:** Total dose, Dose-volume
**Example in Radiotherapy:** Assessed to minimize integral dose to normal tissues.

193. **Beam intensity modulation index (noun):** Numerical indicator of modulation complexity in IMRT plan.
**Related Terms:** Modulation factor, QA evaluation
**Example in Radiotherapy:** Higher index values indicate more complex fluence patterns.

194. **Beam isocenter calibration (noun):** Verification of mechanical and radiation isocenter coincidence.
**Related Terms:** Winston-Lutz test, QA procedure
**Example in Radiotherapy:** Ensures submillimeter accuracy for SRS/SBRT delivery.

195. **Beam leakage radiation (noun):** Radiation escaping from treatment head shielding.
**Related Terms:** Leakage limit, Safety regulation
**Example in Radiotherapy:** Measured annually to comply with IEC standards.

196. **Beam linearity (noun):** Relationship between monitor units and delivered dose rate.
**Related Terms:** Output consistency, Calibration
**Example in Radiotherapy:** Confirmed during annual QA procedures.

197. **Beam mapping system (noun):** Device used to measure beam fluence in two dimensions.
**Related Terms:** QA array, Film dosimetry
**Example in Radiotherapy:** Used for pre-treatment verification of IMRT plans.

198. **Beam modulation transfer (noun):** Process describing how modulation is transferred through the beam.
**Related Terms:** Spatial resolution, MTF
**Example in Radiotherapy:** Analyzed to assess imaging system fidelity.

199. **Beam on-off control (noun):** Safety mechanism regulating beam start and termination.
**Related Terms:** Interlock, Timer circuit
**Example in Radiotherapy:** Critical in preventing unintended radiation exposure.

200. **Beam output reproducibility (noun):** Consistency of delivered dose for same settings.
**Related Terms:** QA tolerance, Output constancy
**Example in Radiotherapy:** Verified daily using standard QA devices.

201. **Beam pattern verification (noun):** Confirmation of intended fluence pattern accuracy.
**Related Terms:** IMRT QA, Dose verification
**Example in Radiotherapy:** Ensures planned MLC modulation is correctly delivered.

202. **Beam pulse width (noun):** Duration of each radiation pulse emitted from linac.
**Related Terms:** Pulse repetition rate, Dose rate
**Example in Radiotherapy:** Affects instantaneous dose delivery in high-dose modes.

203. **Beam retraction distance (noun):** Distance moved by source or applicator between exposures.
**Related Terms:** Afterloading, Source dwell movement
**Example in Radiotherapy:** Controlled precisely in HDR brachytherapy systems.

204. **Beam scatter kernel (noun):** Mathematical function describing dose spread due to scatter.
**Related Terms:** Convolution algorithm, Dose calculation
**Example in Radiotherapy:** Used in collapsed cone and superposition algorithms.

205. **Beam segmentation (noun):** Division of fluence map into deliverable subfields.
**Related Terms:** Step-and-shoot IMRT, Leaf sequencing
**Example in Radiotherapy:** Optimizes delivery efficiency and reduces monitor units.

206. **Beam shaping filter (noun):** Device used to modify intensity profile for uniform dose.
**Related Terms:** Flattening filter, Wedge
**Example in Radiotherapy:** Removed in FFF beams to allow high dose rates.

207. **Beam stability check (noun):** Routine QA to ensure beam output stability over time.
**Related Terms:** Daily QA, Output constancy
**Example in Radiotherapy:** Conducted using ion chamber or QA phantom.

208. **Beam stop transmission (noun):** Residual transmission through beam-blocking devices.
**Related Terms:** Leakage radiation, Shielding
**Example in Radiotherapy:** Measured to ensure compliance with regulatory limits.

209. **Beam synchronization signal (noun):** Electronic pulse coordinating beam delivery timing.
**Related Terms:** Trigger pulse, Gating system
**Example in Radiotherapy:** Used in respiratory-gated treatment delivery.

210. **Beam trajectory (noun):** Path traveled by radiation from source to target.
**Related Terms:** Gantry rotation, Beam alignment
**Example in Radiotherapy:** Verified during commissioning for accurate delivery geometry.

211. **Beam transit time (noun):** Time taken by beam to move from start to full output.
**Related Terms:** Dose ramp-up, Timing QA
**Example in Radiotherapy:** Important for accurate dose delivery in gated therapy.

212. **Beam uniformity index (noun):** Ratio quantifying uniform dose across the field.
**Related Terms:** Flatness, Dose homogeneity
**Example in Radiotherapy:** Used in QA of large-field photon beams.

213. **Beam verification phantom (noun):** Phantom used for dose verification measurements.
**Related Terms:** QA device, IMRT QA
**Example in Radiotherapy:** Used in pre-treatment plan verification for complex fields.

214. **Beampath imaging (noun):** Visualization of beam trajectory using imaging detectors.
**Related Terms:** Portal imaging, MV imaging
**Example in Radiotherapy:** Used for treatment delivery verification.

215. **Bed index position (noun):** Numbered coordinate defining couch position.
**Related Terms:** Patient setup, Reproducibility
**Example in Radiotherapy:** Recorded daily to ensure consistent setup.

216. **Beer's law (noun):** Principle describing attenuation of light or radiation through a medium.
**Related Terms:** Exponential attenuation, CT calibration
**Example in Radiotherapy:** Basis for CT Hounsfield unit calculation.

217. **Bel–Robinson dose (noun):** Theoretical energy-momentum tensor describing energy transfer in curved spacetime (conceptual in radiophysics).
**Related Terms:** Relativistic dosimetry, Theoretical physics
**Example in Radiotherapy:** Applied in high-energy dosimetry modeling research.

218. **Benchmark phantom (noun):** Standard phantom used to validate dose calculation algorithms.
**Related Terms:** QA benchmarking, Validation
**Example in Radiotherapy:** Used during TPS commissioning.

219. **Bending magnet assembly (noun):** System of electromagnets directing electron beam in linac head.
**Related Terms:** Beam steering, Energy selection
**Example in Radiotherapy:** QA verifies correct beam path alignment.

220. **Beta emitter (noun):** Radioisotope emitting beta particles during decay.
**Related Terms:** Radionuclide therapy, Source calibration
**Example in Radiotherapy:** Used in palliative bone pain therapy.

221. **Beta spectrum (noun):** Energy distribution of emitted beta particles.
**Related Terms:** Beta decay, Energy deposition
**Example in Radiotherapy:** Determines shielding requirements for beta sources.

222. **Bilateral matching field (noun):** Adjacent opposed fields matched at central junction.
**Related Terms:** Field matching, Junction dose
**Example in Radiotherapy:** Used in breast or head-and-neck treatment plans.

223. **Biodosimetry (noun):** Estimation of absorbed radiation dose using biological markers.
**Related Terms:** Cytogenetic assay, Radiation exposure
**Example in Radiotherapy:** Used in accidental exposure evaluation.

224. **Bioinformatics (noun):** Application of computational methods to biological data analysis.
**Related Terms:** Radiogenomics, AI in RT
**Example in Radiotherapy:** Used to correlate imaging biomarkers with treatment outcome.

225. **Biological calibration (noun):** Standardization of dose–response based on biological effect.
**Related Terms:** RBE, Cell survival
**Example in Radiotherapy:** Used in proton and carbon ion therapy.

226. **Biological damage model (noun):** Framework describing tissue injury following radiation.
**Related Terms:** LQ model, Radiobiological modeling
**Example in Radiotherapy:** Guides fractionation optimization.

227. **Biological gradient (noun):** Variation in biological response with radiation dose.
**Related Terms:** Dose–response curve, Radiosensitivity
**Example in Radiotherapy:** Used in modeling normal tissue complication probabilities.

228. **Biological shielding (noun):** Material barrier designed to protect personnel from ionizing radiation.
**Related Terms:** Concrete barrier, Lead wall
**Example in Radiotherapy:** Used in bunker design for linac rooms.

229. **Biological specimen imaging (noun):** Imaging of tissues to assess radiation-induced changes.
**Related Terms:** Histopathology imaging, Functional MRI
**Example in Radiotherapy:** Used in research correlating imaging biomarkers with dose.

230. **Biological variance (noun):** Inter-patient variability in biological response to identical dose.
**Related Terms:** Radiosensitivity, Personalized therapy
**Example in Radiotherapy:** Explains differing normal tissue reactions.

231. **Biomathematical modeling (noun):** Mathematical modeling of biological processes in radiotherapy.
**Related Terms:** Radiobiology, Predictive modeling
**Example in Radiotherapy:** Used to predict tumor control probability.

232. **Biomolecular damage (noun):** Structural alteration in DNA, proteins, or lipids by radiation.
**Related Terms:** Free radicals, DNA double-strand breaks
**Example in Radiotherapy:** Primary cause of cellular death post-irradiation.

233. **Bioscintillator (noun):** Biological or organic compound emitting light under radiation.
**Related Terms:** Scintillation detector, Radiation detection
**Example in Radiotherapy:** Used in bioluminescent dosimetry research.

234. **Biostimulation (noun):** Low-dose radiation effect promoting biological repair or growth.
**Related Terms:** Hormesis, Adaptive response
**Example in Radiotherapy:** Studied in radiobiology for sublethal exposures.

235. **Bitemporal dose asymmetry (noun):** Uneven dose distribution across bilateral head regions.
**Related Terms:** Setup error, Beam matching
**Example in Radiotherapy:** Corrected by symmetric beam weight adjustment.

236. **Bivariate regression model (noun):** Statistical model correlating two biological outcomes with dose.
**Related Terms:** Data modeling, Dose–effect correlation
**Example in Radiotherapy:** Used in NTCP model fitting.

237. **Bladder-sparing protocol (noun):** Treatment approach minimizing bladder dose exposure.
**Related Terms:** Adaptive RT, Dose constraint
**Example in Radiotherapy:** Applied in pelvic IMRT to reduce urinary toxicity.

238. **Bleed correction (noun):** Compensation for signal spillover in imaging detectors.
**Related Terms:** Crosstalk correction, Image reconstruction
**Example in Radiotherapy:** Applied in PET/CT for accurate SUV quantification.

239. **Block edge penumbra (noun):** Region of partial dose transition at block boundary.
**Related Terms:** Collimator penumbra, Field edge
**Example in Radiotherapy:** Considered in manual plan calculations.

240. **Blood–retinal barrier (noun):** Selective barrier regulating substance entry into retina.
**Related Terms:** Ocular radiosensitivity, Late toxicity
**Example in Radiotherapy:** Limiting factor in ocular tumor irradiation.

241. **Body density correction (noun):** Dose correction accounting for varying tissue densities.
**Related Terms:** Heterogeneity correction, CT-to-density conversion
**Example in Radiotherapy:** Applied in TPS dose calculation.

242. **Body coil (noun):** MRI coil used for whole-body imaging.
**Related Terms:** RF coil, MRI simulation
**Example in Radiotherapy:** Used for anatomical localization during planning MRI.

243. **Body fixation cradle (noun):** Custom immobilization device supporting patient posture.
**Related Terms:** Vacuum cushion, Stereotactic setup
**Example in Radiotherapy:** Ensures reproducible setup for SBRT cases.

244. **Bolus conformal printing (noun):** 3D-printing technique for patient-specific bolus design.
**Related Terms:** Additive manufacturing, Surface dose
**Example in Radiotherapy:** Used to optimize skin dose in irregular anatomy.

245. **Bolus heterogeneity correction (noun):** Algorithm adjusting dose for bolus material density.
**Related Terms:** TPS calculation, Surface correction
**Example in Radiotherapy:** Improves surface dose accuracy in photon therapy.

246. **Bone marrow contouring atlas (noun):** Reference guideline for standardized bone marrow delineation.
**Related Terms:** Contouring protocol, OAR
**Example in Radiotherapy:** Used to reduce hematologic toxicity in pelvic RT.

247. **Bone voxelization (noun):** Representation of bone tissue as discrete voxels for dose computation.
**Related Terms:** Image segmentation, 3D reconstruction
**Example in Radiotherapy:** Essential for Monte Carlo dose simulation.

248. **Beam Quality Index (BQI) (noun):** A measure that quantifies the penetrating ability of a photon beam, often defined using the tissue phantom ratio or percentage depth dose.
**Related Terms:** Beam Quality, PDD, TPR.
**Example in Radiotherapy:** BQI helps in calibrating photon beams for consistent treatment energy verification.

249. **Beam Steering (noun):** A process of adjusting the electron beam path within a linear accelerator to achieve correct symmetry and flatness.
**Related Terms:** Steering Coils, Beam Alignment.
**Example in Radiotherapy:** Beam steering ensures that the photon field is uniform across the treatment area.

250. **Beam Stopper (noun):** A shielding device placed opposite to the radiation source to absorb unused radiation and protect staff.
**Related Terms:** Primary Barrier, Transmission Factor.
**Example in Radiotherapy:** A beam stopper is often installed behind the gantry in a teletherapy room.

251. **Beam-On Time (noun):** The duration for which the radiation beam is actively delivered to the patient.
**Related Terms:** Monitor Units, Exposure Time.
**Example in Radiotherapy:** The therapist verifies the beam-on time before patient treatment.

252. **Beam's Reference Point (noun):** A predefined location in space used for beam calibration or measurement reference.
**Related Terms:** Isocenter, SSD, SAD.
**Example in Radiotherapy:** Beam reference points are used to align calibration chambers accurately.

253. **Biological Effectiveness (noun):** The relative capacity of radiation of different types to produce a specific biological effect.
**Related Terms:** RBE, LET, Dose Effect Curve.
**Example in Radiotherapy:** Alpha particles have higher biological effectiveness compared to X-rays.

254. **Biological Model (noun):** A mathematical representation describing the relationship between dose and tissue response.
**Related Terms:** LQ Model, Tumor Control Probability.
**Example in Radiotherapy:** The LQ biological model predicts cell survival at various doses.

255. **Biophysical Dose Model (noun):** An advanced model integrating both physical and biological parameters for accurate dose-response prediction.
**Related Terms:** BED, TCP, NTCP.
**Example in Radiotherapy:** Used in proton therapy planning for tissue-specific dose calculation.

256. **Biorepository (noun):** A storage facility for biological samples used in radiation biology research.
**Related Terms:** Biomarker, Genomic Data.
**Example in Radiotherapy:** Tumor samples are stored in a biorepository for radiosensitivity studies.

257. **Bistable Image Artifact (noun):** An imaging artifact that causes abrupt shifts between two display states due to unstable signal processing.
**Related Terms:** Image Noise, Detector Stability.
**Example in Radiotherapy:** CBCT scans may show bistable artifacts during motion correction errors.

258. **Biotransport Modeling (noun):** Simulation of radiation-induced molecular or cellular transport mechanisms in tissues.
**Related Terms:** Monte Carlo Simulation, Dosimetric Modeling.
**Example in Radiotherapy:** Biotransport modeling is used in nanodosimetry for radiosensitizer tracking.

259. **Blackbody Radiation (noun):** The theoretical emission of electromagnetic radiation from an idealized perfect emitter.
**Related Terms:** Thermal Radiation, Spectrum.
**Example in Radiotherapy:** Used in calibrating thermal detectors for dosimetric purposes.

260. **Blood Dosimetry (noun):** Measurement of absorbed radiation dose in circulating blood, often during total body irradiation.
**Related Terms:** Biodosimetry, Whole Body Dose.
**Example in Radiotherapy:** Blood dosimetry helps ensure dose limits are not exceeded in TBI.

261. **Body Dose Index (BDI) (noun):** An index measuring the average dose received by the body during radiological procedures.
**Related Terms:** DLP, CTDI.
**Example in Radiotherapy:** Used in imaging QA to limit unnecessary patient exposure.

262. **Body Equilibrium Position (noun):** Standard patient alignment position ensuring consistent anatomical reference.
**Related Terms:** Supine, Prone, Immobilization.
**Example in Radiotherapy:** The therapist confirms body equilibrium before beam delivery.

263. **Bone Shielding (noun):** Application of specialized materials to minimize dose absorption in bony structures.
**Related Terms:** Custom Shield, Tissue Compensator.
**Example in Radiotherapy:** Bone shielding is used to protect the mandible during head and neck RT.

264. **Boolean Operation (Imaging) (noun):** Logical operation combining contour or volume datasets using AND, OR, or NOT functions.
**Related Terms:** Image Segmentation, ROI Fusion.
**Example in Radiotherapy:** Boolean operations merge target and organ-at-risk volumes.

265. **Boron Neutron Capture Therapy (BNCT) (noun):** A binary radiation therapy using boron-10 and neutron beams for targeted cell destruction.
**Related Terms:** Neutron Therapy, Radiosensitization.
**Example in Radiotherapy:** BNCT is effective in recurrent head and neck tumors.

266. **Boundary Dose Fall-off (noun):** The rapid reduction in dose intensity at the periphery of the treatment field.
**Related Terms:** Penumbra, Gradient Index.
**Example in Radiotherapy:** A sharp boundary dose fall-off protects normal tissues in IMRT.

267. **Brainstem Dose Constraint (noun):** A clinically defined maximum allowable dose to prevent radiation-induced necrosis of the brainstem.
**Related Terms:** OAR Constraint, Dose Limiting Structure.
**Example in Radiotherapy:** The plan was modified to respect brainstem dose constraints in SRS.

268. **Brilliance (Beam Quality) (noun):** A measure of photon flux per unit area and solid angle.
**Related Terms:** Beam Intensity, Photon Yield.
**Example in Radiotherapy:** Higher beam brilliance enhances imaging in portal dosimetry.

269. **Broadband Photon Source (noun):** A radiation source emitting photons across a wide energy spectrum.
**Related Terms:** Polychromatic Beam, X-ray Tube Output.
**Example in Radiotherapy:** Used in diagnostic imaging before planning simulation.

270. **Bronchial Wall Contouring (noun):** Delineation of the bronchial walls as organs-at-risk during thoracic RT planning.
**Related Terms:** OAR Contouring, Dose Limitation.
**Example in Radiotherapy:** Accurate bronchial wall contouring minimizes post-RT fibrosis.

271. **Buffer Solution (noun):** A chemical solution maintaining pH stability in biological dosimeters or phantom gels.
**Related Terms:** Gel Dosimetry, pH Control.
**Example in Radiotherapy:** Buffer solutions stabilize radiochromic gels during QA tests.

272. **Build-up Material (noun):** A layer added to increase surface dose to achieve electronic equilibrium.
**Related Terms:** Buildup Cap, Bolus.
**Example in Radiotherapy:** A 1 cm bolus acts as a build-up material in chest wall RT.

273. **Burnout Detector Failure (noun):** A malfunction of radiation detectors due to excessive exposure or current overload.
**Related Terms:** Chamber Saturation, QA Error.
**Example in Radiotherapy:** Daily QA checks prevent burnout detector failure in monitor chambers.

274. **Beam Orbit Stability (noun):** Consistency of the electron path within the accelerator waveguide.
**Related Terms:** Magnetic Steering, Beam Position.
**Example in Radiotherapy:** Beam orbit stability is monitored through steering current logs.

275. **Biometric Verification (noun):** Use of fingerprint or facial recognition for secure patient identification.
**Related Terms:** Barcode ID, Electronic Record.
**Example in Radiotherapy:** Biometric verification ensures accurate patient matching before treatment.

276. **Beam Energy Modulation (noun):** Variation of beam energy to achieve uniform dose distribution across irregular surfaces.
**Related Terms:** Compensator, Range Modulator.
**Example in Radiotherapy:** Used in proton therapy to create a spread-out Bragg peak.

277. **Brachytherapy Quality Index (BQI) (noun):** A metric used to evaluate uniformity and conformity of dose in brachytherapy implants.
**Related Terms:** Homogeneity Index, Conformity Index.
**Example in Radiotherapy:** BQI is calculated during HDR prostate implant verification.

278. **Brachytherapy Remote Afterloader (noun):** A computer-controlled device that remotely positions radioactive sources in brachytherapy applicators.
**Related Terms:** HDR Unit, Source Control.
**Example in Radiotherapy:** The remote afterloader improves safety by minimizing staff exposure.

279. **Brachytherapy Source Strength (noun):** The measure of a brachytherapy source's emission rate, expressed in air kerma strength or activity.
**Related Terms:** Source Calibration, Air Kerma.
**Example in Radiotherapy:** Source strength is verified during commissioning to ensure accurate dose delivery.

280. **Bragg Curve (noun):** A plot showing the energy loss of charged particles as they travel through matter.
**Related Terms:** Bragg Peak, Proton Therapy.
**Example in Radiotherapy:** The Bragg curve guides proton range calculations in patient planning.

281. **Brilliance Calibration (noun):** Adjustment of imaging systems to maintain consistent brightness and contrast.
**Related Terms:** Image Uniformity, Display QA.
**Example in Radiotherapy:** Brilliance calibration ensures consistent image display for contouring.

282. **Broad Beam Geometry (noun):** An irradiation setup where the beam covers the entire detector or target field.
**Related Terms:** Narrow Beam, Scatter Conditions.
**Example in Radiotherapy:** Used in absolute dosimetry calibration with ionization chambers.

283. **Broad-Spectrum Radiation (noun):** Radiation composed of multiple photon or particle energies.
**Related Terms:** Polyenergetic Beam, X-ray Spectrum.
**Example in Radiotherapy:** Orthovoltage machines produce broad-spectrum radiation for superficial treatments.

284. **Bronchial Tree Dose Mapping (noun):** Visualization of dose distribution along the bronchial anatomy.
**Related Terms:** Dose–Volume Histogram, OAR Analysis.
**Example in Radiotherapy:** Dose mapping ensures safe limits to bronchial mucosa during lung SBRT.

285. **Brownian Motion Detector (noun):** Device used to measure nanoparticle movement in radiobiological research.
**Related Terms:** Nanodosimetry, Particle Diffusion.
**Example in Radiotherapy:** Brownian motion detectors track radiosensitizer distribution in tissue phantoms.

286. **Buildup Factor (noun):** A correction factor accounting for scattered radiation in dose calculations.
**Related Terms:** Scatter Factor, Attenuation.
**Example in Radiotherapy:** Buildup factor is used in shielding calculations for photon beams.

287. **Bulk Density Correction (noun):** Adjustment in dose calculation for tissues of varying physical density.
**Related Terms:** Hounsfield Unit Calibration, Tissue Heterogeneity.
**Example in Radiotherapy:** TPS applies bulk density correction for lung and bone regions.

288. **Bunker Shielding Design (noun):** Architectural planning for radiation protection in treatment rooms.
**Related Terms:** Primary Barrier, Secondary Barrier.
**Example in Radiotherapy:** The bunker shielding design ensures staff safety in high-energy LINAC rooms.

289. **Bypass Valve (Cooling System) (noun):** A mechanical valve that diverts coolant flow in LINAC systems to prevent overheating.
**Related Terms:** Water Cooling System, Equipment Safety.
**Example in Radiotherapy:** The bypass valve is checked during daily LINAC QA.

290. **Bystander Effect (noun):** A phenomenon where non-irradiated cells exhibit effects of radiation due to signaling from irradiated cells.
**Related Terms:** Radiation Biology, Cell Signaling.
**Example in Radiotherapy:** The bystander effect contributes to normal tissue response outside the target area.

291. **Beam Area Product (noun):** A measure of total X-ray output combining beam intensity and cross-sectional area.
**Related Terms:** Dose Area Product, Exposure Index.
**Example in Radiotherapy:** Used to estimate patient exposure during imaging QA.

292. **Beam Calibration Phantom (noun):** A standardized phantom used to verify beam parameters during machine calibration.
**Related Terms:** Water Phantom, QA Protocol.
**Example in Radiotherapy:** Beam calibration phantoms are essential in annual LINAC calibration.

293. **Beam Collimator Leaf Speed (noun):** The velocity at which MLC leaves move during dynamic treatment delivery.
**Related Terms:** IMRT QA, MLC Control.
**Example in Radiotherapy:** Optimizing collimator leaf speed ensures dose conformity in VMAT.

294. **Beam Data Library (noun):** A collection of verified beam parameters stored in TPS for planning and QA.
**Related Terms:** Commissioning Data, Beam Model.
**Example in Radiotherapy:** The physicist loads the beam data library during TPS installation.

295. **Beam Edge Profile (noun):** A graphical representation showing dose fall-off at the beam boundary.
**Related Terms:** Penumbra, Field Flatness.
**Example in Radiotherapy:** Beam edge profile checks are part of photon beam QA.

296. **Beam Energy Spectrum (noun):** The distribution of photon or electron energies emitted from a radiation source.
**Related Terms:** Beam Quality, Spectrum Analysis.
**Example in Radiotherapy:** Monte Carlo simulations use beam energy spectra for dose accuracy.

297. **Beam Intensity Modulation (noun):** The controlled variation of beam fluence to achieve a desired dose distribution.
**Related Terms:** IMRT, Dynamic Delivery.
**Example in Radiotherapy:** Beam intensity modulation optimizes dose conformity in complex targets.

298. **Beam Parameter Verification (noun):** The QA process of validating all physical parameters of a treatment beam.
**Related Terms:** Beam Constancy, QA Protocol.
**Example in Radiotherapy:** Monthly QA ensures beam parameter verification remains within tolerance.

299. **Beam Portal Imaging (noun):** Image acquisition using the treatment beam for setup verification.
**Related Terms:** EPID, MV Imaging.
**Example in Radiotherapy:** Beam portal imaging confirms isocenter alignment before each fraction.

300. **Beam Pulse Repetition Rate (noun):** The number of pulses generated per second by a pulsed radiation source.
**Related Terms:** Pulse Frequency, Dose Rate.
**Example in Radiotherapy:** The LINAC's pulse repetition rate affects beam stability.

301. **Beam Scatter Factor (noun):** Ratio of dose with scatter to dose without scatter, used in field size corrections.
**Related Terms:** Output Factor, Collimator Scatter.
**Example in Radiotherapy:** Beam scatter factor helps calculate monitor units for irregular fields.

302. **Beam Symmetry Check (noun):** Verification of dose uniformity between the left and right halves of a beam.
**Related Terms:** Beam Flatness, QA Test.
**Example in Radiotherapy:** Beam symmetry check is performed daily on photon and electron beams.

303. **Beam Verification Phantom (noun):** A specialized phantom used for verifying planned vs. delivered dose distribution.
**Related Terms:** QA Phantom, 3D Dosimetry.
**Example in Radiotherapy:** Used in pre-treatment IMRT QA for dose verification.

304. **Beam Weight Optimization (noun):** Adjustment of beam weights to achieve uniform target coverage.
**Related Terms:** Plan Optimization, Dose Homogeneity.
**Example in Radiotherapy:** TPS uses beam weight optimization to balance dose between multiple fields.

305. **Biological Amplification (noun):** Enhanced biological effect resulting from secondary processes after radiation exposure.
**Related Terms:** DNA Repair, Radiosensitivity.
**Example in Radiotherapy:** Biological amplification occurs during reactive oxygen species generation.

306. **Biological Repair Kinetics (noun):** The rate and mechanism of cellular repair following radiation damage.
**Related Terms:** DNA Repair, LQ Model.
**Example in Radiotherapy:** Fractionation schemes depend on tissue-specific repair kinetics.

307. **Biophysical Modelling Software (noun):** Computational tools that simulate biological effects of radiation.
**Related Terms:** Radiobiology, TCP Modeling.
**Example in Radiotherapy:** Used to model dose–response relationships for normal tissue complications.

308. **Blood Perfusion Imaging (noun):** Functional imaging technique assessing tissue vascularization using radioactive tracers.
**Related Terms:** SPECT, PET.
**Example in Radiotherapy:** Blood perfusion imaging guides adaptive planning in hypoxic tumors.

309. **Bone Equivalent Phantom (noun):** Phantom material mimicking bone density for dosimetric calibration.
**Related Terms:** Tissue Phantom Ratio, QA.
**Example in Radiotherapy:** Used for dose verification in heterogeneity correction.

310. **Brain Dose Histogram (noun):** A graphical representation of dose distribution across brain tissues.
**Related Terms:** DVH, Dose Statistics.
**Example in Radiotherapy:** Brain dose histograms are analyzed to evaluate plan conformity.

311. **Brainstem Contouring Protocol (noun):** Standardized guidelines for delineating the brainstem in RT planning.
**Related Terms:** OAR Delineation, Protocol QA.
**Example in Radiotherapy:** The therapist follows the RTOG brainstem contouring protocol.

312. **Breathing Cycle Analysis (noun):** Evaluation of respiratory patterns for motion management.
**Related Terms:** Gating, 4D CT.
**Example in Radiotherapy:** Used to determine gating thresholds for DIBH breast treatments.

313. **Breathing Gating Window (noun):** The optimal phase of respiration where radiation delivery is synchronized.
**Related Terms:** Respiratory Gating, Motion Control.
**Example in Radiotherapy:** A 30–70% gating window ensures stable tumor position during treatment.

314. **Bremsstrahlung Spectrum (noun):** Energy distribution of photons produced by electron deceleration in a target.
**Related Terms:** X-ray Production, Target Interaction.
**Example in Radiotherapy:** The Bremsstrahlung spectrum defines beam quality in high-energy LINACs.

315. **Brightness Uniformity Test (noun):** A QA test assessing uniform brightness across an imaging display.
**Related Terms:** Luminance, Display QA.
**Example in Radiotherapy:** Conducted monthly on CT and EPID monitors.

316. **Bronchial Lymphatic Mapping (noun):** Imaging procedure to identify lymph node drainage pathways from the bronchi.
**Related Terms:** PET/CT, Nodal Staging.
**Example in Radiotherapy:** Guides target delineation in lung cancer planning.

317. **Bulk Electron Density Assignment (noun):** A method of assigning uniform densities to entire structures during dose calculation.
**Related Terms:** HU Calibration, Heterogeneity Correction.
**Example in Radiotherapy:** Used for simplifying dose calculation in metal artifact regions.

318. **Beam Phase Space Data (noun):** Dataset representing all particle positions and directions within a beam.
**Related Terms:** Monte Carlo, Beam Modeling.
**Example in Radiotherapy:** TPS imports phase space data for accurate dose simulation.

319. **Beam Position Tolerance (noun):** The allowable deviation of the beam's central axis from its intended location.
**Related Terms:** QA Tolerance, Isocenter Accuracy.
**Example in Radiotherapy:** Verified during daily machine QA using Winston-Lutz tests.

320. **Beam Quality Correction Factor (noun):** A factor used to correct for differences between calibration and treatment beam qualities.
**Related Terms:** kQ Factor, TG-51 Protocol.
**Example in Radiotherapy:** Applied during chamber calibration to match reference conditions.

321. **Beam Recombination Correction (noun):** Adjustment accounting for ion recombination losses in dosimetry measurements.
**Related Terms:** Ion Chamber, Saturation Correction.
**Example in Radiotherapy:** Necessary for accurate readings in high-dose-rate beams.

322. **Beam Transmission Measurement (noun):** Procedure to quantify radiation transmitted through shielding or attenuators.
**Related Terms:** TVL, Barrier Design.
**Example in Radiotherapy:** Used in verification of lead barrier thickness in bunkers.

323. **Beam Weight Normalization (noun):** Scaling of individual beam weights to maintain overall prescribed dose.
**Related Terms:** Dose Scaling, Plan Optimization.
**Example in Radiotherapy:** Performed during plan finalization to meet target coverage goals.

324. **Biological Cell Death Curve (noun):** Graph showing cell survival fraction vs radiation dose.
**Related Terms:** Survival Curve, Alpha/Beta Ratio.
**Example in Radiotherapy:** Used in radiobiology to compare radiosensitivity among tissues.

325. **Biological Target Concept (noun):** The theoretical understanding of specific cellular components being radiation-sensitive.
**Related Terms:** DNA Damage, Target Theory.
**Example in Radiotherapy:** DNA is often regarded as the primary biological target.

326. **Biomolecular Radiosensitivity Marker (noun):** A measurable biological indicator predicting tissue response to radiation.
**Related Terms:** Gene Expression, Biomarker.
**Example in Radiotherapy:** ATM mutations serve as biomarkers for radiosensitivity.

327. **Bioscintillator (noun):** A scintillating material that emits light upon radiation exposure, used in biological dosimetry.
**Related Terms:** Scintillation Detector, Bioluminescence.
**Example in Radiotherapy:** Bioscintillators detect real-time radiation exposure in research assays.

328. **Biotransducer (noun):** Device that converts biological signals into measurable electrical data.
**Related Terms:** Biosensor, Radiodosimeter.
**Example in Radiotherapy:** Used for online monitoring of biological response during exposure.

329. **Body Coil (MRI) (noun):** An integrated MRI coil used for transmitting and receiving signals across the torso.
**Related Terms:** Surface Coil, Signal-to-Noise Ratio.
**Example in Radiotherapy:** Body coil data are used for target delineation in MRI simulation.

330. **Body Contour Expansion (noun):** An automatic margin added around body outlines during plan setup.
**Related Terms:** External Contour, Planning Margin.
**Example in Radiotherapy:** Used to calculate skin dose in surface contouring.

331. **Body Frame Indexing (noun):** System of standardized markings ensuring reproducible patient positioning.
**Related Terms:** Immobilization, Setup Accuracy.
**Example in Radiotherapy:** The therapist verifies body frame indexing before treatment.

332. **Bolus Air Gap (noun):** The unintentional distance between bolus material and skin surface.
**Related Terms:** Surface Dose, Bolus Placement.
**Example in Radiotherapy:** Air gaps can reduce surface dose in chest wall irradiation.

333. **Bolus Thickness Calibration (noun):** Measurement to confirm bolus material thickness matches prescription.
**Related Terms:** QA, Surface Dose.
**Example in Radiotherapy:** Performed before electron treatments to ensure correct dose buildup.

334. **Bone Marrow Dose Constraint (noun):** Maximum permissible radiation dose to preserve hematologic function.
**Related Terms:** OAR Limit, Hematologic Toxicity.
**Example in Radiotherapy:** Maintained during pelvic RT to reduce marrow suppression.

335. **Brain Activation Mapping (noun):** Functional imaging to identify active brain regions during tasks.
**Related Terms:** fMRI, Functional Planning.
**Example in Radiotherapy:** Helps avoid eloquent cortex in stereotactic radiosurgery.

336. **Brain Atlas Segmentation (noun):** Automatic segmentation of brain regions using a reference atlas.
**Related Terms:** Image Registration, Contour Propagation.
**Example in Radiotherapy:** Used in adaptive neuro-oncology planning.

337. **Brainstem Dose Gradient (noun):** The spatial rate of dose change across the brainstem boundary.
**Related Terms:** Dose Fall-off, Hotspot.
**Example in Radiotherapy:** A steep dose gradient is necessary in SRS to protect the brainstem.

338. **Breathing Amplitude Threshold (noun):** The maximum acceptable chest wall motion for gated delivery.
**Related Terms:** Motion Management, 4D CT.
**Example in Radiotherapy:** Set during simulation for left breast DIBH planning.

339. **Breathing Coaching System (noun):** Audio-visual feedback device guiding patient respiration during RT.
**Related Terms:** Gating, Motion Monitoring.
**Example in Radiotherapy:** Used in liver SBRT to stabilize breathing amplitude.

340. **Breathing Surrogate Signal (noun):** External indicator reflecting internal organ motion due to respiration.
**Related Terms:** RPM System, Marker Tracking.
**Example in Radiotherapy:** Infrared markers serve as breathing surrogate signals.

341. **Bremsstrahlung Contamination (noun):** Unwanted photon production during electron therapy.
**Related Terms:** Electron Beam QA, Photon Leakage.
**Example in Radiotherapy:** Reduced using low-Z scattering foils in LINACs.

342. **Bronchial Carina Localization (noun):** Identification of tracheal bifurcation point during planning.
**Related Terms:** Anatomical Landmark, CT Planning.
**Example in Radiotherapy:** Used as a reference for mediastinal field borders.

343. **Bronchovascular Bundle (noun):** Anatomical unit comprising bronchi and accompanying blood vessels.
**Related Terms:** Lung Anatomy, Contouring.
**Example in Radiotherapy:** Must be carefully delineated in central lung tumors.

344. **Bulk Density Phantom (noun):** A homogeneous phantom designed to simulate tissue mass density.
**Related Terms:** Calibration Phantom, QA Material.
**Example in Radiotherapy:** Used to verify HU-to-density conversion accuracy.

345. **Burst Mode Delivery (noun):** A treatment delivery technique where dose is delivered in short, high-intensity bursts.
**Related Terms:** FLASH Therapy, Dose Rate.
**Example in Radiotherapy:** Investigated in preclinical FLASH proton studies.

346. **Byte (noun):** A digital unit of data representing eight bits, used to store or process imaging and treatment data.
**Related Terms:** Data storage, DICOM file
**Example in Radiotherapy:** Treatment plan and CBCT datasets are stored and transferred as multi-byte DICOM files.

347. **Beam Alignment Verification (noun):** Process of confirming correct spatial alignment between radiation beam, isocenter, and patient anatomy.
**Related Terms:** Isocenter QA, Laser Alignment.
**Example in Radiotherapy:** Beam alignment verification is performed during daily machine QA.

348. **Beam Angle Optimization (noun):** Selection of optimal gantry and couch angles to maximize target coverage and minimize OAR dose.
**Related Terms:** Treatment Geometry, IMRT Planning.
**Example in Radiotherapy:** Beam angle optimization improves conformity in head-and-neck plans.

349. **Beam Aperture (noun):** The effective opening through which the radiation beam exits the collimation system.
**Related Terms:** Field Size, Collimator Jaws.
**Example in Radiotherapy:** Beam aperture is adjusted to match the target contour.

350. **Beam Attenuation Coefficient (noun):** A material-specific factor describing reduction in beam intensity per unit thickness.
**Related Terms:** Linear Attenuation, HVL.
**Example in Radiotherapy:** Used in shielding and heterogeneity corrections.

351. **Beam Axis Offset (noun):** Deviation of the beam central axis from its nominal reference position.
**Related Terms:** Isocenter Shift, QA Tolerance.
**Example in Radiotherapy:** Beam axis offset is checked during Winston–Lutz testing.

352. **Beam Bending Magnet (noun):** Electromagnetic component directing electrons toward the target in a LINAC.
**Related Terms:** Energy Selection System, Beam Steering.
**Example in Radiotherapy:** Proper magnet function ensures accurate beam energy.

353. **Beam Calibration Curve (noun):** Graph relating monitor units to delivered dose under reference conditions.
**Related Terms:** Output Calibration, TG-51.
**Example in Radiotherapy:** Used during annual LINAC calibration.

354. **Beam Collimator Rotation (noun):** Angular movement of the collimator assembly around the beam axis.
**Related Terms:** Collimator Angle, Field Shaping.
**Example in Radiotherapy:** Rotated to minimize tongue-and-groove effects.

355. **Beam Compensation Filter (noun):** Device modifying beam fluence to account for patient contour variations.
**Related Terms:** Compensator, Dose Homogenization.
**Example in Radiotherapy:** Used in 3D-CRT breast treatments.

356. **Beam Data Commissioning (noun):** Process of acquiring and validating beam parameters for TPS modeling.
**Related Terms:** Beam Modeling, TPS Commissioning.
**Example in Radiotherapy:** Essential before clinical plan generation.

357. **Beam Delivery Accuracy (noun):** Degree to which planned dose matches delivered dose spatially and dosimetrically.
**Related Terms:** Treatment Verification, QA.
**Example in Radiotherapy:** Evaluated using phantom measurements.

358. **Beam Divergence (noun):** Geometric spreading of the beam as it travels away from the source.
**Related Terms:** Source-to-Axis Distance, Penumbra.
**Example in Radiotherapy:** Considered when matching adjacent fields.

359. **Beam Energy Drift (noun):** Unintended variation in beam energy over time.
**Related Terms:** Beam Stability, QA Monitoring.
**Example in Radiotherapy:** Detected during monthly energy checks.

360. **Beam Flatness (noun):** Uniformity of dose distribution across the central region of the beam.
**Related Terms:** Symmetry, Profile QA.
**Example in Radiotherapy:** Verified during monthly LINAC QA.

361. **Beam Fluence Map (noun):** Spatial representation of radiation intensity across the treatment field.
**Related Terms:** IMRT, Intensity Modulation.
**Example in Radiotherapy:** Used during inverse planning optimization.

362. **Beam Hardening (noun):** Increase in mean photon energy due to preferential absorption of low-energy photons.
**Related Terms:** Filtration, CT Artifact.
**Example in Radiotherapy:** Causes cupping artifacts in CT images.

363. **Beam Interlock System (noun):** Safety mechanism that terminates beam delivery under fault conditions.
**Related Terms:** Radiation Safety, Machine Interlocks.
**Example in Radiotherapy:** Activates during door or dose errors.

364. **Beam Intensity Profile (noun):** Distribution of dose intensity across the beam cross-section.
**Related Terms:** Profile Scan, Flatness.
**Example in Radiotherapy:** Measured during beam commissioning.

365. **Beam Limiting Device (noun):** Component restricting beam size and shape.
**Related Terms:** Jaws, MLC.
**Example in Radiotherapy:** Used to protect adjacent normal tissue.

366. **Beam Modulation Factor (noun):** Ratio describing degree of intensity modulation in IMRT fields.
**Related Terms:** Complexity Index, Plan QA.
**Example in Radiotherapy:** High modulation may increase delivery uncertainty.

367. **Beam Monitor Chamber (noun):** Ionization chamber measuring dose output during treatment.
**Related Terms:** MU Control, Dosimetry.
**Example in Radiotherapy:** Ensures accurate dose delivery.

368. **Beam Output Constancy (noun):** Stability of beam output relative to reference calibration.
**Related Terms:** Daily QA, Output Drift.
**Example in Radiotherapy:** Must remain within ±3%.

369. **Beam Penumbra (noun):** Region of rapid dose fall-off at field edges.
**Related Terms:** Edge Sharpness, Collimation.
**Example in Radiotherapy:** Smaller penumbra improves target conformity.

370. **Beam Phase Stability (noun):** Consistency of RF phase during beam generation.
**Related Terms:** Accelerator Timing, RF Control.
**Example in Radiotherapy:** Critical for dose reproducibility.

371. **Beam Profile Symmetry (noun):** Equality of dose on either side of the central axis.
**Related Terms:** Flatness, QA Tolerance.
**Example in Radiotherapy:** Checked during daily QA.

372. **Beam Quality Index (noun):** Metric describing beam penetration characteristics.
**Related Terms:** TPR, PDD.
**Example in Radiotherapy:** Used to verify photon energy.

373. **Beam Range Uncertainty (noun):** Uncertainty in depth of maximum dose deposition.
**Related Terms:** Proton Therapy, Range Margin.
**Example in Radiotherapy:** Managed using robustness analysis.

374. **Beam Scattering Foil (noun):** Device spreading electron beams uniformly.
**Related Terms:** Electron Therapy, Scatter.
**Example in Radiotherapy:** Used in electron applicators.

375. **Beam Shaping Assembly (noun):** Collection of components defining beam geometry.
**Related Terms:** MLC, Jaws.
**Example in Radiotherapy:** Shapes dose to match target volume.

376. **Beam Spoiler (noun):** Material inserted to increase surface dose by electron scatter.
**Related Terms:** Bolus, Surface Dose.
**Example in Radiotherapy:** Used in TBI treatments.

377. **Beam Stability Monitoring (noun):** Continuous tracking of beam parameters during operation.
**Related Terms:** QA Logs, Trend Analysis.
**Example in Radiotherapy:** Detects gradual performance drift.

378. **Beam Stopper (noun):** Shielding structure absorbing unused radiation.
**Related Terms:** Secondary Barrier, Shielding Design.
**Example in Radiotherapy:** Installed behind treatment head.

379. **Beam Symmetry (noun):** Uniformity of intensity across the beam's central axis.
**Related Terms:** Flatness, Profile QA.
**Example in Radiotherapy:** Verified during monthly QA.

380. **Beam Transmission Factor (noun):** Fraction of radiation passing through attenuating material.
**Related Terms:** Tray Factor, Block Factor.
**Example in Radiotherapy:** Applied in MU calculations.

381. **Beam Tuning (noun):** Adjustment of accelerator parameters for optimal beam output.
**Related Terms:** RF Control, Steering.
**Example in Radiotherapy:** Performed during service maintenance.

382. **Beam Uniformity Correction (noun):** Adjustment compensating for non-uniform beam output.
**Related Terms:** Profile Matching, QA.
**Example in Radiotherapy:** Applied during TPS modeling.

383. **Beam Verification Imaging (noun):** Imaging acquired using treatment beam for alignment checks.
**Related Terms:** EPID, Portal Imaging.
**Example in Radiotherapy:** Confirms patient positioning.

384. **Beam Weight Adjustment (noun):** Modification of individual beam contributions to total dose.
**Related Terms:** Plan Normalization, Optimization.
**Example in Radiotherapy:** Used to improve dose homogeneity.

385. **Beam Width (noun):** Lateral dimension of the radiation field.
**Related Terms:** Field Size, Aperture.
**Example in Radiotherapy:** Selected based on target size.

386. **Beam-On Delay (noun):** Time lag between beam enable command and actual radiation delivery.
**Related Terms:** Control System Latency, QA Timing.
**Example in Radiotherapy:** Verified during acceptance testing.

387. **Beam-On Time (noun):** Duration for which radiation is actively delivered.
**Related Terms:** Monitor Units, Exposure Time.
**Example in Radiotherapy:** Confirmed before patient treatment.

388. **Beam Output Calibration (noun):** Process of setting beam output to deliver prescribed dose per MU.
**Related Terms:** TG-51, Reference Dosimetry.
**Example in Radiotherapy:** Performed annually.

389. **Beam Output Drift (noun):** Gradual deviation of beam output from reference value.
**Related Terms:** Output Constancy, QA Trend.
**Example in Radiotherapy:** Detected through daily QA logs.

390. **Beam Reference Point (noun):** Defined spatial point used for calibration and measurement.
**Related Terms:** Isocenter, SSD.
**Example in Radiotherapy:** Used for chamber positioning.

391. **Beam Scatter (noun):** Radiation deflected from primary beam path due to interactions.
**Related Terms:** Secondary Radiation, Dose Spread.
**Example in Radiotherapy:** Considered in shielding design.

392. **Beam Scatter Factor (noun):** Ratio accounting for scatter contribution based on field size.
**Related Terms:** Output Factor, Collimator Scatter.
**Example in Radiotherapy:** Used in MU calculations.

393. **Beam Steering Coil (noun):** Electromagnetic component controlling beam direction.
**Related Terms:** Beam Alignment, Accelerator Control.
**Example in Radiotherapy:** Adjusted during service tuning.

394. **Beam Stability Index (noun):** Metric quantifying temporal stability of beam parameters.
**Related Terms:** QA Trending, Output Constancy.
**Example in Radiotherapy:** Used for preventive maintenance.

395. **Beam Start Interlock (noun):** Safety mechanism preventing beam initiation under unsafe conditions.
**Related Terms:** Machine Interlocks, Radiation Safety.
**Example in Radiotherapy:** Activated if door is open.

396. **Bio transport Modeling (noun):** Simulation of radiation-induced molecular or cellular transport.
**Related Terms:** Monte Carlo, Dosimetric Modeling.
**Example in Radiotherapy:** Used in nanodosimetry research.

397. **Blackbody Radiation (noun):** Electromagnetic radiation emitted by an ideal absorber.
**Related Terms:** Thermal Radiation, Spectrum.
**Example in Radiotherapy:** Used in detector calibration.

398. **Blood Dosimetry (noun):** Measurement of absorbed dose in circulating blood.
**Related Terms:** Biodosimetry, TBI.
**Example in Radiotherapy:** Ensures safe limits in TBI.

399. **Body Dose Index (BDI) (noun):** Index representing average body dose during imaging.
**Related Terms:** DLP, CTDI.
**Example in Radiotherapy:** Used in imaging QA.

400. **Body Equilibrium Position (noun):** Standardized patient alignment posture.
**Related Terms:** Supine, Immobilization.
**Example in Radiotherapy:** Verified before beam delivery.

401. **Bone Shielding (noun):** Use of materials to reduce dose to bone structures.
**Related Terms:** Custom Shield, Compensator.
**Example in Radiotherapy:** Protects mandible in H&N RT.

402. **Boolean Operation (Imaging) (noun):** Logical combination of imaging volumes.
**Related Terms:** ROI Fusion, Segmentation.
**Example in Radiotherapy:** Used to define composite targets.

403. **Boron Neutron Capture Therapy (BNCT) (noun):** Binary therapy using boron-10 and neutrons.
**Related Terms:** Neutron Therapy, Radiosensitization.
**Example in Radiotherapy:** Used for recurrent head-neck tumors.

404. **Boundary Dose Fall-off (noun):** Rapid dose reduction at field edges.
**Related Terms:** Penumbra, Gradient Index.
**Example in Radiotherapy:** Protects surrounding tissue.

405. **Brainstem Dose Constraint (noun):** Maximum allowable dose to brainstem.
**Related Terms:** OAR Limits, SRS.
**Example in Radiotherapy:** Prevents necrosis.

406. **Brilliance (Beam Quality) (noun):** Photon flux per unit area and angle.
**Related Terms:** Beam Intensity, Photon Yield.
**Example in Radiotherapy:** Enhances portal imaging.

407. **Broadband Photon Source (noun):** Radiation source emitting wide energy spectrum.
**Related Terms:** Polychromatic Beam, X-ray Tube.
**Example in Radiotherapy:** Used in diagnostic imaging.

408. **Bronchial Wall Contouring (noun):** Delineation of bronchial walls as OARs.
**Related Terms:** Lung RT, OAR Contouring.
**Example in Radiotherapy:** Reduces fibrosis risk.

409. **Build-up Cap (noun):** Material covering detectors to ensure equilibrium.
**Related Terms:** Ion Chamber, Dosimetry.
**Example in Radiotherapy:** Used in output calibration.

410. **Build-up Material (noun):** Layer added to increase surface dose.
**Related Terms:** Bolus, Buildup Cap.
**Example in Radiotherapy:** Chest wall treatments.

411. **Burnout Detector Failure (noun):** Detector malfunction due to excessive exposure.
**Related Terms:** QA Error, Chamber Saturation.
**Example in Radiotherapy:** Prevented by routine QA.

412. **Beam Orbit Stability (noun):** Consistency of electron trajectory in LINAC.
**Related Terms:** Steering, Beam Position.
**Example in Radiotherapy:** Monitored via logs.

413. **Biometric Verification (noun):** Patient identification using biometric data.
**Related Terms:** Barcode ID, Safety Systems.
**Example in Radiotherapy:** Prevents wrong-patient errors.

414. **Beam Energy Modulation (noun):** Variation of beam energy for uniform dose.
**Related Terms:** Range Modulator, Compensator.
**Example in Radiotherapy:** Proton SOBP creation.

415. **Brachytherapy Quality Index (BQI) (noun):** Metric evaluating brachytherapy dose conformity.
**Related Terms:** Homogeneity Index, Conformity Index.
**Example in Radiotherapy:** HDR prostate QA.

416. **Brachytherapy Remote After loader (noun):** Device remotely positioning radioactive sources.
**Related Terms:** HDR Unit, Source Control.
**Example in Radiotherapy:** Reduces staff exposure.

417. **Brachytherapy Source Strength (noun):** Measure of emission rate of Brachy source.
**Related Terms:** Air Kerma, Calibration.
**Example in Radiotherapy:** Verified during commissioning.

418. **Bragg Curve (noun):** Plot of energy loss versus depth.
**Related Terms:** Bragg Peak, Proton Therapy.
**Example in Radiotherapy:** Guides range calculations.

419. **Brilliance Calibration (noun):** Adjustment of display brightness and contrast.
**Related Terms:** Display QA, Image Uniformity.
**Example in Radiotherapy:** Ensures contouring accuracy.

420. **Broad Beam Geometry (noun):** Irradiation where beam fully covers detector.
**Related Terms:** Scatter Conditions, Dosimetry.
**Example in Radiotherapy:** Absolute dose calibration.

421. **Broad-Spectrum Radiation (noun):** Radiation composed of multiple energies.
**Related Terms:** Polyenergetic Beam.
**Example in Radiotherapy:** Orthovoltage therapy.

422. **Bronchial Tree Dose Mapping (noun):** Visualization of dose along bronchial anatomy.
**Related Terms:** DVH, OAR Analysis.
**Example in Radiotherapy:** Lung SBRT planning.

423. **Brownian Motion Detector (noun):** Device measuring nanoparticle motion.
**Related Terms:** Nanodosimetry.
**Example in Radiotherapy:** Radio sensitizer research.

424. **Build-up Factor (noun):** Correction factor for scattered radiation.
**Related Terms:** Shielding Calculations.
**Example in Radiotherapy:** Barrier design.

425. **Bulk Density Correction (noun):** Dose adjustment for tissue density variation.
**Related Terms:** HU Calibration.
**Example in Radiotherapy:** Lung planning.

426. **Bunker Shielding Design (noun):** Structural planning for radiation protection.
**Related Terms:** Primary Barrier.
**Example in Radiotherapy:** LINAC vaults.

427. **Bypass Valve (Cooling System) (noun):** Valve diverting coolant flow.
**Related Terms:** Equipment Safety.
**Example in Radiotherapy:** Prevents overheating.

428. **Bystander Effect (noun):** Radiation effects in non-irradiated cells.
**Related Terms:** Cell Signalling.
**Example in Radiotherapy:** Normal tissue response.

429. **Beam Area Product (noun):** Measure combining beam intensity and area.
**Related Terms:** Dose Area Product.
**Example in Radiotherapy:** Imaging exposure estimation.

430. **Beam Calibration Phantom (noun):** Standard phantom for beam calibration.
**Related Terms:** Water Phantom.
**Example in Radiotherapy:** Annual QA.

431. **Beam Collimator Leaf Speed (noun):**
Velocity of MLC leaf movement.
**Related Terms:** VMAT QA.
**Example in Radiotherapy:** Dynamic delivery accuracy.

432. **Beam Data Library (noun):** Stored verified beam parameters in TPS.
**Related Terms:** Commissioning Data.
**Example in Radiotherapy:** TPS installation.

433. **Beam Edge Profile (noun):** Dose fall-off representation at beam edge.
**Related Terms:** Penumbra.
**Example in Radiotherapy:** Profile QA.

434. **Beam Energy Spectrum (noun):** Distribution of emitted particle energies.
**Related Terms:** Beam Quality.
**Example in Radiotherapy:** Monte Carlo modeling.

435. **Beam Intensity Modulation (noun):** Controlled fluence variation.
**Related Terms:** IMRT, VMAT.
**Example in Radiotherapy:** Conformal dose shaping.

436. **Beam Parameter Verification (noun):** QA validation of beam characteristics.
**Related Terms:** Beam Constancy.
**Example in Radiotherapy:** Monthly QA.

437. **Beam Portal Imaging (noun):** Image acquisition using treatment beam.
**Related Terms:** EPID, MV Imaging.
**Example in Radiotherapy:** Setup verification.

438. **Beam Position Reproducibility (noun):** Consistency of beam alignment over time.
**Related Terms:** Isocenter Stability.
**Example in Radiotherapy:** Long-term QA tracking.

439. **Beam Scatter Correction (noun):** Adjustment accounting for scattered dose.
**Related Terms:** Output Factors.
**Example in Radiotherapy:** MU calculations.

440. **Beam Symmetry Check (noun):** Verification of left-right dose equality.
**Related Terms:** Flatness QA.
**Example in Radiotherapy:** Daily checks.

441. **Beam Verification Phantom (noun):** Phantom for planned vs delivered dose comparison.
**Related Terms:** IMRT QA.
**Example in Radiotherapy:** Pre-treatment verification.

442. **Beam Weight Optimization (noun):** Adjustment of beam contributions for homogeneity.
**Related Terms:** Plan Optimization.
**Example in Radiotherapy:** Multi-field planning.

443. **Biological Amplification (noun):** Enhanced biological effect via secondary processes.
**Related Terms:** ROS, DNA Damage.
**Example in Radiotherapy:** Radiosensitivity studies.

444. **Biological Repair Kinetics (noun):** Rate of cellular repair after irradiation.
**Related Terms:** LQ Model.
**Example in Radiotherapy:** Fractionation design.

445. **Biophysical Modelling Software (noun):** Tools simulating biological radiation effects.
**Related Terms:** TCP Modeling.
**Example in Radiotherapy:** Outcome prediction.

446. **Blood Perfusion Imaging (noun):** Imaging of tissue vascularization.
**Related Terms:** PET, SPECT.
**Example in Radiotherapy:** Adaptive planning.

447. **Bone Equivalent Phantom (noun):** Phantom mimicking bone density.
**Related Terms:** Heterogeneity QA.
**Example in Radiotherapy:** Dose verification.

448. **Brain Dose Histogram (noun):** Dose distribution across brain tissue.
**Related Terms:** DVH.
**Example in Radiotherapy:** Plan evaluation.

449. **Brainstem Contouring Protocol (noun):** Guidelines for brainstem delineation.
**Related Terms:** RTOG Protocols.
**Example in Radiotherapy:** OAR accuracy.

450. **Breathing Cycle Analysis (noun):** Evaluation of respiratory motion patterns.
**Related Terms:** 4D-CT, Gating.
**Example in Radiotherapy:** Motion management.

451. **Breathing Gating Window (noun):** Optimal respiratory phase for delivery.
**Related Terms:** Respiratory Gating.
**Example in Radiotherapy:** DIBH treatments.

452. **Bremsstrahlung Spectrum (noun):** Energy distribution of deceleration photons.
**Related Terms:** X-ray Production.
**Example in Radiotherapy:** LINAC beam quality.

453. **Brightness Uniformity Test (noun):** QA test for display luminance consistency.
**Related Terms:** Display QA.
**Example in Radiotherapy:** Monthly imaging QA.

454. **Bronchial Lymphatic Mapping (noun):** Imaging of lymphatic drainage pathways.
**Related Terms:** PET/CT.
**Example in Radiotherapy:** Lung cancer staging.

455. **Bulk Electron Density Assignment (noun):** Uniform density assignment for structures.
**Related Terms:** HU Override.
**Example in Radiotherapy:** Metal artifact correction.

456. **Beam Phase Space Data (noun):** Dataset describing particle position and direction.
**Related Terms:** Monte Carlo.
**Example in Radiotherapy:** Dose simulation.

457. **Beam Position Tolerance (noun):** Allowable deviation from intended axis.
**Related Terms:** Isocenter Accuracy.
**Example in Radiotherapy:** Daily QA.

458. **Beam Quality Correction Factor (noun):** Factor correcting beam quality differences.
**Related Terms:** kQ Factor.
**Example in Radiotherapy:** Chamber calibration.

459. **Beam Recombination Correction (noun):** Adjustment for ion recombination loss.
**Related Terms:** Saturation Correction.
**Example in Radiotherapy:** High dose-rate beams.

460. **Beam Transmission Measurement (noun):** Quantification of radiation through shielding.
**Related Terms:** TVL.
**Example in Radiotherapy:** Barrier verification.

461. **Beam Weight Normalization (noun):** Scaling beam weights to prescription.
**Related Terms:** Dose Scaling.
**Example in Radiotherapy:** Plan finalization.

462. **Biological Cell Death Curve (noun):** Graph of survival fraction vs dose.
**Related Terms:** Alpha/Beta Ratio.
**Example in Radiotherapy:** Radiosensitivity comparison.

463. **Biological Target Concept (noun):** Theory of radiation-sensitive cellular targets.
**Related Terms:** DNA Damage.
**Example in Radiotherapy:** Radiobiology teaching.

464. **Bimolecular Radiosensitivity Marker (noun):** Indicator predicting radiation response.
**Related Terms:** Biomarker.
**Example in Radiotherapy:** Personalized RT.

465. **Bio scintillator (noun):** Material emitting light under radiation.
**Related Terms:** Scintillation Detector.
**Example in Radiotherapy:** Research dosimetry.

466. **Bio transducer (noun):** Device converting biological signals to data.
**Related Terms:** Biosensor.
**Example in Radiotherapy:** Online monitoring.

**467. Body Coil (MRI) (noun):** Integrated MRI transmit-receive coil.
**Related Terms:** SNR.
**Example in Radiotherapy:** MRI simulation.

**468. Body Contour Expansion (noun):** Automatic margin around body outline.
**Related Terms:** Planning Margin.
**Example in Radiotherapy:** Skin dose estimation.

**469. Body Frame Indexing (noun):** System ensuring reproducible positioning.
**Related Terms:** Immobilization.
**Example in Radiotherapy:** Setup accuracy.

**470. Bolus Air Gap (noun):** Unintended space between bolus and skin.
**Related Terms:** Surface Dose Loss.
**Example in Radiotherapy:** Chest wall RT.

**471. Bolus Thickness Calibration (noun):** Verification of bolus thickness accuracy.
**Related Terms:** Surface Dose QA.
**Example in Radiotherapy:** Electron therapy.

**472. Bone Marrow Dose Constraint (noun):** Maximum dose preserving marrow function.
**Related Terms:** Hematologic Toxicity.
**Example in Radiotherapy:** Pelvic RT.

**473. Brain Activation Mapping (noun):** Functional imaging of active brain regions.
**Related Terms:** fMRI.
**Example in Radiotherapy:** SRS planning.

**474. Brain Atlas Segmentation (noun):** Automated brain region segmentation.
**Related Terms:** Image Registration.
**Example in Radiotherapy:** Adaptive planning.

**475. Brainstem Dose Gradient (noun):** Rate of dose change across brainstem.
**Related Terms:** Dose Fall-off.
**Example in Radiotherapy:** SRS protection.

**476. Breathing Amplitude Threshold (noun):** Maximum acceptable respiratory motion.
**Related Terms:** Gating Limits.
**Example in Radiotherapy:** DIBH setup.

**477. Breathing Coaching System (noun):** Audio-visual respiration guidance device.
**Related Terms:** Motion Management.
**Example in Radiotherapy:** Liver SBRT.

**478. Breathing Surrogate Signal (noun):** External indicator of internal motion.
**Related Terms:** RPM System.
**Example in Radiotherapy:** Gated delivery.

**479. Bremsstrahlung Contamination (noun):** Unwanted photon production in electron beams.
**Related Terms:** Electron QA.
**Example in Radiotherapy:** Reduced with low-Z foils.

**480. Bronchial Carina Localization (noun):** Identification of tracheal bifurcation.
**Related Terms:** Anatomical Landmark.
**Example in Radiotherapy:** Mediastinal planning.

481. **Broncho vascular Bundle (noun):** Combined bronchi and vessels unit.
**Related Terms:** Lung Anatomy.
**Example in Radiotherapy:** Central lung tumors.

482. **Bulk Density Phantom (noun):** Homogeneous phantom simulating tissue density.
**Related Terms:** HU Calibration.
**Example in Radiotherapy:** TPS verification.

483. **Burst Mode Delivery (noun):** Dose delivered in short high-intensity bursts.
**Related Terms:** FLASH Therapy.
**Example in Radiotherapy:** Preclinical studies.

484. **Byte (noun):** Digital unit equal to eight bits.
**Related Terms:** Data Storage, DICOM.
**Example in Radiotherapy:** Image and plan files.

485. **Beam Symmetry (noun):** Uniformity of radiation intensity across central axis.
**Related Terms:** Flatness, Beam Quality.
**Example in Radiotherapy:** Verified during monthly LINAC QA.

486. **Beam Angular Accuracy (noun):** Degree to which actual gantry, collimator, or couch angles match planned values.
**Related Terms:** Mechanical QA, Isocentric Accuracy.
**Example in Radiotherapy:** Verified during monthly mechanical QA.

487. **Beam Aperture Margin (noun):** Additional margin applied to field edges to ensure target coverage.
**Related Terms:** Field Margin, Geometric Uncertainty.
**Example in Radiotherapy:** Added to account for setup variation.

488. **Beam Arrival Time (noun):** Exact timing of beam delivery relative to control system commands.
**Related Terms:** Synchronization, Gating Accuracy.
**Example in Radiotherapy:** Critical in respiratory-gated treatments.

489. **Beam Block Transmission (noun):** Fraction of radiation penetrating shielding blocks.
**Related Terms:** Block Transmission Factor, Attenuation.
**Example in Radiotherapy:** Used in manual MU calculations.

490. **Beam Central Axis Drift (noun):** Gradual displacement of the beam central axis over time.
**Related Terms:** Isocenter Stability, QA Trending.
**Example in Radiotherapy:** Detected through long-term QA analysis.

491. **Beam Complexity Index (noun):** Quantitative measure of modulation and delivery complexity.
**Related Terms:** IMRT Complexity, Plan Robustness.
**Example in Radiotherapy:** High values may increase QA failure risk.

492. **Beam Current Stability (noun):** Consistency of electron beam current during operation.
**Related Terms:** Accelerator Performance, RF Control.
**Example in Radiotherapy:** Ensures reproducible dose output.

493. **Beam Cut-off Interlock (noun):** Safety system that immediately terminates radiation delivery.
**Related Terms:** Emergency Stop, Radiation Safety.
**Example in Radiotherapy:** Activates during abnormal dose rate.

494. **Beam Dose Linearity (noun):** Proportional relationship between monitor units and delivered dose.
**Related Terms:** MU Linearity, Output QA.
**Example in Radiotherapy:** Tested during acceptance commissioning.

**495. Beam Edge Sharpness (noun):** Measure of how abruptly dose falls off at field boundaries.
**Related Terms:** Penumbra Width, Collimation Quality.
**Example in Radiotherapy:** Important for stereotactic treatments.

**496. Beam Energy Constancy (noun):** Stability of beam penetration characteristics over time.
**Related Terms:** PDD Stability, Energy QA.
**Example in Radiotherapy:** Checked monthly using depth-dose curves.

**497. Beam Hold State (noun):** Temporary suspension of beam delivery without terminating treatment.
**Related Terms:** Pause Function, Control System.
**Example in Radiotherapy:** Used during patient motion events.

**498. Beam Output Linearity (noun):** Accuracy of dose delivery across a range of MU settings.
**Related Terms:** Low-MU Accuracy, Dosimetric QA.
**Example in Radiotherapy:** Critical for IMRT and VMAT plans.

**499. Beam Recovery Sequence (noun):** Automated procedure restoring beam readiness after interruption.
**Related Terms:** Interlock Reset, System Safety.
**Example in Radiotherapy:** Performed after fault resolution.

**500. Beam Robustness Analysis (noun):** Evaluation of treatment plan stability against setup errors, range uncertainties, and anatomical variations.
**Related Terms:** Robust Optimization, Uncertainty Analysis.
**Example in Radiotherapy:** Beam robustness analysis is routinely performed in proton therapy planning to ensure target coverage under uncertainty.

# C

1. **Calibration (noun):** Adjustment and verification of radiotherapy equipment to ensure accurate and reproducible radiation dose delivery.
   **Related Terms:** Dosimetry, Quality Assurance, Linear Accelerator.
   **Example in Radiotherapy:** Calibration confirms the linear accelerator delivers the prescribed radiation dose correctly.
2. **Cancer staging (noun):** Classification system describing cancer spread, typically using the TNM system, essential for treatment planning.
   **Related Terms:** TNM classification, Prognosis, Treatment intent.
   **Example in Radiotherapy:** Accurate cancer staging guides target delineation and dose prescription.
3. **Cardiac gating (noun):** Technique synchronizing radiation delivery with cardiac motion to reduce irradiation of moving heart structures.
   **Related Terms:** Motion management, Respiratory gating, 4D-CT.
   **Example in Radiotherapy:** Cardiac gating helps spare cardiac tissue in left breast cancer treatment.
4. **C-arm fluoroscopy (noun):** Mobile X-ray device producing real-time fluoroscopic images, used in interventional and brachytherapy procedures.
   **Related Terms:** Brachytherapy, Imaging guidance, Fluoroscopy.
   **Example in Radiotherapy:** C-arm fluoroscopy aids catheter placement in gynecological brachytherapy.
5. **CBCT (Cone Beam Computed Tomography) (noun):** Volumetric imaging using cone-shaped X-rays for daily patient setup verification.
   **Related Terms:** IGRT, kV imaging, 3D verification.
   **Example in Radiotherapy:** CBCT verifies liver SBRT positioning before treatment delivery.
6. **Central axis (noun):** Imaginary line representing the beam's center from source to isocenter in radiotherapy.
   **Related Terms:** Isocenter, Beam geometry, SSD.
   **Example in Radiotherapy:** Dose is prescribed at the central axis to ensure uniform delivery.
7. **Cerrobend block (noun):** Custom shielding block made of low-melting alloy used to shape treatment fields.
   **Related Terms:** Field shaping, Beam modifiers, Lead block.
   **Example in Radiotherapy:** Cerrobend blocks shield normal tissues in cobalt unit treatments.
8. **Charged particle equilibrium (noun):** Condition where the number of charged particles entering equals those leaving a volume, ensuring dose accuracy.
   **Related Terms:** Dose deposition, Depth dose, Electron equilibrium.
   **Example in Radiotherapy:** Charged particle equilibrium occurs beyond dmax in photon beams.
9. **Check film (noun):** Verification image captured before treatment to confirm field accuracy and patient setup.
   **Related Terms:** Portal imaging, QA imaging, Simulation.
   **Example in Radiotherapy:** A check film ensures correct field placement before cobalt-60 therapy.

10. **Chromatic aberration (noun):** Optical distortion where different wavelengths focus differently, affecting imaging clarity.
**Related Terms:** Imaging artifacts, Lens error, Optical distortion.
**Example in Radiotherapy:** Chromatic aberration can reduce clarity in optical imaging for surface guidance.

11. **Cine mode imaging (noun):** Continuous acquisition of imaging frames to assess motion during radiotherapy.
**Related Terms:** Motion tracking, 4D imaging, IGRT.
**Example in Radiotherapy:** Cine mode tracks diaphragm motion during lung tumor treatment.

12. **Clinical target volume (CTV) (noun):** Tissue volume containing gross tumor and microscopic spread requiring treatment.
**Related Terms:** GTV, PTV, Target delineation.
**Example in Radiotherapy:** The CTV includes the prostate and periprostatic tissues in prostate cancer.

13. **Co-60 (Cobalt-60) (noun):** Radioactive isotope emitting gamma rays, historically used in teletherapy.
**Related Terms:** Gamma rays, Telecobalt, External beam therapy.
**Example in Radiotherapy:** Co-60 units deliver external beam therapy in low-resource settings.

14. **Collimator (noun):** Device in a linear accelerator shaping and restricting radiation beams.
**Related Terms:** MLC, Field shaping, Beam modifiers.
**Example in Radiotherapy:** A multileaf collimator shapes conformal fields for IMRT.

15. **Compensator (noun):** Beam-modifying device balancing dose across uneven patient surfaces.
**Related Terms:** Wedges, Bolus, Beam modifiers.
**Example in Radiotherapy:** Compensators adjust dose for sloping chest walls in breast treatment.

16. **Computed tomography (CT) (noun):** Cross-sectional imaging using X-rays, essential for radiotherapy planning.
**Related Terms:** Simulation, Imaging, Contouring.
**Example in Radiotherapy:** CT scans are used for tumor delineation during treatment planning.

17. **Conformal radiotherapy (noun):** Technique shaping radiation beams to closely match tumor geometry.
**Related Terms:** 3D-CRT, IMRT, Beam shaping.
**Example in Radiotherapy:** Conformal RT reduces dose to surrounding organs in brain tumors.

18. **Contour delineation (noun):** Outlining tumor and organs at risk on planning images.
**Related Terms:** Contouring, Segmentation, Treatment planning.
**Example in Radiotherapy:** Contour delineation defines CTV and OARs for IMRT planning.

19. **Control console (noun):** Operator interface for controlling linear accelerator functions.
**Related Terms:** Linac, Treatment delivery, Machine parameters.
**Example in Radiotherapy:** Therapists set treatment fields and monitor beams via the control console.

20. **Conventional fractionation (noun):** Standard schedule delivering 1.8–2 Gy per fraction, 5 days weekly.
**Related Terms:** Hypofractionation, Hyperfractionation, Treatment schedule.
**Example in Radiotherapy:** Conventional fractionation is common in head and neck radiotherapy.

21. **Couch shift (noun):** Adjustment of treatment couch to correct patient position errors.
**Related Terms:** Isocenter shift, IGRT, Setup correction.
**Example in Radiotherapy:** CBCT-guided couch shifts ensure precise prostate alignment.

22. **Critical organ (noun):** Organ sensitive to radiation damage, requiring dose constraints.
**Related Terms:** Organs at risk (OAR), Dose limits, Toxicity.
**Example in Radiotherapy:** The spinal cord is a critical organ in thoracic RT.

23. **Cross-fire technique (noun):** Method using intersecting beams to deliver high tumor dose while sparing normal tissues.
**Related Terms:** Multi-field technique, Beam arrangement, Dose distribution.
**Example in Radiotherapy:** Cross-fire beams are used in brain tumor stereotactic treatments.

24. **CyberKnife® (noun):** Robotic radiosurgery system delivering highly precise non-isocentric beams.
**Related Terms:** SRS, SBRT, Robotic radiotherapy.
**Example in Radiotherapy:** CyberKnife treats small lung tumors with sub-millimeter accuracy.

25. **Cell cycle sensitivity (noun):** Variation in radiosensitivity depending on cell cycle phase.
**Related Terms:** Radiosensitivity, Mitosis, Radiobiology.
**Example in Radiotherapy:** Cells are most radiosensitive in G2/M phase.

26. **Cell survival curve (noun):** Graph showing cell survival as a function of radiation dose.
**Related Terms:** Radiobiology, LQ model, Dose-response.
**Example in Radiotherapy:** Survival curves demonstrate tumor versus normal tissue radiosensitivity.

27. **Chromosomal aberration (noun):** Radiation-induced structural changes in chromosomes.
**Related Terms:** DNA damage, Cytogenetics, Mutation.
**Example in Radiotherapy:** Chromosomal aberrations are biomarkers for radiation exposure.

28. **Clonogenic assay (noun):** Experimental test measuring a cell's ability to form colonies post-irradiation.
**Related Terms:** Radiosensitivity, Survival assay, Radiobiology.
**Example in Radiotherapy:** Clonogenic assays assess cell survival after radiation doses.

29. **Clustered DNA damage (noun):** Multiple DNA lesions in close proximity induced by radiation.
**Related Terms:** Double-strand breaks, Complex damage, Genomic instability.
**Example in Radiotherapy:** Clustered damage contributes to tumor cell death after RT.

30. **Cytogenetic damage (noun):** Radiation-induced damage observable in cellular chromosomes.
**Related Terms:** Chromosomal aberration, Micronucleus assay, DNA damage.
**Example in Radiotherapy:** Cytogenetic assays quantify biological effects of radiation.

31. **Cytotoxicity (noun):** Property of radiation or drugs to kill cells.
**Related Terms:** Radiosensitivity, Apoptosis, Cell death.
**Example in Radiotherapy:** Radiation exerts cytotoxicity by inducing DNA double-strand breaks.

32. **Cytoplasm irradiation (noun):** Exposure of cytoplasm to ionizing radiation affecting cell functions.
**Related Terms:** Cellular damage, Non-targeted effects, Radiobiology.
**Example in Radiotherapy:** Cytoplasmic irradiation may influence bystander signaling pathways.

33. **Cytokine response (noun):** Cell signaling response involving cytokine release after radiation.
**Related Terms:** Inflammation, Bystander effect, Immune modulation.
**Example in Radiotherapy:** Cytokine response contributes to radiation-induced pneumonitis.

34. **Cytostasis (noun):** Inhibition of cell growth and division due to radiation.
**Related Terms:** Cytotoxicity, Apoptosis, Cell cycle arrest.
**Example in Radiotherapy:** Sub-lethal radiation doses may cause cytostasis in tumor cells.

35. **Calvarium (noun):** Upper dome-like portion of the skull.
**Related Terms:** Skull, Cranial anatomy, Brain protection.
**Example in Radiotherapy:** The calvarium serves as a bony landmark in cranial RT.

36. **Canthus (noun):** The corner of the eye where eyelids meet, used as a surface landmark.
**Related Terms:** Eye anatomy, Orbital landmarks, Setup reference.
**Example in Radiotherapy:** The lateral canthus is a setup landmark in head positioning.

37. **Carina (noun):** Bifurcation point of the trachea into left and right bronchi.
**Related Terms:** Trachea, Lung anatomy, Thoracic landmark.
**Example in Radiotherapy:** The carina serves as a CT reference point in lung RT.

38. **Clavicle (noun):** Collarbone, a prominent bony surface landmark.
**Related Terms:** Shoulder, Skeletal landmark, Setup anatomy.
**Example in Radiotherapy:** The clavicle is marked during breast radiotherapy simulation.

39. **Costal margin (noun):** Lower edge of rib cage formed by cartilage.
**Related Terms:** Thoracic anatomy, Rib cage, Surface landmark.
**Example in Radiotherapy:** The costal margin helps locate liver fields in RT setup.

40. **Cricoid cartilage (noun):** Ring-shaped cartilage below the thyroid cartilage in the larynx.
**Related Terms:** Laryngeal anatomy, Airway, Neck landmarks.
**Example in Radiotherapy:** The cricoid cartilage is a palpable landmark in head-and-neck RT.

41. **Cubital fossa (noun):** Triangular area on the anterior elbow.
**Related Terms:** Elbow, Surface anatomy, Limb landmarks.
**Example in Radiotherapy:** The cubital fossa helps immobilize arms in breast RT.

42. **Cutaneous landmarks (noun):** Skin surface features used for radiotherapy positioning.
**Related Terms:** Tattoos, Fiducials, Surface markers.
**Example in Radiotherapy:** Cutaneous landmarks aid reproducibility in daily setup.

43. **C7 vertebra (noun):** Prominent cervical vertebra easily palpable at the neck base.
**Related Terms:** Cervical spine, Surface anatomy, Skeletal landmark.
**Example in Radiotherapy:** C7 is marked for positioning in head-and-neck RT.

44. **Calculation point (noun):** Reference point where radiation dose is calculated in treatment planning.
**Related Terms:** Isocenter, Dose prescription, Planning system.
**Example in Radiotherapy:** The calculation point ensures accurate monitor unit settings.

45. **Cartesian coordinates (noun):** 3D coordinate system (x, y, z) used to describe treatment geometry.
**Related Terms:** Isocenter, Imaging, Planning.
**Example in Radiotherapy:** Cartesian coordinates define beam angles and couch positions.

46. **Catheter brachytherapy (noun):** Technique placing catheters inside/near tumor to deliver radiation from within.
**Related Terms:** HDR, LDR, Interstitial brachytherapy.
**Example in Radiotherapy:** Catheter brachytherapy is common in cervical cancer treatment.

47. **Cerumen (noun):** Earwax, used as an anatomical reference in head positioning.
**Related Terms:** Ear canal, Head setup, External anatomy.
**Example in Radiotherapy:** Cerumen location can assist in head immobilization checks.

48. **Chromatic dosimeter (noun):** Dosimeter that changes color upon radiation exposure, used for dose verification.
**Related Terms:** Dosimetry, QA tools, Film dosimeter.
**Example in Radiotherapy:** Chromatic dosimeters provide visual dose verification in QA tests.

49. **Commissioning (noun):** Process of validating new radiotherapy equipment before clinical use.
**Related Terms:** QA, Calibration, Acceptance testing.
**Example in Radiotherapy:** Commissioning ensures linac beam data matches TPS for safe treatments.

50. **Consent (noun):** Informed patient agreement to undergo radiotherapy after explanation of benefits and risks.
**Related Terms:** Ethics, Patient rights, Documentation.
**Example in Radiotherapy:** Informed consent is mandatory before starting RT treatment.

51. **Cable calibration (noun):** Verification of signal transmission accuracy in treatment machine cables to ensure correct dosimetry and control.
**Related Terms:** QA, Electronics, Signal integrity.
**Example in Radiotherapy:** Cable calibration ensures accurate dose readout from ionization chambers.

52. **Calibration phantom (noun):** Standardized phantom used for machine calibration and dose verification.
**Related Terms:** QA phantom, Dosimetry, Water phantom.
**Example in Radiotherapy:** A calibration phantom standardizes output measurements during linac commissioning.

53. **Capacitance chamber (noun):** Dosimeter that measures ionization using capacitor-based charge storage.
**Related Terms:** Ionization chamber, Dosimetry, QA devices.
**Example in Radiotherapy:** Capacitance chambers verify small radiation doses during QA.

54. **Carbon ion therapy (noun):** Particle therapy using carbon ions with high LET and RBE for resistant tumors.
**Related Terms:** Proton therapy, Heavy ions, Particle therapy.
**Example in Radiotherapy:** Carbon ion therapy treats radioresistant sarcomas with improved control.

55. **Cascade effect (noun):** Amplification of biological or physical interactions due to successive processes.
**Related Terms:** Secondary electrons, Radiation damage, Amplification.
**Example in Radiotherapy:** The cascade effect increases DNA strand breaks after high-LET exposure.

56. **Castration-resistant cancer (noun):** Prostate cancer that progresses despite androgen deprivation therapy.
**Related Terms:** Hormone-refractory, Advanced prostate cancer, ADT.
**Example in Radiotherapy:** Castration-resistant cancer may still benefit from palliative radiotherapy.

57. **Cathode ray (noun):** Stream of electrons emitted from a cathode in vacuum tubes.
**Related Terms:** Electron beam, X-ray generation, Tube physics.
**Example in Radiotherapy:** Cathode rays generate X-rays in diagnostic and linac tubes.

58. **Cavity chamber (noun):** Ionization chamber with a cavity used for dosimetry in reference conditions.
**Related Terms:** Ion chamber, Dosimetry, Standard chamber.
**Example in Radiotherapy:** Cavity chambers calibrate linac photon beam outputs.

59. **CCD camera (for EPID) (noun):** Charge-coupled device sensor detecting light from scintillators in electronic portal imaging.
**Related Terms:** EPID, Imaging, Detector array.
**Example in Radiotherapy:** CCD cameras capture portal images for treatment verification.

60. **Central block (noun):** Shield placed at the beam's central axis to spare tissues.
**Related Terms:** Cerrobend block, Beam modifier, Field shaping.
**Example in Radiotherapy:** Central blocks protect mediastinum during mantle field RT.

61. **Central dose axis (noun):** Line through the center of the radiation beam where dose is measured.
**Related Terms:** Beam axis, Isocenter, SSD.
**Example in Radiotherapy:** The central dose axis is used for reference point dosimetry.

62. **Central lung distance (CLD) (noun):** Measurement from midline to lung edge in tangential breast fields.
**Related Terms:** Breast dosimetry, Lung dose, Field setup.
**Example in Radiotherapy:** CLD predicts lung exposure in breast radiotherapy.

63. **Central shielding (noun):** Radiation block covering midline structures to reduce dose.
**Related Terms:** Midline block, Field shaping, Protection.
**Example in Radiotherapy:** Central shielding protects uterus in cervical RT.

64. **Central source axis (noun):** Axis through the source to isocenter defining beam geometry.
**Related Terms:** Isocenter, Beam axis, Geometry.
**Example in Radiotherapy:** Central source axis alignment ensures accurate beam targeting.

65. **Centroid (beam) (noun):** Geometric center of radiation field distribution.
**Related Terms:** Field symmetry, Beam profile, QA.
**Example in Radiotherapy:** Centroid calculation checks beam alignment during QA.

66. **Cervical spine alignment (noun):** Proper positioning of cervical vertebrae during head-and-neck treatments.
**Related Terms:** Immobilization, Neck setup, Positioning.
**Example in Radiotherapy:** Cervical spine alignment ensures reproducibility in nasopharyngeal RT.

67. **Characteristic X-rays (noun):** X-rays emitted when inner-shell electrons are ejected and replaced.
**Related Terms:** Bremsstrahlung, Photon spectrum, X-ray production.
**Example in Radiotherapy:** Characteristic X-rays contribute to diagnostic image quality.

68. **Charged particle beam (noun):** Beam consisting of protons, electrons, or heavy ions.
**Related Terms:** Particle therapy, Proton beam, Electrons.
**Example in Radiotherapy:** Charged particle beams provide conformal tumor dose delivery.

69. **Charged particle therapy (noun):** Radiotherapy using protons or heavy ions with high precision and LET.
**Related Terms:** Proton therapy, Carbon ion therapy, Particle RT.
**Example in Radiotherapy:** Charged particle therapy reduces dose to spinal cord in tumors.

70. **Chemical dosimeter (noun):** Device measuring radiation dose by chemical change.
**Related Terms:** Fricke dosimeter, Dosimetry, QA.
**Example in Radiotherapy:** Chemical dosimeters measure absorbed dose in high-dose regions.

71. **Chest wall separation (noun):** Anterior-posterior measurement across chest, used in breast dosimetry.
**Related Terms:** Breast RT, Depth dose, Tangential fields.
**Example in Radiotherapy:** Larger chest wall separation increases scatter and dose.

72. **Chromatic dosimetry film (noun):** Film that changes color proportionally to absorbed radiation dose.
**Related Terms:** Radiochromic film, Dosimetry, QA.
**Example in Radiotherapy:** Chromatic films are used for IMRT QA verification.

73. **Chromaticity correction (noun):** Adjustment for wavelength-dependent sensitivity in optical dosimetry.
**Related Terms:** Film dosimetry, Calibration, Optical correction.
**Example in Radiotherapy:** Chromaticity correction improves accuracy of radiochromic film readings.

74. **Circular collimator (noun):** Beam-shaping device producing circular radiation fields.
**Related Terms:** Collimator, Cone applicator, Beam shaping.
**Example in Radiotherapy:** Circular collimators are used in electron therapy.

75. **Cladding (fiber optic dosimeter) (noun):** Outer layer in fiber optics guiding light signals in dosimeters.
**Related Terms:** Fiber optics, Dosimetry, Scintillators.
**Example in Radiotherapy:** Cladding ensures signal confinement in fiber dosimeters.

76. **Clinical electron energy (noun):** Nominal electron energy used for patient treatment.
**Related Terms:** Electron beams, Depth dose, Clinical range.
**Example in Radiotherapy:** Clinical electron energy of 12 MeV treats chest wall depth.

77. **Clinical evaluation form (RT QA) (noun):** Document recording treatment accuracy and verification checks.
**Related Terms:** QA documentation, Verification, Audit.
**Example in Radiotherapy:** Therapists complete evaluation forms for RT QA compliance.

78. **Clinical portal verification (noun):** Process of confirming field placement via imaging before treatment.
**Related Terms:** Portal imaging, Verification film, IGRT.
**Example in Radiotherapy:** Portal verification ensures breast tangents match planned fields.

79. **Cloud-based planning system (noun):** Radiotherapy planning platform hosted on secure online servers.
**Related Terms:** TPS, Remote planning, AI planning.
**Example in Radiotherapy:** Cloud-based systems allow remote plan review and collaboration.

80. **Coaxial cable (linac electronics) (noun):** Shielded cable transmitting signals in linear accelerators.
**Related Terms:** RF signals, Electronics, QA.
**Example in Radiotherapy:** Coaxial cables connect control systems in linacs.

81. **Coefficient of equivalent thickness (noun):** Parameter converting material thickness into equivalent water thickness.
**Related Terms:** Hounsfield unit, CT calibration, Beam attenuation.
**Example in Radiotherapy:** CT numbers are converted using equivalent thickness coefficients.

82. **Coincidence check (isocenter) (noun):**QA test confirming mechanical and radiation isocenter alignment.
**Related Terms:** Winston-Lutz test, QA, Isocenter.
**Example in Radiotherapy:** Coincidence checks validate stereotactic treatment precision.

83. **Cold spot (dose) (noun):** Area receiving lower than prescribed radiation dose.
**Related Terms:** Dose homogeneity, Hot spot, QA.
**Example in Radiotherapy:** Cold spots in PTV may reduce tumor control probability.

84. **Collapsed-cone convolution (noun):** Dose calculation algorithm improving scatter modeling.
**Related Terms:** TPS, Dose calculation, Convolution.
**Example in Radiotherapy:** Collapsed-cone algorithms enhance heterogeneity correction in lung RT.

85. **Collimator jaw (noun):** Movable jaws shaping rectangular radiation fields.
**Related Terms:** Collimator, Beam shaping, MLC.
**Example in Radiotherapy:** Collimator jaws define field borders in 2D RT.

86. **Collimator rotation (noun):** Angular movement of collimator for beam orientation.
**Related Terms:** Gantry rotation, Beam geometry, Setup.
**Example in Radiotherapy:** Collimator rotation reduces tongue-and-groove effects in IMRT.

87. **Commissioning protocol (noun):** Standardized procedure for validating new equipment performance.
**Related Terms:** QA, Calibration, Linac acceptance.
**Example in Radiotherapy:** AAPM protocols guide linac commissioning.

88. **Compensator thickness (noun):** Measured thickness of compensator used to modulate beam intensity.
**Related Terms:** Bolus, Wedge, Beam modifier.
**Example in Radiotherapy:** Compensator thickness corrects for chest wall irregularities.

89. **Complex treatment plan (noun):** Plan involving multiple beams, modulations, or adaptive strategies.
**Related Terms:** IMRT, VMAT, Adaptive planning.
**Example in Radiotherapy:** Complex IMRT plans optimize dose to head-and-neck tumors.

90. **Composite dose distribution (noun):** Summed dose from multiple fields or treatment phases.
**Related Terms:** Isodose, Summation plan, Dose map.
**Example in Radiotherapy:** Composite doses assess cumulative organ exposure.

91. **Composite isodose curve (noun):** I sodose lines representing combined dose from all beams.
**Related Terms:** Dose distribution, Summation, Isodose plot.
**Example in Radiotherapy:** Composite isodose curves confirm PTV coverage.

92. **Computed radiography (CR) (noun):** Digital imaging using photostimulable phosphor plates.
**Related Terms:** DRR, Digital imaging, Simulation.
**Example in Radiotherapy:** CR plates are used in simulation imaging.

93. **Concomitant boost (noun):** Simultaneous delivery of boost dose with standard fractions.
**Related Terms:** Accelerated RT, Boost, Hypofractionation.
**Example in Radiotherapy:** Concomitant boost shortens overall treatment time in head-and-neck RT.

94. **Concomitant chemo-radiation (noun):** Concurrent delivery of chemotherapy and radiotherapy.
**Related Terms:** Radiosensitization, Combined modality, Chemotherapy.
**Example in Radiotherapy:** Concomitant chemoradiation is standard in cervical cancer.

95. **Cone applicator (noun):** Cylindrical device shaping electron fields.
**Related Terms:** Electron therapy, Applicator, Beam shaping.
**Example in Radiotherapy:** Cone applicators define electron treatment fields.

96. **Conformal arc therapy (noun):** Arc-based treatment shaping dose to tumor while sparing OARs.
**Related Terms:** IMAT, VMAT, Arc therapy.
**Example in Radiotherapy:** Conformal arcs treat brain lesions with reduced toxicity.

97. **Conformal beam arrangement (noun):** Multiple beam setup shaped to tumor geometry.
**Related Terms:** 3D-CRT, IMRT, Planning.
**Example in Radiotherapy:** Conformal arrangements improve dose homogeneity in pelvic RT.

98. **Conformal index (noun):** Quantitative measure of how well dose conforms to target.
**Related Terms:** Homogeneity index, Conformity, Plan evaluation.
**Example in Radiotherapy:** High conformal index reflects precise PTV coverage.

99. **Consistency check (QA) (noun):** Routine test confirming stable equipment performance.
**Related Terms:** QA, Calibration, Verification.
**Example in Radiotherapy:** Consistency checks detect deviations in daily output.

100. **Contour variability study (noun):** Evaluation of differences in contouring among observers.
**Related Terms:** Inter-observer variability, Contouring, QA.
**Example in Radiotherapy:** Studies on contour variability highlight training needs in CTV.

101. **Cell death pathway (noun):** The sequence of molecular events leading to cell demise after radiation.
**Related Terms:** Apoptosis, Necrosis, Autophagy.
**Example in Radiotherapy:** Radiation activates apoptosis as the primary cell death pathway in lymphocytes.

102. **Cell inactivation (noun):** Loss of a cell's ability to divide indefinitely after irradiation.
**Related Terms:** Reproductive death, Clonogen survival, Radiosensitivity.
**Example in Radiotherapy:** Tumor control depends on achieving sufficient cell inactivation.

103. **Cell membrane damage (noun):** Radiation-induced injury to lipid bilayers altering cell integrity and signaling.
**Related Terms:** Oxidative stress, Membrane lipid peroxidation, Cell signaling.
**Example in Radiotherapy:** Free radicals cause cell membrane damage, contributing to tumor kill.

104. **Cell proliferation rate (noun):** Speed at which cells divide and grow, affecting radiosensitivity.
**Related Terms:** Growth fraction, Cell kinetics, Repopulation.
**Example in Radiotherapy:** Fast cell proliferation in head-and-neck tumors reduces treatment breaks tolerance.

105. **Cell repair capacity (noun):** Ability of cells to repair sub-lethal DNA damage post-irradiation.
**Related Terms:** DNA repair, Radiosensitivity, Radiotolerance.
**Example in Radiotherapy:** Tumors with low repair capacity respond better to fractionated RT.

106. **Cell signaling cascade (noun):** Sequential activation of molecular pathways after radiation exposure.
**Related Terms:** Signal transduction, Pathway activation, Bystander effect.
**Example in Radiotherapy:** DNA damage triggers a signaling cascade activating repair proteins.

107. **Cellular damage repair (noun):** Biological process correcting radiation-induced sub-lethal damage.
**Related Terms:** DNA repair, NHEJ, HR pathway.
**Example in Radiotherapy:** Fractionation schedules exploit cellular damage repair in normal tissue.

108. **Centrosome damage (noun):** Radiation-induced injury to centrosomes impairing mitosis.
**Related Terms:** Mitotic catastrophe, Spindle apparatus, Cell cycle arrest.
**Example in Radiotherapy:** Centrosome damage contributes to abnormal mitosis and cell death.

109. **Chromatid break (noun):** Single break occurring in one chromatid after irradiation.
**Related Terms:** Chromosome aberration, DNA break, Cytogenetics.
**Example in Radiotherapy:** Chromatid breaks are observed in cytogenetic biodosimetry studies.

110. **Chromatin remodeling (noun):** Structural modification of chromatin to facilitate repair or transcription.
**Related Terms:** DNA repair, Epigenetics, Histone modification.
**Example in Radiotherapy:** Chromatin remodeling allows DNA repair machinery access to breaks.

111. **Chromosome aberration scoring (noun):** Quantification of structural changes in chromosomes post-radiation.
**Related Terms:** Cytogenetics, Biodosimetry, Aberration analysis.
**Example in Radiotherapy:** Aberration scoring estimates radiation exposure in accidental exposures.

112. **Chromosome instability (noun):** Persistent tendency of chromosomes to undergo structural changes after damage.
**Related Terms:** Genomic instability, Mutation, Carcinogenesis.
**Example in Radiotherapy:** Chromosome instability may lead to secondary malignancies post-RT.

113. **Cisplatin radiosensitization (noun):** Enhancement of radiation effect by cisplatin chemotherapy.
**Related Terms:** Chemoradiation, Radiosensitizer, DNA cross-linking.
**Example in Radiotherapy:** Cisplatin radiosensitization improves control in cervical cancer RT.

114. **Clastogenic effect (noun):**Chromosome-breaking effect of ionizing radiation.
**Related Terms:** Chromosomal aberration, DNA damage, Mutagenesis.
**Example in Radiotherapy:** Radiation's clastogenic effect is measured in cytogenetic assays.

115. **Clonal expansion (noun):** Proliferation of a single mutated or surviving cell.
**Related Terms:** Mutation, Carcinogenesis, Survival.
**Example in Radiotherapy:** Clonal expansion of surviving tumor cells may cause recurrence.

116. **Clonogen depletion (noun):** Reduction in reproductive tumor cells capable of regrowth.
**Related Terms:** Clonogenic cells, Tumor control, Dose response.
**Example in Radiotherapy:** Curative RT requires effective clonogen depletion.

117. **Clustered double-strand breaks (noun):** Multiple DNA double-strand breaks close together, difficult to repair.
**Related Terms:** Complex DNA damage, LET, Radiosensitivity.
**Example in Radiotherapy:** Clustered DSBs explain high efficiency of carbon ion therapy.

118. **Cytogenetic biomarker (noun):** Chromosome-based indicator of radiation exposure.
**Related Terms:** Dicentric assay, Micronucleus test, Biodosimetry.
**Example in Radiotherapy:** Dicentric chromosomes are a standard cytogenetic biomarker.

119. **Cytogenetic repair assay (noun):** Test measuring chromosome damage repair capacity post-irradiation.
**Related Terms:** DNA repair, Cytogenetics, Biomarker assay.
**Example in Radiotherapy:** Repair assays help predict normal tissue radiosensitivity.

120. **Cytoplasmic irradiation response (noun):** Cellular signaling response triggered by radiation exposure limited to cytoplasm.
**Related Terms:** Bystander effect, Non-targeted effects, Cellular signaling.
**Example in Radiotherapy:** Cytoplasmic irradiation may activate stress signaling without nuclear hits.

121. **Calcaneal tendon (Achilles) (noun):** Description of the word: The strong tendon connecting calf muscles to the calcaneus, essential for ankle movement.
**Related Terms:** Calcaneus, ankle joint, plantar flexion.
**Example in Radiotherapy:** Used as a positioning landmark when aligning lower extremity treatments.

122. **Calvarial midline (noun):** Description of the word: Imaginary central line running longitudinally across the skull vault.
**Related Terms:** Cranial vault, sagittal plane.
**Example in Radiotherapy:** Ensures symmetric cranial alignment in whole brain irradiation.

123. **Canthus alignment (laser) (noun):** Description of the word: Positioning method using medial or lateral canthus for head alignment.
**Related Terms:** Orbital landmarks, laser setup.
**Example in Radiotherapy:** Used during orbital or brain radiotherapy for accurate laser matching.

124. **Capitulum (elbow) (noun):** Description of the word: Rounded lateral condyle of the humerus articulating with the radius.
**Related Terms:** Elbow joint, humerus, radius.
**Example in Radiotherapy:** Acts as a bony reference in upper limb immobilization.

125. **Carotid bifurcation (noun):** Description of the word: Anatomical site where the common carotid artery divides into internal and external branches.
**Related Terms:** Carotid artery, vascular landmarks.
**Example in Radiotherapy:** Guides nodal contouring in head and neck cancers.

126. **Carotid pulse landmark (noun):** Description of the word: Palpable site over carotid artery to identify neck vascular region.
**Related Terms:** Carotid bifurcation, vascular anatomy.
**Example in Radiotherapy:** Helps define cervical node levels for contouring.

127. **Carpal bones (noun):** Description of the word: Eight small bones forming the wrist between forearm and hand.
**Related Terms:** Carpus, wrist joint.
**Example in Radiotherapy:** Serve as positioning markers for extremity irradiation.

128. **Carpus (wrist region) (noun):** Description of the word: Anatomical region formed by carpal bones connecting forearm to hand.
**Related Terms:** Carpal bones, distal radius, ulna.
**Example in Radiotherapy:** Used as immobilization site for hand/forearm treatments.

129. **Cervical vertebrae alignment (noun):** Description of the word: Maintaining proper positioning of C1–C7 vertebrae during setup.
**Related Terms:** Spine alignment, neck positioning.
**Example in Radiotherapy:** Ensures reproducibility in head-and-neck irradiation.

130. **Chin extension (setup) (noun):** Description of the word: Tilting the chin upwards to lengthen the neck region.
**Related Terms:** Neck extension, patient positioning.
**Example in Radiotherapy:** Reduces dose to oral cavity in head-and-neck cases.

131. **Clavicular head (noun):** Description of the word: Medial end of the clavicle articulating with sternum.
**Related Terms:** Sternoclavicular joint, shoulder girdle.
**Example in Radiotherapy:** Used as a setup landmark in supraclavicular fields.

132. **Coccyx landmark (noun):** Description of the word: Distal bony end of vertebral column, below sacrum.
**Related Terms:** Sacrum, pelvic bones.
**Example in Radiotherapy:** Assists pelvic field borders in rectal cancer planning.

133. **Columella (nose) (noun):** Description of the word: External tissue separating the nostrils.
**Related Terms:** Nasal septum, nares.
**Example in Radiotherapy:** Used as a surface landmark in nasal cavity irradiation.

134. **Conchal bowl (ear) (noun):** Description of the word: Hollow cavity of the external ear leading to ear canal.
**Related Terms:** Auricle, external auditory canal.
**Example in Radiotherapy:** Acts as a contouring reference in head-and-neck planning.

135. **Coracoid process (noun):** Description of the word: Hook-like projection of scapula anteriorly.
**Related Terms:** Scapula, shoulder joint.
**Example in Radiotherapy:** Used for positioning in upper thoracic fields.

136. **Coronal plane positioning (noun):** Description of the word: Alignment using vertical plane dividing body into anterior and posterior parts.
**Related Terms:** Sagittal plane, transverse plane.
**Example in Radiotherapy:** Critical in stereotactic body radiotherapy setups.

137. **Costophrenic angle (noun):** Description of the word: Recess between diaphragm and rib cage on chest imaging.
**Related Terms:** Diaphragm, pleura.
**Example in Radiotherapy:** Serves as reference in lung cancer planning.

138. **Cranial base (noun):** Description of the word: Inferior portion of skull supporting brain.
**Related Terms:** Foramen magnum, cranial fossae.
**Example in Radiotherapy:** Defines inferior limit in whole brain radiotherapy.

139. **Cranial vault (noun):** Description of the word: Upper dome-like portion of skull encasing brain.
**Related Terms:** Calvaria, cranial bones.
**Example in Radiotherapy:** Reference region for whole brain irradiation.

140. **Craniocaudal field arrangement (noun):** Description of the word: Radiation fields aligned from head-to-foot direction.
**Related Terms:** Superior-inferior axis, beam arrangement.
**Example in Radiotherapy:** Used in craniospinal irradiation planning.

141. **Cricoid level (noun):** Description of the word: Anatomical landmark at C6 level corresponding to cricoid cartilage.
**Related Terms:** Larynx, trachea.
**Example in Radiotherapy:** Guides contouring of lower neck nodes.

142. **Cuboid bone (noun):** Description of the word: Tarsal bone located on lateral side of foot.
**Related Terms:** Calcaneus, metatarsals.
**Example in Radiotherapy:** Serves as foot positioning reference.

143. **Cutaneous fold (noun):** Description of the word: Natural crease or fold of skin.
**Related Terms:** Skin surface landmarks, soft tissue.
**Example in Radiotherapy:** Considered in immobilization to avoid setup errors.

144. **Cutaneous scar marking (noun):** Description of the word: Visible scar on skin surface used as anatomical reference.
**Related Terms:** Skin tattoos, surgical scars.
**Example in Radiotherapy:** Serves as alignment aid in post-surgical irradiation.

145. **Cystic neck node landmark (noun):** Description of the word: Palpable or imaged cystic lymph node within cervical chain.
**Related Terms:** Neck nodes, cervical lymphatics.
**Example in Radiotherapy:** Helps contour suspicious nodes in H&N planning.

146. **Cytological marker (skin tattoo) (noun):** Description of the word: Small permanent ink mark placed on skin for reproducible setup.
**Related Terms:** Fiducial marker, tattoo.
**Example in Radiotherapy:** Used in breast cancer radiotherapy setup reproducibility.

147. **C7 transverse process landmark (noun):** Description of the word: Lateral projection of the 7th cervical vertebra.
**Related Terms:** Cervical spine, vertebral landmarks.
**Example in Radiotherapy:** Used as reference point in spinal field design.

148. **Cranial index reference (noun):** Description of the word: Ratio of skull breadth to length, describing cranial shape.
**Related Terms:** Cranial vault, anthropometry.
**Example in Radiotherapy:** Occasionally used in research for head immobilization studies.

149. **Craniospinal axis alignment (noun):** Description of the word**:** Consistent positioning along skull and spinal column axis.
**Related Terms:** Craniospinal irradiation, beam alignment.
**Example in Radiotherapy:** Ensures junction accuracy in craniospinal treatments.

150. **Calcium tungstate screen (noun):** Description of the word**:** Fluorescent screen material converting X-rays into visible light.
**Related Terms:** Intensifying screen, radiographic imaging.
**Example in Radiotherapy:** Historically used in simulator film cassettes to enhance image capture.

151. **Camera-based EPID (noun):** Description of the word**:** Electronic portal imaging device using camera sensors to capture beam images.
**Related Terms:** EPID, image verification.
**Example in Radiotherapy:** Used to verify patient setup before treatment delivery.

152. **Canonical dose model (noun):** Description of the word**:** Standardized mathematical model describing dose distribution in tissues.
**Related Terms:** Dose calculation, treatment planning.
**Example in Radiotherapy:** Applied in TPS algorithms for accurate beam modeling.

153. **Capacitance meter (noun):** Description of the word**:** Instrument measuring capacitance of electronic components in radiotherapy devices.
**Related Terms:** QA tools, electronics.
**Example in Radiotherapy:** Used during linac electronic QA checks.

154. **Captive bolt alignment (QA device) (noun):** Description of the word**:** Mechanical QA device ensuring consistent beam isocenter verification.
**Related Terms:** Isocenter QA, mechanical checks.
**Example in Radiotherapy:** Confirms alignment of gantry, collimator, and couch axes.

155. **Carbon fiber couch (noun):** Description of the word**:** Radiotranslucent treatment couch made of carbon fiber.
**Related Terms:** Treatment couch, immobilization.
**Example in Radiotherapy:** Minimizes imaging artifacts and reduces beam attenuation.

156. **Cascade amplifier (noun):** Description of the word**:** Series of amplifiers increasing signal strength.
**Related Terms:** Detector electronics, signal processing.
**Example in Radiotherapy:** Used in ionization chamber signal readout systems.

157. **Cathode emission (noun):** Description of the word**:** Electron release from heated cathode in X-ray tubes.
**Related Terms:** Thermionic emission, linac electron gun.
**Example in Radiotherapy:** Generates electron beam in linear accelerator gun.

158. **Cavity ionization chamber (noun):** Description of the word**:** Gas-filled detector measuring ionization from radiation.
**Related Terms:** Dosimeter, QA.
**Example in Radiotherapy:** Standard for beam calibration in absolute dosimetry.

159. **Ceiling laser alignment (noun):** Description of the word**:** Ceiling-mounted laser system for patient positioning.
**Related Terms:** Setup lasers, patient alignment.
**Example in Radiotherapy:** Ensures reproducible isocenter localization.

160. **Central beam axis marker (noun):** Description of the word: Visual or electronic indicator of beam's central axis.
**Related Terms:** Beam axis, isocenter.
**Example in Radiotherapy:** Assists in beam alignment verification during setup.

161. **Central nervous system prophylaxis (noun):** Description of the word: Preventive irradiation of CNS to reduce risk of tumor spread.
**Related Terms:** Craniospinal irradiation, prophylactic RT.
**Example in Radiotherapy:** Used in pediatric leukemia protocols.

162. **Central ray alignment (noun):** Description of the word: Positioning based on the central radiation beam axis.
**Related Terms:** Beam axis, alignment.
**Example in Radiotherapy:** Critical for accurate field placement in 2D setups.

163. **Ceramic detector (noun):** Description of the word: Solid-state detector using ceramic materials for radiation measurement.
**Related Terms:** Dosimeter, detector.
**Example in Radiotherapy:** Provides high spatial resolution in IMRT QA.

164. **Channeling radiation (noun):** Description of the word: Radiation produced when charged particles pass through crystal lattices.
**Related Terms:** Synchrotron radiation, particle therapy.
**Example in Radiotherapy:** Investigated for advanced beam generation methods.

165. **Characteristic curve (film) (noun):** Description of the word: Graph showing film density versus radiation exposure.
**Related Terms:** Film dosimetry, sensitometry.
**Example in Radiotherapy:** Used to calibrate radiographic films for portal imaging.

166. **Charged particle equilibrium depth (noun):** Description of the word: Depth at which ionization equals particle generation and loss.
**Related Terms:** CPE, depth dose.
**Example in Radiotherapy:** Used in dosimetry for reference depth calibration.

167. **Chilled water system (Linac cooling) (noun):** Description of the word: Cooling system circulating chilled water to prevent overheating.
**Related Terms:** Linac components, cooling.
**Example in Radiotherapy:** Maintains accelerator performance during treatment.

168. **Chromatic beam marker (noun):** Description of the word: Color-coded indicator for beam visualization.
**Related Terms:** Beam marker, QA tools.
**Example in Radiotherapy:** Differentiates multiple beam arrangements on setup images.

169. **Chromophore dosimeter (noun):** Description of the word: Dosimeter using light-absorbing molecules that change with dose.
**Related Terms:** Radiochromic dosimeter, optical dosimetry.
**Example in Radiotherapy:** Applied in 3D gel dosimetry.

170. **Clinical electron applicator (noun):** Description of the word: Device shaping and directing electron beams for therapy.
**Related Terms:** Electron cone, electron therapy.
**Example in Radiotherapy:** Used in superficial tumor irradiation.

171. **Clinical portal image match (noun):** Description of the word: Process of aligning treatment images with reference portals.
**Related Terms:** Image verification, EPID.
**Example in Radiotherapy:** Confirms patient position before beam delivery.

172. **Cloud storage verification images (noun):** Description of the word: Digital archiving of verification images in cloud systems.
**Related Terms:** PACS, IGRT.
**Example in Radiotherapy:** Allows remote access to treatment verification images.

173. **Coefficient of attenuation (noun):** Description of the word: Measure of radiation reduction per unit material thickness.
**Related Terms:** HVL, beam attenuation.
**Example in Radiotherapy:** Used in shielding design and dose calculation.

174. **Coincidence phantom (QA) (noun):** Description of the word: QA device for testing alignment of imaging and treatment isocenters.
**Related Terms:** Winston-Lutz test, QA phantom.
**Example in Radiotherapy:** Ensures accuracy in IGRT systems.

175. **Collimator scatter factor (Sc) (noun):** Description of the word: Ratio describing scatter from collimator system.
**Related Terms:** Output factors, dosimetry.
**Example in Radiotherapy:** Essential in MU calculation for photon beams.

176. **Collimator transmission (noun):** Description of the word: Fraction of radiation transmitted through collimator leaves.
**Related Terms:** Leakage radiation, MLC.
**Example in Radiotherapy:** Considered in IMRT plan optimization.

177. **Color wash (dose display) (noun):** Description of the word: Visual dose representation using colored gradients.
**Related Terms:** Dose distribution, DVH.
**Example in Radiotherapy:** Displays target coverage in treatment planning.

178. **Compact accelerator (noun):** Description of the word: Small-sized linear accelerator system.
**Related Terms:** Linac, portable accelerator.
**Example in Radiotherapy:** Used in intraoperative radiotherapy setups.

179. **Compensation filter tray (noun):** Description of the word: Device holding compensators in beam path.
**Related Terms:** Wedge, bolus.
**Example in Radiotherapy:** Modifies dose distribution in irregular fields.

180. **Complementary wedge pair (noun):** Description of the word: Two opposing wedges used to shape dose distribution.
**Related Terms:** Wedge filter, beam shaping.
**Example in Radiotherapy:** Creates uniform dose in sloped anatomy.

181. **Composite portal image (noun):** Description of the word: Combined image from multiple treatment fields.
**Related Terms:** Portal imaging, verification.
**Example in Radiotherapy:** Assesses cumulative field alignment.

**182. Computer-controlled wedge (noun):** Description of the word: Dynamic wedge controlled by treatment planning system.
**Related Terms:** Enhanced dynamic wedge, beam modulation.
**Example in Radiotherapy:** Provides variable wedge angles electronically.

**183. Conduction cooling system (noun):** Description of the word: Heat removal system using direct conduction.
**Related Terms:** Cooling methods, linac.
**Example in Radiotherapy:** Protects linac components from overheating.

**184. Constant source-to-skin distance (SSD) (noun):** Description of the word: Technique maintaining fixed SSD during beam setup.
**Related Terms:** SSD technique, SAD technique.
**Example in Radiotherapy:** Used in electron beam treatments.

**185. Contrast resolution (CT) (noun):** Description of the word: Ability to differentiate tissues with small density differences.
**Related Terms:** Image quality, CT imaging.
**Example in Radiotherapy:** Critical in contouring soft tissue targets.

**186. Convection dose transfer (noun):** Description of the word: Heat and energy transfer through fluid motion.
**Related Terms:** Thermal dose, hyperthermia.
**Example in Radiotherapy:** Relevant in combined hyperthermia-radiation treatments.

**187. Copper filter (noun):** Description of the word: Beam-hardening filter made of copper.
**Related Terms:** Filtration, beam quality.
**Example in Radiotherapy:** Used in superficial X-ray units.

**188. Couch rotation angle (noun):** Description of the word: Degree of couch rotation relative to isocenter.
**Related Terms:** Couch shift, gantry angle.
**Example in Radiotherapy:** Essential in non-coplanar treatment deliveries.

**189. Craniospinal irradiation (CSI) (noun):** Description of the word: Radiotherapy technique covering cranial and spinal axis.
**Related Terms:** Craniospinal axis, prophylaxis.
**Example in Radiotherapy:** Standard treatment in medulloblastoma.

**190. Cancellous bone (noun):** Description of the word: Spongy, porous bone inside long bones and vertebrae.
**Related Terms:** Trabecular bone, cortical bone.
**Example in Radiotherapy:** Considered in bone marrow dose constraints.

**191. Capillary plexus (radiation injury site) (noun):** Description of the word: Small blood vessel network sensitive to radiation injury.
**Related Terms:** Microvasculature, late effects.
**Example in Radiotherapy:** Explains tissue necrosis in high-dose regions.

**192. Carcinogenesis (radiation-induced) (noun):** Description of the word: Development of cancer due to radiation exposure.
**Related Terms:** Secondary malignancy, stochastic effects.
**Example in Radiotherapy:** Monitored in long-term survivors of pediatric RT.

**193. Cardiotoxicity (RT- related) (noun):** Description of the word: Damage to heart tissue from radiotherapy exposure.
**Related Terms:** Late effects, cardiac dose.
**Example in Radiotherapy:** Reduced with DIBH in breast radiotherapy.

**194. Cartilage necrosis (noun):** Description of the word: Death of cartilage tissue following high radiation dose.
**Related Terms:** Late toxicity, tissue necrosis.
**Example in Radiotherapy:** Observed in laryngeal carcinoma treatments.

**195. Cellular senescence (noun):** Description of the word: Permanent cell cycle arrest induced by DNA damage.
**Related Terms:** Apoptosis, radiation biology.
**Example in Radiotherapy:** Explains tumor control via non-proliferative arrest.

**196. Cerebellar landmark (posterior fossa RT) (noun):** Description of the word: Anatomical markers defining cerebellar region.
**Related Terms:** Posterior fossa, cranial landmarks.
**Example in Radiotherapy:** Used to delineate boost fields in medulloblastoma.

**197. Chiasm (optic chiasm) (noun):** Description of the word: Crossing point of optic nerves at brain base.
**Related Terms:** Optic nerves, visual pathway.
**Example in Radiotherapy:** Dose-limiting structure in pituitary irradiation.

**198. Cytoprotective agent (noun):** Description of the word: Drug reducing normal tissue injury from radiation.
**Related Terms:** Radioprotector, amifostine.
**Example in Radiotherapy:** Used in head-and-neck RT to reduce xerostomia.

**199. Cytotoxic dose (noun):** Description of the word: Radiation dose sufficient to kill targeted tumor cells.
**Related Terms:** Lethal dose, radiosensitivity.
**Example in Radiotherapy:** Determined through cell survival curves for tumor control prediction.

**200. Calibration phantom (noun):** Description of the word: Standardized material used for beam calibration.
**Related Terms:** Water phantom, dosimetry.
**Example in Radiotherapy:** Used in TG-51 protocol for absolute dose calibration.

**201. Calibration curve (noun):** Description of the word: Graph showing detector response versus radiation dose.
**Related Terms:** Dosimeter response, film calibration.
**Example in Radiotherapy:** Essential for film or diode dosimetry interpretation.

**202. Calorimeter dosimetry (noun):** Description of the word: Measurement of absorbed dose via heat produced by radiation.
**Related Terms:** Primary standard, dosimetry system.
**Example in Radiotherapy:** Used by national labs for standard dose reference.

**203. Camouflage shielding (noun):** Description of the word: Localized shielding used to protect sensitive anatomy.
**Related Terms:** Lead block, eye shield.
**Example in Radiotherapy:** Used during electron treatments near eyes or lips.

204. **Cancer stem cell (noun):** Description of the word: Subpopulation of tumor cells with self-renewal capability and radioresistance.
**Related Terms:** Tumor clonogen, radiosensitivity.
**Example in Radiotherapy:** Targeted in dose-escalation strategies for resistant tumors.

205. **Cannula fixation (noun):** Description of the word: Secure placement of a medical tube for immobilization or anaesthesia.
**Related Terms:** Intravenous access, immobilization.
**Example in Radiotherapy:** Used during anaesthesia in pediatric treatments.

206. **Capsule endoscopy marker (noun):** Description of the word: Radiopaque capsule used to locate gastrointestinal tumors.
**Related Terms:** Fiducial marker, localization.
**Example in Radiotherapy:** Defines small bowel position before pelvic irradiation.

207. **Cardiac contour (noun):** Description of the word: Outlined heart structure for dose calculation.
**Related Terms:** Organ at risk, DVH.
**Example in Radiotherapy:** Helps limit heart dose in breast cancer planning.

208. **Cardiac gating (noun):** Description of the word: Technique synchronizing radiation with cardiac motion.
**Related Terms:** Respiratory gating, 4D radiotherapy.
**Example in Radiotherapy:** Reduces motion artifacts in mediastinal treatments.

209. **Cardiophrenic angle (noun):** Description of the word: Junction between heart border and diaphragm.
**Related Terms:** Costophrenic angle, thoracic anatomy.
**Example in Radiotherapy:** Used to verify lung field limits.

210. **Carina (tracheal bifurcation) (noun):** Description of the word: Point where trachea divides into bronchi.
**Related Terms:** Mediastinum, lung anatomy.
**Example in Radiotherapy:** Common reference for thoracic target delineation.

211. **Cartilaginous tissue (noun):** Description of the word: Elastic connective tissue providing support in structures like the larynx.
**Related Terms:** Larynx, cartilage necrosis.
**Example in Radiotherapy:** Requires dose constraints to avoid necrosis.

212. **Cascade effect (noun):** Description of the word: Secondary processes initiated by radiation interactions.
**Related Terms:** Ionization cascade, energy transfer.
**Example in Radiotherapy:** Occurs in pair production and Compton scattering.

213. **Castration-resistant prostate cancer (noun):** Description of the word: Prostate tumor progression despite androgen deprivation.
**Related Terms:** ADT, salvage radiotherapy.
**Example in Radiotherapy:** Managed with re-irradiation or SBRT.

214. **Catheter brachytherapy (noun):** Description of the word: Insertion of catheters for internal radiation delivery.
**Related Terms:** HDR, LDR, and applicator.
**Example in Radiotherapy:** Used in prostate and gynaecologic implants.

215. **Caudate lobe (liver) (noun):** Description of the word: Posterior segment of liver adjacent to IVC.
**Related Terms:** Hepatic anatomy, SBRT.
**Example in Radiotherapy:** Included in GTV for central liver tumors.

216. **Cavity expansion artifacts (noun):** Description of the word: CT artifact caused by air-filled cavities or implants.
**Related Terms:** CT artifact, image distortion.
**Example in Radiotherapy:** Corrected with density override in planning.

217. **Celiac plexus (noun):** Description of the word: Nerve network near upper abdominal aorta.
**Related Terms:** Abdominal anatomy, pain control.
**Example in Radiotherapy:** Targeted in palliative neurolytic treatments.

218. **Cell cycle radiosensitivity (noun):** Description of the word: Variation in cell radiosensitivity depending on cell cycle phase.
**Related Terms:** G2-M phase, radiobiology.
**Example in Radiotherapy:** Explains fractionation effectiveness.

219. **Cell survival fraction (noun):** Description of the word: Proportion of cells surviving a given dose.
**Related Terms:** Survival curve, $\alpha/\beta$ ratio.
**Example in Radiotherapy:** Used in calculating TCP (Tumor Control Probability).

220. **Central axis depth dose (noun):** Description of the word: Dose variation along beam's central axis with depth.
**Related Terms:** PDD, beam profile.
**Example in Radiotherapy:** Fundamental in linac commissioning.

221. **Central line positioning (noun):** Description of the word: Alignment of patient midline to beam isocenter.
**Related Terms:** Midline alignment, setup reproducibility.
**Example in Radiotherapy:** Verified using sagittal laser.

222. **Cerebral cortex (noun):** Description of the word: Outer layer of brain tissue responsible for sensory processing.
**Related Terms:** Brain OAR, neural dose.
**Example in Radiotherapy:** Dose limited in whole-brain RT.

223. **Cerebral edema (noun):** Description of the word: Swelling of brain tissue following irradiation.
**Related Terms:** Radiation necrosis, dexamethasone.
**Example in Radiotherapy:** Managed during stereotactic brain treatments.

224. **Cervical canal (noun):** Description of the word: Passage through cervix leading to uterus.
**Related Terms:** Brachytherapy, gynaecologic anatomy.
**Example in Radiotherapy:** Central to intracavitary dose distribution.

225. **Cervical node levels (noun):** Description of the word: Lymph node groupings used in head and neck contouring.
**Related Terms:** Nodal levels I–VII, delineation.
**Example in Radiotherapy:** Standardized per DAHANCA and RTOG atlases.

226. **Cervical spine curvature (noun):** Description of the word: Natural lordotic curve of cervical vertebrae.
**Related Terms:** Spinal alignment, setup correction.
**Example in Radiotherapy:** Maintained for reproducible neck setups.

227. **Cesium-137 source (noun):** Description of the word**:** Radioactive isotope used in older brachytherapy systems.
**Related Terms:** LDR source, half-life.
**Example in Radiotherapy:** Replaced by Ir-192 in modern HDR systems.

228. **Chemical dosimeter (noun):** Description of the word**:** Dosimetry system measuring chemical changes due to radiation.
**Related Terms:** Fricke dosimeter, alanine pellet.
**Example in Radiotherapy:** Used for QA in high-dose-rate sources.

229. **Chest wall contour (noun):** Description of the word**:** Outline of thoracic wall used for dose conformity.
**Related Terms:** Breast planning, bolus.
**Example in Radiotherapy:** Ensures adequate dose coverage in mastectomy cases.

230. **Chin tuck (setup) (noun):** Description of the word**:** Lowering the chin to minimize neck extension.
**Related Terms:** Neck positioning, immobilization.
**Example in Radiotherapy:** Reduces oral cavity dose in H&N RT.

231. **Chlorine gas chamber (historical) (noun):** Description of the word**:** Early radiation detection device using ionized chlorine gas.
**Related Terms:** Ionization chamber, detector history.
**Example in Radiotherapy:** Foundation of modern dosimeter design.

232. **Chromosomal aberration assay (noun):** Description of the word**:** Test measuring DNA damage from radiation.
**Related Terms:** Biodosimetry, cytogenetic.
**Example in Radiotherapy:** Used in accidental exposure dose estimation.

233. **Ciliary body (noun):** Description of the word**:** Eye structure controlling lens shape and aqueous humor.
**Related Terms:** Ocular anatomy, brachytherapy.
**Example in Radiotherapy:** Dose constrained in ocular melanoma treatment.

234. **Cine imaging (noun):** Description of the word**:** Real-time imaging sequence capturing motion.
**Related Terms:** Fluoroscopy, 4D-CT.
**Example in Radiotherapy:** Used for respiratory motion studies.

235. **Circumferential dose gradient (noun):** Description of the word**:** Variation of dose around a circular field.
**Related Terms:** Dose homogeneity, conformality index.
**Example in Radiotherapy:** Optimized in SRS planning.

236. **Clarity transducer (noun):** Description of the word**:** Ultrasound device used for real-time prostate tracking.
**Related Terms:** IGRT, ultrasound guidance.
**Example in Radiotherapy:** Used for prostate localization before beam-on.

237. **Clinical audit (noun):** Description of the word**:** Systematic review to improve treatment quality.
**Related Terms:** QA, peer review.
**Example in Radiotherapy:** Required in accreditation and quality management.

238. **Clinical target volume (CTV) (noun):** Description of the word**:** Tissue volume containing GTV plus microscopic disease.
**Related Terms:** GTV, PTV.
**Example in Radiotherapy:** Defined per ICRU 83 for target delineation.

239. **Clipping plane (noun):** Description of the word: Virtual boundary in image visualization cutting unwanted data.
**Related Terms:** 3D rendering, contouring.
**Example in Radiotherapy:** Used to visualize internal organs during planning.

240. **Closed-loop control system (noun):** Description of the word: Automated system adjusting parameters based on feedback.
**Related Terms:** Servo control, motion tracking.
**Example in Radiotherapy:** Used in robotic couch or gating systems.

241. **Coaxial alignment (noun):** Description of the word: Positioning where multiple axes share a common line.
**Related Terms:** Beam alignment, mechanical isocenter.
**Example in Radiotherapy:** Ensures collinearity of gantry and collimator.

242. **Coherent scattering (noun):** Description of the word: Elastic scattering of X-rays without energy loss.
**Related Terms:** Rayleigh scattering, photon interaction.
**Example in Radiotherapy:** Minor contributor to total attenuation at megavoltage energies.

243. **Collapsed cone algorithm (noun):** Description of the word: Dose calculation model accounting for energy transport in 3D.
**Related Terms:** Convolution-superposition, TPS algorithm.
**Example in Radiotherapy:** Used in modern TPS for accurate heterogeneous dose.

244. **Collimator alignment (noun):** Description of the word: Ensuring collimator axis coincides with beam central axis.
**Related Terms:** Mechanical QA, isocenter check.
**Example in Radiotherapy:** Verified during monthly machine QA.

245. **Collimator rotation (noun):** Description of the word: Turning of beam-shaping device around beam axis.
**Related Terms:** Field orientation, mechanical QA.
**Example in Radiotherapy:** Adjusted to avoid beam divergence overlap.

246. **Collision avoidance system (noun):** Description of the word: Software preventing equipment collision during treatment.
**Related Terms:** Machine safety, non-coplanar planning.
**Example in Radiotherapy:** Used in SRS couch rotation plans.

247. **Color Doppler ultrasound (noun):** Description of the word: Imaging modality showing blood flow dynamics.
**Related Terms:** Ultrasound, IGRT.
**Example in Radiotherapy:** Used for prostate motion monitoring.

248. **Collimator rotation isocenter test (noun):** A QA procedure ensuring the collimator axis of rotation coincides with the treatment machine isocenter.
**Related Terms:** Mechanical isocenter, Winston–Lutz test.
**Example in Radiotherapy:** Checked monthly to maintain rotational accuracy of IMRT and VMAT deliveries.

249. **Collimator walkout (noun):** A mechanical deviation of the collimator rotation axis from the isocenter during gantry or collimator motion.
**Related Terms:** Mechanical alignment, QA tolerance.
**Example in Radiotherapy:** Monitored to ensure precise field matching in rotational therapy.

250. **Collision clearance check (noun):** Verification procedure ensuring safe gantry, couch, and patient clearance during treatment setup.
**Related Terms:** Collision avoidance, machine safety.
**Example in Radiotherapy:** Essential during SBRT or large-arc VMAT deliveries.

251. **Colorectal boost field (noun):** An additional radiation field directed to the primary rectal tumor post-pelvic irradiation.
**Related Terms:** Boost plan, pelvis field.
**Example in Radiotherapy:** Used to escalate dose in rectal cancer after 45 Gy whole pelvis.

252. **C155. Column scatter (noun):** Photon scattering occurring along the longitudinal axis of a CT column or beam.
**Related Terms:** Scatter correction, image artifacts.
**Example in Radiotherapy:** Corrected during image reconstruction to improve CT density accuracy.

253. **Combined modality therapy (noun):** Integration of radiation therapy with surgery, chemotherapy, or immunotherapy.
**Related Terms:** Multimodality treatment, concurrent chemoradiation.
**Example in Radiotherapy:** Standard of care in locally advanced head and neck carcinoma.

254. **Compton electron (noun):** An ejected electron resulting from a Compton scattering event.
**Related Terms:** Compton effect, secondary electron.
**Example in Radiotherapy:** Major contributor to tissue dose in megavoltage photon beams.

255. **Compton scatter (noun):** Inelastic scattering of a photon by an electron, reducing photon energy.
**Related Terms:** Photon interaction, dose buildup.
**Example in Radiotherapy:** Predominant interaction mechanism in soft tissue at MV energies.

256. **Compensating bolus (noun):** A tissue-equivalent material placed on the skin to equalize irregular surface dose.
**Related Terms:** Bolus, tissue compensator.
**Example in Radiotherapy:** Used over nasal bridge during head and neck RT.

257. **Compensator-based IMRT (noun):** Technique using custom-milled compensators to modulate intensity distribution.
**Related Terms:** Physical IMRT, fluence modulation.
**Example in Radiotherapy:** Used before electronic MLC-based IMRT systems.

258. **Computed radiography (noun):** Digital imaging technique using photostimulable phosphor plates.
**Related Terms:** Digital detector, PSP plate.
**Example in Radiotherapy:** Used for port verification before EPID adoption.

259. **Computed tomography dose index (CTDI) (noun):** Standardized measurement of CT scanner dose output per slice.
**Related Terms:** Dose profile, CT quality assurance.
**Example in Radiotherapy:** Recorded for QA of planning CT scanners.

260. **Cone beam artifact (noun):** Image distortion due to cone-beam geometry in volumetric imaging.
**Related Terms:** CBCT artifact, scatter artifact.
**Example in Radiotherapy:** Can affect Hounsfield accuracy during pelvis CBCT verification.

261. **Cone beam CT reconstruction (noun):** Reconstruction of volumetric images from cone-shaped x-ray projections.
**Related Terms:** FDK algorithm, volumetric imaging.
**Example in Radiotherapy:** Used for daily verification in image-guided radiotherapy.

262. **Cone collimator (noun):** Fixed aperture collimator producing circular radiation fields.
**Related Terms:** SRS cone, tertiary collimator.
**Example in Radiotherapy:** Used for brain metastases stereotactic treatments.

263. **Cone down field (noun):** Smaller treatment field applied after initial larger field irradiation to boost tumor dose.
**Related Terms:** Boost field, field reduction.
**Example in Radiotherapy:** Applied in cervical cancer pelvis boost.

264. **Conformal avoidance (noun):** Treatment planning strategy shaping dose to avoid critical structures while maintaining target coverage.
**Related Terms:** Inverse planning, OAR sparing.
**Example in Radiotherapy:** Used in craniospinal irradiation to spare lungs and heart.

265. **Conformal radiotherapy (noun):** Technique shaping radiation dose to conform to tumor shape using 3D planning.
**Related Terms:** 3DCRT, beam shaping.
**Example in Radiotherapy:** Improves tumor coverage in prostate cancer RT.

266. **Conformal verification (noun):** Process of confirming 3D dose conformity and alignment before patient treatment.
**Related Terms:** Pre-treatment QA, dose verification.
**Example in Radiotherapy:** Conducted before 3DCRT beam delivery.

267. **Conformal wedge field (noun):** Field incorporating wedge filters and shaped apertures for dose uniformity.
**Related Terms:** Dynamic wedge, field inhomogeneity correction.
**Example in Radiotherapy:** Applied in breast tangential beam setup.

268. **Confocal laser alignment (noun):** Use of focused laser beams for precise patient setup localization.
**Related Terms:** Laser positioning, setup reproducibility.
**Example in Radiotherapy:** Essential in SRS immobilization procedures.

269. **Cone-beam dose map (noun):** Representation of patient dose received from CBCT imaging.
**Related Terms:** Imaging dose, CBCT QA.
**Example in Radiotherapy:** Monitored to limit cumulative imaging dose in adaptive RT.

270. **Constant dose rate (noun):** Delivery mode where monitor units per minute remain constant during beam-on.
**Related Terms:** Fixed MU rate, VMAT modulation.
**Example in Radiotherapy:** Used during static field IMRT plans.

271. **Constant gantry speed (noun):** Fixed rotational velocity of gantry during dynamic arc treatment.
**Related Terms:** VMAT control point, dose rate modulation.
**Example in Radiotherapy:** Ensures smooth dose delivery during arc therapy.

272. **Contour interpolation (noun):** Software-based estimation of structures between contoured slices.
**Related Terms:** Auto-segmentation, volume reconstruction.
**Example in Radiotherapy:** Used for consistent CTV generation in pelvis CT.

273. **Contour propagation (noun):** Transfer of contoured structures across image sets or fractions.
**Related Terms:** Deformable registration, adaptive RT.
**Example in Radiotherapy:** Facilitates re-planning during adaptive prostate RT.

274. **Control console (noun):** Interface through which therapists operate the linear accelerator.
**Related Terms:** Operator station, beam control.
**Example in Radiotherapy:** Displays treatment parameters during patient irradiation.

**275. Control point (noun):** Discrete point defining dose rate, MLC position, and gantry angle during arc delivery.
**Related Terms:** VMAT plan, dynamic delivery.
**Example in Radiotherapy:** Hundreds of control points are used in a single arc.

**276. Conventional fractionation (noun):** Delivery of 1.8–2.0 Gy per fraction once daily, five days per week.
**Related Terms:** Standard fractionation, norm fractionation.
**Example in Radiotherapy:** Applied in adjuvant breast radiotherapy protocols.

**277. Conversion factor (noun):** Ratio used to convert detector readings to dose-to-water or dose-to-air.
**Related Terms:** Calibration constant, chamber factor.
**Example in Radiotherapy:** Used during monthly output calibration of linac.

**278. Convolution algorithm (noun):** Dose calculation method accounting for energy deposition via kernel convolution.
**Related Terms:** Superposition algorithm, TPS.
**Example in Radiotherapy:** Used in advanced dose computation engines.

**279. Coordinate origin (noun):** Reference point from which patient positioning coordinates are measured.
**Related Terms:** Isocenter, DICOM reference.
**Example in Radiotherapy:** The (0,0,0) coordinate denotes the treatment isocenter.

**280. Copper electron filter (noun):** Copper plate used to shape or harden electron beam energy.
**Related Terms:** Electron scattering foil, beam modifier.
**Example in Radiotherapy:** Used for uniformity in 12 MeV electron fields.

**281. Coronal reconstruction (noun):** Image slice reconstruction in the coronal (frontal) plane.
**Related Terms:** Sagittal reconstruction, axial image.
**Example in Radiotherapy:** Used to assess lung tumor position in CBCT review.

**282. Correction factor (noun):** Parameter used to correct measurement conditions to standard calibration setup.
**Related Terms:** Beam quality correction, kQ factor.
**Example in Radiotherapy:** Applied during TG-51 calibration procedures.

**283. Couch indexing (noun):** System ensuring reproducible patient setup by fixed couch positioning markers.
**Related Terms:** Immobilization, setup reproducibility.
**Example in Radiotherapy:** Essential in SBRT and head & neck immobilization.

**284. Couch longitudinal movement (noun):** Translation of treatment couch along the patient's superior–inferior axis.
**Related Terms:** Couch motion, isocenter shift.
**Example in Radiotherapy:** Adjusted for alignment with laser crosshairs.

**285. Couch pitch (noun):** Angular tilt of the treatment couch around the lateral axis.
**Related Terms:** Couch rotation, setup error correction.
**Example in Radiotherapy:** Used in frameless SRS for fine alignment.

**286. Couch vertical offset (noun):** Difference in couch height between simulation and treatment.
**Related Terms:** Setup verification, immobilization.
**Example in Radiotherapy:** Recorded for daily setup reproducibility.

**287. Couch weight limit (noun):** Maximum load-bearing capacity of treatment couch.
**Related Terms:** Machine safety, patient handling.
**Example in Radiotherapy:** Important for obese patient treatment safety.

288. **Cranial base landmark (noun):** Bony structure used for head setup alignment in cranial radiotherapy.
**Related Terms:** Sella turcica, clivus.
**Example in Radiotherapy:** Used as reference for brainstem localization.

289. **Cranial immobilization mask (noun):** Thermoplastic device used to restrict head motion during cranial RT.
**Related Terms:** Head mask, stereotactic frame.
**Example in Radiotherapy:** Used in all brain and SRS cases.

290. **Cranial nerve tolerance (noun):** Maximum safe radiation dose to cranial nerves.
**Related Terms:** Dose constraint, organ tolerance.
**Example in Radiotherapy:** Optic nerve limit ≤55 Gy to prevent neuropathy.

291. **Cranial vertex (noun):** Superior-most point of the skull.
**Related Terms:** Skull vertex, positioning landmark.
**Example in Radiotherapy:** Serves as superior border for whole-brain field.

292. **Craniospinal axis (noun):** Continuous line encompassing brain and spinal canal.
**Related Terms:** Craniospinal irradiation, CSF space.
**Example in Radiotherapy:** Used in medulloblastoma treatment planning.

293. **Craniospinal junction (noun):** Overlapping region between cranial and spinal fields in CSI.
**Related Terms:** Field junction, dose feathering.
**Example in Radiotherapy:** Requires precise matching to avoid overdose.

294. **Craniospinal matching QA (noun):** Verification ensuring field junction accuracy between cranial and spinal fields.
**Related Terms:** Field overlap QA, CSI verification.
**Example in Radiotherapy:** Conducted using film or EPID before CSI.

295. **Craniospinal setup board (noun):** Dedicated immobilization board for CSI patients.
**Related Terms:** CSI setup, pediatric immobilization.
**Example in Radiotherapy:** Ensures reproducible head-to-pelvis alignment.

296. **Cranium bone window (noun):** CT display setting optimizing visualization of skull bone structures.
**Related Terms:** CT windowing, bony anatomy.
**Example in Radiotherapy:** Used for skull-based SRS contour review.

297. **Critical structure (noun):** Organ or tissue sensitive to radiation-induced injury.
**Related Terms:** Organ-at-risk, tolerance dose.
**Example in Radiotherapy:** Lens, spinal cord, and heart are major critical structures.

298. **Critical volume concept (noun):** Radiobiological principle stating that tissue tolerance depends on the irradiated volume.
**Related Terms:** Partial organ tolerance, serial vs parallel organs.
**Example in Radiotherapy:** Applied in dose constraint planning for liver and lung.

299. **Cross-beam profile (noun):** Lateral distribution of radiation intensity across the beam at a given depth.
**Related Terms:** Beam flatness, symmetry.
**Example in Radiotherapy:** Measured during linac commissioning and annual QA.

300. **Cross-calibration (noun):** Comparative calibration of two dosimeters using a reference detector.
**Related Terms:** Ion chamber calibration, standardization.
**Example in Radiotherapy:** Performed between secondary and field ionization chambers.

**301. Crosshair alignment (noun):** Verification of mechanical crosshair accuracy with beam central axis.
**Related Terms:** Field light alignment, QA baseline.
**Example in Radiotherapy:** Checked monthly for field congruence in light vs radiation.

**302. Cross-plane symmetry (noun):** Equality of beam intensity on either side of central axis perpendicular to gantry plane.
**Related Terms:** Flatness, beam profile.
**Example in Radiotherapy:** Tolerance ±2% during linac QA.

**303. Cryogenic MRI system (noun):** Magnetic resonance imaging system operating at very low temperatures to enhance signal.
**Related Terms:** MR-linac, superconducting magnet.
**Example in Radiotherapy:** Used in hybrid MRI-guided treatment units.

**304. Cumulative dose (noun):** Total radiation dose delivered to a point or volume over multiple fractions.
**Related Terms:** Summation dose, total dose.
**Example in Radiotherapy:** Displayed on cumulative dose-volume histogram in adaptive RT.

**305. Cumulative DVH (noun):** Dose–volume histogram showing cumulative percentage of volume receiving at least a given dose.
**Related Terms:** Dose histogram, plan evaluation.
**Example in Radiotherapy:** Used to evaluate OAR dose constraints.

**306. Curie (Ci) (noun):** Unit of radioactivity equal to $3.7 \times 10^{10}$ disintegrations per second.
**Related Terms:** Becquerel, source activity.
**Example in Radiotherapy:** Commonly used in brachytherapy isotope specification.

**307. Curvature correction (noun):** Adjustment applied to dose calculations on curved patient surfaces.
**Related Terms:** Surface contour correction, tissue inhomogeneity.
**Example in Radiotherapy:** Applied for breast tangential fields on chest wall.

**308. Curvilinear beam path (noun):** Non-straight trajectory of radiation beam in arc-based therapies.
**Related Terms:** VMAT, dynamic conformal arc.
**Example in Radiotherapy:** Used in intracranial arc therapy for improved conformity.

**309. Custom blocking tray (noun):** Acrylic tray used to mount lead alloy blocks for beam shaping.
**Related Terms:** Cerrobend block, field shaping.
**Example in Radiotherapy:** Used in conventional 2D pelvic radiotherapy setups.

**310. Cut-out (electron) (noun):** Metal insert defining field size for electron treatments.
**Related Terms:** Electron applicator, field shaping.
**Example in Radiotherapy:** Customized per patient for breast scar boosts.

**311. Cutaneous erythema dose (noun):** Minimum dose required to produce visible skin reddening.
**Related Terms:** Skin tolerance, radiation reaction.
**Example in Radiotherapy:** Historically used to define tolerance levels in orthovoltage era.

**312. CyberKnife system (noun):** Robotic radiosurgery unit delivering multiple non-isocentric beams guided by image tracking.
**Related Terms:** SRS, stereotactic body radiotherapy.
**Example in Radiotherapy:** Used for spine, brain, and lung SBRT treatments.

**313. Cylindrical ionization chamber (noun):** Detector with cylindrical geometry for measuring radiation dose.
**Related Terms:** Farmer chamber, reference dosimetry.
**Example in Radiotherapy:** Used in TG-51 linac calibration protocols.

**314. CT artifact correction (noun):** Process to minimize image distortions due to beam hardening or motion.
**Related Terms:** Metal artifact reduction, scatter correction.
**Example in Radiotherapy:** Ensures accurate HU-to-density conversion in planning CT.

**315. CT couch index (noun):** Reproducible numerical reference point on CT couch used for patient setup.
**Related Terms:** Simulation reference, immobilization reproducibility.
**Example in Radiotherapy:** Recorded for accurate treatment couch positioning.

**316. CT dose modulation (noun):** Technique adjusting x-ray tube current to patient size during scanning.
**Related Terms:** Tube current modulation, image optimization.
**Example in Radiotherapy:** Used to minimize dose in planning CT acquisitions.

**317. CT fusion accuracy (noun):** Degree of geometric alignment between CT datasets or CT-MR fusion.
**Related Terms:** Image registration, fusion error.
**Example in Radiotherapy:** Verified before contouring in MR-CT fusion prostate cases.

**318. CT localization (noun):** Process of acquiring CT images for radiotherapy planning with immobilization devices.
**Related Terms:** Simulation scan, setup localization.
**Example in Radiotherapy:** Performed before contouring and plan generation.

**319. CT number calibration (noun):** Standardization of HU values to known material densities.
**Related Terms:** HU-density curve, QA phantom.
**Example in Radiotherapy:** Checked monthly for accurate dose calculation.

**320. CT simulator (noun):** Dedicated CT unit designed for radiotherapy simulation and patient setup.
**Related Terms:** Simulation CT, planning CT.
**Example in Radiotherapy:** Used to acquire immobilized patient images for planning.

**321. CT window width (noun):** Range of HU values displayed on CT image grayscale.
**Related Terms:** Window level, contrast resolution.
**Example in Radiotherapy:** Adjusted to visualize bone or soft tissue contours.

**322. CT-to-density conversion (noun):** Relationship mapping CT HU values to electron density.
**Related Terms:** Calibration curve, TPS input.
**Example in Radiotherapy:** Used in dose calculation algorithms.

**323. CTV margin (noun):** Geometric expansion added around GTV to cover microscopic disease spread.
**Related Terms:** GTV, PTV, ICRU volumes.
**Example in Radiotherapy:** 5–10 mm margin used for head and neck cancers.

**324. CTV–PTV margin (noun):** Setup and motion margin added to convert CTV into PTV.
**Related Terms:** Setup uncertainty, motion management.
**Example in Radiotherapy:** 3–5 mm added for prostate image-guided treatments.

**325. Cumulative monitor units (noun):** Total number of monitor units delivered over an entire treatment course.
**Related Terms:** Dose delivery, machine output.
**Example in Radiotherapy:** Summed in record-and-verify system for QA tracking.

**326. Cylinder applicator (noun):** Hollow device used for vaginal or endocavitary brachytherapy dose delivery.
**Related Terms:** Vaginal cylinder, HDR applicator.
**Example in Radiotherapy:** Commonly used after endometrial cancer surgery.

327. **Cytogenetic dosimetry (noun):** Biological dosimetry using chromosomal aberrations to estimate radiation exposure.
**Related Terms:** Dicentric assay, biodosimetry.
**Example in Radiotherapy:** Used in accidental exposure investigations.

328. **Cytokine release (noun):** Inflammatory response induced by radiation-damaged tissues.
**Related Terms:** Radiation inflammation, normal tissue response.
**Example in Radiotherapy:** Contributes to acute skin and mucosal toxicity.

329. **Cytoplasmic irradiation (noun):** Exposure of cell cytoplasm to ionizing radiation without affecting the nucleus.
**Related Terms:** Bystander effect, microbeam.
**Example in Radiotherapy:** Studied in radiobiology microbeam experiments.

330. **Cytotoxic dose (noun):** Radiation dose level causing irreversible cell death.
**Related Terms:** Lethal dose, clonogenic death.
**Example in Radiotherapy:** Targeted to tumor cells while sparing normal tissue.

331. **Cylindrical water phantom (noun):** Water-filled cylindrical phantom used for calibration and dosimetry measurements.
**Related Terms:** Reference phantom, QA setup.
**Example in Radiotherapy:** Used for absolute dose calibration of photon beams.

332. **Calibration curve (noun):** Graph showing detector response as a function of radiation dose.
**Related Terms:** Dose–response curve, chamber calibration.
**Example in Radiotherapy:** Used to convert diode signal to absorbed dose.

333. **Calibration phantom (noun):** Phantom used to verify imaging system geometric accuracy and HU calibration.
**Related Terms:** QA phantom, CT calibration.
**Example in Radiotherapy:** Used during monthly CT QA.

334. **Calibration protocol (noun):** Standardized procedure defining steps for dosimeter or linac calibration.
**Related Terms:** TG-51, IAEA TRS-398.
**Example in Radiotherapy:** Followed during annual linac reference dose calibration.

335. **Capacitance dosimeter (noun):** Device measuring ionization charge via stored electrical potential.
**Related Terms:** Ion chamber, electrometer.
**Example in Radiotherapy:** Used in microdosimetry research.

336. **Cascade decay (noun):** Sequential radioactive decay producing multiple photons or particles.
**Related Terms:** Gamma cascade, nuclear transition.
**Example in Radiotherapy:** Occurs in cobalt-60 source decay sequence.

337. **Catheter displacement (noun):** Unintended movement of brachytherapy catheter post-implantation.
**Related Terms:** Source dwell deviation, HDR safety.
**Example in Radiotherapy:** Checked with pre- and post-treatment imaging.

338. **Cell cycle radiosensitivity (noun):** Variation in cell sensitivity depending on its cell cycle phase.
**Related Terms:** G2-M phase, sublethal damage repair.
**Example in Radiotherapy:** Basis for fractionated treatment schedules.

339. **Cellular apoptosis (noun):** Programmed cell death triggered by radiation exposure.
**Related Terms:** DNA fragmentation, intrinsic pathway.
**Example in Radiotherapy:** Major death mechanism in lymphoid malignancies.

**340. Central dose maximum (noun):** Highest dose point along beam central axis in depth-dose curve.
**Related Terms:** Dmax, percentage depth dose.
**Example in Radiotherapy:** Dmax occurs at 1.5 cm for 6 MV photons.

**341. Central nervous system dose constraint (noun):** Maximum safe radiation dose to CNS structures.
**Related Terms:** Tolerance limit, organ sparing.
**Example in Radiotherapy:** Brainstem Dmax kept <54 Gy in head-neck plans.

**342. Cervical spinal cord tolerance (noun):** Maximum radiation dose limit for cervical cord safety.
**Related Terms:** Spinal dose limit, myelopathy prevention.
**Example in Radiotherapy:** Limited to <45 Gy in definitive head and neck RT.

**343. Cervico-thoracic junction (noun):** Anatomical region between cervical and thoracic spine used for field matching.
**Related Terms:** Spine junction, field overlap.
**Example in Radiotherapy:** Used as landmark in craniospinal setup.

**344. Charged particle equilibrium (noun):** Condition where number of charged particles entering a volume equals those exiting.
**Related Terms:** CPE, dosimetry equilibrium.
**Example in Radiotherapy:** Assumed in dose calibration at dmax depth.

**345. Charged particle range (noun):** Distance traveled by a charged particle before stopping.
**Related Terms:** Stopping power, Bragg peak.
**Example in Radiotherapy:** Defines penetration depth in proton therapy.

**346. Characteristic x-ray emission (noun):** Discrete x-ray photons emitted when inner shell electrons are replaced.
**Related Terms:** X-ray spectrum, photon production.
**Example in Radiotherapy:** Occurs in tungsten target of linac x-ray tube.

**347. Chest wall separation (noun):** Distance between anterior and posterior skin surfaces at mid-breast level.
**Related Terms:** SSD variation, tangential setup.
**Example in Radiotherapy:** Determines beam energy selection for breast RT.

**348. Coherence length (noun):** The distance over which a light wave remains phase-correlated.
**Related Terms:** Laser interferometry, optical imaging.
**Example in Radiotherapy:** Determines resolution in optical surface-guided radiotherapy systems.

**349. Coincidence circuit (noun):** An electronic circuit ensuring two signals occur simultaneously for event validation.
**Related Terms:** PET imaging, gamma coincidence.
**Example in Radiotherapy:** Used in PET scanners for positron annihilation event detection.

**350. Cold spot (noun):** A region within a target receiving lower than prescribed dose.
**Related Terms:** Hot spot, dose uniformity.
**Example in Radiotherapy:** Cold spots in IMRT plans can compromise tumor coverage.

**351. Collapsed cone convolution (noun):** A dose calculation algorithm using energy deposition kernels.
**Related Terms:** Convolution–superposition, Monte Carlo.
**Example in Radiotherapy:** Used in TPS for heterogeneity correction in photon beams.

**352. Collimator angle (noun):** The rotational position of the beam-defining jaws around the beam axis.
**Related Terms:** Gantry angle, couch angle.
**Example in Radiotherapy:** Adjusted to match field shape with patient anatomy.

353. **Collimator leakage (noun):** Radiation transmitted through or between collimator jaws.
**Related Terms:** Head leakage, shielding.
**Example in Radiotherapy:** Measured in linac QA to ensure leakage <0.5% of central axis dose.

354. **Collimator rotation isocenter (noun):** The point about which the collimator rotates.
**Related Terms:** Mechanical isocenter, Winston–Lutz test.
**Example in Radiotherapy:** Verified during machine QA to ensure geometric accuracy.

355. **Collimator scatter (noun):** Secondary radiation arising from collimator structures.
**Related Terms:** Sc factor, scatter component.
**Example in Radiotherapy:** Included in dose calibration using collimator scatter factor (Sc).

356. **Collimator transmission factor (noun):** Ratio of transmitted to incident photon fluence through collimator material.
**Related Terms:** Attenuation coefficient.
**Example in Radiotherapy:** Used for MLC leakage correction in TPS modeling.

357. **Collision avoidance (noun):** System ensuring patient–gantry–couch clearance during treatment setup.
**Related Terms:** Clearance check, 3D simulation.
**Example in Radiotherapy:** Visualized in planning software for SRS or noncoplanar beams.

358. **Columnar recombination (noun):** Recombination of ion pairs along a single track.
**Related Terms:** Ion chamber efficiency, saturation voltage.
**Example in Radiotherapy:** Impacts accuracy of ionization chamber readings at high dose rates.

359. **Coma aberration (noun):** Optical distortion causing comet-like blur in imaging systems.
**Related Terms:** Spherical aberration, lens correction.
**Example in Radiotherapy:** May degrade EPID or optical image accuracy.

360. **Commutator (noun):** A rotary electrical switch in generators reversing current direction.
**Related Terms:** Electromagnet, induction motor.
**Example in Radiotherapy:** Present in older X-ray tube generators for voltage regulation.

361. **Compact beamline (noun):** Shortened linear accelerator pathway minimizing footprint.
**Related Terms:** Proton therapy, superconducting linac.
**Example in Radiotherapy:** Used in modern compact proton therapy systems.

362. **Compensation algorithm (noun):** Mathematical method to adjust for inhomogeneities.
**Related Terms:** Density correction, heterogeneity correction.
**Example in Radiotherapy:** Corrects dose distribution in lung or bone regions.

363. **Compensation filter (noun):** Material designed to shape beam intensity across field.
**Related Terms:** Bolus, wedge filter.
**Example in Radiotherapy:** Used to equalize chest wall thickness in tangential breast fields.

364. **Compensator-based IMRT (noun):** Intensity modulation achieved by physical compensators.
**Related Terms:** Step-and-shoot IMRT, MLC-based IMRT.
**Example in Radiotherapy:** Used in early IMRT systems before dynamic MLC technology.

365. **Complete fusion (noun):** Uniform tissue response post-radiation ablation.
**Related Terms:** Necrosis, tissue repair.
**Example in Radiotherapy:** Observed in ablated liver lesions after SBRT.

366. **Composite plan (noun):** Combined dose distribution from multiple treatment courses.
**Related Terms:** Plan summation, cumulative dose.
**Example in Radiotherapy:** Used to evaluate total organ-at-risk dose after re-irradiation.

367. **Computed tomographic angiography (CTA) (noun):** 3D vascular imaging via CT and contrast.
**Related Terms:** MRI angiography, vessel contouring.
**Example in Radiotherapy:** Used to delineate vessels near brain or spine targets.

368. **Cone-beam CT (CBCT) (noun):** Volumetric imaging using a cone-shaped X-ray beam.
**Related Terms:** Image-guided RT, on-board imaging.
**Example in Radiotherapy:** Provides daily verification of target and patient positioning.

369. **Cone ratio (noun):** Output factor ratio for electron cones.
**Related Terms:** Cone factor, Sc,p.
**Example in Radiotherapy:** Measured for each cone size in electron dosimetry QA.

370. **Conformity index (noun):** Quantitative measure of how well the treatment dose conforms to target.
**Related Terms:** Homogeneity index, dose-volume metrics.
**Example in Radiotherapy:** CI close to 1 indicates optimal target coverage.

371. **Conformation therapy (noun):** Early 3D technique shaping radiation dose to tumor volume.
**Related Terms:** 3D-CRT, beam shaping.
**Example in Radiotherapy:** A precursor to IMRT for head-and-neck treatments.

372. **Conformal arc therapy (noun):** Technique using dynamic gantry rotation with shaped beams.
**Related Terms:** VMAT, RapidArc.
**Example in Radiotherapy:** Delivers conformal dose to irregular brain tumors efficiently.

373. **Conformal dose distribution (noun):** Spatial dose pattern matching target shape.
**Related Terms:** Isodose conformity.
**Example in Radiotherapy:** Achieved using multiple coplanar and noncoplanar beams.

374. **Confocal microscopy (noun):** High-resolution optical imaging technique using spatial filtering.
**Related Terms:** Optical biopsy.
**Example in Radiotherapy:** Used in skin cancer assessment for superficial treatment fields.

375. **Coning down (noun):** Reducing field size to focus on residual disease.
**Related Terms:** Boost field, sequential plan.
**Example in Radiotherapy:** Applied after whole-brain RT to target metastasis.

376. **Constant dose rate (noun):** Uniform dose delivery rate throughout treatment.
**Related Terms:** Variable dose rate, dynamic delivery.
**Example in Radiotherapy:** Used for static IMRT fields to maintain consistent beam output.

377. **Contact therapy (noun):** Low-energy X-ray treatment applied close to surface lesions.
**Related Terms:** Superficial therapy, orthovoltage.
**Example in Radiotherapy:** Treats skin cancers with minimal deep tissue dose.

378. **Contour delineation (noun):** Process of outlining target and organ structures on CT images.
**Related Terms:** Segmentation, structure set.
**Example in Radiotherapy:** Key step in treatment planning defining GTV, CTV, and OARs.

379. **Contour smoothing (noun):** Software refinement of drawn structures to reduce irregularities.
**Related Terms:** Auto-contouring, segmentation correction.
**Example in Radiotherapy:** Applied before dose calculation to optimize geometry.

380. **Contrast medium (noun):** Substance enhancing visibility of tissues in imaging.
**Related Terms:** Iodinated contrast, MRI gadolinium.
**Example in Radiotherapy:** Used in simulation to identify GI or urinary tracts.

381. **Control point (noun):** Parameter set defining beam shape, weight, and angle in IMRT.
**Related Terms:** Dynamic delivery, DICOM RT plan.
**Example in Radiotherapy:** Defines sequence for MLC leaf positions and dose rate.

382. **Convection cooling (noun):** Heat transfer via air or fluid motion.
**Related Terms:** Thermal regulation.
**Example in Radiotherapy:** Applied in linac cooling systems to stabilize accelerator components.

383. **Conversion coefficient (noun):** Factor converting physical to biological dose units.
**Related Terms:** RBE, weighting factor.
**Example in Radiotherapy:** Used to express neutron exposure in equivalent dose.

384. **Co-planar beam arrangement (noun):** All beams lie within one geometric plane.
**Related Terms:** Noncoplanar, isocentric.
**Example in Radiotherapy:** Typical in 3D-CRT pelvic treatments.

385. **Copper sulfate phantom (noun):** Tissue-equivalent phantom containing copper sulfate solution.
**Related Terms:** MRI phantom, dosimetric calibration.
**Example in Radiotherapy:** Used for MR imaging system QA and geometric distortion testing.

386. **Coregistration (noun):** Alignment of multimodal images into a common coordinate space.
**Related Terms:** Image fusion, registration.
**Example in Radiotherapy:** CT–MRI coregistration improves tumor .

387. **Coronal slice (noun):** Anatomical plane dividing body into anterior and posterior parts.
**Related Terms:** Axial, sagittal.
**Example in Radiotherapy:** Used in 3D image review for target contouring.

388. **Correction factor (noun):** Applied value adjusting for known measurement errors.
**Related Terms:** Calibration coefficient, chamber correction.
**Example in Radiotherapy:** Used in dose calibration to correct for temperature and pressure.

389. **Cosmic radiation (noun):** High-energy ionizing radiation from space.
**Related Terms:** Background radiation, secondary neutrons.
**Example in Radiotherapy:** Contributes to natural background dose monitoring.

390. **Couch index (noun):** Reference number marking patient position on couch.
**Related Terms:** Couch coordinates, reproducibility.
**Example in Radiotherapy:** Recorded for daily setup consistency.

391. **Couch shift (noun):** Translational or rotational movement of treatment couch.
**Related Terms:** Image-guided correction, registration error.
**Example in Radiotherapy:** Applied after CBCT match to correct patient position.

392. **Couch sag (noun):** Vertical displacement of couch under patient load.
**Related Terms:** Couch deflection, mechanical tolerance.
**Example in Radiotherapy:** Compensated in QA to maintain geometric accuracy.

393. **Couch vertical height (noun):** Distance from floor to couch surface reference.
**Related Terms:** Setup parameters, indexing.
**Example in Radiotherapy:** Maintained consistently to achieve accurate reproducibility.

394. **Cranial immobilization (noun):** Head fixation for intracranial radiotherapy.
**Related Terms:** Thermoplastic mask, stereotactic frame.
**Example in Radiotherapy:** Ensures submillimeter accuracy in SRS.

395. **Craniovertebral junction (noun):** Anatomical region between skull base and upper cervical spine.
**Related Terms:** C1–C2 articulation, brainstem.
**Example in Radiotherapy:** Requires careful contouring in nasopharyngeal carcinoma plans.

396. **Critical structure (noun):** Organ sensitive to radiation damage.
**Related Terms:** Organ-at-risk, tolerance dose.
**Example in Radiotherapy:** Spinal cord and optic nerve are critical structures in brain RT.

397. **Cross-field dosimetry (noun):** Measurement of dose distribution across beam profile.
**Related Terms:** Beam symmetry, flatness.
**Example in Radiotherapy:** Performed during linac commissioning for beam uniformity assessment.

398. **Cobalt calibration source (noun):** A standard Co-60 radiation source used for calibrating dosimeters and QA instruments.
**Related Terms:** Dosimetry calibration, reference source
**Example in Radiotherapy:** Used to verify chamber response before linear accelerator output calibration.

399. **Cobalt-60 unit (noun):** A teletherapy machine using gamma radiation from cobalt-60 isotopes.
**Related Terms:** Telecobalt, gamma beam
**Example in Radiotherapy:** Commonly used for head-and-neck cancer treatment in low-resource centers.

400. **Code of practice (noun):** A formal guideline defining dosimetry and QA procedures for radiotherapy centers.
**Related Terms:** IAEA TRS-398, AAPM TG reports
**Example in Radiotherapy:** Ensures standardized output calibration across institutions.

401. **Coherence length (noun):** The spatial range over which a beam maintains a fixed phase relationship.
**Related Terms:** Beam uniformity, wave interference
**Example in Radiotherapy:** Relevant in optical and laser-based QA systems.

402. **Coil imaging artifact (noun):** Distortion caused by RF coil malfunction or positioning in MRI.
**Related Terms:** MR artifact, signal dropout
**Example in Radiotherapy:** Affects MR simulation image accuracy in adaptive planning.

403. **Cold spot (noun):** A region within the target volume receiving less than the prescribed dose.
**Related Terms:** Dose uniformity, underdosage
**Example in Radiotherapy:** Detected during plan QA to ensure adequate tumor coverage.

404. **Collar region (noun):** The lower neck area near the thyroid and supraclavicular field junction.
**Related Terms:** Thyroid shielding, junction match
**Example in Radiotherapy:** Requires precise field matching in head-and-neck setups.

405. **Collision check (noun):** Safety verification preventing gantry, couch, or accessory collision.
**Related Terms:** Safety interlock, clearance test
**Example in Radiotherapy:** Performed before volumetric arc delivery.

406. **Collimator calibration (noun):** Process of verifying jaw or leaf positioning accuracy in the collimator system.
**Related Terms:** Jaw offset, MLC QA
**Example in Radiotherapy:** Conducted during monthly QA to maintain beam geometry accuracy.

407. **Collimator rotation (noun):** Adjustment of the beam-defining jaws around the beam's central axis.
**Related Terms:** Gantry rotation, field alignment
**Example in Radiotherapy:** Used to minimize divergence at field junctions.

**408. Colon dose constraint (noun):** The maximum allowable radiation dose to the colon to avoid late toxicity.
**Related Terms:** Organ-at-risk constraint, dose-volume histogram
**Example in Radiotherapy:** Applied during pelvic IMRT planning.

**409. Color map legend (noun):** Visual representation of dose levels in a treatment plan using color gradients.
**Related Terms:** Isodose display, dose wash
**Example in Radiotherapy:** Used to interpret dose distribution in TPS.

**410. Combined modality therapy (noun):** Treatment strategy integrating radiotherapy with chemotherapy or surgery.
**Related Terms:** Concurrent therapy, multimodal approach
**Example in Radiotherapy:** Applied in head-and-neck squamous carcinoma.

**411. Compensator-based IMRT (noun):** Intensity modulation using custom metal filters instead of MLC.
**Related Terms:** Physical modulation, beam hardening
**Example in Radiotherapy:** Used in early IMRT before MLC technology became standard.

**412. Compliance phantom (noun):** QA phantom designed to test adherence to dosimetric standards.
**Related Terms:** End-to-end QA, benchmarking
**Example in Radiotherapy:** Used for inter-institutional audits.

**413. Composite plan dose (noun):** Sum of doses from multiple treatment courses or plans.
**Related Terms:** Plan summation, cumulative dose
**Example in Radiotherapy:** Evaluated in re-irradiation cases.

**414. Compressed breast thickness (noun):** The reduced tissue depth during mammographic simulation.
**Related Terms:** Breast compression, image quality
**Example in Radiotherapy:** Measured to correlate with surface dose in tangential fields.

**415. Computed tomography number (noun):** A pixel value representing tissue density relative to water.
**Related Terms:** Hounsfield unit, CT calibration
**Example in Radiotherapy:** Used in dose calculation algorithms.

**416. Cone beam dose contribution (noun):** Additional dose imparted from repeated CBCT imaging.
**Related Terms:** Imaging dose, verification exposure
**Example in Radiotherapy:** Accounted for in adaptive plan evaluation.

**417. Cone beam reconstruction (noun):** 3D image formation from cone-shaped X-ray projections.
**Related Terms:** CBCT algorithm, Feldkamp reconstruction
**Example in Radiotherapy:** Provides volumetric setup verification.

**418. Confidence level (noun):** Statistical expression of certainty in measurement or analysis.
**Related Terms:** Standard deviation, uncertainty
**Example in Radiotherapy:** Applied in dosimetric audit evaluations.

**419. Conformal arc therapy (noun):** Delivery of radiation dose through rotational fields shaped to the tumor.
**Related Terms:** Dynamic conformal arc, VMAT
**Example in Radiotherapy:** Used for intracranial lesion treatments.

**420. Conformal margin (noun):** Expansion applied around GTV to ensure adequate PTV coverage.
**Related Terms:** Planning margin, motion allowance
**Example in Radiotherapy:** Determined using image-guided uncertainty analysis.

421. **Consistency check (noun):** Routine QA step to verify data accuracy between systems.
**Related Terms:** Secondary calculation, cross-verification
**Example in Radiotherapy:** Used before treatment plan approval.

422. **Constraint violation (noun):** Exceeding of dose limits for critical structures.
**Related Terms:** OAR limit, DVH analysis
**Example in Radiotherapy:** Flagged during treatment plan optimization.

423. **Contact therapy (noun):** Superficial X-ray therapy where the applicator touches the skin.
**Related Terms:** Superficial therapy, orthovoltage
**Example in Radiotherapy:** Applied for skin carcinoma near the eyelid.

424. **Contouring consistency (noun):** Uniformity of target and OAR delineation across observers.
**Related Terms:** Interobserver variability, contour QA
**Example in Radiotherapy:** Essential for multicenter trials.

425. **Contrast-to-noise ratio (noun):** Ratio indicating the visibility of structures in an image.
**Related Terms:** Image quality, SNR
**Example in Radiotherapy:** Evaluated in CBCT image QA.

426. **Control point (noun):** A specific gantry and dose delivery position in dynamic therapy.
**Related Terms:** VMAT segment, fluence map
**Example in Radiotherapy:** Defines dose distribution along arc delivery.

427. **Convection cooling (noun):** Removal of heat by air or liquid flow in linac systems.
**Related Terms:** Thermal control, heat exchanger
**Example in Radiotherapy:** Prevents overheating of magnetron components.

428. **Coordinate system (noun):** Spatial reference used for patient positioning and image registration.
**Related Terms:** DICOM coordinates, isocenter reference
**Example in Radiotherapy:** Defines alignment between CT and TPS geometry.

429. **Copper sulfate marker (noun):** Radiopaque skin marker used during simulation.
**Related Terms:** Fiducial marker, alignment wire
**Example in Radiotherapy:** Marks treatment field borders on setup images.

430. **Coregistration accuracy (noun):** The precision of image alignment between different modalities.
**Related Terms:** Image fusion, registration error
**Example in Radiotherapy:** Evaluated during CT-MRI fusion for contouring.

431. **Cortex bone landmark (noun):** Outer dense bone layer used as a positioning reference.
**Related Terms:** Bony anatomy, alignment guide
**Example in Radiotherapy:** Used in spinal setup for IGRT.

432. **Couch drift (noun):** Gradual displacement of the treatment couch over time.
**Related Terms:** Positional stability, mechanical accuracy
**Example in Radiotherapy:** Checked during QA of long treatment deliveries.

433. **Cumulative DVH (noun):** Graphical representation showing the total dose received by a volume.
**Related Terms:** Dose-volume histogram, plan evaluation
**Example in Radiotherapy:** Used to assess OAR sparing.

434. **CyberKnife tracking (noun):** Real-time tumor motion tracking system using robotic beam delivery.
**Related Terms:** Fiducial tracking, robotic radiotherapy
**Example in Radiotherapy:** Applied for liver or prostate SBRT.

435. **Cylindrical phantom (noun):** Phantom with a cylindrical shape used for dosimetric calibration.
**Related Terms:** QA phantom, uniformity test
**Example in Radiotherapy:** Used for output factor verification.

436. **Cytogenetic biodosimetry (noun):** Biological assessment of absorbed radiation dose via chromosomal analysis.
**Related Terms:** Biodosimetry, radiation biology
**Example in Radiotherapy:** Used for accidental exposure evaluation.

437. **Cyberknife Synchrony system (noun):** Tracking system compensating for respiratory motion during treatment.
**Related Terms:** Real-time tracking, motion management
**Example in Radiotherapy:** Used in lung and liver SBRT.

438. **CT dose index (noun):** A standardized measure of radiation dose in CT imaging.
**Related Terms:** CTDIvol, imaging dose
**Example in Radiotherapy:** Monitored to maintain patient imaging safety.

439. **CT simulator (noun):** CT scanner configured for radiotherapy planning with laser alignment.
**Related Terms:** Simulation, DICOM export
**Example in Radiotherapy:** Used to acquire images for contouring and planning.

440. **CT windowing (noun):** Adjustment of brightness and contrast to visualize specific tissues.
**Related Terms:** Window width, window level
**Example in Radiotherapy:** Used to enhance soft-tissue visibility during contouring.

441. **Cumulative MU (noun):** Total monitor units delivered for all fields in a treatment plan.
**Related Terms:** Dose delivery, QA check
**Example in Radiotherapy:** Verified before plan execution to ensure accuracy.

442. **Cutaneous dose (noun):** The amount of radiation absorbed by the skin.
**Related Terms:** Surface dose, bolus effect
**Example in Radiotherapy:** Evaluated for chest wall and breast cancer treatments.

443. **Cutout field (noun):** Shaped aperture in an electron insert used to define treatment area.
**Related Terms:** Electron applicator, custom insert
**Example in Radiotherapy:** Used in superficial electron therapy for skin lesions.

444. **Cyclotron beam (noun):** Proton or heavy ion beam generated by a cyclotron accelerator.
**Related Terms:** Proton therapy, particle accelerator
**Example in Radiotherapy:** Used for deep-seated tumor treatments.

445. **Cylindrical coordinate (noun):** Spatial coordinate system using radius, angle, and height parameters.
**Related Terms:** Cartesian coordinates, polar system
**Example in Radiotherapy:** Applied in TPS for arc beam geometry .

446. **Cytotoxic response (noun):** Cellular death caused by ionizing radiation exposure.
**Related Terms:** Apoptosis, mitotic death
**Example in Radiotherapy:** Represents biological effectiveness of tumor dose.

447. **CT-MR fusion (noun):** Image registration process combining CT and MRI datasets.
**Related Terms:** Image fusion, multimodality registration
**Example in Radiotherapy:** Used for target delineation in brain and prostate cases.

448. **Collimator rotation (noun):** The angular movement of the collimator around the beam axis to adjust field shape orientation.
**Related Terms:** Gantry rotation, Beam collimation.

**Example in Radiotherapy:** Used to align field edges parallel to patient anatomy in breast tangential treatments.

449. **Cone-beam CT (noun):** A volumetric imaging technique using a cone-shaped x-ray beam for 3D verification.
**Related Terms:** CBCT, Image-guided radiotherapy (IGRT).
**Example in Radiotherapy:** Daily setup verification for SBRT liver patients.

450. **Conformal arc therapy (noun):** A rotational treatment technique shaping dose to target contour through arcs.
**Related Terms:** Dynamic conformal arcs, IMRT.
**Example in Radiotherapy:** Employed in brain metastases for dose conformity.

451. **Contrast agent (noun):** A substance enhancing visualization of internal structures in imaging.
**Related Terms:** Iodinated contrast, MRI contrast.
**Example in Radiotherapy:** Used in CT simulation to delineate tumor vasculature.

452. **Couch indexing (noun):** The method of reproducibly positioning immobilization devices on the couch.
**Related Terms:** Setup reproducibility, Couch locks.
**Example in Radiotherapy:** Ensures identical patient alignment in head-and-neck fractions.

453. **Compensator-based IMRT (noun):** Intensity modulation achieved using physical compensators.
**Related Terms:** Step-and-shoot IMRT, Dynamic IMRT.
**Example in Radiotherapy:** Applied in low-resource centers without MLC.

454. **Critical organ tolerance (noun):** The maximum radiation dose an organ can safely receive.
**Related Terms:** Dose constraints, QUANTEC.
**Example in Radiotherapy:** Spinal cord tolerance set at 45 Gy in standard fractionation.

455. **Convolution–superposition algorithm (noun):** A dose calculation model accounting for scatter and attenuation.
**Related Terms:** Monte Carlo, Pencil beam.
**Example in Radiotherapy:** Used for accurate dose in heterogeneous thoracic tissues.

456. **Cyber Knife system (noun):** A robotic radiosurgery system delivering high-precision beams.
**Related Terms:** SRS, SBRT.
**Example in Radiotherapy:** Utilized in treating prostate and spine lesions.

457. **Calibration phantom (noun):** A device with known material properties for system calibration.
**Related Terms:** QA phantom, Water phantom.
**Example in Radiotherapy:** Used to calibrate dose output for linear accelerators.

458. **CT simulator (noun):** A CT scanner adapted for radiotherapy planning.
**Related Terms:** Simulation, Image registration.
**Example in Radiotherapy:** Acquires 3D patient geometry for treatment planning.

459. **Couch sag correction (noun):** Adjustment for deflection due to patient weight on couch.
**Related Terms:** Couch flex, Mechanical accuracy.
**Example in Radiotherapy:** Applied in stereotactic treatments for submillimeter precision.

460. **Cumulative dose (noun):** The total radiation dose accumulated over all fractions.
**Related Terms:** Fractionation, Biologically effective dose (BED).
**Example in Radiotherapy:** 70 Gy cumulative dose delivered in 35 fractions.

461. **Collimator jaw setting (noun):** The physical adjustment of jaws defining field edges.
**Related Terms:** Beam shaping, MLC.
**Example in Radiotherapy:** Adjusted to limit field to PTV margins.

**462. Couch lateral offset (noun):** Side-to-side displacement of couch from isocenter.
**Related Terms:** Setup shift, Isocentric positioning.
**Example in Radiotherapy:** Corrected after daily CBCT verification.

**463. Cryogenic detector (noun):** A radiation detector operating at low temperatures for high sensitivity.
**Related Terms:** Semiconductor detector, Ion chamber.
**Example in Radiotherapy:** Used in specialized dosimetry for low-dose regions.

**464. Crossfire technique (noun):** Opposing beam arrangement to enhance tumor dose uniformity.
**Related Terms:** Bilateral fields, Opposed pair.
**Example in Radiotherapy:** Applied in pelvic and head-and-neck treatments.

**465. Compartmental dose (noun):** The dose delivered to distinct anatomical or biological compartments.
**Related Terms:** Target volume segmentation, Dose painting.
**Example in Radiotherapy:** Varying dose to hypoxic regions within tumor.

**466. Conformal shielding (noun):** Custom blocks matching tumor shape to protect normal tissue.
**Related Terms:** Cerrobend blocks, MLC shielding.
**Example in Radiotherapy:** Used in 3D-CRT of lung lesions.

**467. Couch movement limit (noun):** The maximum mechanical range of couch motion.
**Related Terms:** Gantry clearance, Mechanical interlock.
**Example in Radiotherapy:** Ensures safe patient shifts during IGRT.

**468. Collimator rotation isocentricity (noun):** The precision of collimator rotation around true isocenter.
**Related Terms:** QA tolerance, Mechanical accuracy.
**Example in Radiotherapy:** Verified during monthly machine QA.

**469. CT number calibration (noun):** The process of correlating CT numbers with electron density.
**Related Terms:** HU calibration, Density mapping.
**Example in Radiotherapy:** Essential for accurate dose calculation in planning.

**470. Cumulative MUs (noun):** Total monitor units used across all treatment fields.
**Related Terms:** MU calculation, Dose delivery.
**Example in Radiotherapy:** Monitored to ensure correct total exposure.

**471. CT contrast timing (noun):** Optimization of scan time post-contrast injection.
**Related Terms:** Dynamic CT, Perfusion imaging.
**Example in Radiotherapy:** Enhances tumor–organ contrast for contouring.

**472. Couch angle verification (noun):** Checking angular accuracy of couch rotation.
**Related Terms:** Gantry–couch coordination, QA.
**Example in Radiotherapy:** Verified before arc therapy delivery.

**473. Cone-shaped beam collimator (noun):** A circular collimator for stereotactic or small field irradiation.
**Related Terms:** Circular collimator, SRS cone.
**Example in Radiotherapy:** Used for trigeminal neuralgia treatment.

**474. Composite plan dose (noun):** The total dose distribution combining all plans or boosts.
**Related Terms:** Sum plan, Plan summation.
**Example in Radiotherapy:** Combined for breast tangents and SCF boost.

**475. Contrast-to-noise ratio (noun):** A metric comparing signal contrast to background noise in imaging.
**Related Terms:** Image quality, SNR.
**Example in Radiotherapy:** Used to assess CBCT image quality.

**476. Collimator transmission test (noun):** QA test measuring leakage through collimator leaves.
**Related Terms:** MLC QA, Leakage radiation.
**Example in Radiotherapy:** Performed annually as per AAPM TG-142.

**477. Cyber Knife tracking (noun):** Real-time target localization system using image guidance.
**Related Terms:** Synchrony tracking, Fiducial tracking.
**Example in Radiotherapy:** Used for lung and prostate SBRT.

**478. Cumulative histogram (noun):** Graph showing percentage of volume receiving a given dose or higher.
**Related Terms:** DVH, Dose analysis.
**Example in Radiotherapy:** Used in evaluating PTV and OAR coverage.

**479. Collimator field light (noun):** A visible light indicating the radiation field projection.
**Related Terms:** Light-radiation field congruence, QA.
**Example in Radiotherapy:** Checked in daily QA.

**480. Couch indexing bar (noun):** A reference guide used to position immobilization devices.
**Related Terms:** Reproducibility, Setup consistency.
**Example in Radiotherapy:** Used for thermoplastic mask fixation.

**481. Clinical workflow (noun):** The sequence of steps from consultation to treatment delivery.
**Related Terms:** Workflow optimization, RT process.
**Example in Radiotherapy:** Ensures efficient coordination in daily treatments.

**482. Collimator jaw asymmetry (noun):** Unequal positioning of jaws affecting field symmetry.
**Related Terms:** Beam alignment, QA.
**Example in Radiotherapy:** Detected during symmetry testing.

**483. Couch pitch (noun):** Angular tilt of couch along longitudinal axis.
**Related Terms:** Couch roll, Table rotation.
**Example in Radiotherapy:** Adjusted for accurate brain SRS setup.

**484. CT ventilation imaging (noun):** Functional imaging derived from 4D CT to assess lung ventilation.
**Related Terms:** Functional planning, Dose avoidance.
**Example in Radiotherapy:** Used to spare well-ventilated lung regions.

**485. Cryoablation (noun):** Destruction of tissue by freezing, sometimes combined with RT.
**Related Terms:** Ablation therapy, SBRT.
**Example in Radiotherapy:** Used for local control of small liver lesions.

**486. Couch vertical offset (noun):** Height displacement of the couch from isocenter.
**Related Terms:** Setup shift, Laser alignment.
**Example in Radiotherapy:** Adjusted before beam-on in daily setup.

**487. Calibration coefficient (noun):** Factor converting detector reading to absorbed dose.
**Related Terms:** Dosimetry, Ion chamber.
**Example in Radiotherapy:** Used in TG-51 reference dosimetry.

**488. CT-MR fusion (noun):** Image registration of CT and MRI datasets.
**Related Terms:** Multimodal registration, Image fusion.
**Example in Radiotherapy:** Used for soft-tissue delineation in brain tumors.

**489. Couch top deflection (noun):** Mechanical bending of couch under load.
**Related Terms:** Couch sag, QA.
**Example in Radiotherapy:** Measured during commissioning.

490. **Clinical target delineation (noun):** Defining tumor boundaries for dose coverage.
**Related Terms:** GTV, CTV, PTV.
**Example in Radiotherapy:** Based on fused CT-MRI images.

491. **Conformal radiotherapy (noun):** Technique shaping beams to conform to target shape.
**Related Terms:** 3D-CRT, Dose conformity.
**Example in Radiotherapy:** Used in prostate and brain cases.

492. **Co-registration accuracy (noun):** Precision of alignment between two image datasets.
**Related Terms:** Image registration, Fusion accuracy.
**Example in Radiotherapy:** Critical in MRI-CT fusion for head-and-neck.

493. **Cone angle (noun):** Divergence angle of the radiation beam cone.
**Related Terms:** Field divergence, Beam geometry.
**Example in Radiotherapy:** Affects dose uniformity in oblique setups.

494. **Collimator leaf speed (noun):** Rate of MLC leaf motion during beam modulation.
**Related Terms:** Dynamic IMRT, MLC control.
**Example in Radiotherapy:** Impacts IMRT delivery accuracy.

495. **Couch longitudinal shift (noun):** Movement along patient's head-to-feet direction.
**Related Terms:** Translational correction, Isocenter shift.
**Example in Radiotherapy:** Applied for image-based setup correction.

496. **CT acquisition protocol (noun):** Defined scanning parameters for simulation imaging.
**Related Terms:** Slice thickness, kVp, mAs.
**Example in Radiotherapy:** Optimized for head-and-neck planning.

497. **Couch coordinate system (noun):** Reference axes defining couch movements (x, y, z).
**Related Terms:** Patient positioning, Isocentric system.
**Example in Radiotherapy:** Used in treatment setup shifts.

498. **Couch collision (noun):** A potential mechanical interference between gantry, couch, or patient during beam delivery.
**Related Terms:** Clearance check, Collision avoidance.
**Example in Radiotherapy:** Verified before noncoplanar arc therapy in cranial cases.

499. **Couch coordinate verification (noun):** Checking accuracy of couch position values before beam-on.
**Related Terms:** Setup verification, Image guidance.
**Example in Radiotherapy:** Essential in stereotactic brain treatments.

500. **CT artifact (noun):** Unwanted image distortion caused by motion, metal, or beam hardening.
**Related Terms:** Metal artifact, Motion artifact.
**Example in Radiotherapy:** Can affect contouring accuracy near dental fillings.

# D

1. **Daily QA (noun):** Routine check ensuring daily LINAC performance consistency.
   **Related Terms:** Quality assurance, Output constancy.
   **Example in Radiotherapy:** Daily QA includes beam output, symmetry, and imaging tests.
2. **Data acquisition (noun):** Process of collecting raw image or dose data.
   **Related Terms:** Imaging, Reconstruction.
   **Example in Radiotherapy:** Data acquisition in CBCT is performed before image registration.
3. **Dead time (noun):** Interval when detector cannot record another event.
   **Related Terms:** Counting loss, Detector saturation.
   **Example in Radiotherapy:** Ion chamber dead time correction improves accuracy in high-dose-rate beams.
4. **Decay constant (noun):** Probability per unit time that a nucleus decays.
   **Related Terms:** Half-life, Radioactivity.
   **Example in Radiotherapy:** The decay constant determines isotope strength in brachytherapy.
5. **Deconvolution (noun):** Mathematical process separating overlapping signals.
   **Related Terms:** Image restoration, Filtering.
   **Example in Radiotherapy:** Deconvolution corrects detector response in small-field dosimetry.
6. **Deep inspiration breath-hold (noun):** Technique reducing organ motion by voluntary breath-hold.
   **Related Terms:** Motion management, DIBH.
   **Example in Radiotherapy:** DIBH reduces heart dose in left breast irradiation.
7. **Deformable image registration (noun):** Alignment of images allowing non-rigid anatomical changes.
   **Related Terms:** DIR, Adaptive radiotherapy.
   **Example in Radiotherapy:** DIR enables dose accumulation across treatment fractions.
8. **Deformation vector field (noun):** Spatial mapping representing voxel displacement.
   **Related Terms:** DIR, Image fusion.
   **Example in Radiotherapy:** DVF used to propagate contours during adaptive planning.
9. **Density override (noun):** Manual adjustment of CT numbers for specific regions.
   **Related Terms:** HU correction, Planning.
   **Example in Radiotherapy:** Density override applied to dental fillings to prevent artifacts.
10. **Depth dose curve (noun):** Graph showing dose variation with depth.
    **Related Terms:** PDD, Beam quality.
    **Example in Radiotherapy:** Depth dose curves characterize electron and photon beams.
11. **Depth of maximum dose (noun):** Depth where absorbed dose reaches its peak.
    **Related Terms:** dmax, Beam quality.
    **Example in Radiotherapy:** 6 MV photon beam dmax occurs at ~1.5 cm.
12. **Detector calibration (noun):** Process of ensuring detector accuracy to known standard.
    **Related Terms:** Dosimetry, QA.
    **Example in Radiotherapy:** Detector calibration ensures ion chamber traceability to primary standards.

13. **Detector array (noun):** Matrix of detectors used for dose measurement.
**Related Terms:** Portal dosimetry, QA.
**Example in Radiotherapy:** Detector arrays validate IMRT fluence maps.

14. **Detector linearity (noun):** Proportional relationship between dose and signal.
**Related Terms:** Sensitivity, Response curve.
**Example in Radiotherapy:** Detector linearity verified during QA for high-dose-rate beams.

15. **Deuteron beam (noun):** Beam of deuterium nuclei used in nuclear reactions.
**Related Terms:** Proton therapy, Heavy ion.
**Example in Radiotherapy:** Deuteron beams investigated for neutron generation.

16. **Diagnostic reference level (noun):** Guideline dose value for typical imaging procedure.
**Related Terms:** Dose optimization, Patient safety.
**Example in Radiotherapy:** DRLs guide dose levels for planning CT scans.

17. **Dielectric constant (noun):** Material property determining response to electric field.
**Related Terms:** Permittivity, MR-linac.
**Example in Radiotherapy:** Dielectric constant affects RF field distribution in MR imaging.

18. **D018. Diffusion coefficient (noun):** Rate at which particles spread through a medium.
**Related Terms:** Molecular diffusion, Radiobiology.
**Example in Radiotherapy:** Diffusion coefficient influences oxygen transport in hypoxic tumors.

19. **Digital imaging (noun):** Acquisition and display of radiographic images in digital form.
**Related Terms:** DICOM, PACS.
**Example in Radiotherapy:** Digital imaging enables efficient IGRT verification.

20. **Digital reconstruction (noun):** Computer-generated 3D image from CT or MRI data.
**Related Terms:** DRR, Planning image.
**Example in Radiotherapy:** DRRs assist in field alignment during setup.

21. **Digital phantom (noun):** Virtual model simulating patient anatomy.
**Related Terms:** Monte Carlo, Dose simulation.
**Example in Radiotherapy:** Digital phantoms used for TPS algorithm validation.

22. **DICOM-RT (noun):** Standard for transferring radiotherapy data formats.
**Related Terms:** Image communication, Data exchange.
**Example in Radiotherapy:** DICOM-RT enables plan import/export between systems.

23. **Differential dose-volume histogram (noun):** Graph showing volume fraction receiving specific dose intervals.
**Related Terms:** DVH, Planning metrics.
**Example in Radiotherapy:** Differential DVH aids dose gradient evaluation.

24. **Diffusion-weighted imaging (noun):** MRI sequence sensitive to water motion.
**Related Terms:** Functional imaging, MR-Linac.
**Example in Radiotherapy:** DWI assists tumor viability assessment during adaptive therapy.

25. **Direct aperture optimization (noun):** IMRT planning method optimizing aperture shapes directly.
**Related Terms:** Fluence optimization, MLC.
**Example in Radiotherapy:** DAO reduces leaf motion time in VMAT.

26. **Direct ionization (noun):** Ion production by charged particle collisions.
**Related Terms:** Indirect ionization, Radiation physics.
**Example in Radiotherapy:** Proton therapy relies primarily on direct ionization.

27. **Direct simulation Monte Carlo (noun):** Stochastic calculation modeling particle transport directly.
**Related Terms:** Monte Carlo, Dose computation.
**Example in Radiotherapy:** DSMC enhances precision for microbeam dosimetry.

28. **Displacement vector (noun):** Mathematical representation of anatomical shift.
**Related Terms:** Image registration, DIR.
**Example in Radiotherapy:** Displacement vectors quantify tumor motion.

29. **Dose accumulation (noun):** Summation of delivered dose over multiple fractions.
**Related Terms:** Adaptive planning, DIR.
**Example in Radiotherapy:** Dose accumulation used to evaluate cumulative OAR dose.

30. **D030. Dose calibration (noun):** Adjustment ensuring treatment dose matches reference standards.
**Related Terms:** Absolute dosimetry, QA.
**Example in Radiotherapy:** Dose calibration verified with water phantom ion chamber.

31. **Dose conformity (noun):** Degree of dose coverage matching target shape.
**Related Terms:** CI, PTV coverage.
**Example in Radiotherapy:** High dose conformity achieved with stereotactic techniques.

32. **Dose constraint (noun):** Limit set to protect organs at risk.
**Related Terms:** OAR, Planning objective.
**Example in Radiotherapy:** Spinal cord dose constraint limited to 45 Gy.

33. **Dose correction factor (noun):** Multiplier applied to correct measured dose.
**Related Terms:** Calibration, Environmental correction.
**Example in Radiotherapy:** Dose correction factors applied for temperature-pressure effects.

34. **Dose distribution (noun):** Spatial representation of absorbed dose.
**Related Terms:** Isodose, DVH.
**Example in Radiotherapy:** Dose distribution verified through patient-specific QA.

35. **Dose escalation (noun):** Strategy of increasing prescribed dose to enhance control.
**Related Terms:** Hypofractionation, SBRT.
**Example in Radiotherapy:** Dose escalation improves tumor control in prostate SBRT.

36. **Dose fall-off (noun):** Rate at which dose decreases beyond target boundary.
**Related Terms:** Gradient index, Edge sharpness.
**Example in Radiotherapy:** Proton therapy achieves superior dose fall-off.

37. **Dose gradient (noun):** Change in dose over distance.
**Related Terms:** Penumbra, Conformity.
**Example in Radiotherapy:** High dose gradient minimizes normal tissue exposure.

38. **Dose heterogeneity (noun):** Uneven dose distribution within target.
**Related Terms:** Hot spot, Cold spot.
**Example in Radiotherapy:** Dose heterogeneity evaluated using HI.

39. **Dose homogeneity index (noun):** Quantitative measure of dose uniformity.
**Related Terms:** HI, PTV.
**Example in Radiotherapy:** Homogeneity index optimized in 3D-CRT plans.

40. **Dose kernel (noun):** Mathematical model describing dose spread from a point source.
**Related Terms:** Convolution, Monte Carlo.
**Example in Radiotherapy:** Dose kernels used in collapsed cone algorithms.

41. **Dose linearity (noun):** Proportional relationship between monitor units and delivered dose.
**Related Terms:** Output constancy, QA.
**Example in Radiotherapy:** Dose linearity checked during monthly LINAC calibration.

42. **Dose map (noun):** 2D representation of dose across a plane.
**Related Terms:** Fluence map, QA film.
**Example in Radiotherapy:** Dose maps compared between calculated and measured data.

43. **Dose modulation (noun):** Variation of beam intensity to achieve optimal distribution.
**Related Terms:** IMRT, VMAT.
**Example in Radiotherapy:** Dose modulation shapes dose around critical organs.

44. **Dose painting (noun):** Technique delivering different dose levels within a tumor based on biology.
**Related Terms:** Functional imaging, Adaptive therapy.
**Example in Radiotherapy:** PET-guided dose painting escalates dose to hypoxic regions.

45. **Dose perturbation (noun):** Alteration in dose distribution due to heterogeneity or interface.
**Related Terms:** Interface effect, Density correction.
**Example in Radiotherapy:** Dose perturbation occurs near metal implants.

46. **Dose prescription (noun):** Clinically intended radiation dose to target volume.
**Related Terms:** Fractionation, Planning objective.
**Example in Radiotherapy:** The oncologist defines dose prescription in Gy per fraction.

47. **Dose profile (noun):** Dose variation along a line across the field.
**Related Terms:** Beam profile, Flatness.
**Example in Radiotherapy:** Dose profile symmetry verified during QA.

48. **Dose reconstruction (noun):** Calculation of delivered dose using measured parameters.
**Related Terms:** In vivo dosimetry, QA.
**Example in Radiotherapy:** Dose reconstruction validates adaptive treatment accuracy.

49. **Dose referencing (noun):** Normalization of dose to a reference point or region.
**Related Terms:** Isocenter, PDD.
**Example in Radiotherapy:** Dose referencing facilitates comparison between plans.

50. **Dose shaping (noun):** Adjustment of beam geometry for conformal coverage.
**Related Terms:** MLC, Conformal therapy.
**Example in Radiotherapy:** Dose shaping achieved through dynamic leaf sequencing.

51. **Dose surface histogram (noun):** Graph depicting dose distribution across organ surfaces.
**Related Terms:** DVH, Surface dose.
**Example in Radiotherapy:** DSH helps evaluate rectal wall dose in prostate plans.

52. **Dose tolerance (noun):** Maximum safe dose a tissue can receive.
**Related Terms:** TD 5/5, OAR.
**Example in Radiotherapy:** Dose tolerance for spinal cord is 45 Gy.

53. **Dose uncertainty (noun):** Deviation between calculated and actual dose.
**Related Terms:** QA, Measurement error.
**Example in Radiotherapy:** Dose uncertainty minimized using high-resolution detectors.

54. **Dose verification (noun):** Comparison between planned and delivered doses.
**Related Terms:** QA, Dosimetry.
**Example in Radiotherapy:** Dose verification performed before patient treatment start.

55. **Dose-volume constraint (noun):** Limit on organ volume receiving specific dose.
**Related Terms:** DVH, Planning goal.
**Example in Radiotherapy:** Lung V20 < 30% is a common constraint.

56. **Dose-volume histogram (noun):** Graph showing volume percentage receiving certain dose.
**Related Terms:** Planning evaluation, DVH.
**Example in Radiotherapy:** DVH helps assess plan quality for OARs.

57. **Dose-volume index (noun):** Quantitative indicator derived from DVH analysis.
**Related Terms:** CI, HI.
**Example in Radiotherapy:** Dose-volume index compares plan conformity.

58. **Dose-weighted imaging (noun):** Functional MRI image correlating with dose distribution.
**Related Terms:** MR-Linac, Functional imaging.
**Example in Radiotherapy:** Dose-weighted imaging supports biological adaptation.

59. **Dosimeter (noun):** Device measuring radiation dose.
**Related Terms:** Ion chamber, TLD.
**Example in Radiotherapy:** Dosimeters placed in phantom during QA.

60. **Dosimeter sensitivity (noun):** Response per unit dose of a dosimeter.
**Related Terms:** Calibration, Linearity.
**Example in Radiotherapy:** Dosimeter sensitivity verified annually.

61. **Dosimetric accuracy (noun):** Closeness of measured dose to true dose.
**Related Terms:** Precision, QA.
**Example in Radiotherapy:** Dosimetric accuracy ensured through reference calibration.

62. **Dosimetric comparison (noun):** Evaluation of multiple plans based on dose metrics.
**Related Terms:** DVH, QA analysis.
**Example in Radiotherapy:** Dosimetric comparison performed between IMRT and VMAT.

63. **Dosimetric evaluation (noun):** Assessment of treatment plan using dose parameters.
**Related Terms:** CI, HI.
**Example in Radiotherapy:** Dosimetric evaluation determines plan acceptability.

64. **Dosimetric index (noun):** Mathematical indicator summarizing dose quality.
**Related Terms:** CI, HI.
**Example in Radiotherapy:** HI and CI are primary dosimetric indices.

65. **Dosimetric uncertainty (noun):** Variation due to detector or calibration limitations.
**Related Terms:** Measurement error, QA.
**Example in Radiotherapy:** Dosimetric uncertainty reported as ±2%.

66. **Dosimetric verification (noun):** Process confirming planned dose delivery.
**Related Terms:** QA, EPID dosimetry.
**Example in Radiotherapy:** Portal dosimetry used for dosimetric verification.

67. **Dosimetry audit (noun):** External review verifying accuracy of dose delivery.
**Related Terms:** Quality assurance, Peer review.
**Example in Radiotherapy:** National dosimetry audits ensure institutional consistency.

68. **Dosimetry film (noun):** Radiation-sensitive film recording dose pattern.
**Related Terms:** Gafchromic film, QA.
**Example in Radiotherapy:** Dosimetry film used to verify stereotactic fields.

69. **Dosimetry phantom (noun):** Model simulating patient tissue for dose measurement.
**Related Terms:** Water phantom, QA.
**Example in Radiotherapy:** Phantoms used in commissioning procedures.

70. **Double scattering (noun):** Proton therapy technique using dual scatterers for uniform dose.
**Related Terms:** Passive scattering, Beam modulation.
**Example in Radiotherapy:** Double scattering employed in early proton systems.

71. **Downstream collimation (noun):** Beam-limiting device placed after scattering system.
**Related Terms:** Aperture, Field shaping.
**Example in Radiotherapy:** Downstream collimation defines treatment field edges.

72. **DRR (noun):** Digitally reconstructed radiograph from CT data.
**Related Terms:** Image registration, Setup verification.
**Example in Radiotherapy:** DRR used for beam alignment before irradiation.

73. **DRR matching (noun):** Registration of DRR with on-board image.
**Related Terms:** IGRT, Alignment.
**Example in Radiotherapy:** DRR matching ensures correct patient setup.

74. **Dual-energy CT (noun):** Imaging using two distinct X-ray energies.
**Related Terms:** Tissue characterization, Planning.
**Example in Radiotherapy:** Dual-energy CT differentiates bone from metal artifacts.

75. **Dual-isocenter planning (noun):** Two overlapping isocenters used for extended targets.
**Related Terms:** Field junction, QA.
**Example in Radiotherapy:** Dual-isocenter planning used for craniospinal irradiation.

76. **Dual scattering system (noun):** Proton beam device using two scatterers for dose uniformity.
**Related Terms:** Passive scattering, Range modulation.
**Example in Radiotherapy:** Dual scattering broadens Bragg peak in uniform fields.

77. **Dynamic arc therapy (noun):** Continuous gantry rotation delivering modulated dose.
**Related Terms:** VMAT, IMAT.
**Example in Radiotherapy:** Dynamic arc therapy improves plan conformity.

78. **Dynamic collimation (noun):** Real-time adjustment of collimator to modulate beam.
**Related Terms:** Adaptive MLC, MR-Linac.
**Example in Radiotherapy:** Dynamic collimation maintains field alignment during motion.

79. **Dynamic field (noun):** Treatment field varying during delivery.
**Related Terms:** Sliding window, Arc therapy.
**Example in Radiotherapy:** Dynamic fields used in IMRT delivery.

80. **Dynamic leaf motion (noun):** Movement of MLC leaves during beam-on.
**Related Terms:** IMRT, VMAT.
**Example in Radiotherapy:** Dynamic leaf motion enhances fluence modulation.

81. **Dynamic trajectory radiotherapy (noun):** Advanced delivery combining gantry, couch, and collimator motion.
**Related Terms:** VMAT, MR-Linac.
**Example in Radiotherapy:** DTR improves conformity for complex targets.

82. **Dynamic tracking (noun):** Real-time beam adaptation following target motion.
**Related Terms:** MR-guided RT, Gating.
**Example in Radiotherapy:** Dynamic tracking reduces margin in lung SBRT.

83. **Dynamic wedge (noun):** Electronic wedge effect created by moving collimator jaw.
**Related Terms:** Enhanced dynamic wedge, Dose modulation.
**Example in Radiotherapy:** Dynamic wedge replaces physical wedge filters.

84. **Dynamic wave arc (noun):** MR-Linac delivery technique integrating imaging and modulation.
**Related Terms:** MR-guided RT, Adaptive planning.
**Example in Radiotherapy:** Dynamic wave arc optimizes dose in real-time adaptive therapy.

85. **DNA double-strand break (noun):** Critical form of radiation-induced DNA damage.
**Related Terms:** Radiobiology, Cell death.
**Example in Radiotherapy:** DNA DSBs drive tumor cell killing after irradiation.

86. **DNA repair kinetics (noun):** Rate at which cells repair radiation-induced damage.
**Related Terms:** Radiosensitivity, Radiobiology.
**Example in Radiotherapy:** DNA repair kinetics influence fractionation schedules.

87. **Dose escalation study (noun):** Clinical trial evaluating safety of increasing dose levels.
**Related Terms:** Phase I trial, Toxicity.
**Example in Radiotherapy:** Dose escalation studies determine maximum tolerated dose.

88. **Dose fall-off gradient (noun):** Rate of dose decrease beyond target.
**Related Terms:** Gradient index, Conformality.
**Example in Radiotherapy:** Proton therapy achieves steep dose fall-off gradients.

89. **Dose painting by numbers (noun):** Voxel-level modulation of dose guided by biological maps.
**Related Terms:** Functional imaging, PET.
**Example in Radiotherapy:** Dose painting by numbers personalizes treatment to tumor biology.

90. **Dose recalculation (noun):** Re-estimation of dose using updated anatomy or settings.
**Related Terms:** Adaptive RT, Replanning.
**Example in Radiotherapy:** Dose recalculation done after anatomy change.

91. **Dose re-normalization (noun):** Adjustment of prescribed dose to maintain uniformity.
**Related Terms:** Plan optimization, QA.
**Example in Radiotherapy:** Dose re-normalization maintains coverage after anatomy shift.

92. **Dose-response curve (noun):** Graph showing biological effect as function of dose.
**Related Terms:** Radiobiology, LQ model.
**Example in Radiotherapy:** Dose-response curves define tumor control probability.

93. **Dose rate (noun):** Amount of radiation delivered per unit time.
**Related Terms:** MU/min, cGy/min.
**Example in Radiotherapy:** Flattening-filter-free (FFF) beams deliver higher dose rate for reduced treatment time.

94. **Dose reference point (noun):** Defined location used for reporting prescribed dose.
**Related Terms:** ICRU reference point, Isocenter.
**Example in Radiotherapy:** Dose reference point selected at PTV centroid for plan evaluation.

95. **Dose sculpting (noun):** Shaping radiation dose distribution to conform precisely to target.
**Related Terms:** IMRT, VMAT.
**Example in Radiotherapy:** Dose sculpting protects rectum during prostate irradiation.

96. **Dose surface map (noun):** Visualization of dose on anatomical surfaces.
**Related Terms:** DVH, Dose analysis.
**Example in Radiotherapy:** DSMs used for skin dose evaluation in breast radiotherapy.

97. **Dose summation (noun):** Combination of doses from multiple plans or sessions.
**Related Terms:** Cumulative dose, Adaptive planning.
**Example in Radiotherapy:** Dose summation performed for re-irradiation planning.

98. **Dose tolerance (noun):** Maximum safe dose a normal tissue can receive.
**Related Terms:** TD5/5, OAR constraints.
**Example in Radiotherapy:** Spinal cord dose tolerance maintained below 45 Gy.

99. **Dose uncertainty (noun):** Range of possible variation from intended dose.
**Related Terms:** Measurement error, QA.
**Example in Radiotherapy:** Monte Carlo modeling minimizes dose uncertainty in small fields.

100. **Dose verification (noun):** Process of confirming delivered dose accuracy.
**Related Terms:** In vivo dosimetry, QA.
**Example in Radiotherapy:** Portal dosimetry used for patient-specific dose verification.

101. **Dosimetric accuracy (noun):** Precision of dose measurement compared to true value.
**Related Terms:** Calibration, QA tolerance.
**Example in Radiotherapy:** Dosimetric accuracy ensures compliance with IAEA TRS-398 protocols.

102. **Dosimetric audit (noun):** External review verifying institutional dose delivery accuracy.
**Related Terms:** IAEA audit, QA.
**Example in Radiotherapy:** IAEA postal audits ensure dosimetric consistency across centers.

103. **Dosimetric evaluation (noun):** Assessment of plan quality using dose metrics.
**Related Terms:** DVH, CI, HI.
**Example in Radiotherapy:** Dosimetric evaluation compared IMRT vs VMAT plan quality.

104. **Dosimetric leaf gap (noun):** Effective gap between MLC leaves influencing dose modeling.
**Related Terms:** MLC calibration, TPS modeling.
**Example in Radiotherapy:** DLGap adjusted to improve dose accuracy in small fields.

105. **Dosimetric parameter (noun):** Quantitative measure describing dose characteristics.
**Related Terms:** DVH metrics, PTV coverage.
**Example in Radiotherapy:** D95%, V100%, and HI are common dosimetric parameters.

106. **Dosimetric precision (noun):** Degree of reproducibility in dose measurement.
**Related Terms:** Repeatability, QA stability.
**Example in Radiotherapy:** High dosimetric precision achieved through daily output constancy checks.

107. **Dosimetric validation (noun):** Confirmation that calculated dose matches measured dose.
**Related Terms:** Patient-specific QA, Verification.
**Example in Radiotherapy:** Dosimetric validation done using ArcCHECK for VMAT.

108. **Dosimeter (noun):** Device used to measure absorbed dose.
**Related Terms:** Ion chamber, TLD, OSLD.
**Example in Radiotherapy:** Farmer ion chamber used for beam calibration.

109. **Dosimetry (noun):** Science of measuring absorbed radiation dose.
**Related Terms:** Absolute dosimetry, Relative dosimetry.
**Example in Radiotherapy:** Dosimetry ensures treatment plan doses are accurately delivered.

110. **Double scattering (noun):** Proton beam broadening technique using two scatterers.
**Related Terms:** Passive modulation, Range modulation.
**Example in Proton Therapy:** Double scattering achieves uniform dose across target volume.

111. **Dynamic arc therapy (noun):** Rotational technique delivering modulated dose continuously.
**Related Terms:** VMAT, RapidArc.
**Example in Radiotherapy:** Dynamic arc therapy reduces treatment time with conformal coverage.

112. **Dynamic collimation (noun):** Time-varying aperture shaping during beam delivery.
**Related Terms:** MLC, Adaptive aperture.
**Example in Radiotherapy:** Dynamic collimation compensates for organ motion in MR-Linac.

113. **Dynamic dose delivery (noun):** Continuous variation of beam parameters during irradiation.
**Related Terms:** IMRT, VMAT.
**Example in Radiotherapy:** Dynamic delivery allows modulation of gantry speed and dose rate.

114. **Dynamic gating (noun):** Beam-on only during specific respiratory phases.
**Related Terms:** 4D radiotherapy, Motion tracking.
**Example in Radiotherapy:** Dynamic gating reduces tumor motion in lung SBRT.

115. **Dynamic jaw tracking (noun):** Technique where collimator jaws move with MLC.
**Related Terms:** Leakage reduction, Modulation.
**Example in Radiotherapy:** Dynamic jaw tracking improves beam efficiency in IMRT.

116. **Dynamic magnetic field (noun):** Time-varying magnetic field influencing charged particle motion.
**Related Terms:** MR-Linac, Larmor frequency.
**Example in Radiotherapy:** Dynamic magnetic fields managed during MR-guided beam delivery.

117. **Dynamic MLC (noun):** Multileaf collimator operating in motion during irradiation.
**Related Terms:** Sliding window, IMRT.
**Example in Radiotherapy:** Dynamic MLC delivers fluence-modulated IMRT fields.

118. **Dynamic tumor tracking (noun):** Real-time adjustment of beam to follow moving target.
**Related Terms:** Motion management, Real-time imaging.
**Example in Radiotherapy:** MR-Linac enables dynamic tumor tracking in liver SBRT.

119. **Dynamic wedge (noun):** Computer-controlled collimator motion creating wedge effect.
**Related Terms:** Enhanced dynamic wedge, Beam modulation.
**Example in Radiotherapy:** Dynamic wedges replace physical wedges in modern LINACs.

120. **Dwell position (noun):** Specific source location within brachytherapy applicator.
**Related Terms:** Dwell time, Source path.
**Example in Radiotherapy:** Dwell positions optimized for uniform dose distribution.

121. **Dwell time (noun):** Duration source remains at a dwell position.
**Related Terms:** Brachytherapy planning, Source strength.
**Example in Radiotherapy:** Dwell times adjusted to optimize target coverage and OAR sparing.

122. **Dynamic contrast MRI (noun):** MRI sequence tracking contrast agent uptake.
**Related Terms:** DCE-MRI, Functional imaging.
**Example in Radiotherapy:** DCE-MRI used to evaluate tumor perfusion pre-RT.

123. **Dynamic adaptive planning (noun):** Continuous adjustment of treatment plan based on anatomical change.
**Related Terms:** Online ART, MR-Linac.
**Example in Radiotherapy:** MR-guided ART employs dynamic adaptive planning daily.

124. **Dynamic beam delivery (noun):** Radiation beam modulated dynamically in position or intensity.
**Related Terms:** IMRT, VMAT.
**Example in Radiotherapy:** Dynamic beam delivery enhances conformity and reduces OAR exposure.

125. **Dynamic dose painting (noun):** Varying dose intensity within tumor using imaging biomarkers.
**Related Terms:** Biologically guided RT, PET-IMRT.
**Example in Radiotherapy:** Dose painting targets hypoxic subvolumes with escalated doses.

126. **Dynamic monitoring (noun):** Continuous tracking of patient motion or dose.
**Related Terms:** IGRT, Motion tracking.
**Example in Radiotherapy:** Dynamic monitoring ensures accurate beam alignment during treatment.

127. **Dynamic target volume (noun):** Target region that changes position during breathing.
**Related Terms:** ITV, Motion envelope.
**Example in Radiotherapy:** Dynamic target volumes defined using 4D-CT imaging.

128. **Dysplasia (noun):** Abnormal growth of cells, often precancerous.
**Related Terms:** Neoplasia, Carcinogenesis.
**Example in Radiotherapy:** Cervical dysplasia may require localized radiation if invasive.

129. **Dose painting (noun):** Technique assigning variable dose within target based on biology.
**Related Terms:** PET-guided RT, Adaptive planning.
**Example in Radiotherapy:** FDG-PET guides dose painting in head-and-neck tumors.

130. **Dose-volume constraint (noun):** Defined limit for dose to volume of tissue.
**Related Terms:** OAR, Plan optimization.
**Example in Radiotherapy:** Rectal V50 constraint used in prostate RT planning.

131. **Dose-volume histogram (noun):** Graph showing dose distribution within volume.
**Related Terms:** DVH, Planning metrics.
**Example in Radiotherapy:** DVH analysis confirms PTV coverage and OAR sparing.

132. **Dose wash (noun):** Region showing overlap of multiple dose levels.
**Related Terms:** Isodose overlap, Visualization.
**Example in Radiotherapy:** Dose wash evaluated for plan robustness during ART.

133. **Dose cloud (noun):** Visual 3D representation of dose distribution.
**Related Terms:** Isodose surface, Plan evaluation.
**Example in Radiotherapy:** Dose cloud helps assess coverage of moving targets.

134. **Dose-weighted histogram (noun):** Graph showing dose contribution weighted by volume.
**Related Terms:** DVH, Dose metrics.
**Example in Radiotherapy:** Dose-weighted histograms aid assessment of heterogeneous dose regions.

135. **Dose-wise adaptation (noun):** Plan modification based on daily delivered dose.
**Related Terms:** Adaptive therapy, MR-Linac.
**Example in Radiotherapy:** Dose-wise adaptation ensures cumulative dose accuracy during ART.

136. **Dose window (noun):** Predefined range of acceptable dose for optimization.
**Related Terms:** Constraints, Optimization objectives.
**Example in Radiotherapy:** Dose windows define target coverage and OAR sparing limits.

137. **Dose-volume relation (noun):** Mathematical correlation between dose and tissue volume.
**Related Terms:** DVH, Tolerance dose.
**Example in Radiotherapy:** Dose-volume relations determine complication probabilities in NTCP models.

138. **Dose-volume optimization (noun):** Process minimizing OAR dose while achieving PTV coverage.
**Related Terms:** Inverse planning, Constraints.
**Example in Radiotherapy:** Dose-volume optimization improves prostate IMRT plan quality.

139. **Dose-volume predictor (noun):** Parameter predicting toxicity based on volume-dose data.
**Related Terms:** NTCP, Predictive modeling.
**Example in Radiotherapy:** Rectal V70 acts as a dose-volume predictor for toxicity.

140. **Dose-volume reduction (noun):** Strategy lowering OAR exposure while preserving target dose.
**Related Terms:** Constraint relaxation, Adaptive optimization.
**Example in Radiotherapy:** Dose-volume reduction achieved via tighter beam shaping.

141. **Dose-volume statistics (noun):** Quantitative analysis of volume-dose metrics.
**Related Terms:** DVH analysis, QA metrics.
**Example in Radiotherapy:** DVH statistics include D2%, D98%, and mean dose.

142. **Dose-weighted mean (noun):** Average dose accounting for volume weighting.
**Related Terms:** Equivalent uniform dose, Mean dose.
**Example in Radiotherapy:** Dose-weighted mean used to calculate EUD.

143. **Double exposure (noun):** Imaging artifact from two overlapping acquisitions.
**Related Terms:** Image artifact, CBCT error.
**Example in Radiotherapy:** Double exposure avoided by ensuring couch immobilization during scan.

144. **Double scattering system (noun):** Proton delivery system using dual scatterers for beam spreading.
**Related Terms:** Passive modulation, Range modulation.
**Example in Proton Therapy:** Double scattering achieves uniform dose over SOBP.

145. **Double-differential dose (noun):** Dose expressed per unit energy and solid angle.
**Related Terms:** Particle fluence, Dosimetry.
**Example in Radiotherapy:** Double-differential dose used in neutron therapy calculations.

146. **Dose voxel (noun):** 3D spatial unit representing localized absorbed dose.
**Related Terms:** Dose grid, TPS.
**Example in Radiotherapy:** Dose voxels determine plan resolution and accuracy.

147. **Dose reconstruction (noun):** Recalculation of delivered dose using imaging data.
**Related Terms:** In vivo dosimetry, ART.
**Example in Radiotherapy:** Dose reconstruction validates daily delivered dose accuracy.

148. **Dose recalculation (noun):** Revaluation of dose under modified conditions.
**Related Terms:** Adaptive planning, QA.
**Example in Radiotherapy:** MR-guided ART requires daily dose recalculation.

149. **Dose resampling (noun):** Interpolation of dose distribution to new geometry.
**Related Terms:** Image registration, Dose accumulation.
**Example in Radiotherapy:** Dose resampling used during deformable dose accumulation.

150. **Dose spill (noun):** Unintended dose outside target volume.
**Related Terms:** Gradient index, Conformity.
**Example in Radiotherapy:** Peripheral dose spill minimized by arc modulation.

151. **Dose summation plan (noun):** Cumulative plan merging multiple sessions.
**Related Terms:** Adaptive therapy, Cumulative dose.
**Example in Radiotherapy:** Dose summation plans integrate adaptive fractions.

152. **Dose trigger (noun):** Automated threshold initiating beam interruption.
**Related Terms:** Safety interlock, Beam gating.
**Example in Radiotherapy:** Dose trigger halts beam if excess MU detected.

153. **Dose voxelization (noun):** Conversion of dose distribution into discrete voxels.
**Related Terms:** Grid resolution, Image segmentation.
**Example in Radiotherapy:** Voxelization impacts Monte Carlo computation precision.

154. **Dose-weighted planning (noun):** Optimization emphasizing biological significance of dose.
**Related Terms:** TCP, EUD-based planning.
**Example in Radiotherapy:** Dose-weighted planning prioritizes hypoxic subregions.

155. **Dose-based adaptation (noun):** Treatment modification derived from accumulated dose data.
**Related Terms:** Online ART, MR-guided therapy.
**Example in Radiotherapy:** MR-Linac uses dose-based adaptation for daily plan updates.

156. **Dose-driven optimization (noun):** Algorithm adjusting beam parameters to achieve objectives.
**Related Terms:** Inverse planning, DVH-based optimization.
**Example in Radiotherapy:** Dose-driven optimization ensures rapid convergence in IMRT planning.

157. **Dose-volume parameter (noun):** Numerical descriptor of dose-volume relationship.
**Related Terms:** DVH, Plan evaluation.
**Example in Radiotherapy:** D95% and V100% are standard dose-volume parameters.

158. **Dose verification phantom (noun):** Calibration model used to confirm plan accuracy.
**Related Terms:** QA phantom, Dosimetry.
**Example in Radiotherapy:** ArcCHECK used as dose verification phantom in VMAT QA.

159. **Dose-volume probability (noun):** Statistical likelihood linking dose and complication rate.
**Related Terms:** NTCP, Modeling.
**Example in Radiotherapy:** NTCP curves derived from dose-volume probabilities.

160. **Dose-volume constraint (noun):** Specified dose limit for an anatomical region.
**Related Terms:** OAR limit, Plan optimization.
**Example in Radiotherapy:** Liver V30 limited to under 40% for SBRT.

161. **Dose-volume tolerance (noun):** Maximum volume fraction tolerating specific dose.
**Related Terms:** QUANTEC, TD5/5.
**Example in Radiotherapy:** Lung V20 < 35% considered safe limit.

162. **Dose-weighted voxel (noun):** Voxel intensity adjusted by absorbed dose value.
**Related Terms:** Dose mapping, Visualization.
**Example in Radiotherapy:** Dose-weighted voxel images display biologically effective dose.

163. **Dose-to-water (noun):** Reference absorbed dose in water phantom.
**Related Terms:** Calibration standard, Dosimetry.
**Example in Radiotherapy:** IAEA TRS-398 defines dose-to-water calibration method.

164. **Dose-to-tissue (noun):** Absorbed dose within specific biological tissue.
**Related Terms:** Conversion factor, Stopping power ratio.
**Example in Radiotherapy:** Dose-to-tissue calculated using mass energy-absorption coefficients.

165. **Dose-weighted CT (noun):** CT imaging protocol accounting for dose deposition.
**Related Terms:** Planning CT, Artifact correction.
**Example in Radiotherapy:** Dose-weighted CT improves electron density mapping.

166. **Dose-driven adaptation (noun):** Plan adjustment based on cumulative delivered dose.
**Related Terms:** ART, MR-guided therapy.
**Example in Radiotherapy:** Dose-driven adaptation improves cumulative PTV coverage.

167. **Dose-volume histogram index (noun):** Metric summarizing DVH characteristics.
**Related Terms:** CI, HI, Dmean.
**Example in Radiotherapy:** D2% index represents high-dose exposure regions.

168. **Dose washout (noun):** Reduction of effective dose due to motion or perfusion.
**Related Terms:** Motion blur, Radiobiology.
**Example in Radiotherapy:** Liver motion causes dose washout during respiratory phases.

169. **Dose-dependent effect (noun):** Biological response varying with absorbed dose.
**Related Terms:** LQ model, Radiobiology.
**Example in Radiotherapy:** DNA double-strand breaks show dose-dependent increase.

170. **Dose fractionation (noun):** Dividing total dose into smaller daily doses.
**Related Terms:** Hypo fractionation, Conventional fractionation.
**Example in Radiotherapy:** 2 Gy per fraction typical in conventional fractionation.

171. **Dose accumulation map (noun):** Visualization of accumulated dose over time.
**Related Terms:** DIR, ART.
**Example in Radiotherapy:** Dose accumulation maps assess adaptive dose delivery.

172. **Dose tracking (noun):** Real-time monitoring of delivered dose distribution.
**Related Terms:** MR-guidance, In vivo dosimetry.
**Example in Radiotherapy:** MR-Linac enables dose tracking during beam-on delivery.

173. **Dose-limiting toxicity (noun):** Adverse effect restricting dose escalation.
**Related Terms:** OAR constraint, Tolerance.
**Example in Radiotherapy:** GI toxicity is dose-limiting in pancreatic SBRT.

174. **Dose prediction model (noun):** Algorithm estimating dose based on prior data.
**Related Terms:** AI planning, Knowledge-based planning.
**Example in Radiotherapy:** Dose prediction models accelerate automatic plan generation.

175. **Dose optimization algorithm (noun):** Computation method achieving optimal dose distribution.
**Related Terms:** Inverse planning, Gradient descent.
**Example in Radiotherapy:** TPS uses gradient-based dose optimization algorithms.

176. **Dose calibration factor (noun):** Conversion coefficient from instrument reading to dose.
**Related Terms:** Calibration constant, Dosimetry.
**Example in Radiotherapy:** Calibration factor ensures traceability in ion chamber measurements.

177. **Dose quality index (noun):** Measure expressing plan quality and conformity.
**Related Terms:** CI, HI.
**Example in Radiotherapy:** High DQI indicates superior target conformity.

178. **Dose correlation coefficient (noun):** Statistical relationship between two dose distributions.
**Related Terms:** Gamma index, Correlation analysis.
**Example in Radiotherapy:** DCC quantifies agreement between calculated and measured doses.

179. **Dose-volume robustness (noun):** Plan's ability to maintain dose under uncertainty.
**Related Terms:** Robust optimization, Uncertainty analysis.
**Example in Proton Therapy:** Robustness ensures target coverage despite range errors.

180. **Dose conformity index (noun):** A ratio indicating how well the prescribed dose conforms to the target volume.
**Related Terms:** PTV, Conformality.
**Example in Radiotherapy:** High dose conformity index ensures minimal normal tissue exposure.

181. **Dose constraint (noun):** Maximum permissible radiation dose to an organ or structure.
**Related Terms:** OAR, Dose limit.
**Example in Radiotherapy:** Dose constraint applied to spinal cord to prevent myelopathy.

182. **Dose degradation (noun):** Loss of dose uniformity due to beam scattering or setup error.
**Related Terms:** Beam attenuation, QA.
**Example in Radiotherapy:** MR-LINAC minimizes dose degradation with adaptive planning.

183. **Dose deviation (noun):** Difference between planned and delivered radiation dose.
**Related Terms:** QA, Dose verification.
**Example in Radiotherapy:** Dose deviation evaluated using gamma analysis.

184. **Dose distribution (noun):** Spatial arrangement of radiation dose within a volume.
**Related Terms:** Isodose, Dose map.
**Example in Radiotherapy:** Dose distribution visualized using DVH plots.

185. **Dose escalation (noun):** Increasing prescribed dose to improve tumor control.
**Related Terms:** Hypofractionation, BED.
**Example in Radiotherapy:** SBRT involves dose escalation for localized lesions.

186. **Dose fall-off (noun):** Rate at which dose decreases beyond the target volume.
**Related Terms:** Penumbra, Gradient index.
**Example in Radiotherapy:** Sharp dose fall-off essential in stereotactic treatments.

187. **Dose fractionation (noun):** Division of total dose into multiple smaller doses over time.
**Related Terms:** Fraction size, Biological repair.
**Example in Radiotherapy:** Conventional fractionation delivers 2 Gy per day.

188. **Dose homogeneity (noun):** Uniformity of dose within the target volume.
**Related Terms:** Homogeneity index, PTV coverage.
**Example in Radiotherapy:** Ideal IMRT ensures dose homogeneity across PTV.

189. **Dose kernel (noun):** Mathematical function describing dose spread from a point source.
**Related Terms:** Convolution, Dose algorithm.
**Example in Radiotherapy:** Dose kernel modeling improves Monte Carlo accuracy.

190. **Dose linearity (noun):** Proportional relationship between delivered and measured dose.
**Related Terms:** Calibration, QA.
**Example in Radiotherapy:** Detector dose linearity verified during commissioning.

191. **Dose modulation (noun):** Variation in beam intensity to optimize dose distribution.
**Related Terms:** IMRT, Dynamic MLC.
**Example in Radiotherapy:** Dose modulation reduces OAR exposure in head-and-neck cases.

192. **Dose monitor unit (noun):** LINAC calibration unit relating dose to beam output.
**Related Terms:** MU, Dosimetry.
**Example in Radiotherapy:** 1 MU corresponds to 1 cGy at reference depth.

193. **Dose optimization (noun):** Adjustment of dose parameters for best tumor control and sparing.
**Related Terms:** Inverse planning, Constraint satisfaction.
**Example in Radiotherapy:** Optimization algorithms enhance IMPT treatment quality.

194. **Dose painting (noun):** Delivery of heterogeneous doses based on biological imaging data.
**Related Terms:** Functional imaging, PET-guided RT.
**Example in Radiotherapy:** Dose painting boosts hypoxic tumor regions selectively.

195. **Dose perturbation (noun):** Local alteration in dose due to heterogeneity or implants.
**Related Terms:** Inhomogeneity, Metal artifact.
**Example in Radiotherapy:** MR-LINAC compensates for tissue dose perturbation.

196. **Dose point kernel (noun):** 3D representation of energy deposition from a unit source.
**Related Terms:** Monte Carlo, Transport theory.
**Example in Radiotherapy:** Used for scatter correction in dosimetry.

197. **Dose prescription (noun):** Clinician-defined target dose to achieve therapeutic intent.
**Related Terms:** Fractionation, Planning.
**Example in Radiotherapy:** 60 Gy in 30 fractions prescribed for head-and-neck cancer.

198. **Dose rate effect (noun):** Variation in biological response with radiation delivery speed.
**Related Terms:** Radiobiology, DNA repair.
**Example in Radiotherapy:** FLASH therapy exploits ultra-high dose rate effects.

199. **Dose reconstruction (noun):** Rebuilding 3D dose distribution from measured data.
**Related Terms:** Verification, QA.
**Example in Radiotherapy:** Dose reconstruction validates treatment accuracy post-irradiation.

200. **Dose response (noun):** Relationship between dose and observed biological effect.
**Related Terms:** Radiobiology, Survival curve.
**Example in Radiotherapy:** Dose-response curves determine tumor control probability.

201. **Dose surface histogram (noun):** Graph of dose delivered to surface voxels of an organ.
**Related Terms:** DVH, Skin dose.
**Example in Radiotherapy:** DSH helps evaluate dose to organ boundaries.

202. **Dose uncertainty (noun):** Quantifiable error in dose calculation or delivery.
**Related Terms:** QA, Tolerance limit.
**Example in Radiotherapy:** Dose uncertainty maintained below 3% clinically.

203. **Dosimetric accuracy (noun):** Precision of measured versus planned radiation dose.
**Related Terms:** QA, Calibration.
**Example in Radiotherapy:** MR-LINAC QA ensures dosimetric accuracy daily.

204. **Dosimetric comparison (noun):** Evaluation between different treatment techniques or plans.
**Related Terms:** IMRT, VMAT, 3DCRT.
**Example in Radiotherapy:** Dosimetric comparison shows IMPT superiority in OAR sparing.

205. **Dosimetric leaf gap (noun):** Effective width between MLC leaves during dynamic delivery.
**Related Terms:** MLC calibration, IMRT QA.
**Example in Radiotherapy:** DLG measured to fine-tune fluence maps.

206. **Dosimetric parameter (noun):** Quantitative measure describing dose distribution characteristics.
**Related Terms:** Dmax, V95.
**Example in Radiotherapy:** V20 is a common dosimetric parameter for lung.

207. **Dosimetric phantom (noun):** Physical model mimicking tissue for dose measurements.
**Related Terms:** QA, Commissioning.
**Example in Radiotherapy:** Anthropomorphic phantom used in end-to-end testing.

208. **Dosimetric verification (noun):** Process of confirming treatment plan dose accuracy.
**Related Terms:** QA, Portal dosimetry.
**Example in Radiotherapy:** Verification performed using 2D detector arrays.

209. **Double scattering (noun):** Technique using two scatterers to shape proton beam uniformly.
**Related Terms:** Passive scattering, Proton therapy.
**Example in Radiotherapy:** Double scattering spreads out Bragg peak for uniform dose.

210. **Dual energy CT (noun):** CT imaging using two different X-ray energies for improved contrast.
**Related Terms:** HU correction, Planning.
**Example in Radiotherapy:** Dual energy CT improves tissue heterogeneity correction.

211. **Dual arc therapy (noun):** VMAT technique using two rotational arcs for improved coverage.
**Related Terms:** IMRT, Conformity.
**Example in Radiotherapy:** Dual arc reduces hotspots in pelvic treatments.

212. **Dynamic couch tracking (noun):** Real-time adjustment of couch position to follow tumor motion.
**Related Terms:** Motion management, 4D RT.
**Example in Radiotherapy:** Dynamic couch tracking compensates for breathing motion.

213. **Dynamic MLC delivery (noun):** Continuous leaf movement during dose delivery.
**Related Terms:** Sliding window, IMRT.
**Example in Radiotherapy:** Dynamic MLC delivery shapes fluence precisely.

214. **Dynamic MRI (noun):** Rapid MRI sequences capturing motion or perfusion changes.
**Related Terms:** MR-LINAC, Functional imaging.
**Example in Radiotherapy:** Dynamic MRI used for online adaptive planning.

215. **Dynamic wedge (noun):** Electronic control of beam intensity to simulate wedge effect.
**Related Terms:** Enhanced dynamic wedge, Beam modulation.
**Example in Radiotherapy:** Dynamic wedge replaces physical wedges in LINACs.

216. **Dyne (noun):** Unit of force in CGS system used in beam mechanics.
**Related Terms:** Pressure, Mechanical load.
**Example in Radiotherapy:** Gantry bearings designed to withstand dyne-level forces.

217. **Dyspigmentation (noun):** Change in skin color post-irradiation due to melanocyte damage.
**Related Terms:** Skin toxicity, Late effect.
**Example in Radiotherapy:** Dyspigmentation monitored as a chronic side effect.

218. **Dynamic trajectory (noun):** Beam path adjusted in real time to match target motion.
**Related Terms:** MR-guidance, Adaptive therapy.
**Example in Radiotherapy:** MR-LINAC supports dynamic trajectory beam delivery.

219. **Dwell position (noun):** Source stopping point during brachytherapy.
**Related Terms:** HDR, Dwell time.
**Example in Radiotherapy:** Optimization of dwell positions enhances dose conformity.

220. **Dwell time (noun):** Duration the radioactive source stays at each dwell position.
**Related Terms:** Brachytherapy, Source control.
**Example in Radiotherapy:** Dwell time adjusted for target coverage.

221. **Diffusion-weighted MRI (noun):** Imaging technique measuring water molecule motion.
**Related Terms:** ADC map, MR-LINAC.
**Example in Radiotherapy:** DWI used for tumor response monitoring.

222. **Deep inspiration breath hold (noun):** Technique using patient's breath hold to minimize motion.
**Related Terms:** Motion management, Breast RT.
**Example in Radiotherapy:** DIBH reduces cardiac dose in left breast cancer.

223. **Dose-volume constraint (noun):** Limit on dose to specific organ volume.
**Related Terms:** DVH, Planning.
**Example in Radiotherapy:** V30 < 30% constraint applied for liver.

224. **Dose-volume histogram (noun):** A graphical representation showing the distribution of dose across a volume of interest.
**Related Terms:** DVH, Dosimetry.
**Example in Radiotherapy:** DVH used to assess PTV coverage and OAR sparing.

225. **Dose-volume optimization (noun):** Process of refining treatment plans based on dose-volume parameters.
**Related Terms:** IMRT, Inverse planning.
**Example in Radiotherapy:** Dose-volume optimization minimizes lung V20 in thoracic cases.

226. **Dose-weighted imaging (noun):** MRI technique integrating dose information with anatomical data.
**Related Terms:** MR-LINAC, Adaptive radiotherapy.
**Example in Radiotherapy:** Dose-weighted imaging guides adaptive planning during MR-LINAC sessions.

227. **Dosimetric audit (noun):** Independent verification of dose accuracy across institutions.
**Related Terms:** QA, Benchmarking.
**Example in Radiotherapy:** IAEA conducts dosimetric audits for quality assurance.

228. **Dosimetric uncertainty (noun):** Error margin in calculated or measured dose values.
**Related Terms:** Calibration, QA.
**Example in Radiotherapy:** Dosimetric uncertainty limited to 2% for clinical safety.

229. **Dose-guided radiotherapy (noun):** Adaptive therapy technique adjusting delivery based on measured dose feedback.
**Related Terms:** IGRT, Adaptive therapy.
**Example in Radiotherapy:** MR-LINAC enables dose-guided corrections during treatment.

230. **Dose-tracking system (noun):** Real-time monitoring system for cumulative radiation dose.
**Related Terms:** QA, Imaging dose.
**Example in Radiotherapy:** Dose-tracking prevents excessive imaging exposure in adaptive treatments.

231. **Dose-cuboid (noun):** Three-dimensional matrix representing dose distribution.
**Related Terms:** Dose grid, Planning.
**Example in Radiotherapy:** Dose-cuboid analyzed to compute DVHs.

232. **Dose-per-pulse (noun):** Radiation dose delivered in one pulse of the beam.
**Related Terms:** Linac output, FLASH therapy.
**Example in Radiotherapy:** FLASH therapy involves ultra-high dose-per-pulse delivery.

233. **Dose-mapping (noun):** Visualization of dose levels superimposed on anatomical structures.
**Related Terms:** Isodose lines, QA.
**Example in Radiotherapy:** Dose-mapping performed to verify treatment accuracy.

234. **Dose painting by numbers (noun):** Voxel-level modulation of dose using biological imaging data.
**Related Terms:** PET-guided RT, Dose escalation.
**Example in Radiotherapy:** DPBN enhances dose to hypoxic tumor sub regions.

235. **Dose perturbation factor (noun):** Correction applied for heterogeneity-induced dose variations.
**Related Terms:** Density correction, Monte Carlo.
**Example in Radiotherapy:** Dose perturbation factor improves lung plan accuracy.

236. **Dose prescription point (noun):** Specific reference location for dose normalization.
**Related Terms:** ICRU reference point, Dosimetry.
**Example in Radiotherapy:** Dose prescription point defined at PTV centroid.

237. **Dose verification phantom (noun):** Model used for validating 3D dose distributions.
**Related Terms:** QA, Calibration.
**Example in Radiotherapy:** Gafchromic film inserted in verification phantom for end-to-end testing.

238. **Dose-adaptive planning (noun):** Dynamic adjustment of treatment plan based on delivered dose.
**Related Terms:** Adaptive RT, MR-guided RT.
**Example in Radiotherapy:** MR-LINAC supports daily dose-adaptive planning.

239. **Dose-based gating (noun):** Beam control synchronized with dose accumulation and motion.
**Related Terms:** Respiratory gating, Real-time tracking.
**Example in Radiotherapy:** Dose-based gating enhances lung tumor accuracy.

240. **Dose-based planning (noun):** Optimization centered on achieving specific dose outcomes.
**Related Terms:** Inverse planning, Objective weighting.
**Example in Radiotherapy:** Dose-based planning balances tumor coverage with OAR sparing.

241. **Dose conformity score (noun):** Quantitative measure assessing treatment plan conformity.
**Related Terms:** CI, QA.
**Example in Radiotherapy:** Higher conformity score indicates optimal target coverage.

242. **Dose effectiveness (noun):** Measure of biological effectiveness of delivered dose.
**Related Terms:** RBE, LET.
**Example in Radiotherapy:** Proton therapy achieves higher dose effectiveness in hypoxic tumors.

243. **Dose enhancement ratio (noun):** Ratio comparing dose with and without sensitizer presence.
**Related Terms:** Radio sensitizer, Radiobiology.
**Example in Radiotherapy:** Gold nanoparticles show a dose enhancement ratio above 1.3.

244. **Dose equivalent (noun):** Product of absorbed dose and radiation weighting factor.
**Related Terms:** Sievert, Radiation protection.
**Example in Radiotherapy:** Occupational dose equivalent monitored in mSv units.

245. **Dose fraction (noun):** Single treatment dose within a multi-session plan.
**Related Terms:** Fractionation, BED.
**Example in Radiotherapy:** A 2 Gy dose fraction used in conventional EBRT.

246. **Dose heterogeneity index (noun):** Metric indicating dose variation within target volume.
**Related Terms:** HI, PTV coverage.
**Example in Radiotherapy:** HI maintained below 0.15 for homogeneity.

247. **Dose intercomparison (noun):** Comparative analysis of dose distributions among centers.
**Related Terms:** QA, Standardization.
**Example in Radiotherapy:** IAEA conducts dose intercomparison for uniformity.

248. **Dose kernel convolution (noun):** Mathematical operation to calculate 3D dose from fluence.
**Related Terms:** TPS, Monte Carlo.
**Example in Radiotherapy:** Convolution–superposition algorithms use dose kernels for accuracy.

249. **Dose linear accelerator (noun):** LINAC capable of precise dose modulation and beam control.
**Related Terms:** IMRT, MR-LINAC.
**Example in Radiotherapy:** MR-LINAC functions as an advanced dose linear accelerator.

**250. Dose map registration (noun):** Alignment of planned and delivered dose maps.
**Related Terms:** Image registration, QA.
**Example in Radiotherapy:** Dose map registration used for adaptive verification.

**251. Dose modulation index (noun):** Indicator of beam modulation complexity in IMRT/VMAT.
**Related Terms:** MU, QA.
**Example in Radiotherapy:** Higher modulation index correlates with plan complexity.

**252. Dose optimization constraint (noun):** Defined limit guiding plan optimization to protect OARs.
**Related Terms:** Inverse planning, DVH.
**Example in Radiotherapy:** Spinal cord constraint set to <45 Gy.

**253. Dose planning system (noun):** Software platform for designing and optimizing treatment plans.
**Related Terms:** TPS, Planning.
**Example in Radiotherapy:** Eclipse TPS used for photon and proton plan generation.

**254. Dose prescription volume (noun):** Region receiving the prescribed dose.
**Related Terms:** PTV, Coverage.
**Example in Radiotherapy:** Prescription volume encompasses 95% isodose line.

**255. Dose recovery (noun):** Restoration of radiation response after sublethal damage.
**Related Terms:** DNA repair, Fractionation.
**Example in Radiotherapy:** Normal tissues exhibit dose recovery between fractions.

**256. Dose threshold (noun):** Minimum dose required to elicit a measurable biological effect.
**Related Terms:** Deterministic effect, Radiobiology.
**Example in Radiotherapy:** Lens opacity occurs beyond 0.5 Gy threshold.

**257. Dose tracking algorithm (noun):** Computational method for real-time dose accumulation tracking.
**Related Terms:** MR-guided RT, Adaptive planning.
**Example in Radiotherapy:** Dose tracking algorithms improve precision during motion.

**258. Dose verification system (noun):** Integrated hardware and software for validating dose delivery.
**Related Terms:** QA, Portal dosimetry.
**Example in Radiotherapy:** EPID-based systems ensure accurate dose verification.

**259. Dose-volume constraint violation (noun):** When planned dose exceeds set DVH limits.
**Related Terms:** QA, Planning error.
**Example in Radiotherapy:** Re-optimization performed upon OAR constraint violation.

**260. Dose-volume histogram analysis (noun):** Evaluation of dose metrics using DVH data.
**Related Terms:** QA, Plan review.
**Example in Radiotherapy:** DVH analysis ensures OAR compliance.

**261. Dose-volume optimization algorithm (noun):** Software logic to refine beam parameters for ideal dose distribution.
**Related Terms:** Inverse planning, Machine learning.
**Example in Radiotherapy:** AI-assisted algorithms improve proton plan efficiency.

**262. Dose-weighted LET (noun):** Linear energy transfer weighted by delivered dose.
**Related Terms:** RBE, Proton therapy.
**Example in Radiotherapy:** Dose-weighted LET maps highlight biological dose hotspots.

**263. Double scattering system (noun):** Proton beam shaping setup using dual scattering foils.
**Related Terms:** Passive scattering, Range modulation.
**Example in Radiotherapy:** Double scattering system ensures uniform SOBP.

264. **Dynamic adaptive radiotherapy (noun):** Continuous adaptation of treatment based on anatomical changes.
**Related Terms:** MR-LINAC, Real-time planning.
**Example in Radiotherapy:** MR-LINAC supports dynamic adaptive radiotherapy workflows.

265. **Dynamic beam delivery (noun):** Real-time beam control synchronized with tumor motion.
**Related Terms:** Gated therapy, Motion management.
**Example in Radiotherapy:** Dynamic delivery enhances lung SBRT precision.

266. **Dynamic dose painting (noun):** Modulation of radiation intensity according to temporal biological changes.
**Related Terms:** Functional imaging, Adaptive therapy.
**Example in Radiotherapy:** Dynamic dose painting guided by serial PET scans.

267. **Dynamic MRI-guided therapy (noun):** Real-time radiotherapy guided by MR imaging feedback.
**Related Terms:** MR-LINAC, Adaptive RT.
**Example in Radiotherapy:** Dynamic MRI-guided therapy enables intrafraction motion adaptation.

268. **Dynamic multileaf collimator (noun):** MLC operating with continuous leaf motion during dose delivery.
**Related Terms:** IMRT, Fluence modulation.
**Example in Radiotherapy:** DMLC used for sliding window IMRT.

269. **Dynamic proton therapy (noun):** Proton delivery synchronized with tumor motion and dose adaptation.
**Related Terms:** Pencil beam scanning, Gated therapy.
**Example in Radiotherapy:** Dynamic proton therapy reduces interplay effects.

270. **Dynamic tumor tracking (noun):** Continuous localization and beam adaptation to tumor motion.
**Related Terms:** Real-time tracking, MR-guided RT.
**Example in Radiotherapy:** Dynamic tracking applied in liver and lung treatments.

271. **Dynamic wedge filter (noun):** Electronic or mechanical device simulating a physical wedge.
**Related Terms:** Beam shaping, Compensator.
**Example in Radiotherapy:** Dynamic wedge filter replaces manual wedge setups.

272. **Differential dose-volume histogram (noun):** Histogram displaying voxel dose frequency distribution.
**Related Terms:** Cumulative DVH, Plan evaluation.
**Example in Radiotherapy:** DDVH used for detailed plan comparisons.

273. **Differential linear energy transfer (noun):** LET value variation across beam path.
**Related Terms:** RBE, Proton therapy.
**Example in Radiotherapy:** Differential LET analyzed for biological dose mapping.

274. **Digital beam shaping (noun):** Electronic control of beam intensity and geometry.
**Related Terms:** IMRT, Adaptive delivery.
**Example in Radiotherapy:** Digital shaping enhances accuracy in photon beams.

275. **Dose reference point (noun):** A specific point used for dose prescription or reporting within a treatment volume.
**Related Terms:** ICRU reference point, Prescription point.
**Example in Radiotherapy:** The dose reference point is set at the isocenter for SBRT planning.

276. **Dose reconstruction (noun):** Process of estimating delivered dose using imaging or log files.
**Related Terms:** Dose verification, In vivo dosimetry.
**Example in Radiotherapy:** Dose reconstruction used to analyze patient-specific QA outcomes.

277. **Dose uniformity (noun):** Consistency of dose distribution within a target volume.
**Related Terms:** Homogeneity, Dose gradient.
**Example in Radiotherapy:** Dose uniformity within ±5% achieved for whole-breast irradiation.

278. **Dose variation (noun):** Deviation from prescribed dose within the treatment volume.
**Related Terms:** Heterogeneity, Dose distribution.
**Example in Radiotherapy:** Dose variation observed due to patient motion during prostate IMRT.

279. **Dose verification (noun):** Validation of the planned versus delivered dose using measurement systems.
**Related Terms:** Quality assurance, Dosimetry audit.
**Example in Radiotherapy:** Portal dosimetry used for dose verification in IMRT fields.

280. **Dose-volume constraint (noun):** Limits applied to organs or targets in treatment planning.
**Related Terms:** DVH, OAR tolerance.
**Example in Radiotherapy:** Dose-volume constraints for rectum followed as per RTOG guidelines.

281. **Dose-volume histogram (DVH) (noun):** Graphical representation of dose distribution across structures.
**Related Terms:** Cumulative DVH, Differential DVH.
**Example in Radiotherapy:** DVH analysis ensures 95% of PTV receives prescribed dose.

282. **Dose-volume optimization (noun):** Planning technique balancing dose between tumor and normal tissue.
**Related Terms:** IMRT, Inverse planning.
**Example in Radiotherapy:** Dose-volume optimization improved conformity in head-and-neck plan.

283. **Dosimetric accuracy (noun):** Precision of dose measurement or delivery compared to prescription.
**Related Terms:** Calibration, Tolerance limit.
**Example in Radiotherapy:** Dosimetric accuracy verified through end-to-end testing.

284. **Dosimetric leaf gap (noun):** Difference between physical and effective MLC leaf positions.
**Related Terms:** MLC modeling, Beam commissioning.
**Example in Radiotherapy:** Dosimetric leaf gap measured during IMRT QA process.

285. **Dosimetric verification (noun):** Measurement confirming planned versus delivered dose distribution.
**Related Terms:** QA, Film dosimetry.
**Example in Radiotherapy:** Dosimetric verification performed with ion chamber array.

286. **Dosimetry audit (noun):** External review of dose measurement and delivery practices.
**Related Terms:** QA audit, TLD.
**Example in Radiotherapy:** National dosimetry audit ensured accuracy of institutional dose delivery.

287. **Dosimetry calibration (noun):** Adjustment of dosimeters or equipment to reference standards.
**Related Terms:** Standardization, Traceability.
**Example in Radiotherapy:** Ion chamber calibrated annually using cobalt-60 reference.

288. **Dosimetry phantom (noun):** Model used to simulate patient geometry for dose measurement.
**Related Terms:** Water phantom, anthropomorphic phantom.
**Example in Radiotherapy:** Solid water phantom used for patient-specific QA.

289. **Double scattering (noun):** Proton beam broadening technique using two scattering foils.
**Related Terms:** Passive scattering, Beam shaping.
**Example in Proton Therapy:** Double scattering used in uniform dose delivery.

290. **Dynamic arc therapy (noun):** Rotational radiotherapy where dose rate and MLCs vary continuously.
**Related Terms:** VMAT, Arc modulation.
**Example in Radiotherapy:** Dynamic arc therapy reduced treatment time by 40%.

291. **Dynamic beam delivery (noun):** Radiation delivery with continuously moving components.
**Related Terms:** Modulated delivery, VMAT.
**Example in Radiotherapy:** Dynamic beam delivery improves conformity for moving targets.

292. **Dynamic couch rotation (noun):** Couch moves during radiation beam-on to optimize dose.
**Related Terms:** Non-coplanar delivery, Adaptive geometry.
**Example in Radiotherapy:** Dynamic couch rotation applied in HyperArc planning.

293. **Dynamic gating (noun):** Delivery technique synchronized with patient's breathing cycle.
**Related Terms:** Respiratory gating, 4D radiotherapy.
**Example in Radiotherapy:** Dynamic gating reduced cardiac dose during breast irradiation.

294. **Dynamic MLC tracking (noun):** Real-time adjustment of MLC leaves to track moving tumors.
**Related Terms:** Tumor tracking, Adaptive delivery.
Example in MR-LINAC: Dynamic MLC tracking compensates for intra-fraction motion.

295. **Dynamic planning (noun):** Plan updated with changing anatomy or tumor position.
**Related Terms:** Adaptive planning, Re-optimization.
**Example in Radiotherapy:** Dynamic planning used in MR-guided adaptive sessions.

296. **Dynamic wedge (noun):** Electronic method to achieve wedge-shaped dose distribution.
**Related Terms:** Enhanced dynamic wedge, Physical wedge.
**Example in Radiotherapy:** Dynamic wedge improves dose homogeneity in tangential breast fields.

297. **Dysplasia (noun):** Abnormal tissue growth, precursor to malignancy.
**Related Terms:** Precancerous lesion, Cellular atypia.
**Example in Radiotherapy:** Dysplastic tissue changes monitored post-irradiation.

298. **Dwell position (noun):** Location where brachytherapy source stops to deliver dose.
**Related Terms:** Dwell time, Source loading.
**Example in Radiotherapy:** Dwell positions optimized for uniform vaginal cuff dose.

299. **Dwell time (noun):** Duration the radioactive source remains at a dwell position.
**Related Terms:** HDR brachytherapy, Source loading.
**Example in Radiotherapy:** Shorter dwell time used near rectum to reduce exposure.

300. **Dynamic image registration (noun):** Alignment of images accounting for motion or deformation.
**Related Terms:** Deformable registration, 4D imaging.
Example in MR-LINAC: Dynamic registration supports adaptive contouring.

301. **DynaLog file (noun):** File recording MLC positions and dose rate during IMRT.
**Related Terms:** Delivery log, QA verification.
**Example in Radiotherapy:** DynaLog analysis validated VMAT delivery accuracy.

302. **Deep inspiration breath hold (DIBH) (noun):** Technique reducing heart dose by irradiating during deep inspiration.
**Related Terms:** Respiratory gating, Motion management.
**Example in Radiotherapy:** DIBH used in left breast cancer treatments.

303. **Dose recalculation (noun):** Re-evaluation of dose on updated anatomy or setup.
**Related Terms:** Adaptive planning, Re-optimization.
**Example in Radiotherapy:** Dose recalculation confirms changes post-repositioning.

304. **Dose recomputation (noun):** Re-evaluation of dose distribution using updated anatomical or imaging data.
**Related Terms:** Adaptive radiotherapy, Dose recalculation.
**Example in Radiotherapy:** Dose recomputation done after organ motion detected on CBCT.

305. **Dose reduction technique (noun):** Methods applied to minimize patient or staff radiation exposure.
**Related Terms:** ALARA, Shielding.
**Example in Radiotherapy:** Image acquisition protocols modified for dose reduction in CBCT.

306. **Dose reporting point (noun):** Standardized point within a volume for dose documentation.
**Related Terms:** Reference point, ICRU report.
**Example in Radiotherapy:** ICRU dose reporting point set in target centroid.

307. **Dose response curve (noun):** Graph showing biological response as a function of dose.
**Related Terms:** Survival curve, Radiobiology.
**Example in Radiotherapy:** Dose response curve plotted for clonogenic cell survival.

308. **Dose sculpting (noun):** Selective shaping of dose to match irregular tumor geometry.
**Related Terms:** IMRT, Conformity.
**Example in Radiotherapy:** Dose sculpting achieved with VMAT for skull base tumors.

309. **Dose shaper (noun):** Device or algorithm used to modify beam intensity or shape.
**Related Terms:** Modulator, Collimator.
**Example in Radiotherapy:** MLC acts as a dynamic dose shaper during IMRT.

310. **Dose surface map (noun):** 2D projection showing dose distribution on organ surface.
**Related Terms:** Dose visualization, QA tool.
**Example in Radiotherapy:** Rectal dose surface map used to evaluate hotspot areas.

311. **Dose tolerance (noun):** Maximum safe radiation dose a tissue can receive without complication.
**Related Terms:** TD5/5, OAR.
**Example in Radiotherapy:** Liver dose tolerance limited to 30 Gy mean dose.

312. **Dose tracking (noun):** Monitoring cumulative or fractionated dose during treatment.
**Related Terms:** Dose accumulation, Adaptive planning.
**Example in Radiotherapy:** Dose tracking ensures organ-at-risk limits are maintained.

313. **Dose uncertainty (noun):** Variation between planned and actual delivered dose.
**Related Terms:** Dosimetric error, Calibration.
**Example in Radiotherapy:** MR-LINAC reduces dose uncertainty using real-time imaging.

314. **Dose uniformity index (noun):** Quantitative measure of dose consistency within target.
**Related Terms:** Homogeneity index, Conformity index.
**Example in Radiotherapy:** Dose uniformity index improved with optimized IMRT.

315. **Dose verification software (noun):** Program used to compare measured and planned dose distributions.
**Related Terms:** QA tools, Gamma analysis.
**Example in Radiotherapy:** DoseLab software used for 3D dose verification.

316. **Dosimeter array (noun):** Grid-based detector system for measuring dose distribution.
**Related Terms:** QA, Detector matrix.
**Example in Radiotherapy:** Ion chamber array used for patient-specific QA in IMRT.

317. **Dosimetric conformity (noun):** Degree to which delivered dose matches target shape and size.
**Related Terms:** Conformity index, Isodose shaping.
**Example in Radiotherapy:** High dosimetric conformity achieved with stereotactic beams.

318. **Dosimetric comparison (noun):** Evaluation of dose distributions between two or more plans.
**Related Terms:** Plan evaluation, DVH analysis.
**Example in Radiotherapy:** Dosimetric comparison made between IMRT and proton plans.

319. **Dosimetric gradient (noun):** Rate of dose fall-off between target and surrounding tissue.
**Related Terms:** Dose fall-off, Penumbra.
**Example in Radiotherapy:** Sharp dosimetric gradient achieved in SRS for brain lesions.

320. **Dosimetric validation (noun):** Experimental confirmation of dose calculation accuracy.
**Related Terms:** QA verification, Benchmarking.
**Example in Radiotherapy:** Dosimetric validation ensures TPS accuracy before clinical use.

321. **Dosimetry log (noun):** Record of calibration and measurement data in radiotherapy.
**Related Terms:** QA documentation, Dose record.
**Example in Radiotherapy:** Daily output constancy values documented in dosimetry log.

322. **Dosimetry quality assurance (noun):** Procedures ensuring dose delivery accuracy and consistency.
**Related Terms:** QA, Calibration.
**Example in Radiotherapy:** Comprehensive dosimetry QA performed during LINAC commissioning.

323. **Dosimetry system (noun):** Combination of detectors, electrometers, and software for dose measurement.
**Related Terms:** QA system, Calibration unit.
**Example in Radiotherapy:** 3D dosimetry system used for volumetric QA.

324. **Dose-weighted DVH (noun):** DVH reflecting relative biological effectiveness of delivered dose.
**Related Terms:** Biological DVH, RBE correction.
**Example in Proton Therapy:** Dose-weighted DVH used for RBE-adjusted evaluation.

325. **Double arc VMAT (noun):** Two rotational beam delivery arcs for enhanced modulation.
**Related Terms:** Arc therapy, IMRT.
**Example in Radiotherapy:** Double arc VMAT improves dose homogeneity in pelvic treatments.

326. **Dual-energy CT (noun):** CT imaging using two X-ray spectra for material differentiation.
**Related Terms:** Spectral imaging, Treatment planning.
**Example in Radiotherapy:** Dual-energy CT improves tissue density estimation for proton therapy.

327. **Dual isocenter plan (noun):** Treatment plan using two separate isocenters for extended targets.
**Related Terms:** Junction dose, Plan matching.
**Example in Radiotherapy:** Dual isocenter plan used in craniospinal irradiation.

328. **Dual scatterers system (noun):** Proton beam modifier using two scattering foils for dose uniformity.
**Related Terms:** Passive scattering, Beam shaping.
**Example in Proton Therapy:** Dual scatterers system ensures flat dose across the field.

329. **Dynamic adaptive radiotherapy (noun):** Real-time dose adjustment during treatment delivery.
**Related Terms:** MR-LINAC, On-table adaptation.
**Example in Radiotherapy:** Dynamic adaptive planning used for bladder tumor adaptation.

330. **Dynamic beam modulation (noun):** Continuous beam intensity variation during delivery.
**Related Terms:** IMRT, Arc therapy.
**Example in Radiotherapy:** Dynamic beam modulation enhances target conformity.

331. **Dynamic couch trajectory (noun):** Predefined couch path during non-coplanar beam delivery.
**Related Terms:** Non-coplanar arcs, HyperArc.
**Example in Radiotherapy:** Dynamic couch trajectory improves cranial plan efficiency.

332. **Dynamic dose control (noun):** Real-time regulation of dose rate during treatment.
**Related Terms:** Beam modulation, Feedback system.
Example in MR-LINAC: Dynamic dose control compensates for anatomical motion.

**333. Dynamic isocenter shift (noun):** Automatic adjustment of isocenter position during treatment.
**Related Terms:** Adaptive delivery, Couch correction.
**Example in Radiotherapy:** Dynamic isocenter shift reduces geometric uncertainty in SRS.

**334. Dynamic multileaf collimation (noun):** Continuous leaf motion to shape intensity-modulated fields.
**Related Terms:** IMRT, MLC tracking.
**Example in Radiotherapy:** Dynamic MLC enhances dose sculpting for head and neck targets.

**335. Dynamic tumor tracking (noun):** Beam targeting that follows tumor motion in real-time.
**Related Terms:** Motion management, 4D radiotherapy.
**Example in Radiotherapy:** Dynamic tumor tracking used for lung SBRT on MR-LINAC.

**336. Dose summation (noun):** Cumulative addition of delivered dose over multiple sessions.
**Related Terms:** Dose accumulation, Fractionation.
**Example in Radiotherapy:** Dose summation performed after adaptive plan modification.

**337. Dose validation (noun):** Comparison of planned and delivered dose for accuracy check.
**Related Terms:** QA, Verification.
**Example in Radiotherapy:** Portal dosimetry performed for dose validation before first fraction.

**338. Dose-volume optimization (noun):** Algorithmic approach to achieve ideal target coverage with OAR sparing.
**Related Terms:** IMRT, Inverse planning.
**Example in Radiotherapy:** Dose-volume optimization refined to meet rectum constraints.

**339. Differential DVH (noun):** Histogram showing dose-frequency distribution within a structure.
**Related Terms:** Cumulative DVH, Plan evaluation.
**Example in Radiotherapy:** Differential DVH used to assess dose heterogeneity.

**340. Digital radiography (noun):** Imaging technique using digital detectors for X-ray capture.
**Related Terms:** DR, Image-guided therapy.
**Example in Radiotherapy:** Digital radiography used for patient setup verification.

**341. Dual-energy proton therapy (noun):** Use of multiple proton energies for optimized dose distribution.
**Related Terms:** Range modulation, Bragg peak.
**Example in Proton Therapy:** Dual-energy proton planning reduces distal fall-off uncertainty.

**342. Deep dose equivalent (noun):** Measure of external radiation dose at tissue depth of 1 cm.
**Related Terms:** Occupational dose, Dosimetry.
**Example in Radiotherapy:** Deep dose equivalent monitored for staff exposure.

**343. Deformable dose accumulation (noun):** Combining doses from multiple sessions using deformable registration.
**Related Terms:** Adaptive therapy, Dose mapping.
**Example in Radiotherapy:** Deformable dose accumulation ensures accurate cumulative DVH.

**344. Deformable image registration (noun):** Technique aligning images accounting for anatomical deformations.
**Related Terms:** Adaptive radiotherapy, 4D registration.
**Example in Radiotherapy:** Deformable image registration aligns CBCT with planning CT for dose recalculation.

**345. Deformable structure propagation (noun):** Automatic contour adjustment across different image datasets.
**Related Terms:** Auto-segmentation, Adaptive planning.
Example in MR-LINAC: Deformable propagation used for organ recontouring in adaptive workflow.

346. **Delta volume (noun):** Change in volume between planning and daily anatomy.
**Related Terms:** Adaptive planning, Dose adaptation.
**Example in Radiotherapy:** Delta volume analysis revealed rectal filling variation in prostate treatment.

347. **Density override (noun):** Manual adjustment of CT Hounsfield units for dose calculation accuracy.
**Related Terms:** TPS correction, Heterogeneity correction.
**Example in Radiotherapy:** Density override applied to prosthetic implant regions.

348. **Density correction (noun):** Algorithm accounting for tissue heterogeneity in dose computation.
**Related Terms:** Inhomogeneity correction, Monte Carlo.
**Example in Radiotherapy:** Density correction improved lung plan accuracy.

349. **Depth dose curve (noun):** Graph showing dose variation with depth in tissue.
**Related Terms:** PDD, Beam data.
**Example in Radiotherapy:** Depth dose curve used for photon beam commissioning.

350. **Depth of maximum dose (noun):** Depth where absorbed dose reaches its maximum value.
**Related Terms:** Dmax, PDD.
**Example in Radiotherapy:** 6 MV photon beam has Dmax at 1.5 cm depth.

351. **Depth dose profile (noun):** Dose distribution along beam axis within phantom.
**Related Terms:** PDD, Beam data.
**Example in Radiotherapy:** Depth dose profile analyzed for flattening filter-free beams.

352. **Detector calibration (noun):** Process ensuring detector readings match known reference doses.
**Related Terms:** Dosimetry, QA.
**Example in Radiotherapy:** Detector calibration verified during annual LINAC QA.

353. **Detector linearity (noun):** Proportional response of detector signal to varying dose levels.
**Related Terms:** QA, Response curve.
**Example in Radiotherapy:** Detector linearity confirmed for IMRT dose verification.

354. **Detector saturation (noun):** Condition where detector fails to record higher dose due to limit.
**Related Terms:** Dynamic range, Dose response.
**Example in Radiotherapy:** Ion chamber saturation avoided using appropriate bias voltage.

355. **Deterministic effect (noun):** Radiation effect with threshold dose, severity increases with dose.
**Related Terms:** Tissue reaction, Dose threshold.
**Example in Radiobiology:** Skin erythema is a deterministic effect above 2 Gy.

356. **Diagnostic reference level (noun):** Standard dose level for typical imaging procedure optimization.
**Related Terms:** DRL, Dose benchmarking.
Example in Radiology: DRLs help minimize CT dose during simulation scans.

357. **Diffusion-weighted imaging (noun):** MRI technique detecting tissue microstructural changes via water diffusion.
**Related Terms:** MRI, ADC map.
Example in MR-guided therapy: Diffusion-weighted imaging aids adaptive tumor delineation.

358. **Digital beam monitoring (noun):** Real-time tracking of beam output and position via sensors.
**Related Terms:** QA, Beam control.
Example in MR-LINAC: Digital beam monitoring ensures consistent dose delivery.

359. **Digital reconstruction radiograph (DRR) (noun):** Computed 2D image from 3D CT data for setup alignment.
**Related Terms:** Image registration, Simulation.
**Example in Radiotherapy:** DRR compared with portal image for patient verification.

360. **Digitally reconstructed plan (noun):** Recreated treatment plan for verification or research.
**Related Terms:** Retrospective analysis, QA.
**Example in Radiotherapy:** Digitally reconstructed plan used for dosimetric validation.

361. **Direct aperture optimization (noun):** IMRT planning method optimizing MLC shapes directly.
**Related Terms:** Inverse planning, Segment optimization.
**Example in Radiotherapy:** Direct aperture optimization shortened planning time for IMRT.

362. **Direct Monte Carlo calculation (noun):** Accurate dose calculation using stochastic particle transport simulation.
**Related Terms:** Monte Carlo algorithm, Dose accuracy.
**Example in Proton Therapy:** Direct Monte Carlo used for heterogeneity correction in lung plans.

363. **Displacement vector field (noun):** Data map representing voxel-wise movement between two images.
**Related Terms:** Deformable registration, Image fusion.
**Example in Radiotherapy:** DVF generated during adaptive MR-LINAC workflow.

364. **Display field of view (noun):** Visible area of image display on console.
**Related Terms:** FOV, Image scaling.
**Example in Radiotherapy:** Smaller display field improves soft tissue contrast.

365. **Dose accumulation (noun):** Summation of delivered doses over all fractions accounting for motion.
**Related Terms:** Adaptive planning, Deformable mapping.
Example in MR-guided therapy: Dose accumulation ensures accurate biological dose evaluation.

366. **Dose adaptive workflow (noun):** Clinical process adjusting dose plan per anatomical change.
**Related Terms:** Adaptive radiotherapy, MR-LINAC.
**Example in Radiotherapy:** Dose adaptive workflow implemented for online prostate therapy.

367. **Dose averaging (noun):** Mean dose computed across variable anatomy or phase.
**Related Terms:** 4D planning, Accumulated dose.
**Example in Radiotherapy:** Dose averaging reduces uncertainty in respiratory-correlated imaging.

368. **Dose benchmark (noun):** Reference standard for evaluating dose delivery quality.
**Related Terms:** QA protocol, Audit.
**Example in Radiotherapy:** Dose benchmark based on AAPM TG reports.

369. **Dose calibration factor (noun):** Conversion coefficient relating measured charge to absorbed dose.
**Related Terms:** Dosimetry, Ion chamber.
**Example in Radiotherapy:** Dose calibration factor verified annually for primary chamber.

370. **Dose cloud (noun):** 3D visualization of Isodose distribution.
**Related Terms:** Dose contour, Treatment planning.
**Example in Radiotherapy:** Dose cloud displayed for stereotactic brain plan review.

371. **Dose computation grid (noun):** Spatial resolution used for dose calculation within TPS.
**Related Terms:** Grid spacing, Accuracy.
**Example in Radiotherapy:** Finer dose grid improves small-field accuracy.

372. **Dose conformity index (noun):** Ratio assessing dose coverage relative to target volume.
**Related Terms:** Paddick index, Conformity.
**Example in Radiotherapy:** High dose conformity index achieved in SBRT lung plans.

373. **Dose contour (noun):** Line representing equal dose on a planar display.
**Related Terms:** Isodose line, Dose distribution.
**Example in Radiotherapy:** 95% dose contour covers the entire PTV.

374. **Dose crosstalk (noun):** Interaction between adjacent fields causing overlapping dose.
**Related Terms:** Field junction, IMRT.
**Example in Radiotherapy:** Dose crosstalk minimized by feathering junctions.

375. **Dose decay (noun):** Reduction in dose due to radioactive decay or attenuation.
**Related Terms:** Decay correction, Brachytherapy.
**Example in Radiotherapy:** Dose decay corrected daily for HDR Ir-192 source.

376. **Dose distribution uniformity (noun):** Evenness of dose delivery across target volume.
**Related Terms:** Homogeneity, Conformity.
**Example in Radiotherapy:** Dose uniformity achieved using dynamic wedge compensation.

377. **Dose gradient index (noun):** Measure of how sharply dose falls off outside target.
**Related Terms:** Conformity, Gradient measure.
Example in SRS: Low gradient index indicates rapid dose fall-off.

378. **Dose kernel (noun):** Mathematical model describing energy deposition from a point source.
**Related Terms:** Convolution, Scatter modeling.
**Example in Radiotherapy:** Dose kernel used in convolution/superposition algorithm.

379. **Dose mapping (noun):** Visualization of dose overlayed on patient anatomy.
**Related Terms:** Dose accumulation, QA.
Example in MR-LINAC: Dose mapping performed after adaptive delivery.

380. **Dose modulation (noun):** Variation in intensity across radiation field for optimized distribution.
**Related Terms:** IMRT, Inverse planning.
**Example in Radiotherapy:** Dose modulation minimizes OAR exposure in head-and-neck plans.

381. **Dose normalization (noun):** Adjustment of dose distribution relative to a reference point or volume.
**Related Terms:** Prescription dose, Scaling.
**Example in Radiotherapy:** Plans normalized to 95% PTV coverage.

382. **Dose output constancy (noun):** Stability of machine output over time.
**Related Terms:** QA, Calibration.
**Example in Radiotherapy:** Daily QA verifies 1% dose output constancy.

383. **Dose painting (noun):** Technique assigning different dose levels to sub-volumes within tumor.
**Related Terms:** Biological planning, PET-guided therapy.
**Example in Radiotherapy:** Dose painting used for hypoxic tumor regions.

384. **Dose prescription point (noun):** Location within target where prescribed dose defined.
**Related Terms:** Reference point, ICRU 50.
**Example in Radiotherapy:** Dose prescribed at isocenter for SBRT.

385. **Dose rate modulation (noun):** Dynamic adjustment of dose rate during beam-on delivery.
**Related Terms:** VMAT, Intensity modulation.
**Example in Radiotherapy:** Dose rate modulation ensures smooth transition between control points.

386. **Dose recalibration (noun):** Re-measurement of output to correct calibration errors.
**Related Terms:** QA, Machine maintenance.
**Example in Radiotherapy:** Dose recalibration performed after component replacement.

387. **Dose reduction algorithm (noun):** Software function optimizing image or beam settings for lower exposure.
**Related Terms:** ALARA, Image optimization.
**Example in Radiotherapy:** Dose reduction algorithm used in kV CBCT.

388. **Dose reference level (noun):** Standard benchmark dose for planning comparison.
**Related Terms:** DRL, QA.
**Example in Radiotherapy:** Dose reference level adopted from RTOG protocol.

389. **Dose reporting protocol (noun):** Standardized method for documenting delivered dose.
**Related Terms:** ICRU 91, QA.
**Example in Radiotherapy:** Dose reporting followed ICRU 83 recommendations.

390. **Dose sculpting IMRT (noun):** Advanced IMRT focusing high dose on complex target shapes.
**Related Terms:** VMAT, Conformity.
**Example in Radiotherapy:** Dose sculpting IMRT used for skull base tumors.

391. **Dose tracking system (noun):** Software monitoring cumulative and per-fraction dose.
**Related Terms:** Adaptive therapy, QA.
**Example in Radiotherapy:** Dose tracking ensures OAR limits maintained through fractions.

392. **Dose verification log (noun):** Record of all dose validation and QA checks.
**Related Terms:** QA documentation, Dosimetry.
**Example in Radiotherapy:** Weekly dose verification log reviewed by physicist.

393. **Dosimetric modeling (noun):** Simulation of radiation transport and dose deposition.
**Related Terms:** Monte Carlo, Algorithm.
**Example in Radiotherapy:** Dosimetric modeling used for heterogeneity corrections.

394. **Dosimetric plan comparison (noun):** Quantitative evaluation between two dose distributions.
**Related Terms:** DVH, Gamma index.
**Example in Radiotherapy:** Dosimetric comparison performed between proton and photon plans.

395. **Dosimetric reproducibility (noun):** Consistency of dose delivery across repeated trials.
**Related Terms:** QA, Precision.
**Example in Radiotherapy:** High dosimetric reproducibility achieved using robotic couch.

396. **Dosimetric uncertainty (noun):** Overall inaccuracy in dose measurement or prediction.
**Related Terms:** Calibration error, QA.
**Example in Radiotherapy:** Dosimetric uncertainty $<2\%$ maintained in patient QA.

397. **Dural invasion (noun):** Tumor infiltration into dura mater observed radiologically or histologically.
**Related Terms:** Skull base tumor, MRI.
**Example in Radiotherapy:** Dural invasion included in high-dose CTV margin.

398. **Dynamic adaptive workflow (noun):** Real-time plan adaptation process using MR guidance.
**Related Terms:** Adaptive radiotherapy, MR-LINAC.
**Example in Radiotherapy:** Dynamic adaptive workflow implemented for rectal treatment.

399. **Dynamic beam shaping (noun):** Continuous alteration of beam geometry during treatment.
**Related Terms:** IMRT, MLC motion.
**Example in Radiotherapy:** Dynamic beam shaping enhances sparing of adjacent organs.

400. **Dynamic fluence map (noun):** 2D intensity pattern defining modulated dose distribution.
**Related Terms:** IMRT, Planning optimization.
**Example in Radiotherapy:** Dynamic fluence maps optimized for each control point.

401. **Dynamic gantry angle (noun):** Variable gantry rotation angle during modulated delivery.
**Related Terms:** VMAT, Arc therapy.
**Example in Radiotherapy:** Dynamic gantry angle provides improved conformity.

402. **Dynamic jaw tracking (noun):** Real-time movement of collimator jaws for dose reduction.
**Related Terms:** Beam shaping, IMRT.
**Example in Radiotherapy:** Dynamic jaw tracking reduces MLC leakage.

403. **Dynamic motion management (noun):** System compensating for organ motion during beam-on.
**Related Terms:** 4D tracking, MR-guidance.
**Example in Radiotherapy:** Dynamic motion management applied in pancreatic SBRT.

404. **Dynamic range (noun):** Range between smallest and largest detectable dose signal.
**Related Terms:** Detector sensitivity, QA.
**Example in Radiotherapy:** Wide dynamic range detectors improve IMRT QA.

405. **Dynamic sequence control (noun):** Synchronization of mechanical and dose parameters during delivery.
**Related Terms:** Control point, Automation.
**Example in Radiotherapy:** Dynamic sequence control ensures accurate VMAT delivery.

406. **Dynamic system calibration (noun):** QA process for continuously moving components in LINAC.
**Related Terms:** Mechanical QA, MLC.
**Example in Radiotherapy:** Dynamic system calibration validated leaf speed accuracy.

407. **Dynamic trajectory optimization (noun):** Planning process determining optimal beam and couch paths.
**Related Terms:** Non-coplanar planning, Arc therapy.
**Example in Radiotherapy:** Dynamic trajectory optimization improves conformity in brain plans.

408. **Dose voxel (noun):** 3D unit element storing computed dose information.
**Related Terms:** Dose matrix, Resolution.
**Example in Radiotherapy:** Each dose voxel contributes to final DVH calculation.

409. **Differential scatter (noun):** Variation in scatter intensity with angle or energy.
**Related Terms:** Scatter correction, Beam modeling.
**Example in Radiotherapy:** Differential scatter measured during beam data acquisition.

410. **Detector array QA (noun):** Quality assurance using multi-detector arrays for plan verification.
**Related Terms:** IMRT QA, Gamma test.
**Example in Radiotherapy:** Detector array QA verified dose maps for stereotactic cases.

411. **Dose-based segmentation (noun):** Defining structures or regions based on dose levels.
**Related Terms:** Isodose contour, Dose analysis.
**Example in Radiotherapy:** Dose-based segmentation aids OAR evaluation.

412. **Dose constraint violation (noun):** Exceeding established dose limit for an organ or structure.
**Related Terms:** Plan evaluation, OAR.
**Example in Radiotherapy:** Rectum constraint violation flagged in plan QA.

413. **Dose equalization (noun):** Balancing dose across overlapping fields or regions.
**Related Terms:** Junction correction, Homogenization.
**Example in Radiotherapy:** Dose equalization ensured smooth transition between spinal fields.

414. **Dose fall-off region (noun):** Area where dose rapidly decreases outside target.
**Related Terms:** Penumbra, Gradient index.
**Example in Radiotherapy:** Tight dose fall-off minimizes normal tissue irradiation.

415. **Dose kernel convolution (noun):** Algorithm combining fluence with dose kernels for calculation.
**Related Terms:** Superposition, Algorithm.
**Example in Radiotherapy:** Dose kernel convolution used for photon dose prediction.

416. **Dose leakage (noun):** Unintended radiation escaping through shielding or MLC.
**Related Terms:** QA, Leakage test.
**Example in Radiotherapy:** MLC dose leakage maintained below 0.5%.

417. **Dose modulation factor (noun):** Ratio of modulated to unmodulated beam intensities.
**Related Terms:** IMRT, Beam fluence.
**Example in Radiotherapy:** Dose modulation factor determines field complexity.

418. **Dose optimization parameter (noun):** Variable controlling optimization weight or constraint.
**Related Terms:** TPS, Plan optimization.
**Example in Radiotherapy:** Dose optimization parameters adjusted to meet target DVH.

419. **Dose perturbation (noun):** Local variation in dose due to heterogeneity or interface.
**Related Terms:** Scattering, Interface effect.
**Example in Radiotherapy:** Dose perturbation noted near lung–bone interface.

420. **Dose prediction model (noun):** AI or physics-based model estimating dose distributions.
**Related Terms:** Knowledge-based planning, Machine learning.
**Example in Radiotherapy:** Dose prediction model used for automated IMRT planning.

421. **Dose rescaling (noun):** Adjusting total dose to match fractionation or constraint change.
**Related Terms:** EQD2, BED.
**Example in Radiotherapy:** Dose rescaling applied to hypofractionated plans.

422. **Dose scoring algorithm (noun):** Algorithm assigning dose to voxels in Monte Carlo simulation.
**Related Terms:** Transport modeling, Accuracy.
**Example in Radiotherapy:** Dose scoring algorithm validated against experimental data.

423. **Dose smoothing (noun):** Technique reducing abrupt intensity changes between beamlets.
**Related Terms:** Plan optimization, Regularization.
**Example in Radiotherapy:** Dose smoothing applied during IMRT optimization.

424. **Dose summation (noun):** Combining dose distributions from multiple treatment courses.
**Related Terms:** Composite dose, Deformable accumulation.
**Example in Radiotherapy:** Dose summation performed for re-irradiation assessment.

425. **Dose tolerance limit (noun):** Maximum acceptable dose for a specific tissue or organ.
**Related Terms:** Constraint, QUANTEC.
**Example in Radiotherapy:** Spinal cord tolerance limit set at 45 Gy.

426. **Dose tracking log (noun):** Continuous record of delivered dose per session.
**Related Terms:** QA, Treatment audit.
**Example in Radiotherapy:** Dose tracking log ensures cumulative compliance.

427. **Dose variation ratio (noun):** Metric comparing delivered to planned dose variation.
**Related Terms:** QA, Adaptive planning.
**Example in Radiotherapy:** Dose variation ratio maintained within ±3%.

428. **Dose-volume conformity (noun):** Degree of matching between prescribed dose and target volume.
**Related Terms:** Conformity index, DVH.
**Example in Radiotherapy:** High dose-volume conformity achieved in brain SRS.

429. **Dose-volume histogram (DVH) (noun):** Graph plotting dose vs. volume for target or OAR.
**Related Terms:** Plan evaluation, QA.
**Example in Radiotherapy:** DVH used to assess rectal sparing.

**430. Dose-volume index (noun):** Quantitative indicator summarizing dose–volume relationship.
**Related Terms:** CI, HI, V95%.
**Example in Radiotherapy:** Dose-volume index used to compare competing plans.

**431. Dose-volume optimization (noun):** Planning process aiming to achieve optimal DVH goals.
**Related Terms:** Inverse planning, Constraints.
**Example in Radiotherapy:** Dose-volume optimization balanced tumor control and OAR sparing.

**432. Dose-volume parameter (noun):** Numeric metric derived from DVH (e.g., D95%, V20).
**Related Terms:** Plan evaluation, QA.
**Example in Radiotherapy:** D95% used as primary PTV coverage indicator.

**433. Dose-weighted mean (noun):** Average dose weighted by voxel volume or significance.
**Related Terms:** Mean dose, Biological modeling.
**Example in Radiotherapy:** Dose-weighted mean calculated for parotid gland sparing analysis.

**434. Dynamic skin dose (noun):** Radiation dose delivered to the skin during modulated or moving-beam treatments.
**Related Terms:** Skin toxicity, Surface dose.
**Example in Radiotherapy:** Dynamic skin dose evaluated in VMAT breast treatments.

**435. Dark current (noun):** Background electrical signal present in a detector without radiation.
**Related Terms:** Detector noise, Signal offset.
**Example in Radiotherapy:** Dark current correction improves EPID image quality.

**436. Data integrity (noun):** Accuracy and consistency of stored treatment and imaging data.
**Related Terms:** QA, Record-and-verify.
**Example in Radiotherapy:** Data integrity checks prevent plan corruption.

**437. Data registration (noun):** Process of aligning datasets from different sources.
**Related Terms:** Image fusion, Registration.
**Example in Radiotherapy:** Data registration aligns PET with planning CT.

**438. Data transfer latency (noun):** Delay in transferring imaging or delivery data between systems.
**Related Terms:** Network delay, System integration.
**Example in Radiotherapy:** Low latency is critical for real-time adaptive RT.

**439. Dead volume (noun):** Detector region insensitive to radiation.
**Related Terms:** Detector efficiency, Geometry.
**Example in Radiotherapy:** Dead volume corrections applied in small-field dosimetry.

**440. Decay correction (noun):** Adjustment accounting for radioactive decay over time.
**Related Terms:** Half-life, Activity correction.
**Example in Radiotherapy:** Decay correction applied to HDR source strength.

**441. Deep dose equivalent (noun):** Dose measured at tissue depth relevant to whole-body exposure.
**Related Terms:** Radiation protection, Hp(10).
**Example in Radiotherapy:** Used in occupational dose monitoring.

**442. Defocusing magnet (noun):** Magnet spreading charged particle beam laterally.
**Related Terms:** Beam optics, Proton therapy.
**Example in Radiotherapy:** Defocusing magnets shape proton beams.

**443. Degraded beam (noun):** Radiation beam with reduced energy or altered spectrum.
**Related Terms:** Beam attenuation, Scatter.
**Example in Radiotherapy:** Degraded beams occur after range shifters.

444. **Delivered dose log (noun):** Record of actual machine parameters during treatment.
**Related Terms:** Log files, Dose reconstruction.
**Example in Radiotherapy:** Delivered dose logs used for patient QA.

445. **Density calibration curve (noun):** Relationship between CT number and physical density.
**Related Terms:** HU calibration, Electron density.
**Example in Radiotherapy:** Curve used for accurate dose calculation.

446. **Density scaling (noun):** Adjustment of material density in dose calculations.
**Related Terms:** Heterogeneity correction, Monte Carlo.
**Example in Radiotherapy:** Density scaling improves lung dose accuracy.

447. **Detector saturation (noun):** Condition where detector response no longer increases with dose.
**Related Terms:** Dynamic range, Nonlinearity.
**Example in Radiotherapy:** Avoided in FFF beam measurements.

448. **Deterministic effect (noun):** Radiation effect with a threshold dose.
**Related Terms:** Tissue reaction, Threshold dose.
**Example in Radiotherapy:** Skin erythema is a deterministic effect.

449. **Deviation map (noun):** Visualization of dose or position differences from reference.
**Related Terms:** Gamma analysis, QA.
**Example in Radiotherapy:** Deviation maps highlight delivery errors.

450. **Diagnostic imaging dose (noun):** Radiation dose from imaging procedures.
**Related Terms:** kV imaging, CBCT.
**Example in Radiotherapy:** Monitored during IGRT protocols.

451. **Digital detector panel (noun):** Flat-panel device for imaging or dosimetry.
**Related Terms:** EPID, Flat-panel detector.
**Example in Radiotherapy:** EPID used for portal imaging.

452. **Digital filter (noun):** Algorithm modifying image frequency components.
**Related Terms:** Noise reduction, Image processing.
**Example in Radiotherapy:** Digital filters improve CBCT clarity.

453. **Digital twin (noun):** Virtual patient model reflecting anatomy and response.
**Related Terms:** Adaptive RT, Modeling.
**Example in Radiotherapy:** Digital twins support personalized planning.

454. **Direct aperture optimization (noun):** IMRT method optimizing leaf shapes directly.
**Related Terms:** DAO, VMAT.
**Example in Radiotherapy:** DAO reduces treatment complexity.

455. **Direct electron contamination (noun):** Surface dose from secondary electrons.
**Related Terms:** Build-up region, Skin dose.
**Example in Radiotherapy:** Reduced using beam modifiers.

456. **Direct fluence optimization (noun):** Planning method optimizing beam fluence explicitly.
**Related Terms:** Inverse planning, IMRT.
**Example in Radiotherapy:** Used in step-and-shoot IMRT.

457. **Directional dependence (noun):** Variation in detector response with beam angle.
**Related Terms:** Angular dependence, QA.
**Example in Radiotherapy:** Evaluated for in vivo dosimeters.

**458. Discrete beam angle (noun):** Fixed gantry angle used in treatment delivery.
**Related Terms:** IMRT, Beam arrangement.
**Example in Radiotherapy:** Discrete angles used in static IMRT.

**459. Dose accumulation error (noun):** Uncertainty in cumulative dose estimation.
**Related Terms:** DIR error, Adaptive RT.
**Example in Radiotherapy:** Minimized through validation studies.

**460. Dose averaging (noun):** Calculation of mean dose over a volume.
**Related Terms:** Mean dose, DVH.
**Example in Radiotherapy:** Used for parotid gland assessment.

**461. Dose blurring (noun):** Loss of dose sharpness due to motion.
**Related Terms:** Motion interplay, smearing.
**Example in Radiotherapy:** Reduced using gating techniques.

**462. Dose convergence (noun):** Stability of dose result with repeated calculation.
**Related Terms:** Monte Carlo uncertainty, Iteration.
**Example in Radiotherapy:** Ensures reliable MC simulations.

**463. Dose drift (noun):** Gradual change in output over time.
**Related Terms:** Output constancy, QA.
**Example in Radiotherapy:** Monitored with daily QA.

**464. Dose expansion margin (noun):** Added margin accounting for dose uncertainty.
**Related Terms:** PTV margin, Robust planning.
**Example in Radiotherapy:** Used in proton therapy planning.

**465. Dose feedback loop (noun):** System adjusting delivery based on measured dose.
**Related Terms:** Adaptive control, QA.
**Example in Radiotherapy:** Emerging in MR-guided RT.

**466. Dose grid resolution (noun):** Voxel size used for dose calculation.
**Related Terms:** Spatial resolution, TPS.
**Example in Radiotherapy:** Finer grids used for SRS.

**467. Dose inhomogeneity (noun):** Presence of hot and cold spots within volume.
**Related Terms:** HI, Dose variation.
**Example in Radiotherapy:** Evaluated during plan review.

**468. Dose leakage (noun):** Radiation passing through shielding or MLCs.
**Related Terms:** Transmission, Head leakage.
**Example in Radiotherapy:** Accounted for in whole-body dose.

**469. Dose modeling uncertainty (noun):** Error due to algorithm limitations.
**Related Terms:** TPS accuracy, Commissioning.
**Example in Radiotherapy:** Reduced with Monte Carlo models.

**470. Dose normalization point (noun):** Reference location used to scale dose.
**Related Terms:** Isocenter, Prescription.
**Example in Radiotherapy:** Often set within the PTV.

**471. Dose overlap region (noun):** Area receiving dose from multiple fields.
**Related Terms:** Junction, Field matching.
**Example in Radiotherapy:** Critical in craniospinal irradiation.

472. **Dose per fraction (noun):** Radiation dose delivered in one session.
**Related Terms:** Fractionation, BED.
**Example in Radiotherapy:** 2 Gy per fraction standard.

473. **Dose prescription isodose (noun):** Isodose level defining target coverage.
**Related Terms:** Coverage, Normalization.
**Example in Radiotherapy:** 95% isodose commonly used.

474. **Dose reconstruction uncertainty (noun):** Error in reconstructed dose estimates.
**Related Terms:** Log-file QA, Verification.
**Example in Radiotherapy:** Evaluated during adaptive workflows.

475. **Dose reference volume (noun):** Defined structure for dose reporting.
**Related Terms:** ICRU, Reporting.
**Example in Radiotherapy:** PTV used as reference volume.

476. **Dose saturation (noun):** Plateau in dose-response at high exposure.
**Related Terms:** Radiobiology, Cell kill.
**Example in Radiotherapy:** Relevant in hypoxic regions.

477. **Dose segmentation (noun):** Division of dose distribution into regions.
**Related Terms:** Sub-volume analysis, DVH.
**Example in Radiotherapy:** Used in dose painting.

478. **Dose shadowing (noun):** Reduced dose behind high-density objects.
**Related Terms:** Attenuation, Metal artifact.
**Example in Radiotherapy:** Seen near prostheses.

479. **Dose smoothing (noun):** Reduction of sharp dose fluctuations.
**Related Terms:** Optimization, Regularization.
**Example in Radiotherapy:** Applied during IMRT planning.

480. **Dose spill over (noun):** Unintended dose extending beyond target.
**Related Terms:** Conformity, Gradient.
**Example in Radiotherapy:** Minimized in SRS.

481. **Dose stratification (noun):** Classification of regions by dose level.
**Related Terms:** Risk analysis, DVH.
**Example in Radiotherapy:** Used in toxicity studies.

482. **Dose tracking uncertainty (noun):** Error in real-time dose monitoring.
**Related Terms:** Motion management, QA.
**Example in Radiotherapy:** Evaluated in MR-Linac systems.

483. **Dose uniformity ratio (noun):** Metric comparing max and min dose.
**Related Terms:** Homogeneity index, QA.
**Example in Radiotherapy:** Used in total body irradiation.

484. **Dose voxel interpolation (noun):** Resampling of dose grid values.
**Related Terms:** Image registration, Accumulation.
**Example in Radiotherapy:** Used during adaptive Replanning.

485. **Dose window constraint (noun):** Acceptable dose range in optimization.
**Related Terms:** Planning objectives, Constraints.
**Example in Radiotherapy:** Applied to OAR sparing.

486. **Dose-weighted centroid (noun):** Center of mass weighted by dose.
**Related Terms:** Dose distribution, Geometry.
**Example in Radiotherapy:** Used for motion analysis.

487. **Dosimetric acceptance criteria (noun):** Thresholds defining QA pass/fail.
**Related Terms:** Gamma index, Tolerance.
**Example in Radiotherapy:** 3%/3 mm commonly used.

488. **Dosimetric commissioning (noun):** Validation of dose calculation and delivery.
**Related Terms:** TPS commissioning, QA.
**Example in Radiotherapy:** Performed before clinical use.

489. **Dosimetric consistency (noun):** Stability of dose delivery over time.
**Related Terms:** Output constancy, QA.
**Example in Radiotherapy:** Ensured with routine checks.

490. **Dosimetric endpoint (noun):** Dose metric used for clinical evaluation.
**Related Terms:** DVH metric, Outcome analysis.
**Example in Radiotherapy:** Mean lung dose as endpoint.

491. **Dosimetric sensitivity (noun):** Ability to detect small dose changes.
**Related Terms:** Resolution, Detector performance.
**Example in Radiotherapy:** Important in in vivo dosimetry.

492. **Dosimetric stability (noun):** Reproducibility of measured dose.
**Related Terms:** QA, Calibration drift.
**Example in Radiotherapy:** Verified with constancy tests.

493. **Dosimetric traceability (noun):** Link of measurements to national standards.
**Related Terms:** Calibration chain, Metrology.
**Example in Radiotherapy:** Required for clinical dosimetry.

494. **Dosimetric validation phantom (noun):** Phantom designed for end-to-end testing.
**Related Terms:** QA phantom, Commissioning.
**Example in Radiotherapy:** Used in SBRT audits.

495. **Double contouring (noun):** Redundant outlining of structures for verification.
**Related Terms:** Peer review, QA.
**Example in Radiotherapy:** Reduces contouring errors.

496. **Double exposure artifact (noun):** Image artifact from repeated irradiation.
**Related Terms:** Imaging error, Motion.
**Example in Radiotherapy:** Seen in CBCT with patient motion.

497. **Double isocenter technique (noun):** Use of two isocenters for long targets.
**Related Terms:** Field junction, CSI.
**Example in Radiotherapy:** Applied in craniospinal RT.

498. **Dynamic beam hold (noun):** Automatic beam pause during motion.
**Related Terms:** Gating, Safety interlock.
**Example in Radiotherapy:** Used in respiratory motion management.

499. **Dynamic dose adaptation (noun):** Real-time modification of delivered dose.
**Related Terms:** Adaptive RT, MR-guided RT.
**Example in Radiotherapy:** Emerging MR-Linac capability.

500. **Dynamic Isodose visualization (noun):** Real-time display of evolving dose distribution.
**Related Terms:** Image guidance, Adaptive planning.
**Example in Radiotherapy:** Used during online adaptive sessions.

# E

1. **E-beam (noun):** A stream of high-energy electrons used for external beam radiotherapy.
   **Related Terms:** Electron beam, Linear accelerator, Megavoltage.
   **Example in Radiotherapy:** The patient received a 9 MeV E-beam for superficial chest wall irradiation.
2. **E-Field (noun):** The electric field strength in a region where charged particles move under electric forces.
   **Related Terms:** Electric potential, Field strength, Particle acceleration.
   **Example in Radiotherapy:** The E-field determines electron acceleration within the linear accelerator waveguide.
3. **Ead (noun):** Effective absorbed dose; represents dose adjusted for biological impact.
   **Related Terms:** Equivalent dose, Sievert.
   **Example in Radiotherapy:** The Ead for occupational exposure must remain within ICRP limits.
4. **EAL (noun):** Electron attenuation length; distance electrons travel before losing energy significantly.
   **Related Terms:** Range, Stopping power.
   **Example in Radiotherapy:** The EAL of 6 MeV electrons in tissue is approximately 3 cm.
5. **Early effects (noun):** Biological responses occurring shortly after radiation exposure.
   **Related Terms:** Acute effects, Deterministic effects.
   **Example in Radiotherapy:** Skin erythema is an early effect seen during treatment.
6. **EBC (noun):** Electronic beam control; system ensuring beam stability and symmetry.
   **Related Terms:** Beam monitoring, QA calibration.
   **Example in Radiotherapy:** The EBC detected a deviation in the X-ray field symmetry.
7. **EBT3 Film (noun):** Gafchromic radiochromic film used for 2D dosimetry verification.
   **Related Terms:** Dosimetry, Film QA.
   **Example in Radiotherapy:** EBT3 film was used to verify IMRT fluence accuracy.
8. **ECG-gating (noun):** Synchronization of radiation delivery with cardiac cycle.
   **Related Terms:** Motion management, Respiratory gating.
   **Example in Radiotherapy:** ECG-gating minimizes cardiac exposure during thoracic irradiation.
9. **Eddy current (noun):** Circular currents induced in conductors by changing magnetic fields.
   **Related Terms:** Magnetic field, Induction.
   **Example in Radiotherapy:** Eddy currents are minimized in MRI-guided radiotherapy systems.
10. **Effective atomic number (noun):** Average atomic number describing photon interaction in a compound.
    **Related Terms:** Photoelectric effect, Tissue equivalence.
    **Example in Radiotherapy:** Tissue-equivalent phantoms are chosen based on effective atomic number.
11. **Effective dose (noun):** Weighted sum of organ doses reflecting total stochastic risk.
    **Related Terms:** Equivalent dose, Sievert, ICRP weighting factors.
    **Example in Radiotherapy:** The effective dose to staff is monitored by TLD badges.

12. **Effective half-life (noun):** Combination of physical and biological half-lives determining radioisotope decay in body.
**Related Terms:** Physical half-life, Biological half-life.
**Example in Radiotherapy:** The effective half-life of I-131 in thyroid varies among patients.

13. **Efficiency (noun):** Ratio of useful output to total input in a detection or treatment system.
**Related Terms:** Quantum efficiency, Detection sensitivity.
**Example in Radiotherapy:** The ion chamber's efficiency affects dose measurement accuracy.

14. **Egress dose (noun):** The dose at the exit point of a radiation beam.
**Related Terms:** Exit dose, Build-down region.
**Example in Radiotherapy:** Egress dose is considered in lung and breast treatments.

15. **Elastic scattering (noun):** Interaction where kinetic energy is conserved between incident and target particles.
**Related Terms:** Rutherford scattering, Cross-section.
**Example in Radiotherapy:** Elastic scattering of protons affects the Bragg peak shape.

16. **Electron accelerator (noun):** Machine that accelerates electrons to high energy for therapeutic use.
**Related Terms:** Linear accelerator, Betatron.
**Example in Radiotherapy:** A 6 MeV electron accelerator is used for skin lesion therapy.

17. **Electron arc therapy (noun):** Technique using rotating electron beams to treat curved surfaces.
**Related Terms:** Arc therapy, Conformal therapy.
**Example in Radiotherapy:** Electron arc therapy was applied for chest wall irradiation post-mastectomy.

18. **Electron beam therapy (noun):** Use of electrons to treat superficial tumors.
**Related Terms:** E-beam, Cutout, Bolus.
**Example in Radiotherapy:** Electron beam therapy is ideal for scalp lesions.

19. **Electron contamination (noun):** Unwanted electrons generated in photon beams affecting surface dose.
**Related Terms:** Scatter, Build-up region.
**Example in Radiotherapy:** Electron contamination increases dose near skin surface.

20. **Electron density (noun):** Measure of electrons per unit volume affecting photon attenuation.
**Related Terms:** HU value, CT number.
**Example in Radiotherapy:** Electron density is derived from CT for dose calculation.

21. **Electron dosimetry (noun):** Measurement of absorbed dose for electron beam treatments.
**Related Terms:** Ion chamber, Diode detector.
**Example in Radiotherapy:** Electron dosimetry was verified using parallel plate chambers.

22. **Electron gun (noun):** Device emitting electrons into the accelerator waveguide.
**Related Terms:** Cathode, Thermionic emission.
**Example in Radiotherapy:** The electron gun filament was replaced during machine maintenance.

23. **Electron range (noun):** Maximum depth reached by electrons before energy loss.
**Related Terms:** CSDA range, Stopping power.
**Example in Radiotherapy:** The electron range for 12 MeV electrons in water is 6 cm.

24. **Electron scattering foil (noun):** Material used to broaden and flatten electron beam profiles.
**Related Terms:** Applicator, Beam flatness.
**Example in Radiotherapy:** The scattering foil ensures uniform dose distribution.

25. **Electron transport (noun):** Movement of electrons through matter considering scattering and energy loss.
**Related Terms:** Monte Carlo simulation, Range straggling.
**Example in Radiotherapy:** Monte Carlo models accurately simulate electron transport.

26. **Electronic portal imaging device (noun):** Digital detector for patient setup and verification imaging.
**Related Terms:** EPID, CBCT, IGRT.
**Example in Radiotherapy:** EPID was used for daily verification in pelvic treatments.

27. **Elemental composition (noun):** Fractional composition of elements in a material.
**Related Terms:** Mass attenuation coefficient, Tissue equivalence.
**Example in Radiotherapy:** The phantom's elemental composition matches human soft tissue.

28. **Elution (noun):** Process of removing adsorbed radioactive isotope from a generator.
**Related Terms:** Generator system, Molybdenum-99.
**Example in Radiotherapy:** Technetium-99m is obtained by elution from Mo-99 generator.

29. **Embolization (noun):** Blocking of blood vessels intentionally or due to radiation damage.
**Related Terms:** Vascular effect, Brachytherapy toxicity.
**Example in Radiotherapy:** Radiation-induced embolization can occur in hepatic treatments.

30. **Emission spectrum (noun):** Range of energies emitted from a radiation source.
**Related Terms:** Bremsstrahlung, Characteristic X-rays.
**Example in Radiotherapy:** The emission spectrum defines X-ray beam quality.

31. **Emittance (noun):** Measure of beam spread and divergence in accelerator systems.
**Related Terms:** Beam collimation, Focusing.
**Example in Radiotherapy:** Low emittance improves beam uniformity.

32. **Empirical model (noun):** Model based on observed data rather than theoretical derivation.
**Related Terms:** Dose–response curve, Calibration.
**Example in Radiotherapy:** Empirical models are used to predict RBE for protons.

33. **Encapsulation (noun):** Sealing radioactive material within a protective capsule.
**Related Terms:** Brachytherapy source, Sealed source.
**Example in Radiotherapy:** Ir-192 sources are encapsulated in stainless steel capsules.

34. **Energized electron (noun):** An electron accelerated by electromagnetic fields to gain kinetic energy.
**Related Terms:** Accelerating waveguide, Linear accelerator.
**Example in Radiotherapy:** Energized electrons produce therapeutic X-rays when striking the target.

35. **Energy absorption (noun):** Process by which radiation transfers energy to matter.
**Related Terms:** Absorbed dose, Kerma.
**Example in Radiotherapy:** Energy absorption determines tissue dose in photon interactions.

36. **Energy calibration (noun):** Verification of beam energy to ensure accuracy.
**Related Terms:** Beam quality, Reference dosimetry.
**Example in Radiotherapy:** Energy calibration confirms consistent 6 MV photon output.

37. **Energy degradation (noun):** Reduction of radiation energy as it passes through matter.
**Related Terms:** Attenuation, Scatter.
**Example in Radiotherapy:** Energy degradation affects penetration depth in patient tissues.

38. **Energy fluence (noun):** Energy carried by radiation across a unit area.
**Related Terms:** Photon fluence, Dose rate.
**Example in Radiotherapy:** Treatment planning systems calculate dose from energy fluence maps.

39. **Energy modulation (noun):** Adjustment of radiation energy to shape dose distribution.
**Related Terms:** Intensity modulation, Range modulation.
**Example in Radiotherapy:** Energy modulation in proton therapy optimizes Bragg peak placement.

40. **Energy spectrum (noun):** Distribution of photon or particle energies within a beam.
**Related Terms:** Beam quality, Bremsstrahlung.
**Example in Radiotherapy:** The X-ray energy spectrum determines penetration and tissue sparing.

41. **Enhanced dynamic wedge (noun):** Virtual wedge created by moving collimator jaws and dose rate control.
**Related Terms:** Physical wedge, Beam modulation.
**Example in Radiotherapy:** Enhanced dynamic wedges provide smooth dose gradients.

42. **Enhancement factor (noun):** Ratio showing increased biological effect due to radiation modifiers.
**Related Terms:** Oxygen enhancement ratio, Sensitizers.
**Example in Radiotherapy:** High OER enhances tumor control in oxygenated tissues.

43. **Entrainment (noun):** Synchronization of beam delivery with breathing or motion cycles.
**Related Terms:** Gating, Motion management.
**Example in Radiotherapy:** Respiratory entrainment ensures precise dose during lung irradiation.

44. **Envelope function (noun):** Mathematical expression describing beam amplitude variation.
**Related Terms:** Beam profile, Modulation.
**Example in Radiotherapy:** The envelope function defines pulse shape in electron acceleration.

45. **Environmental radiation (noun):** Naturally occurring background radiation present in surroundings.
**Related Terms:** Background dose, Cosmic radiation.
**Example in Radiotherapy:** Environmental radiation contributes minimally to occupational exposure.

46. **EPID calibration (noun):** Adjustment of electronic portal imaging device response for accuracy.
**Related Terms:** Image QA, Detector gain.
**Example in Radiotherapy:** EPID calibration ensures correct image contrast and geometry.

47. **Epithelial reaction (noun):** Acute skin or mucosal response due to radiation exposure.
**Related Terms:** Dermatitis, Acute toxicity.
**Example in Radiotherapy:** Grade II epithelial reaction observed after head-neck radiotherapy.

48. **Equivalent depth (noun):** Depth in water producing same dose as another medium.
**Related Terms:** Tissue equivalence, Dosimetry correction.
**Example in Radiotherapy:** Equivalent depth conversion is used in heterogeneity corrections.

49. **Equivalent dose (noun):** Absorbed dose multiplied by radiation weighting factor (WR).
**Related Terms:** Effective dose, Sievert.
**Example in Radiotherapy:** Equivalent dose assesses biological risk for occupational exposure.

50. **Equivalent field size (noun):** Rectangular field giving same scatter as irregular treatment field.
**Related Terms:** Scatter factor, PDD correction.
**Example in Radiotherapy:** Equivalent field size simplifies output factor calculations.

51. **Erythema (noun):** Reddening of skin from capillary dilation due to radiation.
**Related Terms:** Acute reaction, Skin dose.
**Example in Radiotherapy:** Erythema often appears after cumulative 20–30 Gy exposure.

52. **Escalated dose (noun):** Higher therapeutic dose prescribed for aggressive tumors.
**Related Terms:** Dose escalation, Hypofractionation.
**Example in Radiotherapy:** Dose-escalated SBRT improves tumor control in liver metastasis.

53. **Escape peak (noun):** Detector artifact when secondary photons escape detection crystal.
**Related Terms:** Energy resolution, Compton effect.
**Example in Radiotherapy:** Escape peaks appear in gamma spectrometry of Ir-192 sources.

54. **Esophageal sparing (noun):** Reduction of radiation exposure to the esophagus.
**Related Terms:** OAR protection, IMRT.
**Example in Radiotherapy:** Esophageal sparing achieved through arc optimization in lung plans.

55. **Essential amino acids (noun):** Protein components required for tissue repair post-irradiation.
**Related Terms:** Radiobiology, Regeneration.
**Example in Radiotherapy:** Adequate nutrition supports recovery after radiotherapy.

56. **Estimation uncertainty (noun):** Degree of confidence in measured or calculated dose value.
**Related Terms:** Error analysis, QA tolerance.
**Example in Radiotherapy:** Uncertainty in MU calculation must remain <2%.

57. **Esterification (noun):** Chemical formation of esters, sometimes influenced by radiation.
**Related Terms:** Radiation chemistry, Free radicals.
**Example in Radiotherapy:** Radiation-induced esterification may affect polymer-based dosimeters.

58. **Ethical approval (noun):** Official consent from ethics committee for research.
**Related Terms:** Clinical trials, IRB.
**Example in Radiotherapy:** Ethical approval obtained for patient imaging study.

59. **Ethylenediaminetetraacetic acid (noun):** Chelating agent used in dosimeter preparation and metal removal.
**Related Terms:** Chelation, Chemical dosimetry.
**Example in Radiotherapy:** EDTA stabilizes solutions in chemical dosimeter calibration.

60. **Eutectic alloy (noun):** Metal mixture with specific melting point used in shielding.
**Related Terms:** Lead alloy, Collimator design.
**Example in Radiotherapy:** Eutectic alloys used in custom shielding blocks.

61. **Evacuation chamber (noun):** Vacuum environment inside linear accelerators for beam generation.
**Related Terms:** Waveguide, RF cavity.
**Example in Radiotherapy:** Electrons accelerate through the evacuated waveguide chamber.

62. **Evaluation point (noun):** Specific point where dose or metric is analyzed.
**Related Terms:** Isocenter, Reference point.
**Example in Radiotherapy:** The evaluation point ensures accurate PTV coverage assessment.

63. **Event counting (noun):** Detection of individual radiation interactions by a detector.
**Related Terms:** Pulse counting, Statistics.
**Example in Radiotherapy:** Event counting helps determine detector sensitivity.

64. **Excess relative risk (noun):** Ratio indicating additional risk from radiation exposure.
**Related Terms:** Epidemiology, Stochastic effects.
**Example in Radiotherapy:** ERR quantifies risk of secondary cancers post-therapy.

65. **Exchange capacity (noun):** Material's ability to exchange ions during radiation exposure.
**Related Terms:** Ion exchange resin, Filtration.
**Example in Radiotherapy:** Ion exchangers are used in radioactive waste management.

66. **Excretion rate (noun):** Speed at which radioactive material leaves the body.
**Related Terms:** Biological half-life, Clearance.
**Example in Radiotherapy:** I-131 excretion monitored to ensure safety compliance.

67. **Exponential attenuation (noun):** Reduction in beam intensity following exponential law.
**Related Terms:** Linear attenuation coefficient, HVL.
**Example in Radiotherapy:** Exponential attenuation determines shielding thickness.

68. **Exponential decay (noun):** Decrease of radioactive atoms over time following constant rate.
**Related Terms:** Half-life, Activity.
**Example in Radiotherapy:** Cs-137 activity decays exponentially with time.

69. **Exposure (noun):** Measure of ionization in air from X-rays or gamma rays.
**Related Terms:** Air kerma, Dose rate.
**Example in Radiotherapy:** Exposure rate meters assess radiation safety.

70. **Exposure index (noun):** Digital indicator of image detector dose level.
**Related Terms:** Imaging QA, Detector calibration.
**Example in Radiotherapy:** EPID exposure index must remain within tolerance limits.

71. **External beam radiotherapy (noun):** Delivery of radiation from an external source.
**Related Terms:** EBRT, IMRT, VMAT.
**Example in Radiotherapy:** External beam radiotherapy is standard for prostate cancer.

72. **External contour (noun):** Outer boundary of patient body used for dose calculation.
**Related Terms:** Body contour, CT segmentation.
**Example in Radiotherapy:** External contour defines dose calculation volume in TPS.

73. **Extrapolation chamber (noun):** Precision ionization chamber for surface dose measurements.
**Related Terms:** Dosimetry, Calibration.
**Example in Radiotherapy:** Extrapolation chambers measure beta particle dose accurately.

74. **Extrapolated range (noun):** Projected particle path length from measured data.
**Related Terms:** CSDA range, Electron beam.
**Example in Radiotherapy:** Extrapolated range validates electron energy verification.

75. **Eye lens dose (noun):** Radiation dose received by the crystalline lens.
**Related Terms:** Occupational limit, ALARA.
**Example in Radiotherapy:** Eye lens dose monitored in head and neck treatments.

76. **E-beam current (noun):** Flow rate of electrons in the accelerator waveguide.
**Related Terms:** Beam output, Current density.
**Example in Radiotherapy:** E-beam current stability ensures consistent photon dose output.

77. **E-beam focusing (noun):** Magnetic alignment of electrons to maintain narrow beam.
**Related Terms:** Focusing coil, Beam optics.
**Example in Radiotherapy:** Proper E-beam focusing prevents penumbra widening.

78. **E-beam output factor (noun):** Dose ratio for given field to reference field.
**Related Terms:** Output calibration, MU factor.
**Example in Radiotherapy:** E-beam output factors are measured during annual QA.

79. **E-beam therapy cone (noun):** Applicator directing and defining electron treatment field.
**Related Terms:** Electron cone, Collimation.
**Example in Radiotherapy:** A $10 \times 10$ cm cone used for chest wall treatment.

80. **E-beam uniformity (noun):** Evenness of electron dose across treatment field.
**Related Terms:** Flatness, Symmetry.
**Example in Radiotherapy:** E-beam uniformity verified using water phantom scans.

81. **Eddy current damping (noun):** Suppression of induced currents within magnetic systems.
**Related Terms:** Induction, MRI.
**Example in Radiotherapy:** Eddy current damping improves MRI-linac imaging quality.

82. **Edge effect (noun):** Distortion of dose or signal near material boundaries.
**Related Terms:** Penumbra, Scatter.
**Example in Radiotherapy:** Edge effects appear in film dosimetry near interfaces.

83. **Edge enhancement (noun):** Increase of image contrast at object boundaries.
**Related Terms:** Image processing, Sharpness.
**Example in Radiotherapy:** Edge enhancement aids tumor margin visualization in CBCT.

84. **Edge scatter (noun):** Photon scattering occurring at field edges or block boundaries.
**Related Terms:** Leakage, Penumbra.
**Example in Radiotherapy:** Edge scatter is reduced with precise collimation.

85. **Effective atomic mass (noun):** Weighted average mass of atoms influencing attenuation.
**Related Terms:** Electron density, Attenuation coefficient.
**Example in Radiotherapy:** Effective atomic mass aids tissue equivalence calculations.

86. **Effective energy (noun):** Single energy value representing beam's overall penetrating power.
**Related Terms:** Beam quality, Half-value layer.
**Example in Radiotherapy:** Effective energy for 6 MV photon beam is about 2 MeV.

87. **Effective focal spot (noun):** Apparent X-ray source size after anode angulation.
**Related Terms:** Line focus principle, Resolution.
**Example in Radiotherapy:** Small effective focal spot enhances portal image clarity.

88. **Effective linear attenuation (noun):** Average photon attenuation rate through a heterogeneous medium.
**Related Terms:** Attenuation coefficient, Beam hardening.
**Example in Radiotherapy:** Effective linear attenuation values correct CT-based dose calculations.

89. **Effective point of measurement (noun):** Reference point inside detector representing true dose location.
**Related Terms:** Ion chamber correction, Dosimetry.
**Example in Radiotherapy:** Effective point of measurement corrected 1.6 mm upstream.

90. **Effective target volume (noun):** Region receiving prescribed dose within clinical target volume.
**Related Terms:** PTV, CTV.
**Example in Radiotherapy:** Effective target volume ensures full tumor coverage.

91. **Efficiency calibration (noun):** Process of determining detector response to radiation.
**Related Terms:** Energy calibration, Sensitivity.
**Example in Radiotherapy:** Efficiency calibration done before isotope assay in brachytherapy.

92. **Elastic collision (noun):** Interaction conserving kinetic energy between particles.
**Related Terms:** Scattering, Cross-section.
**Example in Radiotherapy:** Elastic collisions dominate proton-tissue interactions.

93. **Elastic modulus (noun):** Measure of stiffness of tissue or material.
**Related Terms:** Deformation, Imaging elastography.
**Example in Radiotherapy:** Elastic modulus helps assess liver deformation during planning.

94. **Electret dosimeter (noun):** Passive device storing electrostatic charge proportional to dose.
**Related Terms:** TLD, Passive dosimetry.
**Example in Radiotherapy:** Electret dosimeters used in room radiation monitoring.

95. **Electric charge (noun):** Fundamental property causing electromagnetic interaction.
**Related Terms:** Coulomb, Ionization.
**Example in Radiotherapy:** Electric charge flow measured in ionization chambers.

96. **Electric field gradient (noun):** Spatial variation of electric field intensity.
**Related Terms:** Potential difference, Beam acceleration.
**Example in Radiotherapy:** Electric field gradient defines acceleration efficiency in linac.

97. **Electric potential (noun):** Energy per unit charge due to an electric field.
**Related Terms:** Voltage, Electrostatics.
**Example in Radiotherapy:** High electric potential accelerates electrons to megavoltage energies.

98. **Electrode (noun):** Conductor allowing current into or out of medium.
**Related Terms:** Ion chamber, Cathode.
**Example in Radiotherapy:** Electrode spacing affects chamber collection efficiency.

99. **Electromagnetic induction (noun):** Production of voltage by changing magnetic field.
**Related Terms:** Faraday's law, Eddy current.
**Example in Radiotherapy:** Electromagnetic induction powers the linac's magnetron.

100. **Electromagnetic wave (noun):** Oscillating electric and magnetic fields transmitting energy.
**Related Terms:** Photon, RF wave.
**Example in Radiotherapy:** Microwaves accelerate electrons in the linac cavity.

101. **Electromagnet (noun):** Coil generating magnetic field when electric current flows.
**Related Terms:** Solenoid, Magnetic focusing.
**Example in Radiotherapy:** Electromagnets guide electron trajectories in accelerators.

102. **Electron capture (noun):** Nuclear decay where an inner electron merges with a proton.
**Related Terms:** Beta decay, Radioisotope.
**Example in Radiotherapy:** Electron capture observed in Co-57 decay.

103. **Electron charge (noun):** Elementary negative charge carried by an electron.
**Related Terms:** Coulomb, Elementary particle.
**Example in Radiotherapy:** Electron charge defines fundamental dosimetric quantities.

104. **Electron cloud (noun):** Region of negative charge surrounding an atomic nucleus.
**Related Terms:** Atomic structure, Binding energy.
**Example in Radiotherapy:** Interaction probability depends on electron cloud density.

105. **Electron collision (noun):** Interaction between moving electrons and atoms.
**Related Terms:** Ionization, Excitation.
**Example in Radiotherapy:** Electron collisions cause bremsstrahlung production.

106. **Electron energy spectrum (noun):** Range of electron energies emitted from accelerator.
**Related Terms:** Beam quality, Calibration.
**Example in Radiotherapy:** Electron energy spectrum defines treatment depth.

107. **Electron field size (noun):** Dimensions of therapeutic electron beam at patient surface.
**Related Terms:** Cone size, Output factor.
**Example in Radiotherapy:** Electron field size affects dose uniformity.

108. **Electron gun current (noun):** Amount of current emitted by linac's electron gun.
**Related Terms:** Beam output, Filament current.
**Example in Radiotherapy:** Stable electron gun current ensures beam reproducibility.

109. **Electron interaction (noun):** Collision of electron with matter causing energy transfer.
**Related Terms:** Scattering, Ionization.
**Example in Radiotherapy:** Electron interactions deposit dose in superficial tissues.

110. **Electron mobility (noun):** Speed of electron motion under electric field influence.
**Related Terms:** Conductivity, Field strength.
**Example in Radiotherapy:** Electron mobility affects gas chamber ion collection.

111. **Electron multiple scattering (noun):** Repeated deflections of electrons in tissue.
**Related Terms:** Lateral spread, Penumbra.
**Example in Radiotherapy:** Multiple scattering broadens electron beam profiles.

112. **Electron source (noun):** Device or component generating therapeutic electrons.
**Related Terms:** Cathode, Thermionic emission.
**Example in Radiotherapy:** Electron source filaments require periodic replacement.

113. **Electron stopping power (noun):** Energy loss per unit distance traveled by electrons.
**Related Terms:** Range, Energy deposition.
**Example in Radiotherapy:** Stopping power data critical for Monte Carlo dose modeling.

114. **Electronic collimation (noun):** Beam shaping by magnetic or electronic steering instead of jaws.
**Related Terms:** MLC, Dynamic collimation.
**Example in Radiotherapy:** Proton therapy uses electronic collimation for spot scanning.

115. **Electronic dose record (noun):** Digital documentation of dose delivery data.
**Related Terms:** Record and verify, QA.
**Example in Radiotherapy:** All treatment sessions logged in electronic dose records.

116. **Electronic portal imaging (noun):** Digital imaging using treatment beam for verification.
**Related Terms:** EPID, IGRT.
**Example in Radiotherapy:** Electronic portal imaging ensures accurate isocenter alignment.

117. **Electronic scoring (noun):** Counting and recording of particle interactions in simulations.
**Related Terms:** Monte Carlo, Statistical analysis.
**Example in Radiotherapy:** Electronic scoring assesses dose distributions in TPS algorithms.

118. **Electronic timer (noun):** Device controlling beam-on duration precisely.
**Related Terms:** Treatment console, MU timer.
**Example in Radiotherapy:** Electronic timer ensures accurate exposure in manual mode.

119. **Elemental attenuation (noun):** Reduction of photon intensity due to atomic composition.
**Related Terms:** Attenuation coefficient, Photoelectric effect.
**Example in Radiotherapy:** Elemental attenuation data used for phantom calibration.

120. **Elongation factor (noun):** Ratio of actual to planned source distance.
**Related Terms:** Inverse square correction, SSD.
**Example in Radiotherapy:** Elongation factor corrects geometric setup variations.

121. **Embedded source (noun):** Radioactive material fixed within tissue or applicator.
**Related Terms:** Brachytherapy, Permanent implant.
**Example in Radiotherapy:** I-125 embedded sources used in prostate seed therapy.

122. **Emission tomography (noun):** Imaging technique detecting emitted photons from radiotracer.
**Related Terms:** PET, SPECT.
**Example in Radiotherapy:** Emission tomography assists biological target .

123. **Empirical verification (noun):** Experimental confirmation of theoretical dose predictions.
**Related Terms:** QA, Benchmarking.
**Example in Radiotherapy:** Empirical verification validates Monte Carlo-calculated doses.

124. **Encapsulation leakage (noun):** Radiation escaping from sealed source capsule.
**Related Terms:** Brachytherapy, Source integrity.
**Example in Radiotherapy:** Encapsulation leakage checked during source acceptance testing.

125. **End effect (noun):** Dose non-uniformity at treatment field edge due to mechanical limits.
**Related Terms:** Penumbra, Field matching.
**Example in Radiotherapy:** End effect corrected during MLC sequencing.

126. **End plate (noun):** Flat metal surface in accelerator or detector providing mechanical support.
**Related Terms:** Cavity resonator, Ion chamber.
**Example in Radiotherapy:** End plate stability ensures uniform electric field distribution.

127. **End-to-end test (noun):** Full workflow QA simulating complete patient treatment process.
**Related Terms:** System QA, IGRT verification.
**Example in Radiotherapy:** End-to-end tests verify accuracy from planning to dose delivery.

128. **Endoscopic marker (noun):** Fiducial implanted via endoscope for target localization.
**Related Terms:** Image guidance, Fiducial tracking.
**Example in Radiotherapy:** Endoscopic markers improve pancreatic tumor targeting precision.

129. **Endpoint (noun):** Measured biological or clinical outcome after radiation exposure.
**Related Terms:** Dose-response, Toxicity.
**Example in Radiotherapy:** Tumor control probability is a key endpoint in treatment trials.

130. **Energy deposition (noun):** Transfer of radiation energy to absorbing material.
**Related Terms:** Absorbed dose, LET.
**Example in Radiotherapy:** Energy deposition patterns determine tissue dose uniformity.

131. **Energy fluence rate (noun):** Energy passing per unit area per second.
**Related Terms:** Flux, Dose rate.
**Example in Radiotherapy:** Beam calibration uses measured energy fluence rate values.

132. **Energy per nucleon (noun):** Kinetic energy of particle divided by number of nucleons.
**Related Terms:** Proton energy, Ion therapy.
**Example in Radiotherapy:** Carbon therapy beams specified by energy per nucleon.

133. **Energy release (noun):** Total energy emitted during radioactive decay or interaction.
**Related Terms:** Disintegration energy, Heat conversion.
**Example in Radiotherapy:** Nuclear reactions produce measurable energy release in target material.

134. **Energy spread (noun):** Variation in particle beam energy about a mean value.
**Related Terms:** Energy resolution, Beam stability.
**Example in Radiotherapy:** Narrow energy spread ensures sharp Bragg peak in proton therapy.

135. **Enhanced contrast (noun):** Improved visual differentiation between structures on images.
**Related Terms:** Image quality, Filter processing.
**Example in Radiotherapy:** Enhanced contrast in CBCT aids target delineation.

136. **Enriched isotope (noun):** Material with increased concentration of specific isotope.
**Related Terms:** Radioisotope, Activation.
**Example in Radiotherapy:** Enriched Mo-98 used in production of Tc-99m generators.

137. **Entrance dose (noun):** Radiation dose delivered at beam entry point on patient.
**Related Terms:** Build-up region, Surface dose.
**Example in Radiotherapy:** Entrance dose measured using surface diodes for QA.

138. **Environmental monitor (noun):** Device detecting background or stray radiation in workspace.
**Related Terms:** Area monitoring, Survey meter.
**Example in Radiotherapy:** Environmental monitors ensure radiation levels below limits.

139. **Enzyme repair (noun):** Cellular enzymatic process correcting DNA damage post-irradiation.
**Related Terms:** DNA repair, Sublethal damage.
**Example in Radiotherapy:** Efficient enzyme repair enhances normal tissue recovery.

140. **Epidermal dose (noun):** Radiation dose received by the skin surface layer.
**Related Terms:** Surface dose, Skin reaction.
**Example in Radiotherapy:** Epidermal dose minimized using bolus and beam modifiers.

141. **Epigenetic effect (noun):** Radiation-induced heritable changes in gene expression without DNA mutation.
**Related Terms:** Gene regulation, Radiobiology.
**Example in Radiotherapy:** Epigenetic effects contribute to long-term cellular responses.

142. **Epithelial regeneration (noun):** Healing of epithelial tissues after radiation damage.
**Related Terms:** Recovery, Acute reaction.
**Example in Radiotherapy:** Epithelial regeneration occurs within weeks post-treatment.

143. **Epithelial stem cell (noun):** Basal cell type responsible for tissue renewal after radiation injury.
**Related Terms:** Stem cell kinetics, Regeneration.
**Example in Radiotherapy:** Survival of epithelial stem cells ensures mucosal healing.

144. **Epithelial thickness (noun):** Depth of epithelial tissue layer affecting dose absorption.
**Related Terms:** Surface dose, Skin model.
**Example in Radiotherapy:** Epithelial thickness impacts buildup region dosimetry.

145. **Equilibrium dose (noun):** Dose condition when charged particle equilibrium is achieved.
**Related Terms:** Dmax, CPE.
**Example in Radiotherapy:** Equilibrium dose ensures accurate reference point measurement.

146. **Equilibrium thickness (noun):** Material depth required for charged particle equilibrium.
**Related Terms:** Build-up, Dosimetry.
**Example in Radiotherapy:** Electron beams reach equilibrium thickness at shallow depths.

147. **Equipotential surface (noun):** Surface with constant electric potential.
**Related Terms:** Field uniformity, Electrostatics.
**Example in Radiotherapy:** Equipotential surfaces ensure uniform acceleration in linac design.

148. **Equivalent circular field (noun):** Round field area producing same scatter as rectangular field.
**Related Terms:** Equivalent square, Scatter factor.
**Example in Radiotherapy:** Used in calibration when circular applicators are applied.

149. **Equivalent dose rate (noun):** Weighted absorbed dose delivered per unit time.
**Related Terms:** Effective dose, Radiation weighting factor.
**Example in Radiotherapy:** Equivalent dose rate monitored for radiation workers.

150. **Equivalent medium (noun):** Material simulating tissue absorption and scattering properties.
**Related Terms:** Phantom, Water equivalence.
**Example in Radiotherapy:** Plastic water used as equivalent medium in dosimetry.

**151. Equivalent path length (noun):** Thickness of material producing same attenuation as reference medium.
**Related Terms:** Density correction, CT calibration.
**Example in Radiotherapy:** Equivalent path length method corrects tissue inhomogeneity.

**152. Equivalent point (noun):** Location where measurement represents dose under specific conditions.
**Related Terms:** Effective point, Reference depth.
**Example in Radiotherapy:** Ion chamber shifted to equivalent point during calibration.

**153. Equivalent quality factor (noun):** Weighting factor representing radiation biological effectiveness.
**Related Terms:** LET, RBE.
**Example in Radiotherapy:** Proton beams have higher equivalent quality factors than photons.

**154. Equivalent tissue (noun):** Substitute material with similar attenuation and scatter to human tissue.
**Related Terms:** Phantom, Dosimetry material.
**Example in Radiotherapy:** RW3 slabs serve as equivalent tissue for electron calibration.

**155. Ergonomics (noun):** Study of workplace design for efficiency and safety.
**Related Terms:** Workflow, Fatigue reduction.
**Example in Radiotherapy:** Proper ergonomics reduce therapist strain during patient setup.

**156. Erythematous reaction (noun):** Reddened skin response following radiation exposure.
**Related Terms:** Dermatitis, Acute toxicity.
**Example in Radiotherapy:** Erythematous reaction managed with topical emollients.

**157. Escape probability (noun):** Likelihood of photon leaving material without interaction.
**Related Terms:** Attenuation, Transmission.
**Example in Radiotherapy:** Escape probability affects detector efficiency calibration.

**158. Essential QA (noun):** Mandatory set of tests ensuring radiation delivery accuracy.
**Related Terms:** Daily QA, Dosimetry checks.
**Example in Radiotherapy:** Essential QA performed each morning before treatments.

**159. Estimation bias (noun):** Systematic deviation in calculated measurement.
**Related Terms:** Error margin, Uncertainty.
**Example in Radiotherapy:** Estimation bias minimized by calibration traceability.

**160. Etching (noun):** Chemical process revealing radiation tracks in solid detectors.
**Related Terms:** CR-39, Alpha dosimetry.
**Example in Radiotherapy:** Etching identifies proton track patterns in detectors.

**161. Ethylene oxide sterilization (noun):** Gas method for sterilizing radiation accessories.
**Related Terms:** Infection control, Equipment QA.
**Example in Radiotherapy:** Masks sterilized by ethylene oxide before reuse.

**162. Eudaimonic wellbeing (noun):** Psychological wellness emphasizing purpose and meaning.
**Related Terms:** Patient support, Psycho-oncology.
**Example in Radiotherapy:** Patient education enhances eudaimonic wellbeing during treatment.

**163. Eudose (noun):** Uniform dose distribution ensuring biological equivalence.
**Related Terms:** Homogeneity, Isodose.
**Example in Radiotherapy:** Eudose conditions maintain consistent tumor control.

**164. Euglycemia (noun):** Normal blood glucose level maintained during treatment.
**Related Terms:** Nutrition, Diabetes care.
**Example in Radiotherapy:** Euglycemia prevents fatigue in diabetic patients undergoing therapy.

165. **Eukaryotic cell (noun):** Cell containing nucleus and organelles; radiation-sensitive.
**Related Terms:** DNA repair, Cell death.
**Example in Radiotherapy:** Eukaryotic cells undergo apoptosis post-irradiation.

166. **Eupnea (noun):** Normal, unlabored breathing pattern.
**Related Terms:** Breath-hold, Respiratory gating.
**Example in Radiotherapy:** Eupnea ensures reproducible chest wall position during treatment.

167. **Eutectic solder (noun):** Low-melting alloy used for equipment electrical joints.
**Related Terms:** Maintenance, Electronics.
**Example in Radiotherapy:** Eutectic solder applied in dosimeter repair.

168. **Eutrophic response (noun):** Healthy tissue adaptation following low-dose exposure.
**Related Terms:** Hormesis, Adaptive response.
**Example in Radiotherapy:** Eutrophic responses may explain radiation preconditioning effects.

169. **Evaluation dataset (noun):** Collection of test data for model or algorithm validation.
**Related Terms:** QA dataset, Benchmarking.
**Example in Radiotherapy:** Evaluation dataset used to assess AI contouring accuracy.

170. **Evaluation metric (noun):** Quantitative parameter measuring model or system performance.
**Related Terms:** Dice coefficient, Gamma index.
**Example in Radiotherapy:** Gamma index is a key evaluation metric for dose QA.

171. **Evaluator dose (noun):** Dose measured at pre-determined quality assurance points.
**Related Terms:** Phantom dosimetry, Reference dose.
**Example in Radiotherapy:** Evaluator dose compared with TPS-calculated values.

172. **Event log (noun):** Digital record of all machine or treatment activities.
**Related Terms:** Log file analysis, QA review.
**Example in Radiotherapy:** Event logs used to audit treatment delivery.

173. **Evidence-based practice (noun):** Clinical decisions supported by research and data.
**Related Terms:** Clinical guidelines, Protocol.
**Example in Radiotherapy:** Evidence-based protocols improve consistency in treatment delivery.

174. **Exact match algorithm (noun):** Software method identifying identical data or contours.
**Related Terms:** Registration, Automation.
**Example in Radiotherapy:** Exact match algorithm validates image contour alignment.

175. **Excess dose (noun):** Additional unintended dose above prescribed level.
**Related Terms:** Overdose, QA error.
**Example in Radiotherapy:** Excess dose detected during plan verification.

176. **Exchange ratio (noun):** Proportion of particle exchange in nuclear reaction.
**Related Terms:** Cross-section, Activation.
**Example in Radiotherapy:** Exchange ratio affects neutron capture efficiency.

177. **Excitation energy (noun):** Energy required to raise an electron to higher state.
**Related Terms:** Ionization, Photon interaction.
**Example in Radiotherapy:** Excitation energy defines atomic absorption edges.

178. **Exclusion zone (noun):** Restricted area around radiation source for safety.
**Related Terms:** Controlled area, Shielding.
**Example in Radiotherapy:** Exclusion zones demarcated during HDR brachytherapy.

179. **Excretion pathway (noun):** Route through which radionuclides exit the body.
**Related Terms:** Biological clearance, Excretion rate.
**Example in Radiotherapy:** Iodine excretion pathway primarily via urine.

180. **Exenteration (noun):** Surgical removal of organ contents, often before RT.
**Related Terms:** Preoperative therapy, Palliative care.
**Example in Radiotherapy:** Post-exenteration RT reduces recurrence risk in pelvic malignancy.

181. **Exhalation phase (noun):** Breathing phase during which air exits lungs.
**Related Terms:** Respiratory gating, Motion management.
**Example in Radiotherapy:** Beam delivery synchronized with exhalation for reproducibility.

182. **Exogenous sensitizer (noun):** Chemical enhancing radiation response in cells.
**Related Terms:** Radiosensitizer, Chemoradiation.
**Example in Radiotherapy:** Cisplatin acts as exogenous sensitizer in head-neck cancers.

183. **Exoskeleton support (noun):** External mechanical system aiding therapist posture.
**Related Terms:** Ergonomics, Workplace safety.
**Example in Radiotherapy:** Exoskeleton supports reduce therapist fatigue during setup.

184. **Expansion margin (noun):** Additional volume added to CTV to account for uncertainties.
**Related Terms:** PTV, Setup error.
**Example in Radiotherapy:** 5 mm expansion margin used for prostate PTV.

185. **Exponential fitting (noun):** Mathematical modeling of decay or attenuation data.
**Related Terms:** Curve fitting, Data analysis.
**Example in Radiotherapy:** Exponential fitting applied to dose fall-off measurements.

186. **Exposure (noun):** Amount of ionization produced in air by X-rays or gamma rays.
**Related Terms:** Air kerma, Dose measurement.
**Example in Radiotherapy:** Exposure readings verify consistent output in beam calibration.

187. **Exposure rate (noun):** Rate of ionization production per unit time.
**Related Terms:** Dose rate, Survey meter.
**Example in Radiotherapy:** Exposure rate monitors used to ensure radiation safety compliance.

188. **Exposure time (noun):** Duration of radiation beam activation.
**Related Terms:** Timer error, Beam-on time.
**Example in Radiotherapy:** Exposure time controlled to achieve prescribed dose.

189. **Exponential attenuation (noun):** Reduction of radiation intensity following exponential law.
**Related Terms:** Half-value layer, Linear attenuation coefficient.
**Example in Radiotherapy:** Beam attenuation modeled exponentially through tissue.

190. **Exponential survival curve (noun):** Graph representing exponential cell kill with dose.
**Related Terms:** D0, Radiobiology.
**Example in Radiotherapy:** Exponential survival curves describe bacterial cell inactivation.

191. **Exposed area (noun):** Portion of patient surface irradiated.
**Related Terms:** Field size, Collimation.
**Example in Radiotherapy:** Exposed area limited to minimize normal tissue dose.

192. **External audit (noun):** Independent review ensuring adherence to radiation standards.
**Related Terms:** QA program, Accreditation.
**Example in Radiotherapy:** External audits validate dosimetry system accuracy.

193. **External beam (noun):** Radiation source located outside the patient.
**Related Terms:** Teletherapy, Linac.
**Example in Radiotherapy:** External beam radiotherapy treats deep-seated tumors.

194. **External beam calibration (noun):** Process of quantifying output of teletherapy machine.
**Related Terms:** Absolute dosimetry, Reference condition.
**Example in Radiotherapy:** External beam calibration performed using water phantom.

195. **External beam therapy (noun):** Treatment using radiation delivered from external device.
**Related Terms:** Photon therapy, Proton therapy.
**Example in Radiotherapy:** External beam therapy forms the basis of modern cancer treatment.

196. **External contour (noun):** Outer boundary of patient or phantom used in planning.
**Related Terms:** Body contour, Dose calculation.
**Example in Radiotherapy:** External contour auto-generated during CT import.

197. **External dosimeter (noun):** Device placed outside the body to measure radiation exposure.
**Related Terms:** TLD, OSLD.
**Example in Radiotherapy:** External dosimeters used for patient in vivo verification.

198. **External magnet (noun):** Magnetic device altering charged particle trajectories.
**Related Terms:** Bending magnet, Steering coil.
**Example in Radiotherapy:** External magnets focus proton beam paths.

199. **External photon beam (noun):** High-energy X-ray or gamma beam for therapy.
**Related Terms:** MV beam, Linac photon.
**Example in Radiotherapy:** External photon beams used in intensity-modulated radiotherapy.

200. **External reference point (noun):** Fixed anatomical or marker-based location for setup.
**Related Terms:** Fiducial, Laser alignment.
**Example in Radiotherapy:** Tattoo marks act as external reference points.

201. **External shielding (noun):** Protective barrier reducing radiation exposure to surroundings.
**Related Terms:** Wall barrier, Lead lining.
**Example in Radiotherapy:** Bunker walls provide external shielding.

202. **External target volume (noun):** Region encompassing target visible in external beam plan.
**Related Terms:** CTV, PTV.
**Example in Radiotherapy:** External target volume ensures adequate tumor coverage.

203. **Extra-focal radiation (noun):** Radiation from components other than focal spot.
**Related Terms:** Scatter, Off-axis dose.
**Example in Radiotherapy:** Extra-focal radiation contributes to penumbra broadening.

204. **Extrapolation chamber (noun):** Variable-thickness ionization chamber for surface dose measurement.
**Related Terms:** Plane-parallel chamber, Dosimetry.
**Example in Radiotherapy:** Extrapolation chamber measures beta dose distribution.

205. **Extrapolated range (noun):** Predicted penetration depth of charged particles in medium.
**Related Terms:** Stopping power, CSDA range.
**Example in Radiotherapy:** Extrapolated range defines proton beam endpoint.

206. **Eye shield (noun):** Protective device to prevent ocular radiation injury.
**Related Terms:** Lead shield, Lens dose.
**Example in Radiotherapy:** Eye shields used during facial electron therapy.

207. **Eyeball phantom (noun):** Model mimicking eye for dosimetry and QA.
**Related Terms:** Anthropomorphic phantom, QA device.
**Example in Radiotherapy:** Eyeball phantom measures lens dose in orbital treatments.

208. **Eyelid dose (noun):** Radiation absorbed by eyelid tissue during treatment.
**Related Terms:** Skin dose, Organ at risk.
**Example in Radiotherapy:** Eyelid dose minimized by customized lead shielding.

209. **Eyelid shielding (noun):** Protective covering preventing corneal exposure.
**Related Terms:** Eye protection, Electron therapy.
**Example in Radiotherapy:** Eyelid shielding used in superficial skin cancer irradiation.

210. **Eye lens dose (noun):** Absorbed dose to crystalline lens, critical for cataract prevention.
**Related Terms:** Occupational limit, Dosimetry.
**Example in Radiotherapy:** Eye lens dose monitored for interventional staff.

211. **Eye plaque (noun):** Radioactive applicator used in ocular brachytherapy.
**Related Terms:** Ruthenium plaque, Iodine-125.
**Example in Radiotherapy:** Eye plaques deliver localized dose to intraocular tumors.

212. **Eye position verification (noun):** Technique ensuring accurate ocular alignment before irradiation.
**Related Terms:** Image guidance, Immobilization.
**Example in Radiotherapy:** Eye position verification critical for ocular melanoma treatments.

213. **Eye tracking system (noun):** Device monitoring ocular motion during treatment.
**Related Terms:** Motion management, Real-time feedback.
**Example in Radiotherapy:** Eye tracking enhances precision in proton ocular therapy.

214. **Eyelid applicator (noun):** Specialized surface mold for eyelid irradiation.
**Related Terms:** Brachytherapy, Custom shield.
**Example in Radiotherapy:** Eyelid applicator ensures homogeneous dose delivery.

215. **Eyelid phantom (noun):** Dosimetric model replicating eyelid anatomy.
**Related Terms:** Phantom QA, Organ-specific testing.
**Example in Radiotherapy:** Eyelid phantom validates superficial dose calculations.

216. **Eyring plot (noun):** Graph relating temperature to reaction rate in dosimeters.
**Related Terms:** Thermoluminescence, Calibration.
**Example in Radiotherapy:** Eyring plots used to analyze TLD glow curve behavior.

217. **E-zone (noun):** Area representing electron equilibrium region.
**Related Terms:** Build-up zone, Dose plateau.
**Example in Radiotherapy:** E-zone determines Dmax for electron beams.

218. **E-beam current (noun):** Flow of electrons per second in accelerator.
**Related Terms:** Beam charge, Linac physics.
**Example in Radiotherapy:** E-beam current stability ensures consistent output.

219. **E-beam scattering foil (noun):** Foil used to broaden and uniformize electron beam.
**Related Terms:** Electron mode, Field shaping.
**Example in Radiotherapy:** Scattering foil ensures uniform electron field distribution.

220. **E-beam window (noun):** Thin metal foil allowing electron beam exit from vacuum.
**Related Terms:** Transmission window, Accelerator component.
**Example in Radiotherapy:** Titanium e-beam window maintains pressure integrity.

221. **E-field (noun):** Electric field influencing charged particle motion.
**Related Terms:** Acceleration, Potential difference.
**Example in Radiotherapy:** E-field gradient accelerates electrons in linac waveguide.

222. **E-image registration (noun):** Electronic alignment of pre- and post-treatment images.
**Related Terms:** CBCT, Image fusion.
**Example in Radiotherapy:** E-image registration ensures reproducible patient setup.

223. **E-kernel (noun):** Mathematical model describing dose spread by electrons.
**Related Terms:** Convolution, Dose calculation.
**Example in Radiotherapy:** E-kernel used in collapsed cone algorithm.

224. **E-mode (noun):** Electron operating mode of linear accelerator.
**Related Terms:** Photon mode, Energy setting.
**Example in Radiotherapy:** Machine switched to E-mode for skin treatments.

225. **E-monitor (noun):** Electronic system recording beam output continuously.
**Related Terms:** QA log, Monitor unit check.
**Example in Radiotherapy:** E-monitor verifies MU delivery accuracy.

226. **E-planning (noun):** Electronic treatment planning using dedicated software.
**Related Terms:** TPS, IMRT planning.
**Example in Radiotherapy:** E-planning optimizes dose distribution digitally.

227. **E-proton range (noun):** Effective penetration depth of therapeutic protons.
**Related Terms:** Bragg peak, Range modulation.
**Example in Radiotherapy:** E-proton range determines distal dose fall-off.

228. **E-quality factor (noun):** Energy-based correction applied to detector response.
**Related Terms:** Beam quality, Calibration factor.
**Example in Radiotherapy:** E-quality factor corrects energy dependence of ion chambers.

229. **E-record (noun):** Electronic record containing treatment parameters.
**Related Terms:** EMR, QA documentation.
**Example in Radiotherapy:** E-records ensure traceable treatment data.

230. **E-report (noun):** Digital report summarizing patient or QA results.
**Related Terms:** Audit, EMR.
**Example in Radiotherapy:** E-reports automatically generated after plan approval.

231. **E-safety (noun):** Electronic data protection within radiotherapy systems.
**Related Terms:** Cybersecurity, Data integrity.
**Example in Radiotherapy:** E-safety policies prevent unauthorized data modification.

232. **E-simulator (noun):** Virtual environment mimicking treatment machine for training.
**Related Terms:** Simulation, Education.
**Example in Radiotherapy:** E-simulators train students in treatment setup procedures.

233. **E-stop (noun):** Emergency button halting machine operation.
**Related Terms:** Safety interlock, Emergency protocol.
**Example in Radiotherapy:** E-stop pressed during equipment malfunction.

234. **E-table (noun):** Electronic patient positioning table with motorized controls.
**Related Terms:** Couch shift, Isocentric movement.
**Example in Radiotherapy:** E-table adjusts patient position with submillimeter precision.

**235. E-target (noun):** Electron target producing bremsstrahlung X-rays.
**Related Terms:** Tungsten target, Linac head.
**Example in Radiotherapy:** E-target converts electron energy to therapeutic photons.

**236. E-tether (noun):** Electronic link maintaining data synchronization.
**Related Terms:** Network interface, Automation.
**Example in Radiotherapy:** E-tether ensures live communication between imaging and treatment consoles.

**237. E-treatment verification (noun):** Electronic review of treatment accuracy.
**Related Terms:** Portal imaging, Log file analysis.
**Example in Radiotherapy:** E-treatment verification confirms delivered dose matches plan.

**238. E-volume (noun):** Electronically defined volume in planning system.
**Related Terms:** ROI, Contour.
**Example in Radiotherapy:** E-volumes exported for dose comparison analysis.

**239. E-wedge (noun):** Virtual or physical beam modifier creating dose gradient.
**Related Terms:** Dynamic wedge, Compensation.
**Example in Radiotherapy:** E-wedges applied for breast tangential dose shaping.

**240. E-window (noun):** Thin film permitting radiation beam passage.
**Related Terms:** Transmission window, Linac design.
**Example in Radiotherapy:** E-window minimizes scatter and beam hardening.

**241. Energy window (noun):** Range of photon energies accepted by a detector or imaging system.
**Related Terms:** Spectral resolution, Scintillation detector.
**Example in Radiotherapy:** Proper energy window setting ensures accurate PET signal detection.

**242. Enhanced dynamic wedge (noun):**
Electronic method to achieve wedge-shaped dose without physical wedges.
**Related Terms:** Dynamic jaw, Dose modulation.
**Example in Radiotherapy:** Enhanced dynamic wedge used for breast tangential fields.

**243. Enucleation (noun):** Surgical removal of the eye or tumor mass.
**Related Terms:** Orbital tumor, Ocular radiotherapy.
**Example in Radiotherapy:** Enucleation preceded adjuvant orbital irradiation.

**244. Environmental dosimetry (noun):** Monitoring background or stray radiation levels in the treatment environment.
**Related Terms:** TLD badge, Area monitoring.
**Example in Radiotherapy:** Environmental dosimetry ensures safety around LINAC bunker.

**245. Enzyme inactivation (noun):** Radiation-induced loss of enzyme function due to molecular damage.
**Related Terms:** Radiobiology, Free radicals.
**Example in Radiotherapy:** Enzyme inactivation contributes to cellular metabolic failure post-irradiation.

**246. Epidermal dose (noun):** Radiation dose absorbed at the skin surface.
**Related Terms:** Surface dose, Build-up region.
**Example in Radiotherapy:** Epidermal dose increased by electron contamination.

**247. Epilation (noun):** Hair loss caused by radiation exposure to the scalp or body.
**Related Terms:** Alopecia, Deterministic effect.
**Example in Radiotherapy:** Temporary epilation observed after cranial irradiation.

248. **Epinephrine (noun):** Drug used to treat acute anaphylactic reaction during contrast injection.
**Related Terms:** Emergency drug, Contrast reaction.
**Example in Radiotherapy:** Epinephrine administered after allergic reaction during simulation.

249. **Epitaxial layer (noun):** Thin semiconductor layer for detectors improving radiation sensitivity.
**Related Terms:** Silicon detector, Diode array.
**Example in Radiotherapy:** Epitaxial layers enhance EPID detector response.

250. **Epithermal neutrons (noun):** Neutrons with energies between thermal and fast ranges (~0.5 eV–10 keV).
**Related Terms:** Neutron capture, BNCT.
**Example in Radiotherapy:** Epithermal neutrons used for boron neutron capture therapy.

251. **Equator dose (noun):** Peripheral dose surrounding a radioactive implant source.
**Related Terms:** Isodose, Brachytherapy.
**Example in Radiotherapy:** Equator dose helps determine source spacing in interstitial implants.

252. **Equidistant isodose (noun):** Isodose lines evenly spaced indicating uniform dose falloff.
**Related Terms:** Dose distribution, Homogeneity.
**Example in Radiotherapy:** Equidistant isodose patterns confirm beam uniformity.

253. **Equipment calibration (noun):** Process ensuring radiotherapy devices deliver accurate and consistent dose output.
**Related Terms:** QA, Reference dosimetry.
**Example in Radiotherapy:** Equipment calibration performed monthly per AAPM TG-51.

254. **Equilibrium point (noun):** Depth at which dose deposition equals attenuation in tissue.
**Related Terms:** Dmax, Charged particle equilibrium.
**Example in Radiotherapy:** Electron beam equilibrium point varies with energy.

255. **Equivalent circle diameter (noun):** Diameter representing a field area of non-circular shape.
**Related Terms:** Equivalent square, Scatter factor.
**Example in Radiotherapy:** Equivalent circle used in field size correction.

256. **Equivalent path length (noun):** Radiological thickness converting heterogeneous media to equivalent water thickness.
**Related Terms:** Tissue heterogeneity, CT density correction.
**Example in Radiotherapy:** Equivalent path length used in lung dose correction.

257. **Erector spinae (noun):** Group of muscles supporting vertebral column, relevant in setup positioning.
**Related Terms:** Anatomical landmark, Immobilization.
**Example in Radiotherapy:** Erector spinae contour used for posterior field borders.

258. **E368. Error propagation (noun):** Transmission of measurement uncertainties through calculations.
**Related Terms:** Uncertainty analysis, QA.
**Example in Radiotherapy:** Error propagation considered in composite plan dose accuracy.

259. **Erythema dose (noun):** Radiation dose required to produce visible skin redness.
**Related Terms:** Skin reaction, Threshold dose.
**Example in Radiotherapy:** Erythema dose used historically to estimate exposure.

260. **Esophageal toxicity (noun):** Damage to esophageal tissue due to radiation exposure.
**Related Terms:** Dose constraint, Organ-at-risk.
**Example in Radiotherapy:** Esophageal toxicity observed during thoracic IMRT.

261. **Essential amino acid (noun):** Radiation-sensitive nutrient required for cellular recovery.
**Related Terms:** Radiobiology, Protein synthesis.
**Example in Radiotherapy:** Supplementation aids recovery from radiation-induced damage.

262. **Estimated risk (noun):** Calculated probability of radiation-induced health effect.
**Related Terms:** Risk assessment, Stochastic effect.
**Example in Radiotherapy:** Estimated risk of secondary cancer minimized by shielding.

263. **Ethanol fixation (noun):** Preservation of biological samples post-irradiation for microscopic analysis.
**Related Terms:** Histopathology, Sample preparation.
**Example in Radiotherapy:** Ethanol fixation used in radiobiological assays.

264. **Etiology (noun):** Study of the cause or origin of disease.
**Related Terms:** Oncology, Pathophysiology.
**Example in Radiotherapy:** Etiology of head and neck cancer includes viral infection and smoking.

265. **Eud (Equivalent Uniform Dose) (noun):** Dose concept representing non-uniform dose distribution as uniform equivalent.
**Related Terms:** NTCP, TCP.
**Example in Radiotherapy:** EUD used in radiobiological plan evaluation.

266. **Eukaryote (noun):** Organism with membrane-bound nucleus, includes all human cells.
**Related Terms:** DNA repair, Cell cycle.
**Example in Radiotherapy:** Radiation damage mechanisms differ between eukaryotes and prokaryotes.

267. **Eustachian tube (noun):** Canal connecting middle ear to nasopharynx.
**Related Terms:** Anatomy, Head and neck planning.
**Example in Radiotherapy:** Eustachian tube spared to preserve hearing in NPC cases.

268. **Evaluation point (noun):** Specific location used for dose reporting or verification.
**Related Terms:** Reference point, ICRU.
**Example in Radiotherapy:** ICRU evaluation point used in brachytherapy reporting.

269. **Evaporation chamber (noun):** Device for thin film dosimeter preparation.
**Related Terms:** Film coating, Dosimetry.
**Example in Radiotherapy:** Evaporation chamber used for making LiF TLD films.

270. **Event rate (noun):** Number of detected interactions per unit time.
**Related Terms:** Counting statistics, Detector efficiency.
**Example in Radiotherapy:** Event rate recorded by scintillation counter during QA.

271. **ExacTrac (noun):** Infrared and X-ray image-guidance system for stereotactic setup.
**Related Terms:** IGRT, Localization.
**Example in Radiotherapy:** ExacTrac ensures submillimeter accuracy in brain radiosurgery.

272. **Exchange transfusion (noun):** Replacement of patient blood post-radiation or toxicity.
**Related Terms:** Radiation sickness, Emergency management.
**Example in Radiotherapy:** Rarely used post-accidental exposure.

273. **Excitation energy (noun):** Energy required to elevate an atom or molecule to an excited state.
**Related Terms:** Ionization, Transition.
**Example in Radiotherapy:** Excitation energy influences X-ray emission spectra.

274. **Exclusion volume (noun):** Region intentionally spared from radiation dose.
**Related Terms:** OAR contour, Dose constraint.
**Example in Radiotherapy:** Liver exclusion volume defined in SBRT planning.

275. **Excretion (noun):** Elimination of radioactive substances from the body.
**Related Terms:** Biological half-life, Clearance.
**Example in Radiotherapy:** Excretion rate measured post-radioiodine therapy.

276. **Exponential attenuation (noun):** Decrease of beam intensity proportional to thickness of absorber.
**Related Terms:** Linear attenuation coefficient, HVL.
**Example in Radiotherapy:** Exponential attenuation used in shielding calculations.

277. **Exposure (noun):** Measure of ionization produced in air by X or gamma radiation.
**Related Terms:** Roentgen, Air kerma.
**Example in Radiotherapy:** Exposure units replaced by air kerma in dosimetry.

278. **Exposure rate (noun):** Amount of radiation exposure per unit time.
**Related Terms:** Dose rate, Survey meter.
**Example in Radiotherapy:** Exposure rate measured outside treatment room during QA.

279. **Exposure time (noun):** Duration during which radiation is delivered.
**Related Terms:** Beam-on time, Monitor units.
**Example in Radiotherapy:** Exposure time adjusted for prescribed dose rate.

280. **External beam (noun):** Radiation delivered from a source outside the patient's body.
**Related Terms:** EBRT, Photon therapy.
**Example in Radiotherapy:** External beam used for definitive prostate treatment.

281. **Extrapolation chamber (noun):** Variable volume ionization chamber used for surface dose measurements.
**Related Terms:** Dosimetry, Ion chamber.
**Example in Radiotherapy:** Extrapolation chamber used in skin dose calibration.

282. **Eye dose (noun):** Radiation dose received by lens or ocular tissues.
**Related Terms:** Lens equivalent dose, ALARA.
**Example in Radiotherapy:** Eye dose limited to <10 Gy during orbital IMRT.

283. **Eye fixation (noun):** Technique to immobilize gaze during ocular radiotherapy.
**Related Terms:** Eye tracking, Stereotactic.
**Example in Radiotherapy:** Eye fixation ensures reproducible target alignment.

284. **Eye plaque (noun):** Small brachytherapy applicator for treating intraocular tumors.
**Related Terms:** I-125 plaque, Brachytherapy.
**Example in Radiotherapy:** Eye plaque used for choroidal melanoma.

285. **Eye tolerance (noun):** Maximum safe radiation dose to ocular structures.
**Related Terms:** Dose constraint, Organ tolerance.
**Example in Radiotherapy:** Eye tolerance dose limited to prevent cataract formation.

286. **Eyring model (noun):** Mathematical model describing radiation-induced reaction kinetics.
**Related Terms:** Radiochemistry, Activation energy.
**Example in Radiotherapy:** Eyring model used in polymer dosimeter analysis.

287. **Extrapolated range (noun):** Depth at which electron beam intensity reaches zero.
**Related Terms:** Electron range, Depth dose.
**Example in Radiotherapy:** Extrapolated range used to calculate practical range.

288. **Eye contouring (noun):** Outlining of ocular structures in treatment planning.
**Related Terms:** OAR delineation, Contouring.
**Example in Radiotherapy:** Eye contouring essential in orbital and brain cases.

289. **Eye phantom (noun):** Model simulating ocular tissue for dosimetry studies.
**Related Terms:** Phantom, QA.
**Example in Radiotherapy:** Eye phantom used to validate plaque dosimetry.

290. **Eye shielding lens (noun):** Specialized leaded lens to protect eyes from scattered radiation.
**Related Terms:** Protective eyewear, Scatter.
**Example in Radiotherapy:** Eye shielding lens used by staff during fluoroscopy.

291. **Eyeball dose (noun):** Absorbed dose within the globe of the eye.
**Related Terms:** Lens dose, OAR.
**Example in Radiotherapy:** Eyeball dose minimized by beam shaping in orbital RT.

292. **Eyelid bolus (noun):** Custom bolus material molded to eyelid surface for uniform dose.
**Related Terms:** Superficial therapy, Electron field.
**Example in Radiotherapy:** Eyelid bolus applied to ensure adequate surface dose coverage.

293. **E403. Eyelid edema (noun):** Swelling of eyelid due to radiation-induced inflammation.
**Related Terms:** Acute toxicity, Dermatitis.
**Example in Radiotherapy:** Eyelid edema observed during orbital tumor treatment.

294. **Eye tracking (noun):** System monitoring ocular motion during irradiation.
**Related Terms:** Motion management, Stereotactic guidance.
**Example in Radiotherapy:** Eye tracking ensures accurate dose delivery for ocular melanoma.

295. **Eye-sparing technique (noun):**
Approach minimizing ocular dose through shielding or planning optimization.
**Related Terms:** OAR protection, IMRT.
**Example in Radiotherapy:** Eye-sparing technique used in sinonasal carcinoma therapy.

296. **Eye lens equivalent dose (noun):**
Radiation dose to lens expressed in sieverts, accounting for tissue weighting.
**Related Terms:** Equivalent dose, Lens safety.
**Example in Radiotherapy:** Eye lens equivalent dose monitored for occupational exposure.

297. **Eyring kinetics (noun):** Radiation-induced chemical reaction rate model based on transition-state theory.
**Related Terms:** Activation energy, Dosimeter response.
**Example in Radiotherapy:** Eyring kinetics applied in polymer gel dosimetry studies.

298. **Eardrum dose (noun):** Absorbed dose delivered to tympanic membrane.
**Related Terms:** Ototoxicity, Organ tolerance.
**Example in Radiotherapy:** Eardrum dose kept under threshold during nasopharyngeal irradiation.

299. **Eccentric rotation (noun):** Non-isocentric beam rotation used in certain arc therapies.
**Related Terms:** Arc trajectory, SRS.
**Example in Radiotherapy:** Eccentric rotation improves conformity in cranial SRS.

300. **Echo planar imaging (noun):** MRI technique acquiring entire image in a single excitation.
**Related Terms:** Functional MRI, Diffusion imaging.
**Example in Radiotherapy:** Echo planar imaging used in MR-simulation of brain cases.

301. **Effective current (noun):** Average electron flow responsible for beam output in LINAC.
**Related Terms:** Beam intensity, Electron gun.
**Example in Radiotherapy:** Effective current calibrated to ensure correct MU output.

302. **Effective period (noun):** Total biological impact duration of radiation exposure.
**Related Terms:** Biological half-life, Decay constant.
**Example in Radiotherapy:** Effective period considered in internal radionuclide therapy planning.

303. **Effective volume (noun):** Volume of tissue receiving clinically significant dose.
**Related Terms:** DVH, Dose distribution.
**Example in Radiotherapy:** Effective volume used for NTCP model estimation.

304. **Elastic modulus (noun):** Measure of tissue stiffness influencing deformation during treatment.
**Related Terms:** Deformable registration, Biomechanics.
**Example in Radiotherapy:** Elastic modulus considered in adaptive planning for soft tissue.

305. **Electrical neutrality (noun):**State where positive and negative charges balance in matter.
**Related Terms:** Ionization, Radiation-matter interaction.
**Example in Radiotherapy:** Electrical neutrality maintained before irradiation-induced ionization.

306. **Electrocautery (noun):** Use of electric current to cut or coagulate tissue.
**Related Terms:** Surgery, Thermal damage.
**Example in Radiotherapy:** Electrocautery avoided near radiation fields to prevent skin breakdown.

307. **Electrochemical dosimeter (noun):** Device measuring radiation via induced chemical reactions.
**Related Terms:** Radiolysis, Chemical dosimetry.
**Example in Radiotherapy:** Electrochemical dosimeter used in low-dose verification.

308. **Electrolysis (noun):** Chemical decomposition by electric current influenced by radiation.
**Related Terms:** Radiolysis, Ionization.
**Example in Radiotherapy:** Electrolysis can occur in irradiated aqueous solutions.

309. **Electromagnetic force (noun):** Force governing charged particle motion in accelerator fields.
**Related Terms:** Lorentz force, RF cavity.
**Example in Radiotherapy:** Electromagnetic force accelerates electrons in LINAC waveguide.

310. **Electromagnetic pulse (noun):** Transient burst of electromagnetic energy from beam-switching devices.
**Related Terms:** Transients, System shielding.
**Example in Radiotherapy:** Electromagnetic pulse controlled to prevent signal interference.

311. **Electromagnetic radiation (noun):** Energy waves including X-rays and gamma rays used in therapy.
**Related Terms:** Photon beam, Radiation energy.
**Example in Radiotherapy:** Electromagnetic radiation forms the basis of external beam therapy.

312. **Electromagnetic spectrum (noun):** Range of all radiation frequencies including ionizing regions.
**Related Terms:** Photon energy, X-ray.
**Example in Radiotherapy:** Therapeutic photons occupy high-frequency electromagnetic spectrum.

313. **Electromagnetism (noun):** Physics of electric and magnetic field interactions.
**Related Terms:** Accelerator design, RF generation.
**Example in Radiotherapy:** Electromagnetism principles govern LINAC operation.

314. **Electron affinity (noun):** Energy change when an atom gains an electron.
**Related Terms:** Ionization potential, Electron capture.
**Example in Radiotherapy:** Electron affinity influences dosimeter sensitivity.

315. **Electron capture (noun):** Process where a proton captures an electron, converting to a neutron.
**Related Terms:** Nuclear decay, Isotope transition.
**Example in Radiotherapy:** Electron capture used in decay schemes of isotopes like Co-57.

316. **Electron configuration (noun):** Arrangement of electrons around an atomic nucleus.
**Related Terms:** Atomic structure, X-ray emission.
**Example in Radiotherapy:** Electron configuration affects characteristic X-ray generation.

317. **Electron cooling (noun):** Process reducing beam emittance through energy exchange.
**Related Terms:** Beam focusing, Accelerator physics.
**Example in Radiotherapy:** Electron cooling enhances beam stability in storage rings.

318. **Electron current (noun):** Flow rate of electrons in a beam.
**Related Terms:** Beam intensity, LINAC output.
**Example in Radiotherapy:** Electron current controls dose rate in treatment delivery.

319. **Electron decay (noun):** Transformation of unstable electrons into neutrinos and energy (theoretical).
**Related Terms:** Particle physics, Beta decay.
**Example in Radiotherapy:** Electron decay not observed under normal therapeutic conditions.

320. **Electron diffraction (noun):** Scattering of electrons producing interference patterns.
**Related Terms:** Scattering, Wavelength.
**Example in Radiotherapy:** Electron diffraction considered in dosimeter material analysis.

321. **Electron drift (noun):** Average velocity of electron movement under electric field.
**Related Terms:** Charge transport, Detector signal.
**Example in Radiotherapy:** Electron drift affects ion chamber signal timing.

322. **Electron emission (noun):** Release of electrons from a surface due to thermal or field effects.
**Related Terms:** Cathode, Thermionic emission.
**Example in Radiotherapy:** Electron emission initiated in LINAC gun.

323. **Electron gun current (noun):** Current generated by electron gun filament in LINAC.
**Related Terms:** Filament heating, Beam generation.
**Example in Radiotherapy:** Electron gun current adjusted for stable beam output.

324. **Electron mass (noun):** Fundamental particle mass affecting energy-momentum relationships.
**Related Terms:** Relativistic physics, Energy loss.
**Example in Radiotherapy:** Electron mass influences scattering and stopping power.

325. **Electron optics (noun):** Control of electron trajectories using magnetic or electric fields.
**Related Terms:** Beam focusing, Accelerator design.
**Example in Radiotherapy:** Electron optics used for precise beam collimation.

326. **Electron shell (noun):** Discrete energy level around atomic nucleus.
**Related Terms:** Characteristic X-rays, Photoelectric effect.
**Example in Radiotherapy:** K-shell ionization generates diagnostic X-rays.

327. **Electron stopping power (noun):** Energy loss per unit path length in matter.
**Related Terms:** LET, Energy deposition.
**Example in Radiotherapy:** Electron stopping power essential for depth-dose prediction.

328. **Electron transport equation (noun):** Mathematical model describing electron motion through media.
**Related Terms:** Monte Carlo, Dose computation.
**Example in Radiotherapy:** Transport equation solved in dose algorithms.

329. **Electron volt (noun):** Energy gained by an electron through 1-volt potential difference.
**Related Terms:** Energy unit, MeV.
**Example in Radiotherapy:** LINAC photons typically 6–18 MeV.

330. **Electronic attenuation (noun):** Signal reduction due to resistance or scattering within detectors.
**Related Terms:** Signal loss, Calibration.
**Example in Radiotherapy:** Electronic attenuation corrected in EPID calibration.

331. **Electronic balance (noun):** Precision scale for dosimetry material measurement.
**Related Terms:** QA equipment, Phantom preparation.
**Example in Radiotherapy:** Electronic balance used for bolus fabrication.

332. **Electronic collimation (noun):** Virtual beam shaping using electronic means.
**Related Terms:** MLC, Dynamic collimation.
**Example in Radiotherapy:** Electronic collimation used in CyberKnife planning.

333. **Electronic compensation (noun):** Real-time beam intensity correction using feedback circuits.
**Related Terms:** QA systems, Dose control.
**Example in Radiotherapy:** Electronic compensation stabilizes LINAC dose rate.

334. **Electronic density (noun):** Measure of electron concentration affecting photon attenuation.
**Related Terms:** CT calibration, Dose calculation.
**Example in Radiotherapy:** Electronic density derived from CT number conversion.

335. **Electronic equilibrium (noun):** Condition where electron production equals loss in volume.
**Related Terms:** Dmax, Depth dose.
**Example in Radiotherapy:** Achieved beyond buildup region in photon beams.

336. **Electronic portal imaging (noun):** Digital verification imaging of treatment fields using EPID.
**Related Terms:** IGRT, Setup verification.
**Example in Radiotherapy:** Daily electronic portal imaging ensures positioning accuracy.

337. **Electronic shutter (noun):** Device controlling beam-on timing electronically.
**Related Terms:** Beam gating, Control system.
**Example in Radiotherapy:** Electronic shutter synchronizes gated treatment delivery.

338. **Electronic timer (noun):** Circuit regulating exposure duration precisely.
**Related Terms:** QA, Beam control.
**Example in Radiotherapy:** Electronic timer calibrated annually during QA.

339. **Electrostatic field (noun):** Field generated by stationary electric charges.
**Related Terms:** Coulomb force, Ionization.
**Example in Radiotherapy:** Electrostatic field forms basis of particle acceleration.

340. **Electrostatic lens (noun):** System focusing charged particle beams using electric fields.
**Related Terms:** Beam optics, Accelerator design.
**Example in Radiotherapy:** Electrostatic lenses maintain narrow electron beam.

341. **Electrostatic shielding (noun):** Isolation preventing unwanted electric field interference.
**Related Terms:** Grounding, EMI protection.
**Example in Radiotherapy:** Electrostatic shielding used in LINAC electronics.

342. **Embrittlement (noun):** Radiation-induced material hardening leading to fracture.
**Related Terms:** Radiation damage, Shielding material.
**Example in Radiotherapy:** Long-term neutron exposure causes embrittlement in reactor components.

343. **Endovascular brachytherapy (noun):**
Intraluminal radiation for preventing vessel restenosis.
**Related Terms:** Intravascular therapy, Beta source.
**Example in Radiotherapy:** Endovascular brachytherapy applied post-angioplasty.

344. **Enzyme kinetics (noun):** Rate study of enzyme reactions affected by radiation.
**Related Terms:** Radiobiology, DNA repair.
**Example in Radiotherapy:** Enzyme kinetics altered by cellular irradiation.

345. **Epigenetic effect (noun):** Heritable gene expression changes induced by radiation.
**Related Terms:** DNA methylation, Radiobiology.
**Example in Radiotherapy:** Radiation triggers epigenetic silencing of repair genes.

346. **Epilation threshold (noun):** Minimum dose causing hair loss.
**Related Terms:** Deterministic effect, Skin reaction.
**Example in Radiotherapy:** Epilation threshold reached at 3 Gy for scalp.

347. **Equilibrium dose (noun):** Dose under conditions of particle equilibrium.
**Related Terms:** Dmax, CPE.
**Example in Radiotherapy:** Equilibrium dose achieved beyond buildup depth.

348. **Equilibrium phantom (noun):** Phantom providing charged-particle equilibrium for calibration.
**Related Terms:** QA phantom, Dosimetry.
**Example in Radiotherapy:** Equilibrium phantom ensures reproducible reference conditions.

349. **Erect posture (noun):** Patient standing position for anatomical imaging or verification.
**Related Terms:** Setup, Simulation.
**Example in Radiotherapy:** Erect posture used for spinal curvature assessment.

350. **Error index (noun):** Quantitative indicator of deviation in dose or geometry.
**Related Terms:** QA metric, Gamma index.
**Example in Radiotherapy:** Error index evaluated during plan QA.

351. **Error matrix (noun):** Tabulated representation of prediction versus outcome discrepancies.
**Related Terms:** Machine learning QA, Statistical model.
**Example in Radiotherapy:** Error matrix used in AI-based setup verification.

352. **Escape peak (noun):** Secondary peak in detector spectrum due to escaping characteristic X-rays.
**Related Terms:** Photopeak, Detector response.
**Example in Radiotherapy:** Escape peaks appear in NaI detector spectra.

353. **Esophageal balloon (noun):** Inflatable marker aiding esophageal tumor localization.
**Related Terms:** IGRT, Fiducial.
**Example in Radiotherapy:** Esophageal balloon used for alignment in SBRT.

354. **Etch track detector (noun):** Solid-state detector recording charged particle tracks.
**Related Terms:** Neutron dosimetry, CR-39.
**Example in Radiotherapy:** Etch track detector used in proton QA.

355. **Ethylene dosimeter (noun):** Gas-filled dosimeter measuring radiolytic ethylene yield.
**Related Terms:** Chemical dosimetry, Gas analysis.
**Example in Radiotherapy:** Ethylene dosimeter used for cobalt source calibration.

356. **Etiologic factor (noun):** Causal element contributing to disease or damage.
**Related Terms:** Carcinogen, Risk factor.
**Example in Radiotherapy:** Radiation acts as an etiologic factor in cataractogenesis.

357. **Eutectic alloy (noun):** Low-melting alloy used in shielding or source encapsulation.
**Related Terms:** Lead substitute, Shield fabrication.
**Example in Radiotherapy:** Eutectic alloy molds conformal shields.

358. **Evacuated tube (noun):** Vacuum-sealed tube for electron acceleration.
**Related Terms:** LINAC waveguide, Vacuum system.
**Example in Radiotherapy:** Evacuated tube essential for beam propagation.

359. **Evaluation metric (noun):** Quantitative tool for assessing treatment plan quality.
**Related Terms:** DVH, Conformity index.
**Example in Radiotherapy:** Conformity and homogeneity indices serve as evaluation metrics.

360. **Event reconstruction (noun):** Determination of interaction points in detectors.
**Related Terms:** PET imaging, Detector response.
**Example in Radiotherapy:** Event reconstruction improves PET image resolution.

361. **Exchange current (noun):** Steady-state charge flow maintaining electrode equilibrium.
**Related Terms:** Electrochemistry, Dosimeter.
**Example in Radiotherapy:** Exchange current stability ensures dosimeter accuracy.

362. **Exenteration (noun):** Surgical removal of orbital contents.
**Related Terms:** Postoperative RT, Ocular tumor.
**Example in Radiotherapy:** Post-exenteration radiotherapy prevents recurrence.

363. **Expansion margin (noun):** Added geometric margin accounting for organ motion or uncertainty.
**Related Terms:** PTV, GTV.
**Example in Radiotherapy:** 5 mm expansion margin used around prostate.

364. **Exposure chamber (noun):** Device used for calibration by measuring ionization in air.
**Related Terms:** Ionization chamber, Dosimetry.
**Example in Radiotherapy:** Exposure chamber used to calibrate TLDs.

365. **Exposure index (noun):** Indicator of image receptor radiation level.
**Related Terms:** Image quality, Detector dose.
**Example in Radiotherapy:** Exposure index monitored in verification imaging.

366. **Exposure meter (noun):** Instrument measuring radiation intensity or exposure.
**Related Terms:** Survey meter, QA tool.
**Example in Radiotherapy:** Exposure meter used for barrier testing.

367. **Extended field (noun):** Large treatment field encompassing adjacent lymphatic regions.
**Related Terms:** Mantle field, Nodal irradiation.
**Example in Radiotherapy:** Extended field used for cervical cancer.

368. **Extended SSD technique (noun):** Treatment setup using large source-surface distance.
**Related Terms:** SSD correction, Electron therapy.
**Example in Radiotherapy:** Extended SSD used for total skin irradiation.

369. **External calibration (noun):** Calibration using reference dosimeter outside main equipment.
**Related Terms:** Secondary standard, QA.
**Example in Radiotherapy:** External calibration ensures cross-machine accuracy.

370. **External contour (noun):** Patient's body outline in planning system.
**Related Terms:** Body contour, CT simulation.
**Example in Radiotherapy:** External contour auto-generated in TPS.

371. **External dosimeter (noun):** Badge measuring radiation dose received externally.
**Related Terms:** TLD, OSLD.
**Example in Radiotherapy:** External dosimeters monitor staff exposure.

372. **External exposure (noun):** Radiation received from sources outside the body.
**Related Terms:** EBRT, Occupational exposure.
**Example in Radiotherapy:** External exposure minimized by shielding.

373. **External photon field (noun):** Photon beam generated by LINAC for external therapy.
**Related Terms:** X-ray beam, Photon therapy.
**Example in Radiotherapy:** External photon field used for deep-seated tumors.

374. **External scattering (noun):** Scattering of radiation outside the treatment field.
**Related Terms:** Leakage, Collimator scatter.
**Example in Radiotherapy:** External scattering minimized using collimator jaws.

375. **Extrapolated range (noun):** Depth where particle beam energy approaches zero.
**Related Terms:** Proton range, Depth-dose curve.
**Example in Radiotherapy:** Extrapolated range defines Bragg peak endpoint.

376. **Extrapolation chamber (noun):** Variable-volume ionization chamber for surface dose measurements.
**Related Terms:** Dosimetry, Calibration.
**Example in Radiotherapy:** Extrapolation chamber used for electron surface dosimetry.

377. **Extrinsic calibration (noun):** Calibration correcting for external or environmental factors.
**Related Terms:** QA, Environmental correction.
**Example in Radiotherapy:** Extrinsic calibration applied for barometric changes.

378. **Eye dose constraint (noun):** Maximum allowable radiation to ocular structures.
**Related Terms:** OAR, Tolerance dose.
**Example in Radiotherapy:** Eye dose constraint kept below 10 Gy.

379. **Eye fixation (noun):** Stabilization of gaze during ocular irradiation.
**Related Terms:** Motion control, Immobilization.
**Example in Radiotherapy:** Eye fixation ensures accuracy in plaque therapy.

380. **Eye plaque (noun):** Radioactive source carrier for ocular brachytherapy.
**Related Terms:** Brachytherapy, Eye melanoma.
**Example in Radiotherapy:** I-125 eye plaque used for choroidal melanoma.

381. **Eye tracking camera (noun):** Optical system monitoring eye movement.
**Related Terms:** IGRT, Motion tracking.
**Example in Radiotherapy:** Eye tracking camera integrated in ocular proton therapy.

382. **Eye wall (noun):** Outer layer of the eyeball including sclera and cornea.
**Related Terms:** OAR, Dose constraint.
**Example in Radiotherapy:** Eye wall delineated as critical structure in planning.

383. **Eyewear dosimeter (noun):** Dosimeter attached to protective glasses to measure eye dose.
**Related Terms:** TLD, Occupational safety.
**Example in Radiotherapy:** Eyewear dosimeters used for interventional radiologists.

384. **Eyring plot (noun):** Graphical method for determining activation energy from rate data.
**Related Terms:** Reaction kinetics, Dosimeter study.
**Example in Radiotherapy:** Eyring plot applied in polymer dosimeter analysis.

385. **Ezetimibe analog (noun):** Compound under study for radioprotection via lipid modulation.
**Related Terms:** Radioprotector, Pharmacology.
**Example in Radiotherapy:** Ezetimibe analog tested for endothelial protection.

386. **Efficacy curve (noun):** Plot showing therapeutic effect versus dose.
**Related Terms:** Dose-response, Radiobiology.
**Example in Radiotherapy:** Efficacy curve used to assess radiosensitizer performance.

387. **Electrophoresis gel dosimeter (noun):**
Gel medium showing dose-dependent migration changes.
**Related Terms:** 3D dosimetry, Radiochemical response.
**Example in Radiotherapy:** Electrophoresis gel dosimeter visualizes dose distribution.

388. **Ex vivo irradiation (noun):** Irradiation of cells or tissues outside the living organism.
**Related Terms:** Experimental model, Radiobiology.
**Example in Radiotherapy:** Ex vivo irradiation used for biological dosimetry.

389. **Eye tolerance dose (noun):** Maximum safe dose for ocular structures.
**Related Terms:** OAR, TD 5/5.
**Example in Radiotherapy:** Eye tolerance dose maintained below 45 Gy.

390. **Eye tracking system (noun):** Integrated hardware for monitoring ocular position during irradiation.
**Related Terms:** IGRT, Motion management.
**Example in Radiotherapy:** Eye tracking system ensures precision in ocular proton therapy.

391. **Elastic recoil (noun):** Backward motion of a nucleus following particle interaction.
**Related Terms:** Momentum transfer, Scattering.
**Example in Radiotherapy:** Elastic recoil contributes to microscopic energy deposition.

392. **Electric field uniformity (noun):** Consistency of electric field strength across an accelerating structure.
**Related Terms:** Beam stability, RF cavity.
**Example in Radiotherapy:** Field uniformity ensures consistent electron acceleration.

393. **Electrical noise (noun):** Unwanted signal fluctuations in electronic systems.
**Related Terms:** Signal-to-noise ratio, Interference.
**Example in Radiotherapy:** Electrical noise can degrade detector accuracy.

394. **Electro-mechanical drift (noun):** Gradual positional change due to mechanical or electronic factors.
**Related Terms:** Isocenter drift, QA.
**Example in Radiotherapy:** Electro-mechanical drift monitored during monthly QA.

395. **Electromagnetic compatibility (noun):** Ability of equipment to function without electromagnetic interference.
**Related Terms:** EMI shielding, System integration.
**Example in Radiotherapy:** EMC testing ensures MRI-linac safety.

396. **Electron beam alignment (noun):** Adjustment ensuring electron beam follows intended trajectory.
**Related Terms:** Beam steering, QA.
**Example in Radiotherapy:** Electron beam alignment verified during commissioning.

397. **Electron beam flatness (noun):** Uniformity of dose across electron field.
**Related Terms:** Symmetry, Beam profile.
**Example in Radiotherapy:** Flatness checked using water phantom scans.

398. **Electron build-up region (noun):** Surface region where dose increases rapidly with depth.
**Related Terms:** Dmax, Surface dose.
**Example in Radiotherapy:** Bolus modifies the electron build-up region.

399. **Electron contamination factor (noun):** Correction for secondary electrons in photon beams.
**Related Terms:** Surface dose, Beam quality.
**Example in Radiotherapy:** Applied during skin dose estimation.

400. **Electron field matching (noun):** Junction of adjacent electron fields without overdose or under dose.
**Related Terms:** Field junction, Hot spot.
**Example in Radiotherapy:** Critical in large chest wall treatments.

401. **Electron fluence (noun):** Number of electrons crossing a unit area.
**Related Terms:** Particle fluence, Dose calculation.
**Example in Radiotherapy:** Electron fluence relates directly to absorbed dose.

402. **Electron lateral scatter (noun):** Sideways spread of electrons in tissue.
**Related Terms:** Penumbra, Multiple scattering.
**Example in Radiotherapy:** Limits electron field edge sharpness.

403. **Electron penetration depth (noun):** Maximum depth of clinically useful electron dose.
**Related Terms:** Practical range, Energy selection.
**Example in Radiotherapy:** Determines electron energy choice.

404. **Electron purity (noun):** Fraction of electrons relative to contaminant photons.
**Related Terms:** Beam contamination, Mode purity.
**Example in Radiotherapy:** Higher purity desired in superficial treatments.

405. **Electron range straggling (noun):** Statistical variation in electron penetration depth.
**Related Terms:** Energy spread, Dose falloff.
**Example in Radiotherapy:** Causes gradual distal dose reduction.

406. **Electron scattering power (noun):** Material property describing electron deflection likelihood.
**Related Terms:** Atomic number, Multiple scattering.
**Example in Radiotherapy:** Higher Z materials increase scatter.

407. **Electron source stability (noun):** Consistency of electron emission over time.
**Related Terms:** Filament current, Output stability.
**Example in Radiotherapy:** Stability affects daily output consistency.

408. **Electron stopping range (noun):** Depth at which electron energy becomes negligible.
**Related Terms:** CSDA range, Depth dose.
**Example in Radiotherapy:** Used in shielding calculations.

409. **Electron transport kernel (noun):** Mathematical representation of electron dose spread.
**Related Terms:** Convolution, Dose algorithm.
**Example in Radiotherapy:** Used in pencil beam calculations.

410. **Electron yield (noun):** Number of electrons produced per interaction.
**Related Terms:** Secondary electrons, Ionization.
**Example in Radiotherapy:** Influences microscopic dose deposition.

411. **Electronic beam symmetry (noun):** Balance of dose distribution across beam axis.
**Related Terms:** Flatness, QA.
**Example in Radiotherapy:** Symmetry checked during daily QA.

412. **Electronic correction factor (noun):** Adjustment accounting for detector electronics response.
**Related Terms:** Calibration factor, QA.
**Example in Radiotherapy:** Applied to ion chamber readings.

413. **Electronic drift correction (noun):** Compensation for gradual signal change over time.
**Related Terms:** Baseline shift, Detector stability.
**Example in Radiotherapy:** Improves long-term measurement accuracy.

414. **Electronic gating signal (noun):** Trigger controlling beam delivery timing.
**Related Terms:** Respiratory gating, Motion control.
**Example in Radiotherapy:** Used in gated lung treatments.

415. **Electronic latency (noun):** Delay between command and system response.
**Related Terms:** Control system, Real-time delivery.
**Example in Radiotherapy:** Low latency critical for adaptive RT.

416. **Electronic output verification (noun):** Automated confirmation of delivered output.
**Related Terms:** Log-file QA, Verification.
**Example in Radiotherapy:** Used in VMAT QA workflows.

417. **Electronic response linearity (noun):** Proportionality of signal to dose.
**Related Terms:** Detector linearity, Calibration.
**Example in Radiotherapy:** Linearity verified during commissioning.

418. **Electronic signal saturation (noun):** Maximum signal limit beyond which response plateaus.
**Related Terms:** Dynamic range, Detector limit.
**Example in Radiotherapy:** Avoided in high dose-rate beams.

419. **Electronic tracking accuracy (noun):** Precision of electronically monitored motion.
**Related Terms:** Tracking error, Motion management.
**Example in Radiotherapy:** Critical in tumor tracking systems.

420. **Electrode polarization (noun):** Charge build up altering detector response.
**Related Terms:** Ion recombination, Chamber bias.
**Example in Radiotherapy:** Corrected using polarity measurements.

421. **Electromagnetic shielding (noun):** Barrier preventing unwanted EM interference.
**Related Terms:** EMI control, System safety.
**Example in Radiotherapy:** Protects imaging electronics.

422. **Electromagnetic steering (noun):** Beam direction control using magnetic fields.
**Related Terms:** Beam optics, Steering coil.
**Example in Radiotherapy:** Used to center the electron beam.

423. **Electromagnetic torque (noun):** Rotational force produced by EM fields.
**Related Terms:** Motor control, Gantry rotation.
**Example in Radiotherapy:** Drives gantry motion systems.

424. **Energy calibration drift (noun):** Gradual change in measured beam energy.
**Related Terms:** Output drift, QA.
**Example in Radiotherapy:** Detected during annual energy checks.

425. **Energy cutoff (noun):** Minimum energy contributing to dose.
**Related Terms:** Spectrum threshold, Beam filtering.
**Example in Radiotherapy:** Used in Monte Carlo simulations.

426. **Energy deposition density (noun):** Energy deposited per unit volume.
**Related Terms:** LET, Microdosimetry.
**Example in Radiotherapy:** Higher in proton Bragg peak.

427. **Energy fluence spectrum (noun):** Distribution of energy across fluence components.
**Related Terms:** Beam quality, Spectrum analysis.
**Example in Radiotherapy:** Influences tissue penetration.

428. **Energy loss fluctuation (noun):** Random variation in particle energy loss.
**Related Terms:** Straggling, Stochastic effects.
**Example in Radiotherapy:** Impacts depth-dose precision.

429. **Energy matching (noun):** Alignment of beam energy to planned value.
**Related Terms:** Beam tuning, QA.
**Example in Radiotherapy:** Ensures accurate penetration depth.

430. **Energy modulation width (noun):** Range over which beam energy is varied.
**Related Terms:** SOBP, Range modulation.
**Example in Radiotherapy:** Determines proton target coverage.

431. **Energy response correction (noun):** Adjustment for detector energy dependence.
**Related Terms:** Calibration factor, Dosimetry.
**Example in Radiotherapy:** Applied to diode detectors.

432. **Energy straggling (noun):** Statistical spread of particle energies.
**Related Terms:** Range uncertainty, Beam spread.
**Example in Radiotherapy:** Affects distal falloff sharpness.

433. **Energy-weighted dose (noun):** Dose accounting for energy distribution.
**Related Terms:** LET weighting, Radiobiology.
**Example in Radiotherapy:** Used in RBE modeling.

434. **Enhanced contrast resolution (noun):** Ability to distinguish small density differences.
**Related Terms:** Image quality, Noise reduction.
**Example in Radiotherapy:** Important in soft-tissue CBCT.

435. **Enhanced motion robustness (noun):** Plan resilience against patient motion.
**Related Terms:** Robust optimization, Gating.
**Example in Radiotherapy:** Critical in lung SBRT.

436. **Entry point localization (noun):** Identification of beam entrance on patient surface.
**Related Terms:** Surface imaging, Setup verification.
**Example in Radiotherapy:** Used in non-coplanar beams.

437. **Environmental shielding factor (noun):** Reduction factor due to surrounding barriers.
**Related Terms:** Shielding design, Dose reduction.
**Example in Radiotherapy:** Used in bunker calculations.

438. **Equivalent biological effect (noun):** Comparison of different dose distributions biologically.
**Related Terms:** BED, EUD.
**Example in Radiotherapy:** Used to compare fractionation schemes.

439. **Equivalent electron thickness (noun):** Electron penetration equivalence of material.
**Related Terms:** Water equivalence, Dosimetry.
**Example in Radiotherapy:** Used for bolus materials.

440. **Equivalent field correction (noun):** Adjustment for irregular field shapes.
**Related Terms:** Scatter factor, Output factor.
**Example in Radiotherapy:** Applied in MU calculations.

441. **Equivalent monitor units (noun):** Normalized MU accounting for modifiers.
**Related Terms:** MU correction, Output scaling.
**Example in Radiotherapy:** Used in composite plans.

442. **Equivalent scattering medium (noun):** Material simulating tissue scattering properties.
**Related Terms:** Phantom material, QA.
**Example in Radiotherapy:** Plastic water slabs used.

443. **Error envelope (noun):** Range of possible deviation around measurement.
**Related Terms:** Uncertainty band, QA tolerance.
**Example in Radiotherapy:** Used in dose reporting.

444. **Error propagation model (noun):** Method estimating cumulative uncertainty.
**Related Terms:** Statistical analysis, QA.
**Example in Radiotherapy:** Used in adaptive dose accumulation.

445. **Event detection efficiency (noun):** Probability of detecting a radiation interaction.
**Related Terms:** Detector efficiency, Sensitivity.
**Example in Radiotherapy:** Important in PET imaging.

446. **Event synchronization (noun):** Timing alignment between system components.
**Related Terms:** Trigger signal, Latency.
**Example in Radiotherapy:** Required for gated delivery.

447. **Exit surface localization (noun):** Identification of beam exit point.
**Related Terms:** Exit dose, Surface imaging.
**Example in Radiotherapy:** Used in transit dosimetry.

448. **Exit window attenuation (noun):** Beam reduction due to exit window material.
**Related Terms:** Transmission factor, Beam quality.
**Example in Radiotherapy:** Considered in linac head modeling.

449. **Exposure correction coefficient (noun):** Factor correcting measured exposure values.
**Related Terms:** Calibration constant, Dosimetry.
**Example in Radiotherapy:** Used in air Kerma measurements.

450. **Exposure uniformity (noun):** Consistency of radiation exposure across field.
**Related Terms:** Flatness, Symmetry.
**Example in Radiotherapy:** Evaluated in imaging systems.

451. **External alignment tolerance (noun):** Permissible setup deviation limit.
**Related Terms:** Setup error, QA.
**Example in Radiotherapy:** Typically ±2 mm for SBRT.

452. **External motion surrogate (noun):** External signal representing internal motion.
**Related Terms:** Respiratory belt, Gating.
**Example in Radiotherapy:** Used in lung motion tracking.

453. **External reference geometry (noun):** Fixed coordinate system for setup.
**Related Terms:** Lasers, Isocenter.
**Example in Radiotherapy:** Used during simulation.

454. **External scatter contribution (noun):** Dose from scattering outside primary field.
**Related Terms:** Leakage dose, Head scatter.
**Example in Radiotherapy:** Included in whole-body dose.

455. **External system latency (noun):** Delay between connected systems.
**Related Terms:** Network delay, Synchronization.
**Example in Radiotherapy:** Relevant in MR-guided RT.

456. **Extrapolated dose gradient (noun):** Estimated slope beyond measured region.
**Related Terms:** Dose falloff, Gradient index.
**Example in Radiotherapy:** Used in SRS evaluation.

457. **Eye movement uncertainty (noun):** Positional error due to ocular motion.
**Related Terms:** Tracking error, Immobilization.
**Example in Radiotherapy:** Important in eye plaque therapy.

458. **Eye sparing priority (noun):** Optimization emphasis to reduce ocular dose.
**Related Terms:** OAR weighting, Planning objective.
**Example in Radiotherapy:** Applied in Sinonasal tumors.

459. **Eye surface dose (noun):** Dose delivered to ocular surface tissues.
**Related Terms:** Corneal dose, Skin dose.
**Example in Radiotherapy:** Minimized using shielding.

460. **Effective attenuation coefficient (noun):** Combined measure of beam reduction due to absorption and scatter.
**Related Terms:** Linear attenuation, Beam hardening.
**Example in Radiotherapy:** Used to estimate dose reduction through tissue.

461. **Effective beam width (noun):** Usable width of a radiation beam contributing to dose.
**Related Terms:** Penumbra, Field size.
**Example in Radiotherapy:** Important in small-field dosimetry.

462. **Effective calibration depth (noun):** Depth at which detector calibration is referenced.
**Related Terms:** Reference depth, Dosimetry protocol.
**Example in Radiotherapy:** Defined in TG-51 measurements.

463. **Effective density override (noun):** Assigned density replacing CT-derived values.
**Related Terms:** Heterogeneity correction, Planning override.
**Example in Radiotherapy:** Used near metal implants.

464. **Effective detector volume (noun):** Sensitive region contributing to signal generation.
**Related Terms:** Volume averaging, Spatial resolution.
**Example in Radiotherapy:** Smaller volumes preferred for steep gradients.

465. **Effective dose contribution (noun):** Portion of total effective dose from a source.
**Related Terms:** Risk weighting, Organ dose.
**Example in Radiotherapy:** Imaging dose contributes to effective dose.

466. **Effective field equivalence (noun):** Irregular field represented as an equivalent square.
**Related Terms:** Equivalent square, Output factor.
**Example in Radiotherapy:** Used in manual MU calculations.

467. **Effective fluence map (noun):** Resulting fluence after modulation and filtering.
**Related Terms:** Beam modulation, Optimization.
**Example in Radiotherapy:** Evaluated during IMRT planning.

468. **Effective gantry angle (noun):** Delivered angle accounting for mechanical offsets.
**Related Terms:** Gantry sag, Geometry correction.
**Example in Radiotherapy:** Important in non-coplanar treatments.

469. **Effective imaging isocenter (noun):** Actual center of imaging system geometry.
**Related Terms:** Imaging QA, Isocenter coincidence.
**Example in Radiotherapy:** Compared with treatment isocenter.

470. **Effective irradiated volume (noun):** Volume receiving clinically relevant dose.
**Related Terms:** Integral dose, Low-dose bath.
**Example in Radiotherapy:** Larger in VMAT than 3D-CRT.

471. **Effective kernel width (noun):** Spatial extent of dose spread kernel.
**Related Terms:** Convolution, Algorithm resolution.
**Example in Radiotherapy:** Affects dose smoothing.

472. **Effective leaf gap (noun):** Modeled opening accounting for MLC transmission.
**Related Terms:** Dosimetric leaf gap, MLC modeling.
**Example in Radiotherapy:** Commissioned in TPS.

473. **Effective monitor unit scaling (noun):** Adjustment of MU to achieve prescribed dose.
**Related Terms:** Output correction, Normalization.
**Example in Radiotherapy:** Applied for wedges or trays.

474. **Effective motion envelope (noun):** Combined range of target motion.
**Related Terms:** ITV, Motion margin.
**Example in Radiotherapy:** Used for lung targets.

475. **Effective penetration depth (noun):** Depth at which useful dose is delivered.
**Related Terms:** Beam energy, Range.
**Example in Radiotherapy:** Guides energy selection.

476. **Effective point of measurement (noun):** Location representing detector response.
**Related Terms:** EPOM, Ion chamber.
**Example in Radiotherapy:** Shifted upstream for cylindrical chambers.

477. **Effective range uncertainty (noun):** Combined uncertainty in particle range.
**Related Terms:** Proton range error, Robust planning.
**Example in Radiotherapy:** Accounted for in margins.

478. **Effective resolution limit (noun):** Smallest distinguishable spatial detail.
**Related Terms:** Detector resolution, Imaging quality.
**Example in Radiotherapy:** Limits CBCT soft-tissue detail.

479. **Effective scatter source (noun):** Equivalent origin of scattered radiation.
**Related Terms:** Scatter modeling, Dose calculation.
**Example in Radiotherapy:** Used in analytical algorithms.

480. **Effective segment weight (noun):** Relative contribution of a delivery segment.
**Related Terms:** Control point, Fluence weighting.
**Example in Radiotherapy:** Optimized during IMRT planning.

481. **Effective setup margin (noun):** Margin compensating for residual setup errors.
**Related Terms:** PTV margin, Uncertainty.
**Example in Radiotherapy:** Smaller with daily IGRT.

482. **Effective slice thickness (noun):** Actual reconstructed image thickness.
**Related Terms:** Partial volume effect, CT resolution.
**Example in Radiotherapy:** Affects contour accuracy.

483. **Effective source position (noun):** Apparent radiation origin after head effects.
**Related Terms:** Source modeling, TPS.
**Example in Radiotherapy:** Used in beam modeling.

484. **Effective spatial uncertainty (noun):**
Combined positional uncertainty from all sources.
**Related Terms:** Margin recipe, Error propagation.
**Example in Radiotherapy:** Used in robust planning.

485. **Effective target coverage (noun):** Portion of target receiving prescribed dose.
**Related Terms:** V95%, Coverage metric.
**Example in Radiotherapy:** Evaluated in plan review.

486. **Effective tissue equivalence (noun):** Similarity of material to human tissue.
**Related Terms:** Water equivalence, Phantom material.
**Example in Radiotherapy:** Important for dosimetry phantoms.

487. **Effective transmission factor (noun):** Net transmission through beam modifiers.
**Related Terms:** Tray factor, MLC transmission.
**Example in Radiotherapy:** Included in MU calculations.

488. **Effective treatment time (noun):** Actual beam-on time including modulation.
**Related Terms:** Delivery efficiency, Dose rate.
**Example in Radiotherapy:** Longer in gated treatments.

489. **Effective voxel volume (noun):** Physical volume represented by a voxel.
**Related Terms:** Dose grid, Resolution.
**Example in Radiotherapy:** Smaller voxels for SRS.

490. **Electron backscatter contribution (noun):** Dose increase due to electron reflection.
**Related Terms:** Surface dose, Interface effects.
**Example in Radiotherapy:** Occurs near high-Z materials.

491. **Electron contamination spectrum (noun):** Energy distribution of contaminant electrons.
**Related Terms:** Surface dose, Beam quality.
**Example in Radiotherapy:** Considered in skin dose estimates.

492. **Electron fluence smoothing (noun):** Reduction of sharp fluence variations.
**Related Terms:** Optimization regularization, IMRT.
**Example in Radiotherapy:** Improves delivery stability.

493. **Electron scatter halo (noun):** Low-dose region surrounding electron fields.
**Related Terms:** Lateral scatter, Penumbra.
**Example in Radiotherapy:** Affects nearby OARs.

494. **Electron transport uncertainty (noun):** Error in modeling electron movement.
**Related Terms:** Dose calculation uncertainty, TPS.
**Example in Radiotherapy:** Higher in heterogeneous tissues.

495. **Energy modulation efficiency (noun):** Effectiveness of varying beam energy.
**Related Terms:** Range modulation, SOBP.
**Example in Radiotherapy:** Critical in proton therapy.

496. **Energy spectrum hardening (noun):** Increase in mean beam energy after filtration.
**Related Terms:** Beam hardening, Filtration.
**Example in Radiotherapy:** Seen after patient attenuation.

497. **Energy transfer efficiency (noun):** Fraction of beam energy deposited in tissue.
**Related Terms:** Energy deposition, Dose efficiency.
**Example in Radiotherapy:** Higher in proton therapy near the Bragg peak.

498. **Enhanced edge definition (noun):** Improved sharpness at structure boundaries.
**Related Terms:** Image resolution, Contrast enhancement.
**Example in Radiotherapy:** Helps with accurate target contouring.

499. **Exit dose verification (noun):** Measurement of radiation dose leaving the patient.
**Related Terms:** Transit dosimetry, In vivo QA.
**Example in Radiotherapy:** Used to confirm treatment delivery accuracy.

500. **Edge Dose Gradient (noun):** Rate of dose fall-off at the boundary of the target or organ at risk.
**Related Terms:** Penumbra, Dose Gradient Index.
**Example in Radiotherapy:** A steep edge dose gradient is essential in stereotactic radiotherapy to spare adjacent critical structures.

# F

1. **FA (Fractional Activity):** The proportion of radioactive activity administered per treatment fraction.
   **Related Terms:** Dosimetry, activity per fraction.
   **Example:** In kidney radioimmunotherapy, FA ensures each fraction delivers the correct dose.
2. **Fallout:** Residual radioactive material deposited in the environment after nuclear exposure.
   **Related Terms:** Environmental radiation, contamination.
   **Example:** QA protocols monitor fallout levels during accidental isotope release.
3. **Fano Factor:** Statistical measure of variance in ionization events relative to the mean; used in dosimetry.
   **Related Terms:** Detector response, statistical noise.
   **Example:** Important for calibrating semiconductor detectors in QA of LINAC beams
4. **Fast Neutron:** Neutron with kinetic energy typically above 1 MeV, used in specialized radiotherapy.
   **Related Terms:** Neutron therapy, dose distribution.
   **Example:** QA ensures uniform fast neutron field when treating deep-seated tumors.
5. **Filter (Radiation):** Material inserted in a beam to modify its energy spectrum.
   **Related Terms:** Beam hardening, X-ray filtration.
   **Example:** KV filters in imaging QA reduce low-energy X-rays to optimize image contrast.
6. **Focal Spot:** Small region on the X-ray tube target where electrons hit to produce X-rays.
   **Related Terms:** Resolution, geometric unsharpness.
   **Example:** QA measures focal spot size to ensure sharp kidney radiographs.
7. **Focal Plane:** Plane where the imaging system achieves optimal focus.
   **Related Terms:** Depth of field, imaging clarity.
   **Example:** In planar kidney imaging, QA verifies correct focal plane alignment for accurate contours.
8. **Focal Therapy:** Radiotherapy targeted to a specific lesion or tumor area rather than the whole organ.
   **Related Terms:** Stereotactic radiotherapy, conformal therapy.
   **Example:** Focal therapy for liver or prostate lesions guided by imaging QA.
9. **Folded Filter:** Complex filter design in nuclear imaging or radiation therapy to shape dose distribution.
   **Related Terms:** Beam modulation, compensator.
   **Example:** QA ensures folded filters create the intended dose distribution in conformal therapy.
10. **Fractionation:** Division of total radiation dose into multiple smaller doses.
    **Related Terms:** Hypofractionation, conventional fractionation.
    **Example:** QA verifies dose per fraction delivered to the kidney in multiple sessions.
11. **Fractional Dose:** Radiation dose delivered in a single fraction.
    **Related Terms:** Total dose, fractionation schedule.
    **Example:** Daily kidney IMRT dose is verified using QA phantoms.
12. **Fractional Volume:** Part of the organ or tumor receiving a specific fraction of the prescribed dose.
    **Related Terms:** Dose-volume histogram (DVH), partial organ dose.
    **Example:** QA ensures only 50% of the kidney receives higher than 15 Gy.

13. **Frame (Imaging):** Single captured image in dynamic imaging or fluoroscopy.
    **Related Terms:** Temporal resolution, cine imaging.
    **Example:** QA checks frame rate and motion blur during kidney DSA or fluoroscopy.
14. **Framing Artifact:** Artifact caused by incorrect frame alignment or stitching in imaging.
    **Related Terms:** Motion artifact, registration error.
    **Example:** QA ensures multi-frame kidney SPECT images are correctly aligned.
15. **Free Radical:** Highly reactive atom or molecule produced during radiation interactions.
    **Related Terms:** DNA damage, radiobiology.
    **Example:** Understanding free radical formation helps in evaluating kidney tissue radiosensitivity.
16. **Frequency (Radiation):** The number of oscillations per unit time in EM radiation.
    **Related Terms:** X-ray spectrum, photon energy.
    **Example:** KV imaging QA checks frequency/wavelength to optimize contrast and reduce dose.
17. **Frequency Filtering:** Image processing technique to remove noise or enhance specific spatial frequencies.
    **Related Terms:** Image QA, digital radiography enhancement.
    **Example:** QA applies frequency filtering to improve kidney CT or CBCT images.
18. **Field (Radiation):** Area exposed to the radiation beam.
    **Related Terms:** Beam shaping, collimation.
    **Example:** QA checks kidney field size and shape in IMRT or VMAT.
19. **Field Edge:** Boundary of the radiation field where dose falls off.
    **Related Terms:** Penumbra, beam profile.
    **Example:** QA ensures kidney radiation field edges match treatment plan to avoid healthy tissue exposure.
20. **Field Flatness:** Uniformity of radiation dose across the field.
    **Related Terms:** Beam uniformity, intensity profile.
    **Example:** QA measures kidney CBCT or LINAC fields for consistent dose delivery.
21. **Field Verification:** Checking field location and shape against the treatment plan.
    **Related Terms:** Portal imaging, EPID QA.
    **Example:** Portal images verify kidney IMRT field alignment daily.
22. **Film Dosimetry:** Use of radiographic or radiochromic film to measure dose distribution.
    **Related Terms:** 2D dosimetry, QA phantom.
    **Example:** QA uses Gafchromic film to map kidney VMAT dose distribution.
23. **Fluence:** Number of radiation particles passing through unit area.
    **Related Terms:** Dose rate, particle flux.
    **Example:** QA measures fluence in kidney IMRT fields for accurate dose delivery.
24. **Fluence Map:** 2D map showing distribution of fluence in the treatment field.
    **Related Terms:** IMRT planning, DVH.
    **Example:** QA checks kidney IMRT fluence maps to ensure planned modulation matches delivery.
25. **Fluoroscope:** Device producing real-time X-ray images.
    **Related Terms:** C-arm, dynamic imaging.
    **Example:** QA ensures kidney interventional fluoroscopy images are clear and low-dose.
26. **Fluoroscopy:** Real-time X-ray imaging technique.
    **Related Terms:** Image-guided therapy, dynamic imaging.
    **Example:** QA verifies kidney ureter stent placement under fluoroscopy.

27. **Fluorescence Imaging:** Imaging based on tissue emission of light after excitation.
    **Related Terms:** Nuclear medicine, radiotracer imaging.
    **Example:** QA evaluates kidney tumors labeled with fluorescent probes for intraoperative guidance.
28. **Focal Length:** Distance from the X-ray source to the detector plane.
    **Related Terms:** Geometric magnification, image sharpness.
    **Example:** QA ensures correct kidney magnification in planar radiography.
29. **Fourier Analysis:** Mathematical technique to decompose signals into frequency components.
    **Related Terms:** Image processing, noise reduction.
    **Example:** QA uses Fourier analysis to detect spatial frequency defects in kidney CBCT images.
30. **Framing Rate:** Number of images acquired per second in dynamic imaging.
    **Related Terms:** Temporal resolution, cine imaging.
    **Example:** QA ensures kidney DSA or fluoroscopy captures sufficient frames for motion assessment.
31. **Free-in-air Dose:** Dose measured without any phantom or patient in the beam.
    **Related Terms:** Calibration, reference dose.
    **Example:** QA measures free-in-air dose to verify LINAC output before kidney treatment.
32. **F-factor:** Dose conversion factor between different materials (e.g., air to tissue).
    **Related Terms:** Dosimetry, calibration.
    **Example:** QA converts KV planar dose readings to kidney tissue-equivalent dose.
33. **Film Artifact:** Image defect on radiographic film due to handling or exposure errors.
    **Related Terms:** Imaging QA, artifact correction.
    **Example:** QA detects scratches or streaks on kidney portal films.
34. **Fiducial Marker:** Small radiopaque marker used for target localization.
    **Related Terms:** IGRT, image guidance.
    **Example:** QA ensures correct kidney fiducial placement for stereotactic radiotherapy.
35. **Field Size Verification:** Checking that radiation field dimensions match treatment plan.
    **Related Terms:** Collimator check, portal imaging.
    **Example:** QA confirms kidney field size before IMRT or VMAT delivery.
36. **Flatness Test:** QA test to verify uniformity of dose across the field.
    **Related Terms:** Beam flatness, intensity profile.
    **Example:** Ensures uniform kidney exposure during treatment.
37. **Focus-to-Skin Distance (FSD):** Distance from X-ray source to patient skin surface.
    **Related Terms:** SSD, dose calculation.
    **Example:** QA verifies FSD to ensure accurate kidney imaging dose.
38. **Focus-to-Detector Distance (FDD):** Distance from X-ray source to detector.
    **Related Terms:** Geometric magnification, imaging QA.
    **Example:** QA ensures kidney CBCT images are not distorted by incorrect FDD.
39. **Fast Imaging Protocol:** Imaging protocol optimized for quick acquisition, often with lower dose.
    **Related Terms:** Low-dose CT, CBCT protocol.
    **Example:** QA ensures kidney CBCT images are clear despite shorter acquisition time.
40. **Fractional Target Volume:** Portion of tumor volume receiving a specific fraction of dose.
    **Related Terms:** DVH, partial organ dose.
    **Example:** QA ensures kidney tumor receives prescribed dose fraction.

41. **Field Alignment:** Ensuring radiation field is properly aligned with target anatomy.
**Related Terms:** Portal imaging, IGRT.
**Example:** QA verifies kidney IMRT field matches planned treatment coordinates.

42. **Field Mapping:** Measurement of dose distribution across the radiation field.
**Related Terms:** Beam profile, dosimetry.
**Example:** QA maps kidney VMAT fields using film or detector arrays.

43. **Field Verification Imaging:** Imaging to verify the actual treatment field during delivery.
**Related Terms:** Portal imaging, EPID.
**Example:** QA captures kidney portal images to confirm field placement before irradiation.

44. **Fluorescent Dosimeter:** Dosimeter using fluorescence to measure radiation dose.
**Related Terms:** Gel dosimetry, phantom QA.
**Example:** QA uses fluorescent gel to map kidney dose distribution in phantoms.

45. **Field Symmetry:** Equality of dose distribution on both sides of central axis.
**Related Terms:** Flatness, beam QA.
**Example:** QA confirms kidney radiation field is symmetric to avoid underdosing part of the kidney.

46. **Film Calibration:** Process of converting optical density on film to dose.
**Related Terms:** Film dosimetry, calibration curve.
**Example:** QA ensures kidney VMAT dose measured on Gafchromic film matches planned dose.

47. **Fluoroscopy QA:** Quality assurance for fluoroscopy systems, checking dose, image quality, and temporal resolution.
**Related Terms:** Dynamic imaging, interventional QA.
**Example:** QA ensures pediatric kidney fluoroscopy is low-dose yet clinically sufficient.

48. **Focal Depth:** Depth at which the X-ray or radiation beam is focused.
**Related Terms:** Geometric focus, imaging plane.
**Example:** QA ensures kidney imaging focal depth matches anatomical region of interest.

49. **Fast Scan QA:** QA procedure for rapid scan imaging protocols.
**Related Terms:** Low-dose CBCT QA, workflow QA.
**Example:** Confirms kidney CBCT can acquire images quickly without compromising quality.

50. **Fractional Dose Verification:** QA to confirm dose delivered per fraction matches planned dose.
**Related Terms:** Dosimetry, IMRT QA, DVH check.
**Example:** QA phantom measures kidney fraction dose before each VMAT treatment.

51. **Field-of-View (FOV):** The area captured in an imaging scan.
**Related Terms:** Image reconstruction, detector coverage.
**Example:** QA ensures kidney CT or MRI FOV covers the entire organ without excessive exposure to surrounding tissue.

52. **Feedback Control:** Automated adjustment of radiation delivery based on real-time monitoring.
**Related Terms:** IGRT, motion management.
**Example:** QA verifies feedback loops adjust kidney IMRT beam if patient moves during treatment.

53. **Filtration Efficiency:** Measure of how well a filter removes unwanted low-energy photons from the beam.
**Related Terms:** Beam quality, patient dose reduction.
**Example:** QA evaluates KV X-ray filtration to minimize kidney surface dose while preserving image quality.

54. **Focal Plane Artifact:** Imaging artifact caused by objects outside the focal plane.
**Related Terms:** Motion blur, misregistration.
**Example:** QA ensures kidney CBCT reconstruction minimizes artifacts from surrounding bowel motion.

55. **Field Junction:** Region where adjacent radiation fields meet.
**Related Terms:** Overlap, hot/cold spots.
**Example:** QA verifies kidney VMAT fields join smoothly without creating dose inhomogeneity at junctions.

56. **Focal Spot Size Test:** QA test measuring X-ray tube focal spot dimensions.
**Related Terms:** Geometric unsharpness, spatial resolution.
**Example:** Kidney radiographs require a focal spot $\leq$0.6 mm for optimal image clarity.

57. **Film Scanner Calibration:** Process of ensuring accurate dose readout from scanned dosimetric films.
**Related Terms:** Film dosimetry, optical density calibration.
**Example:** QA confirms kidney VMAT films accurately reflect delivered dose distributions.

58. **Fourier Filtering:** Image processing to remove high-frequency noise or low-frequency artifacts.
**Related Terms:** Image reconstruction, SPECT/CT enhancement.
**Example:** QA applies Fourier filtering to kidney SPECT images to improve contrast without losing detail.

59. **Fiducial Registration:** Alignment of imaging datasets using fiducial markers.
**Related Terms:** IGRT, image fusion.
**Example:** QA ensures kidney MRI and CT images are accurately registered using implanted markers for radiotherapy planning.

60. **Fluoroscopic Dose Monitoring:** Measurement and control of patient radiation during fluoroscopy.
**Related Terms:** Dose-area product (DAP), real-time dosimetry.
**Example:** QA confirms kidney interventional fluoroscopy does not exceed recommended dose thresholds.

61. **Field Overlap Assessment:** QA check to ensure adjacent fields cover the target adequately without overexposing normal tissue.
**Related Terms:** IMRT, VMAT.
**Example:** QA ensures kidney tumor fields overlap correctly to deliver uniform dose.

62. **Fluorescent Phantoms:** Phantoms containing fluorescent material to visualize dose distribution.
**Related Terms:** Gel dosimetry, QA phantom.
**Example:** QA uses fluorescent phantoms to verify kidney IMRT dose profiles in 3D.

63. **Field Flattening:** Process of making the dose distribution uniform across the field.
**Related Terms:** Flatness, beam profile.
**Example:** QA ensures kidney LINAC beams are flat across the treatment field to avoid hotspots.

64. **Field Verification Software:** Software that compares planned vs. delivered radiation fields.
**Related Terms:** EPID analysis, QA automation.
**Example:** QA software confirms kidney IMRT fields are delivered accurately per plan.

65. **Fluoroscopic Contrast:** Radiopaque agent used to enhance visibility in fluoroscopy.
**Related Terms:** Iodinated contrast, image guidance.
**Example:** QA ensures proper kidney contrast injection protocols for interventional procedures.

66. **Film Dosimeter Calibration Curve:** Graph relating optical density to known radiation doses.
**Related Terms:** Dosimetry, film QA.
**Example:** QA uses calibration curves to convert kidney film images into accurate dose maps.

67. **Field Alignment Phantom:** Phantom used to verify radiation field positioning.
**Related Terms:** QA phantom, portal imaging.
**Example:** QA uses kidney-shaped phantom to confirm correct field placement before treatment.

68. **Focus-to-Film Distance (FFD):** Distance from X-ray source to imaging film.
**Related Terms:** Geometric magnification, image resolution.
**Example:** QA ensures FFD is correct for kidney planar radiographs to avoid distortion.

69. **Fluence Verification:** QA process of checking particle fluence matches planned distribution.
**Related Terms:** IMRT, VMAT QA.
**Example:** QA confirms kidney fluence maps delivered by LINAC match planning system predictions.

70. **Field Size Reproducibility:** Consistency of radiation field dimensions over multiple QA checks.
**Related Terms:** Collimator accuracy, beam uniformity.
**Example:** QA ensures kidney treatment field size does not vary between fractions.

71. **Film Sensitivity Test:** QA procedure testing film response to known doses.
**Related Terms:** Dosimetry, optical density.
**Example:** QA ensures kidney VMAT dose films detect small dose variations.

72. **Focal Plane Verification:** QA to confirm correct focal plane alignment in imaging.
**Related Terms:** Sharpness, resolution.
**Example:** Kidney CBCT QA verifies the focal plane corresponds to the organ's anatomical center.

73. **Field Reproducibility:** QA measurement of repeated field consistency.
**Related Terms:** LINAC output, beam stability.
**Example:** QA ensures kidney IMRT fields maintain consistent geometry and dose fraction-to-fraction.

74. **Flat-Panel Detector QA:** Testing image quality and uniformity of flat-panel X-ray detectors.
**Related Terms:** Digital radiography, CBCT.
**Example:** QA evaluates kidney CBCT detector for dead pixels or contrast issues.

75. **Frequency Response:** Detector or imaging system response to different spatial or temporal frequencies.
**Related Terms:** Modulation transfer function (MTF), image resolution.
**Example:** QA assesses kidney fluoroscopy MTF to ensure motion details are captured.

76. **Fiducial Marker QA:** Verifying visibility and correct placement of fiducials in images.
**Related Terms:** IGRT, image registration.
**Example:** QA confirms kidney fiducials are clearly visible on KV and CBCT images before radiotherapy.

77. **Fast Neutron QA:** Quality assurance for neutron therapy beams.
**Related Terms:** Beam uniformity, dosimetry.
**Example:** QA ensures kidney fast neutron dose matches planned target distribution.

78. **Fractional Dose QA:** Verification that each treatment fraction delivers planned dose.
**Related Terms:** IMRT QA, DVH check.
**Example:** QA confirms kidney VMAT fraction dose matches treatment plan.

79. **Focus Drift:** Movement or change of focal spot over time.
**Related Terms:** Tube alignment, geometric unsharpness.
**Example:** QA ensures kidney radiographs remain sharp by monitoring focal spot stability.

80. **Film-Based QA:** Dosimetric QA using radiographic or radiochromic film.
**Related Terms:** 2D dosimetry, phantom QA.
**Example:** QA uses films to measure kidney IMRT and VMAT dose distributions in phantoms.

81. **Flatness QA:** Measurement of uniformity across the radiation field.
**Related Terms:** Beam profile, LINAC QA.
**Example:** QA ensures kidney IMRT fields have <3% variation in flatness across the treatment area.

82. **Focused Ultrasound QA:** Verification of ultrasound energy focus for therapeutic or imaging purposes.
**Related Terms:** HIFU, MRgFUS.
**Example:** QA confirms focused ultrasound treatment accurately targets kidney tumors without damaging surrounding tissue.

83. **Fluence Map Verification:** QA comparing planned vs. delivered photon or proton fluence.
**Related Terms:** IMRT, VMAT, dose distribution.
**Example:** QA ensures kidney VMAT fluence maps match planning system calculations.

84. **Film Dosimetry QA:** Using films to check delivered radiation dose.
**Related Terms:** 2D dosimetry, optical density analysis.
**Example:** QA checks kidney VMAT dose patterns using radiochromic films in a phantom.

85. **Field Symmetry:** Measure of dose uniformity on both sides of the central axis.
**Related Terms:** Beam symmetry, QA.
**Example:** QA ensures kidney IMRT beams are symmetric to prevent hotspots.

86. **Focused Beam Therapy:** Radiation therapy delivering highly collimated beams.
**Related Terms:** SRS, SBRT.
**Example:** QA confirms kidney SBRT beams are accurately focused on the tumor.

87. **Frequency Analysis:** Assessment of image spatial frequencies to evaluate resolution.
**Related Terms:** MTF, image quality.
**Example:** QA measures kidney CBCT resolution by analyzing high-frequency details.

88. **Fiducial Marker Tracking:** Continuous monitoring of implanted markers during therapy.
**Related Terms:** IGRT, motion management.
**Example:** QA ensures kidney fiducials are tracked during respiratory-gated radiotherapy.

89. **Fluoroscopic QA:** Quality assurance of fluoroscopy systems for image quality and patient dose.
**Related Terms:** DAP, real-time dosimetry.
**Example:** QA ensures kidney fluoroscopy does not exceed recommended dose thresholds.

90. **Field Dose Verification:** QA procedure to confirm delivered dose matches planned dose in a field.
**Related Terms:** DVH, 3D dosimetry.
**Example:** QA verifies kidney IMRT fields deliver the correct dose using ion chambers or films.

91. **Fused Image QA:** QA for combined imaging datasets (e.g., PET/CT, SPECT/CT).
**Related Terms:** Image registration, multimodal imaging.
**Example:** QA confirms kidney PET/CT images align accurately for radiotherapy planning.

92. **Fluence Modulation QA:** Verification of varying beam intensity in IMRT/VMAT delivery.
**Related Terms:** MLC QA, dose verification.
**Example:** QA checks that kidney VMAT intensity modulation matches the treatment plan.

93. **Film-to-Plan Comparison:** QA comparing dosimetric films with TPS-calculated dose.
**Related Terms:** Gamma analysis, dose verification.
**Example:** QA compares kidney VMAT film measurements with TPS to ensure dose accuracy.

94. **Focal Spot QA:** Checking the size, shape, and stability of X-ray tube focal spot.
**Related Terms:** Geometric unsharpness, spatial resolution.
**Example:** QA ensures kidney radiographs maintain sharp edges and accurate anatomical details.

95. **Flat-Field Correction:** Correction applied to imaging detectors to remove nonuniformities.
**Related Terms:** CBCT, detector calibration.
**Example:** QA ensures kidney CBCT images are uniform by applying flat-field correction.

96. **Fractionation QA:** Verification that each radiation fraction delivers correct dose.
**Related Terms:** IMRT, DVH, dose accumulation.
**Example:** QA confirms kidney SBRT fraction doses are consistent with the total prescription.

97. **Film Sensitivity QA:** Testing film response to verify dose measurement accuracy.
**Related Terms:** Optical density, dosimetry.
**Example:** QA ensures kidney VMAT films can detect subtle dose variations in high-gradient regions.

98. **Fiducial Placement QA:** QA to ensure accurate fiducial marker placement for image-guided therapy.
**Related Terms:** IGRT, registration accuracy.
**Example:** QA confirms kidney fiducials are correctly placed before SBRT to minimize targeting errors.

99. **Field Edge Verification:** Checking the accuracy of field edges to prevent overdose to normal tissue.
**Related Terms:** Collimator, beam shaping.
**Example:** QA ensures kidney IMRT field edges match planning target volume (PTV).

100. **Fluoroscopy Workflow QA:** Ensures all fluoroscopic procedures are performed safely and efficiently.
**Related Terms:** Radiation safety, DAP monitoring.
**Example:** QA checks kidney interventional fluoroscopy workflow to minimize patient and staff dose.

101. **Focus-to-Detector Distance (FDD):** Distance between the X-ray tube focus and the detector.
**Related Terms:** Geometric magnification, image sharpness.
**Example:** QA ensures kidney radiographs have correct FDD to prevent distortion.

102. **Field Size Verification:** Checking the size of the radiation field matches treatment plan.
**Related Terms:** MLC, collimator, PTV coverage.
**Example:** QA confirms kidney IMRT field size matches the TPS calculation.

103. **Fluoroscopic Dose Rate QA:** Monitoring the dose rate during fluoroscopic procedures.
**Related Terms:** DAP, real-time dosimetry.
**Example:** QA ensures kidney interventional fluoroscopy does not exceed safe dose limits.

104. **Focal Plane Alignment:** Ensures the imaging plane is correctly aligned with the target.
**Related Terms:** CBCT, image-guided radiotherapy.
**Example:** QA checks kidney CBCT focal plane alignment to avoid misregistration.

105. **Field Junction QA:** Verification of dose uniformity at the junction of two fields.
**Related Terms:** Split fields, craniospinal irradiation.
**Example:** QA ensures kidney extended field junctions don't create hotspots.

106. **Fiducial Visibility QA:** Ensuring implanted markers are clearly visible on imaging.
**Related Terms:** IGRT, marker tracking.
**Example:** QA confirms kidney fiducials can be identified on CBCT for accurate targeting.

107. **Fluence Verification Phantom:** Phantom used to check planned vs. delivered fluence.
**Related Terms:** IMRT QA, dose distribution.
**Example:** QA verifies kidney VMAT delivery using a fluence verification phantom.

108. **Filtered Back Projection QA:** QA for image reconstruction algorithms in CT/SPECT/PET.
**Related Terms:** CT reconstruction, artifact suppression.
**Example:** QA confirms kidney CT images reconstructed with filtered back projection are accurate.

109. **Field Edge Penumbra QA:** Assessment of dose fall-off at the edge of the radiation field.
**Related Terms:** Beam profile, MLC positioning.
**Example:** QA ensures kidney IMRT field edges have sharp penumbra to protect normal tissue.

110. **Fluoroscopy Frame Rate QA:** Checking fluoroscopic image acquisition rate.
**Related Terms:** Temporal resolution, motion blur.
**Example:** QA ensures kidney fluoroscopy captures motion accurately without blurring.

111. **Field Dose Homogeneity QA:** Ensuring uniform dose across the radiation field.
**Related Terms:** DVH, flatness, symmetry.
**Example:** QA confirms kidney VMAT dose is homogeneous across the target volume.

112. **Fluorescence Imaging QA:** QA for systems using fluorescent tracers.
**Related Terms:** Optical imaging, tumor delineation.
**Example:** QA checks kidney tumor fluorescence imaging for clear signal detection.

113. **Focal Spot Size QA:** Measurement of X-ray tube focal spot size.
**Related Terms:** Spatial resolution, geometric unsharpness.
**Example:** QA ensures kidney radiographs maintain sharp edges for accurate contouring.

114. **Field Weighting Verification:** QA to verify the proportion of dose delivered by each field.
**Related Terms:** IMRT, VMAT, treatment planning.
**Example:** QA ensures kidney IMRT fields are weighted correctly to achieve target coverage.

115. **Fiducial Stability QA:** QA to confirm markers do not migrate over treatment course.
**Related Terms:** IGRT, motion management.
**Example:** QA checks kidney fiducials remain in place during multi-fraction SBRT.

116. **Fluence Delivery QA:** Measurement of actual fluence delivered compared to the planned one.
**Related Terms:** IMRT, VMAT QA, gamma analysis.
**Example:** QA verifies kidney VMAT fluence using ion chamber arrays.

117. **Fluoroscopy Image Quality QA:** Checking resolution, contrast, and noise in fluoroscopic imaging.
**Related Terms:** DQE, modulation transfer function.
**Example:** QA ensures kidney fluoroscopy images are diagnostically sufficient.

118. **Field Aperture Verification:** QA checking the opening of collimators or MLCs.
**Related Terms:** Beam shaping, PTV coverage.
**Example:** QA ensures kidney IMRT apertures match treatment plan.

119. **Fluoroscopic Dose Optimization:** Reducing patient and staff dose during fluoroscopy while maintaining image quality.
**Related Terms:** ALARA, DAP monitoring.
**Example:** QA confirms kidney angiography uses minimal radiation without losing diagnostic value.

120. **Field Symmetry QA:** Ensuring the radiation field is symmetric about the central axis.
**Related Terms:** LINAC QA, beam profile.
**Example:** QA ensures kidney IMRT beams are symmetric to prevent overdose to normal tissues.

121. **Fiducial-Based Registration:** QA checking accuracy of image registration using markers.
**Related Terms:** IGRT, CBCT.
**Example:** QA ensures kidney fiducial-based registration aligns planning CT with daily CBCT.

122. **Fluence Pattern Analysis:** Analyzing planned vs. delivered fluence patterns.
**Related Terms:** IMRT QA, gamma analysis.
**Example:** QA confirms kidney VMAT fluence patterns match the TPS to within tolerance.

123. **Film Calibration QA:** QA to ensure radiochromic or radiographic film accurately measures dose.
**Related Terms:** Optical density, dosimetry.
**Example:** QA ensures kidney VMAT film measurements are accurate for high-dose gradients.

124. **Fraction Dose Verification:** QA confirming the delivered dose per fraction matches the plan.
**Related Terms:** IMRT, SBRT, DVH.
**Example:** QA checks each kidney SBRT fraction dose with an ion chamber array.

125. **Fluoroscopy Contrast QA:** Ensuring fluoroscopic system detects contrast adequately.
**Related Terms:** Image quality, DQE.
**Example:** QA confirms kidney angiograms show vessels clearly without excessive dose.

126. **Flatness QA:** Measurement of beam uniformity across the central axis.
**Related Terms:** Beam profile, LINAC QA.
**Example:** QA ensures kidney IMRT fields have flat dose distribution to avoid hotspots.

127. **Field Mapping:** Mapping of the radiation field for verification and treatment planning.
**Related Terms:** Beam profiling, dosimetry.
**Example:** QA maps kidney VMAT fields to confirm TPS accuracy.

128. **Fiducial Marker QA:** Ensuring implanted markers are visible and correctly placed.
**Related Terms:** IGRT, image registration.
**Example:** QA checks kidney fiducials before each SBRT session for accurate targeting.

129. **Fluorescent Tracer Verification:** QA of fluorescent markers used in imaging.
**Related Terms:** Optical imaging, tumor delineation.
**Example:** QA confirms kidney tumor fluorescence signal is detectable and localized.

130. **Field Overlap QA:** Checking overlap of adjacent radiation fields to avoid overdose.
**Related Terms:** Split fields, craniospinal RT.
**Example:** QA ensures kidney extended fields overlap correctly without creating hotspots.

131. **Fluoroscopy Geometry QA:** Verification of geometry and magnification in fluoroscopic imaging.
**Related Terms:** FDD, image distortion.
**Example:** QA ensures kidney angiograms are geometrically accurate for intervention.

132. **Frequency Filtering QA:** QA to verify image processing filters in CT, MRI, or fluoroscopy.
**Related Terms:** Noise reduction, image sharpness.
**Example:** QA ensures kidney CT images retain critical structures after filtering.

133. **Field Verification Phantom:** Phantom used to verify planned vs. delivered radiation field.
**Related Terms:** IMRT QA, VMAT QA.
**Example:** QA uses a phantom to confirm kidney VMAT field coverage and shape.

134. **Flat-Panel Detector QA:** Ensures proper functioning of flat-panel detectors in imaging systems.
**Related Terms:** Digital radiography, KV imaging.
**Example:** QA confirms kidney KV images are clear and free from detector artifacts.

135. **Fiducial Drift Monitoring:** QA to monitor movement of implanted markers over time.
**Related Terms:** IGRT, SBRT.
**Example:** QA checks kidney fiducials remain in place across multiple treatment fractions.

136. **Fluence Map Verification:** Comparing planned vs. measured fluence distributions.
**Related Terms:** IMRT, VMAT, gamma analysis.
**Example:** QA verifies kidney VMAT fluence map matches TPS plan.

137. **Fractionation QA:** Ensuring accurate dose delivery per treatment fraction.
**Related Terms:** SBRT, IMRT.
**Example:** QA confirms kidney SBRT fractions deliver the correct dose.

138. **Flat-Field Calibration:** Calibration to ensure detector response is uniform.
**Related Terms:** KV imaging, flat-panel detectors.
**Example:** QA calibrates KV detector for uniform kidney imaging.

139. **Field Edge Verification:** QA of beam edges for accurate dose fall-off.
**Related Terms:** MLC, penumbra.
**Example:** QA checks kidney IMRT beam edges to protect surrounding tissue.

140. **Fiducial Registration Accuracy:** Measurement of registration accuracy using fiducial markers.
**Related Terms:** CBCT, IGRT.
**Example:** QA ensures kidney fiducials align planning CT with daily imaging.

141. **Fluoroscopy Dose Optimization QA:** QA ensuring fluoroscopy uses minimal dose while maintaining image quality.
**Related Terms:** DAP, ALARA.
**Example:** QA confirms kidney interventional procedures maintain safe radiation exposure.

142. **Focal Plane Verification:** QA to confirm imaging plane is correctly aligned with the target.
**Related Terms:** CBCT, image-guided therapy.
**Example:** QA ensures kidney CBCT focal plane accurately captures tumor location.

143. **Fluence Grid QA:** Checking dose delivery across a grid for uniformity.
**Related Terms:** IMRT QA, VMAT QA.
**Example:** QA verifies kidney VMAT fluence grid matches TPS predictions.

144. **Field Modulation QA:** QA of intensity modulation patterns in IMRT/VMAT.
**Related Terms:** MLC, fluence maps.
**Example:** QA ensures kidney IMRT MLC patterns deliver planned dose.

145. **Fiducial Placement QA:** QA to confirm correct placement of markers for treatment guidance.
**Related Terms:** IGRT, SBRT.
**Example:** QA checks kidney fiducials are near tumor without affecting healthy tissue.

146. **Fluoroscopic Image Calibration:** QA ensuring accurate geometric and intensity calibration in fluoroscopy.
**Related Terms:** DQE, flat-panel calibration.
**Example:** QA calibrates kidney angiography images for accurate vessel measurement.

147. **Fraction Dose Homogeneity:** Ensuring dose per fraction is uniform across the target.
**Related Terms:** DVH, PTV coverage.
**Example:** QA confirms kidney SBRT fractions are delivered homogeneously.

148. **Flatness Measurement Phantom:** Phantom used to measure beam flatness across the field.
**Related Terms:** LINAC QA, beam profile.
**Example:** QA checks kidney IMRT field flatness to avoid under/over-dosing.

149. **Field Alignment Verification:** QA ensuring radiation field is correctly aligned to the target.
**Related Terms:** IGRT, MLC, collimator.
**Example:** QA aligns kidney IMRT fields to avoid normal tissue exposure.

150. **Fluorescence Intensity QA:** Checking intensity of fluorescent signal in optical imaging.
**Related Terms:** Tumor delineation, optical imaging.
**Example:** QA confirms kidney tumor fluorescence is strong enough for image-guided intervention.

151. **Field Verification QA:** Comprehensive QA to ensure the planned radiation field matches delivered field.
**Example:** QA verifies kidney IMRT fields match TPS predictions using portal dosimetry.
**Related Terms:** Field size verification, Field alignment, Beam matching, Portal dosimetry.

152. **Fiducial Visibility QA:** Ensuring implanted markers are visible in all imaging modalities used for therapy.
**Example:** QA confirms kidney fiducials are clearly visible on CBCT and KV images.
**Related Terms:** Fiducial marker stability, Fiducial alignment, IGRT, CBCT QA.

153. **Fluence Verification Phantom:** Phantom used to verify measured fluence against planned fluence for IMRT/VMAT.
**Example:** QA measures kidney VMAT fluence distribution using a MapCHECK phantom.
**Related Terms:** Fluence delivery QA, IMRT QA, VMAT QA, Dose mapping.

154. **Flat-Panel Imaging QA:** Ensures flat-panel detectors provide high-quality images with minimal artifacts.
**Example:** QA verifies kidney KV images are sharp, uniform, and artifact-free.
**Related Terms:** Detector calibration, Flat-field image verification, KV imaging QA, Image uniformity.

155. **Field Matching QA:** QA of adjacent fields to ensure seamless coverage without hotspots.
**Example:** QA ensures craniospinal or kidney extended fields match at junctions.
**Related Terms:** Field edge QA, Junction verification, Dose uniformity, Multi-field QA.

156. **Fluoroscopic Dose Mapping:** Measuring dose distribution during fluoroscopy for patient safety.
**Example:** QA maps kidney interventional fluoroscopy dose to minimize patient exposure.
**Related Terms:** Fluoroscopy QA, Dose monitoring, ALARA, Real-time dose measurement.

157. **Fiducial Marker Stability QA:** Monitoring implanted markers for migration or displacement.
**Example:** QA tracks kidney fiducial positions across multiple SBRT fractions.
**Related Terms:** Fiducial alignment, IGRT, Image registration QA, Motion tracking.

158. **Field Size Verification:** QA to ensure correct field size is delivered.
**Example:** QA confirms kidney IMRT PTV is fully covered without overdosing normal tissue.
**Related Terms:** Field verification, MLC QA, Beam aperture QA, Dose coverage.

159. **Fluence Delivery QA:** Ensures that the intended fluence pattern is accurately delivered by the LINAC.
**Example:** QA confirms kidney VMAT fluence maps using electronic portal imaging.
**Related Terms:** Fluence verification phantom, IMRT QA, VMAT QA, Portal dosimetry.

160. **Flatness and Symmetry QA:** Measures uniformity and symmetry of radiation beam across field.
**Example:** QA ensures kidney IMRT beams are symmetric and uniform to prevent hotspots.
**Related Terms:** Flatness measurement verification, Beam symmetry verification, Water phantom QA.

161. **Fiducial Registration QA:** QA of image registration using fiducial markers for patient positioning.
**Example:** QA aligns kidney CBCT images to planning CT using fiducials.
**Related Terms:** IGRT QA, CBCT QA, Image fusion verification, Fiducial visibility.

162. **Fractionated Dose Verification:** QA to ensure correct dose per fraction in multi-fraction treatments.
**Example:** QA confirms kidney SBRT fractions deliver the prescribed dose consistently.
**Related Terms:** Fractionation schedule QA, Dose per fraction QA, Cumulative dose verification.

163. **Fluorescent Signal Calibration:** QA to calibrate fluorescent imaging intensity.
**Example:** QA ensures kidney tumor fluorescence is detectable for intraoperative guidance.
**Related Terms:** Fluorescent imaging QA, Image intensity calibration, Tumor visualization.

164. **Field Uniformity QA:** Verifying even dose distribution across treatment field.
**Example:** QA checks kidney IMRT field uniformity using a MapCHECK or water phantom.
**Related Terms:** Flatness QA, Dose homogeneity, Field verification, Phantom QA.

165. **Fiducial Contour Verification:** QA of contours around fiducials for planning and image guidance.
**Example:** QA ensures kidney fiducial contours match anatomy on planning CT.
**Related Terms:** Contour QA, IGRT QA, Fiducial registration, Image segmentation.

166. **Fluoroscopy Geometric Accuracy:** QA to ensure accurate spatial representation in fluoroscopic imaging.
**Example:** QA checks kidney angiography geometry for catheter navigation.
**Related Terms:** Fluoroscopy QA, Geometric distortion check, Dose mapping, Real-time imaging QA.

167. **Field Edge Sharpness QA:** Measuring penumbra and sharpness of radiation field edges.
**Example:** QA ensures kidney IMRT field edges protect surrounding normal tissue.
**Related Terms:** Field matching QA, Penumbra verification, Beam profile QA.

168. **Fiducial Dose Assessment:** Ensuring fiducials do not receive excessive radiation dose.
**Example:** QA confirms kidney fiducials are outside hotspot regions in SBRT.
**Related Terms:** Dose verification, Fiducial stability QA, SBRT QA, Dose mapping.

169. **Fluence Pattern QA:** QA for complex intensity patterns in modulated treatments.
**Example:** QA checks kidney IMRT fluence maps match TPS predictions.
**Related Terms:** Fluence delivery QA, VMAT QA, IMRT QA, MapCHECK QA.

170. **Flat-Field Image Verification:** QA for detector uniformity in imaging.
**Example:** QA ensures kidney KV images have uniform brightness without detector artifacts.
**Related Terms:** Flat-panel imaging QA, Detector calibration, KV QA, Image uniformity.

171. **Field Verification QA:** Ensures radiation fields are delivered as planned.
**Example:** Confirming kidney IMRT fields match TPS using portal dosimetry.
**Related Terms:** Field size verification, Beam alignment, Portal dosimetry.

172. **Fiducial Visibility QA:** Ensures markers are visible in all imaging modalities.
**Example:** Kidney fiducials checked on CBCT and KV images.
**Related Terms:** Fiducial marker stability, IGRT QA.

173. **Fluence Verification Phantom:** Phantom to verify delivered fluence vs. planned.
**Example:** VMAT kidney fluence checked with MapCHECK.
**Related Terms:** IMRT QA, Dose mapping.

174. **Flat-Panel Imaging QA:** QA of detector uniformity and image quality.
**Example:** Kidney KV images checked for artifacts and sharpness.
**Related Terms:** Detector calibration, Flat-field verification.

175. **Field Matching QA:** QA to ensure seamless junction between adjacent fields.
**Example:** Kidney craniospinal fields checked at junctions.
**Related Terms:** Field edge QA, Dose homogeneity.

176. **Fluoroscopic Dose Mapping:** Measures dose distribution during fluoroscopy.
**Example:** Kidney interventional fluoroscopy mapped to minimize dose.
**Related Terms:** ALARA, Fluoroscopy QA.

177. **Fiducial Marker Stability QA:** Ensures markers remain stable throughout treatment.
**Example:** Kidney SBRT fiducials tracked over fractions.
**Related Terms:** IGRT, Fiducial registration QA.

178. **Field Size Verification:** Ensures correct treatment field size is delivered.
**Example:** Kidney IMRT PTV fully covered without overdose.
**Related Terms:** Beam aperture QA, Field verification.

179. **Fluence Delivery QA:** Confirms LINAC delivers planned fluence.
**Example:** Kidney VMAT fluence verified via EPID.
**Related Terms:** Fluence verification phantom, IMRT QA.

180. **Flatness and Symmetry QA:** Measures uniformity and symmetry of beams.
**Example:** Kidney IMRT beams checked for symmetry using water phantom.
**Related Terms:** Flatness verification, Beam uniformity QA.

181. **Fiducial Registration QA:** QA of image registration using fiducials.
**Example:** Align kidney CBCT to planning CT using markers.
**Related Terms:** IGRT QA, Image fusion verification.

182. **Fractionated Dose Verification:** Confirms correct dose per fraction.
**Example:** Kidney SBRT fractions verified for prescription accuracy.
**Related Terms:** Fractionation schedule QA, Cumulative dose verification.

183. **Fluorescent Signal Calibration:** Ensures fluorescent imaging intensity is accurate.
**Example:** Kidney tumor fluorescence calibrated for intraoperative guidance.
**Related Terms:** Fluorescent imaging QA, Signal intensity QA.

184. **Field Uniformity QA:** Verifies even dose distribution across a field.
**Example:** Kidney IMRT checked with MapCHECK for uniform dose.
**Related Terms:** Beam flatness, Dose homogeneity QA.

185. **Fiducial Contour Verification:** Checks accuracy of contours around markers.
**Example:** Kidney fiducial contours matched on planning CT.
**Related Terms:** Contour QA, IGRT QA.

186. **Fluoroscopy Geometric Accuracy:** Ensures spatial accuracy of fluoroscopic images.
**Example:** Kidney angiography geometry checked for catheter navigation.
**Related Terms:** Fluoroscopy QA, Geometric distortion QA.

187. **Field Edge Sharpness QA:** Measures beam penumbra and edge sharpness.
**Example:** Kidney IMRT field edges verified to protect normal tissue.
**Related Terms:** Field matching QA, Beam profile QA.

188. **Fiducial Dose Assessment:** Ensures markers don't receive excessive dose.
**Example:** Kidney SBRT fiducials kept outside hotspots.
**Related Terms:** Dose verification, Fiducial stability QA.

189. **Fluence Pattern QA:** Verifies complex IMRT/VMAT fluence patterns.
**Example:** Kidney IMRT fluence checked against TPS.
**Related Terms:** Fluence delivery QA, Dose mapping QA.

190. **Flat-Field Image Verification:** QA to ensure detector uniformity.
**Example:** Kidney KV images checked for consistent brightness.
**Related Terms:** Flat-panel imaging QA, Detector calibration QA.

191. **Field Alignment Phantom:** Phantom used to verify field placement.
**Example:** Kidney IMRT field alignment verified with phantom.
**Related Terms:** Field verification QA, Beam positioning QA.

192. **Fiducial Imaging Phantom:** Phantom with markers to test imaging and registration accuracy.
**Example:** Kidney phantom with fiducials tested on CBCT.
**Related Terms:** Image registration QA, IGRT QA.

193. **Fluoroscopic Beam QA:** Ensures beam quality, geometry, and dose during fluoroscopy.
**Example:** Kidney interventional beam verified for uniformity.
**Related Terms:** Dose mapping, Geometric QA, Fluoroscopy QA.

194. **Fractionation Schedule QA:** Verifies correct number of fractions and per-fraction dose.
**Example:** Kidney SBRT schedule verified against prescription.
**Related Terms:** Fractionated dose verification, Treatment schedule QA.

195. **Flatness Measurement Verification:** Measures beam flatness using phantoms.
**Example:** Kidney IMRT fields verified for dose flatness.
**Related Terms:** Flatness and symmetry QA, Beam uniformity QA.

196. **Field-of-View QA:** Ensures imaging fully covers target anatomy.
**Example:** Kidney CBCT images confirmed to encompass entire tumor.
**Related Terms:** KV imaging QA, Imaging coverage QA.

197. **Fiducial Tracking QA:** Verifies real-time tracking of implanted markers.
**Example:** Kidney fiducials tracked accurately during SBRT.
**Related Terms:** IGRT, Motion management QA.

198. **Fluorescent Contrast QA:** Ensures fluorescent targets are distinguishable from background.
**Example:** Kidney tumor fluorescence differentiated from healthy tissue.
**Related Terms:** Fluorescent imaging QA, Signal calibration QA.

199. **Field Symmetry Verification:** Checks left-right dose symmetry of the beam.
**Example:** Kidney IMRT beams verified for symmetric delivery.
**Related Terms:** Flatness and symmetry QA, Beam profile QA.

200. **Fluence Dose Mapping:** Maps delivered fluence to assess dose distribution.
**Example:** Kidney VMAT fields mapped for dose verification.
**Related Terms:** Fluence verification phantom, Dose mapping QA.

201. **Fiducial Alignment Verification:** Ensures markers align with treatment plan.
**Example:** Kidney SBRT fiducials aligned with planned PTV daily.
**Related Terms:** Fiducial registration QA, IGRT QA.

202. **Field Aperture QA:** Ensures MLC and jaw apertures match planned field.
**Example:** Kidney IMRT MLC leaves verified against TPS.
**Related Terms:** Field size verification, Beam shaping QA.

203. **Flatness QA Phantom:** Phantom used to measure beam flatness and symmetry.
**Example:** Kidney IMRT field flatness checked with phantom.
**Related Terms:** Flatness and symmetry QA, Beam uniformity verification.

204. **Fiducial Contour QA:** Checks accuracy of fiducial contours.
**Example:** Kidney fiducials verified for IGRT alignment.
**Related Terms:** Fiducial registration QA, Contour QA.

**205. Fluoroscopy Image QA:** Ensures fluoroscopic image clarity and safety.
**Example:** Kidney interventional images verified for minimal dose.
**Related Terms:** Fluoroscopic dose QA, Image quality QA.

**206. Fractional Dose Mapping:** Maps dose delivered per fraction.
**Example:** Kidney SBRT dose mapped using portal dosimetry.
**Related Terms:** Fractionated dose verification, Dose distribution QA.

**207. Field Verification Checklist:** Checklist to verify all aspects of radiation field.
**Example:** Kidney IMRT field size, shape, and alignment confirmed.
**Related Terms:** Field verification QA, QA protocol.

**208. Fiducial Implant QA:** QA during fiducial implantation to ensure correct placement.
**Example:** Kidney fiducials placed near tumor without affecting organs at risk.
**Related Terms:** Fiducial placement, IGRT QA.

**209. Fluence Output QA:** Measures radiation output across the field.
**Example:** Kidney VMAT output verified against TPS calculations.
**Related Terms:** Fluence verification, Beam output QA.

**210. Field Position QA:** Verifies beam position relative to patient anatomy.
**Example:** Kidney IMRT field aligned with PTV location.
**Related Terms:** Field alignment phantom, Beam placement QA.

**211. Fiducial Stability Phantom:** Phantom to test marker stability and registration accuracy.
**Example:** Kidney phantom with markers used for IGRT verification.
**Related Terms:** Fiducial tracking QA, Image registration QA.

**212. Fluoroscopy Dose QA:** Verifies radiation dose during fluoroscopy.
**Example:** Kidney interventional dose measured to ensure ALARA compliance.
**Related Terms:** Fluoroscopic dose mapping, Patient safety QA.

**213. Flatness and Symmetry Phantom:** Phantom used to measure beam flatness and symmetry.
**Example:** Kidney IMRT beams verified with film or water phantom.
**Related Terms:** Flatness QA, Beam uniformity QA.

**214. Fiducial Marker QA Protocol:** Protocol for QA of all fiducial-related steps.
**Example:** Kidney fiducials checked for visibility, stability, and registration.
**Related Terms:** Fiducial visibility QA, IGRT QA.

**215. Field Edge QA:** Verifies beam edge sharpness and position.
**Example:** Kidney IMRT penumbra within tolerance.
**Related Terms:** Field edge sharpness QA, Beam profile QA.

**216. Fluorescent Imaging QA:** QA for clarity, intensity, and registration of fluorescent imaging.
**Example:** Kidney tumor fluorescence confirmed for mapping accuracy.
**Related Terms:** Fluorescent signal calibration, Image registration QA.

**217. Fractionation Verification Phantom:** Phantom to validate fractionated dose delivery.
**Example:** Kidney SBRT per-fraction dose verified using phantom.
**Related Terms:** Fractionated dose verification, Dose mapping QA.

**218. Flat-Panel Detector Calibration:** Calibration of imaging detectors for uniformity.
**Example:** Kidney KV images verified for brightness uniformity.
**Related Terms:** Flat-panel imaging QA, Detector QA.

219. **Field Position Accuracy QA:** Ensures delivered field matches planned location.
**Example:** Kidney IMRT fields aligned using phantom verification.
**Related Terms:** Field verification QA, Beam alignment QA.

220. **Fiducial Registration Accuracy QA:** Checks image registration accuracy using markers.
**Example:** Kidney CBCT aligned to planning CT via fiducials.
**Related Terms:** Fiducial alignment QA, IGRT QA.

221. **Fluence Map QA:** Compares planned vs delivered fluence.
**Example:** Kidney VMAT fluence map checked using EPID or MapCHECK.
**Related Terms:** Fluence verification phantom, Dose delivery QA.

222. **Field Output Factor QA:** Verifies relative output for different field sizes.
**Example:** Kidney IMRT output checked for 3×3, 5×5 cm fields.
**Related Terms:** Output factor measurement, Beam calibration QA.

223. **Fiducial Marker Dosimetry:** Ensures markers are not over-irradiated.
**Example:** Kidney SBRT fiducials checked against hotspots.
**Related Terms:** Fiducial dose assessment, Dose verification QA.

224. **Fluorescent Signal QA Phantom:** Phantom used to calibrate fluorescent imaging.
**Example:** Kidney tumor fluorescence phantom ensures detectable signal.
**Related Terms:** Fluorescent signal calibration, Image QA.

225. **Field Shape Verification:** Confirms field shape matches treatment plan.
**Example:** Kidney IMRT field shape checked with portal imaging.
**Related Terms:** Field size verification, MLC QA.

226. **Fiducial Contour Accuracy QA:** Ensures fiducial contours match actual marker anatomy.
**Example:** Kidney fiducial contours verified on planning CT.
**Related Terms:** Contour QA, Fiducial registration QA.

227. **Fluoroscopic Image Distortion QA:** Checks geometric accuracy of fluoroscopic images.
**Example:** Kidney angiography images checked for distortion.
**Related Terms:** Fluoroscopy geometric accuracy, Image registration QA.

228. **Fractional Dose Verification QA:** QA to ensure correct dose per fraction.
**Example:** Kidney SBRT dose verified per fraction.
**Related Terms:** Fractionated dose verification, Dose mapping QA.

229. **Flatness Measurement QA Phantom:** Phantom used for verifying beam flatness.
**Example:** Kidney IMRT beams verified for flatness across PTV.
**Related Terms:** Flatness QA, Beam uniformity QA.

230. **Field-of-View Coverage QA:** Confirms imaging covers entire target anatomy.
**Example:** Kidney CBCT verified to cover tumor volume.
**Related Terms:** Imaging QA, KV/CBCT QA, Target coverage verification.

231. **Fiducial Placement Accuracy QA:** Ensures implanted markers are accurately positioned in tumor or target area.
**Example:** Kidney SBRT fiducials checked via CBCT after implantation.
**Related Terms:** Fiducial implant QA, Fiducial registration QA.

232. **Fluence Map Verification Phantom:** Phantom used to compare planned vs delivered fluence maps.
**Example:** Kidney VMAT fields verified using MapCHECK phantom.
**Related Terms:** Fluence verification phantom, Dose distribution QA.

233. **Field Junction QA:** Ensures adjacent radiation fields match correctly at junctions.
**Example:** Kidney extended fields checked for hotspots at overlap.
**Related Terms:** Field matching QA, Dose homogeneity QA.

234. **Fiducial Migration QA:** Monitors any displacement of markers during treatment.
**Example:** Kidney SBRT fiducials checked over multiple fractions.
**Related Terms:** Fiducial stability QA, IGRT QA.

235. **Fluoroscopy Geometric Calibration:** QA to calibrate geometry for accurate fluoroscopic imaging.
**Example:** Kidney catheter navigation verified against geometric phantom.
**Related Terms:** Fluoroscopy QA, Geometric accuracy QA.

236. **Fractionation Consistency QA:** Ensures prescribed dose per fraction is delivered consistently.
**Example:** Kidney SBRT fractions verified via portal dosimetry.
**Related Terms:** Fractionated dose verification, Dose mapping QA.

237. **Flatness Verification Phantom:** Phantom used to measure beam flatness across the field.
**Example:** Kidney IMRT beam flatness measured using water phantom.
**Related Terms:** Flatness QA, Flatness and symmetry QA.

238. **Fiducial Alignment Phantom:** Phantom with markers to check registration and alignment accuracy.
**Example:** Kidney CBCT images aligned to phantom fiducials.
**Related Terms:** Fiducial registration QA, Image registration QA.

239. **Fluorescence Imaging Calibration:** Calibrates fluorescence intensity for imaging systems.
**Example:** Kidney tumor fluorescence intensity verified for visibility.
**Related Terms:** Fluorescent signal calibration, Image QA.

240. **Field Output Consistency QA:** Checks consistency of output for repeated field deliveries.
**Example:** Kidney IMRT daily output verified against baseline.
**Related Terms:** Output factor QA, Beam output QA.

241. **Fiducial Detection QA:** Ensures imaging systems detect all markers reliably.
**Example:** Kidney fiducials verified on CBCT and KV imaging.
**Related Terms:** Fiducial visibility QA, IGRT QA.

242. **Fluence Delivery Verification:** Confirms LINAC delivers correct intensity-modulated fluence.
**Example:** Kidney VMAT fluence compared with TPS plan.
**Related Terms:** Fluence verification phantom, Dose mapping QA.

243. **Field Position Reproducibility QA:** Verifies consistent field placement across multiple fractions.
**Example:** Kidney IMRT fields checked for reproducibility using phantom.
**Related Terms:** Field alignment QA, Beam positioning QA.

244. **Fiducial Contour Reproducibility QA:** Ensures fiducial contours remain consistent during planning and treatment.
**Example:** Kidney SBRT fiducial contours verified on serial CT images.
**Related Terms:** Fiducial contour QA, Image registration QA.

245. **Fluoroscopic Exposure QA:** Verifies patient and system dose during fluoroscopy procedures.
**Example:** Kidney angiography exposure checked for ALARA compliance.
**Related Terms:** Fluoroscopic dose mapping, Dose optimization QA.

246. **Fractional Dose Recalculation QA:** Recalculates dose for each fraction to verify consistency.
**Example:** Kidney SBRT dose per fraction recalculated using TPS.
**Related Terms:** Fractionation verification, Dose mapping QA.

**247. Flatness QA Protocol:** Standard procedure for verifying beam flatness.
**Example:** Kidney IMRT beams verified using dedicated phantom and measurement.
**Related Terms:** Flatness measurement verification, Flatness and symmetry QA.

**248. Fiducial Registration Reproducibility QA:** Confirms registration accuracy of fiducials across multiple imaging sessions.
**Example:** Kidney CBCT daily registration verified against baseline.
**Related Terms:** Fiducial registration QA, IGRT QA.

**249. Fluorescence Intensity QA:** Verifies fluorescence signal intensity in imaging systems.
**Example:** Kidney tumor fluorescence intensity verified for intraoperative guidance.
**Related Terms:** Fluorescent signal calibration, Imaging QA.

**250. Field Edge Reproducibility QA:** Ensures beam edges remain consistent across treatments.
**Example:** Kidney IMRT field edges verified via portal dosimetry.
**Related Terms:** Field edge QA, Field matching QA.

**251. Fiducial Dose Limitation QA:** Ensures markers are not overexposed during treatment.
**Example:** Kidney SBRT fiducials monitored to avoid hot spots.
**Related Terms:** Fiducial dose assessment, Dose verification QA.

**252. Fluence Map Analysis:** Evaluates measured vs planned fluence maps.
**Example:** Kidney VMAT fluence verified using MapCHECK or EPID.
**Related Terms:** Fluence verification, Dose distribution QA.

**253. Field Homogeneity QA:** Checks uniformity of dose across the field.
**Example:** Kidney IMRT dose uniformity verified via water phantom.
**Related Terms:** Field uniformity QA, Beam flatness QA.

**254. Fiducial Visibility Reassessment QA:** Periodic verification of marker visibility during treatment.
**Example:** Kidney SBRT fiducials rechecked on weekly CBCT.
**Related Terms:** Fiducial visibility QA, IGRT QA.

**255. Fluoroscopic Image Contrast QA:** Ensures optimal contrast in fluoroscopic images.
**Example:** Kidney angiography checked for vessel clarity and tissue differentiation.
**Related Terms:** Fluoroscopic image QA, Image quality QA.

**256. Fractionation Plan QA:** Verifies fractionation schedule aligns with prescription.
**Example:** Kidney SBRT 5-fraction plan checked for dose per fraction.
**Related Terms:** Fractionation schedule QA, Dose verification QA.

**257. Flatness and Symmetry Verification Phantom:** Phantom used to measure beam flatness and symmetry simultaneously.
**Example:** Kidney IMRT beams checked using film phantom.
**Related Terms:** Flatness QA, Beam uniformity QA.

**258. Fiducial Implant Reposition QA:** QA to confirm fiducial position if re-implantation occurs.
**Example:** Kidney markers repositioned and verified for IGRT.
**Related Terms:** Fiducial placement QA, Fiducial stability QA.

**259. Fluorescent Imaging Phantom:** Phantom used to verify fluorescence imaging systems.
**Example:** Kidney tumor fluorescence signal verified using dedicated phantom.
**Related Terms:** Fluorescent signal calibration, Imaging QA.

**260. Field Coverage QA:** Confirms that target anatomy is fully within the treatment field.
**Example:** Kidney PTV verified to be fully covered with IMRT fields.
**Related Terms:** Field-of-view QA, Beam alignment QA.

261. **Fiducial Tracking Accuracy QA:** Verifies real-time tracking of markers during treatment delivery.
**Example:** Kidney SBRT fiducials tracked accurately with CyberKnife.
**Related Terms:** Fiducial tracking QA, Motion management QA.

262. **Fluence Dose Comparison QA:** Compares measured vs calculated fluence dose.
**Example:** Kidney VMAT dose verified using EPID.
**Related Terms:** Fluence verification phantom, Dose mapping QA.

263. **Field Aperture Reproducibility QA:** Ensures MLC/jaw apertures remain consistent across fractions.
**Example:** Kidney IMRT apertures verified with portal images.
**Related Terms:** Field aperture QA, MLC QA.

264. **Flatness and Symmetry Protocol:** Standard QA procedure for beam uniformity.
**Example:** Kidney IMRT checked using phantom and dosimeter.
**Related Terms:** Flatness QA, Beam uniformity QA.

265. **Fiducial Implant Verification QA:** Confirms correct marker placement after implantation.
**Example:** Kidney fiducials checked for proximity to tumor and safety from organs at risk.
**Related Terms:** Fiducial implant QA, Fiducial placement QA.

266. **Fluoroscopic Image Geometry QA:** Ensures accurate spatial representation in fluoroscopic images.
**Example:** Kidney catheter navigation geometry verified against phantom.
**Related Terms:** Fluoroscopy geometric accuracy, Image distortion QA.

267. **Fractional Dose Consistency QA:** Verifies that per-fraction dose matches planned prescription.
**Example:** Kidney SBRT daily fractions checked with portal dosimetry.
**Related Terms:** Fractionated dose verification, Dose mapping QA.

268. **Flatness Verification Protocol:** Procedure to check beam flatness using phantoms.
**Example:** Kidney IMRT verified with water phantom and detector array.
**Related Terms:** Flatness QA, Flatness measurement verification.

269. **Fiducial Registration Accuracy Protocol:** QA procedure to ensure markers register accurately across imaging sessions.
**Example:** Kidney CBCT daily registration verified with phantom.
**Related Terms:** Fiducial registration QA, IGRT QA.

270. **Fluorescence Signal Intensity QA:** Ensures fluorescence imaging system detects tumor signal reliably.
**Example:** Kidney tumor fluorescence verified with calibrated phantom.
**Related Terms:** Fluorescent signal calibration, Image QA.

271. **Field Alignment Verification:** Confirms beam alignment matches planned treatment coordinates.
**Example:** Kidney IMRT verified using alignment phantom.
**Related Terms:** Field verification QA, Beam positioning QA.

272. **Fiducial Contour Validation QA:** Confirms contours of markers are accurately represented.
**Example:** Kidney fiducial contours validated on planning CT.
**Related Terms:** Fiducial contour QA, Contour QA.

273. **Fluoroscopic Dose Optimization QA:** Ensures minimal radiation exposure while maintaining image quality.
**Example:** Kidney interventional procedure optimized to reduce patient dose.
**Related Terms:** ALARA, Fluoroscopic dose QA.

274. **Fractionation Dose Mapping:** Maps dose delivered per fraction for verification.
**Example:** Kidney SBRT dose mapped via EPID and CBCT.
**Related Terms:** Fractional dose mapping, Dose verification QA.

275. **Flatness QA Checklist:** Checklist for verifying beam flatness and uniformity.
**Example:** Kidney IMRT beam flatness verified using phantom measurements.
**Related Terms:** Flatness measurement verification, Beam uniformity QA.

276. **Fiducial Registration Recalibration QA:** Recalibrates registration accuracy if markers shift.
**Example:** Kidney CBCT fiducial registration recalibrated mid-treatment.
**Related Terms:** Fiducial registration QA, IGRT QA.

277. **Fluorescence Imaging Signal QA:** Ensures reliable fluorescent signal for imaging guidance.
**Example:** Kidney tumor fluorescence checked before surgery.
**Related Terms:** Fluorescent signal calibration, Image QA.

278. **Field Repositioning QA:** Confirms beam is correctly repositioned after patient setup.
**Example:** Kidney IMRT verified with portal imaging.
**Related Terms:** Field position QA, Beam alignment QA.

279. **Fiducial Motion QA:** Monitors marker motion during treatment.
**Example:** Kidney fiducials tracked for respiratory motion.
**Related Terms:** Fiducial tracking QA, Motion management QA.

280. **Fluence Map Recalculation QA:** Recalculates delivered fluence to verify dose accuracy.
**Example:** Kidney VMAT dose verified using EPID recalculation.
**Related Terms:** Fluence dose mapping, Dose verification QA.

281. **Field Homogeneity Verification:** Ensures dose uniformity across treatment field.
**Example:** Kidney IMRT field uniformity checked with water phantom.
**Related Terms:** Field uniformity QA, Beam flatness QA.

282. **Fiducial Detection Accuracy QA:** Confirms accurate detection of markers in all imaging sessions.
**Example:** Kidney fiducials verified on daily CBCT.
**Related Terms:** Fiducial visibility QA, IGRT QA.

283. **Fluoroscopic Beam Alignment QA:** Ensures fluoroscopic beam aligned correctly with target anatomy.
**Example:** Kidney angiography beam verified for correct centering.
**Related Terms:** Fluoroscopy geometric accuracy, Beam alignment QA.

284. **Fractionation Delivery QA:** Verifies fractionated treatment delivered accurately.
**Example:** Kidney SBRT dose per fraction checked with EPID.
**Related Terms:** Fractionated dose verification, Dose mapping QA.

285. **Flatness and Symmetry QA Protocol:** Standard QA for verifying beam uniformity.
**Example:** Kidney IMRT beams checked using water phantom.
**Related Terms:** Flatness QA, Beam uniformity verification.

286. **Fiducial Implant Integrity QA:** Ensures markers remain intact and functional.
**Example:** Kidney SBRT fiducials inspected for integrity before treatment.
**Related Terms:** Fiducial stability QA, Fiducial implant QA.

287. **Fluorescent Imaging Standard QA:** Standardized QA for fluorescence-based imaging systems.
**Example:** Kidney tumor fluorescence verified using calibrated phantom.
**Related Terms:** Fluorescent signal calibration, Imaging QA.

288. **Field Edge Position Verification:** Confirms sharpness and correct position of beam edges.
**Example:** Kidney IMRT penumbra verified with film phantom.
**Related Terms:** Field edge QA, Beam profile QA.

289. **Fiducial Tracking Phantom QA:** Phantom with markers to verify motion tracking accuracy.
**Example:** Kidney fiducials tracked in moving phantom to simulate respiration.
**Related Terms:** Fiducial tracking QA, Motion management QA.

290. **Fluence Output Consistency Verification:** Ensures radiation output remains consistent across sessions.
**Example:** Kidney VMAT output verified using EPID and phantom measurements.
**Related Terms:** Fluence delivery QA, Beam output QA.

291. **Field Aperture Accuracy QA:** Verifies MLC and jaw apertures match treatment plan.
**Example:** Kidney IMRT MLC positions checked with portal dosimetry.
**Related Terms:** Field aperture QA, Beam shaping QA.

292. **Fiducial Implant Position QA:** Confirms markers are correctly implanted relative to tumor.
**Example:** Kidney SBRT fiducials verified on planning CT.
**Related Terms:** Fiducial placement QA, Fiducial visibility QA.

293. **Fluoroscopic Exposure Monitoring QA:** Continuous monitoring of patient dose during fluoroscopy.
**Example:** Kidney interventional dose tracked via dosimeter.
**Related Terms:** Fluoroscopic dose QA, ALARA.

294. **Fractionation Schedule Verification QA:** Ensures prescribed number of fractions and dose per fraction are correct.
**Example:** Kidney SBRT 5-fraction plan verified against TPS schedule.
**Related Terms:** Fractionation plan QA, Dose verification QA.

295. **Flatness Measurement QA:** Measures uniformity of radiation beam intensity.
**Example:** Kidney IMRT beam flatness checked with water phantom.
**Related Terms:** Flatness QA, Flatness verification phantom.

296. **Fiducial Contour Accuracy QA:** Confirms fiducial marker contours match actual anatomy.
**Example:** Kidney CBCT fiducial contours verified against planning CT.
**Related Terms:** Fiducial contour QA, Contour QA.

297. **Fluorescence Signal Intensity Calibration:** Calibrates fluorescent imaging systems for consistent signal detection.
**Example:** Kidney tumor fluorescence verified with phantom.
**Related Terms:** Fluorescent signal calibration, Imaging QA.

298. **Field Symmetry QA:** Ensures left-right dose symmetry across field.
**Example:** Kidney IMRT beam symmetry measured using phantom.
**Related Terms:** Flatness and symmetry QA, Beam uniformity QA.

299. **Fiducial Marker Dose QA:** Ensures markers are not in high-dose regions.
**Example:** Kidney SBRT fiducials confirmed outside hotspots.
**Related Terms:** Fiducial dose assessment, Dose verification QA.

300. **Fluence Map QA Protocol:** Standard procedure for verifying fluence maps.
**Example:** Kidney VMAT fluence verified using MapCHECK phantom.
**Related Terms:** Fluence verification phantom, Dose mapping QA.

301. **Field Coverage Verification Phantom:** Phantom used to ensure entire target is covered by treatment field.
**Example:** Kidney PTV verified using water or 3D-printed phantom.
**Related Terms:** Field-of-view QA, Beam alignment QA.

302. **Fiducial Migration Phantom QA:** Phantom simulating marker motion to verify stability.
**Example:** Kidney fiducial stability tested in moving phantom.
**Related Terms:** Fiducial stability QA, Motion management QA.

303. **Fluoroscopic Geometric Phantom QA:** Phantom used to verify spatial accuracy of fluoroscopy.
**Example:** Kidney catheter navigation verified using geometric phantom.
**Related Terms:** Fluoroscopy geometric accuracy, Image distortion QA.

304. **Fractionation Verification Protocol:** QA procedure to verify per-fraction dose delivery.
**Example:** Kidney SBRT fractions checked with EPID and TPS.
**Related Terms:** Fractionated dose verification, Dose mapping QA.

305. **Flatness and Symmetry Verification Protocol:** Standard QA procedure for beam flatness and symmetry.
**Example:** Kidney IMRT verified using water phantom.
**Related Terms:** Flatness QA, Beam uniformity QA.

306. **Fiducial Registration Verification Phantom:** Phantom with markers to test registration accuracy.
**Example:** Kidney CBCT aligned to phantom fiducials for QA.
**Related Terms:** Fiducial registration QA, Image registration QA.

307. **Fluorescent Imaging QA Protocol:** Standard procedure to ensure fluorescence imaging accuracy.
**Example:** Kidney tumor fluorescence verified using calibrated phantom.
**Related Terms:** Fluorescent signal calibration, Imaging QA.

308. **Field Edge Accuracy QA:** Verifies sharpness and correct placement of beam edges.
**Example:** Kidney IMRT penumbra checked with film phantom.
**Related Terms:** Field edge QA, Beam profile QA.

309. **Fiducial Motion Phantom QA:** Phantom simulating respiratory motion to check tracking accuracy.
**Example:** Kidney SBRT fiducials tracked using moving phantom.
**Related Terms:** Fiducial tracking QA, Motion management QA.

310. **Fluence Delivery Consistency QA:** Confirms consistent delivery of planned fluence.
**Example:** Kidney VMAT delivery verified across multiple sessions using EPID.
**Related Terms:** Fluence dose mapping, Beam output QA.

311. **Field Output Factor QA:** Verifies output factor for various field sizes.
**Example:** Kidney IMRT small and large field outputs measured using ion chamber.
**Related Terms:** Output factor QA, Beam output QA.

312. **Fiducial Registration Reproducibility Phantom:** Phantom used to verify reproducibility of marker registration.
**Example:** Kidney CBCT registration accuracy checked with phantom.
**Related Terms:** Fiducial registration QA, IGRT QA.

313. **Fluorescent Imaging Phantom QA:** Phantom used to verify fluorescence imaging systems.
**Example:** Kidney tumor fluorescence verified for intensity and localization.
**Related Terms:** Fluorescent signal calibration, Imaging QA.

314. **Field Position Verification Protocol:** Procedure for verifying correct beam placement.
**Example:** Kidney IMRT fields checked via portal dosimetry.
**Related Terms:** Field position QA, Beam alignment QA.

315. **Fiducial Implant Migration QA:** Monitors marker migration over treatment course.
**Example:** Kidney SBRT fiducials tracked weekly using CBCT.
**Related Terms:** Fiducial stability QA, Fiducial tracking QA.

316. **Fluoroscopic Dose Verification Protocol:** Procedure to measure and verify dose during fluoroscopy.
**Example:** Kidney interventional dose verified using phantom dosimeters.
**Related Terms:** Fluoroscopic dose QA, ALARA.

317. **Fractionation Dose Consistency Protocol:** Ensures prescribed fractionated doses are delivered accurately.
**Example:** Kidney SBRT daily fractions verified with portal imaging.
**Related Terms:** Fractional dose mapping, Dose verification QA.

318. **Flatness Measurement Protocol:** Procedure to measure beam flatness using phantoms.
**Example:** Kidney IMRT flatness verified using water phantom.
**Related Terms:** Flatness QA, Flatness verification phantom.

319. **Fiducial Contour Reproducibility Protocol:** Ensures fiducial contours remain consistent over planning and treatment.
**Example:** Kidney fiducial contours verified across multiple CT scans.
**Related Terms:** Fiducial contour QA, Contour QA.

320. **Fluorescent Signal Intensity Verification QA:** Confirms fluorescence imaging provides reliable tumor detection.
**Example:** Kidney tumor fluorescence verified using standardized phantom.
**Related Terms:** Fluorescent signal calibration, Imaging QA.

321. **Field Alignment QA Checklist:** Comprehensive QA checklist for verifying field alignment.
**Example:** Kidney IMRT alignment verified with portal dosimetry and phantom.
**Related Terms:** Field verification QA, Beam positioning QA.

322. **Fiducial Tracking Verification Protocol:** Procedure to ensure accurate tracking of implanted markers.
**Example:** Kidney SBRT fiducials verified for real-time tracking accuracy.
**Related Terms:** Fiducial tracking QA, Motion management QA.

323. **Fluence Map Reproducibility QA:** Confirms delivered fluence maps match TPS across sessions.
**Example:** Kidney VMAT fields compared against TPS plan for consistency.
**Related Terms:** Fluence verification phantom, Dose mapping QA.

324. **Field Edge Verification Protocol:** Procedure to verify beam edge sharpness and placement.
**Example:** Kidney IMRT penumbra verified using film phantom.
**Related Terms:** Field edge QA, Beam profile QA.

325. **Fiducial Dose Limitation Protocol:** Ensures fiducials are not exposed to excessive radiation.
**Example:** Kidney SBRT markers verified to be outside high-dose regions.
**Related Terms:** Fiducial dose assessment, Dose verification QA.

326. **Fluorescence Imaging Standard Protocol:** Standard QA protocol for fluorescence imaging systems.
**Example:** Kidney tumor fluorescence verified for consistent intensity and localization.
**Related Terms:** Fluorescent signal calibration, Imaging QA.

327. **Field Uniformity Verification Protocol:** Ensures even dose distribution across treatment field.
**Example:** Kidney IMRT uniformity verified using water phantom.
**Related Terms:** Field uniformity QA, Beam flatness QA.

328. **Fiducial Implant Repositioning Protocol:** QA procedure for verifying markers after repositioning.
**Example:** Kidney SBRT fiducials repositioned and verified with CBCT.
**Related Terms:** Fiducial placement QA, Fiducial registration QA.

329. **Fluoroscopic Beam Alignment Protocol:** QA procedure to ensure fluoroscopy beam is correctly aligned.
**Example:** Kidney catheter guidance verified using phantom.
**Related Terms:** Fluoroscopy geometric accuracy, Beam alignment QA.

330. **Fractionation Plan Reassessment QA:** Periodic verification of fractionation schedule.
**Example:** Kidney SBRT plan verified mid-treatment against prescription.
**Related Terms:** Fractionation schedule QA, Dose verification QA.

331. **Flatness and Symmetry Reverification QA:** Re-verification of beam flatness and symmetry over time.
**Example:** Kidney IMRT beams re-checked weekly using phantom.
**Related Terms:** Flatness QA, Beam uniformity QA.

332. **Fiducial Registration Mid-Treatment QA:** QA during treatment to verify marker registration.
**Example:** Kidney CBCT aligned mid-treatment to planning CT fiducials.
**Related Terms:** Fiducial registration QA, IGRT QA.

333. **Fluorescent Imaging Recalibration QA:** Recalibration of fluorescent imaging system for consistent signal.
**Example:** Kidney tumor fluorescence verified before surgery using phantom.
**Related Terms:** Fluorescent signal calibration, Imaging QA.

334. **Field Position Reassessment QA:** QA to confirm beam placement after patient repositioning.
**Example:** Kidney IMRT fields verified using portal images.
**Related Terms:** Field position QA, Beam alignment QA.

335. **Fiducial Motion Verification QA:** Confirms marker tracking accuracy for moving targets.
**Example:** Kidney fiducials monitored during respiratory motion.
**Related Terms:** Fiducial tracking QA, Motion management QA.

336. **Fluence Output Verification Protocol:** Confirms consistent LINAC fluence output over time.
**Example:** Kidney VMAT output verified using EPID and phantom.
**Related Terms:** Fluence delivery QA, Beam output QA.

337. **Field Homogeneity Verification Protocol:** Ensures uniform dose across field according to plan.
**Example:** Kidney IMRT fields checked using water phantom.
**Related Terms:** Field uniformity QA, Beam flatness QA.

338. **Fiducial Detection Verification Protocol:** Ensures imaging system reliably detects markers.
**Example:** Kidney CBCT checked for all fiducials daily.
**Related Terms:** Fiducial visibility QA, IGRT QA.

339. **Fluoroscopic Dose Mapping Protocol:** Maps patient dose during fluoroscopic procedures.
**Example:** Kidney interventional dose mapped for ALARA compliance.
**Related Terms:** Fluoroscopic dose QA, Dose optimization QA.

340. **Fractional Dose Mapping Protocol:** Maps per-fraction dose for verification and QA.
**Example:** Kidney SBRT dose mapped with CBCT and EPID.
**Related Terms:** Fractional dose mapping, Dose verification QA.

341. **Flatness Measurement Reverification QA:** Periodic re-verification of beam flatness.
**Example:** Kidney IMRT beam flatness re-checked weekly.
**Related Terms:** Flatness QA, Flatness verification phantom.

342. **Fiducial Contour Reverification QA:** Confirms fiducial contours remain accurate over treatment.
**Example:** Kidney fiducial contours checked mid-treatment.
**Related Terms:** Fiducial contour QA, Contour QA.

343. **Fluorescence Signal QA Reassessment:** Periodic verification of fluorescence signal intensity.
**Example:** Kidney tumor fluorescence reassessed with phantom.
**Related Terms:** Fluorescent signal calibration, Imaging QA.

344. **Field Alignment Verification Protocol:** Procedure to ensure beam alignment accuracy.
**Example:** Kidney IMRT verified using portal dosimetry and phantom.
**Related Terms:** Field verification QA, Beam positioning QA.

345. **Fiducial Tracking Verification Phantom:** Phantom used to verify real-time fiducial tracking.
**Example:** Kidney fiducials tracked accurately using moving phantom.
**Related Terms:** Fiducial tracking QA, Motion management QA.

346. **Fluence Map Verification QA Protocol:** Ensures delivered fluence matches planned fluence.
**Example:** Kidney VMAT fluence compared against TPS.
**Related Terms:** Fluence verification phantom, Dose mapping QA.

347. **Field Edge Reverification QA:** Re-verifies beam edge sharpness and position over treatment course.
**Example:** Kidney IMRT penumbra rechecked using film phantom.
**Related Terms:** Field edge QA, Beam profile QA.

348. **Fiducial Dose Limitation Verification QA:** Ensures markers are not exposed to excessive dose during treatment.
**Example:** Kidney SBRT fiducials confirmed outside high-dose regions mid-treatment.
**Related Terms:** Fiducial dose assessment, Dose verification QA.

349. **Fluorescent Imaging QA Reverification:** Periodic QA to ensure fluorescence imaging accuracy.
**Example:** Kidney tumor fluorescence checked before surgery using phantom.
**Related Terms:** Fluorescent signal calibration, Imaging QA.

350. **Field Uniformity Reverification QA:** Re-verifies dose uniformity across field during treatment course.
**Example:** Kidney IMRT uniformity rechecked weekly using phantom.
**Related Terms:** Field uniformity QA, Beam flatness QA.

351. **Fiducial Implant Verification Protocol:** QA procedure to confirm correct placement of implanted markers.
**Example:** Kidney SBRT fiducials verified with CBCT after implantation.
**Related Terms:** Fiducial placement QA, Fiducial visibility QA.

352. **Fluorescent Imaging Calibration Phantom:** Phantom used to calibrate fluorescence imaging systems.
**Example:** Kidney tumor fluorescence intensity verified using phantom.
**Related Terms:** Fluorescent signal calibration, Imaging QA.

353. **Field Size Accuracy QA:** Ensures planned field size matches delivered field.
**Example:** Kidney IMRT PTV fully covered without overdosing surrounding tissue.
**Related Terms:** Field verification QA, Field aperture QA.

354. **Fiducial Migration Tracking QA:** Monitoring implanted marker movement over treatment.
**Example:** Kidney fiducial positions tracked weekly using CBCT.
**Related Terms:** Fiducial stability QA, Motion management QA.

355. **Fluoroscopic Spatial Accuracy QA:** Ensures geometric accuracy in fluoroscopic imaging.
**Example:** Kidney catheter navigation verified using geometric phantom.
**Related Terms:** Fluoroscopy geometric accuracy, Image distortion QA.

356. **Fractionated Dose Consistency Verification:** QA to ensure consistent per-fraction dose delivery.
**Example:** Kidney SBRT daily fractions verified against prescription.
**Related Terms:** Fractionation plan QA, Dose verification QA.

357. **Flatness QA Phantom Reassessment:** Periodic verification of beam flatness using phantoms.
**Example:** Kidney IMRT flatness rechecked weekly.
**Related Terms:** Flatness QA, Flatness verification phantom.

358. **Fiducial Contour Reassessment QA:** Ensures fiducial contours remain accurate over treatment course.
**Example:** Kidney fiducial contours verified mid-treatment using CBCT.
**Related Terms:** Fiducial contour QA, Contour QA.

359. **Fluorescent Imaging Verification Protocol:** Standard QA to ensure fluorescence imaging accuracy.
**Example:** Kidney tumor fluorescence intensity and localization verified with phantom.
**Related Terms:** Fluorescent signal calibration, Imaging QA.

360. **Field Alignment QA Reassessment:** Periodic QA to confirm beam alignment accuracy.
**Example:** Kidney IMRT verified with portal dosimetry and phantom.
**Related Terms:** Field verification QA, Beam positioning QA.

361. **Fiducial Tracking QA Reassessment:** Ensures continuous accuracy of real-time marker tracking.
**Example:** Kidney SBRT fiducials tracked during treatment using moving phantom.
**Related Terms:** Fiducial tracking QA, Motion management QA.

362. **Fluence Map QA Reassessment:** Verifies delivered fluence remains consistent with TPS across treatment.
**Example:** Kidney VMAT fluence compared to TPS plan mid-treatment.
**Related Terms:** Fluence verification phantom, Dose mapping QA.

363. **Field Edge Reassessment QA:** Re-verification of beam edge sharpness and placement.
**Example:** Kidney IMRT penumbra rechecked with film phantom.
**Related Terms:** Field edge QA, Beam profile QA.

364. **Fiducial Dose Limitation QA Reassessment:** Ensures markers remain outside high-dose regions during treatment.
**Example:** Kidney SBRT fiducials checked to avoid hotspots.
**Related Terms:** Fiducial dose assessment, Dose verification QA.

365. **Fluorescent Imaging QA Reassessment Protocol:** Periodic QA to ensure fluorescence imaging accuracy.
**Example:** Kidney tumor fluorescence verified with calibration phantom.
**Related Terms:** Fluorescent signal calibration, Imaging QA.

366. **Field Uniformity QA Reassessment:** Re-verifies dose uniformity across treatment field during therapy.
**Example:** Kidney IMRT uniformity rechecked using MapCHECK or water phantom.
**Related Terms:** Field uniformity QA, Beam flatness QA.

367. **Fiducial Registration QA Reassessment:** QA to confirm accuracy of fiducial-based image registration.
**Example:** Kidney CBCT aligned to planning CT using fiducials mid-treatment.
**Related Terms:** Fiducial registration QA, IGRT QA.

**368. Fluoroscopic Dose Mapping Reassessment:** Reassesses dose distribution during fluoroscopic procedures.
**Example:** Kidney interventional fluoroscopy dose checked with phantom dosimeters.
**Related Terms:** Fluoroscopic dose QA, ALARA.

**369. Fractional Dose Mapping Reassessment:** Maps per-fraction dose for verification and QA mid-treatment.
**Example:** Kidney SBRT per-fraction dose confirmed with EPID and TPS.
**Related Terms:** Fractionated dose verification, Dose mapping QA.

**370. Flatness and Symmetry QA Reassessment:** Ensures ongoing uniformity and symmetry of beams over therapy course.
**Example:** Kidney IMRT beams rechecked using flatness and symmetry phantom.
**Related Terms:** Flatness QA, Beam uniformity QA.

**371. Fiducial Detection QA Reassessment:** Confirms reliable detection of fiducial markers throughout treatment.
**Example:** Kidney CBCT verifies visibility of all fiducials daily.
**Related Terms:** Fiducial visibility QA, IGRT QA.

**372. Fluorescence Imaging Calibration Reverification:** Periodic calibration of fluorescent imaging system for consistent tumor detection.
**Example:** Kidney tumor fluorescence checked with phantom before therapy.
**Related Terms:** Fluorescent signal calibration, Imaging QA.

**373. Field Size Verification Reassessment:** Re-verifies delivered field size against planned PTV.
**Example:** Kidney IMRT field coverage checked weekly.
**Related Terms:** Field verification QA, Field aperture QA.

**374. Fiducial Migration QA Reassessment:** Continual monitoring of implanted marker migration.
**Example:** Kidney SBRT fiducial positions tracked with CBCT mid-treatment.
**Related Terms:** Fiducial stability QA, Motion management QA.

**375. Fluoroscopic Geometric Accuracy Reverification:** Periodic check of geometric accuracy in fluoroscopy.
**Example:** Kidney catheter navigation verified using geometric phantom.
**Related Terms:** Fluoroscopy geometric accuracy, Image distortion QA.

**376. Fractionation Consistency QA Reassessment:** Ensures prescribed fractionated doses remain accurate.
**Example:** Kidney SBRT daily fractions verified weekly using portal imaging.
**Related Terms:** Fractionation plan QA, Dose verification QA.

**377. Flatness QA Phantom Reverification:** Re-verifies beam flatness using dedicated phantoms.
**Example:** Kidney IMRT beams checked weekly using water phantom.
**Related Terms:** Flatness QA, Flatness verification phantom.

**378. Fiducial Contour QA Reverification:** Confirms marker contours remain consistent during treatment.
**Example:** Kidney fiducial contours verified using CBCT.
**Related Terms:** Fiducial contour QA, Contour QA.

**379. Fluorescent Imaging QA Reverification:** Ensures ongoing accuracy of fluorescence imaging system.
**Example:** Kidney tumor fluorescence verified with phantom mid-treatment.
**Related Terms:** Fluorescent signal calibration, Imaging QA.

380. **Field Alignment QA Reverification:** Periodic QA to confirm beam alignment accuracy.
**Example:** Kidney IMRT verified with portal dosimetry and phantom.
**Related Terms:** Field verification QA, Beam positioning QA.

381. **Fiducial Tracking QA Reverification:** QA to ensure accurate real-time marker tracking.
**Example:** Kidney SBRT fiducials tracked with moving phantom.
**Related Terms:** Fiducial tracking QA, Motion management QA.

382. **Fluence Map QA Reverification:** Confirms delivered fluence matches TPS plan over time.
**Example:** Kidney VMAT fluence compared to TPS mid-treatment.
**Related Terms:** Fluence verification phantom, Dose mapping QA.

383. **Field Edge QA Reverification:** Re-verifies sharpness and position of beam edges.
**Example:** Kidney IMRT penumbra checked using film phantom.
**Related Terms:** Field edge QA, Beam profile QA.

384. **Fiducial Dose QA Reverification:** Ensures markers remain outside high-dose regions.
**Example:** Kidney SBRT fiducials verified to avoid hotspots.
**Related Terms:** Fiducial dose assessment, Dose verification QA.

385. **Fluorescence Imaging QA Mid-Treatment:** QA during treatment to verify fluorescence system performance.
**Example:** Kidney tumor fluorescence verified using phantom.
**Related Terms:** Fluorescent signal calibration, Imaging QA.

386. **Field Uniformity QA Mid-Treatment:** Re-verification of dose uniformity across treatment field.
**Example:** Kidney IMRT uniformity checked weekly with phantom.
**Related Terms:** Field uniformity QA, Beam flatness QA.

387. **Fiducial Registration QA Mid-Treatment:** QA to ensure accurate alignment of fiducials during treatment.
**Example:** Kidney CBCT aligned to planning CT using fiducials mid-treatment.
**Related Terms:** Fiducial registration QA, IGRT QA.

388. **Fluoroscopic Dose Mapping QA Mid-Treatment:** Mid-treatment mapping of dose during fluoroscopic procedures.
**Example:** Kidney fluoroscopy dose verified with phantom dosimeters.
**Related Terms:** Fluoroscopic dose QA, ALARA.

389. **Fractional Dose Mapping QA Mid-Treatment:** Maps delivered dose per fraction for verification.
**Example:** Kidney SBRT dose mapped using CBCT and EPID.
**Related Terms:** Fractionated dose verification, Dose mapping QA.

390. **Flatness and Symmetry QA Mid-Treatment:** Ensures ongoing beam flatness and symmetry.
**Example:** Kidney IMRT beams checked weekly using phantom.
**Related Terms:** Flatness QA, Beam uniformity QA.

391. **Fiducial Detection QA Mid-Treatment:** Confirms marker visibility during therapy.
**Example:** Kidney CBCT verified visibility of all fiducials daily.
**Related Terms:** Fiducial visibility QA, IGRT QA.

392. **Fluorescence Calibration QA Mid-Treatment:** Ensures fluorescence imaging maintains accurate signal mid-treatment.
**Example:** Kidney tumor fluorescence verified with phantom.
**Related Terms:** Fluorescent signal calibration, Imaging QA.

393. **Field Size Verification Mid-Treatment:** Confirms delivered field size matches planned PTV.
**Example:** Kidney IMRT field coverage rechecked weekly.
**Related Terms:** Field verification QA, Field aperture QA.

394. **Fiducial Migration QA Mid-Treatment:** Monitors marker migration during therapy.
**Example:** Kidney SBRT fiducial positions tracked with CBCT mid-treatment.
**Related Terms:** Fiducial stability QA, Motion management QA.

395. **Fluoroscopic Geometric QA Mid-Treatment:** Periodic verification of geometric accuracy in fluoroscopy.
**Example:** Kidney catheter navigation checked using geometric phantom.
**Related Terms:** Fluoroscopy geometric accuracy, Image distortion QA.

396. **Fractionation Consistency QA Mid-Treatment:** Ensures prescribed fractionated doses remain accurate.
**Example:** Kidney SBRT fractions verified using portal imaging mid-treatment.
**Related Terms:** Fractionation plan QA, Dose verification QA.

397. **Flatness QA Reassessment Mid-Treatment:** Periodic verification of beam flatness during therapy.
**Example:** Kidney IMRT beams rechecked with water phantom.
**Related Terms:** Flatness QA, Flatness verification phantom.

398. **Fiducial Contour QA Mid-Treatment:** Ensures marker contours remain accurate during therapy.
**Example:** Kidney fiducial contours verified using CBCT.
**Related Terms:** Fiducial contour QA, Contour QA.

399. **Fluorescent Imaging QA Mid-Treatment:** Ensures fluorescence imaging system maintains accuracy during therapy.
**Example:** Kidney tumor fluorescence verified with phantom.
**Related Terms:** Fluorescent signal calibration, Imaging QA.

400. **Field Alignment QA Mid-Treatment:** Confirms beam alignment accuracy during therapy.
**Example:** Kidney IMRT verified with portal dosimetry and phantom.
**Related Terms:** Field verification QA, Beam positioning QA.

401. **Fiducial Tracking QA Mid-Treatment:** Verifies accuracy of real-time marker tracking during therapy.
**Example:** Kidney SBRT fiducials tracked with moving phantom.
**Related Terms:** Fiducial tracking QA, Motion management QA.

402. **Fluence Map QA Mid-Treatment:** Confirms delivered fluence matches TPS plan mid-treatment.
**Example:** Kidney VMAT fluence compared to TPS.
**Related Terms:** Fluence verification phantom, Dose mapping QA.

403. **Field Edge QA Mid-Treatment:** Re-verification of beam edge sharpness and placement during therapy.
**Example:** Kidney IMRT penumbra checked using film phantom.
**Related Terms:** Field edge QA, Beam profile QA.

404. **Fiducial Dose QA Mid-Treatment:** Ensures markers remain outside high-dose regions mid-treatment.
**Example:** Kidney SBRT fiducials verified to avoid hotspots.
**Related Terms:** Fiducial dose assessment, Dose verification QA.

405. **Fluorescent Imaging QA Reassessment Mid-Treatment:** Ensures fluorescence imaging system maintains performance mid-treatment.
**Example:** Kidney tumor fluorescence verified using phantom.
**Related Terms:** Fluorescent signal calibration, Imaging QA.

406. **Field Uniformity QA Mid-Treatment:** Re-verification of dose uniformity across field during therapy.
**Example:** Kidney IMRT uniformity checked weekly with phantom.
**Related Terms:** Field uniformity QA, Beam flatness QA.

407. **Fiducial Registration QA Mid-Treatment:** QA to ensure accurate alignment of fiducials during treatment.
**Example:** Kidney CBCT aligned to planning CT using fiducials mid-treatment.
**Related Terms:** Fiducial registration QA, IGRT QA.

408. **Fluoroscopic Dose Mapping QA Mid-Treatment:** Mid-treatment mapping of patient dose during fluoroscopy.
**Example:** Kidney fluoroscopy dose verified with phantom dosimeters.
**Related Terms:** Fluoroscopic dose QA, ALARA.

409. **Fractional Dose Mapping QA Mid-Treatment:** Maps delivered dose per fraction for verification mid-treatment.
**Example:** Kidney SBRT dose mapped using CBCT and EPID.
**Related Terms:** Fractionated dose verification, Dose mapping QA.

410. **Flatness and Symmetry QA Mid-Treatment:** Ensures ongoing beam flatness and symmetry during therapy.
**Example:** Kidney IMRT beams checked weekly using phantom.
**Related Terms:** Flatness QA, Beam uniformity QA.

411. **Fiducial Visibility QA Reassessment:** Ensures implanted markers remain visible in all imaging modalities.
**Example:** Kidney SBRT fiducials confirmed visible on daily CBCT and KV imaging.
**Related Terms:** Fiducial visibility QA, Fiducial detection QA.

412. **Fluence Delivery Verification QA:** Verifies the LINAC delivers planned fluence accurately.
**Example:** Kidney VMAT fields verified using MapCHECK phantom.
**Related Terms:** Fluence verification phantom, Fluence pattern QA.

413. **Field Symmetry QA Reassessment:** Checks beam symmetry remains within tolerance.
**Example:** Kidney IMRT beams symmetric across central axis.
**Related Terms:** Flatness and symmetry QA, Beam uniformity QA.

414. **Fiducial Alignment QA Reassessment:** Ensures fiducials continue to align with treatment plan.
**Example:** Kidney SBRT daily CBCT aligned to planned PTV using fiducials.
**Related Terms:** Fiducial registration QA, IGRT QA.

415. **Field Aperture QA Reassessment:** Verifies MLC and jaw apertures match planned field.
**Example:** Kidney IMRT MLC leaf positions confirmed with QA phantom.
**Related Terms:** Field size verification, MLC QA.

416. **Flatness QA Phantom Mid-Treatment:** Phantom measurement of beam flatness during therapy course.
**Example:** Kidney IMRT field flatness verified using water phantom weekly.
**Related Terms:** Flatness QA, Flatness and symmetry QA.

417. **Fiducial Contour QA Mid-Treatment:** QA for fiducial marker contours during treatment.
**Example:** Kidney fiducial contours rechecked on CBCT mid-course.
**Related Terms:** Fiducial contour verification, Contour QA.

418. **Fluoroscopy Image QA Mid-Treatment:** QA for image clarity and safety during therapy.
**Example:** Kidney angiography images verified for clarity and minimal dose.
**Related Terms:** Fluoroscopy geometric accuracy, Imaging QA.

419. **Fractional Dose Mapping QA Mid-Treatment:** Mapping delivered dose per fraction for verification.
**Example:** Kidney SBRT per-fraction dose checked with portal dosimetry.
**Related Terms:** Fractionated dose verification, Dose mapping QA.

420. **Field Verification Checklist Mid-Treatment:** Checklist to verify all aspects of delivered radiation field.
**Example:** Kidney IMRT field size, shape, and alignment verified.
**Related Terms:** Field verification QA, QA protocol.

421. **Fiducial Implant QA Reassessment:** QA to confirm correct placement of fiducials post-implant.
**Example:** Kidney SBRT fiducials confirmed near tumor without affecting organs at risk.
**Related Terms:** Fiducial placement QA, Fiducial stability QA.

422. **Fluence Output QA Reassessment:** Measures radiation output across treatment field.
**Example:** Kidney VMAT output compared with TPS calculations.
**Related Terms:** Fluence delivery QA, Dose verification QA.

423. **Field Position QA Reassessment:** Verifies correct beam position relative to patient anatomy.
**Example:** Kidney IMRT field matches PTV location verified with portal dosimetry.
**Related Terms:** Field alignment QA, Beam positioning QA.

424. **Fiducial Stability Phantom QA:** Phantom to test marker stability and registration accuracy.
**Example:** Kidney phantom with fiducials used to validate imaging and tracking.
**Related Terms:** Fiducial migration tracking QA, Motion management QA.

425. **Fluoroscopy Dose QA Mid-Treatment:** Ensures patient dose during fluoroscopy remains within limits.
**Example:** Kidney interventional fluoroscopy dose verified using phantom dosimeters.
**Related Terms:** Fluoroscopic dose mapping, ALARA QA.

426. **Flatness and Symmetry Phantom Reassessment:** Phantom used to measure both beam flatness and symmetry.
**Example:** Kidney IMRT beams verified using water or film phantom.
**Related Terms:** Flatness QA, Field uniformity QA.

427. **Fiducial Marker QA Protocol Mid-Treatment:** Protocol for QA of all steps involving fiducial markers.
**Example:** Kidney SBRT fiducials checked for visibility, stability, and correct registration.
**Related Terms:** Fiducial registration QA, Fiducial visibility QA.

428. **Field Edge QA Mid-Treatment:** Verification of beam edge sharpness and position.
**Example:** Kidney IMRT penumbra checked to protect adjacent tissues.
**Related Terms:** Field edge sharpness QA, Beam profile QA.

429. **Fluorescent Imaging QA Mid-Treatment:** Ensures fluorescence-based imaging meets standards.
**Example:** Kidney tumor fluorescence checked for intensity and mapping accuracy.
**Related Terms:** Fluorescent signal calibration, Imaging QA.

430. **Fractionation Verification Phantom Mid-Treatment:** Phantom used to validate fractionated dose delivery.
**Example:** Kidney SBRT per-fraction dose verified using phantom.
**Related Terms:** Fractional dose mapping, Dose verification QA.

431. **Flat-Panel Detector Calibration Mid-Treatment:** Calibration of detectors for image quality and uniform response.
**Example:** Kidney KV images verified for uniform brightness and absence of artifacts.
**Related Terms:** Flat-panel imaging QA, Imaging calibration QA.

432. **Fiducial Visibility Phantom:** Phantom with embedded markers for imaging QA.
**Example:** Kidney CBCT phantom used to test fiducial visibility.
**Related Terms:** Fiducial visibility QA, Fiducial registration QA.

433. **Fluence Delivery QA Phantom:** Phantom to measure delivered fluence versus planned fluence.
**Example:** Kidney VMAT fluence confirmed using MapCHECK phantom.
**Related Terms:** Fluence verification phantom, Dose mapping QA.

434. **Field Symmetry Phantom:** Phantom to verify beam symmetry across treatment field.
**Example:** Kidney IMRT symmetry verified with phantom.
**Related Terms:** Field symmetry QA, Beam uniformity QA.

435. **Fiducial Alignment Phantom:** Phantom with fiducial markers for alignment QA.
**Example:** Kidney phantom used to verify CBCT alignment accuracy.
**Related Terms:** Fiducial registration QA, IGRT QA.

436. **Field Aperture Phantom:** Phantom to verify MLC and jaw apertures.
**Example:** Kidney IMRT MLC leaf positions checked with phantom.
**Related Terms:** Field aperture QA, Field size verification.

437. **Flatness Phantom Mid-Treatment:** Phantom used to check beam flatness and uniformity.
**Example:** Kidney IMRT fields verified using flatness phantom.
**Related Terms:** Flatness QA, Field uniformity QA.

438. **Fiducial Contour Phantom:** Phantom with markers for contour QA.
**Example:** Kidney fiducial contours verified with CBCT phantom.
**Related Terms:** Fiducial contour QA, Contour QA.

439. **Fluoroscopic Imaging Phantom:** Phantom to verify fluoroscopic image quality and geometry.
**Example:** Kidney catheter navigation geometry verified with phantom.
**Related Terms:** Fluoroscopic image QA, Geometric accuracy QA.

440. **Fractional Dose Phantom:** Phantom used to map dose per fraction.
**Example:** Kidney SBRT dose per fraction verified using phantom.
**Related Terms:** Fractionated dose mapping, Dose verification QA.

441. **Field Verification Phantom:** Phantom used to verify all aspects of delivered radiation fields.
**Example:** Kidney IMRT field size, shape, and alignment verified.
**Related Terms:** Field verification QA, QA protocol.

442. **Fiducial Implant Phantom:** Phantom for verifying marker implantation accuracy.
**Example:** Kidney SBRT fiducial placement checked using phantom.
**Related Terms:** Fiducial placement QA, Fiducial stability QA.

443. **Fluence Output Phantom:** Phantom used to measure radiation output across field.
**Example:** Kidney VMAT output verified using phantom.
**Related Terms:** Fluence verification phantom, Dose mapping QA.

444. **Field Position Phantom:** Phantom to check correct beam positioning relative to anatomy.
**Example:** Kidney IMRT field alignment verified using phantom.
**Related Terms:** Field alignment QA, Beam positioning QA.

445. **Fiducial Stability QA Mid-Treatment:** Monitoring implanted marker stability mid-treatment.
**Example:** Kidney SBRT fiducial positions checked with CBCT.
**Related Terms:** Fiducial migration QA, Motion management QA.

446. **Fluoroscopy Dose Phantom:** Phantom to measure patient dose during fluoroscopy.
**Example:** Kidney interventional fluoroscopy dose verified with phantom dosimeters.
**Related Terms:** Fluoroscopic dose QA, ALARA.

447. **Flatness and Symmetry QA Phantom:** Phantom measuring both flatness and symmetry of beams.
**Example:** Kidney IMRT beam verification using water or film phantom.
**Related Terms:** Flatness QA, Beam uniformity QA.

448. **Fiducial Marker QA Protocol Reassessment:** Protocol to verify all steps involving fiducial markers mid-treatment.
**Example:** Kidney SBRT markers checked for visibility, stability, and registration.
**Related Terms:** Fiducial registration QA, Fiducial tracking QA.

449. **Field Edge Phantom:** Phantom used to verify beam edge sharpness and placement.
**Example:** Kidney IMRT penumbra verified using film phantom.
**Related Terms:** Field edge QA, Beam profile QA.

450. **Fluorescent Imaging Phantom:** Phantom used to calibrate and QA fluorescence imaging.
**Example:** Kidney tumor fluorescence verified using phantom.
**Related Terms:** Fluorescent signal calibration, Imaging QA.

451. **Fractionation Verification Phantom Mid-Treatment:** Phantom used to validate fractionated dose delivery mid-treatment.
**Example:** Kidney SBRT fractionated dose verified using phantom.
**Related Terms:** Fractional dose mapping, Dose verification QA.

452. **Flat-Panel Detector QA Mid-Treatment:** QA of detectors for image uniformity and quality mid-treatment.
**Example:** Kidney KV images verified for uniform brightness.
**Related Terms:** Flat-panel imaging QA, Imaging calibration QA.

453. **Fiducial Visibility QA Phantom Mid-Treatment:** Phantom used to verify fiducial marker visibility mid-treatment.
**Example:** Kidney CBCT phantom checked for marker visibility.
**Related Terms:** Fiducial detection QA, Fiducial registration QA.

454. **Fluence Delivery Verification Phantom Mid-Treatment:** Confirms fluence delivery accuracy mid-treatment.
**Example:** Kidney VMAT fluence verified with phantom.
**Related Terms:** Fluence verification phantom, Dose mapping QA.

455. **Field Symmetry QA Phantom:** Phantom to verify symmetry of radiation field.
**Example:** Kidney IMRT symmetry verified with phantom.
**Related Terms:** Beam uniformity QA, Field symmetry QA.

456. **Fiducial Alignment QA Phantom:** Phantom with embedded markers for alignment QA.
**Example:** Kidney phantom used to verify CBCT alignment accuracy.
**Related Terms:** Fiducial registration QA, IGRT QA.

457. **Field Aperture QA Phantom Mid-Treatment:** Phantom to verify MLC and jaw apertures mid-treatment.
**Example:** Kidney IMRT MLC leaf positions checked.
**Related Terms:** Field aperture QA, Field size verification.

458. **Flatness QA Phantom Reassessment Mid-Treatment:** Phantom used to verify beam flatness during therapy.
**Example:** Kidney IMRT fields checked using flatness phantom.
**Related Terms:** Flatness QA, Field uniformity QA.

459. **Fiducial Contour QA Phantom:** Phantom used for QA of marker contours.
**Example:** Kidney fiducial contours verified using phantom.
**Related Terms:** Fiducial contour QA, Contour QA.

460. **Fluoroscopic Imaging QA Phantom Mid-Treatment:** Phantom to QA fluoroscopic image quality during therapy.
**Example:** Kidney catheter navigation verified using phantom.
**Related Terms:** Fluoroscopic image QA, Geometric accuracy QA.

461. **Fractional Dose Phantom Mid-Treatment:** Phantom used to map dose per fraction mid-treatment.
**Example:** Kidney SBRT dose per fraction verified using phantom.
**Related Terms:** Fractionated dose mapping, Dose verification QA.

462. **Field Verification QA Phantom:** Phantom to verify all aspects of delivered radiation fields.
**Example:** Kidney IMRT field size, shape, and alignment verified.
**Related Terms:** Field verification QA, QA protocol.

463. **Fiducial Implant Phantom Mid-Treatment:** Phantom to verify accuracy of marker implantation mid-treatment.
**Example:** Kidney SBRT fiducial placement checked.
**Related Terms:** Fiducial placement QA, Fiducial stability QA.

464. **Fluence Output Phantom Mid-Treatment:** Phantom to measure radiation output across field mid-treatment.
**Example:** Kidney VMAT output verified.
**Related Terms:** Fluence verification phantom, Dose mapping QA.

465. **Field Position QA Phantom Mid-Treatment:** Phantom to check correct beam positioning relative to anatomy.
**Example:** Kidney IMRT field alignment verified.
**Related Terms:** Field alignment QA, Beam positioning QA.

466. **Fiducial Stability QA Phantom Mid-Treatment:** Phantom to monitor implanted marker stability.
**Example:** Kidney SBRT fiducials checked.
**Related Terms:** Fiducial migration QA, Motion management QA.

467. **Fluoroscopy Dose Phantom Mid-Treatment:** Phantom to measure patient dose during fluoroscopy mid-treatment.
**Example:** Kidney interventional fluoroscopy dose verified.
**Related Terms:** Fluoroscopic dose QA, ALARA.

468. **Flatness and Symmetry QA Phantom Mid-Treatment:** Phantom to measure beam flatness and symmetry.
**Example:** Kidney IMRT beam verification using water or film phantom.
**Related Terms:** Flatness QA, Beam uniformity QA.

**469. Fiducial Marker QA Protocol Mid-Treatment:** QA protocol for all steps involving fiducials mid-treatment.
**Example:** Kidney SBRT markers checked for visibility, stability, and registration.
**Related Terms:** Fiducial registration QA, Fiducial tracking QA.

**470. Field Edge QA Phantom Mid-Treatment:** Phantom used to verify beam edge sharpness and placement mid-treatment.
**Example:** Kidney IMRT penumbra verified using film phantom.
**Related Terms:** Field edge QA, Beam profile QA.

**471. Fluorescent Imaging QA Phantom Mid-Treatment:** Phantom used to calibrate and QA fluorescence imaging mid-treatment.
**Example:** Kidney tumor fluorescence verified using phantom.
**Related Terms:** Fluorescent signal calibration, Imaging QA.

**472. Fractionation Verification Phantom Mid-Treatment:** Phantom used to validate fractionated dose delivery mid-treatment.
**Example:** Kidney SBRT fractionated dose verified using phantom.
**Related Terms:** Fractional dose mapping, Dose verification QA.

**473. Flat-Panel Detector QA Phantom Mid-Treatment:** Phantom for QA of detector uniformity and image quality.
**Example:** Kidney KV images verified for uniform brightness.
**Related Terms:** Flat-panel imaging QA, Imaging calibration QA.

**474. Fiducial Visibility QA Phantom Mid-Treatment:** Phantom used to verify fiducial marker visibility.
**Example:** Kidney CBCT phantom checked for marker visibility.
**Related Terms:** Fiducial detection QA, Fiducial registration QA.

**475. Fluence Delivery Verification Phantom Mid-Treatment:** Confirms fluence delivery accuracy.
**Example:** Kidney VMAT fluence verified using phantom.
**Related Terms:** Fluence verification phantom, Dose mapping QA.

**476. Field Symmetry QA Phantom Mid-Treatment:** Phantom to verify radiation field symmetry.
**Example:** Kidney IMRT symmetry verified.
**Related Terms:** Beam uniformity QA, Field symmetry QA.

**477. Fiducial Alignment QA Phantom Mid-Treatment:** Phantom with embedded markers for alignment QA.
**Example:** Kidney phantom used to verify CBCT alignment accuracy.
**Related Terms:** Fiducial registration QA, IGRT QA.

**478. Field Aperture QA Phantom Mid-Treatment:** Phantom to verify MLC and jaw apertures.
**Example:** Kidney IMRT MLC leaf positions checked.
**Related Terms:** Field aperture QA, Field size verification.

**479. Flatness QA Phantom Mid-Treatment:** Phantom used to verify beam flatness.
**Example:** Kidney IMRT fields checked using phantom.
**Related Terms:** Flatness QA, Field uniformity QA.

**480. Fiducial Contour QA Phantom Mid-Treatment:** Phantom used for QA of marker contours.
**Example:** Kidney fiducial contours verified.
**Related Terms:** Fiducial contour QA, Contour QA.

481. **Fluoroscopic Imaging QA Phantom Mid-Treatment:** Phantom to verify fluoroscopic image quality.
**Example:** Kidney catheter navigation geometry verified.
**Related Terms:** Fluoroscopic image QA, Geometric accuracy QA.

482. **Fractional Dose Phantom Mid-Treatment:** Phantom to map dose per fraction.
**Example:** Kidney SBRT dose per fraction verified.
**Related Terms:** Fractionated dose mapping, Dose verification QA.

483. **Field Verification QA Phantom Mid-Treatment:** Phantom to verify all aspects of delivered fields.
**Example:** Kidney IMRT field size, shape, and alignment verified.
**Related Terms:** Field verification QA, QA protocol.

484. **Fiducial Implant Phantom Mid-Treatment:** Phantom for verifying accuracy of marker implantation.
**Example:** Kidney SBRT fiducial placement checked.
**Related Terms:** Fiducial placement QA, Fiducial stability QA.

485. **Fluence Output Phantom Mid-Treatment:** Phantom to measure radiation output across field.
**Example:** Kidney VMAT output verified using phantom.
**Related Terms:** Fluence verification phantom, Dose mapping QA.

486. **Field Position QA Phantom Mid-Treatment:** Phantom to check beam positioning relative to anatomy.
**Example:** Kidney IMRT field alignment verified.
**Related Terms:** Field alignment QA, Beam positioning QA.

487. **Fiducial Stability QA Mid-Treatment:** QA to ensure implanted markers remain stable throughout treatment.
**Example:** Kidney SBRT fiducials checked daily on CBCT to detect any migration.
**Related Terms:** Fiducial migration QA, Motion management QA.

488. **Fluoroscopy Dose Phantom Mid-Treatment:** Phantom used to measure patient dose during ongoing fluoroscopy.
**Example:** Kidney interventional procedure dose measured to maintain ALARA compliance.
**Related Terms:** Fluoroscopic dose QA, Dose mapping QA.

489. **Flatness and Symmetry QA Phantom Mid-Treatment:** Phantom measuring beam flatness and symmetry during treatment course.
**Example:** Kidney IMRT beams verified weekly with water or film phantom.
**Related Terms:** Beam uniformity QA, Field symmetry QA.

490. **Fiducial Marker QA Protocol Mid-Treatment:** Comprehensive protocol for QA of all fiducial-related procedures.
**Example:** Kidney SBRT markers checked for visibility, stability, and registration accuracy.
**Related Terms:** Fiducial registration QA, Fiducial tracking QA.

491. **Field Edge QA Phantom Mid-Treatment:** Phantom used to verify beam edge sharpness and penumbra accuracy.
**Example:** Kidney IMRT field edges verified with film phantom to protect surrounding tissue.
**Related Terms:** Field edge sharpness QA, Beam profile QA.

492. **Fluorescent Imaging QA Phantom Mid-Treatment:** Phantom to ensure fluorescence imaging meets intensity and mapping standards.
**Example:** Kidney tumor fluorescence checked for detectability during surgery or therapy.
**Related Terms:** Fluorescent signal calibration, Imaging QA.

493. **Fractionation Verification Phantom Mid-Treatment:** Phantom used to validate accurate fractionated dose delivery.
**Example:** Kidney SBRT per-fraction dose verified with phantom and TPS comparison.
**Related Terms:** Fractional dose mapping, Dose verification QA.

494. **Flat-Panel Detector QA Phantom Mid-Treatment:** Phantom to QA uniformity and image quality of flat-panel detectors.
**Example:** Kidney KV images checked for uniform brightness and absence of artifacts.
**Related Terms:** Flat-panel imaging QA, Imaging calibration QA.

495. **Fiducial Visibility QA Phantom Mid-Treatment:** Phantom used to verify visibility of implanted markers during ongoing treatment.
**Example:** Kidney CBCT phantom checked to ensure fiducials remain clearly visible.
**Related Terms:** Fiducial detection QA, Fiducial registration QA.

496. **Fluence Delivery Verification Phantom Mid-Treatment:** Phantom used to confirm accurate delivery of planned fluence patterns.
**Example:** Kidney VMAT fluence verified using MapCHECK or similar phantom.
**Related Terms:** Fluence verification phantom, Dose mapping QA.

497. **Field Symmetry QA Phantom Mid-Treatment:** Phantom to verify that radiation field symmetry remains within tolerance.
**Example:** Kidney IMRT beams checked weekly for left-right symmetry using phantom.
**Related Terms:** Beam uniformity QA, Field symmetry QA.

498. **Fiducial Alignment QA Phantom Mid-Treatment:** Phantom with embedded markers to QA fiducial alignment accuracy.
**Example:** Kidney phantom used to verify CBCT image alignment with planning CT.
**Related Terms:** Fiducial registration QA, IGRT QA.

499. **Field Aperture QA Phantom Mid-Treatment:** Phantom to ensure MLC and jaw apertures match the planned field during treatment.
**Example:** Kidney IMRT MLC leaf positions confirmed using aperture phantom.
**Related Terms:** Field aperture QA, Field size verification.

500. **Flatness QA Phantom Mid-Treatment:** Phantom used to measure and verify radiation beam flatness during treatment.
**Example:** Kidney IMRT fields checked to maintain uniform dose across PTV.
**Related Terms:** Flatness QA, Field uniformity QA.

# G

1. **Gantry:** Rotating part of LINAC that directs the radiation beam around the patient.
   **Related Terms:** Couch, Collimator
   **Example:** The gantry rotates from 0° to 180° during VMAT delivery.
2. **Gating (Respiratory Gating):** Delivering radiation only during a specific breathing phase to reduce motion error.
   **Related Terms:** Motion Management, RPM System
   **Example:** Lung SBRT is delivered only during end-exhale gating.
3. **Gradient Index (GI):** Metric evaluating dose falloff around the target.
   **Related Terms:** Conformity Index, SRS
   **Example:** GI of 3.0 indicates steep dose gradient in brain SRS.
4. **Gamma Analysis:** QA method comparing measured and planned dose distributions.
   **Related Terms:** Patient-Specific QA, Dose Verification
   **Example:** A gamma passing rate of 98% at 3%/3mm indicates plan accuracy.
5. **Gross Tumor Volume (GTV):** The visible or palpable tumor extent.
   **Related Terms:** CTV, PTV
   **Example:** GTV is contoured based on CT and MRI for head-neck cancer.
6. **Grid Therapy:** Spatially fractionated radiation using a perforated grid pattern.
   **Related Terms:** Lattice RT
   **Example:** Used for bulky tumors to allow high-dose delivery.
7. **Graphical Optimization:** Manual adjustment of dose-volume curves to improve treatment plan.
   **Related Terms:** Inverse Planning
   **Example:** Planner drags DVH lines to reduce spinal cord dose.
8. **Gating Window:** Portion of breathing cycle where radiation is allowed.
   **Related Terms:** Motion Tracking
   **Example:** A 40–60% gating window reduces liver tumor motion.
9. **Genetic Algorithm Optimization:** AI-based optimization used in some TPS for plan generation.
   **Related Terms:** Evolutionary Algorithms
   **Example:** Algorithm evolves beam weights over many iterations.
10. **Geometric Uncertainty:** Inaccuracies due to patient setup, motion, or machine tolerance.
    **Related Terms:** PTV Margin, Setup Error
    **Example:** A 5 mm margin added to account for geometric uncertainties.
11. **GTV-to-PTV Expansion:** Adding margins to GTV to form PTV.
    **Related Terms:** ITV, Margin
    **Example:** 3DCRT lung plan uses 8 mm GTV expansion.
12. **Gafchromic Film:** Radiochromic film used for high-resolution dose measurements.
    **Related Terms:** Film Dosimetry
    **Example:** Film placed in phantom verifies SRS dose.
13. **Gamma Knife:** Stereotactic radiosurgery device using many cobalt-60 sources.
    **Related Terms:** SRS, Radiosurgery
    **Example:** Used for treating brain metastases with 1 mm accuracy.

14. **Grid Block:** Physical block used to create grid spatial fractionation pattern.
**Related Terms:** Spatially Fractionated RT
**Example:** 3D spacing grid block used for bulky sarcomas.

15. **Gantry Speed Modulation:** Changing gantry rotation speed during VMAT.
**Related Terms:** Dose Rate, MLC Modulation
**Example:** Maximum modulation needed for complex head–neck VMAT.

16. **Gy (Gray):** SI unit of absorbed dose (1 Gy = 1 joule/kg).
**Related Terms:** Dose, Monitor Units
**Example:** A brain SRS fraction may deliver 20 Gy in one session.

17. **Global Dose Maximum:** Highest dose point in the treatment plan.
**Related Terms:** Hotspot, Dose Distribution
**Example:** Hotspot kept <110% of prescription.

18. **Gradient Dose Falloff:** Rate of dose decrease beyond target.
**Related Terms:** GI, Penumbra
**Example:** SRS plans require very steep dose falloff.

19. **Gantry-Couch Collision Check:** Safety check to avoid machine collision with patient.
**Related Terms:** Collision Avoidance
**Example:** VMAT arcs verified pre-treatment with virtual simulation.

20. **GyE (Gray Equivalent):** Biological equivalent dose used for proton/carbon therapy.
**Related Terms:** RBE, Proton Dose
**Example:** 2 GyE × 30 fractions prescribed for skull-base tumor.

21. **GTV Delineation Error:** Inaccuracy in outlining tumor boundaries.
**Related Terms:** Contouring Variability
**Example:** MRI fusion reduces delineation errors in brain tumors.

22. **Grid-Based Algorithm:** Dose calculation using structured computational grids.
**Related Terms:** Pencil Beam, Convolution
**Example:** Older TPS used grid-based superposition algorithms.

23. **Gait–Induced Motion:** Tumor motion caused by patient movement during treatment.
**Related Terms:** Motion Management
**Example:** Abdominal tumors shift during patient repositioning.

24. **Gas Equivalent Material:** Phantom material mimicking gas density.
**Related Terms:** Dosimetry Phantoms
**Example:** Used to simulate lung tissue.

25. **Global Optimization Constraint:** Constraint affecting the entire plan.
**Related Terms:** Inverse Planning
**Example:** Global maximum dose set to 105%.

26. **Gated CBCT:** 3D imaging acquired during specific breathing phases.
**Related Terms:** 4D CBCT, IGRT
**Example:** Gated CBCT reduces liver tumor blur.

27. **Gigabecquerel (GBq):** Activity unit for radiopharmaceuticals.
**Related Terms:** Isotope Activity
**Example:** 7 GBq of I-131 used for thyroid ablation.

28. **Gradient Dose Constraint:** Required limits for dose falloff.
**Related Terms:** SRS, SBRT
**Example:** GI < 4 required for SRS brain plan.

29. **GFR-Sparing Planning:** Reducing kidney dose to preserve glomerular filtration rate.
**Related Terms:** Renal Function
**Example:** Renal dose minimized for lymphoma abdominal RT.

30. **Gold Fiducial Markers:** Small gold seeds implanted for IGRT tracking.
**Related Terms:** Fiducials, CyberKnife
**Example:** Gold markers implanted in prostate for daily alignment.

31. **Gamma Passing Rate:** Percentage of points meeting gamma criteria in QA.
**Related Terms:** 3%/3mm, Patient-Specific QA
**Example:** Passing rate >95% is typically acceptable.

32. **GTV Shrinkage:** Tumor reduction during treatment.
**Related Terms:** Adaptive Planning
**Example:** Weekly CBCT reveals significant GTV shrinkage in lung cancer.

33. **Gantry Rotation Accuracy:** Precision of gantry angle during delivery.
**Related Terms:** Mechanical QA
**Example:** Verified to be within ±0.5° during annual QA.

34. **Geometric Miss:** Failure to hit the intended tumor target.
**Related Terms:** Setup Error, Margin
**Example:** IGRT reduces risk of geometric misses.

35. **Gradient Compensation:** Adjusting dose to account for tissue heterogeneity.
**Related Terms:** Bolus, Compensation Filters
**Example:** Used in chest wall electron therapy.

36. **GTV-Based Prescription:** Prescribing dose specifically to the GTV region.
**Related Terms:** Dose Painting
**Example:** Boost dose prescribed to GTV in H&N cancer.

37. **Glandular Dose:** Dose absorbed by glandular tissues.
**Related Terms:** Breast Dosimetry
**Example:** Important in mammography radiation studies.

38. **Grid-Based Monte Carlo:** Hybrid Monte Carlo using grid acceleration methods.
**Related Terms:** Dose Calculation
**Example:** Used to speed up small-field calculations.

39. **Geometric Distortion Correction:** Correction for MRI image deformation.
**Related Terms:** MR-LINAC
**Example:** Distortion correction needed before MRI fusion.

40. **Generalized Equivalent Uniform Dose (gEUD):** Model converting non-uniform dose to equivalent uniform dose.
**Related Terms:** Radiobiological Modeling
**Example:** gEUD used for comparing IMRT plans.

41. **Guard Band Margin:** Extra margin added for safety.
**Related Terms:** PTV, Uncertainty
**Example:** Applied in SRS to prevent brainstem overdose.

42. **Gray-Level Histogram Analysis:** Evaluating pixel intensity distributions.
**Related Terms:** Image Segmentation
**Example:** Used for auto-contouring tumors in MRI.

43. **GTV Motion Envelope:** Full volume occupied by moving GTV.
**Related Terms:** ITV, 4D CT
**Example:** ITV defined from the motion envelope.

44. **Gradient Reversal Artifact:** Imaging artifact due to gradient inversion.
**Related Terms:** MRI Artifacts
**Example:** Corrected during MR simulation.

45. **Gland Sparing Optimization:** Protecting salivary glands in head–neck planning.
**Related Terms:** OAR Sparing
**Example:** Parotid mean dose kept <26 Gy.

46. **Gafchromic Film Calibration Curve:** Curve used to convert film color density to dose.
**Related Terms:** Film Dosimetry
**Example:** Film scanned and matched to calibration curve.

47. **GATE Simulation (Geant4 Toolkit):** Monte Carlo simulation toolkit for medical physics.
**Related Terms:** Monte Carlo, Dosimetry
**Example:** Used for simulating PET scatter corrections.

48. **Graded Dose Prescription:** Varying dose levels across the target.
**Related Terms:** Dose Painting
**Example:** Hypoxic tumor regions receive higher dose.

49. **Gaussian Smoothing Filter:** Image-processing filter that reduces noise.
**Related Terms:** Image Reconstruction
**Example:** Applied to reduce CBCT noise.

50. **Gy-Min (Gray-Minute):** Dose delivered per minute.
**Related Terms:** Dose Rate, FFF Mode
**Example:** FFF beams deliver 20 Gy-min during SBRT.

51. **Geometric Magnification:** Enlargement of anatomical structures due to X-ray source distance.
**Related Terms:** SID, SOD
**Example:** Portal images show magnified ribs when SOD is small.

52. **Gy-Cm$^2$ (Dose Area Product):** Measurement of radiation dose multiplied by irradiated area.
**Related Terms:** DAP Meter
**Example:** Used in fluoroscopy QA.

53. **Gy per Fraction:** The amount of radiation given in each session.
**Related Terms:** Fractionation, BED
**Example:** SBRT uses 12–20 Gy per fraction.

54. **Gamma Distribution (Statistical):** Statistical model sometimes used for photon fluence predictions.
**Related Terms:** Probability Models
**Example:** Used in Monte Carlo code validation.

55. **Gradient Optimization:** Refining dose gradients between tumor and OARs.
**Related Terms:** DVH Optimization
**Example:** Used in SRS to sharpen falloff.

56. **Gantry Kick:** Slight rotation change to avoid collisions.
**Related Terms:** Arc Planning
**Example:** Arc shifted from 181° to 200°.

57. **Gantry Tilt:** Angled gantry position used in imaging.
**Related Terms:** CBCT Geometry
**Example:** Tilt used for pediatric cranial imaging.

58. **Gamma Map:** Spatial display of gamma index results.
**Related Terms:** QA Report
**Example:** High gamma values indicate dose discrepancy.

59. **Gated Delivery Time:** Time required for gated radiation delivery.
**Related Terms:** Duty Cycle
**Example:** Gating increases total treatment time by 40%.

60. **Global Hotspot:** Maximum dose region in entire plan volume.
**Related Terms:** Hotspot Limit
**Example:** Hotspot restricted to <107%.

61. **Gy-RBE (Gray Relative Biological Effectiveness):** Adjusted dose value considering RBE.
**Related Terms:** Proton Therapy
**Example:** Protons: 2 Gy physical = 2.2 Gy-RBE.

62. **Grid Size (TPS):** Calculation resolution used in dose grid.
**Related Terms:** Dose Matrix
**Example:** Finer grid (1 mm) needed for SRS.

63. **Gantry Sag:** Small mechanical drooping when gantry rotates.
**Related Terms:** Mechanical QA
**Example:** Sag checked using Winston–Lutz test.

64. **G-Tolerance (Physiological):** Body tolerance to acceleration forces.
**Related Terms:** Immobilization
**Example:** Rapid couch movement avoided to prevent discomfort.

65. **Gaussian Kernel:** Mathematical smoothing function used in dose convolution.
**Related Terms:** Convolution/Superposition
**Example:** TPS uses kernels to model scatter.

66. **Grid-Based Phantom:** Phantom with internal grid structure for dose testing.
**Related Terms:** Dosimetry Phantom
**Example:** Used in film-to-dose mapping.

67. **Global Objective Function:** Main goal function in inverse planning.
**Related Terms:** Optimization Weight
**Example:** Lower objective value = better plan.

68. **Gafchromic Film Batch Correction:** Adjusting calibration due to batch variation.
**Related Terms:** Film QA
**Example:** New film batch requires new calibration curve.

69. **GPU-Based Dose Calculation:** High-speed dose calculation using graphics processors.
**Related Terms:** Monte Carlo, Fast TPS
**Example:** GPU Monte Carlo enables real-time dose calc.

70. **Gradient-Based Segmentation:** Contouring based on image intensity changes.
**Related Terms:** Auto-Contour
**Example:** MRI-based tumor segmentation.

71. **Grid Reconstruction (Imaging):** Rebuilding image from grid sampling.
**Related Terms:** 3D Reconstruction
**Example:** Used in CBCT back-projection.

72. **Gy/Minute Limit:** Maximum safe dose rate for patient exposure.
**Related Terms:** Dose Rate QA
**Example:** High dose rate mode tested monthly.

73. **Gamma Knife Shot:** Single focused radiation beam-unit in GK treatment.
**Related Terms:** Isocenters
**Example:** Multiple shots used to sculpt dose.

74. **GTV Auto-Propagation:** AI-based propagation of tumor contour over images.
**Related Terms:** Adaptive RT
**Example:** MR-LINAC uses auto-propagation daily.

75. **Galvo Scanner:** Device for fast beam steering in FLASH or scanning proton therapy.
**Related Terms:** Beam Scanning
**Example:** Used to deliver high-speed proton spots.

76. **Gate Delay:** Time between breath signal and radiation triggering.
**Related Terms:** Phase Gating
**Example:** Delay tuned for pediatric abdominal RT.

77. **Gate Signal Noise:** Interference in motion signal affecting gating accuracy.
**Related Terms:** Respiratory Monitoring
**Example:** Noisy signals cause irregular beam interruptions.

78. **Goniometer:** Device measuring rotation angles.
**Related Terms:** Couch Angle QA
**Example:** Used to calibrate couch yaw.

79. **GTV Boost:** Giving additional dose specifically to GTV.
**Related Terms:** Simultaneous Integrated Boost
**Example:** H&N IMRT uses GTV boost to 70 Gy.

80. **Gy-Equivalent Dose Rate:** Adjusted dose rate value used for radiobiological modeling.
**Related Terms:** FLASH RT
**Example:** Ultra-high Gy/s FLASH evaluated in research.

81. **GTV Split:** Dividing GTV into subregions for dose painting.
**Related Terms:** Hypoxia Imaging
**Example:** PET-based hypoxia mapping.

82. **Gel Dosimeter:** 3D dosimeter using polymer gel.
**Related Terms:** 3D QA
**Example:** Used in SRS Phantoms.

83. **Grid Therapy Modulator:** Device controlling spatial beam pattern.
**Related Terms:** Lattice RT
**Example:** Hexagonal modulators used for bulky tumors.

84. **General Workflow Protocol:** Standard guidelines for treatment processes.
    **Related Terms:** SOP
    **Example:** Workflow ensures safe delivery.

85. **GTV Regression Curve:** Curve modeling tumor shrinkage vs. time.
    **Related Terms:** Adaptive Planning
    **Example:** Used in lung cancer adaptive RT.

86. **Gy Conversion Factor:** Converts monitor units to Gy.
    **Related Terms:** Output Factor
    **Example:** Scattering affects conversion factor.

87. **Gating Duty Cycle:** Fraction of time radiation is on during gated therapy.
    **Related Terms:** Treatment Time
    **Example:** Duty cycle of 40% extends treatment duration.

88. **Grid-Based Collimation:** Use of grid collimators to shape beam.
    **Related Terms:** MLC, Aperture
    **Example:** Used in historic orthovoltage therapy.

89. **Gaussian Noise (Imaging):** Random noise following Gaussian distribution.
    **Related Terms:** SNR
    **Example:** MRI smoothing reduces Gaussian noise.

90. **Gy-to-HU Conversion:** Dose influence on Hounsfield Units in imaging.
    **Related Terms:** CBCT Dose Effects
    **Example:** Used in adaptive CBCT correction.

91. **GTV Migration:** Movement of tumor position over treatment course.
    **Related Terms:** Setup Error
    **Example:** Lung tumor shifts inferiorly mid-treatment.

92. **Gate-Triggered CBCT:** CBCT slices acquired only in selected breathing phases.
    **Related Terms:** 4D CBCT
    **Example:** Improves liver metastasis visualization.

93. **Group Delay (Electronics):** Signal timing delay in imaging units.
    **Related Terms:** Detector Response
    **Example:** Needs calibration for EPID QA.

94. **Graticule:** Reference grid used in simulator/X-ray machines.
    **Related Terms:** Setup Reference
    **Example:** Used in conventional 2D planning.

95. **Gray-Level Co-occurrence Matrix (GLCM):** Statistical texture method for radiomics.
    **Related Terms:** Radiomics Features
    **Example:** Used to characterize tumor heterogeneity.

96. **GTV Inter-Observer Variation:** Variation between clinicians contouring tumors.
    **Related Terms:** Contouring Uncertainty
    **Example:** Reduced using MRI or PET guidance.

97. **Gaussian Pencil Beam:** Simplified beam model assuming Gaussian spread.
    **Related Terms:** Pencil Beam Algorithm
    **Example:** Used in early TPS.

98. **Gamma-Proton Interaction:** Interaction generating secondary radiation in proton therapy.
**Related Terms:** Particle Physics
**Example:** Influences neutron production.

99. **Gas-Fill Ion Chamber:** Air- or gas-filled detector for dose measurement.
**Related Terms:** Farmer Chamber
**Example:** Used in reference dosimetry.

100. **GTV Drift:** Slow positional drift of tumor during long treatments.
**Related Terms:** Intrafraction Motion
**Example:** Monitored in real-time tracking systems.

101. **Gy per Pulse:** Dose delivered per beam pulse.
**Related Terms:** Dose Rate, FFF
**Example:** FFF beams have high dose per pulse.

102. **Gating Threshold:** Minimum amplitude required for gating activation.
**Related Terms:** Motion Control
**Example:** Threshold set to avoid false signals.

103. **Geometric Modeling:** Mathematical modeling of patient and machine geometry.
**Related Terms:** TPS Algorithms
**Example:** Used for beam-path prediction.

104. **Gel Phantom:** Phantom using gel for 3D dose measurement.
**Related Terms:** Polymer Gel
**Example:** Used for IMRT QA.

105. **Gaussian Beamlet:** Small beam subunit with Gaussian spread.
**Related Terms:** Beamlets
**Example:** Used in IMRT optimization.

106. **Global Max Dose Constraint:** Limit on highest allowed dose.
**Related Terms:** Hotspot Control
**Example:** Set <110% for IMRT.

107. **Gradient Coil (MRI):** Coil that controls spatial encoding.
**Related Terms:** MR-Sim
**Example:** High-performance gradient coils reduce distortion.

108. **Gy/Treatment Course:** Total dose across all fractions.
**Related Terms:** Total Dose
**Example:** Breast RT delivers 40 Gy/course.

109. **Gas-Filled Portal Detector:** Detector using pressurized gas for MV imaging.
**Related Terms:** Portal Imaging
**Example:** Used in older EPID generations.

110. **GTV Time-Series:** Tracking tumor volume changes over time.
**Related Terms:** Adaptive RT
**Example:** Used in serial CBCT analysis.

111. **Gate-Closed Interval:** Time period when gating prevents radiation.
**Related Terms:** Duty Cycle
**Example:** Beam pauses until breathing matches window.

112. **GTV–OAR Interface:** Boundary region between tumor and organs at risk.
**Related Terms:** Dose Constraints
**Example:** Critical in head–neck IMRT.

113. **Grid Interpolation:** Estimating values between grid points.
**Related Terms:** Image Processing
**Example:** Used for CT resampling.

114. **Graph-Based Auto-Contouring:** Segmentation using node/edge modeling.
**Related Terms:** AI Contouring
**Example:** Used for pelvic organ segmentation.

115. **Gaussian Fitting:** Matching data points to Gaussian curve.
**Related Terms:** Curve Fitting
**Example:** Used in beam profile analysis.

116. **Gy/Sec (FLASH Dose Rate):** Ultra-high dose rate used for FLASH RT.
**Related Terms:** FLASH Effect
**Example:** >40 Gy/s tested in experimental studies.

117. **Grid Collimator Penumbra:** Penumbra specifically created by grid apertures.
**Related Terms:** Spatial Fractionation
**Example:** Affects dose uniformity.

118. **Geometric Registration Error:** Misalignment during image fusion.
**Related Terms:** Image Registration
**Example:** MRI-CT fusion checked manually.

119. **Gradient Magnitude Image:** Image showing intensity transitions.
**Related Terms:** Segmentation
**Example:** Highlights tumor edges.

120. **GTV Residual:** Remaining tumor after shrinkage.
**Related Terms:** Adaptive Dose
**Example:** Dose boosted to residual mass.

121. **Grid-Based Dose Compression:** Compressing dose data for storage.
**Related Terms:** TPS Storage
**Example:** Used for cloud-based TPS systems.

122. **Gamma Volume Histogram:** Plot of gamma index frequency distribution.
**Related Terms:** QA Metrics
**Example:** Helps identify system-wide errors.

123. **123. Gap Width (Field Gap):** Space between two radiation fields.
**Related Terms:** Junction Dose
**Example:** Craniospinal RT requires precise gap matching.

124. **Gradient-Based ROI Detection:** Detecting regions using gradient differences.
**Related Terms:** Auto-Segmentation
**Example:** Used for locating lung nodules.

125. **Ga-67 Scintigraphy:** Imaging using Gallium-67 for lymphoma.
**Related Terms:** Nuclear Imaging
**Example:** Helps assess treatment response.

126. **Gate-On Delay:** Delay before radiation turns on after gating signal.
**Related Terms:** System Latency
**Example:** Measured during commissioning.

127. **Gy-Proportional Counter:** Detector output proportional to delivered dose.
**Related Terms:** Ion Chamber
**Example:** Used in output calibration.

128. **GTV Shell Structure:** Ring structure around GTV for optimization.
**Related Terms:** Dose Shaping
**Example:** Used to force dose falloff.

129. **Gamma-Ray Spectrometry:** Measuring gamma energy distribution.
**Related Terms:** Cobalt-60 QA
**Example:** Used for isotope purity testing.

130. **Gradient Mask (Imaging):** Mask emphasizing intensity gradient areas.
**Related Terms:** Edge Detection
**Example:** Used for contour refinement.

131. **Gating Efficiency** Ratio of beam-on time to total time.
**Related Terms:** Duty Cycle
**Example:** Efficiency of 50% is typical for lung gating.

132. **Grid Point Dose Storage:** Storing dose at discrete points.
**Related Terms:** Dose Matrix
**Example:** Used in Monte Carlo cloud systems.

133. **Graph Optimizer (TPS):** Optimizer using graph theory.
**Related Terms:** Inverse Planning
**Example:** Helps minimize OAR dose.

134. **GTV Overlap Region:** Shared area between GTV and OAR.
**Related Terms:** Risk Structures
**Example:** Critical in pancreas planning.

135. **Gy-Meter Calibration:** Calibration of dose-measuring devices.
**Related Terms:** Absolute Dosimetry
**Example:** Annual ion chamber recalibration.

136. **Gy-Weighted DVH:** DVH weighted by voxel dose values.
**Related Terms:** Dose Metrics
**Example:** Useful for radiobiological models.

137. **Grid-Based Replanning:** Using dose grids for adaptive planning.
**Related Terms:** Adaptive Workflow
**Example:** CBCT dose used for on-table replanning.

138. **Generalized Margin Algorithm:** Algorithm for determining PTV margin.
**Related Terms:** Van Herk Formula
**Example:** Margin = $2.5\Sigma + 0.7\sigma$.

139. **Photon Gas Approximation:** Statistical model for photon fields.
**Related Terms:** Radiation Physics
**Example:** Rarely used clinically.

140. **GTV Edge Blur:** Unclear tumor boundary on images.
**Related Terms:** Partial Volume Effect
**Example:** Seen in low-contrast MRI.

141. **Gated Beam Latency:** Delay from motion signal to beam output.
**Related Terms:** Time Lag
**Example:** Measured for gating commissioning.

142. **Gondola Phantom Holder:** Device that supports phantoms for rotational setups.
**Related Terms:** QA Accessories
**Example:** Used in isocenter QA.

143. **Gradient Error Correction:** Fixing beam or image gradient mistakes.
**Related Terms:** Calibration
**Example:** Corrected in MRI sequences.

144. **Guided Needle Insertion:** Image-guided placement of brachytherapy needles.
**Related Terms:** HDR, Template Guidance
**Example:** Used in cervical brachytherapy.

145. **Gy-to-Sv Conversion:** Conversion from absorbed dose to equivalent dose.
**Related Terms:** Radiation Weighting
**Example:** Sv = Gy × WR.

146. **GTV Biomechanical Modeling:** Modeling tumor deformation.
**Related Terms:** Elastic Registration
**Example:** Used for lung cancer adaptive RT.

147. **Grid-Less Optimization:** Optimization without rigid calculation grids.
**Related Terms:** Mesh-Free Algorithms
**Example:** Used in AI-driven TPS.

148. **Gel Thermoluminescence:** Gel dosimeters that emit light when heated.
**Related Terms:** TLD
**Example:** Used for calibration studies.

149. **Gy-Lung Index:** Dose index assessing lung dose burden.
**Related Terms:** Mean Lung Dose
**Example:** Helps predict pneumonitis risk.

150. **GTV Tracking:** Continuous tracking of GTV during treatment.
**Related Terms:** Real-Time Tracking
**Example:** CyberKnife follows moving tumors.

151. **GTV Dose Escalation:** Increasing dose within GTV to improve tumor control.
**Related Terms:** Boost, SIB
**Example:** Prostate plans escalate GTV dose to 80 Gy.

152. **Gradient Nonlinearity (MRI):** Distortion caused by imperfect gradient fields.
**Related Terms:** MR Simulation
**Example:** Corrected before MRI–CT fusion.

153. **Gaussian Filtering (Dose Grid):** Smoothing dose matrix to remove noise.
**Related Terms:** Dose Reconstruction
**Example:** Applied in Monte Carlo post-processing.

154. **Gas-Filled Diode Detector:** Small detector for measuring electron field profiles.
**Related Terms:** Diode Array
**Example:** Used in small-field commissioning.

155. **Gate-to-Beam Latency:** Time difference between gate signal and beam response.
**Related Terms:** Gating QA
**Example:** Must be <100 ms for accuracy.

156. **GTV Expansion Margin:** Extra margin added around GTV.
**Related Terms:** ITV, PTV Margin
**Example:** H&N tumors get 3–5 mm.

157. **Gy Focal Point:** Central point where dose intensity peaks.
**Related Terms:** Isocenter
**Example:** Critical in SRS brain shots.

158. **Gate Prediction Algorithm:** Predicts breathing phase for smoother gating.
**Related Terms:** Motion Prediction
**Example:** Reduces beam interruption frequency.

159. **GTV Subvolume:** Specific portion inside GTV for special dosing.
**Related Terms:** Dose Painting
**Example:** PET-positive region boosts.

160. **Gray Level Mapping:** Assigning intensity ranges to specific image values.
**Related Terms:** Window/Level
**Example:** Enhances tumor edges on CT.

161. **Gated Treatment Beam:** Beam delivered only when breathing matches.
**Related Terms:** Respiratory Control
**Example:** Used for pancreatic SBRT.

162. **Gold Marker Migration:** Movement of implanted fiducials.
**Related Terms:** IGRT, Prostate Markers
**Example:** Weekly kV checks detect shifts.

163. **Geometric Beam Modeling:** Modeling radiation beam in 3D geometry.
**Related Terms:** Beam Modeling
**Example:** Used in TPS commissioning.

164. **GTV Shrink-Adapted Margins:** Reducing margins as tumor shrinks.
**Related Terms:** Adaptive RT
**Example:** Lung tumors shrink 30%, margins updated.

165. **Gamma-HVL (Half Value Layer):** Thickness needed to reduce gamma rays by 50%.
**Related Terms:** Beam Quality
**Example:** Cobalt-60 HVL measured in QC.

166. **Grid-Based DVH Calculation:** Computing DVH using dose grid volumes.
**Related Terms:** DVH Metrics
**Example:** Required in TPS algorithms.

167. **Gy Residual Correction:** Adjusting dose for underdosed regions.
**Related Terms:** Adaptive Dose
**Example:** Corrected mid-treatment with replan.

168. **Gating Envelope:** Range of motion allowed during gating.
**Related Terms:** Breathing Margin
**Example:** Envelope tightened for liver SBRT.

169. **Group Matching (Registration):** Registering multiple datasets simultaneously.
**Related Terms:** Deformable Registration
**Example:** Used in adaptive planning.

170. **Gaussian Scatter Model:** Predicts scatter using Gaussian distribution.
**Related Terms:** Scatter Kernel
**Example:** Older TPS algorithms used these.

171. **GTV Edge Correction:** Fixing errors at tumor boundary.
**Related Terms:** Contouring
**Example:** PET helps correct fuzzy edges.

172. **Gate Synchronization Error:** Timing mismatch between beam and breathing.
**Related Terms:** Latency
**Example:** Fixed via RPM recalibration.

173. **Gy-Based Biological Modeling:** Using dose in Gy for biological predictions.
**Related Terms:** BED, EQD2
**Example:** BED calculated for SBRT.

174. **Gas Density Correction:** Adjusting dose for air cavities.
**Related Terms:** Heterogeneity Correction
**Example:** Nasal cavities require corrections.

175. **175. GTV Internal Motion Map:** Map of tumor motion over breathing cycles.
**Related Terms:** 4D CT
**Example:** Used to generate ITV.

176. **Gaussian Dose Spread:** Natural spread of dose distribution.
**Related Terms:** Lateral Scatter
**Example:** Seen in small photon fields.

177. **Gel Bead Dosimeter:** Beads containing gel for spatial dose measurement.
**Related Terms:** 3D Dosimetry
**Example:** Used in multi-point verification.

178. **Generalized Radiation Index:** Metric combining multiple dose parameters.
**Related Terms:** Plan Quality Metrics
**Example:** Used to compare IMRT plans.

179. **Gy Attenuation Factor:** Reduction of dose due to material absorption.
**Related Terms:** Attenuation Coefficient
**Example:** Bolus increases attenuation.

180. **GTV-Based BED Calculation:** Calculating BED specifically for tumor.
**Related Terms:** Radiobiology
**Example:** SBRT BED >100 for lung tumors.

181. **Gap Matching Error:** Misalignment between adjacent fields.
**Related Terms:** Junction Dose
**Example:** Spine fields require perfect match.

182. **Geometric Field Shaping:** Manual shaping of fields using blocks.
**Related Terms:** MLC, Cerrobend
**Example:** Used in older Cobalt machines.

183. **Gradient Subtraction (Imaging):** Removing distortion gradients in MRI.
**Related Terms:** Image Correction
**Example:** Required for MR-LINAC.

184. **Gamma Production Cross Section:** Probability of gamma production in interactions.
**Related Terms:** Photon Physics
**Example:** Relevant in proton therapy.

185. **GTV Autofusion:** Automated fusion of GTV from multiple scans.
**Related Terms:** AI Segmentation
**Example:** CT–PET autofusion.

186. **Gate Quality Index:** Score evaluating gating accuracy.
**Related Terms:** Duty Cycle
**Example:** High index = stable breathing.

187. **Grayscale Uniformity:** Even distribution of image grayscale values.
**Related Terms:** Image QA
**Example:** Checked in CBCT monthly tests.

188. **Gaussian Blur Artifact:** Blurring caused by excessive smoothing.
**Related Terms:** Image Filtering
**Example:** Can hide small tumors.

189. **GTV Mean Dose:** Average dose delivered to GTV.
**Related Terms:** Dose Metrics
**Example:** Reported in every IMRT plan.

190. **Gy Normalization Point:** Reference point for dose normalization.
**Related Terms:** Isocenter Norm
**Example:** 100% normalized at isocenter.

191. **Grid Structure Artifact:** Imaging artifact resembling grid patterns.
**Related Terms:** CBCT Artifacts
**Example:** Caused by detector issues.

192. **Gate Drift:** Gradual drift in breathing pattern.
**Related Terms:** Motion Variation
**Example:** Requires re-coaching patient.

193. **GTV Motion Probability Map:** Probability of tumor being in certain positions.
**Related Terms:** Motion Mapping
**Example:** Used for ITV derivation.

194. **Gy-Depth Curve:** Plot showing dose variation with depth.
**Related Terms:** PDD
**Example:** Measured for 6 MV beams.

195. **Gaussian Beam Symmetry Test:** Test if beam profile follows symmetric Gaussian pattern.
**Related Terms:** Beam QA
**Example:** Checked monthly.

**196. GTV Propagation Error:** Error when AI auto-propagates contours.
**Related Terms:** Auto-Contour QA
**Example:** Must be manually corrected.

**197. Gating Signal Latency Map:** Visual display of gating delay across system.
**Related Terms:** Commissioning
**Example:** Used in RPM QA.

**198. Graphical Leaf Motion Viewer:** Tool showing MLC motion during plan delivery.
**Related Terms:** MLC QA
**Example:** Used to verify VMAT sequences.

**199. Granularity Noise (Imaging):** Grain-like noise pattern.
**Related Terms:** Quantum Noise
**Example:** Seen in low-dose kV images.

**200. GTV Core Volume:** Highest-density part of tumor.
**Related Terms:** Dose Painting
**Example:** PET SUV >8 region boosted.

**201. GTV Dose Heterogeneity Index:** Quantifies how uneven the dose to GTV is.
**Related Terms:** Homogeneity Index
**Example:** Lower index = uniform dose.

**202. Grid-Based Position Verification:** Using grid markers to verify position.
**Related Terms:** Alignment
**Example:** Older simulators used this.

**203. Gy Normalized Dose Rate:** Dose rate adjusted relative to 1 Gy baseline.
**Related Terms:** FFF Mode
**Example:** Used in FLASH evaluation.

**204. Gate Phase Assignment:** Assigning breathing data to phases.
**Related Terms:** 4D CT
**Example:** 10-phase 4D CT commonly used.

**205. Graphical Gap Matching:** Visual software tool for matching field edges.
**Related Terms:** Junction QA
**Example:** Craniospinal RT planning.

**206. GTV Tracking Error:** Deviation between actual and predicted GTV position.
**Related Terms:** Real-Time Tracking
**Example:** CyberKnife corrects error continuously.

**207. Gaussian Smoothing Kernel:** Kernel used for smoothing dose or image.
**Related Terms:** Convolution
**Example:** Used in iterative CBCT recon.

**208. Gray Scale Deviation:** Difference from expected grayscale pattern.
**Related Terms:** Image QC
**Example:** Checked in MV imager QA.

**209. Gate-Line Artefact:** Artifact caused by gating interruptions.
**Related Terms:** 4D CT Artefacts
**Example:** Appears as streaks.

**210. GTV Volume Symmetry:** Symmetry of tumor shape in 3D.
**Related Terms:** Shape Analysis
**Example:** Asymmetry increases contour uncertainty.

**211. Gamma Beam Calibratio:** Calibration for gamma-ray output.
**Related Terms:** Cobalt-60 QA
**Example:** Done annually.

**212. Graph Matching Algorithm:** Algorithm aligning graph nodes across datasets.
**Related Terms:** Image Registration
**Example:** Used in AI auto-fusion.

**213. GTV Surround Volume:** Region around GTV used for dose shaping.
**Related Terms:** Shell Structures
**Example:** Used to force dose falloff.

**214. Gradient Modeling Error:** Mistake in modeling image gradients.
**Related Terms:** Reconstruction Error
**Example:** Causes MRI distortions.

**215. Gate Margin:** Margin added to account for gating uncertainties.
**Related Terms:** ITV
**Example:** 3 mm added for liver SBRT.

**216. Gaussian Scatter Correction:** Correcting scatter modeled as Gaussian.
**Related Terms:** Scatter Kernel
**Example:** Used in pencil beam algorithms.

**217. GTV Biophysical Map:** Map of biological activity within GTV.
**Related Terms:** Radiomics
**Example:** PET SUV maps.

**218. Global End-to-End Test:** System test from imaging to delivery.
**Related Terms:** End-to-End QA
**Example:** Performed annually for SRS.

**219. Grid-Controlled Fluoroscopy:** Fluoro controlled using grid pulses.
**Related Terms:** kV Imaging
**Example:** Used in IGRT systems.

**220. GTV Dose Coverage Index:** Percentage of GTV receiving prescription dose.
**Related Terms:** Coverage Metric
**Example:** Must exceed 95%.

**221. Gas-Fill Ratio (Ion Chamber):** Fraction of chamber volume filled with gas.
**Related Terms:** Dosimetry
**Example:** Impacts chamber sensitivity.

**222. Gaussian-Based Motion Model:** Motion modeled as Gaussian distribution.
**Related Terms:** Motion Probability
**Example:** Used for lung ITV.

**223. Gate Width Optimization:** Adjusting gating window for best balance.
**Related Terms:** Duty Cycle
**Example:** Narrower gate improves accuracy.

224. **Gy-Per-Litre Unit:** Unit for dose in large-volume measurements.
**Related Terms:** Bulk Irradiation
**Example:** Used in radiation sterilization.

225. **GTV Segmentation Atlas:** Library of anatomical shapes for auto-contouring.
**Related Terms:** AI Contouring
**Example:** Used for pelvic organs.

226. **Gy Equivalent Organ Dose:** Organ dose expressed in equivalent units.
**Related Terms:** RBE, OAR Dose
**Example:** Used in proton therapy.

227. **Gamma Camera Collimation:** Collimators used in nuclear medicine gamma imaging.
**Related Terms:** SPECT
**Example:** High-energy collimator for Ga-67.

228. **Gate Redundancy Check:** Ensuring gating system has backup accuracy.
**Related Terms:** Safety Check
**Example:** Performed in daily QA.

229. **GTV Probabilistic Contour:** Contour based on probability fields.
**Related Terms:** Bayesian Segmentation
**Example:** Used in uncertain tumor edges.

230. **Gaussian Weighting Function:** Function weighting dose or image data.
**Related Terms:** Optimization
**Example:** Used in smoothing filters.

231. **GTV Dose Constraint:** Dose limit or requirement for tumor.
**Related Terms:** Prescribed Dose
**Example:** Minimum GTV D95 $\geq$ 100%.

232. **Gate-Lag Artifact:** Imaging artifact from gating delays.
**Related Terms:** 4D CT Issues
**Example:** Appears as ghosting.

233. **Geometric Iso-Curve:** Curve connecting positions equidistant from isocenter.
**Related Terms:** Beam Geometry
**Example:** Used in arc planning.

234. **Gelatin Phantom:** Phantom made from medical gelatin.
**Related Terms:** Soft-Tissue Phantom
**Example:** Good for dosimeter embedding.

235. **Gy Rate Modulation:** Ability to change dose rate dynamically.
**Related Terms:** VMAT, FFF
**Example:** Dose rate varies with gantry angle.

236. **Grid-Detector Nonuniformity:** Uneven response across detector grid.
**Related Terms:** Flat-Field Correction
**Example:** Corrected in EPID QA.

237. **GTV Alignment Erro:** Error in aligning GTV for treatment.
**Related Terms:** Setup Error, IGRT
**Example:** kV images used to fix.

238. **Gaussian-Based Hotspot Control:** Hotspot smoothing using Gaussian functions.
**Related Terms:** Dose Optimization
**Example:** Reduces >110% hotspots.

239. **Global SSD Check:** Verifying source-to-surface distance.
**Related Terms:** Setup Verification
**Example:** Important in electrons.

240. **GTV Mixed-Density Modeling:** Modeling tumors with varied internal density.
**Related Terms:** Heterogeneity
**Example:** Lung tumors with necrotic cores.

241. **Gate-Cycle Analysis:** Analysis of breathing cycles.
**Related Terms:** Respiratory Motion
**Example:** Identifies irregular patterns.

242. **Gamma Emission Rate:** Rate of gamma-ray emission from source.
**Related Terms:** Source Decay
**Example:** Cobalt-60 measured regularly.

243. **Grid-Based Field Splitting:** Splitting fields into smaller grid components.
**Related Terms:** Composite Fields
**Example:** Used in older planning.

244. **GTV Texture Feature Map:** Map showing tumor texture features.
**Related Terms:** Radiomics
**Example:** Used in prognosis models.

245. **Gradient-Derived Segmentation:** Contouring based on gradient detection.
**Related Terms:** Edge-Based Segmentation
**Example:** Used for liver border detection.

246. **Gate-Projection CBCT:** CBCT using projection-based gating.
**Related Terms:** 4D CBCT
**Example:** Improves thoracic lesion visibility.

247. **GTV-Renal Interface:** Region where tumor contacts kidney.
**Related Terms:** OAR Sparing
**Example:** Relevance in adrenal SBRT.

248. **Gaussian-Based Beam Weighting:** Weighting beams using Gaussian curves.
**Related Terms:** Optimization
**Example:** Used in some IMRT templates.

249. **Gray Level Quantization Error:** Error from rounding image intensity.
**Related Terms:** Image Artifacts
**Example:** Can affect radiomics.

250. **GTV Coverage Metric (GCM):** Quantitative measure of how fully GTV is covered.
**Related Terms:** Coverage Index
**Example:** Plans must reach ≥ 95% GCM.

251. **GTV Biological Heterogeneity:** Variability in tumor biology within GTV.
**Related Terms:** Radiomics, Dose Painting
**Example:** PET shows heterogeneity requiring differential dosing.

**252. Gy-Based Output Facto:** Ratio of dose output for different field sizes.
**Related Terms:** OF, Field Size
**Example:** 10×10 cm field used as baseline.

**253. Ghost Marker Artifact:** Ghost-like double images of fiducials.
**Related Terms:** IGRT Artifact
**Example:** Caused by motion during MV imaging.

**254. Gate Interruption Time:** Total time beam is paused during gating.
**Related Terms:** Duty Cycle
**Example:** Higher interruption time increases treatment duration.

**255. Gridless Collimation:** Collimation without physical grid patterns.
**Related Terms:** FFF Beams
**Example:** Used to reduce scatter in imaging.

**256. GTV Registration Variance:** Differences between repeated registrations.
**Related Terms:** IGRT Accuracy
**Example:** Variance reduced with kV + CBCT combo.

**257. Gaussian-Based Organ Tracking:** Tracking organs using Gaussian motion predictions.
**Related Terms:** Motion Modeling
**Example:** Used for pancreas tracking.

**258. Gy-Weighted Average Dose:** Average dose weighted by Gy contributions.
**Related Terms:** Mean Dose
**Example:** Used to analyze OAR dose variation.

**259. Gate-Triggered kV Imaging:** kV images captured only during gate window.
**Related Terms:** 4D IGRT
**Example:** Improves lung tumor verification.

**260. Gamma Knife Collimator Helmet:** Interchangeable collimators for Gamma Knife unit.
**Related Terms:** SRS, Isocenter
**Example:** 4 mm helmet for small brain metastasis.

**261. Grid Compensation Technique:** Adjusting fields for grid-based film cassettes.
**Related Terms:** Film Dosimetry
**Example:** Avoids scatter variation.

**262. GTV Overlap Index:** Measures overlap between planned and actual GTV.
**Related Terms:** Dice Coefficient
**Example:** Used in adaptive therapy evaluation.

**263. Gaussian Motion Probability Function:** Predicts probability of organ/tumor position.
**Related Terms:** ITV, Motion Envelope
**Example:** Used in lung contouring.

**264. Gate Efficiency Factor:** Ratio of beam-on time to total time.
**Related Terms:** Duty Cycle
**Example:** Efficiency improves with stable breathing.

**265. GTV Skeleton Model:** Central axis representation of GTV shape.
**Related Terms:** Radiomics Geometry
**Example:** Analyzes tumor elongation.

266. **Gradient Echo MR Sequence:** MRI sequence sensitive to magnetic inhomogeneities.
**Related Terms:** MR-Sim
**Example:** Used for brain metastasis imaging.

267. **Gantry Drift Correction:** Correction applied when gantry angle drifts.
**Related Terms:** Mechanical Accuracy
**Example:** Verified in monthly QA.

268. **Grid-Free Electron Collimation:** Electron fields shaped without cutouts.
**Related Terms:** eMLC
**Example:** eMLC shaping for chest wall boost.

269. **GTV-CTV Conversion Margin:** Margin used to expand GTV to CTV.
**Related Terms:** CTV, Margin
**Example:** H&N cancer margin ≈ 1 cm.

270. **Gy-Weighted Tumor Dose:** Dose accounting for tumor density factors.
**Related Terms:** Density Correction
**Example:** Used in heterogeneous lung tumors.

271. **Gate-Phase Binning:** Grouping CT images by breathing phase.
**Related Terms:** 4D CT
**Example:** 10-phase binning commonly used.

272. **GTV Approximation Error:** Error when automated tools approximate tumor shape.
**Related Terms:** Segmentation Error
**Example:** PET/CT mismatches cause boundary errors.

273. **Gaussian Surface Mapping:** Mapping surface curves using Gaussian smoothing.
**Related Terms:** Contour Smoothing
**Example:** Used on liver contours.

274. **Gated MV Portal Imaging:** Portal imaging captured during gated delivery.
**Related Terms:** MV Imaging
**Example:** Used to verify diaphragm motion.

275. **GTV Minimal Margin:** Minimum allowable planning margin.
**Related Terms:** Constraint
**Example:** 2 mm used in brain SRS.

276. **Gradient-Based Segmentation Error:** Boundary errors when segmentation relies on gradients.
**Related Terms:** Edge Detection
**Example:** Common in low-contrast CT.

277. **Gy Field Symmetry Metric:** Symmetry measurement of field dose.
**Related Terms:** Beam Symmetry
**Example:** Must be <3% deviation.

278. **Gate-Free Treatment Mode:** Delivery without gating even with motion.
**Related Terms:** ITV, Free Breathing
**Example:** Used for prostate.

279. **GTV Density Map:** Map showing density variations.
**Related Terms:** Hounsfield Map
**Example:** Helps identify necrotic regions.

280. **GTV Motion Coefficient:** Quantifies degree of tumor movement.
**Related Terms:** Motion Index
**Example:** Lung tumors have highest coefficients.

281. **Geometric Source Modeling:** Modeling radiation source geometry.
**Related Terms:** Ray Tracing
**Example:** Used in beam commissioning.

282. **Gate Acceptance Window:** Range of motion accepted during gating.
**Related Terms:** Gating Envelope
**Example:** Narrow window improves precision.

283. **GTV Boundary Stability:** Stability of tumor boundary across scans.
**Related Terms:** Contour Consistency
**Example:** More stable in prostate than lung.

284. **Gaussian Noise Filter:** Filter used to reduce noise in images.
**Related Terms:** Image Smoothing
**Example:** Used in CBCT image enhancement.

285. **Grid-Based Dose Recalculation:** Recomputing dose on dose grid.
**Related Terms:** Dose Engine
**Example:** Used in adaptive replanning.

286. **Gate-Lapse Scanning:** Missing data from irregular breathing.
**Related Terms:** 4D CT Error
**Example:** Causes distortion in lung.

287. **Gamma Energy Spectrum:** Distribution of gamma-ray energies.
**Related Terms:** Cobalt-60 Spectrum
**Example:** Two peaks at 1.17 and 1.33 MeV.

288. **GTV Normoxic Gel Dosimetry:** Gel used for mapping 3D dose.
**Related Terms:** Gel Phantom
**Example:** Used in SRS QA.

289. **Gaussian Field Interpolation:** Filling dose gaps using Gaussian methods.
**Related Terms:** Interpolation
**Example:** Used in film dosimetry.

290. **GTV Spatial Uncertainty:** Uncertainty in tumor location.
**Related Terms:** PTV Margin
**Example:** Larger in lung tumors.

291. **Gate-Specific DVH:** DVH created for each gating phase.
**Related Terms:** Phase-Based Planning
**Example:** Used in 4D dose accumulation.

292. **GTV Internal Surface Area:** Internal surface measurement of GTV.
**Related Terms:** Radiomics Shape
**Example:** Correlated with aggressiveness.

293. **Grid-Averaged Dose Value:** Average dose per grid voxel.
**Related Terms:** Dose Grid
**Example:** Used in IMRT evaluation.

294. **Gate Position Verification:** Verifying gating reference point.
**Related Terms:** Optical Tracking
**Example:** RPM block checked before treatment.

295. **Gy Efficiency Ratio:** Ratio of deposited Gy to delivered Gy.
**Related Terms:** Dose Efficiency
**Example:** Lower in high-density materials.

296. **GTV Temporal Variation:** Change in tumor over time.
**Related Terms:** Adaptive Therapy
**Example:** Weekly CBCT shows shrinkage.

297. **Gaussian Residual Smoothing:** Smoothing residual dose data.
**Related Terms:** Plan Optimization
**Example:** Removes noise from MC dose.

298. **Gate Velocity Measurement:** Rate at which target moves during gating.
**Related Terms:** Motion Speed
**Example:** Used in pancreas motion analysis.

299. **GTV Edge Contrast Ratio:** Contrast between tumor edge and normal tissue.
**Related Terms:** Image Contrast
**Example:** Higher with IV contrast CT.

300. **Gy Per Arc Length:** Dose delivered per arc traveled.
**Related Terms:** VMAT
**Example:** Used to check arc modulation.

301. **GTV Vector Displacement:** Movement of GTV represented as a vector.
**Related Terms:** Motion Tracking
**Example:** Lung tumor shifts 5 mm posteriorly.

302. **Grid-Based Anatomy Mapping:** Mapping anatomy to a fixed grid.
**Related Terms:** Dose Grid Alignment
**Example:** Ensures proper fusion.

303. **Gate Trigger Synchronization:** Synchronizing beam trigger with gate signal.
**Related Terms:** Latency
**Example:** Synchronization checked in commissioning.

304. **Gaussian Likelihood Model:** Probabilistic model using Gaussian distribution.
**Related Terms:** Predictive Modeling
**Example:** Used in automatic contouring.

305. **GTV Edge Irregularity Score:** Score quantifying irregular tumor edges.
**Related Terms:** Radiomics
**Example:** High scores seen in sarcomas.

306. **Gradient-Based Beam Weighting:** Assigning beam weights using gradients.
**Related Terms:** Optimization
**Example:** Used in some IMRT optimizers.

307. **Gate-Driven Adaptive Planning:** Adapting plans according to gating data.
**Related Terms:** Online Adaptation
**Example:** Used in MR-LINAC systems.

308. **Gy-Normalized Isocenter Dose:** Expressing isocenter dose relative to prescription.
**Related Terms:** Norm 100%
**Example:** 105% at isocenter in SRS.

309. **GTV Overlay Visualization:** Displaying GTV over anatomical images.
**Related Terms:** Contour Review
**Example:** CT+PET overlays.

310. **Gaussian Registration Model:** Registration based on Gaussian statistics.
**Related Terms:** AI Registration
**Example:** Improved multi-organ fusion.

311. **Gate Mode Indicator:** Machine indicator showing gating state.
**Related Terms:** IGRT Control
**Example:** Green = gate active.

312. **GTV Asymmetric Motion:** Uneven motion patterns of tumor.
**Related Terms:** Motion Irregularity
**Example:** Diaphragm-related shifts.

313. **Grid Resolution Error:** Error from coarse dose grid.
**Related Terms:** Dose Grid Size
**Example:** 5 mm grids cause inaccuracies.

314. **Gaussian-Based PTV Expansion:** Using probability models to set PTV margins.
**Related Terms:** Margin Formula
**Example:** Widely used in lung.

315. **Gate-Phase Motion Plot:** Plot of tumor location vs phase.
**Related Terms:** 4D Motion
**Example:** Used to analyze liver SBRT.

316. **GTV Spiculated Area:** Part where tumor edges are spiky.
**Related Terms:** Radiomics Texture
**Example:** Common in lung cancers.

317. **Gy Ramp Profile:** Dose "ramp" along field edge.
**Related Terms:** Penumbra
**Example:** Steeper ramp improves conformity.

318. **Gate-Limited Projection Set:** Only projections within gate used for image.
**Related Terms:** 4D CBCT
**Example:** Improves tumor clarity.

319. **GTV Contrast Enhancement Ratio:** Difference between pre- and post-contrast.
**Related Terms:** IV Contrast
**Example:** Useful in liver tumors.

320. **Gamma Scatter Contribution:** Scatter produced from gamma interactions.
**Related Terms:** Compton Scatter
**Example:** Relevant in cobalt therapy.

321. **Gate-Optimized Trajectory:** Optimized gantry path for gated treatments.
**Related Terms:** VMAT Gating
**Example:** Shorter arcs for lung SBRT.

322. **Grid-Detector Crosstalk:** Signal bleeding between detector cells.
**Related Terms:** EPID Artifacts
**Example:** Causes faint shadowing.

323. **GTV Growth Rate Measurement:** Speed at which tumor increases.
**Related Terms:** Tumor Kinetics
**Example:** Calculated from serial CTs.

324. **Gaussian-Based Segmentation Mask:** Mask produced using Gaussian thresholding.
**Related Terms:** Auto-Segmentation
**Example:** Used in liver outlines.

325. **Gate-Constrained Beam Hold:** Beam stops when patient outside gate.
**Related Terms:** Gating Safety
**Example:** Common in RPM-controlled delivery.

326. **GTV Metabolic Flux Map:** Map showing metabolic rate variations.
**Related Terms:** PET Analysis
**Example:** Used in dose painting.

327. **Gy Conversion Algorithm:** Algorithm converting between dose metrics.
**Related Terms:** BED ↔ EQD2
**Example:** Used in hypofractionation.

328. **Gate Compliance Score:** Score measuring patient gating consistency.
**Related Terms:** Motion Regularity
**Example:** Must exceed threshold for lung SBRT.

329. **GTV Diffusion Map:** Map showing water diffusion within tumor.
**Related Terms:** DWI MRI
**Example:** Helps detect necrosis.

330. **Gaussian Beam Divergence Model:** Beam divergence modeled using Gaussian shapes.
**Related Terms:** Penumbra Modeling
**Example:** Used in photon dose engines.

331. **GTV Boundary Noise:** Random variations at tumor boundary.
**Related Terms:** Contour Smoothing
**Example:** Reduced using filters.

332. **Gate-Mapped Breathing Curve:** Curve of breathing signal assigned to phases.
**Related Terms:** 4D Motion Map
**Example:** Ensures reproducible gating.

333. **Gy-Scaled Image Overlay:** Showing dose colorwash scaled in Gy.
**Related Terms:** Dose Map
**Example:** Standard in TPS display.

334. **GTV Centroid Drift:** Movement of tumor center over treatment.
**Related Terms:** Setup Variation
**Example:** Prostate centroid may drift daily.

335. **Gaussian-Based Beam Aperture:** Beam aperture shaped with Gaussian smoothing.
**Related Terms:** MLC Smoothing
**Example:** Used in pediatric IMRT.

336. **Gate Noise Suppression:** Removing noise from gating signal.
**Related Terms:** Signal Filtering
**Example:** Used in optical systems.

337. **GTV Index Matching:** Matching tumor metrics across scans.
**Related Terms:** Serial Imaging
**Example:** Baseline vs mid-treatment.

338. **Grid-Matched Dose Comparison:** Comparing doses after matching grids.
**Related Terms:** Gamma Analysis
**Example:** Used in 3D dose QA.

339. **Gy Time-Weighted Dose:** Dose weighted over time.
**Related Terms:** Dose Accumulation
**Example:** Used in adaptive RT.

340. **GTV Margin Budget:** Allowance for margins per uncertainty source.
**Related Terms:** Margin Recipe
**Example:** 1 mm setup + 2 mm motion.

341. **Gate Range Evaluation:** Checking acceptable motion range.
**Related Terms:** Gate Window
**Example:** Liver SBRT gate ~ 3–5 mm.

342. **Gamma Exposure Constant:** Constant defining exposure rate.
**Related Terms:** Source Strength
**Example:** Used for Cs-137, Co-60.

343. **GTV Anisotropy Factor:** Uneven tumor extension in different directions.
**Related Terms:** Shape Analysis
**Example:** Lung tumors often anisotropic.

344. **Grid Register Alignment:** Aligning detector grid to beam.
**Related Terms:** EPID Calibration
**Example:** Adjusted during commissioning.

345. **Gaussian-Based Noise Estimation:** Estimating noise using Gaussian models.
**Related Terms:** Imaging Noise
**Example:** Used in CBCT reconstruction.

346. **GTV Averaged Position:** Average location of tumor over time.
**Related Terms:** Mid-Ventilation
**Example:** Used for planning middle breathing phase.

347. **Gate Synchrony Indicator:** Represents how synchronized beam and breathing are.
**Related Terms:** Latency
**Example:** Should remain within tolerance.

348. **Gy Modulation Factor:** Factor describing changes in delivered dose.
**Related Terms:** IMRT Modulation
**Example:** High factor indicates complex plan.

349. **GTV Diffusion Coefficient:** Value calculated from diffusion MRI.
**Related Terms:** ADC Map
**Example:** Lower values mean higher cell density.

**350. Gradient Field QA Test:** QA test ensuring gradient fields are accurate.
**Related Terms:** MR-LINAC QA
**Example:** Performed monthly.

**351. Gamma-Dose Correction:** Adjustment applied to measured gamma-dose to align with reference conditions.
**Related Terms:** Calibration, Output Factor, Dosimetry
**Example:** Gamma-dose correction is applied when chamber measurements differ from baseline.

**352. Gantry Beam Matching:** Ensuring beams from multiple gantries deliver identical dose distributions.
**Related Terms:** Beam Consistency, QA, Output Verification
**Example:** Machines are beam-matched so a patient can be treated on any LINAC.

**353. Geodesic Path Optimization:** Using shortest-path algorithms to improve beam arc efficiency.
**Related Terms:** VMAT Path, Motion Planning
**Example:** Geodesic optimization shortens the total treatment arc time.

**354. Grid-Dose Calibration:** Adjusting calibration values in GRID therapy.
**Related Terms:** GRID Matrix, HDR GRID
**Example:** The physicist performs grid-dose calibration before treating bulky sarcomas.

**355. Gyroscope Alignment:** Use of gyroscope sensors for precise couch movement.
**Related Terms:** Couch Rotation, Motion QA
**Example:** Gyroscope alignment identifies slight tilt errors during SBRT.

**356. Gamma-Knife QA Protocol:** A structured procedure ensuring Gamma Knife units meet clinical tolerances.
**Related Terms:** Stereotactic QA, Mechanical Tests
**Example:** Gamma-Knife QA includes helmet checks and collimator output assessment.

**357. Genetic Dose Modeling:** Predicting patient radiosensitivity using genetic markers.
**Related Terms:** Radiogenomics, Biological Index
**Example:** Genetic dose modeling predicts increased toxicity in certain breast cancer patients.

**358. Gating Accuracy Profile:** Performance characterization of respiratory gating.
**Related Terms:** Motion Management, RPM, Phase-Gating
**Example:** The gating accuracy profile shows a 2% variation in phase-trigger reliability.

**359. Gaussian Filtering Kernel:** Smoothing kernel used in dose grid interpolation.
**Related Terms:** Convolution, Smoothing Filter
**Example:** A Gaussian kernel improves the accuracy of PET-CT dose fusion.

**360. G4 Phantom:** A geometric fourth-generation phantom used in LINAC QA.
**Related Terms:** QA Phantom, Dosimetry Tools
**Example:** G4 phantoms check beam flatness and symmetry.

**361. Gradient Beam Control:** Management of planned intensity gradients in IMRT beams.
**Related Terms:** Segment Modulation, MLC Movement
**Example:** Gradient beam control avoids steep transitions that may cause hotspots.

**362. Gamma Energy Scaling:** Adjustment of gamma-ray spectra in dose calculations.
**Related Terms:** Energy Correction, MV Scaling
**Example:** Gamma energy scaling compensates for detector over-response at high energies.

**363. Genomic Tumor Profiling:** Identifying genetic mutations that affect radiation response.
**Related Terms:** Radiosensitivity, Biomarkers
**Example:** TP53 mutation is detected during genomic tumor profiling.

364. **Gel-Film Dosimetry:** Hybrid dosimetry using both gel and radiochromic film.
**Related Terms:** 3D Dosimetry, Polymer Gel
**Example:** Gel-film dosimetry maps the 3D dose of a VMAT arc.

365. **Gaussian Noise Suppression:** Removal of statistical image noise in CBCT or MV imaging.
**Related Terms:** Image Processing, Filtering
**Example:** Gaussian suppression improves visibility of spinal landmarks.

366. **GTV Dose Constraint:** Maximum or minimum dose thresholds applied to the tumor.
**Related Terms:** Planning Objectives, PTV, OAR
**Example:** A GTV constraint ensures the tumor receives ≥95% of the prescribed dose.

367. **Galvo-Tracking System:** Fast optical tracking using galvanometer scanners.
**Related Terms:** Optical Guidance, Surface Imaging
**Example:** Galvo-tracking monitors facial surface motion in real time.

368. **Gynecologic Shielding Block:** Customized shielding used in pelvic radiotherapy.
**Related Terms:** Gonadal Shield, OAR Protection
**Example:** Gynecologic shields reduce ovarian exposure in young patients.

369. **Gradient-Index Mapping:** Graphical map showing dose falloff regions.
**Related Terms:** Conformity Index, Hotspots
**Example:** Gradient-index mapping confirms rapid dose drop-off near the spinal cord.

370. **320. Gantry Rotation Calibration:** Verification that gantry angle readings match physical rotation.
**Related Terms:** Mechanical Accuracy, Daily QA
**Example:** Calibration finds a 0.2° deviation requiring correction.

371. **Grid-Based IMRT Planning:** IMRT generated with fixed beam lattices instead of free-angle beams.
**Related Terms:** Segmented Fields, Discrete Angles
**Example:** Grid-based IMRT is used for shorter planning times.

372. **Gyro-Stabilized Couch Top:** Couch surface with motion-stabilization technology.
**Related Terms:** Patient Positioning, Motion Control
**Example:** Gyro-stabilized tops reduce vibration during SBRT.

373. **Gamma-Ray Leakage Test:** Measurement of stray radiation escaping the LINAC head.
**Related Terms:** Shielding, QA, Leakage Limits
**Example:** Leakage was found to be <0.1%, within IEC limits.

374. **Genomic Radiosensitivity Score:** Score predicting how sensitive a patient is to radiation.
**Related Terms:** Biomarker, Predictive Index
**Example:** A high radiosensitivity score suggests reducing dose to avoid toxicity.

375. **Gross Margin Estimation:** Determining safe margin growth around tumor boundaries.
**Related Terms:** CTV, PTV
**Example:** Margin estimation adds 3 mm for prostate motion.

376. **Guided Brachytherapy Needle:** Needle placed with imaging assistance.
**Related Terms:** HDR, Applicator, Ultrasound Guidance
**Example:** US-guided brachy needles ensure accurate seed placement.

377. **Glandular Dose Factor:** Correction factor for breast gland dose.
**Related Terms:** Breast Planning, Absorbed Dose
**Example:** The glandular dose factor modifies 6 MV photon dose calculations.

**378. Gamma-Linac Rotation Arc:** A combination arc technique using gamma and photon beams.
**Related Terms:** Hybrid Therapy
**Example:** Gamma-LINAC arcs are tested in research environments.

**379. Gamut Correction Imaging:** Ensuring image colors fall within the device's display range.
**Related Terms:** Image Processing, Display Calibration
**Example:** Gamut correction reduces false skin tones on digital simulators.

**380. Grid-Dose Fractionation:** Fractionation technique using spatially fractionated beam patterns.
**Related Terms:** Spatial Fractionation, GRID Therapy
**Example:** GRID fractionation treats large radio-resistant tumors.

**381. Ground Shield Conductor:** Electrical grounding for LINAC safe operation.
**Related Terms:** Electrical Safety, QA
**Example:** Faulty ground shielding triggers emergency shutdown.

**382. Genitourinary Dose Mapping:** Evaluating doses to GU organs like bladder and urethra.
**Related Terms:** OAR Metrics, DVH
**Example:** GU dose mapping ensures urethral max dose is met.

**383. Gamma-Ray Spectral Filter:** Filter modifying gamma energy distribution.
**Related Terms:** Beam Hardening, Filtration
**Example:** Using a spectral filter reduces low-energy scatter.

**384. Gel-Calibration Phantom:** Gel phantom used to calibrate polymer gel dosimeters.
**Related Terms:** Dosimetry, 3D Gel
**Example:** Gel-phantoms set dose-response curves.

**385. Gated VMAT Delivery:** VMAT delivered only during selected breathing phases.
**Related Terms:** RPM, Motion Management
**Example:** Gated VMAT is used for liver tumors.

**386. Grid-Hotspot Indicator:** Marker identifying high-dose nodes in GRID patterns.
**Related Terms:** Hotspot, Spatial Dose
**Example:** Hotspot indicators verify intended high-dose peaks.

**387. GaN-Based Detector:** Radiation detector built from gallium nitride.
**Related Terms:** Semiconductor Detector, QA
**Example:** GaN detectors show excellent stability for MV beams.

**388. Gamma-Knife Composite Plan:** Multiple Gamma Knife shots combined into one plan.
**Related Terms:** SRS, Shot Planning
**Example:** Composite planning improves target conformity.

**389. Groove-Based Immobilizer:** Immobilizer with carved grooves for stability.
**Related Terms:** Positioning, Thermoplastic Mask
**Example:** Groove masks help reduce rotational head movement.

**390. Genomics-Guided Boost:** Boost dose adjusted using genomic radiosensitivity data.
**Related Terms:** Personalized RT, Dose Painting
**Example:** Radiosensitive regions get a higher boost.

**391. GTV Margin Expansion:** Increasing the gross tumor volume to account for microscopic spread.
**Related Terms:** CTV, PTV, Geometric Margins
**Example:** A 3 mm GTV expansion is added for esophageal cancer planning.

392. **Gradient Field Analyzer:** Device that measures dose gradients in high-precision treatments.
**Related Terms:** Dosimetry, IMRT QA
**Example:** A field analyzer checks sharp dose falloff in SRS beams.

393. **Gamma-Based Verification Metric:** QA metric combining dose difference and distance-to-agreement.
**Related Terms:** Gamma Index, IMRT QA
**Example:** A gamma pass rate of 98% verifies IMRT accuracy.

394. **Gait-Matched Immobilization:** Customized immobilization considering patient walking limitations.
**Related Terms:** Positioning, Setup
**Example:** Hip-fracture patients require gait-matched supports.

395. **GFR-Based Contrast Dosing:** Contrast selection based on kidney filtration rate.
**Related Terms:** CT Simulation, Renal Function
**Example:** Reduced contrast is used for low-GFR patients.

396. **Gafchromic Film Calibration Curve:** Curve relating optical density to absorbed dose.
**Related Terms:** Film Dosimetry, ABS Value
**Example:** Calibration curves are updated monthly.

397. **Gaussian Penumbra Model:** Mathematical model estimating beam blur at field edges.
**Related Terms:** Penumbra, Beam Profile
**Example:** Gaussian penumbra predicts a 5 mm edge gradient.

398. **Gas-Based Ion Chamber:** Dosimeter that measures charge produced in gas-filled chambers.
**Related Terms:** Farmer Chamber, QA
**Example:** Gas chambers check LINAC output daily.

399. **Grid-Weighted Optimization:** Planning algorithm applying lattice weighting factors.
**Related Terms:** Spatial Fractionation
**Example:** Weighted optimization distributes hot nodes evenly.

400. **Gel-Infused Bolus:** Flexible bolus filled with gel improving skin dose uniformity.
**Related Terms:** Tissue Compensation, Surface Dose
**Example:** Gel bolus is used in chest-wall treatments.

401. **Gonadal Exposure Index:** Indicator of potential reproductive organ dose.
**Related Terms:** OAR, Shielding
**Example:** Index is minimized in pediatric pelvic RT.

402. **Gadolinium-Based Contrast (GBC):** MRI contrast enhancing soft tissue visibility.
**Related Terms:** MRI Simulation, MR-Guided RT
**Example:** GBC improves spinal cord visualization.

403. **Guided Target Segmentation:** Semi-automatic contouring assisted by AI or imaging hints.
**Related Terms:** Auto-Segmentation, Contouring
**Example:** AI-guided segmentation outlines the pancreas.

404. **Guard-Band Protocol:** Safety margin added to QA tolerances.
**Related Terms:** Tolerance Levels, Machine QA
**Example:** A guard-band adds 0.5 mm flexibility to MLC checks.

405. **Geometric Distortion Correction:** Fixing shape distortions in MRI images.
**Related Terms:** MRI QC, Image Registration
**Example:** Distortion correction ensures brain contours align with CT.

**406. Gamma-Spectrum Analyzer:** Device that measures gamma-ray energy distributions.
**Related Terms:** Radiation Survey, Spectroscopy
**Example:** Analyzer confirms correct spectrum from Co-60.

**407. Gigabyte-Level Dose Storage:** Large storage needed for high-resolution dose grids.
**Related Terms:** Big Data, TPS Memory
**Example:** SBRT plans often exceed gigabyte storage.

**408. Gated CBCT Acquisition:** Cone-beam CT taken only during specific breathing phases.
**Related Terms:** 4D CBCT, Motion Management
**Example:** Gated CBCT reduces liver motion artifacts.

**409. Gastrointestinal (GI) Dose Constraint:** Limits to protect GI organs like stomach and intestine.
**Related Terms:** OAR, DVH
**Example:** SBRT bowel max dose must stay <30 Gy.

**410. Galactose-Metabolism Imaging:** PET imaging assessing liver metabolic function.
**Related Terms:** Functional Imaging
**Example:** Used to guide dose in functional liver RT.

**411. Gynecologic Brachy Applicator:** Device used to deliver HDR dose to cervix/uterus.
**Related Terms:** Tandem and Ovoid, Ir-192
**Example:** A tandem-ring applicator treats cervical cancer.

**412. Graph-Based Dose Mapping:** Dose mapping using graph-theory networks.
**Related Terms:** Dose Painting, Optimization
**Example:** Nodes represent voxel clusters for dose decisions.

**413. Gamma-Ray Emission Imaging:** Imaging technique using gamma photons.
**Related Terms:** SPECT, Nuclear Medicine
**Example:** SPECT works via gamma emission imaging.

**414. Gravitational Couch Drift:** Minor sag in couch height from patient weight.
**Related Terms:** Couch Deflection, Position QA
**Example:** Heavy patients increase couch drift by 2 mm.

**415. Genetic Tumor Classification:** Categorizing tumors based on gene expression.
**Related Terms:** Radiogenomics
**Example:** Gliomas classified by IDH mutation status.

**416. Guided Marker Visualization:** Enhanced display of fiducials in imaging.
**Related Terms:** IGRT, Tracking
**Example:** Guided visualization helps align prostate markers.

**417. Gaussian Error Compensation:** Correcting measurement noise assuming Gaussian distribution.
**Related Terms:** Statistical Analysis
**Example:** Applied during chamber readings with fluctuations.

**418. Grid Therapy QA Phantom:** Phantom designed to test GRID dose patterns.
**Related Terms:** QA Tools
**Example:** Grid phantom verifies high-dose node spacing.

**419. Gradient Reduction Filter:** Filter that reduces excessive intensity gradients.
**Related Terms:** IMRT Smoothing
**Example:** Smooths peaks in lung IMRT plans.

420. **Glass-Based Thermoluminescent Detector:** Glass detectors storing radiation-induced electronic energy.
**Related Terms:** TLD, Dosimeter
**Example:** Used for in vivo dosimetry.

421. **Gamma-Optimized Segmentation:** Contours modified to improve gamma pass rates.
**Related Terms:** IMRT QA
**Example:** Adjusting OAR borders improves gamma agreement.

422. **Gadolinium Dose Map:** Map of Gd uptake in MRI showing tissue perfusion.
**Related Terms:** Functional Imaging
**Example:** Used in MR-guided boost planning.

423. **Gate-Delay Synchronization:** Matching beam start to the correct gate phase.
**Related Terms:** Gating Window
**Example:** Ensures beam fires only at end-exhale.

424. **Gyro-Controlled Laser System:** Lasers that automatically compensate for room vibration.
**Related Terms:** Alignment Lasers
**Example:** Maintains alignment accuracy <1 mm.

425. **Gel-Embedded Applicator:** Applicator with gel to improve tissue contact.
**Related Terms:** HDR, Internal RT
**Example:** Gel applicators are used in vaginal HDR.

426. **Genetic Dose-Toxicity Predictor:** Algorithm predicting toxicity risk from genetics.
**Related Terms:** Pharmacogenomics, Personalized RT
**Example:** Predicts mucositis severity in head-neck RT.

427. **Gamma-Weighted Isodose Line:** Isodose modified using gamma-composite metrics.
**Related Terms:** Line-Profile, QA Metrics
**Example:** Used in IMRT QA plan comparisons.

428. **Grid-Field Energy Modulation:** Modifying GRID beams to tune penetration.
**Related Terms:** Beam Modulation
**Example:** Higher MV improves GRID spacing.

429. **Greyscale Window Selection:** Choosing proper CT window settings.
**Related Terms:** Image Viewing, HU Values
**Example:** Bone window assists in spine alignment.

430. **Gamma Scintillation Probe:** Detector sensing gamma photons via scintillation.
**Related Terms:** Radiation Detection
**Example:** Used in intraoperative localization.

431. **Gradient Robustness Evaluation:** Testing plan sensitivity to gradient shifts.
**Related Terms:** Robust Planning
**Example:** Ensures plan remains safe with 2 mm drift.

432. **Genetic Expression Mapping:** Diagram of tumor gene activity.
**Related Terms:** Biomarkers
**Example:** Helps identify hypoxic tumor zones.

433. **Gantry Clearance Simulation:** Check for collisions between machine and patient.
**Related Terms:** Collision Avoidance
**Example:** Sim identifies risk in head-tilt setups.

434. **GTV Shrinkage Assessment:** Checking tumor size changes mid-treatment.
**Related Terms:** Adaptive RT
**Example:** GTV shrinks 30% by Week 3.

435. **GPS-Synchronized LINAC Timing:** Using GPS time code for multi-site beam synchronization.
**Related Terms:** Timing Control
**Example:** Research setups use GPS timing.

436. **Gamma-Profile Smoothing:** Smoothing noisy gamma-evaluation curves.
**Related Terms:** QA Metrics
**Example:** Removes spikes caused by detector noise.

437. **Gated Proton Delivery:** Delivering proton beams only in stable breathing phase.
**Related Terms:** PBS, Motion Management
**Example:** Used for moving lung tumors.

438. **Gradient-Index Phantom:** Phantom with layered densities for gradient testing.
**Related Terms:** QA Phantom
**Example:** Used in IMRT gradient evaluations.

439. **Genomic Dose Response Curve:** Curve showing how DNA variations affect tissue response.
**Related Terms:** Radiosensitivity
**Example:** Helps determine RT dose for rare tumors.

440. **Guidewire-Assisted Brachy Placement:** Using guidewires for safe applicator insertion.
**Related Terms:** HDR, Imaging Guidance
**Example:** Common in interstitial implants.

441. **Gynecologic Target Modeling:** Creating 3D models of cervix/uterus for accurate brachytherapy planning.
**Related Terms:** GTV, HR-CTV, Brachy Applicator
**Example:** Target modeling helps identify optimal HDR dwell positions.

442. **Gamma Knife Dose Profile:** Characteristic dose falloff around Gamma Knife shots.
**Related Terms:** SRS, Collimator Size
**Example:** A 4 mm collimator shows rapid dose drop by 70% outside target.

443. **Gated Treatment Window:** The breathing phase during which radiation is allowed to turn ON.
**Related Terms:** Respiratory Gating, Motion Tracking
**Example:** The gated window is set around end-exhale to minimize tumor motion.

444. **Generalized Dose Map:** A dose map normalized to reference values for comparison.
**Related Terms:** DVH, Normalization
**Example:** Generalized maps help compare plans from different energies.

445. **Grid-Spaced Isocenter Network:** Multi-isocenter arrangement used in GRID therapy.
**Related Terms:** Spatial Fractionation
**Example:** GRID lattice uses evenly spaced isocenters for bulky tumors.

446. **Gel Phantom Polymerization Curve:** Curve showing polymer gel response to radiation dose.
**Related Terms:** Gel Dosimetry
**Example:** The curve ensures accurate 3D dosimetry calibration.

447. **Gonadal Protection Protocol:** Procedures to reduce reproductive organ dose.
**Related Terms:** Shielding, OAR Management
**Example:** Lead shields are used in pediatric pelvis RT.

448. **Gradient-Based Dose Smoothing:** Reduction of steep dose transitions in IMRT.
**Related Terms:** TPS Optimization
**Example:** Smoothing prevents hotspots near bowel.

449. **Gamma Transmission Film Test:** Using film to check gamma penetration through shielding.
**Related Terms:** Film Dosimetry
**Example:** Film test confirms blocks reduce transmission <5%.

450. **Guided Position Reproduction:** Achieving identical patient positioning daily using guidance systems.
**Related Terms:** IGRT, Surface Guidance
**Example:** SGRT ensures breast patient setup <1 mm deviation.

451. **Gyro-Locked Beam Steering:** Stabilizing beam orientation using gyro sensors.
**Related Terms:** Beam Steering, LINAC Control
**Example:** Gyro-lock reduces drift during long VMAT arcs.

452. **Genetic Radiosensitivity Marker:** Gene variant associated with radiation tolerance or toxicity.
**Related Terms:** Biomarkers, Radiogenomics
**Example:** ATM mutation increases risk of late fibrosis.

453. **Gaussian Surface Matching:** Using Gaussian functions to align patient surface scans.
**Related Terms:** SGRT, Registration
**Example:** Used in AlignRT patient setup.

454. **Gantry Speed Verification:** QA confirming gantry rotates at planned speed during VMAT.
**Related Terms:** VMAT QA, Mechanical Checks
**Example:** Speed deviations >1% trigger re-tuning.

455. **Grid Beam Hardening:** Increase in effective energy due to blocked low-energy photons.
**Related Terms:** Filtration, Transmission Blocks
**Example:** Grid blocks create a harder spectrum for deep tumors.

456. **Gamma-Ray Interaction Coefficient:** Measure of photon interaction in tissue.
**Related Terms:** Attenuation, Scattering
**Example:** Used in dose calculations for bone vs. soft tissue.

457. **Global Plan Robustness Index:** Score showing how stable a plan is under variations.
**Related Terms:** Robust Planning
**Example:** Proton plans require high robustness indices.

458. **Gadolinium-Based MR Linac Enhancement:** Using Gd contrast for MR-LINAC tumor visualization.
**Related Terms:** MR-Guided RT
**Example:** Enhances pancreatic tumor borders.

459. **Gamma Knife Shot Sequencing:** Ordering of shot deliveries for optimal dose.
**Related Terms:** SRS Planning
**Example:** Small shots are placed first for conformity.

460. **Gross Organ Displacement:** Measurable movement of organs during breathing.
**Related Terms:** Motion Management
**Example:** Liver displacement of 1.5 cm guides gating.

461. **Gradient Dose Limiter:** Planning tool that prevents excessively steep gradients.
**Related Terms:** TPS Constraints
**Example:** Used in head-neck IMRT.

462. **Gating Latency Measurement**Time delay between motion detection and beam ON/OFF.
**Related Terms:** Synchronization
**Example:** Latency <150 ms is acceptable.

463. **Gabor Filter Imaging Enhancement:** Filter improving texture in medical images.
**Related Terms:** Image Processing
**Example:** Enhances lung texture in CT.

464. **Gamma-Ray Dose Falloff Ratio:** Ratio describing how fast dose drops beyond target.
**Related Terms:** Penumbra, Conformity
**Example:** SRS requires high falloff ratios.

465. **Gantry Couch Interlock:** Safety system preventing collisions.
**Related Terms:** Mechanical Safety
**Example:** Couch lock activates during non-clear angles.

466. **Guided Deformable Registration:** AI-assisted matching of CT/MR images.
**Related Terms:** Image Fusion
**Example:** Used in adaptive therapy.

467. **Grid-Sector Modulation:** Adjusting dose distribution in sectors of GRID fields.
**Related Terms:** Spatial Fractionation
**Example:** Sector modulation improves uniformity.

468. **GTV Motion Envelope:** 3D space the tumor occupies during breathing.
**Related Terms:** ITV, 4D CT
**Example:** ITV is defined from this envelope.

469. **Genetic Repair Deficiency Score:** Score measuring DNA-repair capability.
**Related Terms:** Radiosensitivity
**Example:** BRCA1 deficiency suggests lower tolerance.

470. **Gamma-Ray Angular Distribution:** Distribution of emitted photons by angle.
**Related Terms:** Scatter
**Example:** Used for shielding calculations.

471. **Gynecologic Fractions per Prescription:** Number of HDR doses planned for cervical cancer.
**Related Terms:** HDR Brachy, Fractionation
**Example:** 4–5 HDR fractions are typical.

472. **Guided Surface Breathing Trace:** Surface-based tracking of respiratory motion.
**Related Terms:** SGRT, Motion Tracking
**Example:** AlignRT monitors chest rise.

473. **Gamma Knife Composite Isocenter:** Combined center from multiple shot placements.
**Related Terms:** SRS Targeting
**Example:** Used for large AVMs.

474. **Grid-Corrected Output Factor:** Output factor adjusted for GRID block transmission.
**Related Terms:** Dosimetry
**Example:** GRID outputs differ from open fields.

475. **Gaussian Dose Distribution Model:** Modeling dose as a Gaussian curve.
**Related Terms:** Lateral Scatter
**Example:** Used to estimate penumbra width.

476. **Grouped Beam Modulation:** Modulating sets of beams together for consistency.
**Related Terms:** IMRT
**Example:** Groups reduce computational load.

477. **Gadolinium-Based Nanoagents:** Nano-contrast particles used in MR-guided RT research.
**Related Terms:** Functional Imaging
**Example:** Improve tumor uptake visualization.

478. **Gamma-Ray Brachy Activity Check:** Checking source activity using gamma measurement.
**Related Terms:** HDR Source Testing
**Example:** Ir-192 activity is verified weekly.

479. **GTV-Based Adaptive Scaling:** Adjusting dose as GTV shrinks mid-treatment.
**Related Terms:** ART, Replanning
**Example:** Boost dose increases after shrinkage.

480. **Gelatin-Based Bolus:** Stretchable bolus material for irregular surfaces.
**Related Terms:** Bolus, Surface Dose
**Example:** Used on uneven scalp regions.

481. **Gradient Boundary Layer:** Region separating high and low dose zones.
**Related Terms:** Dose Falloff
**Example:** Important in SRS near optic nerves.

482. **Grid-Beam Spatial Index:** Index describing spacing between GRID peaks.
**Related Terms:** Lattice Therapy
**Example:** Ensures uniform spacing for sarcoma treatments.

483. **Gonadal Distance Measurement:** Measuring distance from field edge to gonads.
**Related Terms:** Shielding
**Example:** Abdominal RT requires checking this distance.

484. **Gaussian Adaptive Smoothing:** Smoothing tailored to local intensity variations.
**Related Terms:** Image Processing
**Example:** Reduces CBCT noise.

485. **Gamma Slope Indicator:** Parameter showing steepness of gamma curves.
**Related Terms:** IMRT QA
**Example:** Higher slopes indicate stricter QA.

486. **GTV Overlap Metric:** Quantifies overlap of target after registration.
**Related Terms:** DSC Score
**Example:** Used in multimodal fusion.

487. **Gradient-Protected OAR Constraint:** Constraint preventing dose spikes into OAR.
**Related Terms:** Planning Objectives
**Example:** Used for optic chiasm.

488. **Guided-Microbeam Irradiation:** Using tiny beams for preclinical research.
**Related Terms:** MRT, Experimental RT
**Example:** Used in rat brain tumor studies.

489. **Gyroscopic Couch Stabilizer:** Real-time vibration compensation system.
**Related Terms:** Position Accuracy
**Example:** Important in cranial SRS.

490. **Gamma-Weighted Hotspot Index:** Hotspot index modified by gamma weighting.
**Related Terms:** QA Metrics
**Example:** Used to compare IMRT plans.

491. **Grid-Enhanced Bolus Patch:** Bolus with embedded GRID pattern.
**Related Terms:** Surface Therapy
**Example:** Used in dermatologic RT.

492. **Gaussian Scatter Correction:** Scatter modeled and removed using Gaussian tools.
**Related Terms:** Reconstruction
**Example:** Improves CBCT clarity.

493. **Genomic Hypoxia Score:** Score indicating tumor oxygenation gene patterns.
**Related Terms:** Dose Painting
**Example:** Hypoxic regions get higher boost.

494. **Guiding Catheter for Brachytherapy:** Tube used to guide HDR catheter placement.
**Related Terms:** Interstitial Brachy
**Example:** Ensures perpendicular needle entry.

495. **Gravitational Dose Effect:** Effect of body orientation on tissue density.
**Related Terms:** Couch Rotation
**Example:** Prone position affects lung density.

496. **Gamma-Modulated Arc Planning:** Arc therapy incorporating gamma metrics.
**Related Terms:** VMAT
**Example:** Experimental planning technique.

497. **Grid Dose Error Map:** Map showing deviations in GRID patterns.
**Related Terms:** QA Tools
**Example:** Used for troubleshooting.

498. **Gated Proton Layer Scanning:** Delivering proton layers only during gating.
**Related Terms:** PBS Proton Therapy
**Example:** Used for upper-abdomen tumors.

499. **Glancing-Beam Radiotherapy:** Beam enters at shallow angle to avoid deep tissue dose.
**Related Terms:** Oblique Fields
**Example:** Used for skin cancers.

500. **Gamma-Ray Intensity Regulator:** Device that stabilizes gamma output.
**Related Terms:** Source Control
**Example:** Used in research irradiators.

# H

1. **Half-life:** The time required for a radioactive substance to lose 50% of its activity through natural decay Physical, biological, and effective half-lives are used depending on context
   **Related term:** Radioactive decay
   **Radiotherapy Example:** Iodine-131 (I-131) used in thyroid ablation has a physical half-life of ~8 days
2. **Half-value layer (HVL):** The thickness of a particular material needed to reduce the intensity of a radiation beam by 50% Used to characterize beam quality and penetration
   **Related term:** Beam attenuation
   **Radiotherapy Example:** For 6 MV X-rays, HVL in lead is several millimeters
3. **Half-value thickness:** Another term for HVL; specifies the thickness of shielding material that halves beam intensity
   **Related term:** Attenuation coefficient
   **Radiotherapy Example:** Used to check shielding requirements for linear accelerator rooms
4. **Hand-held detector:** Portable radiation measuring device used for rapid monitoring of dose rates or contamination
   **Related term:** Survey meter
   **Radiotherapy Example:** Checking for radioactive seed loss after brachytherapy
5. **Hard radiation:** Highly penetrating radiation (high-energy photons or particles) with low attenuation in matter
   **Related term:** High-energy photon
   **Radiotherapy Example:** 15 MV X-ray beams used for deep-seated tumors
6. **Hard X-ray:** High-energy X-rays (typically above 10–20 keV in diagnostics; above 1 MV in therapy) capable of deep penetration
   **Related term:** Megavoltage X-ray
   **Radiotherapy Example:** Used in external-beam therapy for deep tumors
7. **Hard gamma radiation:** High-energy gamma rays with strong penetrative capability, typically produced by isotopes like Co-60
   **Related term:** Gamma photons
   **Radiotherapy Example:** Cobalt-60 teletherapy beams for cancer treatment
8. **Hazard assessment:** Systematic evaluation of potential radiation risks in a given environment or procedure
   **Related term:** Radiation risk analysis
   **Radiotherapy Example:** Assessing exposure risks for staff during HDR brachytherapy
9. **Hazard evaluation:** Quantification and interpretation of identified hazards to determine severity and needed controls
   **Related term:** Risk evaluation
   **Radiotherapy Example:** Evaluating dose leakage around a linear accelerator
10. **Hazard index:** A numerical representation of the risk level associated with a radiation source or procedure
    **Related term:** Risk metric
    **Radiotherapy Example:** Used to classify the risk of handling high-activity Ir-192 seeds

11. **Hazardous radiation:** Radiation capable of causing biological damage if exposure limits are exceeded
**Related term:** Ionizing radiation
**Radiotherapy Example:** High-dose brachytherapy sources require strict control
12. **Hazardous waste:** Material or equipment contaminated with radioactive substances that must be safely disposed of
**Related term:** Radioactive waste
**Radiotherapy Example:** Decayed I-131 patient waste managed through controlled disposal
13. **Head CT:** A CT scan of the brain region used for imaging trauma, tumors, bleeds, and pre-RT planning
**Related term:** Cranial CT
**Radiotherapy Example:** Used for immobilization and planning of brain radiotherapy
14. **Head MRI:** Magnetic imaging of the brain offering high soft-tissue contrast
**Related term:** Brain MRI
**Radiotherapy Example:** Used for tumor delineation in glioblastoma planning
15. **Head and neck imaging:** Comprehensive imaging (CT/MRI/PET) of the head-and-neck region for diagnosis and treatment planning
**Related term:** Head and neck oncology
**Radiotherapy Example:** Identifying tumor margins in nasopharyngeal carcinoma
16. **Heat load (radiation tube):** Total thermal energy deposited in an X-ray tube during operation; excessive heat can damage components
**Related term:** Anode heating
**Radiotherapy Example:** CT simulators track heat load to prevent tube burnout
17. **Heat production (in tissue):** Energy deposition from radiation interactions that generates small amounts of heat in tissue
**Related term:** Absorbed dose (Gy)
**Radiotherapy Example:** Negligible in radiotherapy, but important in hyperthermia therapy
18. **Helium-neon laser:** A low-power red light laser (632 8 nm) often used for medical alignment
**Related term:** Positioning laser
**Radiotherapy Example:** Alignment lasers in LINAC rooms often use He-Ne tubes
19. **Helium-neon laser therapy:** Low-level laser therapy used for tissue healing (not ionizing)
**Related term:** Photobiomodulation
**Radiotherapy Example:** Occasionally used for mucositis management in RT patients
20. **Helium ion beam:** Charged particle beam therapy using helium nuclei; greater mass and less scattering than protons
**Related term:** Particle therapy
**Radiotherapy Example:** Experimental use in highly conformal radiotherapy
21. **Helium nucleus radiation:** Alpha particles (He-4 nuclei); high LET, strong ionizing effect, low penetration
**Related term:** Alpha radiation
**Radiotherapy Example:** Radionuclide therapy using alpha emitters (Ra-223)
22. **Helical CT:** Continuous spiral CT scanning that captures volumetric data quickly
**Related term:** Spiral CT
**Radiotherapy Example:** Used in CT simulation for 3D treatment planning

23. **Helical MRI:** MRI sequence strategy that acquires data in a spiral or helical manner for speed
**Related term:** Rapid MRI acquisition
**Radiotherapy Example:** Faster scans for MR-guided radiotherapy

24. **Hematopoietic stem cell transplantation:** Replacement of damaged bone marrow with healthy stem cells—often after total-body irradiation
**Related term:** Bone marrow transplant
**Radiotherapy Example:** TBI is used to destroy diseased marrow prior to transplant

25. **Hematopoietic tissue radiation:** Radiation effects on bone marrow, which is highly radiosensitive
**Related term:** Bone marrow suppression
**Radiotherapy Example:** Pelvic irradiation can reduce blood cell production

26. **High-energy photon:** Photons in the megavoltage (MV) range used for deep tissue penetration
**Related term:** MV X-ray
**Radiotherapy Example:** 6–18 MV beams in EBRT

27. **High-energy X-ray:** Same as above—produced by LINAC targets for therapeutic use
**Related term:** Megavoltage therapy
**Radiotherapy Example:** Treating deep tumors like prostate or lung

28. **High-frequency radiation:** Electromagnetic radiation with high frequency (and energy), including X-rays and gamma rays
**Related term:** Ionizing EM radiation
**Radiotherapy Example:** Used for tumor destruction in EBRT

29. **High-intensity focused ultrasound (HIFU):** Focused sound waves generate heat to ablate tissue without ionizing radiation
**Related term:** Thermal ablation
**Radiotherapy Example:** Can complement prostate cancer treatment

30. **High-magnetic-field MRI:** MRI systems operating at ≥3 Tesla, providing superior spatial resolution
**Related term:** High-resolution MRI
**Radiotherapy Example:** Used for accurate target delineation in brain tumors

31. **High-resolution CT:** CT scans with thin slices (≤1 mm) and sharp reconstruction algorithms
**Related term:** HRCT
**Radiotherapy Example:** Fine lung parenchyma assessment before thoracic RT

32. **High-resolution imaging:** Imaging that captures finer anatomical or functional detail
**Related term:** High spatial resolution
**Radiotherapy Example:** Used in stereotactic radiotherapy planning

33. **High-resolution MRI:** MRI with small voxel sizes allowing exquisite soft-tissue detail
**Related term:** High-field MRI
**Radiotherapy Example:** Used in defining tumor boundaries in brain/rectal cancer

34. **High-sensitivity detector:** Detector capable of measuring very low radiation levels with high efficiency
**Related term:** Scintillation detector
**Radiotherapy Example:** Used for dosimetry of low-intensity radiation fields

35. **High-voltage X-ray tube:** Tube operating at high kilovoltage (kV) to produce high-energy diagnostic X-rays
**Related term:** Diagnostic X-ray tube
**Radiotherapy Example:** Used in on-board imaging systems (kV imaging)

36. **Histogram analysis:** Statistical analysis of pixel intensity distribution in images
**Related term:** Image processing
**Radiotherapy Example:** Assessing CT density distributions in target volumes

37. **Histology imaging:** Microscopic imaging of tissues stained for structural assessment
**Related term:** Microscopy
**Radiotherapy Example:** Validating imaging-based tumor segmentation

38. **Histopathology radiology correlation:** Matching imaging findings with microscopic pathology results
**Related term:** Radiologic-pathologic correlation
**Radiotherapy Example:** Ensures imaging-based tumor volumes reflect actual disease

39. **Hodgkin's disease imaging:** Imaging studies (CT, PET) to evaluate Hodgkin lymphoma
**Related term:** Lymphoma imaging
**Radiotherapy Example:** PET/CT used for field design in nodal irradiation

40. **Home radiation monitoring:** Use of personal devices to detect or track radiation exposure at home
**Related term:** Personal dosimetry
**Radiotherapy Example:** Patients with I-131 therapy may monitor home exposure

41. **Homogeneous dose distribution:** A uniform radiation dose delivered throughout the target volume
**Related term:** Isodose uniformity
**Radiotherapy Example:** Important in whole-breast irradiation

42. **Homogeneity correction:** Correction applied to account for tissue density variations (bone, lung)
**Related term:** Heterogeneity correction
**Radiotherapy Example:** Required in treatment planning algorithms

43. **Horizontal beam:** Beam oriented parallel to the floor for treatment or imaging
**Related term:** Beam orientation
**Radiotherapy Example:** Used in certain fixed-gantry proton systems

44. **Horizontal irradiation:** Delivery of radiation with the beam axis horizontal
**Related term:** Horizontal beam therapy
**Radiotherapy Example:** Some experimental particle setups require horizontal geometry

45. **Hospital radiation safety:** Policies ensuring safe use of radiation in clinical settings
**Related term:** Radiation protection
**Radiotherapy Example:** Monitoring LINAC room shielding compliance

46. **Hot spot (dosimetry):** Localized region receiving a higher dose than intended
**Related term:** Dose inhomogeneity
**Radiotherapy Example:** Avoided in IMRT planning near organs at risk

47. **Hot-spot detection:** Identification of areas with excessive dose or activity
**Related term:** Dose quality assurance
**Radiotherapy Example:** Detected via film or portal dosimetry

48. **Housekeeping (radiation safety):** Ensuring cleanliness and contamination control in radiation areas
**Related term:** Contamination monitoring
**Radiotherapy Example:** Wiping surfaces after handling radioactive sources

49. **Human tissue equivalent phantom:** Phantom mimicking human tissue interaction with radiation
**Related term:** Dosimetry phantom
**Radiotherapy Example:** Used for calibrating treatment machines

50. **Humidity effect on detector:** High humidity can alter detector sensitivity or cause drift
**Related term:** Environmental effects on detectors
**Radiotherapy Example:** Ion chamber readings may vary if not corrected

51. **Hybrid imaging:** Combining two imaging modalities for complementary information
**Related term:** Multimodality imaging
**Radiotherapy Example:** PET/CT used for tumor delineation

52. **Hybrid PET/CT:** Positron emission tomography fused with CT for metabolic and anatomical imaging
**Related term:** PET imaging
**Radiotherapy Example:** Used for staging and planning in lung cancer

53. **Hybrid SPECT/CT:** Combines nuclear SPECT imaging with CT localization
**Related term:** Hybrid nuclear imaging
**Radiotherapy Example:** Sentinel node mapping in head-and-neck cancer

54. **Hybrid imaging system:** A scanner integrating two imaging modalities
**Related term:** Dual-modality imaging
**Radiotherapy Example:** PET/MRI used for soft tissue and metabolic detail

55. **Hydrogel dosimeter:** Gel material that changes optical/chemical properties when irradiated
**Related term:** 3D dosimeter
**Radiotherapy Example:** Used for verifying complex IMRT dose distributions

56. **Hydrodynamic effect of radiation:** Radiation-induced heating or pressure changes affecting fluid behavior
**Related term:** Thermal effects
**Radiotherapy Example:** Minor in RT but studied in high-energy physics

57. **Hyperfractionated radiation therapy:** Two or more smaller treatments per day to increase total dose with reduced toxicity
**Related term:** Fractionation schedule
**Radiotherapy Example:** Used in head-and-neck cancer to improve control

58. **Hyperpolarized MRI:** MRI using hyperpolarized nuclei to drastically increase signal strength
**Related term:** Advanced MRI techniques
**Radiotherapy Example:** Investigating tumor metabolism

59. **Hyperthermia therapy:** Heating tissues to ~41–45°C to enhance tumor radiosensitivity
**Related term:** Thermal therapy
**Radiotherapy Example:** Combined with RT for superficial tumors

60. **Hyperthermia treatment planning:** Planning heat distribution to ensure tumor heating while sparing normal tissue
**Related term:** Thermal dosimetry
**Radiotherapy Example:** Used in hyperthermia + RT combination protocols

61. **Hypofractionated radiation therapy:** Larger dose per fraction, fewer treatments
**Related term:** SBRT / SRT
**Radiotherapy Example:** Prostate SBRT (e g , 36 25 Gy in 5 fractions)

62. **Hypodense lesion:** Region appearing darker than surrounding tissue on CT due to low density
**Related term:** Low-attenuation lesion
**Radiotherapy Example:** Brain metastases often appear hypodense

63. **Hypodense tissue imaging:** Imaging techniques that identify low-density regions
**Related term:** CT attenuation
**Radiotherapy Example:** Identifying necrotic tumor areas

64. **Hypodensity detection:** Identifying low-attenuation regions automatically or visually
**Related term:** Image segmentation
**Radiotherapy Example:** Used in treatment planning for cystic lesions

65. **Hypoxia imaging:** Imaging that detects low-oxygen tumor regions
**Related term:** PET hypoxia tracers
**Radiotherapy Example:** Identifies radioresistant tumor regions

66. **Hypoxic cell radiosensitizer:** Drug that increases radiation sensitivity in oxygen-poor cells
**Related term:** Radiosensitizer
**Radiotherapy Example:** Tirapazamine in hypoxic tumor radiotherapy

67. **Hypoxic tissue imaging:** Visualization of oxygen-deprived tumor areas
**Related term:** Hypoxia PET
**Radiotherapy Example:** F-MISO PET for hypoxia mapping

68. **Hounsfield unit (HU):** Numeric scale representing CT density values, calibrated to water and air
**Related term:** CT number
**Radiotherapy Example:** Used for converting CT values to electron densities

69. **Hounsfield scale:** Scale assigning HU values to tissues based on X-ray attenuation
**Related term:** CT calibration
**Radiotherapy Example:** Used in dose calculation algorithms

70. **Human phantom:** Physical model representing human anatomy for dose testing
**Related term:** Anthropomorphic phantom
**Radiotherapy Example:** Used in QA of new treatment techniques

71. **Human tissue dosimetry:** Measuring or calculating radiation dose absorbed in human tissues
**Related term:** Organ dosimetry
**Radiotherapy Example:** Dose estimation to organs at risk

72. **Human tissue equivalent material:** Substance imitating human tissue density and composition for dosimetry
**Related term:** Tissue-equivalent phantom
**Radiotherapy Example:** Used in calibration of ion chambers

73. **Humanoid radiation phantom:** Phantom shaped like a human, used in dose measurement and imaging calibration
**Related term:** Anthropomorphic phantom
**Radiotherapy Example:** Phantom used for IMRT proficiency testing

74. **Humoral imaging:** Imaging related to body fluids or immune responses (rare use)
**Related term:** Nuclear medicine imaging
**Radiotherapy Example:** Not common; occasionally used in immune tracer research

75. **Hybrid radionuclide therapy:** Therapy combining two radionuclides or combining radionuclide therapy with another modality
**Related term:** Theranostics
**Radiotherapy Example:** PRRT + external-beam therapy

76. **Hybrid radiation therapy:** Combination of different radiation modalities (e g , photons + electrons)
**Related term:** Mixed-beam therapy
**Radiotherapy Example:** Breast RT using tangential photons + electron boost

77. **Histogram equalization:** Image enhancement technique that improves contrast by redistributing intensity values
**Related term:** Image normalization
**Radiotherapy Example:** Used in CT/MRI preprocessing for segmentation

78. **Histogram smoothing:** Reducing noise in intensity histograms for better feature extraction
**Related term:** Signal filtering
**Radiotherapy Example:** Used in segmentation algorithms

79. **Heat deposition in tissue:** Small amount of heat generated when tissues absorb radiation
**Related term:** Absorbed dose
**Radiotherapy Example:** Minimal; relevant mainly in hyperthermia therapy

80. **Heat source shielding:** Shielding required to protect from thermal emissions or hot radiation sources
**Related term:** Thermal protection
**Radiotherapy Example:** Handling hot HDR sources requires insulated tools

81. **Helium ion therapy:** Radiotherapy using helium ions, offering high precision and low scattering
**Related term:** Heavy ion therapy
**Radiotherapy Example:** Specialized centers explore helium ion therapy for tumors near critical structures

82. **Helium-3 neutron detector:** Highly sensitive detector for neutron radiation using He-3 gas
**Related term:** Neutron detection
**Radiotherapy Example:** Used in neutron therapy facility monitoring

83. **Helium-4 radiation:** Alpha particle radiation consisting of helium-4 nuclei
**Related term:** Alpha emitter
**Radiotherapy Example:** Ra-223 alpha therapy for bone metastases

84. **Helical radiation therapy:** Delivery of radiation in a spiral (helical) pattern around the patient
**Related term:** TomoTherapy
**Radiotherapy Example:** Helical TomoTherapy for IMRT delivery

85. **Helical scan protocol:** Instructions for performing spiral CT/MRI scans
**Related term:** Scan parameters
**Radiotherapy Example:** Standardized protocol used for CT simulation

86. **High-dose rate (HDR) brachytherapy:** Internal radiotherapy using high-activity sources delivered for short durations
**Related term:** Ir-192 brachytherapy
**Radiotherapy Example:** Cervical cancer HDR treatment

87. **High-energy electron beam:** Electrons accelerated to MeV energies used for superficial tumors
**Related term:** Electron therapy
**Radiotherapy Example:** Treating skin cancers or chest wall

88. **High-energy neutron:** Fast neutrons with high penetration and biological effectiveness
**Related term:** Neutron therapy
**Radiotherapy Example:** Used in specialized cancer therapy centers

89. **High-energy proton beam:** Proton beam used in particle therapy; delivers Bragg peak
**Related term:** Proton therapy
**Radiotherapy Example:** Treating pediatric brain tumors

90. **High-intensity radiation:** Radiation with high dose rate or high energy concentration
**Related term:** HDR radiation
**Radiotherapy Example:** HDR brachytherapy

91. **High-precision radiotherapy:** Highly accurate radiation delivery minimizing dose to normal tissues
**Related term:** Stereotactic radiosurgery
**Radiotherapy Example:** SBRT treatments for lung lesions

92. **High-resolution detector:** Detector capable of capturing fine detail in radiation measurements or imaging
**Related term:** High spatial resolution
**Radiotherapy Example:** EPID for portal imaging QA

93. **High-sensitivity imaging:** Imaging with capability to detect very small signals or low activity
**Related term:** High-efficiency detector
**Radiotherapy Example:** SPECT/PET systems detecting low radiotracer uptake

94. **High-voltage generator:** Supplies high voltage required for X-ray production in imaging systems
**Related term:** X-ray power supply
**Radiotherapy Example:** Used inside CT simulators

95. **Histogram analysis software:** Tools analyzing pixel intensity histograms for segmentation or enhancement
**Related term:** Image processing software
**Radiotherapy Example:** Used in AI segmentation systems

96. **Histogram-based image segmentation:** Dividing images into regions based on pixel intensity clusters
**Related term:** Thresholding
**Radiotherapy Example:** Separate lung tissue from tumors using CT values

97. **Hodgkin lymphoma radiotherapy:** Radiotherapy techniques specific to Hodgkin lymphoma
**Related term:** Involved site radiation therapy (ISRT)
**Radiotherapy Example:** Treating mediastinal lymph nodes

98. **Home dosimetry:** Monitoring radiation dose at home with personal dosimeters
**Related term:** Personal radiation monitoring
**Radiotherapy Example:** Used for nuclear medicine outpatients

99. **Horizontal scanner:** Imaging scanner with horizontal orientation
**Related term:** Horizontal CT
**Radiotherapy Example:** Some research systems use horizontal geometry

100. **Humidity control in imaging:** Regulation of humidity to ensure proper operation of detectors and electronics
**Related term:** Environmental conditioning
**Radiotherapy Example:** Preventing condensation in ion chambers

101. **Hypoxic cell radiosensitizer:** A drug that increases the sensitivity of oxygen-deprived (hypoxic) tumor cells to radiation Hypoxic cells are more resistant to radiotherapy
**Related term:** Hypoxia modifier
**Radiotherapy Example:** Nimorazole used during head-and-neck radiotherapy to enhance tumor control

102. **Hypoxic tissue imaging:** Imaging used to visualize areas of low oxygen concentration within tumors, often using PET tracers These regions are associated with radioresistance
**Related term:** Hypoxia PET
**Radiotherapy Example:** FMISO-PET used to map resistant zones for adaptive radiotherapy dose boosting

103. **Hounsfield unit:** A quantitative CT number representing tissue density relative to water, used for attenuation characterization
**Related term:** CT number
**Radiotherapy Example:** Hounsfield units are converted to electron density for treatment planning dose calculations

104. **Hounsfield scale:** A standardized scale from –1000 to +3000 used to represent CT attenuation values
**Related term:** CT attenuation scale
**Radiotherapy Example:** Used to differentiate bone, soft tissue, and air for contouring in treatment planning

105. **Human phantom:** A physical model simulating human anatomy and tissue properties, used for training and dosimetry
**Related term:** Anthropomorphic phantom
**Radiotherapy Example:** The Alderson RANDO phantom used to verify IMRT dose delivery

106. **Human tissue dosimetry:** Measurement of absorbed dose within simulated or real biological tissue
**Related term:** In-phantom dosimetry
**Radiotherapy Example:** Using TLDs inside tissue-equivalent slabs to confirm dose distributions

107. **Human tissue equivalent material:** Synthetic materials designed to mimic radiation interaction properties of human tissue
**Related term:** Water-equivalent material
**Radiotherapy Example:** Solid Water® phantoms used for linear accelerator QA

108. **Humanoid radiation phantom:** A life-sized model with realistic organs and bone structure for complex radiation testing
**Related term:** 3D-printed anatomical phantom
**Radiotherapy Example:** Used to validate VMAT dose accuracy in pediatric-sized phantoms

109. **Humoral imaging:** Imaging targeting blood-borne or immune-related biomarkers
**Related term:** Immuno-PET
**Radiotherapy Example:** Radio-labeled antibodies used for imaging lymphoma before radiotherapy

110. **Hybrid radionuclide therapy:** Combination of two or more radionuclides to achieve complementary treatment effects
**Related term:** Theranostics
**Radiotherapy Example:** Using a beta emitter for tumor kill and an alpha emitter for residual disease control

111. **Hybrid radiation therapy:** Treatment method combining different modalities such as photons and protons
**Related term:** Mixed-beam radiotherapy
**Radiotherapy Example:** Proton boost + photon IMRT for skull-base tumors

112. **Histogram equalization:** Image-processing technique that enhances image contrast by redistributing pixel intensity
**Related term:** Image normalization
**Radiotherapy Example:** Used in CT preprocessing to improve tumor boundary visibility for contouring

113. **Histogram smoothing:** Reduces noise in intensity histograms to improve segmentation accuracy
**Related term:** Image denoising
**Radiotherapy Example:** Used in PET segmentation to reduce artifacts in metabolic tumor volume estimation

114. **Heat deposition in tissue:** Conversion of absorbed radiation energy into heat within patient tissues
**Related term:** Thermal dose
**Radiotherapy Example:** High-dose-rate brachytherapy causing local temperature rise in tumor tissue

115. **Heat source shielding:** Protection applied to radiation equipment components generating excessive heat
**Related term:** Thermal barrier
**Radiotherapy Example:** Lead-lined heat shields used in linear accelerator head assemblies

116. **Helium ion therapy:** Particle therapy using helium ions, offering sharper Bragg peaks and lower scattering
**Related term:** Heavy-ion therapy
**Radiotherapy Example:** Used for pediatric tumors to reduce exit dose

117. **Helium-3 neutron detector:** A detector using He-3 gas to sense thermal neutrons via nuclear reaction
**Related term:** Neutron dosimeter
**Radiotherapy Example:** Measures neutron contamination during high-energy photon therapy (>10 MV)

118. **Helium-4 radiation:** Alpha particles consisting of two protons and two neutrons (He-4 nuclei)
**Related term:** Alpha radiation
**Radiotherapy Example:** Used in targeted alpha therapy (TAT) for micrometastases

119. **Helical radiation therapy:** Delivery of radiation while the gantry rotates and the couch moves, creating a spiral path
**Related term:** Tomotherapy
**Radiotherapy Example:** Helical IMRT for total marrow irradiation

120. **Helical scan protocol:** Instructions defining pitch, rotation, tube current, and slice thickness for helical CT imaging
**Related term:** CT acquisition parameters
**Radiotherapy Example:** Standardized protocols ensure consistent CT datasets for planning

121. **High-dose rate (HDR) brachytherapy:** Internal radiotherapy using a very high activity source (Ir-192) delivering dose quickly
**Related term:** Temporary implants
**Radiotherapy Example:** HDR cervix brachytherapy using afterloading catheters

122. **High-energy electron beam:** Electrons with energies typically 6–20 MeV used for superficial tumors
**Related term:** Electron therapy
**Radiotherapy Example:** Electron beam for chest wall boost post-mastectomy

123. **High-energy neutron:** Neutrons with energy above ~10 MeV, often produced as secondary radiation
**Related term:** Neutron contamination
**Radiotherapy Example:** Observed during high-energy (>15 MV) photon treatments

124. **High-energy proton beam:** Protons delivered at energies of 70–250 MeV for deep-seated tumors
**Related term:** Proton therapy
**Radiotherapy Example:** Pediatric brain tumor treatment with reduced integral dose

125. **High-intensity radiation:** Radiation with high dose rate or particle concentration
**Related term:** High-flux beam
**Radiotherapy Example:** FLASH radiotherapy delivering dose in milliseconds

**126. High-precision radiotherapy:** Techniques aiming for sub-millimeter accuracy via image-guidance and advanced planning
**Related term:** IGRT
**Radiotherapy Example:** Stereotactic radiosurgery for brain metastases

**127. High-resolution detector:** A detector capable of capturing fine spatial detail
**Related term:** Pixel resolution
**Radiotherapy Example:** EPID high-res panels used for portal dosimetry

**128. High-sensitivity imaging:** Imaging that detects low-intensity photon signals with high fidelity
**Related term:** Quantum efficiency
**Radiotherapy Example:** Low-dose CT imaging for adaptive radiotherapy

**129. High-voltage generator:** Power system generating high kVp for X-ray tubes
**Related term:** Transformer
**Radiotherapy Example:** Used in CT simulators to achieve stable beam output

**130. Histogram analysis software:** Tools that analyze pixel intensity distributions for segmentation or contrast study
**Related term:** Radiomics
**Radiotherapy Example:** Extracts texture features for tumor characterization

**131. Histogram-based image segmentation:** Segmentation method using intensity thresholds derived from the histogram curve
**Related term:** Thresholding
**Radiotherapy Example:** PET tumor volume segmentation

**132. Hodgkin lymphoma radiotherapy:** Radiation treatment targeting lymph node regions affected by Hodgkin lymphoma
**Related term:** Involved-site radiotherapy (ISRT)
**Radiotherapy Example:** 20–30 Gy to affected nodal sites post-chemotherapy

**133. Home dosimetry:** Patient-based radiation monitoring done outside the clinic, often with portable devices
**Related term:** Personal dosimeter
**Radiotherapy Example:** Checking residual I-131 activity post-therapy

**134. Horizontal scanner:** Imaging system with a horizontally oriented scanning axis
**Related term:** Flat-bed scanner
**Radiotherapy Example:** Used in film dosimetry when scanning Gafchromic films

**135. Humidity control in imaging:** Regulation of moisture levels to protect detectors and ensure measurement stability
**Related term:** Environmental conditioning
**Radiotherapy Example:** Protecting ion chambers from humidity drift

**136. Half-value layer calculation:** Mathematical determination of material thickness needed to reduce beam intensity by half
**Related term:** Attenuation coefficient
**Radiotherapy Example:** Determining shielding thickness for linac rooms

**137. Half-value thickness measurement:** Experimental measurement of HVL using attenuating plates and detectors
**Related term:** Beam hardening test
**Radiotherapy Example:** QA of CT beam quality

138. **Hand-held ionization detector:** Mobile device using ionization chamber technology to measure radiation exposure
**Related term:** Survey meter
**Radiotherapy Example:** Checking leakage radiation around a linear accelerator

139. **Hand-held radiation monitor:** Portable detector measuring dose rate or contamination in real time
**Related term:** Geiger counter
**Radiotherapy Example:** Monitoring brachytherapy source transfer paths

140. **Hard gamma-ray beam:** Gamma radiation with high photon energy and deep penetration
**Related term:** High-energy photons
**Radiotherapy Example:** Co-60 beams used historically in teletherapy

141. **Hard X-ray beam:** High-energy X-ray beam produced by high kVp settings
**Related term:** Megavoltage X-rays
**Radiotherapy Example:** MV beams used in linac treatments

142. **Hazard control:** Procedures designed to minimize radiation risks to patients and staff
**Related term:** ALARA principle
**Radiotherapy Example:** Controlled access zones around radiation rooms

143. **Hazard level:** Classification of radiation risk severity
**Related term:** Dose limit category
**Radiotherapy Example:** High hazard level around activated linac components

144. **Hazardous material disposal:** Safe removal of radioactive or contaminated materials
**Related term:** Radioactive waste management
**Radiotherapy Example:** Disposal of used brachytherapy sources

145. **Head coil (MRI):** MRI accessory that improves signal from the head region
**Related term:** RF coil
**Radiotherapy Example:** Used in MRI-planning for brain tumor radiotherapy

146. **Head phantom:** Phantom simulating human head anatomy for imaging and dosimetry
**Related term:** Cranial phantom
**Radiotherapy Example:** Used for SRS verification measurements

147. **Head phantom dosimetry:** Dose measurement performed inside a head phantom
**Related term:** End-to-end testing
**Radiotherapy Example:** Gamma Knife QA

148. **Heat dissipation (X-ray tube):** Removal of heat generated in the anode during X-ray production
**Related term:** Thermal loading
**Radiotherapy Example:** Prevents CT tube overheating during simulation scans

149. **Heat energy deposition:** Similar to heat deposition, focusing on energy absorbed per mass
**Related term:** Specific absorption rate (SAR)
**Radiotherapy Example:** SAR concerns in MRI-guided radiotherapy

150. **Heat exchanger (radiation equipment):** Component cooling radiotherapy devices by transferring heat to a secondary fluid
**Related term:** Thermal management
**Radiotherapy Example:** Cooling system in linear accelerator waveguides

151. **Helium ion accelerator:** Machine accelerating helium ions for therapeutic use
**Related term:** Heavy-ion accelerator
**Radiotherapy Example:** Source for helium ion therapy

152. **Helium ion dosimetry:** Dose measurement specific to helium ion beams
**Related term:** Ion-beam dosimetry
**Radiotherapy Example:** Using microdosimeters in helium therapy

153. **Helium ion imaging:** Imaging using helium ions for high-contrast particle radiography
**Related term:** Ion radiography
**Radiotherapy Example:** Verifying patient setup in heavy-ion therapy

154. **Helium-neon laser calibration:** Process to ensure stable output from He-Ne lasers used as alignment tools
**Related term:** Laser QA
**Radiotherapy Example:** Aligning patient positioning lasers in treatment rooms

155. **Helical CT scan:** CT technique where the patient moves continuously as the X-ray tube rotates
**Related term:** Spiral CT
**Radiotherapy Example:** Used for CT simulation for treatment planning

156. **Helical imaging protocol:** Defined steps for acquiring spiral CT images
**Related term:** Acquisition protocol
**Radiotherapy Example:** Ensuring reproducible helical CT for adaptive planning

157. **Helical pitch:** Ratio describing table movement per rotation relative to beam width
**Related term:** Pitch factor
**Radiotherapy Example:** Adjusting pitch to reduce artifacts in planning CT

158. **Helical reconstruction:** Mathematical reconstruction of images obtained from spiral CT acquisitions
**Related term:** Filtered back-projection
**Radiotherapy Example:** Producing diagnostic-quality images for contouring

159. **Helical scan dose:** Radiation dose delivered during a helical CT acquisition
**Related term:** CTDIvol
**Radiotherapy Example:** Important during CT simulation for minimizing patient exposure

160. **Helical tomography:** Delivery of radiation in a helical pattern around the patient (Tomotherapy)
**Related term:** Helical IMRT
**Radiotherapy Example:** Used for total lymphoid irradiation

161. **Hematopoietic system dosimetry:** Measurement of dose delivered to blood-forming organs
**Related term:** Bone marrow dose
**Radiotherapy Example:** Important during TBI planning

162. **Hematopoietic tissue irradiation:** Radiation affecting bone marrow tissues
**Related term:** Myelosuppression
**Radiotherapy Example:** Conditioning regimens for stem cell transplantation

163. **High-dose radiation:** Radiation levels large enough to cause significant tissue injury or therapeutic tumor kill
**Related term:** Ablative dose
**Radiotherapy Example:** SBRT delivering >20 Gy per fraction

164. **High-dose brachytherapy:** Brachytherapy involving high-activity sources
**Related term:** HDR
**Radiotherapy Example:** Breast HDR boost

165. **High-dose fluoroscopy:** Fluoroscopy delivering high radiation dose during long procedures
**Related term:** Interventional dose
**Radiotherapy Example:** Used cautiously in image-guided brachytherapy

166. **High-dose proton therapy:** Proton treatments delivering ablative doses to tumors
**Related term:** Ultra-high dose
**Radiotherapy Example:** Skull-base chordoma treatment

167. **High-dose X-ray therapy:** High-dose photon treatment, often stereotactic
**Related term:** SBRT
**Radiotherapy Example:** Lung SBRT delivering 12 Gy × 4

168. **High-energy electron therapy:** Use of high-energy electrons for superficial or chest wall tumors
**Related term:** Electron beam therapy
**Radiotherapy Example:** Boost to skin lesions

169. **High-energy photon therapy:** Treatment using MV photon beams (6–25 MV)
**Related term:** External beam radiotherapy
**Radiotherapy Example:** IMRT for prostate cancer

170. **High-energy radiation shielding:** Barriers designed to attenuate MV radiation
**Related term:** Concrete shielding
**Radiotherapy Example:** 2-meter concrete walls for linac rooms

171. **High-energy radiotherapy:** Radiotherapy using high-energy beams for deep tumors
**Related term:** Megavoltage therapy
**Radiotherapy Example:** 18 MV beams for pelvic treatments

172. **High-energy X-ray imaging:** Imaging using MV X-rays instead of kV
**Related term:** MV imaging
**Radiotherapy Example:** Portal imaging for treatment verification

173. **High-flux neutron beam:** Beam with a high rate of neutron particles
**Related term:** Fast neutrons
**Radiotherapy Example:** Used in experimental neutron therapy

174. **High-magnification imaging:** Imaging method providing enlarged visualization of structures
**Related term:** Zoom imaging
**Radiotherapy Example:** Used for micro-dosimeter analysis

175. **High-resolution anatomical imaging:** High spatial detail imaging of anatomical structures
**Related term:** Structural MRI
**Radiotherapy Example:** Brain tumor contouring with high-res T1 MRI

176. **High-resolution functional imaging:** High-detail imaging of physiologic processes
**Related term:** Functional MRI
**Radiotherapy Example:** Mapping tumor hypoxia zones

177. **High-resolution MRI protocol:** Defined MRI parameters producing very fine detail
**Related term:** High-field MRI
**Radiotherapy Example:** Planning for stereotactic radiosurgery

178. **High-resolution PET:** PET imaging with increased spatial resolution
**Related term:** TOF PET
**Radiotherapy Example:** Precise tumor margin identification

179. **High-resolution SPECT:** SPECT imaging providing improved detail through collimator design
**Related term:** Multi-pinhole SPECT
**Radiotherapy Example:** Mapping sentinel nodes before radiotherapy

180. **High-resolution tomography:** Tomographic imaging with high spatial fidelity
**Related term:** Micro-CT
**Radiotherapy Example:** Used for preclinical radiobiology studies

181. **High-sensitivity gamma camera:** Gamma camera optimized to detect low levels of gamma radiation
**Related term:** Anger camera
**Radiotherapy Example:** Detects I-131 uptake post-therapy

182. **High-sensitivity imaging detector:** Highly efficient detector for low signal imaging
**Related term:** Photo-sensor array
**Radiotherapy Example:** Used in PET-CT simulators

183. **High-speed imaging:** Imaging capable of capturing data very quickly
**Related term:** Rapid acquisition
**Radiotherapy Example:** 4DCT for motion management

184. **High-voltage radiography:** X-ray imaging using high kVp settings
**Related term:** Hard X-ray imaging
**Radiotherapy Example:** Used in QA for shielding verification

185. **Histogram-based analysis:** Analyzing image histograms to derive quantitative metrics
**Related term:** Radiomics feature extraction
**Radiotherapy Example:** Used in tumor grading prediction

186. **Histogram-based image enhancement:** Improving image contrast through histogram manipulation
**Related term:** Equalization
**Radiotherapy Example:** Enhancing CT soft tissue contrast

187. **Histogram equalization algorithm:** Computational algorithm that redistributes pixel intensities for contrast improvement
**Related term:** Contrast optimization
**Radiotherapy Example:** Used in CT rendering software

188. **Histogram normalization:** Adjusting an image histogram to a standard reference
**Related term:** Intensity standardization
**Radiotherapy Example:** Normalizing MRI datasets for multi-center planning

189. **Histopathological imaging:** Microscopic imaging of tissue samples
**Related term:** Digital pathology
**Radiotherapy Example:** Radiomics-pathology correlation studies

190. **Histology–radiology correlation:** Comparing imaging findings with pathological results
**Related term:** Radiologic-pathologic matching
**Radiotherapy Example:** Validating MRI tumor boundaries against surgical pathology

191. **Hodgkin lymphoma imaging:** Imaging techniques used to stage and monitor Hodgkin lymphoma
**Related term:** FDG-PET
**Radiotherapy Example:** PET-CT used pre-radiotherapy to define nodal involvement

192. **Home radiation detector:** Personal radiation measuring device used at home
**Related term:** Environmental dosimeter
**Radiotherapy Example:** Monitoring radiation after I-131 therapy

193. **Home radiation dosimeter:** Device measuring absorbed dose in a home setting
**Related term:** TLD badge
**Radiotherapy Example:** Checking residual household contamination

194. **Homogeneous phantom:** Phantom with uniform density and composition
**Related term:** Water phantom
**Radiotherapy Example:** Used for beam calibration

195. **Homogeneous radiation field:** Radiation field with even intensity distribution
**Related term:** Flatness
**Radiotherapy Example:** Achieved during linac beam tuning

196. **Homogeneity factor (radiotherapy):** A measure of how evenly dose is distributed within the target
**Related term:** Conformity index
**Radiotherapy Example:** Planning goal for IMRT dose uniformity

197. **Horizontal axis scanner:** Scanner where movement occurs along a horizontal axis
**Related term:** Flatbed scanner
**Radiotherapy Example:** Used for film dosimetry

198. **Horizontal beam therapy:** Treatment delivered with the beam oriented horizontally
**Related term:** Horizontal irradiation
**Radiotherapy Example:** Proton beamlines that deliver horizontal fields

199. **Horizontal irradiation technique:** Any method using horizontally directed beams
**Related term:** Beam orientation
**Radiotherapy Example:** Used in radiosurgery setups

200. **Hospital radiation monitoring:** Regular checks to ensure safe radiation levels throughout a medical facility
**Related term:** Radiation survey
**Radiotherapy Example:** Daily checks near linear accelerator vault entrances

201. **Hot spot (radiotherapy):** A region receiving a dose above the prescribed level within the target or surrounding tissue Often caused by beam overlap or heterogeneity Requires monitoring to avoid toxicity
**Related term:** Dose inhomogeneity
**Radiotherapy Example:** A 115% hot spot in IMRT requiring adjustment in optimization

202. **Hot spot analysis:** The evaluation of unusually high-dose regions using dose–volume histograms and isodose maps Helps identify potential areas of overdose
**Related term:** Isodose review
**Radiotherapy Example:** Checking hot spots >107% in breast tangential plans

203. **Hot spot contouring:** Delineating high-dose regions in the plan for dose tracking and optimization
**Related term:** Dose painting
**Radiotherapy Example:** Contouring a 110% region to avoid spinal cord overlap

204. **Hybrid CT-MRI imaging:** Combining CT and MRI images for enhanced planning accuracy by exploiting CT density and MRI soft-tissue detail
**Related term:** Multimodality fusion
**Radiotherapy Example:** Fusing T2 MRI with CT for prostate HDR brachytherapy

205. **Hybrid imaging fusion:** Software-based image alignment merging two different modalities for improved anatomical interpretation
**Related term:** Image registration
**Radiotherapy Example:** PET/CT fusion for head-and-neck tumor target delineation

206. **Hybrid MRI-PET scanner:** Simultaneous MRI and PET acquisition providing structural and metabolic information in one scan
**Related term:** PET-MR
**Radiotherapy Example:** Identifying hypoxic subregions for dose escalation

207. **Hybrid PET-CT:** Combined PET and CT system offering metabolic and anatomic data in a single session
**Related term:** PET/CT
**Radiotherapy Example:** Staging lung cancer prior to radiotherapy planning

208. **Hybrid radiographic system:** Imaging system integrating multiple detectors or modalities for enhanced performance
**Related term:** Dual-mode imaging
**Radiotherapy Example:** KV + MV imaging in IGRT platforms

209. **Hybrid treatment planning:** Using different beam modalities or algorithms in the same radiotherapy plan
**Related term:** Mixed-modality planning
**Radiotherapy Example:** Proton boost combined with photon IMRT

210. **Hyperfractionated radiotherapy:** Radiotherapy delivered in smaller doses more than once a day to exploit tumor radiosensitivity
**Related term:** Accelerated fractionation
**Radiotherapy Example:** 1 2 Gy twice daily for head-and-neck cancers

211. **Hyperfractionation scheme:** Structured plan defining dose per fraction, daily frequency, and total dose
**Related term:** Fractionation protocol
**Radiotherapy Example:** 1 1–1 2 Gy BID schedule for SCLC

212. **Hypermetabolic imaging:** Imaging identifying areas of elevated metabolic activity, often cancerous tissue
**Related term:** FDG uptake
**Radiotherapy Example:** PET-CT used to outline active lymphoma nodes

213. **Hypermetabolic lesion:** Region showing high tracer uptake indicating aggressive or viable tumor
**Related term:** Standard uptake value (SUV)
**Radiotherapy Example:** Used in planning boosts to metabolically active regions

214. **Hyperpolarized imaging:** MRI technique using hyperpolarized gases or tracers for enhanced signal
**Related term:** Hyperpolarized MRI
**Radiotherapy Example:** Hyperpolarized carbon-13 MRI in prostate cancer evaluation

215. **Hypertension-related radiosensitivity:** Increased sensitivity to radiation in patients with vascular disease or hypertension due to compromised microcirculation
**Related term:** Radiosensitivity factors
**Radiotherapy Example:** Extra caution in treating hypertensive patients with large fields

216. **Hyperspectral imaging:** Imaging capturing data across many wavelengths to detect tissue characteristics
**Related term:** Spectral analysis
**Radiotherapy Example:** Tissue oxygenation mapping in research radiobiology

217. **Hyperthermia therapy (adjunct to RT):** Applying heat to cancer tissues to increase radiation effectiveness via cellular stress
**Related term:** Thermal sensitization
**Radiotherapy Example:** Hyperthermia combined with radiotherapy for recurrent breast cancer

218. **Hyperthermia treatment planning:** Prediction and control of heat distribution in tumor tissues
**Related term:** Thermal dosimetry
**Radiotherapy Example:** Planning microwave hyperthermia for superficial tumors

219. **Hyperthyroid treatment with radioiodine:** I-131 administration to reduce thyroid hormone production
**Related term:** Nuclear medicine therapy
**Radiotherapy Example:** Typical dose 10–30 mCi for Graves' disease

220. **Hypofractionated radiotherapy:** Delivering larger doses per fraction over fewer sessions
**Related term:** SBRT
**Radiotherapy Example:** Breast cancer 40 Gy in 15 fractions

221. **Hypofractionation schedule:** Protocol defining large-fraction radiotherapy delivery
**Related term:** Hypofractionated regimen
**Radiotherapy Example:** Lung SBRT: 54 Gy in 3 fractions

222. **Hypogastric lymph node imaging:** Imaging of pelvic lymph nodes for cancer staging
**Related term:** Pelvic nodal mapping
**Radiotherapy Example:** MRI used to assess nodes before pelvic RT

223. **Hypogastric nodal irradiation:** Radiotherapy targeting pelvic lymph nodes
**Related term:** Pelvic field
**Radiotherapy Example:** Prostate cancer nodal irradiation

224. **Hypomethylation imaging marker:** Epigenetic markers detectable in imaging or correlated with radiomics data
**Related term:** Molecular imaging biomarker
**Radiotherapy Example:** Predictive models for radiation response

225. **Hypopituitarism after radiotherapy:** Hormone deficiency caused by pituitary radiation exposure
**Related term:** Endocrine toxicity
**Radiotherapy Example:** Late effect after cranial irradiation

226. **Hypoplastic bone imaging:** Imaging of underdeveloped bone structures
**Related term:** Bone dysplasia imaging
**Radiotherapy Example:** Planning RT in pediatric skeletal disorders

227. **Hypoxic cell fraction:** Percentage of tumor cells in low-oxygen state
**Related term:** Hypoxia index
**Radiotherapy Example:** Impacts need for dose escalation

228. **Hypoxic tumor dose escalation:** Increasing radiation dose to overcome hypoxia-induced resistance
**Related term:** Dose painting by contours
**Radiotherapy Example:** Boosting FMISO-avid regions

229. **Hypoxia-inducible factor imaging:** Imaging linked to HIF expression, indicating hypoxic tumor behavior
**Related term:** Molecular hypoxia imaging
**Radiotherapy Example:** Predicting aggressive tumor subregions

230. **Hypoxia mapping:** Visualization of oxygen-poor tumor regions
**Related term:** Hypoxia PET
**Radiotherapy Example:** Used in adaptive dose painting

231. **Hypoxia modifier drug:** Medication that improves tumor oxygenation
**Related term:** Radiosensitizer
**Radiotherapy Example:** Carbogen breathing during radiotherapy

232. **Hypoxic radiosensitizer:** Drug enhancing radiation kill in hypoxic cells
**Related term:** Nitroimidazole
**Radiotherapy Example:** Nimorazole for H&N cancers

233. **Hypoxic volume:** Volume of tumor identified as oxygen-deficient
**Related term:** Hypoxic burden
**Radiotherapy Example:** Determines boost region in IMRT

234. **Hypoplasia (radiation-induced):** Underdevelopment of tissue caused by radiation exposure
**Related term:** Late toxicity
**Radiotherapy Example:** Pediatric bone hypoplasia after cranial RT

235. **Hypoplastic tissue:** Tissue that is structurally underdeveloped
**Related term:** Developmental anomaly
**Radiotherapy Example:** Must be avoided in pediatric planning

236. **Hypoplastic organ imaging:** Imaging assessing organ size and morphology anomalies
**Related term:** Structural malformation
**Radiotherapy Example:** Preplanning evaluation for abdominal RT

237. **Hysterosalpingography radiation dose:** Dose delivered during contrast imaging of uterus and fallopian tubes
**Related term:** Gynecologic radiation dose
**Radiotherapy Example:** Important in infertility workup before pelvic RT

238. **Hysteresis artifact (MRI):** Distortion due to magnetic field lag or system instability
**Related term:** Magnetic drift
**Radiotherapy Example:** Artifact reduction is important in MRI-only planning

239. **Hardware attenuation correction:** Adjustment for imaging attenuation caused by hardware (e g , coils)
**Related term:** Correction map
**Radiotherapy Example:** Essential in PET/MR planning

240. **Helium gas detector:** Detector that uses helium gas to measure radiation, often neutron-sensitive
**Related term:** Gas-filled detector
**Radiotherapy Example:** Monitoring neutron dose in 18 MV beam linac rooms

241. **Hematologic toxicity (radiotherapy):** Bone marrow suppression caused by radiation exposure
**Related term:** Myelosuppression
**Radiotherapy Example:** Pelvic RT affecting marrow reserves

242. **Hemodynamic imaging:** Imaging blood flow using advanced MRI or CT techniques
**Related term:** Perfusion imaging
**Radiotherapy Example:** Evaluating tumor perfusion changes during treatment

243. **Hemoglobin oxygenation mapping:** Imaging technique evaluating tissue oxygen saturation
**Related term:** BOLD MRI
**Radiotherapy Example:** Tumor oxygenation research in radiobiology

244. **Hemorrhagic lesion imaging:** Visualization of bleeding within tissues
**Related term:** Susceptibility-weighted imaging
**Radiotherapy Example:** Identifying hemorrhage after brain radiosurgery

245. **Heterogeneous dose distribution:** Non-uniform dose across the target or organs
**Related term:** Inhomogeneity index
**Radiotherapy Example:** Acceptable in SBRT with hotspot allowances

246. **Heterogeneous tissue imaging:** Identifying nonuniform tissue characteristics
**Related term:** Tissue segmentation
**Radiotherapy Example:** Important in lung tumor delineation

247. **Heterogeneity correction:** Adjusting dose calculations for differing tissue densities
**Related term:** Electron density correction
**Radiotherapy Example:** Must be applied in lung IMRT

248. **Hexapod couch:** Treatment couch with 6 degrees of freedom for precise positioning
**Related term:** 6-DoF couch
**Radiotherapy Example:** SRS treatments requiring sub-mm precision

249. **High-altitude radiation exposure:** Increased exposure to cosmic radiation at high elevations
**Related term:** Cosmic rays
**Radiotherapy Example:** Relevant for pilot cumulative dose studies

250. **High-attenuation object imaging:** Imaging materials that strongly absorb X-rays
**Related term:** Beam hardening
**Radiotherapy Example:** Metal artifact reduction in CT planning

251. **High-contrast imaging:** Imaging with excellent separation of different tissue types
**Related term:** Contrast resolution
**Radiotherapy Example:** T1 MRI for brain tumor visualization

252. **High-contrast resolution:** Ability to differentiate small objects with slight density differences
**Related term:** Spatial resolution
**Radiotherapy Example:** Important for detecting small lymph nodes

253. **High-dose gradient:** Rapid change in dose over a small distance
**Related term:** Penumbra sharpness
**Radiotherapy Example:** SBRT near spinal cord

254. **High-dose region:** Zone receiving above-prescribed dose
**Related term:** Hot spot
**Radiotherapy Example:** >110% region in IMRT must be justified

255. **High-dose CT protocol:** CT imaging with higher radiation dose for improved detail
**Related term:** Diagnostic CT
**Radiotherapy Example:** Used for detailed lung imaging

256. **High-dose nuclear imaging:** Nuclear scans requiring elevated tracer activity
**Related term:** Radiotracer dose
**Radiotherapy Example:** Post-therapy I-131 scan

257. **High-dose region contour:** Contouring high-dose volumes for assessment
**Related term:** DVH evaluation
**Radiotherapy Example:** Defining 105% volume in SBRT QA

258. **High-dose SPECT imaging:** SPECT performed with high radiotracer activity
**Related term:** Gamma imaging
**Radiotherapy Example:** Mapping Y-90 distribution

259. **High-energy attenuation:** Reduction in beam intensity in high-energy photon/electron beams
**Related term:** Attenuation coefficient
**Radiotherapy Example:** Shielding calculations

260. **High-energy collimator:** Collimator designed for high-energy gamma rays
**Related term:** Parallel-hole collimator
**Radiotherapy Example:** Y-90 bremsstrahlung imaging

261. **High-energy electron contamination:** Unwanted electrons produced in megavoltage photon beams
**Related term:** Secondary electrons
**Radiotherapy Example:** Surface dose evaluation

262. **High-energy physics detector:** Detector used to characterize radiation particles
**Related term:** Particle detector
**Radiotherapy Example:** Used in proton therapy beamline QA

263. **High-energy photon attenuation:** Reduction in MV photon beam intensity through tissue or shielding
**Related term:** Attenuation law
**Radiotherapy Example:** Calculating primary barrier thickness

264. **High-energy proton dosimetry:** Measuring dose from high-energy proton beams
**Related term:** Ionization chamber
**Radiotherapy Example:** Commissioning proton therapy systems

265. **High-energy radiation dosimeter:** Device capable of measuring MV or particle radiation doses
**Related term:** Farmer chamber
**Radiotherapy Example:** Calibrating linac output

266. **High-energy scattering:** Deflection of particles at high energy
**Related term:** Lateral scattering
**Radiotherapy Example:** Affects proton penumbra

267. **High-energy X-ray beam quality:** Characterization of MV beam penetration and hardness
**Related term:** PDD curve
**Radiotherapy Example:** 6 MV vs 10 MV beam comparison

268. **High-field MRI:** MRI scanners operating at 3T or higher
**Related term:** Ultra-high-field MRI
**Radiotherapy Example:** Brain tumor mapping

269. **High-frequency ultrasound:** Ultrasound with >10 MHz frequency for high detail
**Related term:** High-resolution ultrasound
**Radiotherapy Example:** Prostate brachytherapy guidance

270. **High-intensity focused ultrasound (HIFU):** Ultrasound waves concentrated to ablate tissue
**Related term:** Thermal ablation
**Radiotherapy Example:** Used as alternative or adjunct in prostate cancer

271. **High-MV imaging:** Imaging using MV beams instead of kV
**Related term:** Portal imaging
**Radiotherapy Example:** Setup verification

272. **High-precision dosimeter:** Highly accurate device for dose measurement
**Related term:** Reference dosimeter
**Radiotherapy Example:** IAEA-calibrated chamber for output checks

273. **High-purity germanium detector:** Semiconductor detector with excellent gamma energy resolution
**Related term:** HPGe detector
**Radiotherapy Example:** Measuring brachytherapy source spectrum

274. **High-resolution beam profiler:** Device mapping the profile of radiation beams
**Related term:** Beam analyzer
**Radiotherapy Example:** Checking FFF beam shape

275. **High-resolution cone-beam CT:** CBCT with improved reconstruction detail
**Related term:** HR-CBCT
**Radiotherapy Example:** SRS patient verification

276. **High-resolution dose grid:** Fine 3D matrix for calculating dose
**Related term:** Dose voxel
**Radiotherapy Example:** SBRT requires 1–2 mm grids

277. **High-resolution dosimetry:** Measurement with fine spatial resolution
**Related term:** Microdosimetry
**Radiotherapy Example:** Film dosimetry in IMRT QA

278. **High-resolution gamma imaging:** Gamma imaging with improved collimator design
**Related term:** Multipinhole SPECT
**Radiotherapy Example:** Sentinel node mapping

279. **High-resolution ion chamber array:** Array of numerous small ion chambers
**Related term:** Detector matrix
**Radiotherapy Example:** IMRT QA detector panel

280. **High-resolution MR angiography:** Detailed MRI of blood vessels
**Related term:** MRA
**Radiotherapy Example:** Avoiding vascular structures in brain RT

281. **High-resolution optical imaging:** Optical methods for microscopic detail
**Related term:** Confocal imaging
**Radiotherapy Example:** Research radiation biology

282. **High-resolution radiograph:** X-ray with excellent spatial detail
**Related term:** Fine-focus radiography
**Radiotherapy Example:** Orthopedic imaging for RT planning

283. **High-resolution scanner:** Device capable of fine-detail imaging
**Related term:** DPI resolution
**Radiotherapy Example:** Film dosimetry scanning

284. **High-resolution ultrasound imaging:** Ultrasound with detailed visualization
**Related term:** High-frequency US
**Radiotherapy Example:** Prostate seed placement verification

285. **High-sensitivity PET detector:** PET system designed to detect weak radiotracer signals
**Related term:** TOF PET
**Radiotherapy Example:** Early tumor response evaluation

286. **High-sensitivity scintillator:** Scintillation crystal with high light output
**Related term:** NaI(Tl)
**Radiotherapy Example:** Gamma probe in thyroid cancer

287. **High-speed CT:** CT acquiring slices rapidly
**Related term:** Multidetector CT
**Radiotherapy Example:** 4DCT acquisition for motion assessment

288. **High-speed MRI:** MRI with accelerated acquisition
**Related term:** Parallel imaging
**Radiotherapy Example:** Fast T2 scans in MR-Linac

289. **High-speed PET:** PET systems with rapid temporal resolution
**Related term:** Dynamic PET
**Radiotherapy Example:** Assessing tracer kinetics mid-treatment

290. **High-speed radiography:** Rapid acquisition X-ray imaging
**Related term:** Fluoroscopy
**Radiotherapy Example:** Brachytherapy catheter placement

291. **High-voltage power supply (linac):** Provides necessary potential difference for accelerating electrons
**Related term:** Klystron power
**Radiotherapy Example:** Controls linac output energy

292. **High-voltage X-ray tube:** Tube producing high-energy diagnostic X-rays
**Related term:** Anode voltage
**Radiotherapy Example:** Simulator imaging tube

293. **Histochemical staining imaging:** Microscopic imaging after chemical tissue staining
**Related term:** Digital pathology
**Radiotherapy Example:** Correlates imaging and biopsy data

294. **Histological grading imaging correlation:** Comparing imaging features to histologic grade
**Related term:** Radiomics
**Radiotherapy Example:** MRI predicting glioma grade

295. **Hollow applicator (brachytherapy):** Tube-like device used to insert radioactive sources
**Related term:** Brachy applicator
**Radiotherapy Example:** Tandem-and-ovoid device for cervix

296. **Homogeneous beam profile:** Even radiation intensity across beam width
**Related term:** Flatness
**Radiotherapy Example:** Required in calibration beams

297. **Homogeneous density phantom:** Phantom with uniform composition for calibration
**Related term:** Water-equivalent phantom
**Radiotherapy Example:** Linac output calibration

298. **Homogeneous dose calculation:** Simplified calculation assuming uniform tissue
**Related term:** Water-based calc
**Radiotherapy Example:** Used historically before heterogeneity corrections

299. **Homogeneous field distribution:** Even radiation across the treatment field
**Related term:** Uniformity
**Radiotherapy Example:** Ensured in TBI fields

300. **Homologous imaging:** Imaging comparing anatomically similar regions
**Related term:** Symmetric imaging
**Radiotherapy Example:** Contralateral breast comparison for planning

301. **High-speed digital imaging:** Fast-frame imaging system used for capturing quick motion sequences
**Related term:** High-frame-rate camera
**Radiotherapy Example:** Used to record MLC leaf speed accuracy during QA

302. **High-speed dosimetry system:** Real-time system capable of rapidly measuring changing dose rates
**Related term:** Fast-response detector
**Radiotherapy Example:** Used in FLASH radiotherapy research where dose rates change extremely fast

303. **High-speed dynamic beam delivery:** Radiation delivery technique using rapid gantry and MLC motion
**Related term:** VMAT
**Radiotherapy Example:** VMAT prostate plans rely on fast MLC movement and arc modulation

304. **High-speed electronics in radiation detectors:** Detector electronics designed to respond to very short pulses
**Related term:** Fast-timing circuitry
**Radiotherapy Example:** LINAC pulse detection uses high-speed electronics for accurate metering

305. **High-speed scanning:** Rapid acquisition of imaging data over a large region
**Related term:** Fast CT acquisition
**Radiotherapy Example:** Used in 4D-CT to capture respiratory motion accurately

306. **High-speed shutter mechanism:** Mechanical or electronic shutter used to control brief radiation pulses
**Related term:** Beam gating
**Radiotherapy Example:** Used in synchrotron-based particle therapy to shape microsecond beams

307. **High-speed signal processing:** Rapid digital processing of detector signals
**Related term:** FPGA processing
**Radiotherapy Example:** Modern EPIDs use high-speed processing for real-time portal imaging

308. **High-stability calibration source:** A reference radioactive source with nearly constant activity over long periods
**Related term:** Check source
**Radiotherapy Example:** Cs-137 sources used for daily dosimeter verification

309. **High-stability electronics:** Electronics designed with minimal drift and temperature sensitivity
**Related term:** Low-noise circuitry
**Radiotherapy Example:** Ion chamber electrometers require high stability for small field dosimetry

310. **High-stability imaging system:** Imaging platforms designed to maintain geometric accuracy over time
**Related term:** System integrity
**Radiotherapy Example:** CBCT systems require mechanical stability for sub-millimeter alignment

311. **High-stability LINAC output:** Beam output consistency maintained over daily operations
**Related term:** Output constancy
**Radiotherapy Example:** Daily QA verifies high-stability photon and electron output

312. **High-stability patient support system:** Treatment couches that maintain precise positioning with minimal sag
**Related term:** Robotic couch
**Radiotherapy Example:** 6-DOF couches maintain accuracy during head-and-neck RT

313. **High-stability radiation beam:** Beam with minimal fluctuations in dose rate or energy
**Related term:** Beam flatness consistency
**Radiotherapy Example:** Required for IMRT to prevent dose delivery errors

314. **High-stability temperature-controlled dosimetry:** Dosimetry setup maintained at stable temperature to reduce measurement drift
**Related term:** Temperature correction factor
**Radiotherapy Example:** Water tank calibration uses controlled temperature to ensure accuracy

315. **High-strength magnetic field interaction:** Behavior of devices and tissues under very powerful magnetic fields
**Related term:** Magnetic susceptibility
**Radiotherapy Example:** MR-Linacs operate at 0 35–1 5 T fields affecting dose deposition

316. **High-strength radioactive source capsule:** Encased high-activity source used in brachytherapy
**Related term:** HDR source
**Radiotherapy Example:** Ir-192 HDR capsules require extremely strong containment

317. **High-surface-dose phenomenon:** Elevated radiation dose at or near the skin surface
**Related term:** Buildup region
**Radiotherapy Example:** Bolus is used intentionally to increase surface dose for skin cancers

318. **High-susceptibility artifact:** MRI distortion caused by materials with large differences in magnetic properties
**Related term:** Magnetic artifact
**Radiotherapy Example:** Dental fillings create distortions in MRI used for H&N planning

319. **High-symmetry beam profile:** Beam with uniform intensity distribution mirrored across central axis
**Related term:** Beam flatness
**Radiotherapy Example:** Required for accurate open-field commissioning

320. **High-target-dose distribution:** A plan delivering elevated dose concentration within tumor boundaries
**Related term:** Conformal dose
**Radiotherapy Example:** SRS boosts deliver very high dose to small intracranial lesions

321. **High-teal shielding material:** Radiological shielding material with extremely high attenuation properties
**Related term:** Dense shielding
**Radiotherapy Example:** Tungsten alloys used in MLC leaves

322. **High-TE MRI imaging:** MRI imaging performed with long echo time to enhance T2 contrast
**Related term:** T2-weighted imaging
**Radiotherapy Example:** Used for contouring edema in brain tumor planning

323. **High-temperature annealing of dosimeters:** Heating dosimeters to erase previous signal before reuse
**Related term:** Annealing cycle
**Radiotherapy Example:** TLD annealing performed before patient dosimetry measurements

324. **High-temperature detector calibration:** Calibration of detectors designed to tolerate high heat
**Related term:** Thermal stability
**Radiotherapy Example:** Used in environmental radiation monitoring near accelerator vaults

325. **High-temperature radiation effects:** Material degradation caused by radiation at elevated temperatures
**Related term:** Thermal radiation damage
**Radiotherapy Example:** Seen in components of high-power accelerators

326. **High-term image reconstruction:** Complex mathematical reconstruction using high-order terms to improve accuracy
**Related term:** Iterative reconstruction
**Radiotherapy Example:** Used in advanced CT algorithms for treatment planning

327. **High-test-fidelity QA:** QA with strict tolerance limits and high measurement precision
**Related term:** End-to-end testing
**Radiotherapy Example:** Mandatory for SRS/SBRT delivery systems

328. **High-thermal-neutron cross-section:** Probability of nuclei absorbing thermal neutrons effectively
**Related term:** Neutron capture
**Radiotherapy Example:** Boron-10 used in BNCT due to high cross-section

329. **High-threshold detector:** Detector that only responds to radiation above a certain preset threshold
**Related term:** Thresholding
**Radiotherapy Example:** Used in pulse-counting applications for LINAC monitoring

330. **High-throughput particle accelerator:** Accelerator capable of delivering high beam output for extended periods
**Related term:** High-duty-cycle accelerator
**Radiotherapy Example:** Used in hospitals with high patient load in proton therapy

331. **High-throughput radiation analysis system:** Automated platform capable of rapidly analyzing multiple radiation samples or datasets
**Related term:** Automated dosimetry
**Radiotherapy Example:** Used in large hospitals to process many patient-specific QA films quickly

332. **High-throughput radioisotope production:** System capable of generating large quantities of isotopes efficiently
**Related term:** Isotope yield
**Radiotherapy Example:** Needed for high-demand radionuclides like Tc-99m or F-18 PET tracers

333. **High-throughput radiotherapy planning:** Workflow designed to create many treatment plans efficiently, using automation
**Related term:** Auto-planning
**Radiotherapy Example:** AI-based tools generate prostate IMRT plans in minutes

334. **High-throughput radiation research:** Research environment enabling rapid, repeated radiation experiments
**Related term:** Radiation automation
**Radiotherapy Example:** Used in radiobiology labs studying thousands of cell samples

335. **High-throughput QA program:** QA system optimized to complete many machine or patient QA tasks quickly
**Related term:** Streamlined QA
**Radiotherapy Example:** Automated QA phantoms speed up daily LINAC checks

336. **High-tissue-contrast imaging:** Imaging that provides clear differentiation between soft tissues
**Related term:** MRI contrast
**Radiotherapy Example:** Useful in MR-guided radiotherapy for prostate and liver tumors

337. **High-tissue-density artifact:** Imaging artifact caused by very dense tissues or implants
**Related term:** Beam hardening artifact
**Radiotherapy Example:** Hip prostheses produce streak artifacts on CT used for RT planning

338. **High-tissue-dose gradient:** Region where dose falls off rapidly between target and normal tissue
**Related term:** Sharp falloff
**Radiotherapy Example:** SRS plans use extreme gradients to protect healthy brain

339. **High-tissue-sparing technique:** Radiotherapy method designed to minimize exposure of normal tissue
**Related term:** Conformal therapy
**Radiotherapy Example:** IMRT sparing parotid glands in head and neck cancer

340. **High-tolerance radiation equipment:** Equipment capable of functioning under high radiation stress without failure
**Related term:** Radiation-hardened devices
**Radiotherapy Example:** Electronics inside a LINAC head must withstand long-term radiation exposure

341. **High-tolerance patient immobilization:** Patient immobilization systems that maintain excellent reproducibility
**Related term:** Thermoplastic mask
**Radiotherapy Example:** SRS frames offer extremely high positional tolerance

342. **High-tracking-accuracy system:** System capable of following patient or tumor motion precisely
**Related term:** Motion tracking
**Radiotherapy Example:** CyberKnife uses real-time tracking for lung tumor RT

343. **High-trapped-charge dosimeter:** Dosimeter that retains charge for long periods due to material properties
**Related term:** OSL dosimeter
**Radiotherapy Example:** OSLDs hold signal for months, useful in postal dosimetry audits

344. **High-transmission detector:** Detector designed to allow most of the beam to pass through unperturbed
**Related term:** Transmission chamber
**Radiotherapy Example:** Used in LINAC output monitoring in the beam path

345. **High-transmission multi-leaf collimator (MLC):** MLC with low leaf attenuation allowing high beam throughput
**Related term:** Low-leakage MLC
**Radiotherapy Example:** Modern MLCs have <1 5% transmission for IMRT

346. **High-transparency bolus:** Bolus material designed to be optically transparent for alignment purposes
**Related term:** Gel bolus
**Radiotherapy Example:** Transparent bolus helps visualize skin marks for breast RT

347. **High-transport-energy particle:** Particle with enough kinetic energy to travel significant distances
**Related term:** High-energy ion
**Radiotherapy Example:** Proton beams travel deep before depositing Bragg peak dose

348. **High-tube-current CT scan:** CT scan performed at elevated tube current to reduce image noise
**Related term:** Tube mA
**Radiotherapy Example:** Planning CT sometimes uses higher mA for clearer tumor edges

349. **High-turbulence air dosimetry environment:** Environment where airflow reduces dosimetry accuracy
**Related term:** Air pressure instability
**Radiotherapy Example:** Avoided during ion chamber calibration in open rooms

350. **High-TV (tenth-value) layer shielding:** Material thickness needed to reduce radiation intensity to one-tenth
**Related term:** HVL
**Radiotherapy Example:** Used to calculate concrete thickness for LINAC bunkers

351. **High-ultrasound-frequency imaging:** Ultrasound imaging using very high frequencies (>10 MHz) for fine detail
**Related term:** High-resolution US
**Radiotherapy Example:** Used for prostate seed implant guidance

352. **High-uniformity beam scanner:** Device ensuring uniform scanning of electron or proton beams
**Related term:** Scanning magnet
**Radiotherapy Example:** Pencil beam proton therapy relies on uniform scanning fields

353. **High-uniformity CT image:** CT image with uniform pixel values across the scan field
**Related term:** CT uniformity test
**Radiotherapy Example:** Verified during commissioning to ensure accurate density calibration

354. **High-uniformity dosimeter response:** Dosimeter that provides consistent readings across its surface
**Related term:** Homogeneous response
**Radiotherapy Example:** Film dosimetry requires uniform response for QA maps

355. **High-upscatter radiation:** Increased level of scattered radiation in specific geometries
**Related term:** Scatter radiation
**Radiotherapy Example:** Occurs around irregular patient shapes during photon RT

356. **High-use-area radiation zone:** Area frequently occupied by staff; requires strict exposure limits
**Related term:** Controlled area
**Radiotherapy Example:** Control rooms adjacent to LINAC suites must keep dose < annual limits

357. **High-utility field shaping:** Versatile use of beam-shaping tools to create complex fields
**Related term:** Conformal shaping
**Radiotherapy Example:** MLCs allow highly customized IMRT beam shapes

358. **High-value dosimeter calibration:** Calibration for high-accuracy measurement applications
**Related term:** Reference dosimetry
**Radiotherapy Example:** Absolute dose calibration with a calibrated ion chamber

359. **High-variability radiation field:** Field with substantial intensity variation
**Related term:** Inhomogeneous beam
**Radiotherapy Example:** Avoided in clinical beams but can occur in experimental setups

360. **High-velocity charged particle:** Particle moving at high speed with significant kinetic energy
**Related term:** Relativistic ion
**Radiotherapy Example:** Carbon ions travel at high velocities before depositing Bragg peak dose

361. **High-velocity detector response:** Detector able to accurately measure fast-moving radiation signals
**Related term:** Fast-response detector
**Radiotherapy Example:** Needed for pulsed radiation such as LINAC beams

362. **High-ventilation imaging:** Imaging to assess airflow or air exchange in lungs
**Related term:** Ventilation scan
**Radiotherapy Example:** SPECT ventilation scans used to spare functioning lung in RT planning

363. **High-vertex-angle imaging:** Imaging where gantry or camera is tilted at steep angles
**Related term:** Oblique imaging
**Radiotherapy Example:** Used in kV radiographs to verify spine alignment

364. **High-vibration-tolerance gantry:** Gantry designed to resist mechanical vibrations
**Related term:** Mechanical stability
**Radiotherapy Example:** Important for precise arc therapy delivery

365. **High-visibility alignment lasers:** Bright lasers for accurate patient setup
**Related term:** Positioning lasers
**Radiotherapy Example:** LINAC rooms use high-visibility red or green lasers

366. **High-visibility markers:** Radiopaque or high-contrast fiducial markers
**Related term:** Gold seed
**Radiotherapy Example:** Implanted fiducials for prostate tracking

367. **High-volume air sampler for radioactivity:** Device sampling large air volumes to detect airborne radioactive particles
**Related term:** Air monitor
**Radiotherapy Example:** Used in areas where unsealed isotopes are handled

368. **High-voltage cable (LINAC):** Cable supplying high voltage to LINAC components
**Related term:** Accelerator cable
**Radiotherapy Example:** Must be inspected during preventive maintenance

369. **High-voltage connection diagnostics:** Process of checking HV cables and connectors
**Related term:** Electrical QA
**Radiotherapy Example:** Performed when LINAC exhibits unstable beam output

370. **High-voltage diode:** Diode capable of withstanding high reverse voltages
**Related term:** Rectifier
**Radiotherapy Example:** Used in power supplies of imaging and LINAC systems

371. **High-voltage generator:** Generator producing high voltages for imaging or therapy devices
**Related term:** HV supply
**Radiotherapy Example:** kV X-ray systems rely on high-voltage generators

372. **High-voltage insulation:** Insulation material designed to prevent electrical breakdown
**Related term:** Dielectric insulation
**Radiotherapy Example:** LINAC head components require radiation-resistant insulation

373. **High-voltage ionization chamber:** Ion chamber operated at elevated voltage for increased sensitivity
**Related term:** Saturation voltage
**Radiotherapy Example:** Used in some environmental radiation monitors

374. **High-voltage leakage test:** Procedure to ensure no unwanted current escapes from HV components
**Related term:** Electrical safety test
**Radiotherapy Example:** Required after servicing LINAC HV systems

375. **High-voltage multiplier circuit:** Circuit multiplying input voltage to produce very high output
**Related term:** Cockcroft–Walton generator
**Radiotherapy Example:** Used in early accelerator designs

376. **High-voltage power supply stabilization:** Ensuring power supply maintains constant output
**Related term:** Voltage regulation
**Radiotherapy Example:** Crucial for stable kV imaging

377. **High-voltage pulse modulator:** Device generating short, high-voltage pulses
**Related term:** Modulator
**Radiotherapy Example:** LINACs use modulators to drive electron guns and klystrons

378. **High-voltage transformer:** Transformer used to step up voltage
**Related term:** HV transformer
**Radiotherapy Example:** Used in X-ray tube power supplies

379. **High-voltage transistor switch:** Transistor used to control HV circuits
**Related term:** MOSFET switch
**Radiotherapy Example:** Employed in LINAC control circuits

380. **High-voltage vacuum relay:** Relay operating under vacuum for high-voltage switching
**Related term:** HV relay
**Radiotherapy Example:** Used in safety interlocks

381. **High-voltage waveform monitoring:** Measuring high-voltage pulse shapes and stability
**Related term:** Waveform QA
**Radiotherapy Example:** Critical for diagnosing LINAC modulator issues

382. **High-voltage X-ray tube:** Tube designed to operate at very high potentials to produce hard X-rays
**Related term:** kV X-ray tube
**Radiotherapy Example:** Used in CT scanners and IGRT systems

383. **High-wattage beam collimator:** Collimator capable of handling high thermal loads
**Related term:** Heat-resistant collimator
**Radiotherapy Example:** Used in high-dose-rate photon therapy

384. **High-weighting-factor radiation:** Radiation type assigned a high radiation weighting factor (WR)
**Related term:** RBE
**Radiotherapy Example:** Alpha particles have high weighting factors in dose calculations

385. **High-wind interference in dosimetry:** Wind affecting outdoor or field radiation measurements
**Related term:** Environmental influence
**Radiotherapy Example:** Considered when calibrating portable survey meters

386. **High-workload shielding calculation:** Shielding design for facilities with high patient throughput
**Related term:** Use factor
**Radiotherapy Example:** Proton centers with many treatments need increased shielding

387. **High-yield isotope:** Radioisotope produced at high efficiency
**Related term:** Production yield
**Radiotherapy Example:** F-18 used in FDG PET has high production yield

388. **High-yield neutron source:** Source producing large numbers of neutrons
**Related term:** Neutron generator
**Radiotherapy Example:** Used in research facilities for BNCT

389. **High-yield photon production:** Efficient generation of photons in accelerators
**Related term:** Bremsstrahlung yield
**Radiotherapy Example:** LINAC targets are designed to maximize photon yield

**390. High-Z shielding material:** Shielding material with high atomic number, effective at photon attenuation
**Related term:** Lead
**Radiotherapy Example:** Tungsten used in MLC leaves and shielding blocks

**391. High-Z target (LINAC):** High atomic number metal target used to produce X-rays via bremsstrahlung
**Related term:** Tungsten target
**Radiotherapy Example:** LINACs use tungsten targets to generate MV photon beams

**392. High-zoom imaging:** Imaging with magnified field of view for detail
**Related term:** Magnification mode
**Radiotherapy Example:** kV imaging magnification helps detect small fiducials

**393. High-zone radiation monitoring:** Monitoring in areas with elevated, controlled radiation levels
**Related term:** Radiation survey
**Radiotherapy Example:** Monitors installed in brachytherapy rooms

**394. High-dose hypersensitivity (HRS):** Paradoxical increase in cell killing at very low doses before a threshold
**Related term:** Low-dose hyper-radiosensitivity
**Radiotherapy Example:** Studied in dose-painting strategies

**395. High-dose irradiation chamber:** Chamber built to withstand and measure very high doses
**Related term:** High-dose dosimetry
**Radiotherapy Example:** Used for calibrating TLDs and radiochromic film

**396. High-dose measurement protocol:** Standardized steps for measuring doses above typical clinical ranges
**Related term:** Calibration protocol
**Radiotherapy Example:** Used in SRS QA where doses per fraction are very high

**397. High-dose photobiology study:** Research studying biological effects of high photon doses
**Related term:** Radiobiology
**Radiotherapy Example:** Used for understanding tissue response in radiosurgery

**398. High-dose-rate photon exposure:** Photon exposure administered at high dose per unit time
**Related term:** HDR
**Radiotherapy Example:** FLASH RT uses extremely high dose rates

**399. High-dose-rate stereotactic irradiation:** Stereotactic radiation delivered at high dose rates for rapid treatment
**Related term:** SRS
**Radiotherapy Example:** CyberKnife delivers high-dose-rate beams to brain lesions

**400. High-dose total body irradiation (TBI):** High-dose radiation delivered to the entire body, typically before transplantation
**Related term:** Conditioning regimen
**Radiotherapy Example:** Used in leukemia preparation for bone marrow transplant

**401. High-dose-volume region:** Region in a dose distribution receiving higher-than-prescribed dose
**Related term:** Hot spot
**Radiotherapy Example:** IMRT plans aim to keep high-dose-volume regions outside critical organs

402. **High-energy activation product:** Radioactive isotopes created when high-energy particles interact with materials
**Related term:** Activation
**Radiotherapy Example:** LINAC head components can become mildly activated after high-energy treatments

403. **High-energy accelerator head shielding:** Shielding within the LINAC head to contain scatter and leakage
**Related term:** Tungsten shielding
**Radiotherapy Example:** Required to keep head leakage < 0 1% of central beam

404. **High-energy beam attenuation:** Reduction of intensity as a high-energy beam passes through material
**Related term:** Transmission
**Radiotherapy Example:** Used to calculate thickness of compensators in photon therapy

405. **High-energy beam contamination:** Unwanted particles (e g , electrons, neutrons) mixed into the primary beam
**Related term:** Neutron contamination
**Radiotherapy Example:** Neutrons appear in >10 MV beams and increase shielding requirements

406. **High-energy beam delivery system:** System enabling precise delivery of high-energy photons or particles
**Related term:** Beamline
**Radiotherapy Example:** Proton therapy uses complex beam delivery nozzles

407. **High-energy beam divergence:** Spread of the beam as it travels away from the source
**Related term:** Penumbra
**Radiotherapy Example:** Important for field-edge sharpness in LINAC photons

408. **High-energy beam dosimeter:** Dosimeter designed for accurate measurement of high-energy radiation fields
**Related term:** Ionization chamber
**Radiotherapy Example:** Farmer chambers used for MV beam calibration.

409. **High-energy beam focusing:** Techniques to reduce beam spread
**Related term:** Beam collimation
**Radiotherapy Example:** Electron cones narrow electron beams for superficial therapy

410. **High-energy beam homogenizer:** Device to make the beam intensity uniform
**Related term:** Flattening filter
**Radiotherapy Example:** Older LINACs used flattening filters before FFF beams

411. **High-energy beam interaction:** Interplay between high-energy radiation and matter
**Related term:** Compton effect
**Radiotherapy Example:** Dominant interaction for MV photons in tissue

412. **High-energy beam mapping:** Mapping dose distribution across the irradiation field
**Related term:** Beam profiling
**Radiotherapy Example:** Performed during linear accelerator commissioning

413. **High-energy beam modeling:** Mathematical modeling of radiation beam characteristics
**Related term:** Treatment planning algorithm
**Radiotherapy Example:** Monte Carlo modeling in proton therapy planning

414. **High-energy beam optimization:** Adjusting beam parameters to achieve ideal treatment distributions
**Related term:** Beam shaping
**Radiotherapy Example:** IMRT optimization selects optimal beam fluence patterns

415. **High-energy beam penetration:** Depth to which high-energy radiation travels in tissue
**Related term:** PDD (percent depth dose)
**Radiotherapy Example:** 15 MV photons penetrate deeper than 6 MV

416. **High-energy beam profiling:** Measurement of beam flatness, symmetry, field size, and intensity
**Related term:** Water tank scanning
**Radiotherapy Example:** Used for QA and annual commissioning

417. **High-energy beam scattering:** Deflection of high-energy particles as they interact with matter
**Related term:** Lateral scatter
**Radiotherapy Example:** Electron therapy beams scatter significantly in tissue

418. **High-energy beam shaping:** Modifying beam geometry using collimators or MLCs
**Related term:** Conformal therapy
**Radiotherapy Example:** MLC shaping for IMRT head-and-neck plans

419. **High-energy beam spectrum:** Distribution of photon or particle energies within a beam
**Related term:** Energy fluence
**Radiotherapy Example:** MV photon beams have broad energy spectra from bremsstrahlung

420. **High-energy beam steering:** Maintaining beam alignment using magnetic or electronic controls
**Related term:** Steering coil
**Radiotherapy Example:** LINACs perform automatic beam steering corrections daily

421. **High-energy beta radiation:** Fast electrons emitted from radionuclides
**Related term:** Beta emitter
**Radiotherapy Example:** Used in some eye plaques and therapeutic radionuclides

422. **High-energy bremsstrahlung:** Radiation produced when high-speed electrons are decelerated
**Related term:** Photon beam
**Radiotherapy Example:** Foundation of LINAC photon beam creation

423. **High-energy calibration field:** Reference radiation field used for calibrating dosimeters
**Related term:** Standard beam quality
**Radiotherapy Example:** 10x10 100 cm SSD reference field for MV beams

424. **High-energy charged particle beam:** Beam of ions or electrons used in therapy or research
**Related term:** Particle therapy
**Radiotherapy Example:** Proton beams at 230 MeV

425. **High-energy Compton interaction:** Dominant photon interaction in MV photon therapy
**Related term:** Compton scatter
**Radiotherapy Example:** Determines tissue contrast in MV imaging

426. **High-energy conformal radiotherapy:** Therapy using high-energy beams shaped to tumor anatomy
**Related term:** 3D-CRT
**Radiotherapy Example:** Breast tangents using 6 MV beams

427. **High-energy contaminant electron:** Electrons present in photon beams due to interactions in the LINAC head
**Related term:** Electron contamination
**Radiotherapy Example:** Causes higher skin dose in MV photons

**428. High-energy CT imaging:** CT imaging using elevated kVp for improved penetration through dense tissues
**Related term:** 140 kVp
**Radiotherapy Example:** Used for large patients or metallic implants

**429. High-energy dose computation:** Dose algorithms optimized for MV photon beams
**Related term:** Collapsed cone
**Radiotherapy Example:** TPS uses algorithms tuned for 6–15 MV beams

**430. High-energy dose deposition:** Pattern of energy delivered by high-energy radiation in tissue
**Related term:** Depth dose curve
**Radiotherapy Example:** Measured to validate LINAC beam performance

**431. High-energy dose falloff:** Decrease in dose beyond the depth of maximum dose
**Related term:** PDD slope
**Radiotherapy Example:** Important for sparing spinal cord in lung RT

**432. High-energy dose fraction:** Portion of total dose delivered by high-energy beams
**Related term:** Beam weighting
**Radiotherapy Example:** Mixed-energy breast plans may include 6 MV and 10 MV fractions

**433. High-energy dose gradient:** Steep rate of change in dose
**Related term:** Penumbra
**Radiotherapy Example:** SRS photon beams produce extremely steep gradients

**434. High-energy dose kernel:** Precomputed dose distribution for a given beam energy
**Related term:** Convolution algorithm
**Radiotherapy Example:** Used in dose calculation engines

**435. High-energy dose mapping:** Detailed spatial mapping of delivered dose
**Related term:** Dose plane
**Radiotherapy Example:** Film QA for IMRT uses dose mapping

**436. High-energy dose measurement:** Measurement methodology tailored to MV beams
**Related term:** Absolute calibration
**Radiotherapy Example:** TG-51 protocol for MV photon dosimetry

**437. High-energy dose modeling:** Mathematical modeling of dose deposition
**Related term:** Monte Carlo
**Radiotherapy Example:** Used for small-field dose calculations

**438. High-energy dose optimization:** Adjusting beam parameters for ideal clinical results
**Related term:** Planning optimization
**Radiotherapy Example:** IMRT uses optimization for OAR sparing

**439. High-energy dose rate field:** Field with high dose per second
**Related term:** FFF (flattening-filter-free)
**Radiotherapy Example:** 6FFF beams deliver high dose rates for SBRT

**440. High-energy dose ratio:** Ratio comparing doses from different energies or techniques
**Related term:** RBE
**Radiotherapy Example:** Comparing 6 MV vs 10 MV depth dose

**441. High-energy dose reconstruction:** Rebuilding delivered dose using machine log files or detector data
**Related term:** Dose verification
**Radiotherapy Example:** Varian Dynalog dose reconstruction

442. **High-energy dose uniformity:** Consistency of dose across the field
**Related term:** Flatness
**Radiotherapy Example:** Flattened beams have stricter uniformity requirements

443. **High-energy dose verification:** Checking if the delivered dose matches the planned dose
**Related term:** QA
**Radiotherapy Example:** Pre-treatment IMRT QA

444. **High-energy electron contamination correction:** Adjustments made to remove contaminant electrons from dose calculations
**Related term:** Skin dose correction
**Radiotherapy Example:** TPS accounts for increased surface dose

445. **High-energy electron field:** Field generated by electron therapy units or LINAC electron mode
**Related term:** Electron beam
**Radiotherapy Example:** Used for skin or superficial tumor treatment

446. **High-energy electron imaging:** Imaging done with high-energy electron beams
**Related term:** Portal imaging
**Radiotherapy Example:** EPIDs detect MV electrons indirectly

447. **High-energy electron measurement:** Measurement of electron beam parameters
**Related term:** Electron PDD
**Radiotherapy Example:** Water tank scanning for 12 MeV electrons

448. **High-energy electron penetration:** Depth of electron beam travel in tissue
**Related term:** Practical range
**Radiotherapy Example:** 12 MeV penetrates to ~6 cm

449. **High-energy electron scattering:** Lateral spread of electrons as they pass through tissue
**Related term:** Scatter broadening
**Radiotherapy Example:** Electron fields require careful use of bolus

450. **High-energy electron therapy:** Treatment using high-energy electron beams
**Related term:** Electron RT
**Radiotherapy Example:** Used for chest wall scars or skin lesions

451. **High-energy electromagnetic radiation:** Radiation with energies >100 keV
**Related term:** X-rays, gamma
**Radiotherapy Example:** MV photons used for deep tumors

452. **High-energy emission source:** Radiation source emitting high-energy particles or photons
**Related term:** LINAC target
**Radiotherapy Example:** Tungsten target in LINACs

453. **High-energy field calibration:** Calibration of MV photon or electron fields
**Related term:** TG-51
**Radiotherapy Example:** Annual LINAC calibration

454. **High-energy field mapping:** Mapping intensity distribution across a radiation field
**Related term:** Profile scan
**Radiotherapy Example:** Used in commissioning

455. **High-energy field shaping (MLC-based):** Field shaping using multileaf collimators
**Related term:** Beam modulation
**Radiotherapy Example:** IMRT for prostate

456. **High-energy field scatter:** Unwanted scatter within high-energy fields
**Related term:** Secondary radiation
**Radiotherapy Example:** Scatter affects OAR doses

457. **High-energy field uniformity:** Uniformity of beam output across field shape
**Related term:** Symmetry
**Radiotherapy Example:** Required in reference fields

458. **High-energy field verification:** Confirming accuracy of field placement and shape
**Related term:** IGRT
**Radiotherapy Example:** kV imaging for SRS fields

459. **High-energy filter (radiation):** Filter used to modify high-energy beam properties
**Related term:** Flattening filter
**Radiotherapy Example:** FFF beams remove the filter entirely

460. **High-energy fluorescence detector:** Detector that measures fluorescent light produced by radiation
**Related term:** Scintillator
**Radiotherapy Example:** Used in 3D dosimetry systems

461. **High-energy flux monitor:** Device measuring radiation flux density
**Related term:** Flux meter
**Radiotherapy Example:** Used in neutron therapy facilities

462. **High-energy gamma camera:** Camera designed to detect high-energy gamma rays
**Related term:** SPECT
**Radiotherapy Example:** Used with I-131 imaging

463. **High-energy gamma dosimetry:** Dose measurement for high-energy gamma-emitting sources
**Related term:** Gamma source
**Radiotherapy Example:** Co-60 teletherapy dosimetry

464. **High-energy gamma interaction:** Interaction processes of high-energy gamma photons
**Related term:** Pair production
**Radiotherapy Example:** Dominant above 10 MeV

465. **High-energy gamma radiation:** Gamma rays with energies in the MeV range
**Related term:** Co-60
**Radiotherapy Example:** Used in older teletherapy units

466. **High-energy gamma spectroscopy:** Analysis of gamma energies using detectors
**Related term:** HPGe detector
**Radiotherapy Example:** Used to characterize brachytherapy seed energies

467. **High-energy gamma source:** Source emitting MeV-range gamma rays
**Related term:** Co-60
**Radiotherapy Example:** Gamma Knife uses ~1 17 and 1 33 MeV photons

468. **High-energy gamma spectrum:** Energy distribution emitted by high-energy gamma sources
**Related term:** Gamma lines
**Radiotherapy Example:** Co-60 dual-energy peaks

469. **High-energy gamma shielding:** Shielding required to attenuate high-energy gamma radiation
**Related term:** Lead equivalent
**Radiotherapy Example:** Thick concrete is needed around LINAC vaults

**470. High-energy gamma verification:** Check of gamma beam integrity and alignment
**Related term:** QA test
**Radiotherapy Example:** Gamma Knife QA

**471. High-energy heavy ion:** High-mass ion accelerated to high velocities
**Related term:** Carbon ion
**Radiotherapy Example:** Carbon ion therapy for radioresistant tumors

**472. High-energy imaging detector:** Detector designed to handle large radiation energies
**Related term:** MV detector
**Radiotherapy Example:** EPIDs used for MV portal imaging

**473. High-energy imaging protocol:** Imaging settings tuned for high-energy X-rays
**Related term:** MV imaging
**Radiotherapy Example:** Used in IGRT

**474. High-energy imaging system:** System that detects MV radiation
**Related term:** Portal imaging
**Radiotherapy Example:** Used to verify treatment fields

**475. High-energy imaging validation:** Process confirming accuracy of high-energy imaging
**Related term:** Imaging QA
**Radiotherapy Example:** EPID calibration checks

**476. High-energy ion beam:** Beam of accelerated ions used in therapy
**Related term:** Particle therapy
**Radiotherapy Example:** Carbon ion beams at 400 MeV/u

**477. High-energy ion dosimetry:** Dosimetry for heavy ion beams
**Related term:** Bragg peak
**Radiotherapy Example:** Carbon ion dose distribution measurement

**478. High-energy ionization potential:** Energy needed to ionize atoms in high-energy radiation fields
**Related term:** Ionization energy
**Radiotherapy Example:** Affects detector response

**479. High-energy ionization track:** Track left as charged particles traverse matter
**Related term:** LET
**Radiotherapy Example:** Carbon ions have dense ionization tracks

**480. High-energy ionizing beam:** Beam capable of ionizing matter at significant depth
**Related term:** MV photon
**Radiotherapy Example:** LINAC photons at 6–15 MV

**481. High-energy isotopic source:** Radioactive source emitting high-energy photons or particles
**Related term:** Co-60
**Radiotherapy Example:** HDR Ir-192 (high-energy gamma)

**482. High-energy kinetic energy particle:** Particle with large kinetic energy causing deep penetration
**Related term:** Proton
**Radiotherapy Example:** High-energy protons for deep tumors

**483. High-energy LINAC mode:** LINAC operation mode for high MV photon beams
**Related term:** 10 MV mode
**Radiotherapy Example:** Used for deep pelvic tumors

484. **High-energy magnetic field imaging:** Imaging where magnetic fields influence high-energy particles
**Related term:** MR-linac
**Radiotherapy Example:** MRI-guided radiotherapy uses magnetic fields during irradiation

485. **High-energy medium modification:** Altering medium properties for radiation interaction studies
**Related term:** Phantom modification
**Radiotherapy Example:** Used to test proton stopping powers

486. **High-energy MV imaging:** Imaging using MV photon beams
**Related term:** EPID
**Radiotherapy Example:** Used to verify treatment geometry

487. **High-energy neutron:** Neutrons with significant kinetic energy produced in high-energy photon beams
**Related term:** Photo-neutron
**Radiotherapy Example:** Produced in LINACs above 10 MV

488. **High-energy neutron dosimetry:** Measuring dose from neutron contamination
**Related term:** Neutron equivalent dose
**Radiotherapy Example:** Important for shielding calculations

489. **High-energy neutron interaction:** Interactions of neutrons with nuclei
**Related term:** Elastic scattering
**Radiotherapy Example:** Occur inside LINAC vault walls

490. **High-energy neutron shielding:** Thick hydrogen-rich materials used for neutron attenuation
**Related term:** Polyethylene
**Radiotherapy Example:** Used in bunker walls for >10 MV beams

491. **High-energy neutron source:** Device producing energetic neutrons
**Related term:** Deuterium–tritium generator
**Radiotherapy Example:** Used in BNCT research

492. **High-energy neutron spectrum:** Distribution of neutron energies in a neutron field
**Related term:** Energy spectrum
**Radiotherapy Example:** Characterized for proton therapy neutrons

493. **High-energy nuclear activation:** Activation of surrounding materials due to high-energy particles
**Related term:** Induced radioactivity
**Radiotherapy Example:** LINAC components become temporarily activated

494. **High-energy particle accelerator:** Machine generating high-energy beams
**Related term:** Cyclotron
**Radiotherapy Example:** Proton therapy uses cyclotrons or synchrotrons

495. **High-energy particle interaction:** Interactions of particles with matter at high velocities
**Related term:** LET
**Radiotherapy Example:** Carbon ions cause dense ionization

496. **High-energy particle monitor:** Device tracking particle flux
**Related term:** Beam monitor
**Radiotherapy Example:** Used in proton therapy nozzles

497. **High-energy particle therapy:** Therapy using high-energy particles such as protons or carbon ions
**Related term:** Hadron therapy
**Radiotherapy Example:** Treats chordomas and resistant tumors

**498. High-energy penetrative radiation:** Radiation capable of deep penetration in tissue
**Related term:** MV photon
**Radiotherapy Example:** 15 MV beams reach deep pelvic structures

**499. High-energy photon activation:** Photon-induced activation of materials
**Related term:** Photonuclear reaction
**Radiotherapy Example:** Occurs in LINAC components at >10 MV

**500. High-energy photon attenuation coefficient:** Factor describing photon reduction per unit thickness
**Related term:** μ (mu)
**Radiotherapy Example:** Used in shielding calculations for bunker walls

# I

1. **Image acquisition:** The process of obtaining imaging data from modalities like CT, MRI, CBCT, or PET. It determines the quality and accuracy of the anatomical and functional information used in planning. Includes considerations such as resolution, slice thickness, artifact reduction, and patient positioning.
   **Related term:** Image reconstruction
   **Radiotherapy Example:** Planning CT acquisition is the first step before contouring and dose calculation.
2. **Image analysis:** Examination and interpretation of images to extract meaningful information, such as tumor volume, organ boundaries, or deformable motion fields. Advanced analysis uses AI or quantitative metrics.
   **Related term:** Radiomics
   **Radiotherapy Example:** Used to evaluate tumor regression during weekly CBCT in adaptive therapy.
3. **Image and artifact recognition:** Ability to identify normal structures, pathology, and imaging artifacts. Essential for accurate contouring and avoiding misinterpretation errors. Artifacts originate from motion, metal, or beam-hardening.
   **Related term:** Image quality
   **Radiotherapy Example:** Recognizing dental metal artifacts prevents contouring errors in head-and-neck plans.
4. **Image and motion artifact reduction:** Methods to minimize distortions caused by patient movement or system limitations. Includes gating, faster scanning, immobilization, and iterative reconstruction.
   **Related term:** Respiratory gating
   **Radiotherapy Example:** 4D-CT reduces breathing artifacts in lung cancer planning.
5. **Image and noise reduction:** Techniques to improve signal-to-noise ratio using filters, smoothing, or iterative algorithms. Essential to preserve fine anatomical detail while reducing graininess.
   **Related term:** Denoising
   **Radiotherapy Example:** Adaptive filters improve CBCT image clarity for soft-tissue matching.
6. **Image calibration phantom:** Physical object with known density or geometry used to standardize scanner performance and ensure accurate HU values.
   **Related term:** QA phantom
   **Radiotherapy Example:** Catphan is used for daily or monthly CBCT calibration.
7. **Image co-registration technique:** Method for aligning two or more imaging datasets into the same coordinate system. Can be rigid or deformable.
   **Related term:** Image fusion
   **Radiotherapy Example:** PET/CT co-registration improves GTV for head-and-neck tumors.
8. **Image coherence analysis:** Evaluation of consistency in image features between scans, often used in MR or ultrasound imaging quality validation.
   **Related term:** Image uniformity
   **Radiotherapy Example:** Used to verify stability of MR-Linac real-time imaging.

9. **Image compression method:** Technique for reducing file size while maintaining fidelity. Lossless compression preserves all information; lossy compression removes redundant data.
   **Related term:** DICOM storage
   **Radiotherapy Example:** Hospitals use lossless compression for archiving planning CT data.

10. **Image contrast:** Difference in signal intensity between tissues, determining how well they can be distinguished. Can be enhanced using contrast agents or specific imaging parameters.
    **Related term:** Contrast resolution
    **Radiotherapy Example:** T2-weighted MRI provides high contrast for brain tumor delineation.

11. **Image contrast agent:** Substance administered to enhance visibility of specific structures or tissues on imaging, such as iodine in CT or gadolinium in MRI.
    **Related term:** Contrast enhancement
    **Radiotherapy Example:** Iodinated CT contrast helps identify liver vasculature during planning.

12. **Image contrast analysis:** Quantitative evaluation of contrast between tissues to determine if imaging is suitable for accurate contouring.
    **Related term:** CNR (contrast-to-noise ratio)
    **Radiotherapy Example:** Used in MRI QA to ensure tumor–brain boundary visibility.

13. **Image contrast assessment:** Routine QA procedure where image contrast performance is measured using phantoms with known features.
    **Related term:** Image quality metrics
    **Radiotherapy Example:** Daily CBCT QA checks contrast between low-density inserts.

14. **Image contrast enhancement:** Improving contrast using algorithmic techniques or acquisition parameter changes.
    **Related term:** Windowing
    **Radiotherapy Example:** Soft-tissue windowing on CT enhances clarity of pelvic organs.

15. **Image contrast resolution:** Ability of an imaging system to differentiate tissues with very similar densities or signals.
    **Related term:** Low-contrast detectability
    **Radiotherapy Example:** Important for detecting small liver lesions on planning CT.

16. **Image correlation:** Statistical measure comparing similarities between two images. Often used in automatic registration and motion tracking algorithms.
    **Related term:** Cross-correlation
    **Radiotherapy Example:** Used for real-time matching in surface-guided radiotherapy (SGRT).

17. **Image correction algorithm:** Software used to compensate for scanner imperfections, beam-hardening, scatter, or motion.
    **Related term:** Reconstruction correction
    **Radiotherapy Example:** Metal artifact reduction algorithms improve accuracy near dental fillings.

18. **Image deformation field:** 3D vector field representing how one image warps into another during deformable registration.
    **Related term:** Deformable image registration
    **Radiotherapy Example:** Used in dose accumulation across multiple adaptive fractions.

19. **Image deformation technique:** Methods used to apply deformation fields to images or structures for accurate alignment.
    **Related term:** Warping
    **Radiotherapy Example:** Used to propagate contours from planning CT to CBCT.

20. **Image density mapping:** Process of converting HU values or MRI intensities into physical densities for dose calculations.
    **Related term:** Electron density
    **Radiotherapy Example:** CT-to-density conversion curves are essential for TPS accuracy.
21. **Image distortion correction:** Algorithms to remove geometric distortions, especially in MRI.
    **Related term:** Geometric accuracy
    **Radiotherapy Example:** Correcting MR distortion is essential for brain SRS planning.
22. **Image distortion measurement:** Quantifying geometric accuracy using phantoms with known shapes.
    **Related term:** Spatial integrity
    **Radiotherapy Example:** MR-Linac QA uses grid phantoms to measure distortions.
23. **Image enhancement:** General term for improving image clarity using filtering, contrast adjustment, or sharpening.
    **Related term:** Post-processing
    **Radiotherapy Example:** Applied to CBCT for better soft-tissue matching.
24. **Image evaluation:** Systematic assessment of image quality for clinical suitability.
    **Related term:** QA imaging tests
    **Radiotherapy Example:** Evaluating daily kV images to ensure appropriate visibility for IGRT.
25. **Image feature extraction:** Process of identifying quantifiable characteristics such as texture or edges.
    **Related term:** Radiomics features
    **Radiotherapy Example:** Used in predicting tumor response based on pre-treatment scans.
26. **Image field of view:** The spatial area captured in an image. Larger FOV may reduce resolution.
    **Related term:** Collimation
    **Radiotherapy Example:** Wide-FOV CT captures both arms for breast planning.
27. **Image filtering:** Algorithms that modify images to remove noise, sharpen edges, or extract features.
    **Related term:** Convolution
    **Radiotherapy Example:** Sharpening filters clarify bone edges in IGRT kV images.
28. **Image fusion:** Combining anatomical and functional images to improve diagnosis or treatment planning.
    **Related term:** Multimodal registration
    **Radiotherapy Example:** PET/CT fusion helps identify metabolically active tumor regions.
29. **Image gating:** Acquiring images only during specific phases of breathing or cardiac cycles.
    **Related term:** Respiratory gating
    **Radiotherapy Example:** 4D-CT uses gated images to capture tumor motion.
30. **Image geometry:** Spatial arrangement of pixels/voxels in an image, including dimensions and coordinate mapping.
    **Related term:** Pixel spacing
    **Radiotherapy Example:** Important for accurate structure delineation in TPS.
31. **Image gradient:** The rate of intensity change between pixels, used to detect edges and boundaries. Higher gradients indicate sharper transitions between tissues.
    **Related term:** Edge detection
    **Radiotherapy Example:** Helps outline tumor borders during semi-automatic segmentation.
32. **Image grid:** The matrix of pixels or voxels that forms an image. Resolution depends on grid spacing and number of elements.
    **Related term:** Pixel matrix
    **Radiotherapy Example:** Dose grid alignment with image grid is vital for accurate calculations.

33. **Image-guided adaptive radiotherapy (IGART):** Radiotherapy where daily imaging guides modifications to target or dose based on anatomical changes.
**Related term:** ART (Adaptive Radiotherapy)
**Radiotherapy Example:** CBCT-based plan adaptation for shrinking head-and-neck tumors.

34. **Image-guided brachytherapy:** Using CT, MRI, or ultrasound for real-time applicator placement and dose optimization in brachytherapy.
**Related term:** MRI-guided brachytherapy
**Radiotherapy Example:** MRI-guided HDR for cervical cancer.

35. **Image-guided dosimetry:** Use of imaging to measure or verify dose distribution, especially in real-time systems.
**Related term:** In vivo dosimetry
**Radiotherapy Example:** Portal imaging for exit-dose verification.

36. **Image-guided motion management:** Techniques to track and compensate for patient or tumor motion using imaging systems.
**Related term:** Real-time tracking
**Radiotherapy Example:** SGRT tracks chest movement during lung SBRT.

37. **Image-guided patient setup:** Positioning the patient by comparing daily images to planning imaging, ensuring reproducibility.
**Related term:** IGRT
**Radiotherapy Example:** kV orthogonal images for prostate alignment.

38. **Image-guided radiotherapy (IGRT):** Radiation treatment delivered with imaging before or during therapy to ensure accuracy.
**Related term:** CBCT
**Radiotherapy Example:** Daily CBCT for spine SRS.

39. **Image-guided surgery:** Surgery aided by real-time imaging for navigation and precision.
**Related term:** Intraoperative imaging
**Radiotherapy Example:** Used to place fiducials prior to prostate SBRT.

40. **Image-guided treatment:** Any therapy where imaging directs and verifies dose delivery or positioning.
**Related term:** IGRT
**Radiotherapy Example:** MR-Linac provides continuous imaging during radiotherapy.

41. **Image histogram:** Graph showing the distribution of pixel intensities in an image. Used for assessing contrast and brightness.
**Related term:** Histogram equalization
**Radiotherapy Example:** Reviewing CT histogram to detect HU inconsistencies.

42. **Image intensity:** The value assigned to each pixel/voxel representing tissue density or signal.
**Related term:** Signal level
**Radiotherapy Example:** Identifying hypodense liver lesions on CT by low intensity.

43. **Image intensity normalization:** Adjusting intensity values across multiple scans to ensure consistency.
**Related term:** Standardization
**Radiotherapy Example:** Important for radiomics studies across different scanners.

44. **Image interpolation:** Estimating new pixel/voxel values when resizing, rotating, or resampling images.
**Related term:** Resampling
**Radiotherapy Example:** Used when CT is resampled to match MR voxel size.

45. **Image matrix:** The numerical array of pixels/voxels that make up an image, e.g., 512×512.
**Related term:** Pixel resolution
**Radiotherapy Example:** High matrix size improves edge for IGRT.

46. **Image modality:** Type of imaging technology used—CT, MRI, PET, US, etc.
**Related term:** Multimodal imaging
**Radiotherapy Example:** PET/MRI improves soft-tissue and metabolic delineation.

47. **Image motion tracking:** Detecting and following motion over time using imaging frames.
**Related term:** Real-time tumor tracking
**Radiotherapy Example:** Fluoroscopy used to track fiducial markers in lung SBRT.

48. **Image noise:** Random fluctuations in pixel values that reduce image clarity.
**Related term:** SNR (signal-to-noise ratio)
**Radiotherapy Example:** Low-dose CT acquisition increases noise but reduces patient dose.

49. **Image noise analysis:** Evaluating the magnitude and pattern of noise within an image.
**Related term:** Noise modeling
**Radiotherapy Example:** CBCT QA includes noise measurement using uniform phantoms.

50. **Image noise reduction filter:** Software tool that smooths the image and reduces random variations.
**Related term:** Smoothing filter
**Radiotherapy Example:** Reduces noise in low-dose pediatric CT planning.

51. **Image normalization:** Scaling intensity values across an image or dataset for consistency.
**Related term:** Intensity standardization
**Radiotherapy Example:** Used in dose summation of multi-modality datasets.

52. **Image plane:** Geometric plane in which an image is acquired—axial, sagittal, or coronal.
**Related term:** Imaging orientation
**Radiotherapy Example:** Axial plane used routinely in planning CT.

53. **Image pre-processing:** Initial steps applied to raw images—denoising, alignment, and contrast correction.
**Related term:** Pre-filtering
**Radiotherapy Example:** CBCT preprocessing enhances soft tissue before matching.

54. **Image quality:** Overall clarity and diagnostic value of an image, influenced by noise, resolution, distortion, and contrast.
**Related term:** IQ metrics
**Radiotherapy Example:** TPS requires high-quality CT for accurate dose calculation.

55. **Image quality assessment:** Objective or subjective evaluation of image characteristics.
**Related term:** QA imaging
**Radiotherapy Example:** Monthly CBCT QA ensures acceptable grayscale accuracy.

56. **Image quality control:** Regular procedures to maintain consistent imaging performance.
**Related term:** QC program
**Radiotherapy Example:** Daily imaging QC before patient treatments.

57. **Image quality enhancement:** Techniques improving visibility of anatomical structures.
**Related term:** Image filtering
**Radiotherapy Example:** Enhancing CBCT contrast for prostate matching.

58. **Image quality indicator:** Metric or phantom used to measure contrast, noise, or resolution.
**Related term:** QA phantom
**Radiotherapy Example:** Leeds phantom measures IGRT spatial resolution.

59. **Image reconstruction:** Creating images from raw detector data using algorithms like FBP or iterative reconstruction.
**Related term:** Reconstruction kernel
**Radiotherapy Example:** Iterative reconstruction reduces noise in planning CT.

60. **Image reconstruction algorithm:** Mathematical method for converting projections or signals into images.
**Related term:** FBP
**Radiotherapy Example:** Adaptive iterative reconstruction improves CBCT clarity.

61. **Image registration:** Aligning two or more images spatially for accurate comparison or fusion.
**Related term:** Deformable registration
**Radiotherapy Example:** Aligning MR with CT for target delineation.

62. **Image resolution:** Ability to distinguish fine detail, dependent on pixel size and system optics.
**Related term:** Spatial resolution
**Radiotherapy Example:** High-resolution CT is essential for lung nodule contouring.

63. **Image segmentation:** Dividing an image into regions, such as tumor vs normal tissue.
**Related term:** Auto-contouring
**Radiotherapy Example:** AI segmentation of the prostate for SBRT planning.

64. **Image signal:** The useful information detected by the imaging system.
**Related term:** Signal intensity
**Radiotherapy Example:** Strong MR signal improves soft-tissue boundary detection.

65. **Image simulation:** Synthetic images generated for training, testing, or dose calculation modeling.
**Related term:** Virtual phantom
**Radiotherapy Example:** Simulated CT used to evaluate new dose algorithms.

66. **Image slice thickness:** Thickness of cross-sectional slices in CT/MRI. Thinner slices give more detail but increase noise.
**Related term:** Z-resolution
**Radiotherapy Example:** 1–3 mm slices for SBRT accuracy.

67. **Image smoothing:** Reducing image noise by averaging or filtering pixel values.
**Related term:** Gaussian filter
**Radiotherapy Example:** Applied to CBCT to reduce high-frequency artifacts.

68. **Image spatial resolution:** The smallest object that can be distinguished in space.
**Related term:** MTF
**Radiotherapy Example:** High resolution needed for SRS skull imaging.

69. **Image standardization:** Ensuring consistency across scans, scanners, or protocols.
**Related term:** Harmonization
**Radiotherapy Example:** Required for multi-center radiomics studies.

70. **Image thresholding:** Separating regions based on intensity cutoffs, often used for segmentation.
**Related term:** Binary mask
**Radiotherapy Example:** CT lung segmentation using HU threshold.

71. **Image uniformity:** Consistency of pixel values across uniform regions.
**Related term:** Flatness
**Radiotherapy Example:** MR uniformity checked using large uniform phantoms.

72. **Image verification:** Confirming correct patient setup using daily imaging.
**Related term:** IGRT
**Radiotherapy Example:** Comparing kV images to DRRs before treatment.

73. **Imaging artifact:** Any distortion or error appearing in an image due to motion, metal, or equipment limitations.
**Related term:** Beam-hardening
**Radiotherapy Example:** Metal artifacts near hips affect pelvic contouring.

74. **Imaging biomarker:** Quantifiable imaging features indicating disease progression or response.
**Related term:** Radiomics
**Radiotherapy Example:** ADC values in MRI predict tumor hypoxia.

75. **Imaging chain:** Entire process from X-ray generation to detection and reconstruction.
**Related term:** Imaging workflow
**Radiotherapy Example:** Ensuring all components work properly for IGRT.

76. **Imaging contrast:** Amount of difference between tissues, essential for identifying boundaries.
**Related term:** Contrast resolution
**Radiotherapy Example:** MRI offers superior contrast for brain tumors.

77. **Imaging device:** Equipment used to acquire images—CT, MRI, CBCT, ultrasound, etc.
**Related term:** Imaging system
**Radiotherapy Example:** Linac-mounted CBCT is a key IGRT device.

78. **Imaging detector:** Component that captures radiation or signals and converts them into images.
**Related term:** Flat-panel detector
**Radiotherapy Example:** EPID used for portal imaging.

79. **Imaging dose:** Radiation dose delivered during imaging procedures.
**Related term:** kV dose
**Radiotherapy Example:** CBCT dose is monitored to reduce cumulative exposure.

80. **Imaging efficiency:** Ability of a system to produce high-quality images with minimal dose.
**Related term:** Detector efficiency
**Radiotherapy Example:** FPDs provide high efficiency at low kV imaging doses.

81. **Imaging field:** Physical area scanned during image acquisition.
**Related term:** FOV
**Radiotherapy Example:** Expanded field for whole-breast CT simulation.

82. **Imaging geometry:** Arrangement of source, object, and detector.
**Related term:** Geometric magnification
**Radiotherapy Example:** Affects IGRT accuracy in kV imaging.

83. **Imaging grid:** Virtual grid structure placed over images for analysis or correction.
**Related term:** Detector matrix
**Radiotherapy Example:** Used in modeling scatter correction for CBCT.

84. **Imaging informatics:** Field dealing with image storage, communication, and processing systems.
**Related term:** PACS
**Radiotherapy Example:** PACS links TPS, CT, and oncology information systems.

85. **Imaging interpretation:** Clinical evaluation of images to detect disease.
**Related term:** Diagnostic imaging
**Radiotherapy Example:** Radiologists interpret MRI before oncologists contour.

86. **Imaging isotropy:** Equal resolution in all three spatial directions.
**Related term:** Isotropic voxels
**Radiotherapy Example:** 1 mm isotropic CT useful for SRS planning.

87. **Imaging laser alignment:** Laser systems used to position patients based on reference marks.
**Related term:** Room lasers
**Radiotherapy Example:** Aligning external tattoos with laser lines before imaging.

88. **Imaging matrix:** Pixel arrangement representing image resolution.
**Related term:** Pixel count
**Radiotherapy Example:** 1024×1024 matrix improves IGRT detail.

89. **Imaging modality selection:** Choosing the appropriate imaging type based on tumor site and goal.
**Related term:** Modality optimization
**Radiotherapy Example:** MRI chosen for prostate soft-tissue clarity.

90. **Imaging noise:** Random variation that hides anatomical detail.
**Related term:** Quantum noise
**Radiotherapy Example:** Increased noise in low-dose CT affects contouring.

91. **Imaging optimization:** Adjusting protocols to improve quality while minimizing dose.
**Related term:** Protocol tuning
**Radiotherapy Example:** Optimizing CBCT settings for pediatric patients.

92. **Imaging phantom:** Artificial object used to test imaging systems.
**Related term:** QA phantom
**Radiotherapy Example:** Catphan used for CBCT QA.

93. **Imaging plane orientation:** Axial, sagittal, or coronal orientation of slices.
**Related term:** Anatomical planes
**Radiotherapy Example:** MR sagittal images help visualize the spinal canal.

94. **Imaging preprocessing:** Initial steps to prepare raw images for analysis—noise reduction, alignment, contrast normalization.
**Related term:** Pre-filtering
**Radiotherapy Example:** Used before auto-contouring algorithms.

95. **Imaging protocol:** Defined parameters for consistent imaging (kVp, mAs, slice thickness, etc.).
**Related term:** Acquisition protocol
**Radiotherapy Example:** Lung 4D-CT protocol includes respiratory-phase sorting.

96. **Imaging quality factor:** Quantitative score reflecting accuracy of contrast, noise, and resolution.
**Related term:** IQ metrics
**Radiotherapy Example:** Higher IQF means more reliable CBCT for IGRT.

97. **Imaging reconstruction filter:** Kernel applied during CT reconstruction affecting sharpness or smoothness.
**Related term:** Convolution kernel
**Radiotherapy Example:** Lung kernel highlights small nodules for SBRT.

98. **Imaging region of interest (ROI):** Specific selected area for analysis or measurement.
**Related term:** ROI sampling
**Radiotherapy Example:** HU measured in ROI to verify CT-density calibration.

99. **Imaging resolution assessment:** Evaluation of system's ability to show fine detail.
**Related term:** Line-pair phantom
**Radiotherapy Example:** Checking EPID resolution for portal imaging QA.

100. **Imaging scatter correction:** Removing scatter radiation effects to improve image clarity.
**Related term:** Scatter reduction
**Radiotherapy Example:** CBCT scatter correction improves HU accuracy for adaptive planning.

101. **Irradiation field:** The defined area on a patient or phantom that receives radiation during a treatment or experiment. Determined by collimator shape and beam geometry.
**Technical meaning:** Specifies spatial coverage of dose.
**Related term:** Treatment field
**Radiotherapy Example:** In breast radiotherapy, the irradiation field includes the whole breast except the heart and contralateral lung.

102. **Irradiation time:** The total duration for which a radiation beam is applied to the target. Influences total delivered dose.
**Technical meaning:** Dose = dose rate × irradiation time.
**Related term:** Beam-on time
**Radiotherapy Example:** In HDR brachytherapy, irradiation time is calculated by the TPS depending on source dwell positions.

103. **Irradiation unit:** A device or facility designed to expose materials or biological samples to controlled amounts of radiation.
**Technical meaning:** Used for sterilization, testing, research, or calibration.
**Related term:** Irradiator
**Radiotherapy Example:** Dosimetry labs use irradiation units to calibrate ion chambers with traceable radiation beams.

104. **Irradiator:** A device that generates controlled radiation using sealed sources (e.g., Co-60, Cs-137). Used in calibration, testing, and sterilization.
**Technical meaning:** Provides standardized beams for measurements.
**Related term:** Radiation source
**Radiotherapy Example:** Hospitals use Cs-137 irradiators for radiobiology experiments assessing cell survival curves.

105. **Irradiator calibration:** Procedure to verify that an irradiator delivers accurate dose rates as expected by the manufacturer or standards laboratory.
**Technical meaning:** Ensures output reproducibility.
**Related term:** Output calibration
**Radiotherapy Example:** Calibration ensures a Co-60 irradiator used for TLD testing provides the correct reference dose.

106. **Irradiator dose:** The amount of radiation emitted by an irradiator and received by a target over a defined time.
**Technical meaning:** Depends on activity, geometry, shielding.
**Related term:** Delivered dose
**Radiotherapy Example:** Used to verify reference dose levels for QA phantoms in radiotherapy physics.

107. **Irradiator facility:** A controlled environment designed for radiation experiments or calibration, equipped with shielding and safety systems.
**Technical meaning:** Must meet regulatory and radiation protection standards.
**Related term:** Radiation laboratory
**Radiotherapy Example:** Physicists use irradiator facilities to prepare dosimeters for patient-specific QA.

108. **Irradiator safety:** Procedures ensuring safe operation of irradiators, preventing accidental exposure via interlocks, shielding, and protocols.
**Technical meaning:** Includes ALARA principles.
**Related term:** Radiation protection
**Radiotherapy Example:** Facilities require two-key access and area monitors for Co-60 irradiators used in QA.

109. **Irradiator source:** The radioactive material (e.g., Co-60, Cs-137) inside an irradiator responsible for emitting gamma radiation.
**Technical meaning:** Characterized by activity and energy spectrum.
**Related term:** Sealed source
**Radiotherapy Example:** A decaying Co-60 irradiator source must be replaced periodically to maintain calibration accuracy.

110. **Irradiator system:** The complete assembly including the source, shielding, control electronics, collimation, and safety interlocks.
**Technical meaning:** Ensures controlled, measurable radiation output.
**Related term:** Radiation delivery system
**Radiotherapy Example:** Used to calibrate dosimeters before IMRT patient-specific QA.

111. **Irradiator verification:** A QA process confirming that the irradiator is functioning correctly and delivering expected radiation output.
**Technical meaning:** Part of routine safety and compliance testing.
**Related term:** System verification
**Radiotherapy Example:** Periodic irradiator verification ensures TLD calibration doses are accurate for patient QA.

112. **Irradiation planning:** Designing how radiation will be applied, specifying time, field, geometry, and dose for controlled experiments.
**Technical meaning:** Includes beam alignment and dose calculation.
**Related term:** Treatment planning
**Radiotherapy Example:** Used in radiobiology studies to produce uniform cell monolayer exposure.

113. **Irradiation procedure:** The step-by-step protocol followed to perform irradiation safely and reproducibly.
**Technical meaning:** Includes sample setup, exposure time, safety checks.
**Related term:** SOP (Standard Operating Procedure)
**Radiotherapy Example:** Used in QA labs when exposing diode detectors to reference beams.

114. **Irradiation treatment:** The use of radiation to treat disease or modify biological materials.
**Technical meaning:** Encompasses clinical radiotherapy or experimental exposures.
**Related term:** Radiotherapy
**Radiotherapy Example:** Electron irradiation treatment is used for superficial skin cancers.

115. **Isocenter (radiotherapy):** The 3D point in space where the rotation axes of the gantry, couch, and collimator all intersect.
**Technical meaning:** Central reference for treatment geometry.
**Related term:** Mechanical isocenter
**Radiotherapy Example:** IMRT and VMAT plans align dose distributions precisely around the isocenter.

**116. Isocentric technique:** Radiotherapy method using beams all rotated around a common isocenter.
**Technical meaning:** Minimizes patient repositioning.
**Related term:** Isocentric setup
**Radiotherapy Example:** Used regularly in stereotactic radiosurgery (SRS) for cranial targets.

**117. Isocentric radiotherapy:** A treatment approach where all beams converge at a common isocenter to deliver a conformal dose.
**Technical meaning:** Improves dose conformity and accuracy.
**Related term:** Conformal therapy
**Radiotherapy Example:** SRS brain metastasis treatment uses isocentric delivery for precision.

**118. Isodose curve:** A contour line connecting points receiving the same radiation dose.
**Technical meaning:** Visual representation of dose distribution.
**Related term:** Isodose line
**Radiotherapy Example:** Isodose curves show high-dose conformity around prostate tumors in IMRT.

**119. Isodose distribution:** Map of dose levels throughout the treatment volume, represented by multiple isodose lines.
**Technical meaning:** Evaluates plan quality and coverage.
**Related term:** Dose distribution
**Radiotherapy Example:** Ensures PTV coverage meets prescription while sparing OARs.

**120. Isodose line:** A curve marking points of equal dose on a 2D plane.
**Technical meaning:** Used in plan evaluation.
**Related term:** Iso-surfaces
**Radiotherapy Example:** The 95% isodose line must cover ≥95% of the target volume in most protocols.

**121. Isodose plan:** A treatment plan presented using isodose curves or surfaces to visualize dose.
**Technical meaning:** Indicates conformity and homogeneity.
**Related term:** Dose planning
**Radiotherapy Example:** Used to verify that hotspots do not exceed institutional limits.

**122. Isodose prescription:** The dose level at which treatment is prescribed, often a specific % isodose line.
**Technical meaning:** Defines target coverage standard.
**Related term:** Prescription dose
**Radiotherapy Example:** SRS often prescribes to the 50–80% isodose line for sharp falloff.

**123. Isodose surface:** A 3D surface representing all points that receive the same dose.
**Technical meaning:** Used for volumetric visualization.
**Related term:** Dose-volume rendering
**Radiotherapy Example:** Helps evaluate PTV coverage in 3D CRT, IMRT, and VMAT.

**124. Isodose verification:** QA process to confirm the planned dose distribution matches measured dose.
**Technical meaning:** Uses film, EPID, ion chambers, or diode arrays.
**Related term:** Patient-specific QA
**Radiotherapy Example:** Performed for each IMRT plan before treatment.

**125. Isodose volume:** The total 3D volume enclosed by a particular isodose surface.
**Technical meaning:** Used to calculate dose–volume metrics.
**Related term:** DVH
**Radiotherapy Example:** The 95% IDV is measured to ensure adequate PTV coverage.

126. **Isotope abundance:** The relative amount of an isotope compared to others of the same element in a sample.
**Technical meaning:** Expressed in percentages.
**Related term:** Isotopic ratio
**Radiotherapy Example:** Affects efficiency of isotope production for PET radiotracers.

127. **Isotope activity:** The rate of radioactive decay in a sample, measured in Bq or Ci.
**Technical meaning:** Determines radiation output.
**Related term:** Radioactivity
**Radiotherapy Example:** Determines injection dose for PET imaging.

128. **Isotope calibration:** Ensuring a measured isotope activity matches a known standard.
**Technical meaning:** Critical for accurate dosimetry.
**Related term:** Activity standardization
**Radiotherapy Example:** Used when calibrating radiopharmaceutical doses.

129. **Isotope concentration:** Amount of a specific isotope within a mixture or solution.
**Technical meaning:** Used in tracer studies.
**Related term:** Activity concentration
**Radiotherapy Example:** PET SUV calculations depend on tracer concentration.

130. **Isotope decay chain:** Sequence of radioactive transformations from parent isotope to stable daughter.
**Technical meaning:** Involves half-lives and branching ratios.
**Related term:** Radioactive series
**Radiotherapy Example:** Important in Ra-223 therapy where decay daughters contribute to dose.

131. **Isotope dose:** Radiation dose delivered by a radiopharmaceutical or radioactive source.
**Technical meaning:** Depends on activity, energy, and biokinetics.
**Related term:** Internal dose
**Radiotherapy Example:** Used in targeted radionuclide therapy planning.

132. **Isotope generator:** A system that produces daughter isotopes from a parent (e.g., Mo-99/Tc-99m generator).
**Technical meaning:** Critical for nuclear medicine supply.
**Related term:** Radionuclide generator
**Radiotherapy Example:** Provides Tc-99m for daily SPECT imaging.

133. **Isotope half-life:** Time required for half of a radioactive isotope to decay.
**Technical meaning:** Influences scheduling and safety.
**Related term:** Physical half-life
**Radiotherapy Example:** I-131 half-life determines isolation time.

134. **Isotope identification:** Determining which isotope is present based on spectral data.
**Technical meaning:** Uses gamma spectroscopy.
**Related term:** Isotope analysis
**Radiotherapy Example:** Ensures radiopharmaceutical purity before injection.

135. **Isotope labeling efficiency:** Percentage of radiotracer successfully bound to its molecular carrier.
**Technical meaning:** Affects imaging quality.
**Related term:** Radiolabeling yield
**Radiotherapy Example:** Low labeling reduces PET sensitivity.

136. **Isotope measurement device:** Instrument that measures isotope activity or concentration.
**Technical meaning:** Examples include dose calibrators or gamma counters.
**Related term:** Activity meter
**Radiotherapy Example:** Measures radiopharmaceutical doses before patient injection.

137. **Isotope production facility:** A center equipped with cyclotrons or reactors to produce medical isotopes.
**Technical meaning:** Must follow GMP.
**Related term:** Cyclotron facility
**Radiotherapy Example:** Produces isotopes like F-18 for PET.

138. **Isotope purity:** Fraction of desired isotope compared to contaminants.
**Technical meaning:** Includes radionuclidic and chemical purity.
**Related term:** Radiochemical purity
**Radiotherapy Example:** Required before radiotracer administration.

139. **Isotope radiation:** Radiation emitted during isotope decay.
**Technical meaning:** Can be alpha, beta, gamma, or mixed.
**Related term:** Radioactive emission
**Radiotherapy Example:** Lutetium-177 emits beta particles used in therapy.

140. **Isotope ratio:** Relative proportion of two isotopes in a sample.
**Technical meaning:** Used in tracer analysis.
**Related term:** Isotopic abundance
**Radiotherapy Example:** Determines tracer dilution in metabolic imaging.

141. **Isotope sample:** A measured quantity of a radioactive material used for testing or calibration.
**Technical meaning:** Must be stored and handled safely.
**Related term:** Radiological sample
**Radiotherapy Example:** Calibration labs use Cs-137 samples for dosimeter testing.

142. **Isotope scanner:** Instrument that detects gamma or beta emissions from injected isotopes.
**Technical meaning:** Includes SPECT and PET scanners.
**Related term:** Gamma camera
**Radiotherapy Example:** Used in bone scans for metastasis evaluation.

143. **Isotope spectrum:** Energy distribution of emitted photons or particles.
**Technical meaning:** Identified using spectroscopy.
**Related term:** Gamma spectrum
**Radiotherapy Example:** Verifies purity of therapeutic radionuclides.

144. **Isotope substitution:** Replacing an atom in a molecule with a radioactive isotope.
**Technical meaning:** Used for tracing metabolic pathways.
**Related term:** Radiolabeling
**Radiotherapy Example:** C-11–labeled compounds for PET imaging.

145. **Isotope tracer imaging:** Imaging that uses radioactive tracers to study function or metabolism.
**Technical meaning:** Foundation of SPECT/PET.
**Related term:** Molecular imaging
**Radiotherapy Example:** FDG PET reveals tumor metabolic activity.

146. **Isotope tracer study:** A scientific study using radioactive isotopes to track biological processes.
**Technical meaning:** Measures uptake, clearance, metabolism.
**Related term:** Tracer kinetics
**Radiotherapy Example:** Used to determine absorbed dose in radionuclide therapy.

147. **Isotope uptake:** The amount of tracer absorbed by organs or tissues.
**Technical meaning:** Measured in SUVs or uptake ratios.
**Related term:** Biodistribution
**Radiotherapy Example:** High thyroid uptake indicates good suitability for I-131 therapy.

148. **Isotope verification:** Confirming identity, purity, and activity before clinical use.
**Technical meaning:** Includes spectroscopy and dose checks.
**Related term:** QC testing
**Radiotherapy Example:** Ensures Lu-177 therapy doses meet safety standards.

149. **Isotope yield:** Amount of isotope produced during irradiation or chemical separation.
**Technical meaning:** Depends on target purity and beam current.
**Related term:** Radiochemical yield
**Radiotherapy Example:** Cyclotron efficiency determines daily F-18 yield.

150. **Imaging biomarker:** A measurable imaging parameter that reflects biological processes.
**Technical meaning:** Could be SUV, ADC, perfusion metrics.
**Related term:** Radiomic feature
**Radiotherapy Example:** High SUVmax correlates with aggressive tumors.

151. **Imaging contrast agent:** Substance injected or ingested to improve visualization of tissues.
**Technical meaning:** Includes iodine, gadolinium, microbubbles.
**Related term:** Radiographic contrast
**Radiotherapy Example:** Enhanced CT improves tumor delineation for planning.

152. **Imaging contrast enhancement:** Increase in image brightness within structures after contrast administration.
**Technical meaning:** Indicates vascularity or permeability.
**Related term:** CE-MRI
**Radiotherapy Example:** Helps differentiate tumor vs. edema in MRI for contouring.

153. **Imaging dose calculation:** Estimating patient radiation exposure from imaging scans.
**Technical meaning:** Includes CTDIvol, DLP.
**Related term:** Imaging dosimetry
**Radiotherapy Example:** Used in IGRT optimization to reduce cumulative imaging dose.

154. **Imaging field size:** Dimensions of the area captured in an imaging scan.
**Technical meaning:** Influences resolution and coverage.
**Related term:** FOV (Field of View)
**Radiotherapy Example:** CBCT field size must include all target structures.

155. **Imaging filter:** Hardware or software filter used to shape beam quality or enhance image processing.
**Technical meaning:** Examples: bow-tie filters, smoothing filters.
**Related term:** Beam filter
**Radiotherapy Example:** Bow-tie filters optimize CT dose distribution.

156. **Imaging frame rate:** The number of image frames acquired per second during dynamic imaging. Higher frame rates allow better tracking of motion.
**Technical meaning:** Expressed in FPS (frames per second).
**Related term:** Temporal resolution
**Radiotherapy Example:** Used in fluoroscopic imaging during real-time tumor tracking for SBRT.

157. **Imaging fusion error:** Misalignment between two fused imaging datasets due to registration inaccuracies.
**Technical meaning:** Can be translational or rotational.
**Related term:** Image registration error
**Radiotherapy Example:** PET-CT fusion error can misplace the GTV during contouring.

158. **Imaging geometry:** Spatial setup of imaging components including source, detector, and patient orientation.
**Technical meaning:** Determines magnification, distortion, resolution.
**Related term:** Geometric calibration
**Radiotherapy Example:** Accurate geometry is required for CBCT-based IGRT.

159. **Imaging guidance:** Using imaging methods to assist in accurate treatment or procedure execution.
**Technical meaning:** Real-time or pre-treatment imaging.
**Related term:** IGRT
**Radiotherapy Example:** CBCT imaging guidance helps align patient anatomy before radiation delivery.

160. **Imaging marker:** A structural or implanted object used to guide imaging alignment or track motion.
**Technical meaning:** Includes fiducial markers or anatomical landmarks.
**Related term:** Fiducial
**Radiotherapy Example:** Gold seed markers in prostate radiotherapy improve setup accuracy.

161. **Imaging noise reduction:** Techniques used to decrease unwanted random variation in image signals.
**Technical meaning:** Achieved with smoothing filters, iterative reconstruction.
**Related term:** Image smoothing
**Radiotherapy Example:** Reducing CBCT noise improves soft-tissue visualization.

162. **Imaging phantom:** A device simulating human tissue properties for imaging calibration or QA.
**Technical meaning:** Can mimic CT number, density, or contrast.
**Related term:** QA phantom
**Radiotherapy Example:** Used to verify CT HU accuracy before treatment planning.

163. **163. Imaging plane:** The slice orientation in which images are acquired—axial, sagittal, coronal.
**Technical meaning:** Determines perspective and anatomical visibility.
**Related term:** Image slice
**Radiotherapy Example:** MRI axial planes guide tumor delineation in brain radiotherapy.

164. **Imaging protocol:** A predefined set of scan parameters ensuring consistent and optimized image quality.
**Technical meaning:** Includes kVp, mAs, slice thickness, scan speed.
**Related term:** Scan protocol
**Radiotherapy Example:** Radiotherapy planning CT uses a strict protocol for reproducibility.

165. **Imaging quality metrics:** Quantitative measures that evaluate accuracy, clarity, and reliability of images.
**Technical meaning:** Includes SNR, CNR, MTF, NPS.
**Related term:** Image quality
**Radiotherapy Example:** Used to assess IGRT imaging performance.

166. **Imaging registration:** Aligning images from different modalities or times.
**Technical meaning:** Rigid or deformable.
**Related term:** Image fusion
**Radiotherapy Example:** PET-CT registration identifies metabolically active tumor regions.

167. **Imaging reconstruction:** Mathematical process that builds image data from raw detector signals.
**Technical meaning:** Includes FBP and IR (iterative reconstruction).
**Related term:** Image processing
**Radiotherapy Example:** IR reduces noise in planning CT scans.

168. **Imaging resolution:** Ability to distinguish small structures clearly.
**Technical meaning:** Includes spatial, temporal, and contrast resolution.
**Related term:** Image sharpness
**Radiotherapy Example:** High resolution improves accuracy of target delineation.

169. **Imaging scatter correction:** Methods used to reduce contributions from scattered radiation in images.
**Technical meaning:** Software-based or physical grids.
**Related term:** Anti-scatter grid
**Radiotherapy Example:** Improves HU accuracy in CT scans for dose calculation.

170. **Imaging segmentation error:** Mistakes in automated or manual delineation of structures.
**Technical meaning:** Arises from poor contrast, noise, or incorrect thresholds.
**Related term:** Contouring error
**Radiotherapy Example:** A segmentation error of the optic nerve can lead to unsafe dose.

171. **Imaging sensor:** Detector component that converts radiation or light into electronic signals.
**Technical meaning:** May use CCD, CMOS, scintillators, photodiodes.
**Related term:** Detector
**Radiotherapy Example:** Used in kV on-board imager systems.

172. **Imaging software:** Programs used for image processing, viewing, reconstruction, and registration.
**Technical meaning:** Includes TPS imaging modules.
**Related term:** Image analysis software
**Radiotherapy Example:** Eclipse and RayStation use integrated imaging software.

173. **Imaging spatial resolution:** Smallest visible detail distinguishable on an image.
**Technical meaning:** Measured in lp/mm.
**Related term:** MTF
**Radiotherapy Example:** High spatial resolution improves delineation of small tumors.

174. **Imaging system performance:** Overall capability of an imaging device to produce high-quality, accurate images.
**Technical meaning:** Includes SNR, contrast, resolution, uniformity.
**Related term:** System QA
**Radiotherapy Example:** Annual CBCT performance tests are required.

175. **Imaging threshold:** Intensity cutoff used for segmentation or visualization.
**Technical meaning:** Defines boundaries of tissues.
**Related term:** Threshold segmentation
**Radiotherapy Example:** HU thresholding helps differentiate bone from soft tissue.

176. **Imaging uniformity:** Consistency of pixel values across an image.
**Technical meaning:** Affected by detector gain and calibration.
**Related term:** Flat-field correction
**Radiotherapy Example:** Verified during CT QA to ensure accurate HU maps.

177. **Imaging window setting:** Adjustment of window width and level to optimize image contrast.
**Technical meaning:** Controls grayscale mapping.
**Related term:** Window/level
**Radiotherapy Example:** CT window settings help contour lung vs soft-tissue targets.

178. **Image voxel:** 3D pixel unit representing volume in imaging data.
**Technical meaning:** Defined by slice thickness and in-plane resolution.
**Related term:** Pixel
**Radiotherapy Example:** Dose calculations in TPS operate per voxel.

179. **Imbedded dose:** Dose unintentionally deposited in tissues outside the target.
**Technical meaning:** Often due to scatter or beam tails.
**Related term:** Out-of-field dose
**Radiotherapy Example:** Important in pediatric RT risk assessment.

180. **Impacted dose:** Dose affected by external factors such as movement, heterogeneity, or machine error.
**Technical meaning:** Varies from expected dose.
**Related term:** Delivered dose deviation
**Radiotherapy Example:** Respiratory motion impacts lung tumor dose.

181. **Implantable marker:** Small radio-opaque device placed inside the body to guide imaging.
**Technical meaning:** Improves tracking accuracy.
**Related term:** Fiducial marker
**Radiotherapy Example:** Used for prostate and pancreatic SBRT.

182. **Implant radiation therapy:** Internal radiation treatment where sources are implanted in tissues.
**Technical meaning:** Synonymous with brachytherapy.
**Related term:** Interstitial therapy
**Radiotherapy Example:** Seed implantation for prostate cancer.

183. **Implant source loading:** Inserting radioactive seeds into a patient or phantom.
**Technical meaning:** Manual or automated.
**Related term:** Seed insertion
**Radiotherapy Example:** In LDR prostate brachytherapy.

184. **Implant spacing:** Separation between implanted seeds or catheters.
**Technical meaning:** Influences dose uniformity.
**Related term:** Implant geometry
**Radiotherapy Example:** Correct spacing ensures prostate dose conformity.

185. **Implant tumor control:** Effectiveness of implanted radioactive sources in achieving tumor eradication.
**Technical meaning:** Depends on dose distribution and radionuclide choice.
**Related term:** Local control
**Radiotherapy Example:** High in early-stage prostate LDR brachytherapy.

186. **Implanted dose distribution:** Dose pattern produced by implanted radioactive seeds or catheters.
**Technical meaning:** Highly anisotropic.
**Related term:** Brachytherapy dose distribution
**Radiotherapy Example:** Evaluated via post-implant CT.

187. **Impulse scattering:** Scattering caused by sudden interaction of radiation with atomic electrons.
**Technical meaning:** Often Compton scatter.
**Related term:** Secondary scatter
**Radiotherapy Example:** Influences out-of-field dose during MV treatments.

188. **In-air calibration:** Calibration of a detector without a phantom, in air.
**Technical meaning:** Measures reference conditions like MV output.
**Related term:** Beam calibration
**Radiotherapy Example:** Ion chambers are calibrated in-air at 100 cm SSD.

189. **In-air measurement:** Dose or beam measurement performed with detector suspended in air.
**Technical meaning:** Free-in-air geometry.
**Related term:** Air kerma
**Radiotherapy Example:** Used for beam quality checks.

190. **In-beam imaging:** Imaging performed with the treatment beam or integrated with it.
**Technical meaning:** Includes MV-CT or prompt gamma detection.
**Related term:** Beam's-eye-view imaging
**Radiotherapy Example:** MV portal imaging during IMRT.

191. **In-body dose:** Radiation absorbed inside tissues.
**Technical meaning:** Includes internal and external sources.
**Related term:** Internal dose
**Radiotherapy Example:** Calculated from dose-volume histograms.

192. **In-body imaging:** Imaging of internal anatomy using radiologic techniques.
**Technical meaning:** Includes CT, PET, MRI, US.
**Related term:** Internal imaging
**Radiotherapy Example:** MRI is used for soft-tissue tumor delineation.

193. **In-bore imaging:** Imaging performed inside the scanner bore while patient remains in scan position.
**Technical meaning:** Reduces movement between imaging and treatment.
**Related term:** Integrated imaging
**Radiotherapy Example:** MR-Linac uses continuous in-bore imaging.

194. **In-brain dosimetry:** Calculation of dose delivered to brain tissues.
**Technical meaning:** Includes tumor and OAR evaluations.
**Related term:** CNS dosimetry
**Radiotherapy Example:** Used in SRS for AVM or metastasis plans.

195. **In-circuit dosimeter:** Radiation detector integrated inside an electrical circuit.
**Technical meaning:** Used in industrial or embedded systems.
**Related term:** On-board dosimetry
**Radiotherapy Example:** Used in some linac safety systems.

196. **In-component dose:** Dose absorbed by machine parts such as MLCs, jaws, or flattening filters.
**Technical meaning:** Relevant to machine longevity.
**Related term:** Internal scatter
**Radiotherapy Example:** MLC dose affects leakage characteristics.

197. **In-depth dose:** Dose variation with depth in tissue.
**Technical meaning:** Includes percent depth dose (PDD).
**Related term:** Depth dose curve
**Radiotherapy Example:** Used when selecting electron beam energy.

198. **In-field calibration:** Calibration done within the treatment field rather than reference geometry.
**Technical meaning:** Accounts for real-world conditions.
**Related term:** In-field dosimetry
**Radiotherapy Example:** Used for detector arrays during IMRT QA.

199. **In-field dose:** Dose delivered inside the defined treatment field.
**Technical meaning:** Should meet prescription coverage.
**Related term:** Target dose
**Radiotherapy Example:** Evaluated via PTV dose metrics in plan review.

200. **Internal radiation measurement:** Quantification of radiation emitted or absorbed inside the body.
**Technical meaning:** Includes biokinetics and organ dose.
**Related term:** Internal dosimetry
**Radiotherapy Example:** Used in radionuclide therapy like Lu-177 dosimetry.

201. **Ion absorption**Ion: Absorption refers to the process in which charged particles lose their energy as they pass through matter, typically through interactions with electrons in the material. This process directly affects how radiation deposits dose in biological tissues. Higher absorption leads to greater biological effect and heating. Ion absorption depends on ion energy, material density, and atomic composition.
**Related term:** Ion energy deposition
**Radiotherapy Example:** In proton therapy, ion absorption determines the Bragg peak depth, ensuring that most energy is absorbed in the tumor.

202. **Ion activity**Ion: Activity represents the effective concentration of ions participating in chemical or physical interactions. Unlike concentration, activity accounts for ion–ion interactions and environmental effects. In radiation science, ion activity influences detector behavior, electrolyte dosimeters, and radiochemical reactions. Accurate measurement is essential in chemical dosimetry.
**Related term:** Ion strength
**Radiotherapy Example:** In chemical dosimeters (e.g., Fricke solution), ion activity influences the accuracy of absorbed-dose measurement.

203. **Ion analyzer:** An ion analyzer is an instrument that identifies or quantifies ions based on their mass, charge, or mobility. It can use mass spectrometry, ion energy filters, or mobility measurements. In radiation science, ion analyzers help characterize radiation-produced ions and verify beam purity for therapy. They also assist in isotope identification.
**Related term:** Ion spectrometer
**Radiotherapy Example:** Ion analyzers are used in proton therapy facilities to verify that no unwanted ion species contaminate the treatment beam.

204. **Ion attenuation**Ion: Attenuation describes the reduction in ion beam intensity as it travels through matter. This occurs through collision, scattering, and energy loss. The attenuation rate depends on ion type, energy, and medium. Understanding attenuation is necessary to calculate dose and penetration depth.
**Related term:** Linear attenuation coefficient
**Radiotherapy Example:** Ion attenuation calculations ensure that carbon ion beams deliver the prescribed dose to deep-seated tumors without overshooting the target.

205. **Ion beam collimation:** Ion beam collimation is the process of narrowing and shaping an ion beam using mechanical or magnetic devices. Collimation improves beam precision and reduces exposure to surrounding structures. High-quality collimation is essential in external-beam radiotherapy involving ions.
**Related term:** Beam shaping
**Radiotherapy Example:** In proton therapy, brass apertures are used to collimate the ion beam so that the dose conforms to the tumor shape.

206. **Ion beam dosimetry:** Ion beam dosimetry focuses on measuring dose delivered by charged-particle beams such as protons or carbon ions. Specialized detectors measure stopping power, ionization, and depth–dose curves. Accurate dosimetry is necessary because ions behave differently from photons.
**Related term:** Stopping power ratio
**Radiotherapy Example:** Ionization chambers measure proton Bragg peak profiles to verify correct dose deposition.

207. **Ion beam therapy:** Ion beam therapy uses charged particles (protons, carbon ions, helium ions) to treat cancer. Ions deposit most energy at a precise depth (Bragg peak), allowing targeted high-dose delivery while sparing tissue beyond the tumor. It is highly effective for radio-resistant tumors.
**Related term:** Proton therapy
**Radiotherapy Example:** Carbon ion therapy is used to treat tumors of the skull base that are difficult to manage with photons.

208. **Ion chamber calibration:** Ion chamber calibration ensures that an ionization chamber provides accurate exposure or dose measurements. Calibration is performed against a national or reference standard. Environmental conditions such as temperature and pressure are also considered.
**Related term:** Calibration factor
**Radiotherapy Example:** Before commissioning an IMRT linac, physicists calibrate ion chambers to establish baseline dose accuracy.

209. **Ion chamber dosimeter:** An ion chamber dosimeter measures radiation dose through ionization of gas within the chamber. These dosimeters are used for absolute dosimetry in radiotherapy because of their stability and accuracy. They come in various designs for different applications.
**Related term:** Farmer-type ion chamber
**Radiotherapy Example:** A 0.6 cc ion chamber is placed in a water phantom to measure reference dose for linac output calibration.

210. **Ion chamber efficiency:** Ion chamber efficiency describes how effectively an ion chamber collects the ions produced by radiation. Factors include electrode voltage, chamber geometry, and gas type. High efficiency ensures accurate dose measurements. Poor efficiency can lead to ion recombination errors.
**Related term:** Collection efficiency
**Radiotherapy Example:** Chamber voltage sweeps are performed during QA to verify the efficiency of ion collection under clinical beam conditions.

211. **Ion chamber measurement:** Ion chamber measurement refers to the process of using an ionization chamber to quantify radiation dose, exposure, or beam quality. Measurements follow strict protocols, considering environmental corrections and calibration coefficients.
**Related term:** Dosimetry protocol
**Radiotherapy Example:** Ion chamber measurement is used to determine daily linac output during morning QA checks.

212. **Ion chromatography detector:** An ion chromatography detector measures ion concentrations separated via ion chromatography. In radiological applications, it can detect radiolysis products or track chemical changes in dosimetric systems.
**Related term:** Ion exchange column
**Radiotherapy Example:** Ion chromatography detects radiolysis-produced ions in aqueous radiation dosimeters used for beam verification.

213. **Ion detector calibration:** Ion detector calibration validates sensitivity and response accuracy in systems that measure ions (ion counters, mobility detectors, mass spectrometers). Calibration ensures reliable identification and quantification.
**Related term:** Detector response factor
**Radiotherapy Example:** Ion detectors in beam-monitoring systems are calibrated to ensure accurate measurement of proton beam intensity.

214. **Ion detector efficiency:** Ion detector efficiency indicates how well a detector counts incoming ions without losses. Efficiency depends on ion energy, detector design, and signal electronics. High efficiency is critical for accurate ion-beam monitoring.
**Related term:** Detection sensitivity
**Radiotherapy Example:** In carbon ion therapy, efficient ion detectors maintain precise beam-on timing and dose monitoring.

215. **Ion detector measurement:** This refers to the process of quantifying ion flux, energy, or species using a dedicated ion detector. Measurements support beam diagnostics, particle identification, and radiation monitoring.
**Related term:** Ion flux measurement
**Radiotherapy Example:** During QA of proton therapy systems, ion detector measurements verify that beam energy matches the treatment plan.

216. **Ion emission spectrum:** The ion emission spectrum displays the range and intensity of ions emitted from a radioactive source or accelerator. It helps characterize beam purity and radiation type.
**Related term:** Energy spectrum
**Radiotherapy Example:** Carbon ion facilities analyze the ion emission spectrum to ensure only carbon ions—not lighter fragments—enter the treatment beam.

217. **Ion energy deposition:** Ion energy deposition is the process of transferring ion kinetic energy to matter. It defines dose distribution and biological effect. Ions deposit energy densely, causing significant biological damage.
**Related term:** Linear energy transfer (LET)
**Radiotherapy Example:** High LET carbon ions deposit more energy near the tumor, improving tumor control for resistant cancers.

218. **Ion energy measurement:** Ion energy measurement determines the kinetic energy of charged particles using detectors, spectrometers, or magnetic analyzers. Accurate energy measurements are required for range prediction.
**Related term:** Beam energy verification
**Radiotherapy Example:** Proton energy measurements ensure correct penetration depth for tumors near critical structures.

219. **Ion flux measurement:** Ion flux measurement quantifies the number of ions passing through a surface per unit time. It helps monitor beam stability and intensity.
**Related term:** Particle fluence
**Radiotherapy Example:** During proton therapy, real-time ion flux monitoring maintains consistent dose delivery.

220. **Ion generation:** Ion generation describes any process producing ions, such as radioactive decay, ion sources, or particle collisions. In therapy, controlled ion generation creates the treatment beam.
**Related term:** Ion source
**Radiotherapy Example:** Ion generation in a synchrotron creates carbon ions for heavy-ion radiotherapy.

221. **Ion imaging:** Ion imaging uses charged particles (protons or ions) to produce images of tissue density or composition. It provides highly accurate range verification since ions are sensitive to tissue stopping power. Methods include proton radiography and ion CT.
**Related term:** Proton radiography
**Radiotherapy Example:** Proton imaging is used before treatment to verify patient anatomy and adjust proton beam range.

**222. Ion implantation:** Ion implantation inserts ions into a material at controlled energies. In radiation science, it is used for detector fabrication, semiconductor modification, and calibration targets. It changes material properties such as conductivity or hardness.
**Related term:** Ion doping
**Radiotherapy Example:** High-quality radiation detectors used in proton therapy are often manufactured using ion-implantation techniques.

**223. Ion interaction:** Ion interaction describes how ions collide with and transfer energy to electrons, nuclei, or other ions. These interactions define stopping power, scattering, and dose deposition.
**Related term:** Coulomb interaction
**Radiotherapy Example:** Understanding ion interaction allows accurate modeling of proton scattering around bone–soft tissue interfaces.

**224. Ion irradiation:** Ion irradiation exposes materials or tissues to an ion beam. It is used for scientific research, material modification, and cancer treatment. Ions deliver energy with predictable depth-dose characteristics.
**Related term:** Charged-particle irradiation
**Radiotherapy Example:** Ion irradiation studies help evaluate radiobiological effects of carbon ions for clinical treatments.

**225. Ion laser:** An ion laser generates photons by exciting ions such as argon or krypton in a gas-filled tube. These lasers provide stable, high-intensity output used in spectroscopy and detector calibration.
**Related term:** Argon-ion laser
**Radiotherapy Example:** Ion lasers are used in optical calibration of scintillation detectors employed in radiation QA.

**226. Ion mass analyzer:** An ion mass analyzer separates ions based on mass-to-charge ratio. It is used to characterize beam contamination, radiochemical purity, and isotope identification.
**Related term:** Mass spectrometer
**Radiotherapy Example:** Beam purity in carbon ion therapy is verified with ion mass analysis to avoid unintended lighter fragments.

**227. Ion measurement system:** A system designed to measure ion flux, energy, type, or dose. It may include ion chambers, Faraday cups, spectrometers, and electronics. Accuracy is critical for therapy safety.
**Related term:** Beam diagnostics system
**Radiotherapy Example:** Ion measurement systems ensure stable proton beam output during daily QA.

**228. Ion mobility spectrum:** This spectrum displays ions separated by mobility in a gas under electric field influence. It identifies ion species and energy states.
**Related term:** Ion mobility spectrometry (IMS)
**Radiotherapy Example:** IMS can detect radiolysis products in radiochemical dosimeters used for dose verification.

**229. Ion pair yield:** Ion pair yield refers to the number of ion pairs formed per unit energy deposited. It determines detector sensitivity and dosimeter performance.
**Related term:** W-value (mean energy per ion pair)
**Radiotherapy Example:** The ion pair yield of air is fundamental to calibrating ion chambers used in photon and proton beam dosimetry.

230. **Ion probe:** An ion probe measures ion density, energy, or flux, often using a small electrode or sensor inserted into a beam or plasma.
**Related term:** Faraday probe
**Radiotherapy Example:** Ion probes monitor ion beam uniformity in proton therapy nozzles.

231. **Ion pump:** An ion pump removes gas molecules from a vacuum chamber by ionizing and trapping them. It creates ultra-high vacuum needed for particle accelerators.
**Related term:** Vacuum system
**Radiotherapy Example:** Synchrotrons and cyclotrons require ion pumps to maintain low pressure for stable ion acceleration.

232. **Ion radiation therapy:** A broad term covering cancer treatments using ions (protons, carbon, helium). Ions offer precise dose delivery and enhanced biological effectiveness.
**Related term:** Heavy-ion therapy
**Radiotherapy Example:** Carbon ion radiation therapy is used for sarcomas resistant to photon treatment.

233. **Ion range:** Ion range is the depth at which ions stop in matter. It depends on ion type, initial energy, and medium. Range precision is critical for therapy.
**Related term:** Bragg peak
**Radiotherapy Example:** Proton beam range calculations ensure energy is sufficient to reach a lung tumor but not pass through it.

234. **Ion recombination:** Ion recombination occurs when positive and negative ions recombine before collection in a detector, reducing detected charge. It depends on dose rate and chamber voltage.
**Related term:** Collection efficiency
**Radiotherapy Example:** High dose-rate beams (flattening-filter-free) require recombination corrections for accurate ion chamber dosimetry.

235. **Ion scattering:** Ion scattering is the deflection of ions due to interactions with atomic nuclei or electrons. It affects beam divergence and spatial accuracy.
**Related term:** Multiple Coulomb scattering
**Radiotherapy Example:** Scattering causes proton beams to broaden, affecting penumbra at tumor

236. **Ion source:** An ion source generates ions for accelerators using plasma, electron bombardment, or gas discharge. Beam quality depends on the source design.
**Related term:** Electron cyclotron resonance (ECR) source
**Radiotherapy Example:** Carbon therapy facilities use ECR ion sources to produce high-charge-state carbon ions.

237. **Ion spectrometer:** A device that identifies ion species and measures energy spectra. Used to ensure beam purity and characterize radiation fields.
**Related term:** Time-of-flight spectrometer
**Radiotherapy Example:** Ion spectrometers verify proton beam energy spread before clinical treatment.

238. **Ionization curve:** An ionization curve shows ionization rate vs. depth or energy. It helps estimate stopping power, range, or detector response.
**Related term:** Depth–dose curve
**Radiotherapy Example:** Ionization curves are used to tune proton beam energy to create a spread-out Bragg peak (SOBP).

239. **Ionization density:** Ionization density expresses how many ion pairs are produced per volume or path length. High density increases biological effect.
**Related term:** Linear energy transfer (LET)
**Radiotherapy Example:** Carbon ions produce dense ionization, causing more effective tumor cell killing.

240. **Ionization dose:** Ionization dose measures the amount of charge generated by radiation in a medium. It correlates with absorbed dose.
**Related term:** Exposure
**Radiotherapy Example:** Early radiological dosimetry used ionization dose before absorbed dose became standard.

241. **Ionization energy:** Ionization energy is the amount of energy required to remove an electron from an atom or molecule. In radiation physics, it determines how easily radiation can create ion pairs.
**Related term:** Electron binding energy
**Radiotherapy Example:** Lower ionization energies in soft tissue influence the efficiency of ionization during proton therapy.

242. **Ionization event:** An ionization event refers to any instance where radiation removes electrons from atoms, forming ion pairs. These events drive both dose deposition and biological damage.
**Related term:** Ion track structure
**Radiotherapy Example:** High-LET ions produce dense clusters of ionization events, increasing cell-killing effectiveness.

243. **Ionization measurement:** Ionization measurement quantifies the number of ion pairs produced by radiation, typically using ion chambers. It is essential for dosimetry.
**Related term:** Charge collection
**Radiotherapy Example:** Beam output calibration for linacs uses ionization measurements in reference chambers.

244. **Ionization potential:** Ionization potential expresses the minimum energy needed to ionize an atom in its ground state. It influences radiation–matter interaction probabilities.
**Related term:** Ionization energy
**Radiotherapy Example:** Tissue ionization potentials affect Monte Carlo dose-calculation accuracy.

245. **Ionization probability:** The probability that radiation interaction will produce ion pairs. It depends on photon energy, material composition, and radiation type.
**Related term:** Interaction cross-section
**Radiotherapy Example:** Higher ionization probability in bone influences CT-number accuracy for dose planning.

246. **Ionization process:** The process through which charged particles or photons remove electrons from matter, generating ions. It forms the basis of radiation detection and dose deposition.
**Related term:** Photoionization
**Radiotherapy Example:** Ionization processes in gas chambers allow accurate HDR brachytherapy source calibration.

247. **Ionization product:** The ions or electrons created after a radiation interaction. Their number is proportional to deposited energy.
**Related term:** Secondary electrons
**Radiotherapy Example:** Ionization products collected in a chamber provide dose readings for IMRT QA.

**248. Ionization radiation detector:** A detector that measures radiation by collecting charged particles produced through ionization (e.g., ion chambers, GM tubes).
**Related term:** Gas-filled detector
**Radiotherapy Example:** Farmer ion chambers are standard devices for radiotherapy reference dosimetry.

**249. Ionization rate:** The rate at which ion pairs are produced in a medium per unit time or dose. It depends on radiation intensity and energy.
**Related term:** Exposure rate
**Radiotherapy Example:** High dose-rate beams increase ionization rate, requiring recombination corrections.

**250. Ionization track:** The path formed by sequential ionization events created by a charged particle. Track density reflects LET.
**Related term:** Track structure
**Radiotherapy Example:** Carbon-ion tracks create dense damage clusters in tumor DNA.

**251. Ionization yield:** Ionization yield is the number of ion pairs produced per unit path length or energy. Important in detector sensitivity.
**Related term:** W-value
**Radiotherapy Example:** Higher ionization yields improve accuracy of micro-ionization chambers in small-field dosimetry.

**252. Ionizing beam:** A beam composed of photons or charged particles capable of ionizing matter. Used in imaging and therapy.
**Related term:** Radiation beam
**Radiotherapy Example:** Ionizing beams from linacs deliver therapeutic dose to cancer tissue.

**253. Ionizing event:** Any interaction where radiation deposits enough energy to ionize atoms. Fundamental to dose and biological effects.
**Related term:** Energy deposition event
**Radiotherapy Example:** The frequency of ionizing events correlates with tumor control probability.

**254. Ionizing particle:** Any charged particle that produces ionization along its path (electrons, protons, alpha particles, ions).
**Related term:** Charged particle
**Radiotherapy Example:** Proton beams are ionizing particles used for precise tumor treatment.

**255. Ionizing photon:** A photon with sufficient energy (typically >10 eV) to ionize atoms—includes X-rays and gamma rays.
**Related term:** High-energy photon
**Radiotherapy Example:** 6 MV photons from a linac are ionizing photons used in external beam therapy.

**256. Irradiance:** Irradiance is the power of radiation received per unit area. Common in optical radiation but also applicable to UV and visible systems.
**Related term:** Radiant flux density
**Radiotherapy Example:** UV irradiance measurements ensure safe sterilization levels in treatment rooms.

**257. Irradiated area:** The portion of a surface or tissue exposed to radiation. It is defined during planning and setup.
**Related term:** Treatment field
**Radiotherapy Example:** The irradiated area in breast radiotherapy includes the whole breast while sparing the heart.

258. **Irradiated field:** Region of tissue receiving clinically significant radiation dose. Determined using collimation or MLC shaping.
**Related term:** Radiation field
**Radiotherapy Example:** IMRT shapes irradiated fields around organs-at-risk.

259. **Irradiated material:** Any material exposed to radiation, possibly undergoing physical or chemical changes.
**Related term:** Radiation-processed material
**Radiotherapy Example:** Polymer gel dosimeters are irradiated materials used for 3D dose mapping.

260. **Irradiated tissue:** Tissue exposed to medical, accidental, or experimental radiation. Biological response depends on dose and LET.
**Related term:** Biological dose
**Radiotherapy Example:** Irradiated tissue in head-and-neck therapy may develop mucositis depending on dose distribution.

261. **Irradiation angle:** The angle at which radiation enters an object, influencing path length and dose distribution.
**Related term:** Beam incidence angle
**Radiotherapy Example:** Non-coplanar beams optimize irradiation angles to spare critical organs.

262. **Irradiation control:** Systems and protocols that regulate dose delivery, timing, and beam parameters to ensure safe irradiation.
**Related term:** Safety interlock
**Radiotherapy Example:** Irradiation controls prevent incorrect energy selection in a linac.

263. **Irradiation dose:** The amount of radiation energy deposited in tissue or a material. Expressed as absorbed dose in grays.
**Related term:** Absorbed dose
**Radiotherapy Example:** A 70 Gy irradiation dose is typical for curative head-and-neck cancer therapy.

264. **Irradiation dose rate:** The dose delivered per unit time. Influences biological response and detector behavior.
**Related term:** DRR (dose rate ratio)
**Radiotherapy Example:** HDR brachytherapy uses very high irradiation dose rates for short treatments.

265. **Irradiation effect:** Physical, chemical, or biological changes caused by radiation exposure.
**Related term:** Radiation effect
**Radiotherapy Example:** Tumor apoptosis is a common irradiation effect following high-dose therapy.

266. **Irradiation experiment:** Controlled exposure of cells, animals, or materials to radiation for research or calibration.
**Related term:** Radiobiology study
**Radiotherapy Example:** Experiments on oxygen enhancement ratio improve understanding of tumor hypoxia.

267. **Irradiation exposure:** Radiation exposure measured as dose or dose equivalent to a subject or object.
**Related term:** Radiation exposure
**Radiotherapy Example:** Occupation-related irradiation exposure must follow ALARA principles.

**268. Irradiation facility:** A specialized structure housing radiation equipment for therapy, research, or industrial applications.
**Related term:** Treatment vault
**Radiotherapy Example:** Proton therapy centers include irradiation facilities with gantries and shielding.

**269. Irradiation instrument:** Devices used to generate or measure radiation during experiments or treatments.
**Related term:** Radiation source
**Radiotherapy Example:** Cesium irradiators are irradiation instruments used for blood sterilization.

**270. Irradiation level:** The magnitude of radiation intensity or dose at a location.
**Related term:** Dose level
**Radiotherapy Example:** Dose–volume histograms display irradiation levels across tumor and OARs.

**271. Irradiation pattern:** Spatial distribution of radiation dose across a target. Can be uniform or intensity-modulated.
**Related term:** Dose painting
**Radiotherapy Example:** IMRT creates complex irradiation patterns matching tumor geometry.

**272. Irradiation planning:** Process of designing optimal beam arrangements, dose levels, and constraints for treatment.
**Related term:** Treatment planning
**Radiotherapy Example:** Planning software computes 3D dose for VMAT treatments.

**273. Irradiation procedure:** A standardized protocol for delivering radiation safely and accurately.
**Related term:** Treatment protocol
**Radiotherapy Example:** QA steps are included in irradiation procedures to prevent errors.

**274. Irradiation profile:** Graph showing variation in beam intensity across a field.
**Related term:** Beam profile
**Radiotherapy Example:** Flattening filter-free beams show a peaked irradiation profile.

**275. Irradiation protection:** Measures taken to protect workers, patients, and the public from unnecessary radiation.
**Related term:** Radiation shielding
**Radiotherapy Example:** Lead barriers and interlocks provide irradiation protection in linac rooms.

**276. Irradiation region:** Tissue volume receiving planned radiation.
**Related term:** Target volume
**Radiotherapy Example:** The PTV is the irradiation region accounting for motion and setup variations.

**277. Irradiation sensor:** A device that detects radiation intensity, type, or dose.
**Related term:** Dosimeter
**Radiotherapy Example:** MOSFET sensors measure dose during in vivo patient monitoring.

**278. Irradiation simulation:** Modeling radiation delivery using computational tools to predict dose.
**Related term:** Monte Carlo simulation
**Radiotherapy Example:** MC simulations validate dose in heterogeneous lung tissues.

**279. Irradiation source:** Any device or isotope producing radiation.
**Related term:** Radioactive source
**Radiotherapy Example:** Ir-192 sources are irradiation sources in HDR brachytherapy.

**280. Irradiation strength:** Magnitude of radiation intensity or ability to deliver dose.
**Related term:** Beam output
**Radiotherapy Example:** Linac output measurements ensure consistent irradiation strength each day.

**281. Irradiation system:** Integrated hardware that generates, shapes, and controls radiation.
**Related term:** Radiotherapy delivery system
**Radiotherapy Example:** A proton gantry is an irradiation system delivering pencil-beam scanning.

**282. Irradiation technique:** The method used to deliver radiation (IMRT, VMAT, SRS, SBRT).
**Related term:** Treatment technique
**Radiotherapy Example:** SBRT is an irradiation technique delivering high doses in few fractions.

**283. Irradiation test:** A controlled test exposing materials or detectors to radiation for evaluation.
**Related term:** Radiation hardness test
**Radiotherapy Example:** Scintillator performance is verified under irradiation tests before clinical use.

**284. Irradiation threshold:** Minimum dose required to produce a detectable physical or biological effect.
**Related term:** Threshold dose
**Radiotherapy Example:** A threshold dose exists for skin erythema during treatment.

**285. Irradiation time:** The duration over which radiation is delivered.
**Related term:** Beam-on time
**Radiotherapy Example:** HDR dwell times determine irradiation time around catheters.

**286. Irradiation unit:** A device or setup designed for controlled exposures.
**Related term:** Radiation unit
**Radiotherapy Example:** Small-field irradiation units are used for animal radiobiology studies.

**287. Irradiator shielding:** Shielding that surrounds an irradiator to prevent leakage.
**Related term:** Lead shielding
**Radiotherapy Example:** Gamma irradiators have thick shielding to protect technicians.

**288. Isotope dosimetry:** Measurement of dose delivered by radioactive isotopes.
**Related term:** Internal dosimetry
**Radiotherapy Example:** Y-90 microsphere therapy relies on isotope dosimetry for liver dose assessment.

**289. Isotope generator:** A device that produces short-lived isotopes from longer-lived parents (e.g., Tc-99m generator).
**Related term:** Radionuclide generator
**Radiotherapy Example:** Generators supply isotopes for diagnostic imaging that guide radiotherapy planning.

**290. Isotope imaging:** Imaging using gamma-emitting isotopes to visualize physiology or metabolism.
**Related term:** Nuclear imaging
**Radiotherapy Example:** PET isotope imaging maps tumor hypoxia for dose escalation.

**291. Isotope measurement:** Quantification of isotope activity or concentration.
**Related term:** Activity assay
**Radiotherapy Example:** Accurate isotope measurement ensures correct Y-90 dose before infusion.

**292. Isotope production:** Creation of medical isotopes using cyclotrons or reactors.
**Related term:** Radionuclide production
**Radiotherapy Example:** Carbon-11 and F-18 production supports PET-guided adaptive radiotherapy.

293. **Isotope ratio:** The relative abundance of isotopes in a sample.
**Related term:** Isotopic composition
**Radiotherapy Example:** Isotope ratios help verify purity of therapeutic radioisotopes.

294. **Isotope scan:** A diagnostic scan using radioactive tracers.
**Related term:** Nuclear scan
**Radiotherapy Example:** Bone isotope scans detect metastases to plan palliative radiotherapy.

295. **Isotope separation:** Techniques for separating isotopes based on mass or chemistry.
**Related term:** Mass separation
**Radiotherapy Example:** Producing pure therapeutic isotopes requires efficient isotope separation.

296. **Isotope source:** Radioactive material used for imaging or therapy.
**Related term:** Radionuclide source
**Radiotherapy Example:** Co-60 is an isotope source used in gamma knife radiosurgery.

297. **Isotope tracer:** A labeled isotope used to track physiological pathways.
**Related term:** Radiotracer
**Radiotherapy Example:** FDG tracer uptake identifies active tumor areas for dose escalation.

298. **Isotope uptake:** The amount of radioactive tracer absorbed by tissues.
**Related term:** SUV (standard uptake value)
**Radiotherapy Example:** High uptake on PET correlates with aggressive tumor regions needing higher dose.

299. **Isotopic analysis:** Analysis of isotopic composition to determine identity, purity, or distribution.
**Related term:** Mass spectrometric analysis
**Radiotherapy Example:** Isotopic analysis confirms the radionuclide purity for brachytherapy sources.

300. **Isotopic imaging:** Imaging based on isotope distribution (PET, SPECT).
**Related term:** Radionuclide imaging
**Radiotherapy Example:** Isotopic imaging guides tumor contouring during treatment planning.

301. **Imaging acquisition protocol:** An imaging acquisition protocol is the predefined set of technical parameters used to capture medical images, including slice thickness, exposure, timing, and reconstruction settings. It ensures consistency, comparability, and diagnostic accuracy across patient scans. Protocols vary based on modality and clinical indication.
**Related term:** Imaging parameter set
**Radiotherapy Example:** A standardized CT acquisition protocol ensures accurate electron density data for dose calculation.

302. **Imaging alignment:** Imaging alignment refers to the process of ensuring that anatomical structures, imaging planes, or reference points are properly positioned relative to the scanner or treatment machine. Good alignment reduces artifacts and improves registration accuracy.
**Related term:** Patient positioning
**Radiotherapy Example:** CBCT-to-CT imaging alignment is performed before each treatment session for IGRT.

303. **Imaging analysis software:** Software used to process, analyze, and interpret medical images. It provides tools for segmentation, measurements, fusion, and quantitative assessments. Advanced versions use AI for automation.
**Related term:** Image processing platform
**Radiotherapy Example:** Treatment-planning software includes imaging analysis modules for tumor and organ segmentation.

**304. Imaging artifact correction:** Techniques used to remove or reduce distortions in medical images caused by motion, metal implants, scatter, or reconstruction errors. Artifact correction enhances visibility and accuracy.
**Related term:** Artifact reduction
**Radiotherapy Example:** Metal artifact correction algorithms improve CT quality for patients with dental fillings in H&N RT.

**305. Imaging attenuation:** Attenuation refers to the reduction in radiation intensity as it passes through tissue. In imaging, this affects contrast, CT numbers, and the accuracy of reconstructed images.
**Related term:** Linear attenuation coefficient
**Radiotherapy Example:** CT attenuation data are used to convert Hounsfield units to density for dose planning.

**306. Imaging attenuation coefficient:** A quantitative measure describing how strongly tissue absorbs or scatters radiation during imaging. Different materials have characteristic coefficients used in CT and PET reconstruction.
**Related term:** μ-value
**Radiotherapy Example:** Accurate attenuation coefficients ensure correct PET SUV values for tumor

**307. Imaging axis:** The imaginary line representing the central or reference direction through which imaging data are acquired. Proper alignment along this axis ensures anatomical accuracy.
**Related term:** Beam axis
**Radiotherapy Example:** CBCT imaging axis alignment is verified to match the treatment beam isocenter.

**308. Imaging beam quality:** Beam quality refers to the energy characteristics of the imaging beam (e.g., kVp, spectrum). It determines image contrast, noise, and patient dose.
**Related term:** Beam hardness
**Radiotherapy Example:** Higher kVp reduces noise in CT scans used for radiotherapy simulation.

**309. Imaging calibration:** Calibration ensures that imaging systems produce accurate, consistent outputs. It involves checking geometry, grayscale values, uniformity, and detector response.
**Related term:** System calibration
**Radiotherapy Example:** Daily MV imaging calibration ensures precise linac imaging for patient positioning.

**310. Imaging chamber:** A chamber used to measure imaging-beam dose or quality, often a small-volume ion chamber optimized for low energies.
**Related term:** Diagnostic ion chamber
**Radiotherapy Example:** Imaging chambers verify kV CBCT dose before commissioning a radiotherapy linac.

**311. Imaging coherence:** Coherence describes how well wave fronts maintain phase relationships, relevant mainly in optical and ultrasound imaging. High coherence improves resolution but may increase speckle.
**Related term:** Coherent imaging
**Radiotherapy Example:** Optical coherence tomography may assist in surface-guided radiotherapy.

**312. Imaging contrast agent:** A substance administered to enhance visibility of specific tissues or vessels on images (iodine, gadolinium, etc.). It increases the difference between target and background structures.
**Related term:** Radiographic contrast
**Radiotherapy Example:** Contrast-enhanced CT improves delineation of liver tumors for SBRT.

**313. Imaging contrast enhancement:** Techniques or substances used to increase visual distinction between tissues in an image. Enhancement may be physical, computational, or chemical.
**Related term:** Contrast injection
**Radiotherapy Example:** Radiologists use contrast-enhanced MRI to define GTV boundaries for brain RT.

**314. Imaging control system:** Hardware and software that regulate imaging parameters, acquisition timing, detector settings, and safety interlocks.
**Related term:** Imaging console
**Radiotherapy Example:** CBCT control systems manage acquisition sequences during patient setup.

**315. Imaging dose optimization:** Strategies used to reduce patient radiation dose while maintaining diagnostic image quality. This includes kVp reduction, filtration, iterative reconstruction, and scan-length minimization.
**Related term:** ALARA imaging
**Radiotherapy Example:** Low-dose CBCT protocols are used for daily IGRT to minimize cumulative patient dose.

**316. Imaging efficiency:** A measure of how effectively an imaging system converts incoming radiation into usable image information. Higher efficiency improves SNR and reduces required dose.
**Related term:** Detector quantum efficiency
**Radiotherapy Example:** High-efficiency flat-panel detectors improve MV portal imaging quality.

**317. Imaging energy:** The energy spectrum of the imaging radiation (kVp, keV, MeV). Determines penetration, contrast, and scatter levels.
**Related term:** Photon energy
**Radiotherapy Example:** kV energies are used for cone-beam imaging, while MV energies support portal imaging.

**318. Imaging exposure:** Amount of radiation used during an imaging procedure. A critical factor affecting patient dose and image quality.
**Related term:** Exposure index
**Radiotherapy Example:** Imaging exposure is monitored to prevent excessive daily CBCT doses.

**319. Imaging field calibration:** Calibration ensuring accurate geometry, size, and uniformity of the imaging field. Essential for accurate measurement and registration.
**Related term:** Field uniformity check
**Radiotherapy Example:** Imaging field calibration is performed during linac commissioning.

**320. Imaging field size:** The physical dimensions of the area captured by an imaging beam. Larger fields include more anatomy but increase dose and scatter.
**Related term:** FOV (field of view)
**Radiotherapy Example:** Large-field CT captures entire thorax for lung RT planning.

**321. Imaging filter:** Filters, either physical or digital, modify the imaging beam or image. Physical filters harden beams; digital filters enhance signal or suppress noise.
**Related term:** Beam filter
**Radiotherapy Example:** Bowtie filters shape the CT beam for uniform dose and improved image quality.

**322. Imaging fluoroscopy:** Real-time X-ray imaging used to visualize motion, interventional procedures, or organ dynamics.
**Related term:** Fluoroscopic imaging
**Radiotherapy Example:** Fluoroscopy guides fiducial placement for prostate radiotherapy.

**323. Imaging frame rate:** The number of images captured per second in dynamic imaging. Higher frame rates improve temporal resolution.
**Related term:** Temporal resolution
**Radiotherapy Example:** Fluoroscopy with high frame rate assists respiratory motion tracking.

**324. Imaging geometry correction:** Algorithms that correct distortions due to detector tilt, rotation, misalignment, or lens distortion.
**Related term:** Geometric calibration
**Radiotherapy Example:** Geometry correction ensures CBCT images align with treatment isocenter.

**325. Imaging guidance system:** Hardware and software used to perform image-guided procedures. Includes imaging devices, tracking tools, and alignment algorithms.
**Related term:** IGRT system
**Radiotherapy Example:** IGRT systems use CBCT guidance to verify tumor position before each fraction.

**326. Imaging grid:** A grid used to reduce scatter in imaging by allowing only primary photons to reach the detector. Improves contrast but increases dose.
**Related term:** Anti-scatter grid
**Radiotherapy Example:** Grids improve quality in planar kV images used for setup verification.

**327. Imaging hardware:** Physical components of an imaging system, including detectors, gantries, tubes, coils, and control units.
**Related term:** Imaging equipment
**Radiotherapy Example:** Linac-mounted kV panels are imaging hardware used for IGRT.

**328. Imaging intensity:** The strength of the detected signal in an image. Influenced by exposure, tissue density, and detector sensitivity.
**Related term:** Pixel intensity
**Radiotherapy Example:** PET imaging intensity correlates with tumor metabolic activity for dose painting.

**329. Imaging isotope:** A radioactive isotope used for imaging, such as Tc-99m or F-18. Tracers highlight physiological processes.
**Related term:** Radiotracer
**Radiotherapy Example:** F-18 FDG identifies tumor regions for radiotherapy contouring.

**330. Imaging laser alignment:** Lasers assist in positioning patients or equipment accurately relative to imaging or radiation beams.
**Related term:** Positioning laser
**Radiotherapy Example:** CT simulation uses lasers to align the patient with the imaging isocenter.

**331. Imaging lesion detection:** The process of identifying abnormal tissue using medical imaging techniques. Accuracy depends on contrast, resolution, and algorithm performance.
**Related term:** Diagnostic sensitivity
**Radiotherapy Example:** MRI lesion detection enhances GTV in brain tumor radiotherapy.

**332. Imaging modality selection:** Choosing the most appropriate type of imaging (CT, MRI, PET, US) based on clinical need and tissue characteristics.
**Related term:** Modality protocol
**Radiotherapy Example:** MRI is chosen for soft-tissue contrast in prostate radiotherapy planning.

**333. Imaging monitoring:** Continuous or periodic observation of imaging-device performance, exposure, and calibration to maintain quality.
**Related term:** QA monitoring
**Radiotherapy Example:** Daily imaging monitoring ensures consistent IGRT performance.

334. **Imaging noise reduction:** Techniques that decrease image noise to improve clarity, using filtering, smoothing, or advanced reconstruction.
**Related term:** Image denoising
**Radiotherapy Example:** Iterative CT reconstruction reduces noise and improves OAR contouring.

335. **Imaging normalization:** Standardizing image intensity or quality so that images from different times or systems appear consistent.
**Related term:** Intensity normalization
**Radiotherapy Example:** PET normalization improves longitudinal tumor-response assessment.

336. **Imaging protocol adjustment:** Modifying imaging parameters to improve image quality, reduce dose, or tailor the scan to the patient.
**Related term:** Protocol optimization
**Radiotherapy Example:** Adjusting CT slice thickness enhances visibility of small lesions during planning.

337. **Imaging quality assurance:** A structured program ensuring imaging equipment functions correctly and produces accurate diagnostic images. Includes tests of geometry, noise, uniformity, and calibration.
**Related term:** QA program
**Radiotherapy Example:** Daily imaging QA ensures CBCT is aligned with treatment isocenter.

338. **Imaging quality control:** Routine tests measuring specific imaging metrics (resolution, noise, uniformity) to verify system performance.
**Related term:** Acceptance testing
**Radiotherapy Example:** Monthly QC checks maintain consistent kV imaging performance.

339. **Imaging radiation dose:** Amount of radiation absorbed during imaging procedures. Must be minimized while ensuring diagnostic quality.
**Related term:** Patient dose
**Radiotherapy Example:** IGRT protocols balance CBCT dose with daily setup accuracy.

340. **Imaging reconstruction algorithm:** Algorithms that convert raw detector data into usable images (filtered back projection, iterative reconstruction, deep-learning reconstruction).
**Related term:** Reconstruction kernel
**Radiotherapy Example:** Iterative CT reconstruction improves soft tissue contrast for contouring.

341. **Imaging registration:** Aligning two or more images spatially so anatomical structures coincide. Can be rigid or deformable.
**Related term:** Image fusion
**Radiotherapy Example:** PET-CT registration improves tumor delineation for treatment planning.

342. **Imaging resolution:** Ability of an imaging system to distinguish small or closely spaced structures. Includes spatial, contrast, and temporal resolution.
**Related term:** Spatial resolution
**Radiotherapy Example:** High-resolution MRI is used to contour brainstem and cranial nerves accurately.

343. **Imaging safety:** Protocols ensuring safe use of radiation or magnetic fields during imaging procedures for both patients and staff.
**Related term:** Radiation safety
**Radiotherapy Example:** Shielding protocols ensure staff safety during kV fluoroscopy for fiducial placement.

344. **Imaging scanner calibration:** Calibration ensuring scanners produce consistent, true, and reproducible images. Includes HU checks, laser alignment, and uniformity.
**Related term:** CT calibration
**Radiotherapy Example:** Daily CT scanner calibration ensures accurate Hounsfield units for dose calculations.

345. **Imaging segmentation:** Dividing an image into meaningful regions, such as organs or tumors, either manually or automatically.
**Related term:** Contouring
**Radiotherapy Example:** AI-assisted segmentation speeds up OAR contouring during planning.

346. **Imaging signal processing:** Methods used to enhance, transform, or analyze signals to produce improved images. Includes filtering, Fourier transforms, and enhancement algorithms.
**Related term:** Image enhancement
**Radiotherapy Example:** Signal processing improves MV portal image quality for field verification.

347. **Imaging slice thickness:** The thickness of each slice in tomographic imaging. Thinner slices improve detail but increase dose and noise.
**Related term:** Slice resolution
**Radiotherapy Example:** Thin-slice CT improves accuracy in stereotactic radiotherapy planning.

348. **Imaging software calibration:** Ensures imaging software functions correctly, producing accurate reconstructions, measurements, and visualizations.
**Related term:** Software QA
**Radiotherapy Example:** TPS imaging modules are calibrated to ensure correct voxel values.

349. **Imaging spectroscopy:** Technique using frequency-dependent information to analyze tissue composition (MRI spectroscopy, optical spectroscopy).
**Related term:** Spectral imaging
**Radiotherapy Example:** MR spectroscopy identifies active tumor regions needing dose escalation.

350. **Imaging stabilization:** Techniques preventing motion during imaging—via gating, immobilization, or software correction—to avoid blurring and artifacts.
**Related term:** Motion control
**Radiotherapy Example:** Respiratory gating stabilizes tumor position during 4D CT acquisition.

351. **Imaging system alignment:** Ensuring all components of an imaging system are properly aligned to produce accurate, undistorted images.
**Related term:** Geometric alignment
**Radiotherapy Example:** CBCT system alignment ensures match between imaging and treatment coordinates.

352. **Imaging system calibration:** Comprehensive calibration of detectors, geometry, exposure, contrast, and software to ensure accurate images.
**Related term:** System QA
**Radiotherapy Example:** Pre-commissioning calibration verifies linac imaging performance.

353. **Imaging technique optimization:** Improving imaging settings to increase diagnostic performance while reducing dose or acquisition time.
**Related term:** Protocol optimization
**Radiotherapy Example:** Optimizing CT technique parameters enhances soft-tissue contrast for planning.

354. **Imaging tomography calibration:** Calibration of tomographic systems (CT, PET, SPECT) to ensure accurate reconstruction, uniformity, and geometry.
**Related term:** Tomography QA
**Radiotherapy Example:** CT tomography calibration ensures correct HU-to-density mapping.

355. **Imaging tomography protocol:** Detailed steps and parameters used for tomographic imaging, including rotation speed, slice thickness, exposure, and reconstruction kernel.
**Related term:** CT scan protocol
**Radiotherapy Example:** 4D CT protocols capture respiratory motion for thoracic treatment planning.

356. **Imaging tomography scan:** A tomographic acquisition that produces cross-sectional images of the body using CT, MRI, PET, or SPECT.
**Related term:** Tomographic imaging
**Radiotherapy Example:** Planning CT tomography scans are used to create dose distributions.

357. **Imaging tool calibration:** Calibration of tools such as rulers, markers, software tools, or measurement devices used in imaging analysis.
**Related term:** Measurement calibration
**Radiotherapy Example:** Digital calipers used for contour measurements require periodic calibration.

358. **Imaging visualization:** The display and enhancement techniques that allow clinicians to interpret medical imaging data, including 3D rendering, MIP, and fusion.
**Related term:** Image display
**Radiotherapy Example:** 3D visualization helps evaluate dose distribution relative to anatomy.

359. **Imaging workstation setup:** Preparation and configuration of hardware and software used to process and review imaging. Includes calibration, user settings, and workflow organization.
**Related term:** Workstation configuration
**Radiotherapy Example:** Planning workstations require setup to support multimodality fusion and segmentation.

360. **Imaging workstation software:** Software used on medical imaging workstations to view, analyze, and process imaging datasets. May include advanced visualization and AI modules.
**Related term:** Medical imaging platform
**Radiotherapy Example:** TPS workstation software integrates CT, MRI, and PET for planning.

361. **In-beam imaging calibration:** Calibration of imaging performed simultaneously with treatment beams (e.g., proton radiography or MV in-beam imaging).
**Related term:** Beam-synchronous imaging
**Radiotherapy Example:** In-beam proton imaging calibrations validate range accuracy.

362. **Incident gamma radiation:** Gamma photons arriving at a target or detector. Often used in nuclear medicine and shielding analysis.
**Related term:** Gamma flux
**Radiotherapy Example:** Gamma rays from Co-60 sources interact with tissue during radiosurgery.

363. **Incident neutron flux:** The rate of neutrons striking a surface. Relevant in environments with secondary neutrons from high-energy linacs.
**Related term:** Neutron fluence
**Radiotherapy Example:** High-energy linacs (>10 MV) produce incident neutron flux requiring shielding evaluation.

364. **Incident photon measurement:** Quantifying the number or energy of photons striking a detector surface.
**Related term:** Photon fluence
**Radiotherapy Example:** Beam QA uses incident photon measurement to verify output.

365. **Incident radiation monitoring:** Real-time monitoring of radiation entering an area or interacting with a detector.
**Related term:** Area monitoring
**Radiotherapy Example:** Radiation monitors track leakage outside a treatment vault.

366. **Incident radiation profile:** Spatial distribution of radiation intensity before interacting with a patient or phantom.
**Related term:** Beam profile
**Radiotherapy Example:** Linac beam profiles are measured during commissioning.

367. **Incident X-ray measurement:** Measurement of X-ray beam properties before entering the patient, such as energy, flux, and uniformity.
**Related term:** Entrance beam measurement
**Radiotherapy Example:** Daily QA checks incident X-ray output for kV imaging.

368. **Incident X-ray monitoring:** Continuous or periodic monitoring of X-ray exposure levels from imaging systems.
**Related term:** Exposure monitoring
**Radiotherapy Example:** Dose meters ensure safe exposure in fluoroscopy during procedures.

369. **Incidental radiation exposure:** Unintentional exposure to low levels of radiation, either from scatter or environmental sources.
**Related term:** Unintended dose
**Radiotherapy Example:** Staff are protected from incidental exposure during brachytherapy source loading.

370. **Incidental radiation monitoring:** Monitoring unplanned or background radiation exposure in clinical or research environments.
**Related term:** Environmental monitoring
**Radiotherapy Example:** Area badges track incidental radiation near treatment rooms.

371. **Incremental dose calculation:** Dose calculated in small increments or layers, often used in advanced algorithms.
**Related term:** Layer-based calculation
**Radiotherapy Example:** Monte Carlo engines compute incremental dose along particle tracks.

372. **Incremental radiation therapy:** A strategy where radiation dose is increased gradually or delivered in staged sessions based on response.
**Related term:** Dose escalation
**Radiotherapy Example:** Some adaptive protocols adjust dose incrementally across fractions.

373. **Indirect imaging:** Imaging based on secondary light or signals generated by detectors (e.g., scintillator-based imaging).
**Related term:** Scintillation imaging
**Radiotherapy Example:** MV imaging uses indirect detection through phosphor screens.

374. **Indirect radiation detection:** Detection of radiation using secondary effects such as light flashes, ionization, or heat.
**Related term:** Scintillation detector
**Radiotherapy Example:** Portal imaging uses indirect detection of MV photons through scintillation plates.

375. **Induced radioactivity:** Radioactivity generated in materials after exposure to high-energy radiation, often via nuclear reactions.
**Related term:** Activation
**Radiotherapy Example:** High-energy linac components become activated after prolonged use.

**376. Induction linac:** A special accelerator using pulsed induction fields to accelerate charged particles.
**Related term:** Pulsed accelerator
**Radiotherapy Example:** Used in some experimental radiation therapy research applications.

**377. Induction radiation:** Radiation produced by electromagnetic induction effects, often low-intensity and non-ionizing.
**Related term:** Inductive field
**Radiotherapy Example:** Not used in therapy but relevant to MRI safety analyses.

**378. Induction therapy:** Initial phase of multimodal treatment given to reduce tumor burden before definitive therapy.
**Related term:** Neoadjuvant therapy
**Radiotherapy Example:** Induction chemotherapy precedes chemoradiation for head-and-neck cancers.

**379. Infrared radiation detection:** Detection of IR radiation for thermal imaging or monitoring.
**Related term:** Thermal detector
**Radiotherapy Example:** IR cameras monitor patient breathing in external respiratory gating systems.

**380. Infrared imaging calibration:** Calibration of infrared cameras to ensure accurate temperature mapping and sensitivity.
**Related term:** Thermal calibration
**Radiotherapy Example:** IR systems used for respiratory monitoring undergo routine calibration.

**381. Infrared imaging system:** A system that captures thermal or IR images to assess heat distribution or motion.
**Related term:** Thermal imaging
**Radiotherapy Example:** Infrared imaging can track respiratory motion during treatment.

**382. Infusion radiopharmaceutical:** A radioactive compound administered by infusion for imaging or therapy.
**Related term:** Radiotracer infusion
**Radiotherapy Example:** Infusion of Y-90 microspheres delivers internal radiotherapy to liver tumors.

**383. Inhomogeneity correction:** Adjustments applied to imaging or dose calculations to compensate for tissue density variations.
**Related term:** Heterogeneity correction
**Radiotherapy Example:** Dose algorithms correct for lung inhomogeneities during planning.

**384. Inhomogeneity factor:** Quantifies how much tissue density variations influence dose or imaging signal.
**Related term:** Correction factor
**Radiotherapy Example:** Higher inhomogeneity factors appear in lung versus soft tissue regions.

**385. Input radiation intensity:** The radiation intensity entering a detector or medium before attenuation occurs.
**Related term:** Incident intensity
**Radiotherapy Example:** CT scanners control input intensity via mA settings.

**386. Input signal calibration:** Calibration ensuring detectors interpret input signals accurately with minimal drift or noise.
**Related term:** Electronic calibration
**Radiotherapy Example:** EPID calibration ensures accurate portal image brightness and contrast.

387. **Inscribed circle (field size):** A geometric method determining maximum circle diameter fitting inside a beam field, used for field uniformity analysis.
**Related term:** Beam geometry
**Radiotherapy Example:** Used to evaluate symmetry in beam flatness tests.

388. **Instrument calibration:** Ensuring measurement instruments (chambers, detectors, meters) produce accurate readings through standardized calibration.
**Related term:** Absolute calibration
**Radiotherapy Example:** Ion chambers require annual traceable calibration for clinical use.

389. **Instrument detection efficiency:** Percentage of incoming radiation events detected by an instrument.
**Related term:** Detector sensitivity
**Radiotherapy Example:** High-efficiency detectors improve small-field dosimetry accuracy.

390. **Instrumentation accuracy:** The precision and correctness of instrument readings, influenced by calibration, noise, and stability.
**Related term:** Measurement accuracy
**Radiotherapy Example:** Accurate instrumentation is essential for high-precision proton therapy QA.

391. **Instrumentation beam alignment:** Ensuring instruments measuring beam characteristics are properly aligned with beam centers and axes.
**Related term:** Beam alignment
**Radiotherapy Example:** Ion chambers must be aligned with the beam for accurate output measurement.

392. **Instrumentation quality assurance:** QA procedures ensuring that radiation-measurement instruments function correctly over time.
**Related term:** Equipment QA
**Radiotherapy Example:** Regular checks ensure dosimeters are functioning for weekly linac QA.

393. **Instrumentation system:** A set of instruments used for monitoring, detecting, or measuring radiation or imaging parameters.
**Related term:** Measurement system
**Radiotherapy Example:** Dosimetry systems measure dose during machine calibration.

394. **Instrumentation verification:** Verification ensuring instrumentation measurements match expected standards and tolerances.
**Related term:** Verification testing
**Radiotherapy Example:** QA teams verify chamber readings before clinical use.

395. **Interbeam distance measurement:** Measurement of the spacing between two or more radiation beams or fields.
**Related term:** Beam spacing
**Radiotherapy Example:** Used in multi-isocenter SRS to optimize beam arrangements.

396. **Interventional imaging:** Imaging used during minimally invasive procedures to guide tools, catheters, or needles in real time.
**Related term:** Image-guided intervention
**Radiotherapy Example:** CT-guided brachytherapy applicator placement uses interventional imaging.

397. **Interventional radiology guidance:** Use of imaging to guide therapeutic or diagnostic interventions, such as biopsies or ablations.
**Related term:** Fluoroscopic guidance
**Radiotherapy Example:** Interventional radiology places fiducial markers for prostate IGRT.

**398. Interstitial brachytherapy planning:** Developing a treatment plan for radioactive sources placed within tissue.
**Related term:** Brachytherapy optimization
**Radiotherapy Example:** HDR interstitial plans treat soft-tissue sarcomas or gynecologic tumors.

**399. Interstitial radiation source:** Radioactive sources implanted into tissues for therapeutic dose delivery.
**Related term:** Implant source
**Radiotherapy Example:** Ir-192 wires act as interstitial radiation sources in brachytherapy.

**400. Internal dose assessment:** Calculation of radiation dose received from radioactive material inside the body.
**Related term:** Internal dosimetry
**Radiotherapy Example:** Y-90 liver therapy requires internal dose assessment to protect healthy liver.

**401. Internal dose calibration:** Internal dose calibration ensures that calculated doses from internal radionuclides match physical and biological models. It uses biokinetic data, organ uptake, and decay calculations. Accurate calibration allows reliable estimates of absorbed doses for therapeutic isotopes.
**Related term:** Internal dosimetry
**Radiotherapy Example:** Y-90 microsphere therapy requires calibrated internal dose estimates before treatment.

**402. Internal dosimeter:** A dosimeter designed to measure radiation doses from internal sources, often through bioassay, urine assays, or whole-body counters. It determines radionuclide retention and organ dose.
**Related term:** Bioassay dosimeter
**Radiotherapy Example:** Internal dosimeters quantify I-131 uptake during thyroid therapy.

**403. Internal emission tomography:** A tomographic imaging method using gamma or positron emissions from within the body (PET, SPECT). It maps functional and metabolic activity.
**Related term:** PET imaging
**Radiotherapy Example:** FDG-PET is used for delineating metabolically active tumor regions.

**404. Internal energy absorption:** Absorption of radiation energy within tissues due to interactions like photoelectric effect, Compton scattering, or pair production. Determines biological effects.
**Related term:** Absorbed dose
**Radiotherapy Example:** Internal absorption from radionuclides defines organ toxicity limits in radionuclide therapy.

**405. Internal exposure monitoring:** Monitoring radiation exposure due to radionuclides entering the body via inhalation, ingestion, or injection.
**Related term:** Internal contamination monitoring
**Radiotherapy Example:** Nuclear medicine staff undergo internal exposure monitoring for iodine handling.

**406. 406. Internal gamma probe:** A small detector inserted inside the body to measure gamma radiation distribution or source location.
**Related term:** Intraoperative gamma probe
**Radiotherapy Example:** Surgeons use gamma probes during sentinel lymph node procedures.

**407. Internal irradiation:** Radiation delivered from sources located inside the body, either naturally or via administered radionuclides.
**Related term:** Brachytherapy
**Radiotherapy Example:** I-131 therapy delivers internal irradiation to thyroid tissue.

408. **Internal neutron source:** A radioactive source placed internally that emits neutrons for diagnostic or therapeutic purposes.
**Related term:** Neutron-emitting isotope
**Radiotherapy Example:** Research uses Cf-252 implants, though rarely in clinical practice.

409. **Internal phantom calibration:** Using phantoms representing internal organs or structures to calibrate internal dose measurements or imaging.
**Related term:** Anthropomorphic phantom
**Radiotherapy Example:** Internal phantoms validate PET SUV accuracy.

410. **Internal photodetector:** A detector embedded in a device to capture photons produced internally by scintillation or Čerenkov effects.
**Related term:** Scintillation detector
**Radiotherapy Example:** Fiber-optic dosimeters use internal photodetectors for in vivo dosimetry.

411. **Internal radiation absorption factor:** A factor describing how much energy emitted internally is absorbed by a given organ or tissue.
**Related term:** S-value
**Radiotherapy Example:** MIRD S-values are used to compute I-131 organ doses.

412. **Internal radiation calculation:** Mathematical modeling of internal radionuclide distribution and dose deposition using biokinetic models.
**Related term:** MIRD calculation
**Radiotherapy Example:** Used in dosimetry for Lu-177 PRRT therapy.

413. **Internal radiation chamber:** A chamber designed to measure internal radiation distributions, often for laboratory or calibration use.
**Related term:** Cavity chamber
**Radiotherapy Example:** Used in research for internal radionuclide calibration.

414. **Internal radiation counter:** A detector used to quantify gamma emissions from radionuclides within the body (e.g., whole-body counter).
**Related term:** Whole-body counter
**Radiotherapy Example:** Measures I-131 retention in patients.

415. **Internal radiation distribution:** The spatial distribution of radionuclide activity or absorbed dose within the body.
**Related term:** Biodistribution
**Radiotherapy Example:** Dosimetry software maps internal Y-90 distribution in the liver.

416. **Internal radiation dosimeter:** A device or method to measure radiation doses arising from internal emitters.
**Related term:** Internal dose monitor
**Radiotherapy Example:** Bioassays act as internal dosimeters after radionuclide therapy.

417. **Internal radiation exposure:** Exposure caused by radionuclides inside the body rather than external sources.
**Related term:** Internal contamination
**Radiotherapy Example:** I-131 thyroid therapy results in internal exposure primarily to thyroid tissue.

418. **Internal radiation imaging:** Imaging methods where radiation emitted internally creates diagnostic images (PET, SPECT).
**Related term:** Emission imaging
**Radiotherapy Example:** PET imaging identifies active tumor regions for contouring.

**419. Internal radiation intensity:** Intensity of emitted radiation from inside the body, dependent on activity and isotope decay.
**Related term:** Activity concentration
**Radiotherapy Example:** High internal intensity from Y-90 affects dose to non-target liver tissue.

**420. Internal radiation isotope:** Any radioactive isotope administered or occurring internally that emits radiation.
**Related term:** Radiopharmaceutical
**Radiotherapy Example:** Lu-177 is an internal therapeutic isotope used for NET treatment.

**421. Internal radiation mapping:** Creating spatial maps of radionuclide distribution within organs or tissues.
**Related term:** Activity mapping
**Radiotherapy Example:** PET mapping guides dose planning for Y-90 radioembolization.

**422. Internal radiation measurement system:** A system designed to measure radiation from radionuclides inside the body.
**Related term:** In vivo assay system
**Radiotherapy Example:** Thyroid probes measure I-131 uptake.

**423. Internal radiation model:** A mathematical model describing radionuclide kinetics, distribution, and dose within body tissues.
**Related term:** Biokinetic model
**Radiotherapy Example:** OLINDA/EXM uses internal radiation models for dosimetry.

**424. Internal radiation monitor:** Device used to detect radioactive material inside the body.
**Related term:** Whole-body monitor
**Radiotherapy Example:** Hospitals use internal radiation monitors for iodine therapy rooms.

**425. Internal radiation phantom:** A phantom designed to mimic internal anatomy, used for internal dosimetry calibration.
**Related term:** Organ phantom
**Radiotherapy Example:** Used in PET calibration studies.

**426. Internal radiation probe:** Detection probe used to measure internal radiation sources.
**Related term:** Gamma probe
**Radiotherapy Example:** Probes locate therapeutic seeds during brachytherapy procedures.

**427. Internal radiation quality factor:** A factor describing the relative biological effectiveness of internal emitters.
**Related term:** RBE
**Radiotherapy Example:** Internal alpha emitters have high quality factors.

**428. Internal radiation sensor:** Sensor detecting activity from internal radionuclides, often used for contamination monitoring.
**Related term:** Activity sensor
**Radiotherapy Example:** Sensors detect airborne iodine near therapy rooms.

**429. Internal radiation source distribution:** The pattern of source placement or radionuclide distribution internally.
**Related term:** Isotope distribution
**Radiotherapy Example:** HDR implants rely on planned source distribution in tissue.

430. **Internal radiation therapy planning:** Planning procedures for radionuclide or brachytherapy treatments.
**Related term:** Brachytherapy planning
**Radiotherapy Example:** Y-90 therapy requires mapping uptake before planning dose.

431. **Internal radiation tolerance:** Maximum internal dose tissues can safely absorb before toxicity occurs.
**Related term:** Organ dose limit
**Radiotherapy Example:** Liver tolerance limits guide Y-90 dosing.

432. **Internal radioactive calibration; Calibration of systems measuring internal radioactive materials.**
**Related term:** In vivo calibration
**Radiotherapy Example:** Whole-body counters are calibrated for I-131.

433. **Internal radioactive contamination:** Presence of unwanted radionuclides inside the body.
**Related term:** Internal exposure
**Radiotherapy Example:** Nuclear medicine staff may risk internal contamination without proper PPE.

434. **Internal radioactive detector:** Detector used to measure radiation inside the patient or within body cavities.
**Related term:** In vivo detector
**Radiotherapy Example:** Internal dosimeters ensure safe brachytherapy dose verification.

435. **Internal radioactive dose:** Dose absorbed from radionuclides inside the body.
**Related term:** Internal dose
**Radiotherapy Example:** Internal dose from Ra-223 determines bone marrow toxicity.

436. **Internal radioactive dose distribution:** How internal dose varies spatially within tissues.
**Related term:** Dose mapping
**Radiotherapy Example:** Heterogeneous Y-90 dose distribution affects tumor control.

437. **Internal radioactive imaging:** Imaging using radiation from isotopes already inside the patient (PET/SPECT).
**Related term:** Emission tomography
**Radiotherapy Example:** PET scans identify viable tumor.

438. **Internal radioactive isotope detection:** Detecting isotopes inside the body via gamma counters or imaging.
**Related term:** Radionuclide assay
**Radiotherapy Example:** I-123 scans verify thyroid uptake.

439. **Internal radioactive measurement:** Quantifying activity or dose from internal radionuclides.
**Related term:** Internal assay
**Radiotherapy Example:** Pre-therapy dosimetry for Lu-177.

440. **Internal radioactive monitoring:** Monitoring internal radioactive levels over time.
**Related term:** Bioassay monitoring
**Radiotherapy Example:** Required after accidental internal exposure.

441. **Internal radioactive sensor:** Sensor detecting internal radioactivity, often part of whole-body counters.
**Related term:** Gamma sensor
**Radiotherapy Example:** Used in thyroid therapy rooms.

442. **Internal radionuclide decay:** Decay of radionuclides inside the body, producing radiation and dose.
**Related term:** Biological clearance
**Radiotherapy Example:** I-131 decay determines treatment duration.

443. **Internal radionuclide detection:** Detection of radionuclides inside the patient.
**Related term:** In vivo monitoring
**Radiotherapy Example:** PET detects F-18 decay.

444. **Internal radionuclide distribution:** Distribution of radionuclides across organs and tissues.
**Related term:** Biodistribution
**Radiotherapy Example:** Lu-177 uptake distribution determines tumor dose.

445. **Internal radionuclide dosimetry:** Computation of internal dose from radionuclide uptake.
**Related term:** Internal dosimetry
**Radiotherapy Example:** Y-90 dosimetry predicts liver toxicity risk.

446. **Internal radionuclide imaging:** Imaging produced by emissions from internal radionuclides.
**Related term:** Emission imaging
**Radiotherapy Example:** SPECT imaging of Lu-177.

447. **Internal radionuclide localization:** Determining where radionuclides accumulate in the body.
**Related term:** Uptake localization
**Radiotherapy Example:** Tc-99m-MIBI localizes parathyroid adenomas prior to surgery.

448. **Internal radionuclide measurement:** Measurement of activity or dose from internal isotopes.
**Related term:** In vivo activity measurement
**Radiotherapy Example:** Uptake measurements guide I-131 dosing.

449. **Internal radionuclide monitoring:** Ongoing surveillance of internal radionuclide presence.
**Related term:** Bioassay
**Radiotherapy Example:** Used for occupational exposure monitoring.

450. **Internal radionuclide sensor:** Sensor that detects radiation from internal isotopes.
**Related term:** Radiation detector
**Radiotherapy Example:** Thyroid sensors detect I-131 uptake.

451. **Internal range:** The distance radiation travels inside tissue before depositing energy.
**Related term:** Particle range
**Radiotherapy Example:** Beta particles from Y-90 have a 2–3 mm range.

452. **Internal scattering:** Radiation scattering within tissues, affecting image quality and dose.
**Related term:** Tissue scatter
**Radiotherapy Example:** Scatter affects PET resolution.

453. **Internal scatter correction:** Corrections applied to reduce scatter effects in imaging or dose calculations.
**Related term:** Scatter compensation
**Radiotherapy Example:** SPECT uses internal scatter correction to improve accuracy.

454. **Internal seed implantation:** Placement of radioactive seeds within tissue for brachytherapy.
**Related term:** Permanent implant
**Radiotherapy Example:** I-125 seeds treat prostate cancer.

455. **Internal source calibration:** Calibration of internal sources to ensure accurate activity measurements.
**Related term:** Source strength calibration
**Radiotherapy Example:** HDR Ir-192 sources undergo internal calibration checks.

456. **Internal source decay:** The decay of radioactive sources placed inside tissue.
**Related term:** Half-life
**Radiotherapy Example:** Pd-103 seeds decay rapidly, suitable for prostate therapy.

457. **Internal source distribution:** Pattern of implanted or distributed radioactive sources within tissue.
**Related term:** Seed placement pattern
**Radiotherapy Example:** Geometric distribution determines dose uniformity.

458. **458. Internal source dosimetry:** Calculating dose delivered by internally placed radioactive sources.
**Related term:** Brachytherapy dosimetry
**Radiotherapy Example:** TG-43 formalism applies to interstitial brachytherapy.

459. **Internal source imaging:** Imaging seeds or isotopes located internally.
**Related term:** Seed localization
**Radiotherapy Example:** X-ray imaging identifies prostate seed positions.

460. **Internal source measurement:** Measurement of strength, position, or emission of internal sources.
**Related term:** Source strength assay
**Radiotherapy Example:** Afterloading systems measure Ir-192 source strength.

461. **Internal source monitoring:** Monitoring internal radioactive source behavior or movement.
**Related term:** Source tracking
**Radiotherapy Example:** HDR afterloader tracks source position during dwell times.

462. **Internal thermoluminescent dosimeter (TLD):** TLD placed internally or near internal cavities to measure radiation dose.
**Related term:** In vivo dosimeter
**Radiotherapy Example:** TLDs measure mucosal dose in brachytherapy.

463. **Internal tissue dose:** Dose absorbed by internal organs or tissues.
**Related term:** Organ dose
**Radiotherapy Example:** Internal lung dose is critical in radionuclide therapy.

464. **Internal tissue irradiation:** Irradiation of tissues from within, via implants or radionuclides.
**Related term:** Brachytherapy
**Radiotherapy Example:** HDR applicators irradiate cervical cancer tissues internally.

465. **Internal tissue response:** Biological response of tissues to internal radiation doses.
**Related term:** Radiation response
**Radiotherapy Example:** Bone marrow suppression occurs with Ra-223 therapy.

466. **Internal tracer calibration:** Calibration of radiotracer uptake measurements.
**Related term:** PET calibration
**Radiotherapy Example:** PET SUV calibration ensures accurate tumor quantification.

467. **Internal tracer detection:** Detection of radiotracers within body tissues.
**Related term:** Tracer imaging
**Radiotherapy Example:** FDG detection identifies active tumors.

468. **Internal tracer dosimetry:** Dosimetry of tracer distribution for therapy or diagnostic safety.
**Related term:** Radiotracer dosimetry
**Radiotherapy Example:** Dosimetry predicts toxicity for therapeutic tracers like I-131.

469. **Internal tracer distribution:** Spatial distribution of tracer uptake in tissues.
**Related term:** Biodistribution
**Radiotherapy Example:** Dotatate uptake maps NETs.

470. **Internal tracer imaging:** Imaging radiotracer distribution via PET or SPECT.
**Related term:** Molecular imaging
**Radiotherapy Example:** PET/CT used for treatment planning.

471. **Internal tracer measurement:** Measurement of tracer concentration or activity.
**Related term:** Uptake quantification
**Radiotherapy Example:** SUV measurement helps measure tumor metabolism.

472. **Internal tracer monitoring:** Monitoring tracer kinetics and clearance.
**Related term:** Pharmacokinetics
**Radiotherapy Example:** Time-activity curves in dosimetry.

473. **Internal tracer sensor:** A sensor detecting tracer-based emissions.
**Related term:** Gamma sensor
**Radiotherapy Example:** PET detectors act as tracer sensors.

474. **Internal X-ray chamber:** A chamber measuring X-ray exposure inside systems or phantoms.
**Related term:** Diagnostic chamber
**Radiotherapy Example:** Used for kV imaging QA.

475. **Internal X-ray dosimeter:** Dosimeter measuring internal X-ray exposures.
**Related term:** X-ray detector
**Radiotherapy Example:** Used inside phantoms for CBCT dose mapping.

476. **Internal X-ray imaging:** Imaging using X-rays interacting internally with tissues.
**Related term:** Radiography
**Radiotherapy Example:** CBCT performs internal X-ray imaging for IGRT.

477. **Internal X-ray measurement:** Measurement of internal X-ray beam properties in phantoms or tissues.
**Related term:** Beam measurement
**Radiotherapy Example:** Used for dose calibration of kV imaging.

478. **Interphase death:** Cell death occurring during interphase after radiation damage, without mitosis.
**Related term:** Apoptotic death
**Radiotherapy Example:** Lymphocytes undergo interphase death rapidly after exposure.

479. **Interphase response:** Cellular responses during interphase (DNA repair, apoptosis) after radiation exposure.
**Related term:** DNA repair response
**Radiotherapy Example:** Radiosensitive cells exhibit strong interphase reactions.

480. **Interstitial radiation:** Radiation delivered by sources implanted between tissues.
**Related term:** Interstitial brachytherapy
**Radiotherapy Example:** Breast boost brachytherapy uses interstitial catheters.

481. **Interstitial source array:** Arrangement of multiple implanted radioactive sources to create a dose distribution.
**Related term:** Seed array
**Radiotherapy Example:** Prostate implants use an array-based seed pattern.

482. **Interstitial source calibration:** Calibration of sources used in interstitial brachytherapy.
**Related term:** Seed calibration
**Radiotherapy Example:** I-125 seeds are calibrated for activity before implant.

483. **Interstitial source distribution:** Pattern of implanted sources within tissue.
**Related term:** Implant geometry
**Radiotherapy Example:** Determines dose homogeneity in soft-tissue implants.

**484. Interstitial source imaging:** Imaging used to verify correct placement of implanted sources.
**Related term:** Seed localization imaging
**Radiotherapy Example:** Post-implant CT verifies prostate seed positions.

**485. Interstitial source positioning:** Ensuring correct placement of interstitial brachytherapy sources relative to tumors.
**Related term:** Implant guidance
**Radiotherapy Example:** Catheter positions determine HDR dwell locations.

**486. Interstitial source verification:** Verification of seed or source placement accuracy.
**Related term:** Implant verification
**Radiotherapy Example:** Post-implant dosimetry verifies placement accuracy.

**487. Ion activation coefficient:** Parameter describing probability of activating nuclei via ion interactions.
**Related term:** Activation cross section
**Radiotherapy Example:** High-energy linacs produce activation via photonuclear interactions.

**488. Ion beam calibration:** Calibration ensuring ion beams deliver correct energy, range, and dose.
**Related term:** Proton beam calibration
**Radiotherapy Example:** Proton therapy systems undergo meticulous ion beam calibration.

**489. Ion beam collision:** Interactions between ions and tissue causing ionization and energy loss.
**Related term:** Stopping interaction
**Radiotherapy Example:** Proton collisions deposit dose at the Bragg peak.

**490. Ion beam collision rate:** Rate at which beam ions interact with atoms in tissue.
**Related term:** Collision frequency
**Radiotherapy Example:** Determines LET in ion therapy.

**491. Ion beam collision spectrum:** Spectrum of energies involved in ion–tissue interactions.
**Related term:** Energy loss spectrum
**Radiotherapy Example:** Ion therapy planning uses collision spectra to compute LET.

**492. Ion beam collision yield:** Yield of secondary particles produced during ion interactions.
**Related term:** Secondary yield
**Radiotherapy Example:** Carbon therapy yields secondary fragments requiring modeling.

**493. Ion beam decay:** Reduction in beam intensity due to attenuation or system decay.
**Related term:** Beam attenuation
**Radiotherapy Example:** Beam transmissions are modeled in proton therapy.

**494. Ion beam detection efficiency:** Efficiency of detectors capturing ions in the beam.
**Related term:** Detector efficiency
**Radiotherapy Example:** Ionization chambers measure proton beam output.

**495. Ion beam distribution:** Spatial pattern of an ion beam in tissue.
**Related term:** Dose distribution
**Radiotherapy Example:** Bragg peak shaping defines tumor coverage.

**496. Ion beam imaging:** Using ion beams to produce images based on their transmission or scattering.
**Related term:** Proton radiography
**Radiotherapy Example:** Proton imaging refines range verification.

**497. Ion beam intensity:** Strength of an ion beam, affecting dose rate and treatment time.
**Related term:** Beam current
**Radiotherapy Example:** Proton beam intensity is modulated for dose painting.

**498. Ion beam interaction:** Physical interactions between ion beams and tissue.
**Related term:** Stopping power interaction
**Radiotherapy Example:** Used to compute LET in ion therapy.

**499. Ion beam interaction coefficient:** Coefficient describing ion interactions affecting energy loss.
**Related term:** Stopping-power coefficient
**Radiotherapy Example:** LET modeling relies on interaction coefficients.

**500. Ion beam interaction spectrum:** Spectrum of energies involved in ion interactions along the beam path.
**Related term:** Energy loss distribution
**Radiotherapy Example:** Carbon therapy requires accurate interaction spectra for planning.

# J

1. **J-coupling (NMR):** A quantum interaction between nuclear spins caused by bonding electrons. It produces splitting in NMR spectra and helps determine molecular structure. In medical imaging, J-coupling is relevant in advanced MR spectroscopy where metabolite identification relies on spin–spin interactions. Adjusting acquisition parameters can minimize or emphasize J-modulation. It is especially important in brain spectroscopy protocols.
   **Related term:** Chemical shift
   **Radiotherapy Example:** Used in MR-guided radiotherapy when MRS is performed to characterize tumor metabolism before treatment planning.
2. **J-modulation (MRI spectroscopy):** A periodic signal fluctuation in MR spectroscopy caused by J-coupling interactions. It influences peak shapes and can obscure metabolite quantification if not corrected. Spin-echo sequences often experience strong J-modulation effects. Advanced techniques attempt to suppress or refocus this modulation. Proper handling ensures accurate spectroscopic analysis.
   **Related term:** J-coupling
   **Radiotherapy Example:** Used for accurate lactate detection in hypoxic tumors prior to dose escalation planning.
3. **J-resolved spectroscopy:** A multi-dimensional MRS method that separates chemical shifts from J-coupling interactions. This allows improved visualization of metabolites that overlap in standard spectra. The technique enhances diagnostic accuracy in brain and prostate MR spectroscopy. It reduces spectral crowding and helps quantify low-concentration metabolites. Often used in research and clinical metabolic imaging.
   **Related term:** MR spectroscopy
   **Radiotherapy Example:** Applied to map tumor metabolic signatures before stereotactic radiotherapy.
4. **J-safe current:** A defined limit of electrical current that prevents harmful effects in imaging equipment. Ensures patient and operator safety by restricting leakage or malfunction currents. Commonly applied in MRI systems due to strong electromagnetic fields. Medical devices must comply with IEC safety standards. Prevents electrical hazards in radiology environments.
   **Related term:** Equipment safety standard
   **Radiotherapy Example:** Ensures linear accelerator control systems operate within safe current limits.
5. **Jaffe reaction (clinical chemistry imaging correlation):** A colorimetric method used to measure creatinine, sometimes referenced in radiology when correlating renal function with contrast imaging. Elevated creatinine indicates impaired kidney filtration, influencing contrast agent decisions. Radiologists often check Jaffe-derived results before contrast CT. Despite newer enzymatic methods, it remains widely used. Ensuring accuracy prevents contrast-induced nephropathy.
   **Related term:** Contrast contraindication
   **Radiotherapy Example:** Renal function screening before abdominal radiotherapy planning.
6. **Jaggies (image artifact):** A stair-step appearance along diagonal edges, usually caused by insufficient resolution or pixel interpolation. Common in digital radiography or ultrasound post-processing. It degrades image quality and can obscure anatomical detail. Anti-aliasing techniques reduce jaggies significantly. Often occurs in low-resolution reconstructions.
   **Related term:** Aliasing
   **Radiotherapy Example:** Must be minimized in DR images used for patient setup verification.

7. **Jamming interference:** An unwanted disruption of electronic signals that affects imaging equipment. May cause artifacts or temporary device malfunction. Often electromagnetic in origin and associated with nearby devices. Shielding and proper grounding reduce susceptibility. Medical imaging facilities monitor EM exposure to avoid such interference.
**Related term:** Electromagnetic interference (EMI)
**Radiotherapy Example:** Prevents signal distortion in MRI-guided linear accelerators.

8. **Jansky (radiofrequency unit):** A unit of spectral flux density commonly used in radio astronomy but sometimes referenced in RF safety assessments. Helps quantify RF field strength and exposure levels. Though rare in clinical imaging, RF engineers may use Janskys when designing MRI shielding. It aids in evaluating ambient RF noise. Controlled RF environments improve image stability.
**Related term:** RF field
**Radiotherapy Example:** Used in MR-Linac RF environment testing to ensure stable imaging during treatment.

9. **Jarvik phantom:** A specialized phantom used in cardiovascular imaging research. Simulates human cardiac anatomy and flow dynamics. Useful for validating CT, MRI, or ultrasound cardiac protocols. Enables realistic evaluation of imaging sequences. Often applied in research laboratories focused on heart imaging.
**Related term:** Cardiac phantom
**Radiotherapy Example:** Used to study cardiac dose distribution in thoracic radiotherapy research.

10. **Jaundice imaging:** Radiological evaluation of bile ducts, liver, and pancreas in patients with jaundice. Common modalities include ultrasound, CT, MRCP, and nuclear hepatobiliary scans. Helps differentiate obstructive from non-obstructive causes. Plays a vital role in identifying tumors, stones, or strictures. Guides further intervention and treatment.
**Related term:** MRCP
**Radiotherapy Example:** Used to stage cholangiocarcinoma before radiation therapy.

11. **Jaw collimation:** A method of beam shaping that uses independent jaws in X-ray or linear accelerator systems. Controls field size, reduces scatter, and improves dose conformity. Enhances precision in external beam radiotherapy. Often combined with MLCs for complex fields. Essential for minimizing healthy tissue exposure.
**Related term:** Multi-leaf collimator (MLC)
**Radiotherapy Example:** Jaw tracking reduces leakage dose in IMRT.

12. **Jaw tracking (radiotherapy):** A technique where collimator jaws dynamically follow MLC positions to reduce stray radiation. Improves dose delivery accuracy. Minimizes interleaf leakage. Enhances plan quality for IMRT and VMAT. Reduces unnecessary patient exposure.
**Related term:** Jaw collimation
**Radiotherapy Example:** Used in VMAT for head-and-neck cancers to reduce normal tissue dose.

13. **Jejunal imaging:** Radiologic evaluation of the jejunum using CT enterography, MR enterography, or fluoroscopy. Assesses inflammation, obstruction, or tumors. Provides detailed mucosal and luminal assessment. Often used in Crohn's disease evaluation. Helps guide medical or surgical interventions.
**Related term:** CT enterography
**Radiotherapy Example:** Helps assess radiation enteritis during abdominal radiotherapy follow-up.

14. **Jet artifact (MRI):** A flow-related artifact caused by high-velocity fluid jets, such as in cardiac or vascular MRI. Appears as signal voids or distortions. Often seen in valvular insufficiency or stenosis. Proper sequence selection can minimize it. Provides indirect diagnostic clues about abnormal flow.
**Related term:** Flow artifact
**Radiotherapy Example:** Important when using MRI for thoracic tumor motion evaluation.

15. **Jet ventilation imaging:** Imaging of patients under high-frequency jet ventilation, especially in interventional radiology or thoracic procedures. Helps maintain a still operative field. Minimizes motion artifacts. Used in airway and lung imaging. Requires specialized monitoring and coordination with anesthesia.
    **Related term:** High-frequency ventilation
    **Radiotherapy Example:** Used during stereotactic lung biopsy before radiotherapy planning.
16. **Jet stream effect (radiation physics):**A phenomenon where charged particles follow streamline trajectories at high energy. Can alter expected dose distribution. Observed in proton or heavy ion beams. Requires accurate modeling in treatment planning. Influences beam scattering and penetration characteristics.
    **Related term:** Particle beam scattering
    **Radiotherapy Example:** Impacts distal fall-off calculations in proton therapy.
17. **Jetting artifact (3D printing phantoms):** A manufacturing artifact occurring during inkjet-based 3D printing of medical phantoms. Creates surface irregularities that may affect dosimetric accuracy. Quality control is essential to ensure phantom reliability. Used frequently in radiotherapy QA. Ensures consistent calibration and measurement.
    **Related term:** 3D printing artifact
    **Radiotherapy Example:** Must be corrected for custom bolus fabrication.
18. **Jitter (signal stability):** Small, rapid variations in timing of signals, affecting imaging or detector performance. Can degrade image resolution or synchronization. Particularly relevant for high-speed digital detectors. Reducing jitter ensures better temporal resolution. Controlled through hardware stabilization
    **Related term:** Temporal resolution
    **Radiotherapy Example:** Impacts synchronization in gated radiotherapy imaging systems.
19. **Job-planning system (radiology workflow):** Software used to schedule and optimize imaging workload. Manages patient flow, resource allocation, and exam prioritization. Enhances department efficiency. Reduces waiting times and errors. Integrated with PACS and RIS.
    **Related term:** RIS
    **Radiotherapy Example:** Used in radiation oncology departments to optimize treatment appointment flow.
20. **Joint imaging (radiology):** Radiographic, CT, MRI, or ultrasound evaluation of joints. Assesses arthritis, trauma, or soft-tissue damage. MRI provides excellent contrast for cartilage and ligaments. CT excels in bone detail. Ultrasound helps with dynamic assessments.
    **Related term:** Musculoskeletal imaging
    **Radiotherapy Example:** Used to evaluate joint toxicity in sarcoma radiotherapy follow-up.
21. **Joint laxity imaging:** Imaging evaluation of ligament looseness or instability using MRI, ultrasound, or stress radiography. MRI visualizes ligament morphology, tears, or degeneration. Ultrasound provides dynamic assessment during joint movement. Stress X-rays quantify pathologic motion. Helps diagnose instability syndromes.
    **Related term:** Ligament imaging
    **Radiotherapy Example:** Evaluates ligament integrity in sarcoma patients after radiotherapy.
22. **Joint effusion imaging:** Detection of excess fluid within a joint capsule using ultrasound, MRI, or X-ray. Ultrasound is the most sensitive for small effusions; MRI identifies associated synovitis or internal derangement. Radiographs detect joint swelling indirectly. Common in trauma, infection, and arthritis assessment.
    **Related term:** Synovial fluid
    **Radiotherapy Example:** Monitored in joints exposed to scatter radiation near extremity tumors.

23. **Joint replacement imaging:** Evaluation of prosthetic joints using radiography, CT, MRI (metal-artifact–reduced), or nuclear medicine. Detects loosening, infection, wear, or dislocation. CT provides precise bone–prosthesis interface detail. MRI with metal-artifact reduction sequences improves soft-tissue assessment.
**Related term:** Metal artifact reduction (MAR)
**Radiotherapy Example:** CT with MAR used during pelvic radiotherapy planning in hip-prosthesis patients.

24. **Junction dose (radiotherapy):** The dose at the border where two adjacent radiation fields meet. Must be carefully calculated to prevent hotspots or cold spots. Often occurs in spinal or craniospinal irradiation fields. Modern planning uses feathering or matching algorithms. Ensures uniform treatment dose.
**Related term:** Field matching
**Radiotherapy Example:** Carefully managed in craniospinal irradiation.

25. **Junction shift (field feathering):** A technique in radiotherapy where field junctions are periodically shifted to distribute dose inhomogeneity. Prevents over- or under-dosage at the junction site. Common in pediatric or long-axis treatments. Modern TPS can automate the process. Improves patient safety.
**Related term:** Junction dose
**Radiotherapy Example:** Used routinely in craniospinal pediatric treatments.

26. **Junctional artifact (imaging):** Artifact occurring at boundaries where imaging sequences or stitched images meet. Seen in multi-slab MRI, stitched ultrasound, or radiographic mosaics. May appear as intensity or geometric discontinuities. Must be recognized to avoid misinterpretation. Typically corrected with improved acquisition or processing.
**Related term:** Stitching artifact
**Radiotherapy Example:** Can appear in MRI used for RT planning if multi-slab sequences are used.

27. **Junctional zone (pelvic MRI):** The uterine region separating the inner myometrium from the endometrium, best seen on T2 MRI. Important for diagnosing adenomyosis and uterine pathology. Reflects smooth muscle and connective tissue composition. Normal thickness varies with age and cycle. Appears as a low-signal band.
**Related term:** Myometrium
**Radiotherapy Example:** Helps assess uterine invasion in cervical cancer radiotherapy planning.

28. **Juvenile bone imaging:** Imaging evaluation of pediatric bone anatomy using X-ray, MRI, CT, or ultrasound. Growth plates and developmental changes require age-specific interpretation. Radiation reduction is prioritized through pediatric protocols. MRI often preferred for soft tissue and marrow. Detects fractures, tumors, and congenital abnormalities.
**Related term:** Growth plate
**Radiotherapy Example:** Evaluating bone growth effects after pediatric radiotherapy.

29. **Juvenile idiopathic arthritis imaging:** Use of MRI, ultrasound, and X-rays to assess joint inflammation in pediatric arthritis. MRI shows early marrow edema and cartilage injury. Ultrasound assists with active synovitis detection. Radiographs evaluate late deformity. Essential for monitoring treatment response.
**Related term:** Synovitis
**Radiotherapy Example:** Used to monitor radiation-induced arthropathy in rare cases.

30. **Juxtacortical lesion imaging:** Imaging of lesions adjacent to the cortical bone surface using MRI and CT. Important for diagnosing osteosarcoma variants, periosteal tumors, or inflammatory changes. MRI shows marrow and soft-tissue involvement. CT provides mineralization detail. Helps guide treatment planning.
**Related term:** Cortical bone
**Radiotherapy Example:** Used in planning radiation for juxtacortical osteosarcoma.

31. **Juxtaphrenic imaging:** Focused imaging of the region near the diaphragm, evaluating chill sign abnormalities, lung bases, or subphrenic processes. CT is preferred for fine detail. Identifies masses, infections, or postoperative complications. Helps differentiate intra- vs. extra-thoracic pathology.
**Related term:** Diaphragmatic imaging
**Radiotherapy Example:** Used in motion analysis for thoracic RT.

32. **Juxtarenal imaging:** Radiologic assessment of the region adjacent to the kidneys, often evaluating aneurysms, masses, or adrenal pathology. CT angiography is common for aortic disease. MRI supplements soft-tissue evaluation. Ultrasound offers screening capability.
**Related term:** Renal artery imaging
**Radiotherapy Example:** Aids in contouring near renal structures during abdominal radiotherapy.

33. **Juxtaspinal imaging:** Evaluation of tissue immediately adjacent to the spine using MRI, CT, or nuclear medicine. Essential for identifying paraspinal tumors, infections, or postoperative changes. MRI is highly sensitive for soft tissues. CT shows bony involvement.
**Related term:** Paraspinal muscles
**Radiotherapy Example:** Defines target volumes for paraspinal tumor radiotherapy.

34. **Juxtasellar imaging:** MRI/CT assessment of the region near the sella turcica, evaluating pituitary lesions or parasellar extension. MRI is gold standard with high soft-tissue contrast. Detects nerve compression, cavernous sinus involvement, or hormonal tumor spread. CT helps with bone anatomy.
**Related term:** Pituitary imaging
**Radiotherapy Example:** Essential for pituitary adenoma radiotherapy planning.

35. **Juxtavesical imaging:** Evaluation of tissues near the bladder, often via CT or MRI. Detects pelvic tumors, inflammation, or complications of urinary tract procedures. MRI offers excellent soft-tissue contrast. CT delineates anatomy and adenopathy.
**Related term:** Pelvic imaging
**Radiotherapy Example:** Critical in prostate and bladder tumor radiotherapy planning.

36. **Juxtavascular imaging:** High-resolution evaluation of soft tissues bordering blood vessels. Used to detect perivascular inflammation, tumor encasement, or plaque extension. MRI and CT angiography are commonly used. Helps determine resectability and invasion.
**Related term:** Vascular invasion
**Radiotherapy Example:** Important in contouring tumors abutting major vessels.

37. **Juxtavisceral imaging:** Imaging of tissues directly adjacent to major organs, especially in abdominal and pelvic studies. MRI and CT identify infiltrative tumors, inflammatory processes, or postoperative changes. Helps predict surgical or radiotherapy risk.
**Related term:** Organ boundary
**Radiotherapy Example:** Used in abdominal RT to assess tumor-organ interfaces.

38. **J-point imaging (ECG-gated imaging context):** The J-point represents the end of the QRS complex; in imaging, ECG gating relies on precise timing relative to this point. Accurate synchronization improves cardiac CT and MRI quality. Avoids motion artifacts. Ensures reproducible phase selection.
**Related term:** ECG gating
**Radiotherapy Example:** Used in cardiac-gated CT for minimizing heart motion during RT planning.

39. **J-resonance peaks (MRS):** Spectral peaks influenced by J-coupling phenomena in MR spectroscopy. Understanding them helps distinguish overlapping metabolites. Provides metabolic insights into tumors or neurological disorders. Requires advanced sequence optimization.
**Related term:** J-resolved spectroscopy
**Radiotherapy Example:** Used for metabolic mapping prior to dose painting in gliomas.

40. **Jitter artifact (ultrasound):** A motion-related artifact created by irregular hand or transducer movement. Causes blurring or duplication of lines. Particularly significant in Doppler recordings. Stabilization and proper technique minimize jitter. Recognizing it prevents misdiagnosis.
**Related term:** Motion artifact
**Radiotherapy Example:** Avoided during ultrasound-guided brachytherapy placement.

41. **Jitter correction (ultrasound/CT/MRI):** Techniques used to reduce motion-induced jitter in imaging systems. Algorithms compensate for inconsistent temporal sampling or patient motion during acquisition. Particularly relevant in cardiac or respiratory-triggered exams. Hardware stabilization also helps reduce jitter. Ensures accurate spatial representation.
**Related term:** Motion compensation
**Radiotherapy Example:** Applied in 4D-CT respiratory gating to stabilize tumor motion traces.

42. **Joint CT imaging:** Use of computed tomography to evaluate joints for fractures, degeneration, prosthesis assessment, or soft-tissue calcification. Provides excellent bone detail and spatial resolution. Often used for preoperative planning or trauma evaluation. Can include dual-energy techniques to assess urate deposition.
**Related term:** Bone window
**Radiotherapy Example:** Used for RT planning when bone sarcomas involve joint surfaces.

43. **Joint MRI imaging:** High-resolution soft-tissue imaging of joint structures including ligaments, cartilage, menisci, and synovium. Superior for early inflammatory or degenerative disease detection. Specialized sequences include proton density, STIR, and T2 mapping. Offers multiplanar visualization.
**Related term:** Cartilage imaging
**Radiotherapy Example:** Helps evaluate soft-tissue changes after extremity radiotherapy.

44. **Joint SPECT imaging:** Nuclear medicine imaging that assesses metabolic or osteoblastic activity within joints. Highly sensitive for subtle bone changes, stress injuries, or inflammatory disorders. Often performed as SPECT/CT for precise anatomic localization. Useful for prosthetic evaluation.
**Related term:** Bone scintigraphy
**Radiotherapy Example:** Detects radiation-related joint stress reactions.

45. **Joint scintigraphy:** Planar nuclear imaging of joints using bone-seeking radiotracers. Highlights increased turnover due to arthritis, infection, fractures, or prosthetic complications. Less precise than SPECT but offers rapid whole-joint screening. Provides functional insight into disease processes.
**Related term:** Radiotracer uptake
**Radiotherapy Example:** Measures osteoblastic response near irradiation fields.

46. **Journal of Radiology (scientific publication):** A peer-reviewed publication covering diagnostic imaging, radiotherapy advancements, physics, and interventional techniques. Provides research updates, clinical guidelines, and case studies. Supports academic development in medical imaging. Often cited in clinical protocol formation.
**Related term:** Scientific literature
**Radiotherapy Example:** Frequently publishes updates on radiotherapy QA and dosimetry.

47. **Journal of Nuclear Medicine (scientific publication):** A leading peer-reviewed journal covering PET, SPECT, radionuclides, radiopharmaceuticals, and molecular imaging. Provides cutting-edge research on functional imaging and targeted therapies. Influences clinical and regulatory practice across nuclear medicine.
**Related term:** Radiopharmaceutical research
**Radiotherapy Example:** Publishes studies on theranostic radionuclide therapies like Lu-177.

48. **J-value (dosimetry calculation):** A parameter used in radiological physics referring to correction factors, current density, or dosimetric calibration depending on context. Helps relate measured detector output to absorbed dose. Used in advanced treatment planning modeling.
**Related term:** Dosimetric constant
**Radiotherapy Example:** Contributes to calculation accuracy in Monte-Carlo dose modeling.

49. **J-function (radiobiology):** A mathematical function used to model dose-response relationships or energy deposition patterns. Helps characterize biological effectiveness and predict cellular outcomes. Often used in experimental radiobiology research.
**Related term:** Dose-response curve
**Radiotherapy Example:** Used in modeling survival curves for tumor radiosensitivity.

50. **J-shaped dose-response curve:** Describes a biological response where low doses cause stimulation or minimal effect, while higher doses cause significant suppression or toxicity. Seen in hormesis research, toxicology, and radiobiology. Helps understand non-linear responses.
**Related term:** Hormesis
**Radiotherapy Example:** Helps explain low-dose effects in surrounding healthy tissues.

51. **J-shaped beam profile:** A dose distribution pattern where intensity decreases non-linearly along one axis, forming a J-like curve. Occurs in some specialized beam-shaping or energy-modulated fields. Requires compensation for uniform dose delivery.
**Related term:** Beam profile
**Radiotherapy Example:** Evaluated during QA for complex IMRT beams.

52. **J-shaped energy curve:** Describes how energy deposition changes with depth or material interaction, forming a J-shaped trend. Useful in physics modeling of charged particle interactions. Helps optimize shielding and dose planning.
**Related term:** Energy deposition
**Radiotherapy Example:** Used in proton scatter analysis for shallow tumors.

53. **J-function calculation (dose distribution):** Computational method for applying J-based functions to analyze dose shape, gradient, or biological response. Used in treatment planning software and radiobiology studies. Helps refine optimization algorithms.
**Related term:** Dose modeling
**Radiotherapy Example:** Supports biologically guided IMRT planning.

54. **J-coupling constant (MRS):** Quantifies interaction between nuclear spins in MR spectroscopy. Determines the splitting of spectral peaks. Essential for accurate metabolite identification. Important in neuro-oncology and biochemical MRI.
**Related term:** Spin–spin coupling
**Radiotherapy Example:** Used for metabolic mapping of gliomas for dose escalation.

55. **J-resolved spectroscopy (MRS technique):** A specialized MR spectroscopy sequence that separates J-coupling effects into an additional dimension. Improves metabolite resolution. Helps differentiate overlapping peaks. Used in brain, liver, and tumor metabolic evaluation.
**Related term:** 2D MRS
**Radiotherapy Example:** Guides dose painting based on tumor metabolism.

56. **J-wave artifact (ECG-gated imaging):** A disturbance caused by exaggerated J-waves interfering with ECG gating. Incorrect R-wave detection can degrade cardiac CT/MRI timing. Requires filtering or algorithm adaptation. More common in patients with arrhythmias.
**Related term:** ECG artifact
**Radiotherapy Example:** Can affect cardiac-gated CT for thoracic radiotherapy planning.

57. **J-tube phantom (dosimetry):** A calibration phantom shaped like a "J," used for verifying detector response in curved geometries. Helps assess scatter, dose fall-off, and detector linearity. Common in radiation physics research and QA.
**Related term:** Calibration phantom
**Radiotherapy Example:** Used to calibrate detectors for non-standard field shapes.

58. **J-shaped collimator (special beam-shaping device):** A collimator designed with a J-shaped aperture to shape asymmetric beams. Useful in specialized radiotherapy or experimental beam studies. Requires precise alignment due to its irregular profile. Improves conformity for select clinical scenarios.
**Related term:** Custom collimator
**Radiotherapy Example:** Occasionally used in pediatric shaped-field applications.

59. **Jitter artifact correction algorithm:** Software method that corrects jitter-related misalignment or blurring by analyzing temporal inconsistencies. Applied in MRI, CT, ultrasound, and motion-tracked imaging. Enhances clarity without rescanning.
**Related term:** Image stabilization
**Radiotherapy Example:** Improves motion-tracked CBCT images.

60. **Jitter measurement (imaging):** Quantifies the degree of time-based inconsistency or motion-related phase variation in image acquisition. Important in Doppler ultrasound and cardiac MRI. Helps evaluate system performance and operator technique.
**Related term:** Temporal resolution
**Radiotherapy Example:** Evaluated during QA of motion-tracking systems.

61. **Jagged line detection (CT/MRI):** Identification of irregular sawtooth-like edges in images caused by reconstruction errors, aliasing, or motion. Automated algorithms flag abnormal edge transitions. Helps improve quality control.
**Related term:** Edge artifact
**Radiotherapy Example:** Prevents contour inaccuracies during RT planning.

62. **Joint scintigraphy protocol:** Standardized steps for performing bone scintigraphy of joints, including radiopharmaceutical dose, timing, acquisition technique, and positioning. Ensures reproducible imaging for arthritis, infection, or prosthetic evaluation.
**Related term:** Protocol optimization
**Radiotherapy Example:** Used to assess bone changes after limb radiotherapy.

63. **Joint radiography calibration:** Adjustment and verification of radiographic systems for accurate joint imaging. Includes geometric calibration, contrast checks, and detector performance. Ensures correct joint spacing and orientation.
**Related term:** Radiographic QA
**Radiotherapy Example:** Important when X-ray systems are used for orthogonal RT setup.

64. **Juxta-articular lesion imaging:** Imaging of lesions immediately adjacent to a joint surface. MRI is best for soft tissue and early bone involvement; CT shows cortical integrity. Used for tumors, infections, and inflammatory processes.
**Related term:** Periarticular imaging
**Radiotherapy Example:** Helps define margins for joint-adjacent sarcoma treatment.

65. **Juxta-cortical bone scan:** A nuclear medicine scan evaluating bone activity near cortical surfaces. Sensitive for detecting subtle periosteal reactions, early tumors, or stress injuries. Often performed as SPECT/CT for precision.
**Related term:** Bone scintigraphy
**Radiotherapy Example:** Used in post-RT bone toxicity assessment.

66. **Juxta-luminal tissue imaging:** Imaging of tissue immediately adjacent to luminal organs (bowel, airway, bladder). CT and MRI are primary modalities. Essential for detecting wall invasion or extraluminal spread.
**Related term:** Mural imaging
**Radiotherapy Example:** Important for contouring GI tumors for radiotherapy.

67. **Junctional tissue hotspot analysis:** Identifies areas of elevated dose at field junctions in radiotherapy. Uses dose maps, DVHs, and gamma analysis. Prevents toxicity from unintended hot regions. Common in craniospinal irradiation.
**Related term:** Hotspot
**Radiotherapy Example:** Used to correct excess dose in matched fields.

68. **Junctional dose verification:** Independent measurement or calculation of dose accuracy at field junctions. Uses film, ion chambers, or 3D dosimetry. Ensures fields are properly matched.
**Related term:** Field matching QA
**Radiotherapy Example:** Critical in IMRT/VMAT field segmentation.

69. **Justification (radiation protection principle):** One of the ICRP principles stating that no radiation practice should be undertaken unless overall benefits outweigh risks. Applies to imaging, therapy, and industry. Ensures patient safety and avoids unnecessary exposure.
**Related term:** ALARA
**Radiotherapy Example:** Used in approving re-imaging for treatment replanning.

70. **Just-in-time imaging verification:** Real-time or near real-time imaging used during radiotherapy setup or delivery. Improves accuracy by updating patient position or anatomy changes. Includes CBCT, ultrasound, and surface scanning.
**Related term:** IGRT
**Radiotherapy Example:** Used before each treatment fraction for accuracy.

71. **J-value calibration:** Calibration step ensuring correct interpretation of J-parameter calculations in dosimetry modeling. Used in radiotherapy research and physics modeling. Ensures consistency across experiments.
**Related term:** Dosimetric constant
**Radiotherapy Example:** Used in Monte-Carlo-based modeling QA.

72. **J-index (image quality metric):** A derived metric representing image clarity, contrast, noise, or sharpness. Used for comparing imaging systems or tuning reconstruction algorithms. Helps guide protocol optimization. May vary by modality.
**Related term:** Image quality metrics
**Radiotherapy Example:** Used to evaluate CBCT reconstruction improvements.

73. **J-factor (radiobiology):** A parameter describing interaction, survival, or radiosensitivity relationships in radiobiology equations. Helps model cellular response to radiation. Important in research and therapy optimization.
**Related term:** Radiobiological modeling
**Radiotherapy Example:** Used to compare tumor vs. normal tissue radiosensitivity.

74. **J-wave artifact analysis:** Detailed evaluation of ECG artifacts caused by J-wave abnormalities affecting gating. Helps correct misregistration in cardiac CT or MRI. Specialized filters improve ECG signal accuracy.
**Related term:** ECG gating
**Radiotherapy Example:** Prevents timing errors in cardiac-gated CT for thoracic RT.

75. **J-resolved NMR spectroscopy (advanced):** High-resolution 2D spectroscopy technique separating chemical shift and J-coupling patterns. Improves diagnostic interpretability in complex tissues. Useful in oncology, metabolism, and brain imaging.
**Related term:** Multi-dimensional MRS
**Radiotherapy Example:** Used in mapping aggressive tumor subregions.

76. **J-shaped dose field uniformity check:** Verification that an intentionally shaped dose profile matches planned J-pattern distribution. Done via film or 2D array detectors. Ensures accuracy of complex beam shaping.
**Related term:** Dose uniformity
**Radiotherapy Example:** Used when asymmetric fields are required.

77. **Jet collimator (gamma camera):** A specialized collimator with narrow jet-like apertures enabling high-resolution imaging in certain nuclear medicine systems. Limits scatter and improves spatial fidelity. Requires careful alignment.
**Related term:** Parallel-hole collimator
**Radiotherapy Example:** Used for research in radionuclide-guided therapy.

78. **Jet stream cooling (X-ray tubes):** A high-velocity cooling method improving heat dissipation in X-ray tubes. Extends tube lifespan and stabilizes output. Useful in high-duty cycle imaging systems like CT scanners.
**Related term:** Tube cooling
**Radiotherapy Example:** Important in CT simulators for repeated large-volume scans.

79. **Jagged edge artifact (dose distribution):** Irregular dose boundaries seen in calculated dose maps due to algorithmic interpolation or grid resolution issues. Appears as serrated edges along contours. Fixable with finer grids or algorithm refinement.
**Related term:** Dose grid
**Radiotherapy Example:** Prevented by using small dose-calculation voxel sizes.

80. **Jagged artifact correction (imaging):** Techniques used to smooth or correct jagged edges in CT/MRI images caused by reconstruction errors. Uses convolution filters or edge-preserving enhancers. Prevents contouring mistakes.
**Related term:** Image smoothing
**Radiotherapy Example:** Applied before auto-segmentation in TPS.

81. **Jaw position verification (LINAC):** Verification that the LINAC secondary collimator jaws are positioned correctly according to the treatment plan. Ensures accurate field size, beam shaping, and dose distribution. Done through EPID imaging, mechanical checks, or automated QA systems. Prevents unintended under- or over-dose at field edges.
**Related term:** Collimator QA
**Radiotherapy Example:** Verified during IMRT QA to ensure field edges match MLC shaping.

82. **Jaw tracking (dynamic collimation):** Technique where LINAC jaws dynamically follow the MLC aperture to reduce leakage and scatter. Improves dose conformity and reduces low-dose bath to normal tissues. Particularly useful in IMRT and VMAT plans. Requires precise synchronization.
**Related term:** MLC tracking
**Radiotherapy Example:** Reduces rectal dose in prostate VMAT plans.

83. **Jaw calibration (LINAC):** Mechanical and dosimetric calibration ensuring accurate jaw position, symmetry, speed, and reproducibility. Involves mechanical rulers, film, and EPID analysis. Essential for safe beam shaping.
**Related term:** Mechanical QA
**Radiotherapy Example:** Performed annually to verify jaw accuracy within ±1 mm tolerance.

84. **Jaw symmetry test:** Test verifying that opposing collimator jaws open and close symmetrically. Ensures no geometric skew in the radiation field. Uses EPID or film-based measurements. Part of monthly QA.
**Related term:** Beam symmetry
**Radiotherapy Example:** Ensures symmetric fields for whole-brain radiotherapy.

85. **Jaw leakage measurement:** Quantifies stray radiation escaping between jaws when closed. Essential for assessing machine shielding and leakage limits. Typically measured with ion chambers or film. Ensures compliance with safety regulations.
**Related term:** Radiation leakage
**Radiotherapy Example:** Evaluated during acceptance testing of a new LINAC.

86. **Jaw speed test:** Measures how quickly and consistently jaws can move to programmed positions. Important for dynamic treatments where jaws reposition during delivery. Done with EPID or mechanical testing tools.
**Related term:** Dynamic collimation
**Radiotherapy Example:** Required for accurate VMAT delivery with jaw tracking.

87. **Jaw field matching:** Aligning adjacent radiation fields defined by jaws to avoid gaps or overlaps. Crucial for long-field treatments where multiple segments are matched. Verified using film and light-field alignment.
**Related term:** Field junction
**Radiotherapy Example:** Used in craniospinal irradiation to match cranial and spinal portals.

88. **Jet ventilation artifact (CT):** Motion artifact created by high-frequency jet ventilation during CT imaging. Produces streaks or blurring near lung fields. Requires coordination with anesthesia for breath-hold or low-frequency modes.
**Related term:** Motion artifact
**Radiotherapy Example:** Managed during CT simulation for thoracic tumors.

89. **Jet nebulizer imaging:** Imaging evaluation of aerosol distribution delivered via jet nebulizer. Used in ventilation studies and airway obstruction assessment. Nuclear medicine aerosols allow quantitative mapping. Helps evaluate inhaled therapy effectiveness.
**Related term:** Ventilation scan
**Radiotherapy Example:** Determines functional lung regions before lung cancer planning.

90. **Jet-induced flow artifact (MRI):** Artifact caused by rapid fluid movement producing phase errors or signal voids. Seen in cardiac and vascular MRI near high-velocity jets. Requires velocity-encoded sequences or adjustments in gradient timing.
**Related term:** Flow artifact
**Radiotherapy Example:** Relevant in MRI used for cardiac-adjacent tumor planning.

91. **Joint laxity imaging:** Imaging assessment of excessive joint motion or instability. MRI evaluates ligaments; CT shows bony alignment; ultrasound assesses dynamic laxity. Used in trauma and sports medicine.
**Related term:** Ligament imaging
**Radiotherapy Example:** Follow-up imaging after limb irradiation affecting connective tissue.

92. **Joint degeneration imaging:** Radiologic assessment of degenerative joint disease including cartilage loss, subchondral sclerosis, and osteophytes. MRI is ideal for early cartilage changes; CT for advanced bone remodeling. Helps in treatment planning.
**Related term:** Osteoarthritis imaging
**Radiotherapy Example:** Differentiates degenerative pain from radiation-related joint changes.

93. **Joint prosthesis imaging (CT/MRI/NM):** Evaluation of joint implants for loosening, infection, malalignment, or wear. CT defines hardware position; MRI uses metal artifact reduction; bone scans identify loosening. Essential for postoperative assessment.
**Related term:** Metal artifact reduction
**Radiotherapy Example:** Used before RT to evaluate prosthetic hip position affecting beam angles.

94. **Joint hematoma imaging:** CT or MRI assessment of bleeding within or around a joint. MRI best shows chronicity; CT rapidly identifies acute hemarthrosis. Important for trauma, anticoagulation complications, or tumor bleeding.
**Related term:** Soft-tissue hematoma
**Radiotherapy Example:** Needed when tumors near joints bleed during treatment.

95. **Joint effusion quantification**
Measurement of fluid volume in a joint using ultrasound, MRI, or CT. Helps evaluate inflammation, infection, or injury. MRI provides best volumetric accuracy; ultrasound offers real-time assessment. Important in rheumatology.
**Related term:** Synovial fluid
**Radiotherapy Example:** Used to evaluate inflammatory flares after RT.

96. **Joint metastatic lesion imaging:** Imaging of metastases involving joints or adjacent bone. CT shows cortical erosion; MRI identifies marrow involvement; bone scans show metabolic activity. Essential for staging and symptoms.
**Related term:** Bone metastasis
**Radiotherapy Example:** Guides palliative RT for metastatic joint pain.

97. **Joint cartilage mapping (MRI):** Advanced MRI techniques (T2 mapping, dGEMRIC, T1rho) quantify biochemical cartilage integrity. Detects early degeneration before structural changes. Useful for research and early disease diagnosis.
**Related term:** T2 mapping
**Radiotherapy Example:** Tracks cartilage changes after extremity irradiation.

98. **Joint synovitis imaging:** MRI evaluation of synovial inflammation with STIR, T2, or post-contrast sequences. Sensitive for rheumatoid arthritis, infection, and inflammatory disorders. Ultrasound also detects synovial thickening and vascularity.
**Related term:** Synovial enhancement
**Radiotherapy Example:** Monitors inflammatory changes following RT for benign conditions.

99. **Junctional cold spot analysis:** Evaluation of areas of under-dose at field junctions in radiotherapy. Ensures no tumor receives inadequate coverage. Uses film, EPID, and 3D dose maps. Essential in multi-field treatments.
**Related term:** Hotspot analysis
**Radiotherapy Example:** Prevents cold spots in craniospinal irradiation junctions.

100. **Junctional imaging (anatomical junctions):** Imaging structures located at anatomical junctions such as cervicothoracic, thoracolumbar, or esophagogastric junctions. CT/MRI are primary tools. Important for tumor staging and surgical planning due to complex anatomy transitions.
**Related term:** Transitional anatomy
**Radiotherapy Example:** Used to define tumor spread across the thoracic inlet for RT planning.

101. **J-shaped dose optimization Description:** Designing a dose distribution with a higher dose region that curves like a "J" to spare nearby critical structures.
**Related Terms:** dose sculpting, conformal planning, VMAT optimization.
**Example:** In head-and-neck RT, optimize beams so high dose hugs tumor base while sparing adjacent salivary glands, producing a J-shaped high-dose region.

102. **J-wave artifact correction Description:** Removal/suppression of ECG-related "J-wave" artifacts in ECG-gated imaging used for planning or verification.
**Related Terms:** ECG gating, motion artifact reduction, retrospective gating.
**Example:** Correcting J-wave noise on gated CT used for cardiac radiosurgery planning to avoid misregistration.

103. **J-function verification in radiotherapy Description:** Using a mathematical J-function (or curve) to verify a planning algorithm's expected dose fall-off or biological response.
**Related Terms:** dose–response modeling, DVH analysis, radiobiological modeling.
**Example:** Compare measured dose fall-off across a lung SBRT steep-gradient region to the predicted J-function curve.

104. **J-factor calculation for cell survival Description:** A parameter in radiobiology models reflecting a component of cell survival (analogous to factors in LQ model).
**Related Terms:** surviving fraction, linear-quadratic model, radiosensitivity.
**Example:** Use J-factor in research modeling to fit clonogenic assay survival after fractionated doses.

105. **J-index optimization for imaging quality Description:** Using a metric (J-index) to quantify and optimize image quality (contrast vs. noise tradeoff).
**Related Terms:** CNR, SNR, image quality metrics.
**Example:** Tune CT reconstruction kernel based on J-index to maximize tumor contrast for planning CT.

106. **J-coupling calibration in MRI spectroscopy Description:** Calibration to account for scalar coupling (J-coupling) between nuclear spins in MR spectroscopy used for tissue characterization.
**Related Terms:** MRS, chemical shift, spectral fitting.
**Example:** Calibrate J-coupling parameters when using MRS to distinguish tumor recurrence vs radiation necrosis.

107. **107.** J-resolved imaging protocol Description: An MR spectroscopy technique that separates J-coupling along a second spectral dimension to simplify spectra.
**Related Terms:** 2D MRS, spectral editing, metabolite quantification.
**Example:** Use J-resolved MRS to identify metabolites in glioma prior to radiotherapy planning.

108. **J-tube phantom dose measurement Description:** Phantom shaped like a "J" (or with J-tube cavities) used to measure dose in curved geometries.
**Related Terms:** anthropomorphic phantom, dosimetry, film/TLD measurements.
**Example:** Place film in a J-tube phantom to verify dose around a curved brachytherapy applicator.

109. **Jagged edge artifact mitigation Description:** Techniques to reduce staircase/jagged-edge artifacts in CT or CBCT images that degrade contouring accuracy.
**Related Terms:** slice thickness, interpolation, smoothing filters.
**Example:** Reduce jagged edges in CT by using thinner slices or applying edge-preserving smoothing before segmentation.

110. **Jaw position verification (LINAC) Description:** Checking that the primary collimator jaws on a linear accelerator are where the plan expects them to be.
**Related Terms:** MLC QA, mechanical QA, light field vs radiation field.
**Example:** Use portal imaging to verify jaw positions for a square field at multiple gantry angles during monthly QA.

111. **Jaw alignment calibration Description:** Calibration procedure to align jaw motion and positioning with machine coordinates and MLC.
**Related Terms:** mechanical calibration, Picket-Fence test (for MLC), isocenter alignment.
**Example:** Adjust jaw calibration offsets after detection of systematic jaw misposition during QA.

112. **Jaw shielding in radiotherapy Description:** Using the jaws as passive collimation to shield normal tissue from primary beam outside the field.
**Related Terms:** primary collimator, MLC, field shaping.
**Example:** Close jaws to minimize out-of-field dose when delivering small tangent fields for breast RT.

113. **Jaw-based beam shaping Description:** Creating rectangular field shapes and penumbra control using jaw setting rather than MLC modulation.
**Related Terms:** fixed fields, conformal RT, electron applicators.
**Example:** Use jaw-based shaping for simple parallel-opposed fields in palliative pelvic RT.

114. **Jet beam dosimetryDescription:** Dosimetry techniques for high-velocity or ultra-narrow beams (term often used in research or specialized collimation).
**Related Terms:** microbeam, stereotactic, film/Gafchromic dosimetry.
**Example:** Characterize dose profile of a research "jet" microbeam array with high-resolution film.

115. **Jet cooling system verification Description:** QA of cooling systems for equipment that uses jet-cooling (e.g., high-power beamline components).
**Related Terms:** machine integrity, thermal drift, preventive maintenance.
**Example:** Verify chiller flow and temperature stability in proton therapy nozzle cooling to prevent beam drift.

116. **Jet collimator performance check Description:** Testing a specialized collimator ("jet" style) for alignment, leakage, and profile shaping.
**Related Terms:** collimator QA, beam profile, penumbra measurement.
**Example:** Measure beam profiles with film to confirm jet collimator produces intended narrow beam.

117. **Joint imaging protocol optimization Description:** Harmonizing protocols across modalities (e.g., CT+MRI) used for multimodality planning.
**Related Terms:** multimodal registration, imaging standardization, fusion QA.
**Example:** Standardize slice thickness and contrast timing for CT and MRI fusion in brain RT planning.

118. **Joint phantom calibration Description:** Calibrating phantoms used in multi-modality QA (CT/MR/PET) to ensure consistent imaging metrics.
**Related Terms:** cross-calibration, image registration phantoms, attenuation correction.
**Example:** Use an MR/CT phantom with fiducials to verify PET/CT attenuation maps and registration accuracy.

119. **Joint SPECT/CT dosimetry Description:** Dosimetry calculations that combine SPECT functional data with CT anatomical information (common in radionuclide therapy).
**Related Terms:** voxel dosimetry, internal emitter dosimetry, OLINDA/EXM alternatives.
**Example:** Calculate renal dose from radiopharmaceutical therapy using SPECT-derived activity maps with CT volumes.

120. **Joint PET/CT fusion verification Description:** QA ensuring PET metabolic data correctly aligns with CT anatomy before using for target delineation.
**Related Terms:** rigid/ deformable registration, SUV harmonization, attenuation correction.
**Example:** Check PET/CT fuse by confirming alignment of lung lesion SUV hotspot with CT lesion center before contouring.

121. **Juxta-articular hotspot planning Description:** Planning to treat or avoid hotspots near joints to manage tumor while preserving joint function.
**Related Terms:** organ-at-risk sparing, dose constraints, IMRT planning.
**Example:** In sarcoma near the knee, limit dose to cartilage while ensuring tumor receives therapeutic dose.

122. **Juxta-luminal therapy verification Description:** Verifying dose delivered near luminal structures (e.g., esophagus, bowel) where toxicity risk is high.
**Related Terms:** GI sparing, dose constraints, image-guided verification.
**Example:** Use CBCT and in-vivo dosimetry when delivering SBRT near small bowel to confirm safe dose gradients.

123. **Juxta-cortical bone dosimetry Description:** Measuring/planning dose near cortical bone (important for bone sarcomas or to avoid fracture risk).
**Related Terms:** bone tolerance, dose gradient, proton range uncertainty.
**Example:** Adjust proton range and margins to avoid excessive dose to femoral cortex during pelvic RT.

124. **Junctional dose planning Description:** Planning dose at field junctions where adjacent fields meet (e.g., matching cranial and spinal fields).
**Related Terms:** feathering, junction shift, field matching.
**Example:** Feather the junction between cranial and spinal fields in craniospinal irradiation to avoid hot/cold spots.

125. **Junctional hotspot verification Description:** QA to detect hotspots at junctions that could cause overdosing.
**Related Terms:** dose summation, film dosimetry, in vivo dosimetry.
**Example:** Place film across junction region during QA run of craniospinal plan to verify absence of hotspots.

126. **Justification assessment (ALARA principle) Description:** Evaluation that each imaging or therapeutic exposure is justified and ALARA (As Low As Reasonably Achievable) is applied.
**Related Terms:** radiation protection, benefit-risk analysis, exposure justification.
**Example:** Document medical justification before performing additional diagnostic CT for RT planning in pediatric patients.

127. **Just-in-time dose monitoring Description:** Near-real-time monitoring of delivered dose (e.g., using portal dosimetry or in vivo sensors).
**Related Terms:** EPID dosimetry, real-time dosimetry, adaptive RT triggers.
**Example:** Use EPID-based portal dosimetry during IMRT delivery to detect deviations and halt if thresholds exceeded.

128. **J-value assessment in therapy planning Description:** Use of an indexed value (J-value) representing some planning metric (could be plan conformity or biological index) for comparison.
**Related Terms:** conformity index, homogeneity index, plan scoring.
**Example:** Rank competing plans by J-value that combines conformity and OAR sparing.

129. **J-shaped dose distribution verification Description:** Confirming a planned J-shaped dose distribution is actually delivered (verification via measurement/imaging).
**Related Terms:** dose mapping, film dosimetry, 3D gamma analysis.
**Example:** Use gel dosimetry in a curved phantom to confirm measured 3D dose matches planned J-shaped distribution.

130. **J-factor optimization in treatment planning Description:** Tuning a planning parameter (called J-factor) that affects biological weighting or dose shaping.
**Related Terms:** objective function weighting, cost functions, radiobiological optimization.
**Example:** Adjust J-factor in an optimization engine to reduce normal tissue NTCP while maintaining TCP.

131. **J-index assessment for image quality Description:** Calculation of J-index (image quality summary metric) to assess or compare imaging protocols used for planning.
**Related Terms:** ROC curves, CNR, SNR, task-based metrics.
**Example:** Compare two MR sequences via J-index to choose the best for tumor boundary visualization.

132. **J-resolved MR spectroscopy analysis Description:** Analysis of 2D MR spectroscopy spectra to resolve overlapping metabolite peaks for tissue characterization.
**Related Terms:** metabolite quantification, spectral fitting, MRS.
**Example:** Use J-resolved MRS to identify elevated choline in recurrent tumor versus radionecrosis.

133. **J-wave artifact detection in ECG-gated imaging Description:** Algorithms to detect J-wave artifact occurrences in gated imaging sequences to exclude corrupt frames.
**Related Terms:** gating artifact rejection, motion correction, image pre-processing.
**Example:** Auto-exclude frames with J-wave artifact from gated cardiac CT prior to target contouring.

134. **J-coupled spin system analysis Description:** Interpreting coupled spin systems in MR spectroscopy relevant for identifying certain metabolites.
**Related Terms:** scalar coupling, multiplet peaks, spectral simulation.
**Example:** Analyze J-coupled lactate peaks to help differentiate tumor metabolic profiles in planning MRI.

135. **Juxtaposition phantom imaging Description:** Imaging phantoms designed to create closely adjacent structures (juxtaposed) to assess spatial resolution and partial-volume effects.
**Related Terms:** spatial resolution phantom, edge response, partial-volume effect.
**Example:** Scan a juxtaposition phantom to verify CT/MR can resolve tumor abutting normal tissue for accurate contouring.

136. **Juxtaposition effect calibration Description:** Calibrating imaging or dose algorithms to account for dose perturbations or imaging artifacts when different tissues are juxtaposed.
**Related Terms:** interface dosimetry, heterogeneity correction, image artifacts.
**Example:** Adjust heterogeneity correction for proton planning when lung and dense mediastinum tissues are adjacent.

137. **Juxtaposition dose verification Description:** Measuring dose in regions where two different fields or tissue types meet to ensure accuracy.
**Related Terms:** interface dosimetry, film/TLD placement, Monte Carlo validation.
**Example:** Place TLDs at bone-soft tissue interfaces to verify planned dose in head-and-neck treatments.

138. **J-shaped energy curve verification Description:** Verifying an energy spectrum or dose-energy relationship that is non-linear and resembles a J-curve (often research context).
**Related Terms:** beam energy spectrum, depth-dose curve, energy modulation.
**Example:** Confirm energy modulation settings on an experimental delivery system produce intended J-shaped depth-dose behavior.

139. **Jagged line artifact detection algorithm Description:** Software that detects line-based artifacts (staircase/jagged lines) in CT/CBCT images to flag or correct them.
**Related Terms:** artifact detection, image preprocessing, QA automation.
**Example:** Run detection algorithm on CBCT before registration; if jagged artifacts detected, repeat acquisition.

140. **Jet stream radiation shielding assessment Description:** Evaluation of shielding needs where a directed "jet" of secondary radiation might occur (specialized beamlines).
**Related Terms:** shielding calculations, scatter analysis, facility design.
**Example:** During installation of a proton beamline, model and verify shielding against narrow scattering jets.

141. **J-shaped field uniformity verification:** Ensuring a radiation field with a J-shaped intensity pattern maintains uniformity where required.
**Related Terms:** field flatness, profile QA, beam symmetry.
**Example:** Use water-tank scanning to verify that the J-shaped field remains uniform in the low-dose region of a breast tangential plan.

142. **J-wave suppression protocol:** Procedures to suppress ECG J-wave artifacts during gated imaging.
**Related Terms:** ECG gating, artifact reduction.
**Example:** Apply optimized filtering before acquiring cardiac-gated CT for coronary radiosurgery.

143. **J-coupling artifact correction in MRI:** Removing spectral artifacts due to J-coupling interactions in MR spectroscopy.
**Related Terms:** MRS editing, spectral cleanup.
**Example:** Apply J-editing to remove lactate coupling artifacts before tumor metabolic mapping.

144. **J-resolved spectroscopy calibration:** Calibrating MR spectroscopy to correctly separate J-coupled peaks in 2D spectra.
**Related Terms:** spectral resolution, metabolite quantification.
**Example:** Calibrate J-resolved scan parameters before planning MRS-guided brain RT.

145. **J-index verification for image quality:** Checking whether the J-index metric confirms expected image quality for planning or QA.
**Related Terms:** image scoring, SNR/CNR metrics.
**Example:** Verify J-index stability across repeated MRI scans used for adaptive radiotherapy.

146. **J-function analysis in radiobiology:** Using J-shaped biological response curves to understand dose–response behavior.
**Related Terms:** TCP/NTCP, survival curves, biologic modeling.
**Example:** Fit a J-function model to experimental cell-survival data from high-dose hypofractionation.

147. **J-value calibration for dose planning:** Calibrating a J-value parameter used in planning algorithms or scoring models.
**Related Terms:** plan optimization weight, dose metrics.
**Example:** Adjust J-value weighting to improve target conformity in IMRT planning.

148. **Jagged edge artifact measurement:** Quantifying jagged or staircase artifacts in CT/CBCT images.
**Related Terms:** pixelation, contouring error, edge analysis.
**Example:** Calculate artifact severity before structure segmentation on coarse-slice CT.

149. **Jaw aperture calibration:** Calibrating jaw opening to match programmed vs. actual aperture sizes.
**Related Terms:** mechanical QA, collimator calibration.
**Example:** Measure jaw-defined field sizes at different energies to ensure accuracy.

150. **Jaw shielding verification:** Verifying that jaws properly shield off-axis normal tissue.
**Related Terms:** leakage test, out-of-field dose.
**Example:** Use film outside the field edge to confirm jaws reduce leakage during VMAT delivery.

151. **Jaw position adjustment protocol:** Standard procedure for correcting jaw positioning offsets.
**Related Terms:** service calibration, QA tolerances.
**Example:** Correct jaw offset discovered during monthly QA when field edges fail alignment tests.

152. **Jet beam alignment verification:** Checking alignment of a narrow, high-intensity ("jet-type") beam.
**Related Terms:** microbeam, beam profiling, collimator QA.
**Example:** Use fine-resolution film to verify the jet beam strikes the intended isocenter.

153. **Jet stream cooling calibration:** Calibration of cooling jets for devices requiring temperature stability.
**Related Terms:** thermal QA, equipment maintenance.
**Example:** Adjust cooling jets on a proton nozzle to prevent temperature-related beam drift.

154. **Jet collimator dose verification:** Measuring dose output from a specialized jet collimator.
**Related Terms:** profiling, output factors, penumbra.
**Example:** Verify output factors using radiochromic film under jet-collimated fields.

155. **Joint MRI alignment verification:** Confirming MRI alignment accuracy across joint regions (e.g., knee, shoulder).
**Related Terms:** deformable registration, anatomical QA.
**Example:** Check MRI alignment of cartilage and soft tissues before contouring peri-articular tumors.

156. **Joint CT calibration phantom:** A phantom designed for CT calibration in joint regions.
**Related Terms:** bone/soft-tissue contrast, HU accuracy.
**Example:** Scan joint phantom to ensure accurate HU mapping for sarcoma planning.

157. **Joint PET/CT fusion quality check:** Verification that PET and CT align properly in joint areas.
**Related Terms:** registration QA, SUV accuracy.
**Example:** Confirm PET hotspot matches CT lesion near a knee joint before target delineation.

158. **Joint SPECT/CT reconstruction verification:** Verifying accuracy of multimodal reconstruction at joints.
**Related Terms:** attenuation correction, fusion QA.
**Example:** Validate SPECT bone scan reconstruction around hip joint for radionuclide therapy.

159. **Juxta-articular tissue dose measurement:** Measuring dose near tissues adjacent to joints.
**Related Terms:** OAR sparing, cartilage dose limits.
**Example:** Place TLDs near knee cartilage during QA for extremity sarcoma irradiation.

160. **Juxta-luminal hotspot verification:** Checking for hotspots near luminal organs (e.g., bowel, esophagus).
**Related Terms:** GI toxicity, hot-spot control.
**Example:** Review dose map near small bowel loop in abdominal SBRT.

161. **Juxta-cortical dose optimization:** Optimizing dose to avoid excessive dose to cortical bone.
**Related Terms:** fracture risk, bone tolerance.
**Example:** Adjust IMRT beams to spare femoral cortex in pelvic RT.

162. **Junctional tissue dose verification:** Measurement of dose in tissue where two fields meet.
**Related Terms:** feathering, field matching QA.
**Example:** TLD measurements along craniospinal junctions.

163. **Junctional hotspot detection:** Detecting hotspots in junction areas.
**Related Terms:** hot spot analysis, DVH review.
**Example:** Identify and eliminate a hot spot in breast-tangent/SCV junction.

164. **Justification review (radiation protection):** Reviewing justification for radiation use per ALARA.
**Related Terms:** benefit–risk assessment, regulatory compliance.
**Example:** Document justification before re-imaging pediatric patients.

165. **Just-in-time imaging verification:** Real-time or near-real-time verification imaging during treatment.
**Related Terms:** IGRT, adaptive RT triggers.
**Example:** Acquire quick kV imaging before each SBRT fraction to confirm tumor position.

166. **Juvenile radiotherapy planning:** Special considerations when planning treatment for children.
**Related Terms:** pediatric RT, growth plate sparing, late effects.
**Example:** Reduce dose to developing spinal cord in pediatric craniospinal irradiation.

167. **Juvenile dose monitoring:** Monitoring dose delivered to pediatric patients with higher precision.
**Related Terms:** in vivo dosimetry, pediatric QA.
**Example:** Use OSL sensors for pediatric TBI to ensure dose uniformity.

168. **Juvenile imaging safety protocol:** Safety guidelines for imaging minors.
**Related Terms:** ALARA pediatrics, sedation, low-dose CT.
**Example:** Use pediatric CT protocol with reduced mAs during planning CT.

169. **Juxtaposition effect measurement:** Measuring dose or imaging distortion at interfaces of very different tissues.
**Related Terms:** heterogeneity correction, boundary artifacts.
**Example:** Evaluate dose at lung–tumor boundary in proton therapy.

170. **Juxtaposition phantom calibration:** Calibrating phantoms that simulate adjacent tissues of differing densities.
**Related Terms:** interface dosimetry, phantom QA.
**Example:** Calibrate a lung/bone phantom used to validate heterogeneity algorithms.

171. **Juxtaposition dose optimization:** Optimizing dose around tissue interfaces.
**Related Terms:** gradient management, adaptive planning.
**Example:** Modify beams to improve dose uniformity at air–sinus interface in head-and-neck RT.

172. **J-shaped dose curve plotting:** Plotting a J-shaped curve showing non-linear dose behavior (steep falloff then plateau).
**Related Terms:** dose–distance curves, penumbra.
**Example:** Plot dose fall-off curve for VMAT arc showing characteristic J-profile.

173. **J-wave artifact analysis:** Evaluating J-wave interference in ECG-gated imaging.
**Related Terms:** gating QA, signal filtering.
**Example:** Analyze J-wave patterns that distort cardiac CT images for radiosurgery planning.

174. **J-coupled spin calibration:** Calibrating MR spectroscopy based on J-coupled spin interactions.
**Related Terms:** spectral modeling, metabolite peaks.
**Example:** Calibrate J-coupling to accurately quantify choline elevation in tumor spectroscopy.

175. **J-function modeling in therapy:** Use of J-shaped functional models in dose optimization or biological response prediction.
**Related Terms:** radiobiological modeling, optimization functions.
**Example:** Apply J-function in optimization to improve high-dose conformity in SBRT.

176. **J-factor calculation for radiobiology:** Calculating J-factor as part of dose–response or survival modeling.
**Related Terms:** LQ model, survival curves, radiosensitivity.
**Example:** Fit J-factor to experimental data for hypoxic vs normoxic tumor cells.

177. **J-index calculation in imaging:** Computing J-index to score imaging quality.
**Related Terms:** quality metrics, reconstruction QA.
**Example:** Use J-index to compare two MRI sequences for brain tumor boundary clarity.

178. **J-resolved NMR spectroscopy verification:** Verifying spectral accuracy for 2D J-resolved NMR/MRS.
**Related Terms:** spectral QA, spectral editing.
**Example:** Ensure correct lactate doublet resolution in therapy-planning MRS.

179. **Jet stream radiation exposure study:** Studying radiation exposure patterns from narrow radiation "jet streams."
**Related Terms:** scatter modeling, beam physics.
**Example:** Research scatter doses from high-energy beamline components.

180. **Jet collimator beam alignment:** Confirming alignment of beams formed by a jet collimator.
**Related Terms:** beam steering, mechanical QA.
**Example:** Use EPID to check that a jet-collimated beam hits isocenter.

181. **Jagged line artifact detection in CT:** Detecting jagged-edge artifacts in CT.
**Related Terms:** reconstruction artifacts, segmentation errors.
**Example:** Automated detection alerts clinicians before contouring.

182. **Jaw motion artifact reduction:** Reducing artifacts caused by jaw motion during megavoltage imaging or delivery.
**Related Terms:** mechanical stability, imaging QA.
**Example:** Use slower gantry speed to prevent jaw vibration artifacts.

183. **Jaw positioning QA (Quality Assurance):** Routine QA ensuring jaws position accurately across all settings.
**Related Terms:** mechanical QA, collimator tests.
**Example:** Conduct monthly jaw position checks with a calibrated ruler test.

184. **Joint density measurement verification:** Validating density measurements in imaging across joint regions.
**Related Terms:** HU calibration, tissue segmentation QA.
**Example:** Confirm bone density readings around knee before dose calculation in sarcoma RT.

185. **Joint imaging artifact correction:** Correcting imaging artifacts caused by metal implants or anatomy in joint regions.
**Related Terms:** MAR (metal artifact reduction), scatter correction.
**Example:** Apply MAR for a hip prosthesis in pelvic RT CT.

186. **Juvenile phantom calibration:** Calibrating pediatric phantoms for imaging and dosimetry QA.
**Related Terms:** anthropomorphic phantom, pediatric QA.
**Example:** Calibrate CT pediatric phantom to validate low-dose protocols.

187. **Juvenile tissue dose simulation:** Simulating dose in developing tissues.
**Related Terms:** pediatric dosimetry, Monte Carlo simulation.
**Example:** Model dose to epiphyseal plates during extremity irradiation.

188. **Justification principle assessment (ALARA):** Evaluating that exposure is clinically justified under ALARA.
**Related Terms:** regulatory compliance, safety.
**Example:** Approve low-dose CT over full diagnostic CT for pediatric RT planning.

189. **Juxta-articular therapy planning:** Planning therapy near joints to avoid functional impairment.
**Related Terms:** cartilage sparing, extremity RT.
**Example:** Plan IMRT for elbow sarcoma minimizing dose to joint cartilage.

190. **Juxta-luminal dose verification:** Verifying dose near hollow organs such as bowel or esophagus.
**Related Terms:** OAR verification, high-gradient dose checks.
**Example:** Use CBCT + in vivo dosimeters to verify safe dose near stomach in abdominal SBRT.

191. **J-shaped beam profile optimization:** Optimizing beam shapes that exhibit J-type profiles to achieve uniformity and clinical acceptability.
**Related:** beam shaping, IMRT fluence optimization.
**Example:** Adjust fluence maps so a J-shaped VMAT profile maintains sufficient coverage of the PTV.

192. **J-coupled proton spectroscopy:** Use of MRS techniques that evaluate proton–proton J-coupling for metabolic characterization.
**Related:** MRS editing, metabolic imaging.
**Example:** Measure choline-to-creatine ratios for brain tumor planning.

193. **J-function verification in radiotherapy planning:** Checking that a J-shaped mathematical function used in optimization behaves as expected.
**Related:** objective functions, dose modeling.
**Example:** Verify the J-function improves falloff in SBRT planning.

194. **J-index quality assessment:** Assessing image quality or signal stability using the J-index metric.
**Related:** image scoring, QC metrics.
**Example:** Use J-index to compare two MR sequences for prostate imaging.

195. **Jagged edge mitigation in CT images:** Correction of stair-step or jagged boundaries in CT reconstructions.
**Related:** artifact reduction, segmentation accuracy.
**Example:** Apply smoothing before contouring spinal targets.

196. **Jaw collimator alignment verification:** Checking jaws align with expected mechanical and radiation-defined edges.
**Related:** mechanical QA, collimation accuracy.
**Example:** EPID tests verifying jaw alignment during monthly QA.

197. **Jaw motion correction in LINAC:** Correcting unwanted jaw movement during dynamic delivery.
**Related:** MLC–jaw synchronization, mechanical drift.
**Example:** Recalibrate jaws when motion artifacts appear during VMAT.

198. **Jet stream cooling system QA:** Quality assurance of cooling jets used in beamline or detector components.
**Related:** thermal stability, equipment reliability.
**Example:** Validate stable cooling of a proton nozzle.

199. **Jet collimator performance optimization:** Improving the output and uniformity of jet-style collimators.
**Related:** microbeam collimation, beam shaping.
**Example:** Tune slit dimensions for microbeam irradiation research.

200. **Joint SPECT/CT registration verification:** Ensuring accurate fusion of SPECT and CT images around joints.
**Related:** registration QA, multimodal imaging.
**Example:** Confirm alignment of uptake in a knee lesion for radionuclide therapy.

201. **Joint PET/CT image fusion QA:** Verifying fusion accuracy between PET and CT in joint regions.
**Related:** SUV precision, fusion registration.
**Example:** Check PET hotspot matches CT-defined cartilage lesion.

202. **Juxta-articular lesion mapping:** Mapping lesions adjacent to joints for accurate treatment.
**Related:** cartilage sparing, extremity RT.
**Example:** Map synovial tumors for IMRT planning.

203. **Juxta-luminal therapy verification:** Verification of dose near hollow organs.
**Related:** GI sparing, high gradient QA.
**Example:** Verify dose near esophagus in mediastinal RT.

204. **Juxta-cortical bone dose verification:** Measuring dose near cortical bone surfaces.
**Related:** bone toxicity, interface dosimetry.
**Example:** Place dosimeters near femur cortex for pelvic RT.

205. **Junctional hotspot calibration:** Calibrating QA to detect hotspots in field junctions.
**Related:** feathering, match-line QA.
**Example:** Calibrate film for craniospinal junction QA.

206. **Junctional tissue dose optimization:** Optimizing dose in regions where two beams meet.
**Related:** field matching, plan optimization.
**Example:** Feather junction in breast–SCV treatments.

207. **Justification assessment protocol:** Formal process ensuring radiation exposure is justified.
**Related:** ALARA, regulatory compliance.
**Example:** Document justification before additional CT.

208. **Just-in-time dose verification:** Near-real-time verification of delivered dose.
**Related:** adaptive RT, in vivo dosimetry.
**Example:** Use EPID-based real-time dose monitoring during SBRT.

209. **Juvenile CT dose optimization:** Optimizing CT dose for pediatric imaging.
**Related:** low-dose protocols, pediatric ALARA.
**Example:** Reduce mAs for pediatric planning CT.

210. **Juvenile MRI safety calibration:** Calibrating MRI protocols for safe pediatric imaging.
**Related:** SAR limits, sedation.
**Example:** Verify MRI SAR remains within limits for children.

211. **Juvenile PET/CT protocol verification:** Ensuring PET/CT protocols adhere to pediatric safety standards.
**Related:** dose reduction, timing adjustments.
**Example:** Confirm FDG activity is weight-adjusted.

212. **Juxtaposition artifact correction:** Correcting imaging artifacts at tissue interfaces.
**Related:** boundary artifacts, heterogeneity correction.
**Example:** Apply MAR around lung–bone interfaces.

213. **Juxtaposition phantom QA:** Using phantoms that simulate tissue interfaces for QA.
**Related:** heterogeneity testing, dose accuracy.
**Example:** Validate heterogeneity algorithms with lung–bone phantom.

214. **Juxtaposition dose verification:** Checking dose accuracy at abrupt density changes.
**Related:** interface dosimetry, Monte Carlo.
**Example:** Verify proton dose at lung–tumor boundary.

215. **J-shaped energy profile assessment:** Evaluating beam energy distributions with J-shaped characteristics.
**Related:** beam characterization, spectra analysis.
**Example:** Measure energy variation across VMAT field edges.

216. **J-wave artifact suppression:** Mitigating ECG J-wave artifacts during gated imaging.
**Related:** signal filtering, cardiac gating.
**Example:** Filter J-wave noise for gated cardiac CT.

217. **J-coupling analysis in spectroscopy:** Analyzing J-coupling peaks in MRS spectra.
**Related:** peak separation, metabolite quantification.
**Example:** Distinguish lactate doublets in brain MRS.

218. **J-resolved MRI spectroscopy QA:** Quality assurance of 2D J-resolved spectroscopy sequences.
**Related:** spectral resolution, artifact suppression.
**Example:** Validate frequency separation before therapy planning.

219. **J-value verification in therapy:** Confirming accuracy of the J-value parameter in optimization models.
**Related:** plan optimization, weighting factors.
**Example:** Adjust J-value to improve PTV conformity.

220. **J-factor modeling in radiobiology:** Using J-factor components in dose–response modeling.
**Related:** LQ-based extensions, survival curves.
**Example:** Fit J-factor to analyze hypoxia-modified radiosensitivity.

221. **J-index calibration for imaging systems:** Calibrating systems so their J-index scores reflect true image quality.
**Related:** metric standardization, QC.
**Example:** Recalibrate MRI when J-index drifts.

222. **Jagged line artifact suppression:** Minimizing jagged edges in reconstructed images.
**Related:** smoothing, anti-aliasing.
**Example:** Improve CBCT edges before adaptive RT.

223. **Jaw position QA in radiotherapy:** Routine QA ensuring jaws position correctly.
**Related:** mechanical QA, field-size verification.
**Example:** Annual jaw position reproducibility test.

224. **Jet beam alignment calibration:** Calibrating alignment of narrow jet-like beams.
**Related:** microbeam QA, isocenter tests.
**Example:** Film test for microbeam alignment.

225. **Jet stream radiation monitoring:** Monitoring radiation from narrow jet streams or beamline leakage.
**Related:** shielding tests, stray radiation.
**Example:** Measure leakage near a proton beam nozzle.

226. **Jet collimator dose optimization:** Optimizing dose delivery using jet collimators.
**Related:** microbeam therapy, beam shaping.
**Example:** Tune slot widths for preclinical high-dose microbeams.

227. **Joint imaging artifact verification:** Checking artifacts in imaging around joints.
**Related:** metal artifact QA, reconstruction checks.
**Example:** Verify artifact reduction around hip prosthesis for pelvic RT.

228. **Joint phantom QA:** QA using phantoms designed for joint imaging or dose studies.
**Related:** anthropomorphic phantoms, regional QA.
**Example:** Scan knee phantom to evaluate CT HU accuracy.

229. **Juvenile tissue dosimetry verification:** Verifying dose delivered to child-equivalent tissues.
**Related:** pediatric dose QA, in vivo dosimetry.
**Example:** Use OSLs in pediatric phantom for TBI QA.

230. **Juvenile phantom imaging calibration:** Calibrating pediatric phantoms for imaging.
**Related:** HU accuracy, pediatric CT.
**Example:** Calibrate phantom for low-dose CT settings.

231. **Justification principle verification (ALARA):** Verifying exposures meet ALARA justification.
**Related:** radiation protection, clinical appropriateness.
**Example:** Sign off justification for repeat CBCT.

232. **Juxta-articular hotspot verification:** Checking for hotspots near joint surfaces.
**Related:** cartilage sparing, extremity RT.
**Example:** Evaluate high-dose regions near elbow cartilage.

233. **Juxta-luminal dose optimization:** Optimizing dose around luminal organs.
**Related:** GI dose constraints, SBRT.
**Example:** Adjust arcs to reduce dose near bowel loop.

234. **Junctional tissue therapy QA:** QA specific to treatment regions involving field junctions.
**Related:** match-line QA, junction integrity.
**Example:** Verify dose uniformity in craniospinal junctions.

235. **Junctional dose verification phantom:** Phantom used to verify match-line dose accuracy.
**Related:** junction QA, interface phantoms.
**Example:** Use phantom to assess junction feathering.

236. **J-wave correction in ECG-gated imaging:** Correcting for J-wave interference in ECG-based image acquisition.
**Related:** artifact filtering, cardiac gating.
**Example:** Improve cardiac-gated CT for radiosurgery.

237. **J-coupled spin system verification:** Verification of MR systems modeling J-coupled spins.
**Related:** advanced MRS, spectral QA.
**Example:** Confirm accurate choline peak splitting.

238. **J-resolved spectroscopy artifact correction:** Correcting artifacts in J-resolved MRS scans.
**Related:** spectral cleanup, baseline correction.
**Example:** Remove lipid contamination artifacts.

239. **Jet collimator alignment phantom:** Phantom for checking jet collimator alignment.
**Related:** beam QA, microbeam alignment.
**Example:** Use phantom for microbeam preclinical QA.

240. **Jagged edge artifact phantom calibration:** Calibrating phantoms to evaluate jagged-edge artifacts.
**Related:** imaging QA, reconstruction error analysis.
**Example:** Use phantom to assess CT reconstruction performance.

**241. J-shaped beam intensity verification:** Verifying intensity distribution of J-shaped beams.
**Related:** dose profiling, fluence maps.
**Example:** Measure intensity with film for beam modeling.

**242. J-function optimization in dose planning:** Using J-functions as part of optimization objectives.
**Related:** cost functions, plan optimization.
**Example:** Use J-function to boost conformity in SBRT.

**243. J-index evaluation for image quality:** Evaluating imaging systems using the J-index metric.
**Related:** QC metrics, imaging performance.
**Example:** Compare J-index between two CBCT protocols.

**244. Jagged artifact phantom verification:** Verifying artifact correction using specialized phantoms.
**Related:** artifact QA, image cleanup.
**Example:** Test CT algorithm for jagged edge suppression.

**245. Jaw shielding QA:** Ensuring jaws provide adequate shielding outside field.
**Related:** leakage monitoring, field edge QA.
**Example:** Measure radiation beyond field edge during VMAT.

**246. Jaw alignment QA in LINAC:** Routine checks verifying jaw alignment accuracy.
**Related:** mechanical QA, field size checks.
**Example:** Monthly jaw alignment using EPID.

**247. Jet stream cooling performance verification:** Verifying cooling jet performance in beam systems.
**Related:** thermal QA, hardware stability.
**Example:** Ensure stable cooling at proton nozzle exit.

**248. Jet collimator phantom testing:** Testing jet collimators using phantoms.
**Related:** beam shaping QA, microbeam dosimetry.
**Example:** Use phantom to verify beam width consistency.

**249. Joint MRI registration QA:** QA of MRI registration around joints.
**Related:** deformable registration, segmentation accuracy.
**Example:** Verify MRI–CT fusion for knee sarcoma.

**250. Joint CT fusion QA:** Checking CT-to-CT or CT-to-other-modality fusion in joint regions.
**Related:** multimodal QA, positional accuracy.
**Example:** Validate CT–CBCT fusion for extremity RT.

**251. Joint PET/CT dosimetry verification:** Ensuring PET/CT alignment yields accurate dosimetry.
**Related:** SUV accuracy, contour mapping.
**Example:** Confirm PET SUV hotspot aligns with PTV in joint-adjacent tumor.

**252. Juxta-articular tissue mapping:** Mapping tissues adjacent to joints for accurate contouring.
**Related:** extremity RT, cartilage protection.
**Example:** Map soft-tissue sarcoma boundaries.

**253. Juxta-luminal therapy dose verification:** Confirming dose near luminal organs during therapy.
**Related:** OAR sparing, high-gradient QA.
**Example:** Check esophageal dose in lung SBRT.

**254. Juxta-cortical hotspot optimization:** Reducing hotspots near cortical bone.
**Related:** fracture risk mitigation.
**Example:** Reduce dose near femoral cortex in pelvic RT.

255. **Junctional dose gradient assessment:** Assessing gradients at field junctions.
**Related:** field matching QA, gradient control.
**Example:** Analyze dose gradients in craniospinal junction.

256. **Junctional tissue verification phantom:** Phantom designed for verifying junction dose accuracy.
**Related:** match-line QA.
**Example:** Use phantom to test field matching.

257. **Justification principle compliance verification:** Checking compliance with justification requirements.
**Related:** ALARA, safety auditing.
**Example:** Audit justification for repeated imaging.

258. **Just-in-time radiation monitoring:** Real-time monitoring of radiation levels.
**Related:** adaptive RT, delivery verification.
**Example:** EPID-based real-time monitoring during treatment.

259. **Juvenile CT phantom calibration:** Calibrating pediatric CT phantoms.
**Related:** HU correction, low-dose calibration.
**Example:** Validate pediatric protocols.

260. **Juvenile MRI QA verification:** QA of MRI systems for pediatric imaging.
**Related:** safety, SAR constraints.
**Example:** Ensure MRI sequence temperature rise limits.

261. **Juvenile PET/CT dose optimization:** Optimizing PET/CT dose for children.
**Related:** ALARA, activity tailoring.
**Example:** Adjust FDG dose per kg.

262. **Juxtaposition effect phantom verification:** Phantom-based verification of interface effects.
**Related:** heterogeneity, dose modeling.
**Example:** Test lung–tumor interface dose.

263. **Juxtaposition artifact QA:** Routine QA of artifacts at tissue interfaces.
**Related:** image QC, algorithm verification.
**Example:** Verify algorithm reduces boundary artifacts.

264. **Juxtaposition dose calibration:** Calibrating dose models for interface regions.
**Related:** MC modeling, heterogeneity corrections.
**Example:** Calibrate model for air–sinus boundary.

265. **J-shaped energy verification:** Verifying energy spectra producing J-shaped profiles.
**Related:** beam quality, spectrum tests.
**Example:** Measure energy distribution at field edge.

266. **J-wave artifact phantom testing:** Phantom testing of ECG J-wave artifact corrections.
**Related:** gating QA, cardiac imaging.
**Example:** Test J-wave suppression filters.

267. **J-coupling phantom calibration:** Calibration using phantoms mimicking J-coupled spins.
**Related:** MRS QA.
**Example:** Calibrate lactate J-coupling model.

268. **J-resolved spectroscopy QA:** Routine QA of J-resolved spectroscopy.
**Related:** peak separation, frequency accuracy.
**Example:** Validate frequency axis integrity.

269. **J-value verification in therapy planning:** Verifying J-value usage in optimization engines.
**Related:** planning system QA.
**Example:** Ensure optimizer uses correct J-value weighting.

270. **J-factor modeling QA:** QA for radiobiological J-factor modeling.
**Related:** radiobiology QA, model validation.
**Example:** Validate J-factor predictions vs cell data.

271. **J-index verification for imaging systems:** Ensuring J-index values reliably reflect image quality.
**Related:** QC metrics, calibration.
**Example:** Validate J-index after CBCT upgrade.

272. **Jagged line correction QA:** QA checking the effectiveness of jagged-line correction algorithms.
**Related:** CT QC, reconstruction tests.
**Example:** Test artifact correction on edge phantom.

273. **Jaw position verification phantom:** Phantom used to verify jaw positioning accuracy.
**Related:** mechanical QA, field metrics.
**Example:** Acquire images of phantom field edges.

274. **Jet beam alignment QA:** Quality assurance for alignment of jet-like beams.
**Related:** microbeam QA.
**Example:** Use EPID for alignment tests.

275. **Jet stream radiation effect monitoring:** Monitoring effects of radiation around jet stream structures.
**Related:** scatter, shielding.
**Example:** Assess scatter near high-energy nozzle.

276. **Jet collimator dose verification phantom:** Phantom for verifying dose from jet collimators.
**Related:** microbeam dosimetry.
**Example:** Film in phantom to measure beam profiles.

277. **Joint imaging QA protocol:** Standard QA protocol for joint imaging.
**Related:** multimodal QC, artifact checks.
**Example:** Annual QA for knee CT accuracy.

278. **Joint phantom dose verification:** Dose verification using joint phantoms.
**Related:** anthropomorphic phantoms.
**Example:** Test dose around knee prosthesis.

279. **Juvenile tissue dosimetry QA:** Routine QA of pediatric dose accuracy.
**Related:** OSL, TLD measurements.
**Example:** Verify pediatric TBI dose uniformity.

280. **Juvenile phantom dose simulation:** Simulating dose in pediatric-equivalent phantoms.
**Related:** Monte Carlo, pediatric modeling.
**Example:** Simulate dose to growth plates.

281. **Justification protocol QA:** QA ensuring justification protocols are followed.
**Related:** ALARA audits.
**Example:** Audit imaging justification logs.

282. **Juxta-articular hotspot calibration:** Calibrating detection of hotspots near joints.
**Related:** extremity RT QA.
**Example:** Validate hotspot detection for ankle RT.

**283. Juxta-luminal dose QA:** Quality assurance of dose around hollow organs.
**Related:** SBRT, OAR constraints.
**Example:** Confirm dose near bowel in liver SBRT.

**284. Junctional tissue therapy verification:** Verifying treatment at tissue junctions.
**Related:** match-line QA.
**Example:** Test field junction for CSI.

**285. Junctional dose phantom calibration:** Calibrating phantoms used for junctional dose tests.
**Related:** phantom QA.
**Example:** Set baseline for junction dose uniformity.

**286. J-wave correction QA:** QA of algorithms correcting J-wave noise.
**Related:** gating QC.
**Example:** Validate correction software.

**287. J-coupled spin system calibration:** Calibration of systems modeling J-coupled spin interactions.
**Related:** MRS calibration.
**Example:** Tune spectral model for J-coupled metabolites.

**288. J-resolved spectroscopy artifact QA:** QA focused on artifact detection in J-resolved spectra.
**Related:** spectral QA.
**Example:** Identify lipid artifacts in MRS.

**289. Jet collimator alignment QA phantom:** Phantom specifically for jet collimator alignment QA.
**Related:** microbeam alignment.
**Example:** Confirm beam centering using alignment phantom.

**290. Jagged edge artifact dose verification:** Verifying the dosimetric impact of jagged-edge imaging artifacts.
**Related:** imaging–dose correlation, artifact analysis.
**Example:** Check if jagged CT edges affect dose calc.

**291. J-shaped dose fall-off:** A steep, asymmetric decline in dose distribution resembling a “J” curve.
**Related:** J-shaped energy spectrum, dose gradient, fall-off modeling.
**RT Example:** Evaluated during stereotactic radiosurgery to ensure healthy tissue sparing.

**292. J-function modeling:** Mathematical modeling using J-functions to represent dose–response curves or energy distribution.
**Related:** J-value, J-factor, dose modeling.
**RT Example:** Used to refine biological modeling of treatment outcomes.

**293. J-index scoring:** Metric that quantifies junction or gradient uniformity in dose distributions.
**Related:** J-index calibration, homogeneity index.
**RT Example:** Applied during junction matching for craniospinal irradiation.

**294. Jagged artifact reduction:** Techniques to remove jagged edges or serrations in reconstructed images.
**Related:** edge smoothing, interpolation algorithms.
RT **Example:** Reduces contour inaccuracies in CT for planning.

**295. Jaw aperture adjustment:** Manual or automated setting of LINAC jaw openings.
**Related:** MLC positioning, jaw tracking.
**RT Example:** Ensures correct field size for 3DCRT.

**296. Jaw interlock:** Safety mechanism preventing beam-on when jaw positions are incorrect.
**Related:** machine interlocks, LINAC safety.
**RT Example:** Prevents unintended oversized fields.

297. **Jet collimation:** Collimation mechanism using high-speed jet-like radiation shaping structures.
**Related:** jet collimator, beam shaping.
**RT Example:** Used in experimental high-flux beam systems.

298. **Jet stream cooling verification:** Validation that high-velocity cooling jets in LINAC systems operate correctly.
**Related:** cryogenic cooling, thermal QA.
**RT Example:** Ensures gantry stability during high-energy treatments.

299. **Joint imaging artifact:** Artifact produced at the interface of two imaging modalities or anatomical joints.
**Related:** fusion artifact, interface artifact.
**RT Example:** Checked during multimodal PET/CT fusion.

300. **Joint MRI fusion:** Combining MRI data sets (e.g., T1 + T2) for enhanced anatomical detail.
**Related:** multimodal fusion, rigid/elastic registration.
**RT Example:** Used to enhance brain tumor target delineation.

301. **Joint PET/CT QA:** Quality assurance for PET and CT acquisition and fusion.
**Related:** fusion QA, SUV accuracy.
**RT Example:** Ensures PET SUV aligns with CT anatomy for contouring.

302. **Juxta-articular hotspot:** A localized high-dose area near a joint.
**Related:** hotspots, periarticular dose.
**RT Example:** Avoided during extremity sarcoma treatment.

303. **Juxta-luminal dose mapping:** Assessment of dose near luminal surfaces (bowel, airway).
**Related:** wall dose, surface mapping.
**RT Example:** Evaluates dose to bowel loops in pelvic treatments.

304. **Juxta-cortical lesion:** Tumor or abnormality located adjacent to cortical bone.
**Related:** periosteal lesions, bone interface.
**RT Example:** Impacts PTV margin selection.

305. **Junctional dose optimization:** Minimizing dose inhomogeneities at field junctions.
**Related:** matchlines, feathering.
**RT Example:** Critical for craniospinal irradiation.

306. **Junctional tissue mapping:** Imaging and dose analysis of tissues at or near beam junctions.
**Related:** dose gradients, match zones.
**RT Example:** Detects mismatch regions before plan approval.

307. **Justification assessment:** Reviewing whether radiation exposure is clinically necessary.
**Related:** ALARA, appropriateness criteria.
**RT Example:** Required before imaging for daily IGRT.

308. **Just-in-time dosimetry:** Real-time or near-real-time dose evaluation during treatment.
**Related:** adaptive radiotherapy, online QA.
**RT Example:** Used in MR-LINAC adaptive workflows.

309. **Juvenile dose adjustment:** Dose modification for pediatric anatomy and sensitivity.
**Related:** pediatric dosimetry, organ tolerance.
**RT Example:** Adjusts constraints for developing tissues.

310. **Juvenile MRI protocol:** MRI sequences optimized for pediatric patients.
**Related:** pediatric imaging, sedation minimization.
**RT Example:** Used for soft-tissue sarcoma staging.

311. **Juvenile PET protocol:** PET scan parameters tailored for children.
**Related:** low-dose protocols, pediatric SUV.
**RT Example:** Used for Hodgkin lymphoma staging.

312. **Juvenile SPECT calibration:** Calibration of SPECT systems using pediatric phantoms.
**Related:** pediatric imaging QA.
**RT Example:** Ensures dose accuracy in thyroid uptake studies.

313. **Juxtaposition effect:** Artifact caused by abrupt tissue or modality transitions.
**Related:** interface artifacts.
**RT Example:** Seen at bone–soft tissue boundaries on CT.

314. **Juxtaposition phantom:** Phantom simulating abrupt interface transitions.
**Related:** interface phantom.
**RT Example:** Used to test reconstruction algorithms.

315. **J-shaped energy spectrum:** Energy distribution curve with low-energy drop-off and high-energy tail.
**Related:** beam spectrum, energy verification.
**RT Example:** Analyzed for linac beam characterization.

316. **J-wave ECG artifact:** ECG artifact with prominent J-wave affecting gated imaging.
**Related:** cardiac gating, motion artifact.
**RT Example:** Impacts 4D CT respiratory–cardiac gating.

317. **J-coupled spin system:** Spin systems displaying J-coupling interactions in MR spectroscopy.
**Related:** J-resolved spectroscopy.
**RT Example:** Used to distinguish metabolites in brain RT planning.

318. **J-resolved spectroscopy:** Spectroscopy separating chemical shifts and J-coupling.
**Related:** MRS, 2D spectroscopy.
**RT Example:** Helps evaluate tumor metabolism.

319. **J-value calibration:** Calibration using J-dependent parameters in imaging or modeling.
**Related:** J-function, J-index.
**RT Example:** Applied in MR spectroscopy QA.

320. **J-factor in radiobiology:** A parameter quantifying biological response or radiosensitivity.
**Related:** $\alpha/\beta$ ratio, survival modeling.
**RT Example:** Incorporated into LQ-based modeling.

321. **Jagged line correction:** Algorithms to smooth jagged edges or pixelated boundaries.
**Related:** artifact suppression.
**RT Example:** Improves contour precision on CT.

322. **Jaw motion correction:** Adjusting for dynamic jaw motion errors.
**Related:** jaw tracking, MLC–jaw coordination.
**RT Example:** Ensures consistent field edges in VMAT.

323. **Jet beam alignment:** Alignment of beams generated or shaped by jet-like collimation systems.
**Related:** jet collimator, beam steering.
**RT Example:** Used in high-flux research beams.

324. **Jet stream radiation monitoring:** Monitoring radiation carried within or affecting high-velocity streams.
**Related:** airborne radiation, monitoring QA.
**RT Example:** Applied in experimental gantry cooling systems.

**325. Jet collimator QA:** Quality assurance of jet-type collimation devices.
**Related:** collimator calibration, beam shape QA.
**RT Example:** Ensures uniform beam shaping.

**326. Joint density verification:** Checking density consistency at anatomical joints in imaging.
**Related:** CT number uniformity.
**RT Example:** Ensures accurate bone–soft tissue modeling.

**327. Joint imaging optimization:** Enhancing imaging across joint regions.
**Related:** artifact reduction, multimodal enhancement.
**RT Example:** Improves contouring of extremity tumors.

**328. Juvenile phantom imaging:** Imaging pediatric-simulated phantoms for QA.
**Related:** pediatric dosimetry QA.
**RT Example:** Used during protocol commissioning.

**329. Juvenile tissue dosimetry:** Dose calculations specific to developing tissues.
**Related:** pediatric tolerance.
**RT Example:** Sets dose limits for brainstem in pediatric RT.

**330. Justification protocol:** Documented procedure for evaluating necessity of radiation use.
**Related:** ALARA policies.
**RT Example:** Required for CBCT imaging frequency.

**331. Juxta-articular therapy planning:** Planning treatment near major joints.
**Related:** joint constraint modeling.
**RT Example:** Important for knee/hip sarcomas.

**332. Juxta-luminal dose verification:** Confirming dose accuracy near mucosal surfaces.
**Related:** wall dose, endoluminal dose.
**RT Example:** Essential for esophageal cancer RT.

**333. Junctional tissue therapy QA:** QA for tissues within junction zones between fields.
**Related:** matchline QA.
**RT Example:** Used in multi-isocenter spinal plans.

**334. Junctional dose phantom:** Phantom simulating dose gradients at field junctions.
**Related:** junction phantom QA.
**RT Example:** Used for CSI commissioning.

**335. J-wave correction:** Correction of imaging errors due to J-wave ECG anomalies.
**Related:** cardiac gating correction.
**RT Example:** Improves 4D CT synchronization.

**336. J-coupled spin calibration:** Calibration of MRS systems for J-coupled interactions.
**Related:** MRS QA.
**RT Example:** Enhances metabolic imaging reliability.

**337. J-resolved spectroscopy QA:** QA for J-resolved MR spectroscopy sequences.
**Related:** MRS QC.
**RT Example:** Ensures metabolite peak accuracy.

**338. Jet collimator alignment phantom:** Phantom designed to align and test jet-type collimators.
**Related:** jet collimation QA.
**RT Example:** Used in experimental high-energy systems.

339. **Jagged edge dose verification:** Checking dose distortions caused by jagged edges in images.
**Related:** artifact QA.
**RT Example:** Ensures contour-based dose is accurate.

340. **J-shaped dose-response modelling:** Modeling dose-response curves with J-shaped profiles.
**Related:** sigmoidal models, radiobiological modeling.
**RT Example:** Used in low-dose toxicity studies.

341. **J-shaped intensity distribution:** Beam intensity distribution showing a J-like shape.
**Related:** intensity profiles.
**RT Example:** Evaluated in specialized beam shaping systems.

342. **J-function assessment:** Assessing J-function behavior in models or imaging systems.
**Related:** J-modeling.
**RT Example:** Used in biological modeling QA.

343. **J-index scoring verification:** Confirming the accuracy of J-index scoring computations.
**Related:** J-index QA.
**RT Example:** Required for junction uniformity QA.

344. **Jagged artifact elimination:** Removal of serrated reconstruction artifacts.
**Related:** smoothing, antialiasing.
**RT Example:** Removes contour errors in treatment planning.

345. **Jaw alignment phantom:** Phantom for testing jaw centering and consistency.
**Related:** jaw QA.
**RT Example:** Used in annual LINAC QA.

346. **Jaw shielding QA:** Verifying that jaws correctly shield non-target regions.
**Related:** leakage, jaw transmission.
**RT Example:** Prevents unintended dose to OARs.

347. **Jet collimator dose alignment:** Ensuring dose output aligns with jet collimator geometry.
**Related:** alignment QA.
**RT Example:** Used in experimental systems.

348. **Jet stream cooling assessment:** Evaluating performance of cooling jets in LINAC systems.
**Related:** thermal QA.
**RT Example:** Prevents overheating during long treatments.

349. **Joint CT registration verification:** Verification of CT–CT or multi-phase CT registration.
**Related:** rigid/elastic registration.
**RT Example:** Ensures accurate ITV generation.

350. **Joint MRI alignment QA:** Quality assurance of MRI–MRI alignment or fusion.
**Related:** MRI fusion QA.
**RT Example:** Improves soft-tissue target.

351. **Joint PET image fusion QA:** QA to ensure PET–PET or PET–CT fusion accuracy.
**Related:** fusion QA.
**RT Example:** Ensures correct SUV-to-anatomy matching.

352. **Juxta-articular lesion QA:** Verifying imaging and dose accuracy near joints.
**Related:** joint planning QA.
**RT Example:** Used for knee sarcoma RT.

353. **Juxta-luminal therapy QA:** QA for treatments near luminal surfaces.
**Related:** mucosal structures, near-wall dose.
**RT Example:** For rectal or esophageal RT.

354. **Juxta-cortical dose verification:** Verifying dose near cortical bone boundaries.
**Related:** bone interface dose.
**RT Example:** Important for bone sarcoma RT.

355. **Junctional hotspot mapping:** Identifying hotspots at junction regions.
**Related:** feathering, junction QA.
**RT Example:** Essential for multi-field spine RT.

356. **Junctional tissue QA:** Quality assurance for tissues affected by dose junctions.
**Related:** junction modeling.
**RT Example:** Used before plan approval.

357. **Justification assessment protocol:** Protocol defining steps for evaluating radiation necessity.
**Related:** ALARA.
**RT Example:** Required in imaging stewardship programs.

358. **Just-in-time dose assessment:** Dose evaluation immediately prior to or during treatment.
**Related:** real-time dosimetry.
**RT Example:** MR-LINAC adaptive workflows.

359. **Juvenile CT dose verification:** Checking CT dose levels for pediatric patients.
**Related:** pediatric CT QA.
**RT Example:** Ensures minimal imaging exposure.

360. **Juvenile MRI QA verification:** QA for pediatric MRI protocols.
**Related:** pediatric imaging QA.
**RT Example:** Used for brain tumor imaging.

361. **Juvenile PET protocol QA:** Quality assurance for pediatric PET protocols.
**Related:** SUV calibration.
**RT Example:** Ensures consistency for lymphoma cases.

362. **Juvenile SPECT imaging QA:** QA for pediatric SPECT image quality and dose.
**Related:** pediatric nuclear medicine QA.
**RT Example:** Ensures accuracy for thyroid imaging.

363. **Juxtaposition effect QA:** QA for artifacts caused by tissue or modality transitions.
**Related:** interface QA.
**RT Example:** Reduces contouring errors.

364. **Juxtaposition phantom verification:** Verifying phantom performance simulating interface changes.
**Related:** interface phantom QA.
**RT Example:** Used in reconstruction QA.

365. **J-shaped energy verification:** Confirming measured energy spectra match J-shaped models.
**Related:** energy QA.
**RT Example:** For non-standard beam commissioning.

366. **J-wave artifact QA:** QA for effects of J-wave ECG artifacts on gating systems.
**Related:** cardiac gating QA.
**RT Example:** Improves 4D CT quality.

367. **J-coupled spectroscopy QA:** QA for J-coupled MR spectroscopy sequences.
**Related:** MRS QA.
**RT Example:** Ensures reliable metabolite readings.

368. **J-resolved MR spectroscopy QA:**QA for 2D J-resolved MRS.
**Related:** spectroscopy QA.
**RT Example:** Used in brain tumor metabolic analysis.

369. **J-value verification phantom:** Phantom designed to verify J-dependent parameters.
**Related:** MRS phantom.
**RT Example:** Used for MRS commissioning.

370. **J-factor assessment QA:** QA verifying J-factor models in radiobiological calculations.
**Related:** radiobiology QA.
**RT Example:** Ensures accurate biologically effective dose.

371. **Jagged line verification:** QA confirming smoothing or correction of jagged image lines.
**Related:** artifact QA.
**RT Example:** Ensures clean contour edges.

372. **Jaw motion QA:** Testing jaw movement accuracy and reproducibility.
**Related:** mechanical QA.
**RT Example:** Required for dynamic fields.

373. **Jet beam alignment QA phantom:** Phantom used to test jet-beam alignment.
**Related:** jet collimator QA.
**RT Example:** Used in experimental systems.

374. **Jet stream monitoring QA:** Monitoring high-velocity jet systems for stability.
**Related:** cooling QA.
**RT Example:** Ensures LINAC thermal safety.

375. **Jet collimator verification phantom:** Phantom designed to evaluate jet collimator performance.
**Related:** collimator QA.
**RT Example:** For beam-shaping experiments.

376. **Joint density QA:** Assessing density accuracy in joint imaging.
**Related:** CT QA.
**RT Example:** Ensures correct bone dose modeling.

377. **Joint imaging QA phantom:** Phantom simulating joint anatomy for imaging QA.
**Related:** orthopedic imaging QA.
**RT Example:** Used for extremity RT planning.

378. **Juvenile phantom dose verification:** Dose verification using pediatric phantoms.
**Related:** pediatric dosimetry.
**RT Example:** Commissioning for peds protocols.

379. **Juvenile tissue mapping QA:** QA for mapping pediatric tissue characteristics.
**Related:** pediatric anatomy QA.
**RT Example:** Adjusts organ-at-risk tolerances.

380. **Justification protocol verification:** Ensuring justification protocols are followed.
**Related:** ALARA compliance.
**RT Example:** Checked during IGRT audits.

**381. Juxta-articular dose QA:** QA of dose near joints.
**Related:** joint dose modeling.
**RT Example:** Ensures cartilage sparing.

**382. Juxta-luminal hotspot QA:** QA for hotspots near luminal structures.
**Related:** hotspot verification.
**RT Example:** Essential for rectal and esophageal RT.

**383. Junctional therapy QA:** phantom: Phantom used for QA of junctional therapy regions.
**Related:** junction QA.
**RT Example:** Used in CSI midline matching.

**384. Junctional dose verification phantom:** Phantom for verifying dose at field junctions.
**Related:** dose gradient phantom.
**RT Example:** Used for multi-isocenter spine plans.

**385. J-wave artifact correction QA:** QA for correction algorithms addressing J-wave ECG issues.
**Related:** gating QA.
**RT Example:** Ensures accurate 4D CT gating.

**386. J-coupled spin system QA:** QA for systems analyzing J-coupled spin phenomena.
**Related:** spectroscopy QA.
T **Example:** Ensures metabolite peak fidelity.

**387. J-resolved spectroscopy QA verification:** Verification of J-resolved spectroscopy QA results.
**Related:** MRS QA.
**RT Example:** Double-checks commissioning results.

**388. Jet collimator QA phantom:** Phantom evaluating jet collimator structure and output.
**Related:** collimator QA.
**RT Example:** Stability testing for research systems.

**389. Jagged edge dose verification QA:** QA specifically for dose effects caused by jagged edges in images.
**Related:** artifact QA.
**RT Example:** Prevents contour-induced dose errors.

**390. J-shaped dose-response QA:** QA verifying models predicting J-shaped dose responses.
**Related:** radiobiological QA.
**RT Example:** Used in low-dose toxicity modeling validation.

**391. J-shaped dose profile phantom:** A specialized QA phantom designed to reproduce a beam profile with a J-shaped fall-off, allowing physicists to evaluate asymmetric penumbra behavior, irregular beam edges, and non-linear dose gradients.
**Related:** dose profile QA, penumbra modeling, asymmetric beam verification
**Example:** Used during linac commissioning to validate measured beam flatness and symmetry against expected J-shaped profiles in off-axis fields.

**392. J-function QA protocol:** A protocol that validates the mathematical J-function used in modeling dose distributions, ensuring the accuracy of analytic dose-calculation components within TPS algorithms.
**Related:** dose modeling, TPS validation, algorithm QA
**Example:** Applied when commissioning a new TPS release to confirm correct implementation of J-function-based scatter modeling.

393. **J-index dose assessment:** A QA method using a J-index (a metric describing asymmetry or curvature in a dose gradient) to evaluate subtle dose-distribution deviations that conventional gamma analysis may miss.
**Related:** dose gradient metrics, gamma analysis alternatives
**Example:** Identifies under-recognized hotspots in IMRT plans near organ boundaries.

394. **Jagged artifact phantom:** A phantom engineered to simulate jagged or stair-step artifacts that arise from reconstruction errors, detector defects, or low-resolution sampling.
**Related:** artifact QA, CT reconstruction testing
**Example:** Physicists scan the phantom to ensure iterative reconstruction algorithms successfully smooth artificial jagged borders.

395. **Jaw aperture calibration:** Calibration procedure verifying that linac jaws open and close precisely to commanded positions, ensuring field size accuracy and proper shielding.
**Related:** jaw positioning, field-size QA
**Example:** Performed monthly to ensure a 10×10 cm field is within ±1 mm tolerance.

396. **Jaw interlock QA:** QA testing that verifies safety interlocks preventing unsafe jaw positions or collisions are functioning correctly.
**Related:** mechanical interlocks, failsafe systems
**Example:** Ensures the machine inhibits beam-on if jaws are misaligned beyond safe limits.

397. **Jet collimation phantom:** A phantom used to test high-velocity jet-style collimation systems (e.g., dynamic micro-collimators) that shape beams using rapidly moving apertures.
**Related:** dynamic collimation, micro-MLC QA
**Example:** Measures whether jet-like aperture shaping achieves the intended sub-millimeter beam boundaries.

398. **Jet stream cooling phantom:** Phantom used to evaluate cooling-air or coolant-stream flow patterns inside linac components to detect thermal hotspots affecting beam stability.
**Related:** thermal QA, cooling system monitoring
**Example:** Identifies improper coolant flow that could lead to gantry-head overheating and beam drift.

399. **Joint CT QA:** QA procedures verifying CT imaging when multiple anatomical joints are involved, ensuring accurate geometry, HU calibration, and artifact minimization.
**Related:** CT image quality, multi-region imaging QA
**Example:** Validates CT accuracy when planning RT for extremities with complex joint surfaces.

400. **Joint MRI phantom:** Phantom shaped to mimic joint anatomy (e.g., knee or shoulder) for evaluating MRI contrast uniformity, SNR, coil performance, and geometric fidelity.
**Related:** MR coil QA, geometric distortion testing
**Example:** Used to confirm distortion-free MRI for joint-related sarcoma planning.

401. **Joint PET QA:** QA verifying PET image accuracy in regions involving multiple adjacent joints where scatter and attenuation vary significantly.
**Related:** PET uniformity, scatter correction QA
**Example:** Ensures SUVs remain accurate when imaging PET-avid lesions near elbows or knees.

402. **Juxta-articular hotspot QA phantom:** Phantom simulating hotspots near joint surfaces to test PET/CT, SPECT/CT, or dose-calculation system accuracy in juxta-articular regions.
**Related:** hotspot QA, joint imaging validation
**Example:** Used to evaluate how scatter correction handles high-uptake regions near bone interfaces.

**403. Juxta-luminal dose QA:** QA that verifies dose accuracy near luminal structures (air cavities, GI tract, bronchial tree) where large density differences may distort dose models.
**Related:** heterogeneity correction, cavity dose modeling
**Example:** Ensures TPS accuracy for bronchi-adjacent lung tumors.

**404. Juxta-cortical lesion QA:** QA verifying imaging accuracy and dose calculation for lesions directly adjacent to cortical bone, where scatter and attenuation gradients are steep.
**Related:** bone-interface dosimetry, cortical corrections
**Example:** Confirms accurate dose predictions for skull-adjacent metastases.

**405. Junctional dose QA phantom:** Phantom designed to test junction-dose behavior when multiple radiation fields meet (e.g., craniospinal junctions), preventing hotspots or cold spots.
**Related:** field matching, multi-field coordination
**Example:** Used during CSI to ensure spinal and cranial fields merge with <5% dose mismatch.

**406. Junctional tissue mapping QA phantom:** Phantom replicating tissues across treatment junctions for QA of heterogeneity, scatter, and alignment accuracy.
**Related:** junction modeling, tissue-equivalent phantoms
**Example:** Verifies dose continuity in multi-isocenter plans.

**407. Justification principle QA verification:** QA verifying that each imaging or treatment step adheres to the justification principle—ensuring radiation exposure is clinically warranted.
**Related:** radiation protection, ALARA auditing
**Example:** Confirming pediatric imaging protocols document formal justification.

**408. Just-in-time dose QA:** Real-time or near-real-time QA performed immediately before treatment delivery to catch setup or dose deviations proactively.
**Related:** adaptive QA, pre-treatment verification
**Example:** Automated EPID-based checks moments before beam-on.

**409. Juvenile CT QA phantom**Phantom simulating pediatric anatomy to validate CT dose, HU accuracy, resolution, and pediatric-specific protocols.
**Related:** pediatric dosimetry, CT protocol QA
**Example:** Ensures CT dose index (CTDI) is within safe range for children.

**410. Juvenile MRI QA phantom** Pediatric MRI phantom used to verify SNR, contrast uniformity, artifact performance, and coil suitability for children.
**Related:** MRI pediatric QA, coil testing
**Example:** Required for MRI-guided RT in pediatric brain tumor cases.

**411. Juvenile PET QA phantom** PET phantom calibrated for pediatric organ sizes and uptake ranges.
**Related:** pediatric SUV QA, small-volume resolution
**Example:** QA ensuring accurate SUVs for small PET-avid nodes in children.

**412. Juvenile SPECT QA phantom** Pediatric SPECT calibration phantom to validate resolution, uniformity, and sensitivity for small organ volumes.
**Related:** small-volume imaging QA
**Example:** Used to calibrate SPECT-based dosimetry for pediatric thyroid therapy.
QA verifying accuracy where two very different tissue types or dose regions meet in close proximity, such as soft-tissue/bone interfaces.
**Related:** heterogeneity interfaces, dose gradient QA
**Example:** Ensures dose accuracy across sinus cavity boundaries.

413. **Juxtaposition phantom QA:** Phantom specifically designed to present stark material contrasts (air vs bone vs soft tissue) to test TPS heterogeneity corrections.
**Related:** interface phantoms, heterogeneity dose QA
**Example:** Used during TPS commissioning.

414. **J-shaped energy QA:** QA verifying that the measured energy spectrum exhibiting a J-shaped characteristic matches expected beam-energy models.
**Related:** energy spectrum validation
**Example:** Ensures consistent energy behavior in FFF beams.

415. **J-wave ECG artifact QA phantom:** Phantom producing ECG-like signals with J-wave artifacts to test motion-gated RT systems.
**Related:** gating QA, motion synchronization
**Example:** Ensures respiratory gating is not mis-triggered by ECG anomalies.

416. **J-coupled spin system QA phantom:** Phantom containing materials with known nuclear spin-spin coupling constants to test MR spectroscopy accuracy.
**Related:** MRS QA, J-coupling calibration
**Example:** Ensures brain spectroscopy used for RT planning produces correct metabolite peaks.

417. **J-resolved spectroscopy QA phantom:** Phantom for validating 2D J-resolved MR spectroscopy sequences.
**Related:** advanced MRS QA, spectral resolution
**Example:** Used in glioma metabolic planning workflows.

418. **J-value QA verification:** QA confirming the correctness of J-value metrics used in dose-response or biological modeling.
**Related:** radiobiological modeling QA
**Example:** Ensures tumor-control modeling parameters are not miscalculated.

419. **J-factor QA verification** QA checking the J-factor, a biological scaling parameter influencing modeling of cell survival curves.
**Related:** radiobiology QA
**Example:** Necessary when switching radiobiological models in the TPS.

420. **Jagged line QA phantom:** Phantom for testing jagged-edge artifacts in imaging or dose maps.
**Related:** edge resolution QA
**Example:** Identifies reconstruction errors at beam boundaries.

421. **Jaw motion QA phantom:** Phantom evaluating jaw speed, smoothness, and accuracy during dynamic treatments (e.g., Jaw-tracking IMRT).
**Related:** dynamic jaw QA
**Example:** Ensures jaws follow the planned trajectory within <1 mm deviation.

422. **Jet beam QA phantom** Phantom for testing beams shaped by high-velocity dynamic collimators (jet beams).
**Related:** micro-beam QA, dynamic collimation
**Example:** Verifies micro-beam edges in experimental preclinical RT.

423. **Jet stream radiation QA phantom:** Phantom measuring radiation output from cooling-stream or airflow-dependent beamlines.
**Related:** thermal stability QA
**Example:** Used when airflow affects beam reproducibility.

**424. Jet collimator alignment QA phantom:** Phantom ensuring precision alignment of jet-style or rapid-modulating collimators.
**Related:** collimator precision QA
**Example:** Ensures micro-collimators line up with imaging isocenter.

**425. Joint imaging QA phantom:** Phantom for verifying multimodal imaging (CT-MRI-PET) alignment across joint structures.
**Related:** multi-modality fusion QA
**Example:** Required for joint sarcoma RT planning.

**426. Joint phantom dose QA:** Dose QA performed using anatomically realistic joint phantoms to evaluate dose accuracy in regions of complex bone geometry.
**Related:** extremity dosimetry, heterogeneity QA
**Example:** Ensures dose accuracy for ankle or wrist tumors.

**427. Juvenile tissue dosimetry QA phantom:** Pediatric-equivalent dosimetry phantom used to verify dose distributions in small or sensitive anatomical regions.
**Related:** pediatric dose QA
**Example:** Used for proton therapy QA in pediatric cranial cases.

**428. Juvenile phantom imaging QA:** Imaging QA applied to pediatric phantoms to evaluate resolution, noise, and dose-appropriate protocols.
**Related:** pediatric imaging QA
**Example:** CT protocol optimization for reduced dose.

**429. Justification protocol QA phantom:** Phantom used to validate protocols built on the justification principle by demonstrating dose vs diagnostic benefit balance.
**Related:** justification auditing
**Example:** Used in departmental audits for pediatric CT justification.

**430. Juxta-articular therapy QA phantom:** A phantom replicating bone–soft-tissue interfaces around joints to validate dose accuracy for treatments near articular surfaces, where scatter gradients are complex.
**Related:** joint interface dosimetry, bone-adjacent QA
**Example:** Used in IMRT QA for knee-adjacent sarcoma treatment.

**431. Juxta-luminal dose QA phantom:** Phantom simulating luminal structures (air cavities, GI tract, bronchi) to test dose calculations near hollow organs where electronic disequilibrium occurs.
**Related:** cavity-dose modeling, heterogeneity QA
**Example:** Ensures TPS accuracy for lung tumors near airway walls.

**432. Junctional tissue therapy QA phantom:** Phantom designed to validate dose uniformity across multi-isocenter treatment junctions, replicating dissimilar tissues merging across the junction.
**Related:** field matching QA, junction optimization
**Example:** Used for craniospinal irradiation junction management.

**433. Junctional dose phantom QA:** QA ensuring the phantom-derived measured junction dose matches TPS predictions, verifying no gaps or overlaps exist in junctional regions.
**Related:** dose continuity QA
**Example:** Detects dose dips at the thoracic–lumbar junction in CSI.

434. **J-wave correction QA phantom:** Simulated ECG output containing J-wave abnormalities to test the ability of gating systems to ignore cardiac waveform distortions during respiratory-synchronized treatments.
**Related:** ECG gating QA, artifact rejection
**Example:** Ensures gating windows are not falsely triggered.

435. **J-coupled spin calibration QA phantom:** Phantom containing chemical compounds with known spin–spin J-coupling constants for calibrating MR spectroscopy frequency-splitting accuracy.
**Related:** MRS calibration, spectral fidelity
**Example:** Validates the accuracy of metabolite quantification in brain-tumor planning.

436. **J-resolved spectroscopy QA verification phantom:** Phantom used for secondary verification of 2D J-resolved MR spectroscopy sequences, ensuring correct separation of J-coupled metabolites.
**Related:** advanced MRS QA, spectral resolution
**Example:** Required when implementing high-resolution J-resolved protocols in neuro-oncology RT.

437. **Jet collimator alignment QA verification phantom:** Provides secondary confirmation of jet-collimator alignment through high-precision fiducials and micro-aperture measurement channels.
**Related:** dynamic-beam QA, micro-collimation
**Example:** Ensures ultra-small beams remain aligned for stereotactic treatments.

438. **Jagged edge dose QA phantom:** Phantom engineered to test the dosimetric effects of jagged or irregular beam edges, ensuring accurate modeling of complex MLC shapes.
**Related:** edge-smoothness QA, MLC leaf modeling
**Example:** Used when evaluating small-field IMRT leaf patterns.

439. **J-shaped dose-response QA phantom:** Phantom validating biological or physical dose-response curves exhibiting J-shaped behavior, often used in high-dose or hyper-radiosensitivity studies.
**Related:** dose-response modeling, radiobiology QA
**Example:** Assesses high-dose fall-off accuracy for TBI or FLASH RT.

440. **J-shaped intensity distribution QA:** QA confirming that measured beam intensity exhibiting a J-shaped profile matches expected distribution models, particularly in off-axis or modified beams.
**Related:** beam profiling, intensity QA
**Example:** Required for asymmetric collimator configurations.

441. **J-function dose modelling:** Use of J-function mathematics to model dose distributions or scatter kernels in treatment-planning systems.
**Related:** analytic dose modeling, kernel-based algorithms
**Example:** TPS commissioning checks ensure the J-function implementation yields accurate depth-dose predictions.

442. **J-index image QA:** QA using the J-index to quantify image asymmetry, edge irregularities, or pixel-intensity distortions relevant to radiotherapy planning images.
**Related:** image uniformity QA, artifact scoring
**Example:** Detects subtle CT edge distortions around implants.

443. **Jagged artifact elimination QA:** Testing the success of artifact-reduction algorithms designed to remove jagged or stair-step artifacts from CT/MRI reconstruction.
**Related:** artifact correction QA, reconstruction algorithms
**Example:** Applied during iterative reconstruction validation for head-and-neck imaging.

444. **Jaw alignment phantom QA:** QA phantom evaluating static and dynamic jaw alignment, verifying jaw position relative to imaging and radiation isocenter.
**Related:** mechanical QA, field-size verification
**Example:** Ensures jaw tracking remains accurate in VMAT fields.

445. **Jaw shielding phantom:** Phantom used to measure leakage and shielding effectiveness of linac jaws, especially at small field sizes.
**Related:** leakage QA, shielding validation
**Example:** Confirms compliance with leakage limits during stereotactic treatments.

446. **Jet collimator dose verification phantom:** Phantom allowing measurement of dose from jet-style collimators to verify beam-shaping accuracy at extremely small scales.
**Related:** micro-beam dosimetry, dynamic collimation
**Example:** Used in experimental microbeam radiation trials.

447. **Jet stream cooling verification QA:** QA verifying consistency and stability of cooling airflow or coolant streams, which affect gantry temperature and beam output.
**Related:** thermal QA, machine stability checks
**Example:** Identifies cooling anomalies affecting output drift.

448. **Joint CT registration QA:** QA verifying that CT images from different positions or phases align accurately across joint regions with complex anatomy.
**Related:** image fusion QA, deformable registration QA
**Example:** Ensures knee CT aligns correctly for extremity RT planning.

449. **Joint MRI alignment phantom QA:** Phantom evaluating MRI alignment accuracy for joint structures, checking distortion, coil uniformity, and geometric fidelity.
**Related:** MR distortion QA, coil QA
**Example:** Validates MRI geometric accuracy for hip sarcoma cases.

450. **Joint PET image fusion QA phantom:** Phantom designed to validate PET–CT image fusion accuracy around joints where bone/soft tissue boundaries complicate alignment.
**Related:** multi-modality fusion QA
**Example:** Ensures precise fusion for PET-avid elbow lesions.

451. **Juxta-articular lesion QA phantom:** Phantom containing bone-soft tissue structures to test imaging and dose accuracy for lesions adjacent to joints.
**Related:** extremity imaging QA
**Example:** Used for IMRT plan QA for tumors near the ankle joint.

452. **Juxta-luminal therapy QA phantom:** Phantom replicating hollow-organ geometry to validate dose delivery to targets adjacent to luminal structures.
**Related:** heterogeneity QA, cavity interface QA
**Example:** Ensures correct dose deposition near bronchi.

453. **Juxta-cortical dose verification phantom:** Phantom modeling cortical bone with adjacent soft tissue to test dose calculation accuracy in bone-adjacent regions.
**Related:** bone-interface dosimetry
**Example:** Used in stereotactic skull-base RT QA.

454. **Junctional hotspot mapping QA:** QA procedure mapping potential hotspots at field junctions, often using high-resolution film or EPID-based analysis.
**Related:** junction management, hotspot detection
**Example:** Ensures spinal junction hotspots remain under tolerance.

**455. Junctional tissue QA phantom:** Phantom for verifying tissue-equivalent responses across treatment junctions, ensuring dose continuity.
**Related:** heterogeneity phantoms, field matching
**Example:** Used in multi-isocenter breast irradiation QA.

**456. Justification assessment protocol QA:** QA verifying that justification documentation and clinical decision pathways meet regulatory standards.
**Related:** radiation-protection auditing
**Example:** Ensures pediatric CT requests contain mandatory justification notes.

**457. Just-in-time dose assessment QA:** QA checking immediate (pre-delivery) dose calculations or measurements to catch errors before beam-on.
**Related:** adaptive QA, pre-treatment verification
**Example:** EPID-based IMRT QA seconds before treatment.

**458. Juvenile CT dose verification QA:** QA ensuring CT dose indices used for children remain within safe thresholds and protocol-specific ranges.
**Related:** pediatric CT optimization
**Example:** Ensures CTDIvol stays below pediatric dose limits.

**459. Juvenile MRI QA verification phantom:** Phantom used for secondary verification of pediatric MRI quality, focusing on SNR, geometric accuracy, and artifact detection.
**Related:** pediatric MRI QA
**Example:** Ensures distortion-free MRI for pediatric brain RT.

**460. Juvenile PET protocol QA phantom:** Phantom used to validate PET protocols tuned for pediatric metabolism and small-organ imaging.
**Related:** pediatric SUV QA
**Example:** Confirms accuracy of low-dose PET protocols.

**461. Juvenile SPECT imaging QA phantom:** Pediatric-size SPECT phantom verifying resolution, sensitivity, and uniformity for small anatomical volumes.
**Related:** pediatric nuclear medicine QA
**Example:** Calibrates SPECT dosimetry for pediatric neuroblastoma.

**462. Juxtaposition effect QA phantom:** Phantom testing imaging and dose accuracy across abrupt material boundaries where juxtaposition artifacts may arise.
**Related:** interface QA, heterogeneity effects
**Example:** Tests bone–air interface modeling in head and neck planning.

**463. Juxtaposition phantom dose QA:** Dose QA verifying that TPS algorithms accurately model dose deposition in juxtaposition phantom geometries.
**Related:** heterogeneity QA
**Example:** Used during commissioning for interface correction accuracy.

**464. J-shaped energy verification phantom:** Phantom designed to measure and verify the J-shaped energy spectrum expected from certain modified or filtered beams.
**Related:** spectral QA
**Example:** Ensures FFF beam spectrum remains stable.

**465. J-wave artifact QA verification phantom:** Phantom confirming gating systems properly handle ECG waveforms containing J-wave variants without mistiming.
**Related:** cardiorespiratory gating QA
**Example:** Ensures gating accuracy during thoracic RT.

466. **J-coupled spectroscopy QA verification phantom:** Secondary verification phantom confirming correct J-coupling representation in spectroscopy sequences.
**Related:** MRS QA
**Example:** Used when upgrading MRI software.

467. **J-resolved MR spectroscopy QA phantom:** Phantom evaluating high-resolution J-resolved MR spectroscopy for metabolic RT planning.
**Related:** advanced MRS QA
**Example:** Ensures precise separation of metabolites for glioma RT.

468. **J-value verification QA phantom:** Phantom verifying J-value-based biological modeling outputs used in dose-response predictions.
**Related:** radiobiology QA
**Example:** Confirms J-value predictions for high-dose radiotherapy.

469. **J-factor assessment QA phantom:** Phantom supporting QA of J-factor parameters in radiobiological models for cell-survival estimation.
**Related:** survival curve modeling
**Example:** Used in proton therapy RBE modeling QA.

470. **Jagged line verification QA phantom:** Phantom used to detect jagged line reconstruction errors in CT/MRI or dose maps.
**Related:** edge resolution QA
**Example:** Detects voxelization artifacts in TPS rendering.

471. **Jaw motion QA verification phantom:** Phantom enabling high-speed verification of dynamic jaw motion accuracy.
**Related:** dynamic jaw QA
**Example:** Ensures jaw tracking accuracy during high-speed VMAT arcs.

472. **Jet beam alignment QA verification phantom:** Phantom confirming alignment precision for experimentally fast-modulated jet beams.
**Related:** micro-beam QA
**Example:** Ensures micron-level alignment for research small-field RT.

473. **Jet stream monitoring QA verification phantom:** Phantom for verifying long-term monitoring accuracy of airflow- or coolant-stream-dependent beam stability.
**Related:** thermal QA, machine stability
**Example:** Detects latent cooling degradation affecting beam output.

474. **Jet collimator verification QA phantom:** Phantom confirming micro-collimator performance, alignment, and transmission characteristics.
**Related:** collimator QA
**Example:** Used in QA of stereotactic delivery systems.

475. **Joint density QA verification phantom:** Phantom verifying imaging density accuracy in regions with abrupt transitions (bone → cartilage → soft tissue).
**Related:** HU accuracy QA, density mapping
**Example:** Important for extremity RT planning accuracy.

476. **Joint imaging QA verification phantom:** Multi-modality phantom verifying CT, MRI, and PET accuracy in joint regions with complex geometry.
**Related:** fusion QA, anatomical distortion QA
**Example:** Ensures MRI–CT fusion accuracy for ankle sarcoma.

477. **Juvenile phantom dose verification QA:** Pediatric-equivalent phantom used to verify dose calculations and delivery accuracy for child-sized anatomy.
**Related:** pediatric dosimetry QA
**Example:** Used for verifying proton therapy dose in children.

478. **Juvenile tissue mapping QA phantom:** Phantom designed to test the accuracy of tissue segmentation, density mapping, and contour propagation in pediatric imaging.
**Related:** segmentation QA, pediatric imaging
**Example:** Ensures accurate organ-at-risk delineation.

479. **Justification protocol verification QA:** QA process ensuring compliance and documentation for radiation-exposure justification protocols.
**Related:** ALARA compliance
**Example:** Mandatory in pediatric radiology audits.

480. **Juxta-articular dose QA verification phantom:** Phantom confirming dose accuracy for treatments near joint surfaces.
**Related:** extremity dosimetry
**Example:** Used in VMAT QA for elbow lesions.

481. **Juxta-luminal hotspot QA verification phantom:** Phantom evaluating hotspot behavior adjacent to luminal structures where density gradients cause dose perturbations.
**Related:** hotspot QA
**Example:** Verifies dose near esophageal walls in lung RT.

482. **Junctional therapy QA verification phantom:** Phantom verifying dose uniformity at therapy-field junctions across heterogeneous tissues.
**Related:** CSI junction QA
**Example:** Ensures junction stability under patient motion.

483. **Junctional dose verification QA phantom:** Phantom validating TPS calculations and measured dose for junctional regions in multi-isocenter treatments.
**Related:** dose continuity QA
**Example:** Ensures no overdose at breast boost–whole breast junction.

484. **J-wave artifact correction QA verification phantom:** Phantom confirming gating and monitoring systems correctly filter and compensate for J-wave ECG artifacts.
**Related:** cardiac gating QA
**Example:** Ensures no false beam interruptions.

485. **J-coupled spin system QA verification phantom:** Phantom for high-precision verification of J-coupled MR spectroscopy sequences.
**Related:** spectroscopy calibration
**Example:** Ensures accuracy in metabolite-based treatment planning.

486. **J-resolved spectroscopy QA verification phantom:** Phantom for tertiary verification of J-resolved spectral separation and peak accuracy.
**Related:** MRS QA
**Example:** Used when adding metabolic RT planning workflows.

487. **Jet collimator QA verification phantom:** Phantom validating the full QA chain for jet-style collimators—accuracy, speed, shape fidelity, transmission.
**Related:** dynamic collimator QA
**Example:** Ensures stable beam shaping for cutting-edge RT systems.

488. **Jagged edge dose verification QA phantom:** Phantom ensuring dose accuracy along irregular dose edges, identifying TPS smoothing or modeling limitations.
**Related:** edge-dose QA
**Example:** Detects small-field dose inaccuracies.

489. **J-shaped dose-response QA verification phantom:982**

490. Phantom designed to validate measurements of J-shaped dose-response curves, often used in biological dose-response calibration or advanced beam modeling.
**Related:** radiobiological verification
**Example:** Used in high-dose radiobiology studies supporting RT protocol development.

491. **Jaw calibration (noun):** Adjustment ensuring collimator jaws align with planned field edges.
**Related Terms:** Beam collimation, QA.
**Example in Radiotherapy:** Jaw calibration verified during monthly QA.

492. **Jaw positioning accuracy (noun):** Precision of jaw placement relative to the beam axis.
**Related Terms:** Field definition, Mechanical accuracy.
**Example in Radiotherapy:** Critical for large-field treatments.

493. **Jaw transmission factor (noun):** Fraction of radiation passing through closed jaws.
**Related Terms:** Leakage radiation, Head scatter.
**Example in Radiotherapy:** Included in dose modeling.

494. **Junction dose uniformity (noun):** Consistency of dose across field junctions.
**Related Terms:** Field matching, Hot spot avoidance.
**Example in Radiotherapy:** Important in craniospinal irradiation.

495. **Junction shift technique (noun):** Method of moving field junctions between fractions.
**Related Terms:** Feathering, Dose smoothing.
**Example in Radiotherapy:** Reduces overdose at junctions.

496. **Junction uncertainty (noun):** Dose variation arising from junction misalignment.
**Related Terms:** Setup error, Margin design.
**Example in Radiotherapy:** Managed with overlap regions.

497. **Justification principle (noun):** Requirement that radiation exposure provides net benefit.
**Related Terms:** Radiation protection, Optimization.
**Example in Radiotherapy:** Applied when approving imaging frequency.

498. **Jaw-defined field edge (noun):** Beam boundary determined by collimator jaws.
**Related Terms:** Penumbra, Field size.
**Example in Radiotherapy:** Used in 3D conformal planning.

499. **Jaw travel limit (noun):** Maximum physical range of jaw motion.
**Related Terms:** Mechanical constraint, Linac design.
**Example in Radiotherapy:** Considered for large targets.

500. **Jaw synchronization (noun):** Coordinated motion of opposing jaws.
**Related Terms:** Control system, Beam shaping.
**Example in Radiotherapy:** Required for dynamic jaw techniques.

501. **Jitter correction (noun):** Compensation for small, rapid positional fluctuations.
**Related Terms:** Mechanical noise, Stability.
**Example in Radiotherapy:** Improves precision in high-resolution delivery.

# K

1. **K-edge:** The sudden increase in X-ray attenuation that occurs when photon energy exceeds the binding energy of the K-shell electrons of an atom.
   **Related Terms:** Photoelectric effect, attenuation jump, contrast enhancement, monoenergetic imaging.
   **Radiotherapy Example:** Used in kV imaging and dual-energy CT to enhance visibility when iodinated contrast agents (with a K-edge at 33.2 keV) are used for target or organ-at-risk delineation.
2. **K-shell electron:** An electron occupying the innermost atomic shell (principal quantum level n=1).
   **Related Terms:** Binding energy, characteristic radiation, photoelectric absorption.
   **Radiotherapy Example:** K-shell ionization is responsible for characteristic X-rays used in imaging detectors and affects attenuation characteristics used in dose calculations for kV beams.
3. **K-alpha radiation:** Characteristic X-ray emitted when an L-shell electron fills a vacancy in the K-shell.
   **Related Terms:** Characteristic X-rays, electron transitions, atomic emission spectra.
   **Radiotherapy Example:** Detected during X-ray tube output; its spectral lines contribute to beam quality and imaging contrast in kV radiographs.
4. **K-beta radiation:** Characteristic X-ray emitted when an M-shell electron fills a vacancy in the K-shell.
   **Related Terms:** K-series radiation, bremsstrahlung, emission lines.
   **Radiotherapy Example:** Seen in X-ray tube spectral analysis and used in QA of beam quality for kV imaging systems.
5. **K-capture (Electron capture):** A mode of radioactive decay in which the nucleus captures an inner (K-shell) electron.
   **Related Terms:** Radioisotope decay, PET radionuclides, nuclear transitions.
   **Radiotherapy Example:** Radionuclides such as I-123 and Ga-67 used in diagnostic imaging undergo electron capture, affecting the emitted photon energies used for SPECT.
6. **K-radiation:** General term referring to all X-ray emissions involving transitions to the K-shell.
   **Related Terms:** Kα, Kβ, characteristic peaks, atomic emission spectra.
   **Radiotherapy Example:** Seen in X-ray tube spectra and relevant for determining filtration and energy selection in image-guided radiotherapy.
7. **K-line emission:** Sharp spectral lines produced by K-shell transitions.
   **Related Terms:** Spectral peaks, characteristic lines, atomic physics.
   **Radiotherapy Example:** Used during kV system calibration; K-lines help identify target material characteristics in an X-ray tube.
8. **K-factor:** A proportionality factor used in various radiologic physics contexts—commonly relating exposure, dose, or calibration constants.
   **Related Terms:** Calibration coefficient, dose scaling, conversion factors.
   **Radiotherapy Example:** Applied during dose calibration of imaging systems or converting measured exposure into absorbed dose for kV QA.

9. **K-space:** Frequency domain data used in MRI image reconstruction.
**Related Terms:** Fourier transform, MR acquisition grid, spatial frequency mapping.
**Radiotherapy Example:** Understanding k-space behavior is crucial during MRI-based target delineation and QA of MRI simulators.

10. **K-value:** Generic term representing a constant or coefficient in physical formulas involving attenuation, kinetic parameters, or calibration.
**Related Terms:** Scaling constant, system parameter, calibration coefficient.
**Radiotherapy Example:** Used when describing attenuation coefficients or calibration factors in kV energy selection for CT imaging.

11. **Kinetics imaging:** Imaging method that analyzes how tracer concentrations change over time.
**Related Terms:** Dynamic PET, time–activity curves, perfusion imaging.
**Radiotherapy Example:** Used in PET-based evaluation of tumor metabolism before adaptive radiotherapy.

12. **Kinetic modeling:** Mathematical modeling of tracer uptake and clearance in tissues.
**Related Terms:** Compartment models, dynamic imaging, biochemical kinetics.
**Radiotherapy Example:** Improves tumor characterization in PET-based radiotherapy planning for dose painting.

13. **Kinetic parameter:** Quantitative variables describing uptake, flow, or transport of radiotracers.
**Related Terms:** K1, k2, k3 parameters, rate constants, uptake fraction.
**Radiotherapy Example:** Used in quantitative PET to refine metabolic tumor volume for dose escalation.

14. **Kinetic tracer:**A radioactive tracer used to study biological flow or uptake dynamics.
**Related Terms:** FDG, perfusion tracers, dynamic SPECT/PET.
**Radiotherapy Example:** Dynamic PET tracers help evaluate tumor hypoxia or perfusion for biological adaptive planning.

15. **Kinetic energy transfer:** Energy transferred from radiation to charged particles during interactions.
**Related Terms:** LET, dose deposition, stopping power.
**Radiotherapy Example:** Drives understanding of microscopic dose in proton therapy and impacts RBE modeling.

16. **Kinetochore imaging:** Imaging of the protein structure that anchors chromosomes during cell division.
**Related Terms:** Mitotic imaging, fluorescence microscopy, cellular imaging.
**Radiotherapy Example:** Research use—helps understand radiation-induced chromosome damage mechanisms.

17. **Kidney scintigraphy:** Nuclear medicine imaging of renal function using gamma-emitting tracers.
**Related Terms:** MAG3 scan, DTPA scan, renal function imaging.
**Radiotherapy Example:** Used to assess renal baseline before planning treatments involving renal dose sensitivity (e.g., TBI or radionuclide therapy).

18. **Kidney SPECT:** 3D nuclear imaging of kidney perfusion, filtration, or uptake.
**Related Terms:** SPECT/CT, quantitative SPECT, renal imaging.
**Radiotherapy Example:** Supports dosimetry for radionuclide therapies such as Lu-177 where renal uptake determines dose limits.

19. **Kidney PET:** PET imaging of renal perfusion or metabolism using positron-emitting tracers.
**Related Terms:** PET/CT, dynamic PET, functional renal imaging.
**Radiotherapy Example:** Useful for evaluating kidney function in radiation plans where kidneys are critical organs (e.g., abdominal IMRT).

20. **Kidney CT:** CT imaging of the kidneys for structure and pathology.
**Related Terms:** Contrast CT, abdominal CT, kV imaging.
**Radiotherapy Example:** Used for kidney contouring and dose constraints during planning for abdominal or retroperitoneal tumors.

21. **Kidney MRI:** MRI imaging of renal anatomy and perfusion.
**Related Terms:** T1/T2 MRI, diffusion MRI, functional MRI.
**Radiotherapy Example:** Used to improve soft-tissue delineation of kidneys when CT boundaries are unclear.

22. **Kidney ultrasound:** Ultrasound imaging used to evaluate size, flow, and obstruction.
**Related Terms:** Doppler flow, echogenicity, sonography.
**Radiotherapy Example:** May be used for post-treatment monitoring of renal toxicity after high-dose abdominal radiotherapy.

23. **Kidney dose calculation:** The process of determining the absorbed radiation dose to the kidneys.
**Related Terms:** DVH, OAR constraints, Monte Carlo.
**Radiotherapy Example:** Critical for IMRT/VMAT plans near kidneys, and essential in radionuclide therapy dosimetry.

24. **Kidney shielding:** Use of shielding or beam arrangement to reduce kidney exposure.
**Related Terms:** Blockers, beam avoidance sectors, organ sparing.
**Radiotherapy Example:** Employed during TBI to limit renal dose using kidney blocks or VMAT avoidance arcs.

25. **Kidney uptake:** Amount of radioactive tracer absorbed by kidney tissue.
**Related Terms:** Time–activity curves, tracer kinetics, organ-specific uptake.
**Radiotherapy Example:** Used in radionuclide treatments to determine maximum tolerable kidney dose.

26. **Kidney perfusion:** Blood flow to the kidneys measured via dynamic imaging.
**Related Terms:** Perfusion MRI, dynamic CT, flow quantification.
**Radiotherapy Example:** Baseline perfusion imaging can assess sensitivity to radiation-induced nephropathy.

27. **Kidney segmentation:** Automated or manual delineation of kidney boundaries on imaging.
**Related Terms:** Contouring, auto-segmentation, atlas-based segmentation.
**Radiotherapy Example:** Accurate segmentation ensures proper dose constraints in abdominal radiotherapy.

28. **Kidney volume measurement:** Quantifying renal volume for clinical assessment.
**Related Terms:** Organ morphometry, segmentation, volumetry.
**Radiotherapy Example:** Used in dose–volume constraint evaluations and toxicity prediction models.

29. **Kidney artifact:** Imaging artifacts affecting kidney visualization (motion, metal, streaks).
**Related Terms:** Motion artifact, beam hardening, reconstruction artifacts.
**Radiotherapy Example:** Artifacts may distort kidney contours, altering DVH accuracy during planning.

30. **Kidney phantom:** A physical model simulating kidney anatomy for imaging or dosimetry calibration.
**Related Terms:** Anthropomorphic phantom, QA phantom, functional phantom.
**Radiotherapy Example:** Used in SPECT/CT QA to validate quantitative renal imaging for radionuclide dosimetry.

31. **Kidney contrast:** Use of contrast agents to enhance kidney visibility in CT or MRI.
**Related Terms:** Iodinated contrast, gadolinium contrast, enhancement.
**Radiotherapy Example:** Improves kidney boundary during CT simulation for precise segmentation.

32. **Kidney attenuation correction:** Correction applied in nuclear imaging to compensate for tissue attenuation around kidneys.
**Related Terms:** SPECT attenuation maps, CT-based correction, quantitative imaging.
**Radiotherapy Example:** Essential when performing SPECT/CT renal dosimetry for radionuclide therapy.

33. **Kidney planar imaging:** 2D nuclear imaging of kidneys using gamma cameras.
**Related Terms:** Renogram, scintigraphy, time–activity imaging.
**Radiotherapy Example:** Used to assess renal function prior to high-dose treatments (e.g., TBI).

34. **Kidney fusion imaging:** Combining multiple modalities (CT/MRI/PET/SPECT) for kidney evaluation.
**Related Terms:** Image registration, multimodality imaging, hybrid imaging.
**Radiotherapy Example:** PET/CT improves visualization for functional kidney sparing in advanced treatment planning.

35. **Kidney dynamic imaging:** Time-dependent imaging to measure renal flow, uptake, and excretion.
**Related Terms:** MAG3 renogram, dynamic PET, perfusion imaging.
**Radiotherapy Example:** Identifies early renal injury patterns during follow-up after abdominal radiotherapy.

36. **Kidney functional imaging:** Imaging used to assess physiological kidney function (filtration, perfusion).
**Related Terms:** SPECT/CT function, PET perfusion, dynamic MRI.
**Radiotherapy Example:** Helps protect high-functioning kidney regions in IMRT dose optimization.

37. **Kidney radiotracer:** Radiopharmaceuticals used specifically for renal imaging.
**Related Terms:** MAG3, DTPA, DMSA, FDG.
**Radiotherapy Example:** Radiotracers are used to determine safe renal dose levels before radionuclide therapies.

38. **Kidney dosimetry:** Assessment of absorbed dose to kidneys.
**Related Terms:** S-values, MIRD formalism, voxel dosimetry.
**Radiotherapy Example:** Critical in radionuclide therapy (Lu-177, Y-90) because kidneys are dose-limiting organs.

39. **Kidney dose distribution:** Spatial distribution of radiation dose across kidney volume.
**Related Terms:** DVH, OAR mapping, heterogeneous dose.
**Radiotherapy Example:** Used to ensure tolerance constraints ($<18$ Gy mean dose in many protocols).

40. **Kidney hotspot:** Localized region within kidney receiving higher dose than desired.
**Related Terms:** Hot voxel, dose spikes, dose inhomogeneity.
**Radiotherapy Example:** Must be minimized in IMRT/VMAT plans to reduce nephropathy risk.

41. **Kidney voxel analysis:** Voxel-based evaluation of kidney dose, function, or uptake.
**Related Terms:** Voxel dosimetry, voxel S-values, quantitative imaging.
**Radiotherapy Example:** Used in personalized radionuclide therapy to predict renal toxicity.

42. **Kidney image registration:** Alignment of kidney images from different modalities.
**Related Terms:** Rigid registration, deformable registration, fusion imaging.
**Radiotherapy Example:** Needed for matching functional (PET/SPECT) and anatomical (CT) kidney images for planning.

43. **Kidney histogram analysis:** Statistical analysis of pixel or voxel values in kidney imaging.
**Related Terms:** Intensity histogram, texture analysis, radiomics.
**Radiotherapy Example:** Radiomics features can predict radiation-induced renal damage.

44. **Kidney segmentation QA:** Quality assurance ensuring kidney contours are accurate and reproducible.
**Related Terms:** Contour review, auto-segmentation validation, organ delineation QA.
**Radiotherapy Example:** Prevents contouring errors that would otherwise misrepresent renal dose.

45. **Kidney PET/CT QA:** Quality assurance of PET/CT imaging specifically for kidney evaluation.
**Related Terms:** Calibration, SUV accuracy, attenuation correction QA.
**Radiotherapy Example:** Ensures accurate functional imaging for renal dose assessment in radionuclide planning.

46. **Kidney MRI QA:** Quality assurance of MRI protocols used for kidney visualization.
**Related Terms:** Image uniformity, distortion correction, sequence QA.
**Radiotherapy Example:** Avoids geometric distortion in MRI-based kidney delineation.

47. **Kidney SPECT QA:** QA procedures for renal SPECT imaging systems.
**Related Terms:** Uniformity, resolution, sensitivity QA.
**Radiotherapy Example:** Ensures accurate quantitative SPECT dosimetry for radionuclide therapies.

48. **Kidney dose verification:** Independent verification of calculated kidney dose.
**Related Terms:** Secondary check, QA verification, dose audit.
**Radiotherapy Example:** Used before delivering high-dose abdominal VMAT to ensure kidney constraints are satisfied.

49. **Kidney therapy planning:** Planning radiation therapy while optimizing kidney sparing.
**Related Terms:** OAR constraints, optimization objectives, IMRT sparing.
**Radiotherapy Example:** Essential in treatments such as retroperitoneal sarcoma or pancreatic radiotherapy.

50. **Kidney internal dosimetry:** Calculating absorbed dose to kidneys from internally administered radiopharmaceuticals.
**Related Terms:** MIRD, S-values, voxel-based dosimetry.
**Radiotherapy Example:** Dose-limiting step in therapies such as 177Lu-DOTATATE or 131I-MIBG.

51. **Kidney external dosimetry:** Dosimetry of kidney exposure from external radiation fields (photons, electrons, protons).
**Related Terms:** DVH analysis, organ-at-risk dosimetry, external beam dose.
**Radiotherapy Example:** Critical when planning IMRT/VMAT for abdominal tumors to ensure the mean kidney dose stays below tolerance.

52. **Kidney functional mapping:** Mapping spatial variations in kidney function using PET, SPECT, or MRI.
**Related Terms:** Parametric imaging, functional segmentation, differential function mapping.
**Radiotherapy Example:** Guides functional kidney sparing IMRT by avoiding high-dose beams through high-function regions.

53. **Kidney toxicity modeling:** Predictive modeling of radiation-induced kidney injury.
**Related Terms:** NTCP models, dose-response curves, machine-learning toxicity prediction.
**Radiotherapy Example:** Used to evaluate risk of nephropathy in high-dose abdominal radiotherapy planning.

54. **Kidney NTCP modeling:** Normal Tissue Complication Probability modeling specific to kidneys.
**Related Terms:** Lyman-Kutcher-Burman (LKB), probit models, dose constraints.
**Radiotherapy Example:** Predicts probability of renal toxicity given DVH parameters from IMRT plans.

55. **Kidney radiobiology:** Study of biological responses of kidney tissue to radiation.
**Related Terms:** Late effects, radiosensitivity, microvascular damage.
**Radiotherapy Example:** Helps set clinical dose limits (<18 Gy mean dose) to minimize long-term renal damage.

56. **Kidney deformation modeling:** Modeling how kidneys move or deform due to breathing or patient motion.
**Related Terms:** Deformable registration, 4D imaging, motion modeling.
**Radiotherapy Example:** Used in adaptive planning to account for kidney shifts between fractions.

57. **Kidney motion compensation:** Correcting for kidney displacement during imaging or treatment.
**Related Terms:** Gating, breath-hold, motion tracking.
**Radiotherapy Example:** Breath-hold techniques reduce kidney motion during abdominal SBRT.

58. **Kidney motion tracking:** Real-time or recorded monitoring of kidney movement.
**Related Terms:** 4D CT, ultrasound tracking, fiducial tracking.
**Radiotherapy Example:** Ensures accurate beam delivery in proton therapy where motion affects range.

59. **Kidney motion artifact:** Imaging artifacts caused by kidney movement, usually respiratory.
**Related Terms:** Ghosting, blurring, phase mismatch.
**Radiotherapy Example:** Reduces accuracy of kidney segmentation in CT simulation unless 4D CT is used.

60. **Kidney boundary detection:** Algorithms or techniques to identify kidney edges in imaging.
**Related Terms:** Edge detection, segmentation, intensity gradients.
**Radiotherapy Example:** Supports auto-contouring systems used during CT simulation.

61. **Kidney contouring protocol:** Standardized guideline for delineating kidneys in radiotherapy planning.
**Related Terms:** RTOG/EORTC guidelines, OAR contour templates.
**Radiotherapy Example:** Ensures consistent contours across planners to meet clinical kidney dose limits.

62. **Kidney contouring atlas:** A visual guide showing standardized kidney segmentation across slices.
**Related Terms:** Atlas-based segmentation, educational contouring, OAR atlas.
**Radiotherapy Example:** Used in training and peer review for abdominal radiotherapy.

63. **Kidney CT simulation protocol:** Standard CT acquisition procedure for optimal kidney visualization during sim.
**Related Terms:** Scan parameters, contrast timing, slice thickness.
**Radiotherapy Example:** Helps ensure reproducible kidney contours for IMRT/VMAT plans.

64. **Kidney MR simulation:** Use of MRI during radiotherapy simulation to improve kidney boundary detection.
**Related Terms:** MR-sim, soft-tissue contrast, MR-only planning.
**Radiotherapy Example:** Used when CT contrast is contraindicated but high kidney contrast is needed.

65. **Kidney dose constraint:** Set clinical limits on allowable kidney radiation dose.
**Related Terms:** OAR constraints, tolerance dose, QUANTEC.
**Radiotherapy Example:** QUANTEC suggests mean kidney dose <18 Gy to avoid renal dysfunction.

66. **Kidney isodose mapping:** Overlaying isodose lines across kidneys in a treatment plan.
**Related Terms:** Dose distribution, plan evaluation, OAR sparing.
**Radiotherapy Example:** Helps identify hotspots during plan review.

67. **Kidney DVH evaluation:** Reviewing the dose-volume histogram for kidney sparing quality.
**Related Terms:** DVH metrics, V20, mean dose.
**Radiotherapy Example:** Essential before approving any abdominal VMAT plan.

68. **Kidney dose-volume limit:** Specific numerical limits applied to kidney DVH parameters.
**Related Terms:** V10, V20, mean dose, NTCP.
**Radiotherapy Example:** Many protocols limit kidney V20 < 32%.

69. **Kidney function preservation:** Strategies to minimize post-radiation kidney injury.
**Related Terms:** Functional avoidance, adaptive sparing, dose reduction.
**Radiotherapy Example:** Plans intentionally reduce dose to the better-functioning kidney.

70. **Kidney adaptive planning:** Adjusting treatment plans based on kidney movement, deformation, or function.
**Related Terms:** ART (adaptive radiation therapy), re-planning, daily adaptation.
**Radiotherapy Example:** Used in MR-Linac workflows when kidneys shift day to day.

71. **Kidney metabolic imaging:** PET-based analysis of kidney metabolism.
**Related Terms:** FDG-PET, glucose metabolism, dynamic PET.
**Radiotherapy Example:** Provides functional information for adaptive sparing.

72. **Kidney radiomics:** Extraction of quantitative imaging features from kidney images.
**Related Terms:** Texture analysis, machine learning, feature engineering.
**Radiotherapy Example:** Predicts susceptibility to radiation-induced nephropathy.

73. **Kidney deformation vector field:** Map describing voxel-by-voxel displacement of kidneys across images.
**Related Terms:** DVF, deformable registration, motion analysis.
**Radiotherapy Example:** Used for dose accumulation in adaptive radiotherapy.

74. **Kidney cumulative dose:** Total accumulated dose to kidneys across all fractions.
**Related Terms:** Dose summation, adaptive dose accumulation, DVF-based accumulation.
**Radiotherapy Example:** Ensures kidney tolerance is not exceeded after re-planning.

75. **Kidney dose heterogeneity:** Variation in dose received across kidney tissue.
**Related Terms:** Dose uniformity, hotspots, gradient.
**Radiotherapy Example:** Excess heterogeneity increases risk of renal toxicity.

76. **Kidney dose gradient:** Rate at which dose falls off around the kidney.
**Related Terms:** Sharp fall-off, dose drop-off, conformality.
**Radiotherapy Example:** High-dose-gradient IMRT helps protect kidneys adjacent to tumors.

77. **Kidney SBRT evaluation:** Assessment specific to kidney dose constraints in SBRT plans.
**Related Terms:** Hypofractionation, high-dose per fraction, late toxicity.
**Radiotherapy Example:** Essential for adrenal or para-aortic SBRT.

78. **Kidney photon optimization:** Photon beam arrangement to minimize kidney dose.
**Related Terms:** Beam shaping, IMRT/VMAT optimization, OAR avoidance.
**Radiotherapy Example:** Avoidance sectors are used to reduce dose to the ipsilateral kidney.

79. **Kidney proton therapy sparing:** Using proton therapy's Bragg peak to reduce kidney dose.
**Related Terms:** Range stopping, LET distribution, proton plan optimization.
**Radiotherapy Example:** Protons often reduce kidney mean dose in pediatric abdominal tumors.

80. **Kidney LET evaluation:** Assessing linear energy transfer to kidney tissue in proton or ion therapy.
**Related Terms:** RBE, dose weighting, high-LET effects.
**Radiotherapy Example:** Important for predicting renal toxicity in carbon-ion therapy.

81. **Kidney RBE modeling:** Modeling relative biological effectiveness for kidney tissue.
**Related Terms:** RBE-weighted dose, proton/carbon RBE, radiobiological models.
**Radiotherapy Example:** RBE variations impact kidney risk in proton beam planning.

82. **Kidney PET kinetic analysis:** Quantitative modeling of renal PET tracer kinetics.
**Related Terms:** Compartment modeling, dynamic imaging, uptake rates.
**Radiotherapy Example:** Assesses longitudinal kidney function after abdominal radiotherapy.

83. **Kidney SPECT quantification:** Quantitative analysis of SPECT uptake per voxel.
**Related Terms:** Calibration, SUV-SPECT, quantitative SPECT/CT.
**Radiotherapy Example:** Crucial for kidney dosimetry in Lu-177 radionuclide therapy.

84. **Kidney filtration imaging:** Imaging of glomerular filtration using radiotracers.
**Related Terms:** DTPA, GFR estimation, renal clearance imaging.
**Radiotherapy Example:** Evaluates baseline renal function to determine safe dose levels.

85. **Kidney clearance imaging:** Assessment of tracer washout from kidneys.
**Related Terms:** Renogram curves, transit time, excretion imaging.
**Radiotherapy Example:** Helps predict long-term renal tolerance to radiation.

86. **Kidney perfusion mapping:** Spatial mapping of blood perfusion through kidney tissue.
**Related Terms:** Dynamic PET, perfusion MRI, CT perfusion.
**Radiotherapy Example:** Guides regions to be preferentially spared in IMRT.

87. **Kidney dose–response curve:** Relationship between dose level and probability of renal injury.
**Related Terms:** NTCP curve, threshold dose, response modeling.
**Radiotherapy Example:** Used in clinical protocols to set renal dose limits.

88. **Kidney cortical imaging:** Imaging specifically highlighting renal cortex.
**Related Terms:** DMSA imaging, cortical function, differential function.
**Radiotherapy Example:** Helps identify vulnerable cortical regions for sparing in planning.

89. **Kidney medullary imaging:** Imaging of renal medulla physiology.
**Related Terms:** Perfusion imaging, T2 MRI, tracer kinetics.
**Radiotherapy Example:** Investigates differential sensitivity between cortex and medulla to radiation.

90. **Kidney region-of-interest analysis:** Assessment of specific kidney subregions using ROI tools.
**Related Terms:** ROI segmentation, quantitative analysis, regional function assessment.
**Radiotherapy Example:** Used to distinguish high-functioning vs low-functioning kidney areas.

91. **Kidney SUV analysis:** Evaluation of standardized uptake value in kidney PET images.
**Related Terms:** SUVmax, SUVmean, PET quantification.
**Radiotherapy Example:** Helps diagnose renal inflammation after radiation exposure.

92. **Kidney nuclear medicine QA:** QA for renal nuclear medicine procedures and equipment.
**Related Terms:** Sensitivity QA, calibration checks, uniformity QA.
**Radiotherapy Example:** Ensures accurate renal uptake values for radionuclide therapy dosimetry.

93. **Kidney renal cortex segmentation:** Segmentation focused on isolating kidney cortex from medulla.
**Related Terms:** Sub-organ segmentation, tissue differentiation, parametric mapping.
**Radiotherapy Example:** Enables detailed functional avoidance in IMRT.

94. **Kidney differential function analysis:** Quantifying how much each kidney contributes to total renal function.
**Related Terms:** MAG3 renogram, split function, differential uptake.
**Radiotherapy Example:** Plans may prioritize sparing the more functional kidney.

95. **Kidney time–activity analysis:** Plotting tracer concentration over time for renal function curves.
**Related Terms:** TAC curves, dynamic PET/SPECT, clearance rates.
**Radiotherapy Example:** Monitoring function decline after high-dose treatments.

96. **Kidney voxel-based dosimetry:** Calculating dose in small voxels for highly precise renal dosimetry.
**Related Terms:** 3D S-values, voxel kernels, absorbed dose mapping.
**Radiotherapy Example:** Used in individualized radionuclide therapy planning.

97. **Kidney Monte Carlo simulation:** Using Monte Carlo codes to model kidney dose or imaging.
**Related Terms:** Particle transport, stochastic simulation, dose modeling.
**Radiotherapy Example:** Provides high accuracy in kidney dose calculation for proton or radionuclide therapy.

98. **Kidney partial-volume correction:** Correcting for underestimation of true tracer activity due to limited spatial resolution.
**Related Terms:** PVC algorithms, resolution modeling, quantitative SPECT/PET.
**Radiotherapy Example:** Required for accurate kidney dosimetry in Lu-177 therapy.

99. **Kidney segmentation refinement:** Fine-tuning kidney contours using advanced algorithms.
**Related Terms:** Smoothing, active contours, CNN-based refinement.
**Radiotherapy Example:** Reduces contour variability between clinicians.

100. **Kidney AI segmentation:** Automatic segmentation of kidneys using AI/deep learning.
**Related Terms:** CNNs, U-Net, auto-contouring.
**Radiotherapy Example:** Commonly integrated into treatment planning systems to speed kidney contouring before IMRT planning.

101. **Kidney AI contour validation:** Process of checking AI-generated kidney contours for accuracy before clinical use.
**Related Terms:** Auto-contouring QA, segmentation validation, AI performance review.
**Radiotherapy Example:** A dosimetrist reviews AI-generated kidney contours before approving a VMAT plan.

102. **Kidney segmentation benchmarking:** Comparing segmentation methods (manual vs AI vs atlas).
**Related Terms:** Performance metrics, Dice coefficient, contour accuracy.
**Radiotherapy Example:** Clinics benchmark AI contouring to ensure kidneys are consistently outlined for IMRT planning.

103. **Kidney insertion phantom:** A physical phantom with artificial kidneys for imaging and dosimetry training.
**Related Terms:** Anthropomorphic phantom, QA phantom, organ inserts.
**Radiotherapy Example:** Used to verify kidney visibility in CT sim protocols.

104. **Kidney deformable phantom:** Phantom that mimics kidney motion and deformation for motion studies.
**Related Terms:** Dynamic phantom, 4D phantom, respiratory motion simulation.
**Radiotherapy Example:** Used for validating 4DCT accuracy for kidney movement.

105. **Kidney 4D CT analysis:** Evaluation of kidney motion across respiratory phases using 4DCT.
**Related Terms:** Phase binning, respiratory gating, motion envelope.
**Radiotherapy Example:** Critical for abdominal SBRT where organ motion affects coverage.

106. **Kidney gated imaging:** Acquiring imaging synchronized with respiratory phase to reduce motion.
**Related Terms:** Breath-hold imaging, gating systems, motion reduction.
**Radiotherapy Example:** Improves kidney boundary accuracy before IMRT.

107. **Kidney breath-hold imaging:** Capturing CT/MR images during voluntary or assisted breath-holds.
**Related Terms:** Deep inspiration breath-hold, BH CT, respiratory control.
**Radiotherapy Example:** Used for reproducible kidney positions in proton therapy.

108. **Kidney functional avoidance planning:** IMRT/VMAT planning that avoids high-function kidney regions identified via imaging.
**Related Terms:** Differential function, functional maps, adaptive sparing.
**Radiotherapy Example:** Avoids perfused renal cortex regions shown in SPECT.

109. **Kidney inter-fraction variation:** Day-to-day changes in kidney position and shape across fractions.
**Related Terms:** Setup variability, adaptive therapy, organ drift.
**Radiotherapy Example:** Tracked during MR-Linac treatments.

110. **Kidney intra-fraction motion:** Kidney movement occurring during treatment delivery itself.
**Related Terms:** Real-time motion, tracking, gating.
**Radiotherapy Example:** Impacts proton Bragg peak positioning.

111. **Kidney planning organ-at-risk volume (PRV):** Expanded margin around kidneys to accommodate motion or uncertainties.
**Related Terms:** PRV margin, geometric uncertainties, robust planning.
**Radiotherapy Example:** PRV used in IMRT abdominal treatments.

112. **Kidney robust optimization:** Radiotherapy optimization that accounts for uncertainties such as motion or range.
**Related Terms:** Robust planning, worst-case scenario, proton robustness.
**Radiotherapy Example:** Proton plans protect kidneys under multiple breathing scenarios.

113. **Kidney end-to-end QA:** Full-workflow QA from imaging to delivery for kidney-sparing plans.
**Related Terms:** Treatment chain QA, phantom testing, clinical workflow QA.
**Radiotherapy Example:** Conducted before commissioning pediatric kidney-sparing protocols.

114. **Kidney contrast-enhanced CT protocol:**CT protocol designed to optimize contrast visibility of kidneys.
**Related Terms:** Arterial phase, venous phase, timing bolus.
**Radiotherapy Example:** Enhances cortical delineation for contouring.

115. **Kidney dose accumulation:** Summing delivered dose across all fractions considering organ motion.
**Related Terms:** Deformable registration, cumulative dose, ART.
**Radiotherapy Example:** Determines true kidney dose in adaptive RT.

116. **Kidney perfusion SPECT:** SPECT imaging to evaluate renal perfusion and function.
**Related Terms:** MAG3, DTPA, functional imaging.
**Radiotherapy Example:** Helps identify which kidney requires maximum sparing.

117. **Kidney toxicity threshold:** Dose level where renal injury risk significantly increases.
**Related Terms:** LD50, tolerance dose, QUANTEC criteria.
**Radiotherapy Example:** Mean dose >18 Gy increases risk of renal impairment.

**118. Kidney tailored dose planning:** Radiotherapy planning that customizes kidney constraints per patient.
**Related Terms:** Personalized planning, patient-specific constraints.
**Radiotherapy Example:** Adjusting limits for patients with pre-existing kidney disease.

**119. Kidney spatial dose mapping:** Mapping dose distribution across subregions of the kidney.
**Related Terms:** Spatial DVH, sub-region analysis, voxel mapping.
**Radiotherapy Example:** Detects local hotspots near cortex.

**120. Kidney dose prediction modeling:** AI or statistical modeling predicting kidney dose before planning.
**Related Terms:** Knowledge-based planning, DVH prediction.
**Radiotherapy Example:** Helps planners decide optimal beam configurations.

**121. Kidney motion envelope:** The full spatial boundary of kidney motion during respiration.
**Related Terms:** ITV, motion range, 4D envelope.
**Radiotherapy Example:** Used to define margins in 4D planning.

**122. Kidney 3D segmentation model:** Model used to generate 3D kidney structures from imaging.
**Related Terms:** AI models, deep learning, 3D morphometry.
**Radiotherapy Example:** Integrated into treatment planning systems.

**123. Kidney voxel-based NTCP modeling:** Using voxel-specific dose/functional data for toxicity prediction.
**Related Terms:** Radiomics NTCP, spatial NTCP, biological NTCP.
**Radiotherapy Example:** Predicts localized renal injury.

**124. Kidney deformation uncertainty:** Uncertainty in how kidneys deform across scans.
**Related Terms:** Anatomical variability, registration error.
**Radiotherapy Example:** Impacts adaptive prostate/abdominal plans.

**125. Kidney autocontour QA:** Validation workflow for automatic kidney contours.
**Related Terms:** AI QA, consistency checks.
**Radiotherapy Example:** Ensures accurate contours before planning.

**126. Kidney cumulative DVH:** DVH representing total accumulated dose after adaptive changes.
**Related Terms:** Dose summation, ART DVH.
**Radiotherapy Example:** Used to verify constraints across the whole course.

**127. Kidney Monte Carlo validation:** Validating kidney dose calculations using Monte Carlo simulations.
**Related Terms:** Particle transport verification.
**Radiotherapy Example:** Often required in proton therapy QA.

**128. Kidney radiopharmaceutical dosimetry:** Internal dose calculation for radionuclides accumulated in kidneys.
**Related Terms:** MIRD schema, internal dosimetry, S values.
**Radiotherapy Example:** Key for Lu-177 peptide therapy where kidneys are dose-limiting.

**129. Kidney clearance modeling:** Mathematical modeling of kidney tracer clearance.
**Related Terms:** Pharmacokinetics, TAC analysis.
**Radiotherapy Example:** Used for radionuclide therapy dosimetric planning.

**130. Kidney S-value calculation:** Computation of S-values for kidney internal dosimetry.
**Related Terms:** MIRD, absorbed fraction, target–source modeling.
**Radiotherapy Example:** Used in dosimetry of Lu-177 DOTATATE.

131. **Kidney region-specific radiosensitivity:** Variation in radiation sensitivity across kidney regions.
**Related Terms:** Biological heterogeneity, cortex sensitivity.
**Radiotherapy Example:** Drives functional avoidance strategies.

132. **Kidney perfusion MRI:** MRI technique measuring renal perfusion.
**Related Terms:** ASL, DCE-MRI, perfusion mapping.
**Radiotherapy Example:** Identifies functional regions for IMRT sparing.

133. **Kidney DCE-CT:** Dynamic contrast-enhanced CT evaluating vascularity.
**Related Terms:** Time-attentuation curves, perfusion CT.
**Radiotherapy Example:** Assesses microvascular injury post-RT.

134. **Kidney nuclear medicine segmentation:** Segmenting kidneys on SPECT/PET images for dosimetry.
**Related Terms:** Thresholding, quantitative segmentation.
**Radiotherapy Example:** Needed for accurate Lu-177 dosimetry.

135. **Kidney dose washout modeling:** Modeling how absorbed dose changes due to biological clearance.
**Related Terms:** Biological half-life, washout kinetics.
**Radiotherapy Example:** Internal dosimetry for radionuclide therapy.

136. **Kidney range uncertainty:** Uncertainty in proton range when aiming to spare kidneys.
**Related Terms:** Stopping power error, anatomical variability.
**Radiotherapy Example:** Affects pediatric abdominal proton plans.

137. **Kidney ULD CT imaging:** Ultra-low-dose CT adapted for kidney visualization.
**Related Terms:** Low-dose imaging, noise optimization.
**Radiotherapy Example:** Used in children receiving repeated imaging.

138. **Kidney HU calibration:** Calibration of kidney Hounsfield Units for accurate dose calculations.
**Related Terms:** CT calibration, electron density mapping.
**Radiotherapy Example:** Ensures correct dose in abdominal IMRT.

139. **Kidney segmentation uncertainty:** Variability in kidney contouring from person to person or algorithm to algorithm.
**Related Terms:** Inter-observer variability.
**Radiotherapy Example:** Mitigated by contouring protocols.

140. **Kidney motion QA:** QA procedures ensuring accurate kidney motion characterization.
**Related Terms:** 4D CT QA, motion phantom QA.
**Radiotherapy Example:** Required for lung/liver/kidney SBRT.

141. **Kidney DWI MRI mapping:** Diffusion-weighted MRI used to map kidney microstructure.
**Related Terms:** ADC maps, diffusion imaging.
**Radiotherapy Example:** Possible biomarker for early radiation damage.

142. **Kidney displacement vector:** Vector quantifying kidney movement between scans.
**Related Terms:** Motion field, displacement mapping.
**Radiotherapy Example:** Used to create motion margins.

143. **Kidney pre-treatment dose review:** Final check of kidney doses before treatment begins.
**Related Terms:** Plan review, OAR check.
**Radiotherapy Example:** Ensures constraints are met before first fraction.

144. **Kidney dose flagging system:** Automated alert when kidney dose approaches limits.
**Related Terms:** QA alerts, threshold warnings.
**Radiotherapy Example:** Alerts planners if mean kidney dose approaches QUANTEC limits.

145. **Kidney renogram curve analysis:** Analysis of renal time-activity curves from nuclear medicine studies.
**Related Terms:** MAG3 curves, differential function.
**Radiotherapy Example:** Used to determine pre-RT kidney health.

146. **Kidney micro-dosimetry:** Dosimetry at microscopic scales within kidney tissue.
**Related Terms:** Sub-cellular dosimetry, nano-dosimetry.
**Radiotherapy Example:** Relevant to alpha-particle therapies.

147. **Kidney risk-adapted planning:** Customization of constraints based on predicted risk.
**Related Terms:** NTCP-driven planning, personalized sparing.
**Radiotherapy Example:** High-risk patients get stricter kidney dose limits.

148. **Kidney perfusion PET mapping:** PET used to map kidney blood flow.
**Related Terms:** Dynamic PET, perfusion tracer.
**Radiotherapy Example:** Helps identify vulnerable functional regions.

149. **Kidney motion tracking ultrasound:** Ultrasound used to track kidney motion in real time.
**Related Terms:** US gating, real-time imaging.
**Radiotherapy Example:** Used to guide gating in abdominal RT.

150. **Kidney functional NTCP:** NTCP model incorporating functional imaging data.
**Related Terms:** fNTCP, hybrid NTCP, functional avoidance.
**Radiotherapy Example:** Provides more accurate risk estimates in IMRT plans.

151. **K-edge beam filtration:** Using materials with K-edge absorption to shape x-ray spectra.
**Related Terms:** Spectral shaping, beam hardening.
**Radiotherapy Example:** Enhances contrast for kidney imaging in kV radiographs.

152. **K-edge dual-energy CT:** Dual-energy imaging exploiting K-edge differences of materials.
**Related Terms:** Material decomposition, spectral CT.
**Radiotherapy Example:** Improves kidney contrast for contouring.

153. **K-edge contrast imaging:** Imaging method using contrast agents with strong K-edge characteristics.
**Related Terms:** Gold nanoparticles, iodine K-edge.
**Radiotherapy Example:** Enhances tumor–kidney differentiation.

154. **K-shell vacancy modeling:** Modeling atomic transitions after K-shell ionization.
**Related Terms:** Auger effect, characteristic x-rays.
**Radiotherapy Example:** Relevant to Auger-emitting radionuclides near kidneys.

155. **K-shell radiative yield analysis:** Quantifying probability of x-ray emission after K-shell ionization.
**Related Terms:** Fluorescence yield.
**Radiotherapy Example:** Important for radionuclide dosimetry near kidneys.

156. **K-edge attenuator design:** Design of attenuators exploiting K-edge jumps to fine-tune beam energy.
**Related Terms:** Spectral modulators.
**Radiotherapy Example:** Used in photon imaging systems.

157. **K-edge subtraction imaging:** Technique subtracting images above and below K-edge to isolate elements.
**Related Terms:** Spectral subtraction, dual-energy.
**Radiotherapy Example:** Helps distinguish iodine in kidney vasculature.

158. **K-edge material decomposition:** Algorithm decomposing tissues based on K-edge responses.
**Related Terms:** Multi-material decomposition.
**Radiotherapy Example:** Improves kidney contouring quality.

159. **K-edge dose enhancement:** Dose amplification due to photoelectric absorption near K-edge energies.
**Related Terms:** High-Z agents, nanoparticle dose enhancement.
**Radiotherapy Example:** Gold nanoparticles may locally enhance renal dose.

160. **K-edge imaging optimization:** Tuning imaging parameters to maximize K-edge signal.
**Related Terms:** Spectral shaping, dual-energy optimization.
**Radiotherapy Example:** Enhances kidney vessel visualization.

161. **K-shell fluorescence modeling:** Predicting characteristic x-ray emissions from K-shell transitions.
**Related Terms:** Fluorescence yield, atomic relaxation.
**Radiotherapy Example:** Relevant to internal dosimetry for radionuclide kidneys uptake.

162. **K-shell electron capture modeling:** Modeling electron capture into a K-shell vacancy during decay.
**Related Terms:** EC decay, Auger processes.
**Radiotherapy Example:** Influences internal dose in renal radionuclide imaging.

163. **K-shell photoelectric cross-section modeling:** Computing photoelectric interaction probabilities at K-edge energies.
**Related Terms:** Atomic cross-sections, dose modeling.
**Radiotherapy Example:** Used in treatment-planning physics engines.

164. **K-shell ionization cross-section verification:** Experimental validation of modeled K-shell interaction data.
**Related Terms:** Atomic QA, photon interaction QA.
**Radiotherapy Example:** Ensures dose calculation accuracy in kV imaging.

165. **K-edge phantom calibration:** Calibration phantom containing K-edge materials.
**Related Terms:** Spectral phantom, contrast phantom.
**Radiotherapy Example:** Validates dual-energy CT performance.

166. **K-edge filter QA:** Quality assurance of filters designed for K-edge spectral shaping.
**Related Terms:** Filter thickness QA, material QA.
**Radiotherapy Example:** Ensures consistent CT imaging for kidneys.

167. **K-edge imaging QA:** Full QA process for K-edge–based imaging systems.
**Related Terms:** Spectral CT QA, material-specific QA.
**Radiotherapy Example:** Ensures reliable kidney contrast imaging.

168. **K-edge modeling in Monte Carlo:** Monte Carlo simulation including detailed K-edge physics.
**Related Terms:** Photon transport modeling.
**Radiotherapy Example:** Used to simulate kidney dose with high-Z contrast.

169. **K-shell fluorescence yield calibration:** Calibration of photon emission probabilities after K-shell events.
**Related Terms:** Atomic calibration.
**Radiotherapy Example:** Improves internal dosimetry calculations.

170. **K-edge detector calibration:** Calibrating detectors for accurate K-edge energy measurement.
**Related Terms:** Spectral detector QA.
**Radiotherapy Example:** Ensures stable dual-energy CT imaging.

171. **K-edge CT reconstruction:** Specialized CT reconstruction techniques exploiting K-edge differences.
**Related Terms:** Material decomposition reconstruction.
**Radiotherapy Example:** Enhances kidney tissue segmentation.

172. **K-edge contrast enhancement modeling:** Modeling how contrast agents amplify K-edge signals.
**Related Terms:** Dose-contrast modeling.
**Radiotherapy Example:** Predicts how iodine impacts kidney CT visibility.

173. **K-edge image segmentation:** Segmenting tissues using K-edge material properties.
**Related Terms:** Spectral segmentation.
**Radiotherapy Example:** Helps isolate kidney vasculature.

174. **K-edge dose mapping:** Mapping dose where K-edge interactions enhance deposition.
**Related Terms:** Spectral dose mapping.
**Radiotherapy Example:** Used in enhanced dose imaging research.

175. **K-edge filtered back-projection:** FBP adapted for K-edge spectral CT datasets.
**Related Terms:** Spectral reconstruction.
**Radiotherapy Example:** Produces clearer kidney images for contouring.

176. **K-edge spectral weighting:** Weighting projections to emphasize K-edge energy ranges.
**Related Terms:** Spectral CT tuning.
**Radiotherapy Example:** Improves kidney cortex contrast.

177. **K-edge micro-CT imaging:**High-resolution CT using K-edge contrast agents.
**Related Terms:** Pre-clinical imaging.
**Radiotherapy Example:** Used in kidney micro-dosimetry studies.

178. **K-edge internal dosimetry:** Dosimetry accounting for K-edge absorption of internal radionuclides.
**Related Terms:** Auger dosimetry.
**Radiotherapy Example:** Important for kidney uptake in radionuclide therapy.

179. **K-edge photon counting imaging:** Photon-counting detectors that identify energies near K-edge thresholds.
**Related Terms:** PCD-CT, energy-resolved detection.
**Radiotherapy Example:** Enables precise kidney contrast imaging.

180. **K-edge nano-contrast imaging:** Use of nanoparticles with strong K-edge signatures for enhanced imaging.
**Related Terms:** GNP contrast, spectral enhancement.
**Radiotherapy Example:** Investigated for kidney perfusion mapping.

181. **K-shell Auger cascade modeling:** Simulation of cascading Auger emissions after K-shell ionization.
**Related Terms:** Auger electron emission.
**Radiotherapy Example:** Important for nano-dosimetry in kidney tissue.

182. **K-shell characteristic radiation mapping:** Mapping characteristic x-rays emitted from K-shell relaxations.
**Related Terms:** Fluorescence mapping.
**Radiotherapy Example:** Used in micro-dosimetry research.

183. **K-edge dose amplification modeling:** Predicting dose enhancement near K-edge materials.
**Related Terms:** High-Z effects.
**Radiotherapy Example:** Relevant for gold nanoparticle dose physics.

184. **K-shell atomic relaxation modeling:** Modeling full sequence of atomic relaxation after a K-shell vacancy.
**Related Terms:** X-ray emission, Auger cascades.
**Radiotherapy Example:** Needed for radionuclide dosimetry in kidneys.

185. **K-shell photon emission calibration:** Calibration related to characteristic photon emission spectra.
**Related Terms:** X-ray spectroscopy calibration.
**Radiotherapy Example:** Used in imaging system commissioning.

186. **K-shell electron yield analysis:** Quantitative evaluation of emitted Auger electrons after K-shell ionization.
**Related Terms:** Auger yield.
**Radiotherapy Example:** Critical in modeling nano-scale kidney damage.

187. **K-edge Monte Carlo benchmark phantom:** Phantom designed for validating K-edge modeling in Monte Carlo.
**Related Terms:** Spectral phantom.
**Radiotherapy Example:** Used to test contrast-enhanced CT accuracy.

188. **K-edge imaging validation phantom:** Phantom ensuring accurate K-edge CT imaging performance.
**Related Terms:** Calibration phantom.
**Radiotherapy Example:** Used in dual-energy CT commissioning.

189. **K-edge CT artifact analysis:** Study of artifacts unique to K-edge imaging.
**Related Terms:** Beam-hardening artifacts.
**Radiotherapy Example:** Ensures kidney contrast images remain artifact-free.

190. **K-edge detector QA phantom:** Phantom for calibrating K-edge-sensitive energy detectors.
**Related Terms:** PCD QA.
**Radiotherapy Example:** Used for spectral CT QA.

191. **K-shell atomic model QA:** QA for models predicting K-shell interactions.
**Related Terms:** Atomic data validation.
**Radiotherapy Example:** Important in dose engines using detailed physics.

192. **K-shell absorption coefficient modeling:** Computing absorption coefficients near K-edge transitions.
**Related Terms:** $\mu(E)$ modeling.
**Radiotherapy Example:** Influences CT-based dose calculations.

193. **K-shell ionization yield mapping:** Spatial mapping of K-shell ionization probabilities.
**Related Terms:** Interaction mapping.
**Radiotherapy Example:** Used in micro-beam imaging research.

194. **K-edge CT contrast stability:** Monitoring consistency of K-edge contrast performance over time.
**Related Terms:** Imaging QA stability.
**Radiotherapy Example:** Ensures stable kidney contrast imaging.

195. **K-edge contrast phantom QA:** Phantom used to test contrast response in K-edge CT.
**Related Terms:** DECT QA phantom.
**Radiotherapy Example:** Used before implementing new contrast protocols.

196. **K-edge fluence mapping:** Mapping photon fluence through materials near the K-edge.
**Related Terms:** Spectral fluence, energy mapping.
**Radiotherapy Example:** Helps understand dose deposition near kidneys.

197. **K-edge micro-dosimetry phantom:** Phantom for micro-scale dose studies using K-edge materials.
**Related Terms:** High-resolution phantom.
**Radiotherapy Example:** Used for kidney nanoparticle dose research.

198. **K-edge reconstruction QA:** QA verifying correct spectral reconstruction in K-edge CT.
**Related Terms:** Reconstruction fidelity.
**Radiotherapy Example:** Ensures reliable images for kidney contouring.

**199. K-edge spectral response curve:** Response curve describing detector sensitivity across K-edge energies.
**Related Terms:** Detector characterization.
**Radiotherapy Example:** Used to calibrate spectral CT hardware.

**200. K-edge calibration workflow:** Full workflow for calibrating K-edge imaging systems.
**Related Terms:** Spectral calibration, QA program.
**Radiotherapy Example:** Commissioned before clinical use of kidney contrast imaging.

**201. KVP setting:** Peak voltage applied to the x-ray tube, controlling photon energy.
**Related Terms:** Tube potential, kV, beam quality.
**Radiotherapy Example:** KV imaging of kidneys uses 80–120 kVp for optimal contrast.

**202. KV imaging:** Imaging using kilovoltage x-rays, typically for localization.
**Related Terms:** Image-guided RT, planar imaging, CBCT.
**Radiotherapy Example:** KV planar imaging ensures kidney is outside high-dose regions in abdominal RT.

**203. KV radiography:** 2D x-ray imaging using kV beams.
**Related Terms:** Planar imaging, image guidance.
**Radiotherapy Example:** Daily KV radiographs verify patient setup before kidney-sparing treatments.

**204. KV calibration:** Process of calibrating kV imaging systems for accurate energy and output.
**Related Terms:** QA, detector calibration.
**Radiotherapy Example:** Ensures KV images provide correct Hounsfield Units for kidney delineation.

**205. KV linearity test:** Verifies linear response of kV detector over dose range.
**Related Terms:** Detector QA, dose-response linearity.
**Radiotherapy Example:** Confirms kidney imaging intensity is proportional to dose.

**206. KV image quality:** Assessment of resolution, contrast, and noise in kV imaging.
**Related Terms:** CNR, MTF, SNR.
**Radiotherapy Example:** Ensures clear kidney edges for contouring.

**207. KV dose measurement:** Measurement of patient or phantom dose from kV imaging.
**Related Terms:** Dose monitoring, image dose, OAR dose.
**Radiotherapy Example:** Ensures kidney dose from imaging is within safe limits.

**208. KV artifact:** Imaging distortions like streaks or beam hardening.
**Related Terms:** Motion artifact, scatter, noise.
**Radiotherapy Example:** Motion artifacts in kidney images can mislead contouring.

**209. KV phantom:** Physical model for testing and calibrating KV imaging systems.
**Related Terms:** QA phantom, calibration phantom.
**Radiotherapy Example:** Ensures kidney visualization quality.

**210. KV exposure:** Total radiation delivered during kV imaging.
**Related Terms:** mAs, dose per image.
**Radiotherapy Example:** Optimized to reduce kidney imaging dose.

**211. KV safety check:** Ensuring KV imaging system operates safely.
**Related Terms:** Radiation safety QA.
**Radiotherapy Example:** Protects kidneys and other organs during daily imaging.

212. **KV protocol:** Standardized imaging parameters for a procedure.
**Related Terms:** Imaging protocol, CBCT protocol.
**Radiotherapy Example:** Pediatric kidney scans follow low-dose KV protocols.

213. **KV optimization:** Adjusting kV parameters for image quality vs dose.
**Related Terms:** Dose optimization, image optimization.
**Radiotherapy Example:** Balances kidney contrast and minimal dose.

214. **KV scan parameter:** Settings like kVp, mAs, rotation for KV CT or CBCT.
**Related Terms:** Imaging acquisition, scan settings.
**Radiotherapy Example:** 100 kVp, 80 mAs for kidney localization.

215. **KV beam uniformity:** Consistency of photon fluence across field.
**Related Terms:** Flatness, homogeneity.
**Radiotherapy Example:** Uniform kidney imaging for accurate dose mapping.

216. **KV field verification:** Ensuring beam field matches planned dimensions.
**Related Terms:** Collimator check, field size QA.
**Radiotherapy Example:** Confirms kidney is within imaging FOV.

217. **KV image contrast:** Ability to distinguish tissues based on x-ray attenuation.
**Related Terms:** CNR, contrast resolution.
**Radiotherapy Example:** Contrast distinguishes renal cortex from tumor.

218. **KV spatial resolution:** Ability to resolve small structures.
**Related Terms:** MTF, line-pair resolution.
**Radiotherapy Example:** Resolves kidney calyces for precise contouring.

219. **KV modulation:** Adjusting x-ray output during scan to optimize image quality.
**Related Terms:** Auto mA, dose modulation.
**Radiotherapy Example:** Reduces kidney dose while maintaining image quality.

220. **KV attenuation:** Reduction of x-ray intensity due to absorption/scattering.
**Related Terms:** Beam hardening, tissue attenuation.
**Radiotherapy Example:** Corrected during KV CT to accurately depict kidney density.

221. **KV dose optimization:** Minimizing imaging dose while keeping quality adequate.
**Related Terms:** ALARA, dose reduction.
**Radiotherapy Example:** Daily KV verification for kidney-sparing plans.

222. **KV QA test:** Routine quality assurance tests for KV imaging.
**Related Terms:** Annual QA, monthly QA, AAPM TG-142.
**Radiotherapy Example:** Checks kidney image contrast and resolution.

223. **KV imaging system:** Hardware and software for kilovoltage imaging.
**Related Terms:** On-board imager, CBCT.
**Radiotherapy Example:** Used for kidney localization prior to treatment.

224. **KV detector calibration:** Ensuring detector output matches expected photon response.
**Related Terms:** Gain calibration, flat-field correction.
**Radiotherapy Example:** Accurate kidney imaging depends on correct detector calibration.

225. **KV beam alignment:** Ensuring kV imaging beam is aligned with treatment beam.
**Related Terms:** Iso-center QA, coincidence check.
**Radiotherapy Example:** Align kidney with planned treatment field.

226. **KV collimator check:** Verification of collimator positions and shapes.
**Related Terms:** Field shaping, jaw check.
**Radiotherapy Example:** Ensures kidney is entirely within imaging field.

227. **KV generator QA:** Quality assurance for KV x-ray tube generator.
**Related Terms:** Output, voltage, exposure time verification.
**Radiotherapy Example:** Prevents imaging dose fluctuations to kidneys.

228. **KV exposure mapping:** Measurement of dose distribution across the imaging field.
**Related Terms:** Dose profile, field mapping.
**Radiotherapy Example:** Confirms kidney does not receive high imaging dose.

229. **KV patient dose:** Dose delivered to patient during KV imaging.
**Related Terms:** Entrance dose, skin dose.
**Radiotherapy Example:** Monitored in pediatric kidney imaging.

230. **KV beam hardening:** Increase in mean beam energy as low-energy photons are absorbed.
**Related Terms:** Artifact, CT correction.
**Radiotherapy Example:** Corrected to avoid kidney CT artifacts.

231. **KV scan quality:** Overall image quality including noise, contrast, resolution.
**Related Terms:** QA metrics, imaging performance.
**Radiotherapy Example:** Kidney visibility must meet planning standards.

232. **KV imaging artifact:** Distortions like streaks, shading, or noise in images.
**Related Terms:** Beam hardening, motion, metal artifact.
**Radiotherapy Example:** Avoids miscontouring of kidney edges.

233. **KV imaging phantom:** Physical model for evaluating KV imaging performance.
**Related Terms:** QA phantom, contrast phantom.
**Radiotherapy Example:** Tests kidney image contrast and resolution.

234. **KV dose assessment:** Evaluation of imaging dose delivered to patient.
**Related Terms:** Dosimetry, dose monitoring.
**Radiotherapy Example:** Ensures cumulative kidney dose remains safe.

235. **KV dose distribution:** Mapping of dose across the imaging field.
**Related Terms:** Dose profile, dose map.
**Radiotherapy Example:** Confirms no hotspots over kidneys.

236. **KV scan verification:** Confirmation that imaging system produces expected quality.
**Related Terms:** QA test, performance verification.
**Radiotherapy Example:** Ensures kidney contours are clearly visualized.

237. **KV exposure correction:** Adjusting exposure to correct over- or underexposure.
**Related Terms:** Auto-exposure, dose optimization.
**Radiotherapy Example:** Reduces imaging dose to kidneys.

238. **KV image analysis:** Evaluation of image metrics (contrast, noise, artifacts).
**Related Terms:** QA review, quantitative analysis.
**Radiotherapy Example:** Confirms kidney edges are suitable for contouring.

239. **KV workflow:** Standardized sequence for performing KV imaging.
**Related Terms:** Imaging protocol, QA workflow.
**Radiotherapy Example:** Ensures consistent kidney localization daily.

**240. KV system QA:** Comprehensive QA for KV imaging system.
**Related Terms:** Daily QA, monthly QA, annual QA.
**Radiotherapy Example:** Ensures kidney image quality and dose consistency.

**241. KV image acquisition:** Process of capturing kV images.
**Related Terms:** Imaging protocol, acquisition parameters.
**Radiotherapy Example:** Daily kidney imaging for verification.

**242. KV beam profile:** Measurement of beam intensity across field.
**Related Terms:** Flatness, uniformity, symmetry.
**Radiotherapy Example:** Ensures uniform kidney imaging dose.

**243. KV image optimization:** Adjusting parameters for best image quality.
**Related Terms:** CNR, noise reduction, contrast enhancement.
**Radiotherapy Example:** Clear kidney images while minimizing dose.

**244. KV scan parameter adjustment:** Fine-tuning KV settings like mAs or kVp for image quality.
**Related Terms:** Protocol modification, dose adjustment.
**Radiotherapy Example:** Adjusted for pediatric kidneys with low-dose requirement.

**245. KV radiation safety:** Measures to minimize unnecessary patient exposure.
**Related Terms:** ALARA, shielding, safety checks.
**Radiotherapy Example:** Lead shielding used during kidney imaging.

**246. KV scan QA:** QA testing of scan performance and image quality.
**Related Terms:** Image QA, exposure QA.
**Radiotherapy Example:** Confirms kidney images meet clinical standards.

**247. KV image registration:** Aligning KV images to planning CT for verification.
**Related Terms:** IGRT, rigid registration, fusion.
**Radiotherapy Example:** Ensures kidney is correctly aligned before RT.

**248. KV histogram analysis:** Analysing intensity distributions for quality or segmentation.
**Related Terms:** Image statistics, QA metrics.
**Radiotherapy Example:** Detects artifacts affecting kidney contouring.

**249. KV modulation QA:** QA of automatic tube current modulation.
**Related Terms:** Dose optimization, mA modulation.
**Radiotherapy Example:** Prevents excess kidney exposure during CBCT.

**250. KV image fusion:** Combining KV images with planning CT/MR for verification.
**Related Terms:** Multi-modality registration.
**Radiotherapy Example:** Confirms kidney position relative to treatment fields.

**251. KV beam QA:** Quality assurance of the kV x-ray beam for flatness, symmetry, and output.
**Related Terms:** Beam uniformity, field verification.
**Radiotherapy Example:** Ensures kidney imaging beam does not overexpose one side.

**252. KV detector QA:** Quality assurance of the kV detector performance (linearity, noise, uniformity).
**Related Terms:** Detector calibration, image quality QA.
**Radiotherapy Example:** Accurate kidney contours depend on detector QA.

**253. KV exposure phantom:** Phantom used to measure and map kV exposure.
**Related Terms:** Dose phantom, QA phantom.
**Radiotherapy Example:** Confirms safe kidney imaging dose distribution.

254. **KV dose verification phantom:** Phantom to verify dose delivered during kV imaging.
**Related Terms:** Dosimetry, QA phantom.
**Radiotherapy Example:** Checks kidney entrance dose during CBCT.

255. **KV scan phantom:** Physical model for testing KV scan protocols and image quality.
**Related Terms:** Imaging phantom, QA tool.
**Radiotherapy Example:** Tests kidney visibility and contrast for low-dose scans.

256. **KV linearity verification:** Ensuring detector response is linear with exposure.
**Related Terms:** Detector QA, dose-response check.
**Radiotherapy Example:** Confirms kidney intensity is proportional to delivered dose.

257. **KV uniformity test:** Test of beam and image uniformity across FOV.
**Related Terms:** Flatness, homogeneity.
**Radiotherapy Example:** Ensures kidney appears evenly without artificial bright or dark spots.

258. **KV field QA:** Verification of beam dimensions, position, and alignment.
**Related Terms:** Collimator check, FOV verification.
**Radiotherapy Example:** Ensures kidney is fully captured in the imaging field.

259. **KV image contrast phantom:** Phantom to assess contrast resolution in KV imaging.
**Related Terms:** Contrast-detail phantom, QA phantom.
**Radiotherapy Example:** Distinguishes kidney cortex and tumor for planning.

260. **KV artifact correction:** Techniques to reduce or remove imaging artifacts.
**Related Terms:** Beam hardening correction, motion artifact reduction.
**Radiotherapy Example:** Minimizes streaks that could distort kidney contours.

261. **KV image calibration:** Adjustment of image intensity and geometric accuracy.
**Related Terms:** Flat-fielding, HU calibration.
**Radiotherapy Example:** Ensures kidney CT densities are accurate for dose calculations.

262. **KV imaging workflow:** Standardized process from acquisition to review.
**Related Terms:** QA workflow, protocol adherence.
**Radiotherapy Example:** Daily kidney imaging follows consistent workflow for reproducibility.

263. **KV detector alignment:** Ensuring detector is aligned with beam axis.
**Related Terms:** Coincidence, isocenter check.
**Radiotherapy Example:** Kidney location in KV image matches treatment isocenter.

264. **KV image uniformity:** Assessment of evenness in image intensity across FOV.
**Related Terms:** Flatness, homogeneity.
**Radiotherapy Example:** Even kidney intensity avoids contouring errors.

265. **KV beam alignment phantom:** Phantom to verify alignment between KV beam and treatment beam.
**Related Terms:** Iso-center phantom, coincidence QA.
**Radiotherapy Example:** Ensures kidney target aligns with treatment plan.

266. **KV scan alignment:** Verification of correct positioning and alignment of KV scan.
**Related Terms:** QA check, patient setup.
**Radiotherapy Example:** Kidney isocenter matches planning CT.

267. **KV spatial resolution QA:** Evaluation of detector ability to resolve small structures.
**Related Terms:** MTF, line pair phantom.
**Radiotherapy Example:** Resolves small renal lesions for treatment planning.

268. **KV modulation verification:** Checks correct functioning of automatic tube current modulation.
**Related Terms:** Dose optimization, mA modulation QA.
**Radiotherapy Example:** Prevents kidney overexposure during CBCT.

269. **KV dose mapping:** Measurement of dose distribution across imaging field.
**Related Terms:** Exposure map, dosimetry QA.
**Radiotherapy Example:** Confirms kidney remains below safe dose limit.

270. **KV exposure optimization:** Adjusting scan parameters to minimize dose while maintaining image quality.
**Related Terms:** ALARA, low-dose imaging.
**Radiotherapy Example:** Pediatric kidney CBCT uses optimized exposure.

271. **KV phantom study:** Use of phantom to assess imaging performance.
**Related Terms:** QA study, calibration phantom.
**Radiotherapy Example:** Evaluates kidney image quality before clinical scans.

272. **KV imaging QA phantom:** Phantom designed for comprehensive KV QA.
**Related Terms:** Multi-test phantom, dose and image QA.
**Radiotherapy Example:** Ensures kidney visibility and safe dose delivery.

273. **KV image verification:** Checking that acquired image meets QA standards.
**Related Terms:** Image QA, protocol check.
**Radiotherapy Example:** Confirms kidney contours are clearly visible.

274. **KV workflow verification:** Verification of imaging protocol adherence.
**Related Terms:** QA audit, standardization.
**Radiotherapy Example:** Kidney imaging performed consistently daily.

275. **KV image quality assessment:** Evaluation of contrast, noise, and resolution.
**Related Terms:** CNR, SNR, spatial resolution.
**Radiotherapy Example:** Ensures kidney edges are clear for planning.

276. **KV scan calibration:** Adjustment to ensure correct image intensity and geometry.
**Related Terms:** HU calibration, geometric calibration.
**Radiotherapy Example:** Kidney CT values match planned dose calculation.

277. **KV exposure QA test:** Verification of exposure accuracy.
**Related Terms:** Dose measurement, mAs check.
**Radiotherapy Example:** Confirms kidney imaging dose is within safe limits.

278. **KV detector QA phantom:** Phantom specifically for detector QA tests.
**Related Terms:** Flat-field phantom, resolution phantom.
**Radiotherapy Example:** Ensures accurate kidney imaging for contouring.

279. **KV image fusion QA:** Verification of multi-modality image registration quality.
**Related Terms:** CT-MRI fusion, PET/CT fusion QA.
**Radiotherapy Example:** Ensures kidney PET/CT alignment for dose planning.

280. **KV alignment QA:** Overall verification of beam and detector alignment.
**Related Terms:** Isocenter QA, beam coincidence.
**Radiotherapy Example:** Kidney is aligned with treatment plan isocenter.

281. **KV radiation measurement:** Measurement of radiation output from KV system.
**Related Terms:** Dosimetry, output QA.
**Radiotherapy Example:** Confirms kidney dose from imaging is acceptable.

282. **KV generator calibration:** Ensures accurate kV and mA output from generator.
**Related Terms:** QA test, tube output calibration.
**Radiotherapy Example:** Stable generator output ensures kidney imaging consistency.

283. **KV beam profile QA:** Evaluation of beam flatness, symmetry, and uniformity.
**Related Terms:** Beam verification, field uniformity.
**Radiotherapy Example:** Ensures kidney imaging dose distribution is even.

284. **KV system calibration:** Comprehensive calibration of KV system for geometry and dose.
**Related Terms:** QA, performance verification.
**Radiotherapy Example:** Ensures accurate kidney imaging for treatment planning.

285. **KV field mapping:** Measurement of imaging field coverage and uniformity.
**Related Terms:** Exposure mapping, dose distribution.
**Radiotherapy Example:** Confirms kidney is fully included in KV FOV.

286. **KV imaging standardization:** Ensuring imaging protocols produce consistent results.
**Related Terms:** Protocol adherence, QA.
**Radiotherapy Example:** Kidney imaging reproducible across multiple sessions.

287. **KV scan quality check:** Routine check of scan quality metrics.
**Related Terms:** QA, image verification.
**Radiotherapy Example:** Kidney edges are clearly visible and artifact-free.

288. **KV exposure distribution:** Mapping of exposure levels across FOV.
**Related Terms:** Dose mapping, uniformity.
**Radiotherapy Example:** Confirms kidneys are not overexposed during CBCT.

289. **KV linearity phantom:** Phantom used to check detector linearity over dose range.
**Related Terms:** Detector QA, response check.
**Radiotherapy Example:** Ensures kidney image intensity is proportional to exposure.

290. **KV dose verification study:** Study to confirm imaging dose delivered matches expected.
**Related Terms:** Dosimetry, QA study.
**Radiotherapy Example:** Ensures cumulative kidney dose remains safe.

291. **KV beam verification phantom:** Phantom used to verify beam alignment and flatness.
**Related Terms:** Beam QA, uniformity phantom.
**Radiotherapy Example:** Confirms kidney is in correct imaging field.

292. **KV image artifact QA:** QA test to detect and minimize imaging artifacts.
**Related Terms:** Artifact reduction, quality check.
**Radiotherapy Example:** Reduces streaks that may distort kidney contours.

293. **KV scan uniformity:** Evaluation of intensity consistency across imaging FOV.
**Related Terms:** Flatness, homogeneity.
**Radiotherapy Example:** Kidney appears evenly illuminated for accurate contouring.

294. **KV detector calibration phantom:** Phantom for routine detector calibration.
**Related Terms:** Flat-field, QA phantom.
**Radiotherapy Example:** Accurate kidney imaging depends on detector calibration.

295. **KV beam modulation QA:** QA test for automatic tube current modulation.
**Related Terms:** mA modulation, dose optimization.
**Radiotherapy Example:** Avoids high kidney dose during CBCT scans.

296. **KV image registration QA:** QA of image registration accuracy with planning CT or MR.
**Related Terms:** Fusion verification, IGRT QA.
**Radiotherapy Example:** Ensures kidney is correctly aligned with treatment plan.

297. **KV patient dose assessment:** Evaluation of dose received by patient from imaging.
**Related Terms:** Dosimetry, dose monitoring.
**Radiotherapy Example:** Monitors kidney imaging dose for safety.

298. **KV histogram QA:** Analysis of intensity distribution for image QA.
**Related Terms:** Image statistics, artifact detection.
**Radiotherapy Example:** Confirms kidney images are uniform and artifact-free.

299. **KV scan optimization:** Adjusting scan parameters to balance image quality and dose.
**Related Terms:** Low-dose imaging, ALARA.
**Radiotherapy Example:** Optimized kidney CBCT reduces radiation exposure.

300. **KV image resolution phantom:** Phantom to evaluate spatial resolution of KV imaging system.
**Related Terms:** Line-pair phantom, MTF.
**Radiotherapy Example:** Ensures small kidney structures are clearly visualized.

301. **KV planar imaging:** Acquisition of single-plane x-ray images using a kV source.
**Related Terms:** Radiography, 2D imaging.
**Radiotherapy Example:** Kidney portal imaging to verify patient setup.

302. **KV imaging correction:** Process of adjusting images for geometric or intensity errors.
**Related Terms:** Flat-fielding, artifact correction.
**Radiotherapy Example:** Correcting streaks in kidney CBCT images.

303. **KV phantom QA:** Use of phantom to perform routine KV QA tests.
**Related Terms:** QA phantom, dosimetry phantom.
**Radiotherapy Example:** Ensures kidney imaging system produces accurate and consistent images.

304. **KV imaging protocol:** Standardized parameters for KV imaging (kV, mA, exposure time).
**Related Terms:** Scan settings, workflow.
**Radiotherapy Example:** Pediatric kidney scans follow low-dose protocol for safety.

305. **KV exposure QA phantom:** Phantom designed specifically to measure KV exposure and dose distribution.
**Related Terms:** Dosimetry phantom, exposure mapping.
**Radiotherapy Example:** Confirms safe kidney entrance dose during CBCT.

306. **KV detector QA verification:** Routine verification of detector performance against standards.
**Related Terms:** Detector calibration, image quality check.
**Radiotherapy Example:** Ensures kidney images have accurate contrast and intensity.

307. **KV scan dose QA:** Measurement and verification of patient dose during KV scans.
**Related Terms:** Dosimetry, ALARA principle.
**Radiotherapy Example:** Confirms cumulative kidney imaging dose remains safe.

308. **KV image contrast QA:** Evaluation of contrast quality in KV images.
**Related Terms:** CNR, lesion visibility.
**Radiotherapy Example:** Differentiates kidney tumor from surrounding tissue for contouring.

309. **KV beam uniformity phantom:** Phantom used to assess uniformity of KV x-ray beam.
**Related Terms:** Flatness test, dose distribution.
**Radiotherapy Example:** Ensures kidney imaging beam delivers uniform exposure.

310. **KV imaging performance QA:** Comprehensive testing of system for image quality and consistency.
**Related Terms:** Resolution, contrast, artifact check.
**Radiotherapy Example:** Confirms kidney imaging system produces reliable images daily.

311. **KV workflow QA:** Quality assurance of imaging workflow and adherence to protocol.
**Related Terms:** Process verification, standardization.
**Radiotherapy Example:** Ensures kidney CBCT scans follow standard setup for reproducibility.

312. **KV radiation safety QA:** Testing and verification to ensure patient and staff safety from KV radiation.
**Related Terms:** Shielding, exposure limits.
**Radiotherapy Example:** Confirms kidney scans comply with ALARA dose limits.

313. **KV exposure verification phantom:** Phantom designed to check KV exposure during scans.
**Related Terms:** Dosimetry phantom, QA tool.
**Radiotherapy Example:** Ensures kidney entrance dose is within planned range.

314. **KV image calibration QA:** Routine QA to ensure image intensity and geometry are accurate.
**Related Terms:** HU calibration, geometric correction.
**Radiotherapy Example:** Kidney CT Hounsfield Units are consistent for dose calculation.

315. **KV generator QA:** Quality assurance of KV x-ray generator output (kV, mA, timing).
**Related Terms:** Tube output verification, calibration.
**Radiotherapy Example:** Stable output ensures reproducible kidney imaging.

316. **KV beam alignment QA phantom:** Phantom used to verify alignment of the KV beam to isocenter.
**Related Terms:** Iso-center QA, coincidence verification.
**Radiotherapy Example:** Ensures kidney is correctly positioned in treatment beam path.

317. **KV image uniformity phantom:** Phantom used to evaluate uniformity of image intensity across the detector.
**Related Terms:** Flat-field phantom, QA tool.
**Radiotherapy Example:** Kidney image appears even without artificial bright or dark regions.

318. **KV imaging system QA phantom:** Comprehensive phantom for assessing overall KV imaging system performance.
**Related Terms:** Multi-test phantom, QA assessment.
**Radiotherapy Example:** Checks kidney imaging resolution, contrast, and dose delivery.

319. **KV scan verification phantom:** Phantom used to verify accuracy of KV scan parameters.
**Related Terms:** QA phantom, scan assessment.
**Radiotherapy Example:** Ensures kidney scan parameters match planning specifications.

320. **KV image acquisition QA:** QA procedure to verify the process of acquiring KV images.
**Related Terms:** Workflow QA, protocol verification.
**Radiotherapy Example:** Confirms kidney CBCT images are captured correctly without artifacts.

321. **KV detector performance QA:** Assessment of detector response, noise, linearity, and resolution.
**Related Terms:** Detector QA, image quality verification.
**Radiotherapy Example:** Ensures kidney contours are accurately captured for planning.

322. **KV linearity QA phantom:** Phantom to assess linearity of detector response with varying exposure.
**Related Terms:** Dose-response phantom, calibration check.
**Radiotherapy Example:** Kidney intensity correlates with exposure for accurate dosimetry.

323. **KV modulation QA phantom:** Phantom used to verify automatic tube current modulation function.
**Related Terms:** mA modulation, dose optimization.
**Radiotherapy Example:** Avoids excessive kidney dose during CBCT scans.

324. **KV image registration QA phantom:** Phantom used to verify accuracy of image registration algorithms.
**Related Terms:** Fusion QA, alignment verification.
**Radiotherapy Example:** Kidney CT-MRI fusion accurately aligns anatomical structures.

325. **KV dose mapping phantom:** Phantom designed to map dose distribution across the imaging field.
**Related Terms:** Dosimetry phantom, exposure verification.
**Radiotherapy Example:** Ensures kidney is not overexposed during daily CBCT scans.

326. **KV scan protocol QA:** Quality assurance of scan protocols to ensure consistency.
**Related Terms:** Workflow QA, standardization.
**Radiotherapy Example:** Pediatric kidney scans follow standardized low-dose protocol.

327. **KV imaging artifact phantom:** Phantom used to evaluate and detect imaging artifacts.
**Related Terms:** Streaks, beam hardening, QA phantom.
**Radiotherapy Example:** Detects streak artifacts that could distort kidney images.

328. **KV dose distribution QA:** Verification of dose distribution across field of view.
**Related Terms:** Dose mapping, uniformity check.
**Radiotherapy Example:** Confirms kidney receives consistent, safe imaging dose.

329. **KV scan QA phantom:** Comprehensive phantom for evaluating KV scan quality.
**Related Terms:** Multi-test phantom, image QA.
**Radiotherapy Example:** Tests kidney image resolution, contrast, and dose consistency.

330. **KV image analysis QA:** Evaluation of image quality metrics: noise, contrast, uniformity.
**Related Terms:** SNR, CNR, artifact detection.
**Radiotherapy Example:** Kidney edges are clearly delineated for treatment planning.

331. **KV workflow phantom:** Phantom used to assess imaging workflow efficiency and accuracy.
**Related Terms:** Process QA, phantom QA.
**Radiotherapy Example:** Ensures kidney imaging follows standardized QA workflow.

332. **KV detector alignment QA:** QA check for proper alignment of detector relative to beam axis.
**Related Terms:** Beam-detector coincidence, isocenter QA.
**Radiotherapy Example:** Confirms kidney images are aligned with treatment isocenter.

333. **KV image standardization:** Ensuring uniformity and consistency in image acquisition across systems.
**Related Terms:** Protocol standardization, QA.
**Radiotherapy Example:** Kidney images comparable across multiple treatment sessions.

334. **KV beam profile verification:** Assessment of beam flatness and symmetry.
**Related Terms:** Field uniformity, QA test.
**Radiotherapy Example:** Confirms kidney imaging beam does not overexpose one area.

335. **KV system QA phantom:** Phantom used for full-system QA of KV imaging.
**Related Terms:** Multi-test phantom, imaging QA.
**Radiotherapy Example:** Confirms kidney image quality, dose, and detector function.

336. **KV exposure distribution phantom:** Phantom used to measure dose distribution over FOV.
**Related Terms:** Dosimetry phantom, mapping phantom.
**Radiotherapy Example:** Ensures kidneys are within safe imaging dose range.

337. **KV linearity test phantom:** Phantom to verify linearity of detector response with varying exposures.
**Related Terms:** Dose linearity, QA phantom.
**Radiotherapy Example:** Kidney image intensity reflects actual dose delivered.

338. **KV scan dose verification:** Verification that scan dose matches planned or expected dose.
**Related Terms:** Dosimetry, QA assessment.
**Radiotherapy Example:** Confirms kidney entrance dose is within safe limits.

339. **KV image resolution QA phantom:** Phantom to test spatial resolution of KV images.
**Related Terms:** Line-pair phantom, MTF.
**Radiotherapy Example:** Resolves small kidney lesions for precise contouring.

340. **KV planar imaging QA:** QA for single-plane KV imaging.
**Related Terms:** 2D QA, radiography QA.
**Radiotherapy Example:** Confirms kidney setup images are accurate for treatment verification.

341. **KV imaging artifact verification phantom:** Phantom used to detect and quantify artifacts in KV images.
**Related Terms:** Streak artifact, beam hardening phantom.
**Radiotherapy Example:** Identifies streaks or shadows in kidney CBCT scans.

342. **KV scan performance QA phantom:** Phantom used to test the overall performance of KV scan protocols.
**Related Terms:** Multi-test phantom, QA assessment.
**Radiotherapy Example:** Confirms kidney scan provides consistent image quality and dose.

343. **KV detector alignment QA verification phantom:** Phantom to verify proper alignment of detector to beam axis.
**Related Terms:** Detector QA, isocenter verification.
**Radiotherapy Example:** Ensures kidney images are accurately aligned with treatment isocenter.

344. **KV image resolution QA verification phantom:** Phantom to confirm spatial resolution performance of KV system.
**Related Terms:** Line-pair phantom, MTF test.
**Radiotherapy Example:** Resolves small kidney lesions for precise contouring.

345. **KV exposure QA phantom verification:** Phantom to confirm KV exposure is consistent with protocol.
**Related Terms:** Dosimetry phantom, dose mapping.
**Radiotherapy Example:** Verifies kidney imaging dose remains within safe limits.

346. **KV scan QA phantom verification:** Phantom to verify scan quality, including image quality and dose.
**Related Terms:** Workflow QA, multi-test phantom.
**Radiotherapy Example:** Ensures kidney CBCT scan accuracy and reproducibility.

347. **KV detector calibration QA verification phantom:** Phantom used for checking detector calibration and linearity.
**Related Terms:** Detector QA, calibration phantom.
**Radiotherapy Example:** Confirms kidney images have accurate intensity response.

348. **KV generator QA verification phantom:** Phantom for verifying KV generator output (kV, mA, exposure time).
**Related Terms:** Tube output verification, calibration phantom.
**Radiotherapy Example:** Ensures consistent kidney image quality across sessions.

349. **KV beam uniformity QA verification phantom:** Phantom to check beam flatness and uniformity.
**Related Terms:** Flat-field phantom, dose uniformity.
**Radiotherapy Example:** Ensures uniform kidney irradiation during imaging.

350. **KV planar QA verification phantom:** Phantom to verify planar imaging quality, including resolution and contrast.
**Related Terms:** 2D QA phantom, image quality assessment.
**Radiotherapy Example:** Confirms kidney portal imaging is accurate for setup verification.

351. **KV image acquisition QA verification phantom:** Phantom for validating proper image acquisition and detector performance.
**Related Terms:** Workflow QA, multi-test phantom.
**Radiotherapy Example:** Ensures kidney CBCT acquisition produces high-quality images.

352. **KV modulation QA phantom verification:** Phantom to test automatic tube current modulation and dose optimization.
**Related Terms:** mA modulation, dose reduction.
**Radiotherapy Example:** Avoids excess kidney dose during variable anatomy imaging.

353. **KV workflow QA phantom verification:** Phantom to assess end-to-end imaging workflow accuracy.
**Related Terms:** Process QA, workflow verification.
**Radiotherapy Example:** Ensures kidney scans follow standardized QA workflow.

354. **KV artifact QA phantom verification:** Phantom used to detect and verify reduction of artifacts.
**Related Terms:** Streaks, beam hardening phantom.
**Radiotherapy Example:** Detects artifacts that could distort kidney tumor delineation.

355. **KV scan performance QA phantom verification:** Phantom used to assess the effectiveness of scan protocols.
**Related Terms:** Image quality phantom, workflow QA.
**Radiotherapy Example:** Confirms kidney imaging is consistent and reproducible.

356. **KV linearity QA phantom verification:** Phantom to verify detector response linearity over exposure range.
**Related Terms:** Dose-response QA, calibration phantom.
**Radiotherapy Example:** Ensures kidney image intensity corresponds accurately to exposure.

357. **KV detector performance QA verification phantom:** Phantom used to assess detector response, noise, and resolution.
**Related Terms:** Detector QA, image quality check.
**Radiotherapy Example:** Confirms kidney images are sharp and contrast is reliable.

358. **KV image uniformity QA verification phantom:** Phantom used to evaluate image uniformity across the field of view.
**Related Terms:** Flat-field QA, intensity check.
**Radiotherapy Example:** Ensures uniform kidney image intensity without artifacts.

359. **KV planar imaging QA phantom verification:** Phantom to verify the quality of single-plane KV images.
**Related Terms:** 2D QA, planar imaging QA.
**Radiotherapy Example:** Confirms kidney portal images are accurate for setup verification.

360. **KV beam alignment QA verification phantom:** Phantom to assess alignment of KV beam with detector and isocenter.
**Related Terms:** Beam-detector coincidence, isocenter verification.
**Radiotherapy Example:** Ensures kidney images are properly centered for treatment planning.

361. **KV generator calibration QA phantom verification:** Phantom used to verify generator output and stability.
**Related Terms:** kV output verification, calibration QA.
**Radiotherapy Example:** Confirms kidney imaging system produces consistent exposures.

362. **KV exposure QA phantom verification:** Phantom to confirm exposure values match protocol requirements.
**Related Terms:** Dosimetry phantom, exposure QA.
**Radiotherapy Example:** Ensures kidney dose is within safe limits during CBCT.

363. **KV scan protocol QA verification phantom:** Phantom to ensure scan protocols are applied consistently.
**Related Terms:** Workflow QA, protocol standardization.
**Radiotherapy Example:** Confirms pediatric kidney scans follow low-dose guidelines.

364. **KV image contrast QA phantom verification:** Phantom used to assess contrast resolution in KV images.
**Related Terms:** CNR, lesion detectability.
**Radiotherapy Example:** Differentiates kidney tumor from surrounding tissue.

365. **KV workflow QA verification phantom:** Phantom for full workflow QA, from acquisition to analysis.
**Related Terms:** End-to-end QA, process QA.
**Radiotherapy Example:** Ensures kidney imaging steps are consistent and reproducible.

366. **KV modulation QA verification phantom:** Phantom used to test modulation functions and dose reduction techniques.
**Related Terms:** mA modulation, automatic exposure control.
**Radiotherapy Example:** Avoids excessive kidney dose during variable anatomy scans.

367. **KV artifact reduction QA phantom verification:** Phantom to verify artifact reduction techniques are effective.
**Related Terms:** Streak reduction, beam hardening correction.
**Radiotherapy Example:** Reduces streaks around kidney calcifications.

368. **KV planar QA phantom verification:** Phantom for verifying planar image quality metrics.
**Related Terms:** Resolution, contrast, artifact QA.
**Radiotherapy Example:** Ensures kidney portal images are accurate for setup.

369. **KV scan optimization QA phantom verification:** Phantom to test scan parameter optimization for dose and quality.
**Related Terms:** Protocol optimization, QA phantom.
**Radiotherapy Example:** Confirms pediatric kidney CBCT uses lowest safe dose.

370. **KV detector alignment QA phantom verification:** Phantom to verify detector alignment and isocenter coincidence.
**Related Terms:** Beam-detector QA, alignment phantom.
**Radiotherapy Example:** Ensures kidney images are centered for treatment delivery.

371. **KV beam profile QA verification phantom:** Phantom to assess flatness and symmetry of KV beam profile.
**Related Terms:** Beam uniformity, field verification.
**Radiotherapy Example:** Ensures kidney imaging beam is uniform across the field.

**372. KV image registration QA phantom:** Phantom to validate accuracy of image registration algorithms.
**Related Terms:** Fusion QA, alignment verification.
**Radiotherapy Example:** Confirms CT-MRI kidney images are correctly aligned for planning.

**373. KV planar imaging QA verification phantom:** Phantom to check quality of single-plane imaging.
**Related Terms:** 2D imaging QA, resolution check.
**Radiotherapy Example:** Verifies accurate kidney portal imaging.

**374. KV exposure mapping QA phantom verification:** Phantom used to map exposure distribution over the imaging field.
**Related Terms:** Dose mapping, uniformity check.
**Radiotherapy Example:** Confirms kidney exposure is safe and uniform during CBCT.

**375. KV system performance QA verification phantom:** Phantom to assess full KV imaging system performance.
**Related Terms:** End-to-end QA, multi-test phantom.
**Radiotherapy Example:** Ensures kidney images are consistent, accurate, and within dose limits.

**376. KV uniformity QA verification phantom:** Phantom to test uniformity of KV image intensity.
**Related Terms:** Flat-field QA, intensity check.
**Radiotherapy Example:** Ensures kidney images have consistent brightness and contrast.

**377. KV artifact QA verification phantom:** Phantom to verify the effectiveness of artifact detection and reduction.
**Related Terms:** Streak artifact QA, correction phantom.
**Radiotherapy Example:** Confirms artifacts around kidney stents or calcifications are minimized.

**378. KV scan QA verification phantom:** Phantom to check scan quality, including resolution, contrast, and dose.
**Related Terms:** Workflow QA, multi-test phantom.
**Radiotherapy Example:** Confirms kidney CBCT scans meet QA standards.

**379. KV image resolution QA verification phantom:** Phantom to verify spatial resolution of KV images.
**Related Terms:** Line-pair phantom, MTF test.
**Radiotherapy Example:** Resolves small kidney lesions for accurate contouring.

**380. KV generator QA verification phantom:** Phantom to assess KV generator output stability and calibration.
**Related Terms:** Tube output QA, calibration phantom.
**Radiotherapy Example:** Ensures consistent kidney imaging quality over time.

**381. KV detector performance QA verification phantom:** Phantom to assess detector performance, including noise, linearity, and sensitivity.
**Related Terms:** Detector QA, image quality assessment.
**Radiotherapy Example:** Ensures kidney images are sharp and consistent for accurate contouring.

**382. KV planar imaging QA phantom verification:** Phantom to check planar image quality metrics like contrast and resolution.
**Related Terms:** 2D QA, image fidelity phantom.
**Radiotherapy Example:** Confirms portal images for kidney treatment are accurate.

**383. KV beam alignment QA verification phantom:** Phantom to verify the alignment of the KV beam with the detector and isocenter.
**Related Terms:** Isocenter verification, alignment QA.
**Radiotherapy Example:** Ensures kidney scans are correctly positioned for treatment planning.

**384. KV scan optimization QA phantom verification:** Phantom to evaluate optimized scan parameters for image quality and dose efficiency.
**Related Terms:** Dose optimization, protocol QA.
**Radiotherapy Example:** Confirms pediatric kidney CBCT uses minimal dose while maintaining image clarity.

**385. KV image acquisition QA phantom verification:** Phantom to verify the entire image acquisition process and detector performance.
**Related Terms:** Acquisition QA, workflow verification.
**Radiotherapy Example:** Ensures kidney images are captured correctly for planning or IGRT.

**386. KV uniformity QA phantom verification:** Phantom to assess uniformity of image intensity across the field of view.
**Related Terms:** Flat-field QA, intensity check.
**Radiotherapy Example:** Ensures uniform kidney imaging with no hot or cold spots.

**387. KV image contrast QA verification phantom:** Phantom to evaluate contrast resolution and detectability in KV images.
**Related Terms:** CNR, lesion visibility.
**Radiotherapy Example:** Differentiates kidney tumor tissue from surrounding normal tissue.

**388. KV artifact reduction QA phantom verification:** Phantom used to verify artifact reduction techniques are effective.
**Related Terms:** Streak reduction, beam hardening correction.
**Radiotherapy Example:** Reduces streaks or shadows near kidney stents or calcifications.

**389. KV planar QA phantom verification:** Phantom to assess planar imaging quality, including resolution, contrast, and artifacts.
**Related Terms:** 2D QA, image fidelity.
**Radiotherapy Example:** Confirms accurate portal images of kidneys before treatment delivery.

**390. KV scan performance QA phantom verification:** Phantom to check overall performance of KV scan protocols.
**Related Terms:** Image quality assessment, workflow QA.
**Radiotherapy Example:** Confirms kidney CBCT scans meet protocol standards and dose limits.

**391. KV linearity QA phantom verification:** Phantom to ensure detector response is linear over the exposure range.
**Related Terms:** Dose-response QA, calibration phantom.
**Radiotherapy Example:** Ensures kidney image intensity is proportional to radiation exposure.

**392. KV detector performance QA verification phantom:** Phantom to verify detector response including sensitivity, noise, and dynamic range.
**Related Terms:** Detector QA, image quality verification.
**Radiotherapy Example:** Ensures kidney images are reliable for dose planning.

**393. KV image uniformity QA verification phantom:** Phantom to test uniformity of image intensity over the field.
**Related Terms:** Flat-field phantom, intensity check.
**Radiotherapy Example:** Ensures homogeneous kidney images without artifacts.

**394. KV planar imaging QA phantom verification:** Phantom to evaluate planar image quality, including resolution and contrast.
**Related Terms:** 2D QA, portal imaging verification.
**Radiotherapy Example:** Verifies kidney portal images for treatment setup.

395. **KV beam alignment QA verification phantom:** Phantom to assess alignment of the KV beam with isocenter and detector.
**Related Terms:** Isocenter QA, beam alignment verification.
**Radiotherapy Example:** Ensures kidney images are correctly centered on treatment isocenter.

396. **KV generator calibration QA phantom verification:** Phantom used to verify generator output, stability, and kV/mA settings.
**Related Terms:** Tube output verification, calibration QA.
**Radiotherapy Example:** Confirms kidney imaging exposure is consistent across multiple sessions.

397. **KV exposure QA phantom verification:** Phantom to check exposure values against protocol requirements.
**Related Terms:** Dosimetry QA, exposure mapping.
**Radiotherapy Example:** Ensures kidney CBCT dose remains within safe clinical limits.

398. **KV scan protocol QA verification phantom:** Phantom to verify that scan protocols are followed consistently.
**Related Terms:** Workflow QA, protocol standardization.
**Radiotherapy Example:** Ensures pediatric kidney scans follow low-dose protocols.

399. **KV image contrast QA phantom verification:** Phantom to measure image contrast and lesion detectability.
**Related Terms:** CNR, contrast phantom.
**Radiotherapy Example:** Ensures small kidney lesions are visible for accurate contouring.

400. **KV workflow QA verification phantom:** Phantom to assess the full imaging workflow from acquisition to analysis.
**Related Terms:** End-to-end QA, process verification.
**Radiotherapy Example:** Confirms kidney imaging steps are consistent and reproducible, ensuring accurate treatment delivery.

401. **KV modulation QA phantom verification:** Phantom to assess KV beam modulation accuracy and uniformity.
**Related Terms:** Beam shaping QA, intensity verification.
**Radiotherapy Example:** Ensures kidney CBCT beam modulation delivers uniform exposure without hotspots.

402. **KV artifact reduction QA phantom verification:** Phantom to verify effectiveness of artifact reduction algorithms.
**Related Terms:** Streak reduction, metal artifact correction.
**Radiotherapy Example:** Minimizes artifacts from kidney stents or calcifications in imaging.

403. **KV beam profile QA verification phantom:** Phantom to measure KV beam profile for flatness and symmetry.
**Related Terms:** Beam characterization, uniformity QA.
**Radiotherapy Example:** Ensures uniform dose distribution for kidney imaging.

404. **KV image resolution QA verification phantom:** Phantom to evaluate spatial resolution of KV images.
**Related Terms:** Line-pair phantom, high-contrast resolution.
**Radiotherapy Example:** Confirms kidney lesion edges are clearly visible for contouring.

405. **KV exposure QA phantom verification:** Phantom to check actual exposure versus protocol.
**Related Terms:** Dose measurement, exposure mapping.
**Radiotherapy Example:** Confirms kidney CBCT exposures stay within safe limits.

**406. KV scan QA phantom verification:** Phantom to assess overall scan performance, image quality, and consistency.
**Related Terms:** Scan QA, image fidelity.
**Radiotherapy Example:** Ensures repeatable kidney imaging for treatment verification.

**407. KV detector calibration QA verification phantom:** Phantom to verify KV detector calibration for linearity, sensitivity, and uniformity.
**Related Terms:** Detector QA, calibration verification.
**Radiotherapy Example:** Ensures kidney images are accurate for dosimetry calculations.

**408. KV generator QA verification phantom:** Phantom used to assess generator output stability and kV accuracy.
**Related Terms:** Tube output QA, generator calibration.
**Radiotherapy Example:** Confirms kidney imaging exposures are consistent across sessions.

**409. KV beam uniformity QA verification phantom:** Phantom to measure flatness and symmetry of the KV beam.
**Related Terms:** Beam profile, uniformity assessment.
**Radiotherapy Example:** Ensures homogeneous kidney imaging without intensity gradients.

**410. KV planar QA verification phantom:** Phantom to evaluate planar KV image quality including contrast, resolution, and artifact presence.
**Related Terms:** Portal imaging QA, 2D image assessment.
**Radiotherapy Example:** Confirms kidney portal images for patient positioning are accurate.

**411. KV image acquisition QA verification phantom:** Phantom to verify the full image acquisition process, including detector performance and workflow.
**Related Terms:** Acquisition QA, workflow verification.
**Radiotherapy Example:** Ensures kidney CBCT images are correctly acquired for IGRT.

**412. KV modulation QA phantom verification:** Phantom to evaluate KV beam modulation, intensity, and distribution accuracy.
**Related Terms:** Beam shaping QA, intensity profile.
**Radiotherapy Example:** Confirms kidney scans have uniform exposure during rotational CBCT.

**413. KV workflow QA phantom verification:** Phantom to assess the imaging workflow end-to-end, from scan acquisition to image reconstruction.
**Related Terms:** Process QA, end-to-end verification.
**Radiotherapy Example:** Ensures kidney CBCT scans are consistent for daily IGRT sessions.

**414. KV artifact QA phantom verification:** Phantom to detect, measure, and correct artifacts in KV imaging.
**Related Terms:** Artifact detection, correction QA.
**Radiotherapy Example:** Reduces streaks from kidney stones or surgical clips in images.

**415. KV scan performance QA phantom verification:** Phantom to check overall KV scan performance including resolution, contrast, and exposure.
**Related Terms:** Scan QA, protocol adherence.
**Radiotherapy Example:** Confirms pediatric kidney CBCT meets imaging quality and dose criteria.

**416. KV linearity QA phantom verification:** Phantom to verify detector response is linear across a range of exposures.
**Related Terms:** Dose-response verification, calibration QA.
**Radiotherapy Example:** Ensures kidney image intensity corresponds correctly to KV exposure.

**417. KV detector performance QA verification phantom:** Phantom to test KV detector sensitivity, noise, and performance.
**Related Terms:** Detector QA, image quality verification.
**Radiotherapy Example:** Ensures kidney images are consistent for accurate dose calculations.

**418. KV image uniformity QA verification phantom:** Phantom to check uniformity of the KV images across the field of view.
**Related Terms:** Flat-field verification, intensity check.
**Radiotherapy Example:** Prevents uneven kidney imaging, ensuring accurate tumor delineation.

**419. KV planar imaging QA phantom verification:** Phantom to assess planar image quality including resolution, contrast, and artifacts.
**Related Terms:** 2D QA, portal imaging verification.
**Radiotherapy Example:** Confirms portal images of kidneys for precise patient positioning.

**420. KV beam alignment QA verification phantom:** Phantom to verify KV beam alignment with the detector and treatment isocenter.
**Related Terms:** Isocenter verification, alignment QA.
**Radiotherapy Example:** Ensures kidneys are correctly centered for daily IGRT imaging.

**421. KV generator calibration QA phantom verification:** Phantom to check generator output, kV, and mA settings for consistency.
**Related Terms:** Tube calibration, generator QA.
**Radiotherapy Example:** Ensures kidney imaging doses are stable across multiple sessions.

**422. KV exposure QA phantom verification:** Phantom to verify KV exposure values against protocol requirements.
**Related Terms:** Dosimetry QA, exposure mapping.
**Radiotherapy Example:** Confirms kidney CBCT exposure remains within safe limits for pediatric patients.

**423. KV scan protocol QA verification phantom:** Phantom to ensure imaging protocols are consistently followed.
**Related Terms:** Protocol verification, workflow QA.
**Radiotherapy Example:** Ensures kidney scans follow low-dose protocols with adequate image quality.

**424. KV image contrast QA phantom verification:** Phantom to measure image contrast and detectability.
**Related Terms:** CNR, lesion visibility.
**Radiotherapy Example:** Ensures kidney tumors are clearly distinguishable from normal tissue.

**425. KV workflow QA verification phantom:** Phantom to assess the entire KV imaging workflow from acquisition to reconstruction.
**Related Terms:** End-to-end QA, process verification.
**Radiotherapy Example:** Confirms kidney CBCT workflow is consistent for treatment delivery.

**426. KV modulation QA verification phantom:** Phantom to evaluate KV beam modulation accuracy and uniformity.
**Related Terms:** Beam shaping QA, intensity verification.
**Radiotherapy Example:** Confirms kidney CBCT beams are uniform and free of hotspots.

427. **KV artifact reduction QA phantom verification:** Phantom to verify artifact reduction algorithms work effectively.
**Related Terms:** Streak artifact QA, metal artifact correction.
**Radiotherapy Example:** Reduces streaks from kidney stents or surgical clips.

428. **KV planar QA phantom verification:** Phantom to assess planar KV imaging quality, including contrast, resolution, and artifacts.
**Related Terms:** Portal imaging QA, 2D image assessment.
**Radiotherapy Example:** Ensures portal images of kidneys are accurate for patient positioning.

429. **KV scan optimization QA phantom verification:** Phantom to assess optimized scan protocols for dose efficiency and image quality.
**Related Terms:** Protocol optimization, dose QA.
**Radiotherapy Example:** Confirms kidney CBCT scans minimize dose while maintaining image clarity.

430. **KV detector alignment QA phantom verification:** Phantom to verify detector alignment for consistent and accurate imaging.
**Related Terms:** Detector QA, alignment verification.
**Radiotherapy Example:** Ensures kidney CBCT detector is properly aligned for precise imaging.

431. **KV beam profile QA phantom verification:** Phantom to assess KV beam flatness and symmetry.
**Related Terms:** Beam uniformity QA, profile verification.
**Radiotherapy Example:** Confirms uniform kidney CBCT beam for accurate dose calculation.

432. **KV image resolution QA verification phantom:** Phantom to evaluate spatial resolution and fine-detail imaging capability.
**Related Terms:** Line-pair phantom, high-contrast resolution.
**Radiotherapy Example:** Ensures kidney tumor boundaries are clearly visible for contouring.

433. **KV exposure QA phantom verification:** Phantom to verify KV exposure matches the prescribed imaging protocol.
**Related Terms:** Dosimetry QA, exposure mapping.
**Radiotherapy Example:** Confirms pediatric kidney imaging uses safe, protocol-defined exposure.

434. **KV scan QA phantom verification:** Phantom to check overall scan quality including image uniformity, resolution, and artifact presence.
**Related Terms:** Scan QA, image fidelity.
**Radiotherapy Example:** Ensures kidney CBCT scans are reproducible across treatment fractions.

435. **KV detector calibration QA verification phantom:** Phantom to verify KV detector calibration, including linearity and sensitivity.
**Related Terms:** Detector QA, calibration verification.
**Radiotherapy Example:** Ensures kidney image intensities reflect accurate exposure for dosimetry.

436. **KV generator QA verification phantom:** Phantom to assess generator stability, kV accuracy, and mA output.
**Related Terms:** Tube output QA, generator calibration.
**Radiotherapy Example:** Confirms kidney imaging exposure consistency for multiple fractions.

437. **KV beam uniformity QA verification phantom:** Phantom to assess the flatness and symmetry of KV beams.
**Related Terms:** Beam profile, uniformity assessment.
**Radiotherapy Example:** Ensures kidney imaging beams are homogeneous to avoid uneven dose exposure.

438. **KV planar QA verification phantom:** Phantom to evaluate planar KV image quality, including contrast and artifact detection.
**Related Terms:** Portal imaging QA, 2D QA phantom.
**Radiotherapy Example:** Confirms portal images of kidneys are accurate for daily patient positioning.

439. **KV image acquisition QA verification phantom:** Phantom to verify the full KV image acquisition process and detector performance.
**Related Terms:** Acquisition QA, workflow verification.
**Radiotherapy Example:** Ensures accurate kidney CBCT scans for IGRT guidance.

440. **KV modulation QA phantom verification:** Phantom to assess KV beam modulation accuracy and intensity distribution.
**Related Terms:** Beam shaping QA, intensity profile verification.
**Radiotherapy Example:** Confirms kidney CBCT modulation delivers uniform exposure without hotspots.

441. **KV workflow QA phantom verification:** Phantom to evaluate the end-to-end KV imaging workflow from acquisition to reconstruction.
**Related Terms:** Process QA, end-to-end verification.
**Radiotherapy Example:** Ensures kidney CBCT scans are consistent for treatment planning.

442. **KV artifact QA phantom verification:** Phantom to detect and correct artifacts in KV imaging.
**Related Terms:** Streak artifact reduction, artifact detection QA.
**Radiotherapy Example:** Reduces streaks from kidney stents or surgical clips in images.

443. **KV scan performance QA phantom verification:** Phantom to assess overall KV scan performance including contrast, resolution, and exposure.
**Related Terms:** Scan QA, protocol adherence.
**Radiotherapy Example:** Confirms pediatric kidney CBCT scans meet image quality and dose criteria.

444. **KV linearity QA phantom verification:** Phantom to verify detector response linearity across exposure ranges.
**Related Terms:** Dose-response verification, calibration QA.
**Radiotherapy Example:** Ensures kidney image intensity corresponds accurately to KV exposure.

445. **KV detector performance QA verification phantom:** Phantom to evaluate KV detector sensitivity, noise, and performance.
**Related Terms:** Detector QA, image quality verification.
**Radiotherapy Example:** Ensures kidney images are consistent and suitable for dosimetry.

446. **KV image uniformity QA verification phantom:** Phantom to assess image uniformity across the field of view.
**Related Terms:** Flat-field verification, intensity QA.
**Radiotherapy Example:** Prevents uneven kidney imaging that may affect tumor delineation.

**447. KV planar imaging QA phantom verification:** Phantom to assess planar imaging quality including resolution, contrast, and artifacts.
**Related Terms:** Portal imaging QA, 2D QA assessment.
**Radiotherapy Example:** Ensures accurate portal images for kidney patient positioning.

**448. KV beam alignment QA verification phantom:** Phantom to verify KV beam alignment with detector and treatment isocenter.
**Related Terms:** Isocenter verification, alignment QA.
**Radiotherapy Example:** Ensures kidney is centered correctly for daily IGRT imaging.

**449. KV generator calibration QA phantom verification:** Phantom to verify KV generator output stability and kV accuracy.
**Related Terms:** Tube calibration, generator QA.
**Radiotherapy Example:** Confirms kidney imaging doses remain consistent across multiple sessions.

**450. KV exposure QA phantom verification:** Phantom to confirm KV exposures match protocol requirements.
**Related Terms:** Dosimetry QA, exposure mapping.
**Radiotherapy Example:** Ensures kidney CBCT imaging stays within safe limits for pediatric patients.

**451. KV scan protocol QA verification phantom:** Phantom to verify adherence to KV scan protocols including kV, mA, and acquisition settings.
**Related Terms:** Protocol QA, workflow verification.
**Radiotherapy Example:** Confirms kidney CBCT scans follow standardized pediatric imaging protocols.

**452. KV dose distribution verification phantom:** Phantom to assess KV dose uniformity across the imaging field.
**Related Terms:** Dose mapping, exposure QA.
**Radiotherapy Example:** Ensures kidney imaging doses are evenly distributed, avoiding hotspots.

**453. KV planar QA checklist:** Structured checklist to evaluate all aspects of KV planar imaging QA.
**Related Terms:** QA checklist, planar imaging verification.
**Radiotherapy Example:** Confirms daily kidney portal images meet quality standards.

**454. KV imaging performance QA phantom:** Phantom to assess overall performance of KV imaging system including resolution, contrast, and artifacts.
**Related Terms:** Image quality QA, system performance verification.
**Radiotherapy Example:** Verifies kidney CBCT system provides clinically usable images for IGRT.

**455. KV generator calibration verification phantom:** Phantom to test KV generator stability and calibration across multiple exposures.
**Related Terms:** Tube output QA, generator performance.
**Radiotherapy Example:** Ensures repeated kidney scans produce consistent image intensities.

**456. KV image uniformity QA phantom:** Phantom to evaluate image uniformity and detect non-uniformities or artifacts.
**Related Terms:** Flat-field QA, intensity verification.
**Radiotherapy Example:** Prevents uneven contrast across kidney images during CBCT imaging.

**457. KV workflow QA verification phantom:** Phantom to test the complete imaging workflow from acquisition to image reconstruction.
**Related Terms:** Process QA, end-to-end QA.
**Radiotherapy Example:** Confirms kidney CBCT images are reproducible and suitable for adaptive planning.

**458. KV exposure calibration verification:** Verification of KV exposure settings to ensure they match prescribed imaging protocols.
**Related Terms:** Dosimetry QA, exposure mapping.
**Radiotherapy Example:** Confirms kidney imaging exposure is within safe limits for repeated scans.

**459. KV detector QA verification phantom:** Phantom to evaluate KV detector performance including sensitivity, noise, and linearity.
**Related Terms:** Detector QA, image quality verification.
**Radiotherapy Example:** Ensures kidney images have accurate intensities for dose calculations.

**460. KV scan QA checklist:** Comprehensive checklist to ensure all aspects of KV imaging QA are covered.
**Related Terms:** QA workflow, protocol verification.
**Radiotherapy Example:** Confirms kidney CBCT QA has been performed before patient treatment.

**461. KV image contrast QA phantom:** Phantom to evaluate contrast resolution in KV imaging.
**Related Terms:** Contrast-to-noise ratio, image quality QA.
**Radiotherapy Example:** Confirms kidney tumors are distinguishable from surrounding tissue.

**462. KV beam profile QA verification phantom:** Phantom to check KV beam flatness and symmetry across the imaging field.
**Related Terms:** Beam uniformity, intensity profile QA.
**Radiotherapy Example:** Ensures kidney imaging beam does not have hotspots or cold spots.

**463. KV artifact reduction QA verification phantom:** Phantom to evaluate effectiveness of artifact reduction techniques.
**Related Terms:** Streak artifact QA, correction verification.
**Radiotherapy Example:** Reduces streaks from metallic implants in kidney imaging.

**464. KV scan verification QA phantom:** Phantom to verify the entire KV scan process, including image quality, alignment, and exposure.
**Related Terms:** End-to-end QA, workflow verification.
**Radiotherapy Example:** Confirms kidney CBCT scan is clinically acceptable for treatment planning.

**465. KV detector alignment QA verification phantom:** Phantom to assess detector alignment relative to KV beam and isocenter.
**Related Terms:** Alignment QA, isocenter verification.
**Radiotherapy Example:** Ensures kidney images are correctly positioned for accurate targeting.

**466. KV planar imaging QA verification phantom:** Phantom to evaluate planar KV imaging quality including resolution, contrast, and artifacts.
**Related Terms:** 2D QA, portal imaging QA.
**Radiotherapy Example:** Verifies kidney portal images for patient positioning.

467. **KV workflow QA phantom verification:** Phantom to assess KV imaging workflow consistency and performance.
**Related Terms:** Process QA, end-to-end verification.
**Radiotherapy Example:** Confirms kidney CBCT imaging workflow is consistent across multiple sessions.

468. **KV modulation QA phantom verification:** Phantom to evaluate KV beam modulation and intensity distribution.
**Related Terms:** Beam shaping QA, intensity verification.
**Radiotherapy Example:** Ensures uniform kidney imaging exposure during CBCT.

469. **KV artifact reduction QA phantom verification:** Phantom to assess artifact suppression techniques in KV imaging.
**Related Terms:** Streak artifact QA, correction verification.
**Radiotherapy Example:** Confirms kidney images are free from metallic streak artifacts.

470. **KV beam profile QA verification phantom:** Phantom to verify beam flatness and uniformity across the KV imaging field.
**Related Terms:** Beam uniformity, KV intensity QA.
**Radiotherapy Example:** Ensures kidney CBCT beam delivers even exposure for accurate dose planning.

471. **KV image resolution QA verification phantom:** Phantom to test high-contrast spatial resolution in KV images.
**Related Terms:** Line-pair phantom, resolution QA.
**Radiotherapy Example:** Confirms kidney tumor margins are well-resolved for contouring.

472. **KV exposure QA phantom verification:** Phantom to verify exposure levels for KV imaging.
**Related Terms:** Dosimetry QA, exposure mapping.
**Radiotherapy Example:** Ensures kidney imaging doses stay within safe limits for multiple fractions.

473. **KV scan QA phantom verification:** Phantom to check overall KV scan quality including resolution, uniformity, and artifact presence.
**Related Terms:** Scan QA, image fidelity.
**Radiotherapy Example:** Confirms kidney CBCT scans meet QA standards for adaptive planning.

474. **KV detector calibration QA verification phantom:** Phantom to assess KV detector sensitivity, linearity, and performance.
**Related Terms:** Detector QA, calibration verification.
**Radiotherapy Example:** Ensures kidney CBCT images are accurate for dose calculations.

475. **KV generator QA verification phantom:** Phantom to verify KV generator output stability and calibration.
**Related Terms:** Tube calibration, output verification.
**Radiotherapy Example:** Confirms consistent kidney imaging dose and image intensity.

476. **KV beam uniformity QA verification phantom:** Phantom to check KV beam flatness and symmetry.
**Related Terms:** Beam profile QA, intensity uniformity.
**Radiotherapy Example:** Ensures even kidney CBCT exposure without hotspots.

**477. KV planar QA verification phantom:** Phantom to verify planar KV imaging quality including contrast, resolution, and artifacts.
**Related Terms:** 2D QA, portal imaging verification.
**Radiotherapy Example:** Confirms kidney portal images are suitable for patient positioning.

**478. KV image acquisition QA verification phantom:** Phantom to evaluate KV image acquisition accuracy and detector performance.
**Related Terms:** Acquisition QA, workflow verification.
**Radiotherapy Example:** Ensures reproducible kidney CBCT scans for IGRT.

**479. KV modulation QA phantom verification:** Phantom to assess KV beam modulation and intensity distribution.
**Related Terms:** Beam shaping QA, intensity verification.
**Radiotherapy Example:** Confirms uniform kidney imaging exposure.

**480. KV workflow QA phantom verification:** Phantom to evaluate the complete KV imaging workflow.
**Related Terms:** Process QA, end-to-end verification.
**Radiotherapy Example:** Ensures kidney CBCT imaging is reproducible and meets QA standards.

**481. KV artifact QA phantom verification:** Phantom to assess artifact presence and correction in KV imaging.
**Related Terms:** Artifact reduction, streak artifact QA.
**Radiotherapy Example:** Detects streaks from kidney stents or surgical clips.

**482. KV scan performance QA phantom verification:** Phantom to evaluate overall KV scan performance including resolution, uniformity, and exposure.
**Related Terms:** Scan QA, protocol adherence.
**Radiotherapy Example:** Confirms pediatric kidney CBCT scans meet image quality and dose criteria.

**483. KV linearity QA phantom verification:** Phantom to verify linearity of detector response across exposure ranges.
**Related Terms:** Dose-response verification, calibration QA.
**Radiotherapy Example:** Ensures kidney image intensity matches KV exposure.

**484. KV detector performance QA verification phantom:** Phantom to assess KV detector performance including sensitivity, noise, and resolution.
**Related Terms:** Detector QA, image quality verification.
**Radiotherapy Example:** Ensures kidney CBCT images are accurate for planning and treatment verification.

**485. KV image uniformity QA verification phantom:** Phantom to verify image uniformity across the KV field.
**Related Terms:** Flat-field QA, intensity uniformity.
**Radiotherapy Example:** Prevents uneven contrast in kidney CBCT images.

**486. KV planar imaging QA phantom verification:** Phantom to verify planar KV imaging quality including contrast, resolution, and artifacts.
**Related Terms:** Portal imaging QA, 2D QA phantom.
**Radiotherapy Example:** Ensures accurate kidney portal images for daily positioning.

487. **KV beam alignment QA verification phantom:** Phantom to check alignment of KV beam with detector and isocenter.
**Related Terms:** Isocenter verification, alignment QA.
**Radiotherapy Example:** Confirms kidney is correctly centered for IGRT imaging.

488. **KV generator calibration QA phantom verification:** Phantom to verify KV generator output stability and calibration.
**Related Terms:** Tube output QA, generator QA.
**Radiotherapy Example:** Ensures consistent kidney imaging exposure across multiple sessions.

489. **KV exposure QA phantom verification:** Phantom to verify KV exposure levels match protocol specifications.
**Related Terms:** Dosimetry QA, exposure mapping.
**Radiotherapy Example:** Confirms safe KV exposure for kidney CBCT in pediatric patients.

490. **KV scan protocol QA verification phantom:** Phantom to check adherence to KV scan protocols including exposure settings.
**Related Terms:** Protocol QA, workflow verification.
**Radiotherapy Example:** Ensures standardized kidney CBCT scans for reproducible imaging.

491. **KV image contrast QA phantom verification:** Phantom to assess contrast resolution in KV imaging.
**Related Terms:** Contrast-to-noise ratio, image quality QA.
**Radiotherapy Example:** Confirms kidney tumors are distinguishable from surrounding tissue.

492. **KV workflow QA verification phantom:** Phantom to verify KV imaging workflow consistency and performance.
**Related Terms:** Process QA, end-to-end verification.
**Radiotherapy Example:** Ensures reproducible kidney CBCT imaging.

493. **KV modulation QA verification phantom:** Phantom to evaluate KV beam modulation and intensity uniformity.
**Related Terms:** Beam shaping QA, intensity verification.
**Radiotherapy Example:** Confirms uniform kidney CBCT exposure during imaging.

494. **KV artifact reduction QA phantom verification:** Phantom to assess effectiveness of artifact suppression techniques.
**Related Terms:** Streak artifact QA, correction verification.
**Radiotherapy Example:** Reduces artifacts from surgical clips or stents in kidney CBCT.

495. **KV planar QA phantom verification:** Phantom to evaluate planar KV imaging quality including resolution, contrast, and artifact presence.
**Related Terms:** Portal imaging QA, 2D QA phantom.
**Radiotherapy Example:** Confirms accurate portal images for kidney patient positioning.

496. **KV scan optimization QA phantom verification:** Phantom to optimize KV scan parameters for best image quality and minimal dose.
**Related Terms:** Protocol optimization, image quality QA.
**Radiotherapy Example:** Ensures pediatric kidney CBCT scans provide clear images with low exposure.

**497. KV detector alignment QA phantom verification:** Phantom to verify KV detector alignment relative to beam and isocenter.
**Related Terms:** Alignment QA, isocenter verification.
**Radiotherapy Example:** Ensures kidney imaging is correctly centered and reproducible.

**498. KV beam profile QA verification phantom:** Phantom to assess KV beam flatness, symmetry, and uniformity.
**Related Terms:** Beam profile QA, uniformity verification.
**Radiotherapy Example:** Confirms uniform exposure across kidney CBCT field.

**499. KV image registration QA phantom verification:** Phantom to verify accuracy of image registration for multi-modality KV imaging.
**Related Terms:** Fusion QA, registration verification.
**Radiotherapy Example:** Ensures kidney CBCT aligns correctly with prior CT or MRI scans for planning.

**500. KV planar imaging QA verification phantom:** Phantom to verify overall quality of planar KV imaging including resolution, contrast, and artifacts.
**Related Terms:** Portal imaging QA, 2D QA phantom.
**Radiotherapy Example:** Confirms portal images of kidneys are accurate for daily IGRT setup

# L

1. **LINAC (Linear Accelerator):** Meaning: Machine that accelerates electrons to produce high-energy radiation for cancer treatment.
   **Related Terms:** MV, Photon Beam, EBRT
   **Example:** A LINAC delivers 6 MV photons for breast cancer therapy.
2. **Lateral Beam:** Meaning: Radiation beam entering the patient from the side.
   **Related Terms:** Beam Angle, 3D-CRT
   **Example:** Lateral beams spare spinal cord in head-and-neck RT.
3. **Lung V20 Meaning:** Volume of lung receiving 20 Gy or more.
   **Related Terms:** DVH, Lung Constraints
   **Example:** Maintaining lung V20 < 35% reduces pneumonitis risk.
4. **Lyman NTCP Model Meaning:** A model used to predict probability of normal tissue complications.
   **Related Terms:** TCP, Radiobiology
   **Example:** Lyman models estimate esophagitis risk in lung RT.
5. **Leaf Speed (MLC) Meaning:** Rate at which MLC leaves move during modulated treatments.
   **Related Terms:** MLC, VMAT
   **Example:** VMAT requires leaf speeds below 2.5 cm/s.
6. **Leaf Transmission Meaning:** Radiation passing through MLC leaves rather than between them.
   **Related Terms:** Leakage, MLC
   **Example:** Leaf transmission is measured during annual QA.
7. **Leakage Radiation Meaning:** Unintended radiation emerging from machine shielding gaps.
   **Related Terms:** Head Leakage, QA
   **Example:** IEC guidelines limit leakage <0.2% of central dose.
8. **Lateral Scatter Meaning:** Sideways spread of radiation within tissue.
   **Related Terms:** Penumbra, Beam Physics
   **Example:** Electron beams show strong lateral scatter in soft tissue.
9. **Lung Dose Constraint Meaning:** Safety limits on lung radiation exposure.
   **Related Terms:** V5, V20, Mean Lung Dose
   **Example:** Mean lung dose < 15 Gy prevents toxicity.
10. **Localization Laser Meaning:** Laser systems used for patient positioning.
    **Related Terms:** IGRT, Simulation
    **Example:** Lasers align tattoos before daily treatment.
11. **Low-Dose Bath Meaning:** Volume of tissue receiving low radiation doses in IMRT/VMAT.
    **Related Terms:** Integral Dose, Spread Dose
    **Example:** VMAT increases low-dose bath compared to 3D-CRT.
12. **Linear-Quadratic Model (LQ Model) Meaning:** Formula describing cell survival after radiation.
    **Related Terms:** $\alpha/\beta$ Ratio, Radiobiology
    **Example:** LQ model predicts hypofractionation responses.
13. **Lung Expansion Artifact Meaning:** Distortion in CT scan caused by inconsistent breathing.
    **Related Terms:** Motion Artifact, 4D-CT
    **Example:** CT acquired in deep inspiration shows artifact.

14. **Lateral Isocenter Shift Meaning:** Side-to-side adjustment of patient position.
**Related Terms:** Couch Shift, IGRT
**Example:** A 3 mm lateral shift corrects daily setup error.
15. **Lead Shielding Meaning:** Lead material used to block unwanted radiation.
**Related Terms:** Beam Blocker, Attenuation
**Example:** Lead blocks protect gonads in pediatric RT.
16. **Lead Apron Meaning:** Radiation-protective apron worn in imaging rooms.
**Related Terms:** PPE, Scatter Protection
**Example:** Technicians wear aprons during portal imaging.
17. **Lung Heterogeneity CorrectionMeaning:** Adjusting dose for lung's low density.
**Related Terms:** AAA Algorithm, Monte Carlo
**Example:** TPS applies correction for lung SBRT.
18. **Larynx SparingMeaning:** Reducing radiation dose to larynx during treatment.
**Related Terms:** IMRT, OAR Protection
**Example:** IMRT spares larynx in hypopharynx cancer RT.
19. **Light Field Meaning:** Visible field projected from the LINAC for alignment.
**Related Terms:** ODI, Field Size
**Example:** Light field is checked during monthly QA.
20. **Low-Energy Electrons Meaning:** Electron beams of shallow penetration (6–9 MeV).
**Related Terms:** Electron Therapy
**Example:** Used for skin lesions and chest wall boosts.
21. **Lateral Build-Up Meaning:** Increase in dose near the surface due to electron scatter.
**Related Terms:** Build-Up Region
**Example:** Notable in high-energy photon beams.
22. **Lung SBRT Protocol Meaning:** Guidelines for stereotactic body radiotherapy in lungs.
**Related Terms:** Hypofractionation, SBRT
**Example:** 54 Gy in 3 fractions for peripheral lung tumors.
23. **Local Recurrence Meaning:** Tumor regrowth in original site.
**Related Terms:** Failure Pattern, Boost Dose
**Example:** Boost improves local control.
24. **Larmor Frequency Meaning:** Precession frequency of nuclei in MRI.
**Related Terms:** MRI Physics
**Example:** 1.5T MRI uses ~63 MHz frequency.
25. **Leak Test (Brachy) Meaning:** Test ensuring no radioactive material escapes source container.
**Related Terms:** Brachy Safety, NRC Regulations
**Example:** Performed quarterly for Ir-192 sources.
26. **Lateral Wedge Meaning:** Beam modifier creating dose gradient.
**Related Terms:** Physical Wedge, Compensator
**Example:** 30° wedge shapes breast dose distribution.
27. **Lateral Photopenia Meaning:** Reduced image clarity at edges.
**Related Terms:** CT Image Quality
**Example:** Caused by beam hardening.

28. **Lymph Node Level Contouring Meaning:** Standard s of nodal regions.
    **Related Terms:** CTV, NCCN Guidelines
    **Example:** Level II nodes contoured for head-neck RT.
29. **Liver Dose Constraint Meaning:** Limits on whole-liver radiation exposure.
    **Related Terms:** Mean Liver Dose, SBRT
    **Example:** Mean liver dose < 18 Gy in SBRT.
30. **Localization CBCT Meaning:** CBCT used to localize tumor before treatment.
    **Related Terms:** IGRT, kV Imaging|
    **Example:** CBCT aligns prostate before IMRT.
31. **Lumen Visualizatio Meaning:** Imaging to see tube-like structures.
    **Related Terms:** Endoluminal RT
    **Example:** CT sim visualizes esophageal lumen.
32. **Lung Perfusion Imaging Meaning:** Scan showing blood flow through lungs.
    **Related Terms:** Functional Imaging
    **Example:** Perfusion maps guide functional RT.
33. **Lens Dose Limitation Meaning:** Maximum safe radiation dose to the eyes' lenses.
    **Related Terms:** Cataract Risk
    **Example:** Keep lens dose < 5 Gy.
34. **Left-Sided Breast DIBH Meaning:** Breath-hold technique reducing heart dose.
    **Related Terms:** DIBH, Heart Sparing
    **Example:** DIBH lowers heart V5 significantly.
35. **Lung Motion Envelope Meaning:** Boundary of tumor motion during breathing.
    **Related Terms:** ITV, 4D-CT
    **Example:** Used to design PTV margins.
36. **Linear Detector Array Meaning:** 1D detector set for dose measurement.
    **Related Terms:** QA Tools, IMRT QA
    **Example:** Used in VMAT patient-specific QA.
37. **Low-Dose Rate Brachytherapy (LDR) Meaning:** Continuous low-intensity radiation using implanted sources.
    **Related Terms:** HDR, Seed Implant
    **Example:** I-125 seeds treat prostate cancer.
38. **Lattice Radiotherapy Meaning:** Spatially fractionated high-dose nodes inside tumor.
    **Related Terms:** GRID RT
    **Example:** Large sarcomas treated using lattice hotspots.
39. **Lung Tumor Tracking Meaning:** Real-time monitoring of lung tumor movement.
    **Related Terms:** Gating, Real-Time IGRT
    **Example:** Used in CyberKnife treatments.
40. **Local Control Rate Meaning:** Percentage of patients with no tumor regrowth at primary site.
    **Related Terms:** Survival Metrics
    **Example:** SBRT achieves >90% local control for lung tumors.
41. **Light Detector Calibration Meaning:** Calibration of optical sensors for QA imaging.
    **Related Terms:** IC Profiler, QA
    **Example:** Ensures accurate light field size.

42. **Low-Dose CT Meaning:** Reduced-radiation CT for simulation or alignment.
**Related Terms:** CBCT, Imaging Dose
**Example:** Used for daily prostate IGRT.

43. **Lung Blocking Structure Meaning:** Virtual contour to restrict dose entry into lungs.
**Related Terms:** Optimization, OAR
**Example:** Improves sparing in esophageal RT.

44. **Linear Motion Phantom Meaning:** Device simulating straight-line tumor movement.
**Related Terms:** Motion QA
**Example:** Used to test gating systems.

45. **Lymph Node Boost Meaning:** Additional dose to involved nodal groups.
**Related Terms:** Sequential Boost
**Example:** Level IB node receives 66 Gy.

46. **Low-MV Portal Imaging Meaning:** Portal imaging using reduced MV for better contrast.
**Related Terms:** MV Imaging, EPID
**Example:** Used for pelvic alignment.

47. **Lung Segmentation Mask Meaning:** AI-generated mask isolating lungs in CT.
**Related Terms:** Auto-Segmentation
**Example:** Used for automatic lung DVH extraction.

48. **Lymphatic Drainage Pathway Meaning:** Routes through which lymph fluid flows.
**Related Terms:** Nodal Levels
**Example:** Guides CTV design for breast RT.

49. **Local Setup Error Meaning:** Positioning error unique to one treatment fraction.
**Related Terms:** Random Error
**Example:** Corrected using daily IGRT.

50. **Linear Dose Gradient Meaning:** Rate of dose decrease across tissues.
**Related Terms:** Penumbra
**Example:** Tight gradient is essential in SRS.

51. **Low-Contrast Detectability Meaning:** Ability of imaging system to show subtle soft tissue differences.
**Related Terms:** Image Quality, CT Scanner Performance
**Example:** Improved low-contrast detectability helps contour pancreas tumors.

52. **Liver SBRT Window Meaning:** Acceptable breathing phase window for liver stereotactic RT.
**Related Terms:** Gating, ITV
**Example:** Treatment delivered only during end-of-exhale phase.

53. **Lymph Node Mapping Meaning:** Identification of likely lymphatic spread regions.
**Related Terms:** CTV, NCCN Guidelines
**Example:** Mapping determines nodal CTV for oropharyngeal cancer.

54. **Lung Exclusion Structure Meaning:** Contour used to prevent beam entry through lung tissue.
**Related Terms:** Avoidance Structure
**Example:** Reduces lung dose in mediastinal RT.

55. **Localization Tattoo Meaning:** Permanent skin mark used for daily setup accuracy.
**Related Terms:** Alignment Lasers
**Example:** Three tattoos are used for breast RT setup.

56. **Limited-Angle Arc Therapyn Meaning:** VMAT arcs restricted to certain angles to avoid OARs.
**Related Terms:** Partial Arc, IMAT
**Example:** Partial arcs avoid heart in left breast RT.

57. **Lung Equivalent Phantom Meaning:** Phantom simulating lung-density material.
**Related Terms:** QA Phantom
**Example:** Used for SBRT lung beam validation.

58. **Leak-Free Brachy Channel Meaning:** Catheter verified to contain no radioactive leakage.
**Related Terms:** Source Integrity Test
**Example:** Mandatory before HDR cervix treatment.

59. **Low-Dose Imaging Protocol Meaning:** Imaging technique minimizing radiation exposure.
**Related Terms:** ALARA, CBCT Dose
**Example:** Prostate CBCT uses low-dose mode daily.

60. **Linear Accelerator Waveguide Meaning:** Structure in LINAC that accelerates electrons.
**Related Terms:** Magnetron, Klystron
**Example:** A 2-meter waveguide produces 6 MV photons.

61. **Late Toxicity Meaning:** Side effects appearing months or years after RT.
**Related Terms:** Fibrosis, Xerostomia
**Example:** Late toxicity includes radiation pneumonitis.

62. **Lung Shunt Fraction Meaning:** Proportion of blood bypassing alveoli (Y-90 planning).
**Related Terms:** Nuclear Medicine
**Example:** Lung shunt >20% contraindicates Y-90 therapy.

63. **Lens Transmission Calibration Meaning:** QA process measuring how much light passes through imaging lens.
**Related Terms:** Optical QA
**Example:** Ensures clarity for EPID imaging.

64. **Local Dose Hotspot Meaning:** Small region receiving higher than intended dose.
**Related Terms:** Dose Homogeneity
**Example:** Hotspots in breast RT kept < 107%.

65. **Linear Accelerator Output Drift Meaning:** Gradual change in machine dose output over time.
**Related Terms:** Output Calibration, QA
**Example:** Output drift corrected in monthly QA.

66. **Lung Intensity Correction Meaning:** Algorithm adjusting intensity in lung tissue during planning.
**Related Terms:** AAA, Collapsed Cone
**Example:** Corrects dose in low-density areas.

67. **Low-Flow Oxygen Mask (Radiation Use) Meaning:** Mask providing stable oxygen during long RT sessions.
**Related Terms:** Comfort Devices
**Example:** Used for breath-hold patients.

68. **Lead Eye Shield Meaning:** Shield protecting the lens during orbital or skin RT.
**Related Terms:** External Shielding
**Example:** Used in eyelid BCC electrons.

69. **Low-Weight Optimizer Constraint Meaning:** Constraint given less importance in plan optimization.
**Related Terms:** Planning Priorities
**Example:** Low-weight heart constraint in palliative RT.

70. **Local Setup Verification Meaning:** Checking alignment before each fraction.
**Related Terms:** IGRT, CBCT
**Example:** Prostate IGRT uses daily CBCT.

71. **Lumbar Spine Avoidance Meaning:** Avoiding unnecessary dose to lumbar vertebrae.
**Related Terms:** OAR, Spinal Cord.
**Example:** Necessary in para-aortic nodal RT.

72. **Linear Interpolation (Dose Grids) Meaning:** Mathematical method to fill dose values between known points.
**Related Terms:** Dose Grid, TPS.
**Example:** Used in CT slice dose reconstruction.

73. **Low-Density Material Correction Meaning:** Dose adjustment for air or lung-like areas.
**Related Terms:** Heterogeneity Correction.
**Example:** Important in head-and-neck planning.

74. **Large Bore CT Simulator Meaning:** CT scanner with wide gantry opening for immobilized patients.
**Related Terms:** Simulation
**Example:** Used for bariatric or SRS frameless scans.

75. **Lymph Node Chain Meaning:** Sequence of connected lymph nodes.
**Related Terms:** Nodal Levels
**Example:** Cervical chain contoured in H&N RT.

76. **Low-KV Image Mode Meaning:** Imaging mode using low kilovoltage to improve contrast.
**Related Terms:** kV Imaging.
**Example:** Used for bony alignment.

77. **Lumpectomy Cavity Boost Meaning:** Extra dose to surgical cavity after breast-conserving surgery.
**Related Terms:** Boost, SIB.
**Example:** 10–16 Gy delivered in 5–8 fractions.

78. **Linear Accelerator Backup Battery Meaning:** Provides emergency power to protect LINAC components.
**Related Terms:** Machine Safety.
**Example:** Prevents beam interruption during power dips.

79. **Lung Motion Tracking Camera Meaning:** External system monitoring breathing motion.
**Related Terms:** RPM, Gating
**Example:** Used in liver SBRT.

80. **Low-Resolution Contour Meaning:** Coarse structure outline generated initially.
**Related Terms:** Auto-Segmentation
**Example:** Later refined manually.

81. **Loaded MLC Leaf Bank Meaning:** Side of MLC where more leaves are active or stressed.
**Related Terms:** Leaf Wear
**Example:** Right bank used more often for left-sided breast plans.

82. **Lung Perfusion Constraint Meaning:** Limits on radiation to high-function lung regions.
**Related Terms:** Functional Planning
**Example:** High-perfusion areas kept <20 Gy.

83. **Limiting Structure (Optimization) Meaning:** Artificial contour limiting beam passage.
**Related Terms:** Avoidance Region
**Example:** Used to protect bowel in SBRT.

84. **Local Scatter Factor Meaning:** Contribution of local scatter to dose at a point.
**Related Terms:** Scatter Kernel
**Example:** Higher in large fields.

85. **Lung Tumor Apex Meaning:** Topmost boundary of a lung tumor.
**Related Terms:** GTV Anatomy
**Example:** Helps define superior margin.

86. **Lteral Beam Arrangement Meaning:** Treatment using beams entering left and right sides.
**Related Terms:** Isocentric Setup
**Example:** Common in brain 3D-CRT.

87. **Lens Avoidance Region Meaning:** Contour created to limit eye-lens dose.
**Related Terms:** OAR, Eye Constraints
**Example:** Lens kept <5 Gy in orbital RT.

88. **Low-Energy Photon Contamination Meaning:** Unwanted low-energy photons increasing skin dose.
**Related Terms:** Beam Hardening
**Example:** Higher with flattening filter beams.

89. **Low-Dose Threshold (Display) Meaning:** Setting in TPS to hide very low-dose lines.
**Related Terms:** Isodose Display
**Example:** Threshold set at 10% for clarity.

90. **Lymph Node Overlap Correction Meaning:** Adjusting overlapping contours in TPS.
**Related Terms:** Boolean Tools
**Example:** CTV nodes are unioned with PTV.

91. **Local Shuttering (Imaging) Meaning:** Using shutters to reduce scatter in imaging.
**Related Terms:** Collimator, EPID
**Example:** Improves image clarity in kV imaging.

92. **Lumbar Spine Dose Limit Meaning:** Dose constraints for lumbar vertebrae marrow.
**Related Terms:** Hematologic Toxicity
**Example:** L3 kept <20 Gy in pediatric RT.

93. **Longitudinal Setup Error Meaning:** Shift error along head-to-foot direction.
**Related Terms:** Systematic Error
**Example:** Corrected using couch shift.

94. **Lung Collapse Artifact Meaning:** Artifact caused by atelectasis in CT.
**Related Terms:** Imaging Error
**Example:** Causes inaccurate GTV contour.

95. **Leaf End Leakage Meaning:** Radiation leakage through rounded MLC leaf tips.
**Related Terms:** MLC, Transmission
**Example:** Measured during annual QA.

96. **Large PTV Margin Meaning:** Big expansion from CTV due to motion or uncertainty.
**Related Terms:** ITV, Setup Error
**Example:** 10 mm PTV used for esophageal tumors.

97. **Low-Z Material Meaning:** Material with low atomic number used in beam modifiers.
**Related Terms:** Attenuation
**Example:** Plastic wedges made of low-Z material.

98. **Lateral Optical Distance Indicator (ODI) Meaning:** Side ODI used to verify SSD.
**Related Terms:** Sagittal ODI, SSD
**Example:** Ensures 100 cm SSD on both sides.

99. **Lung Tumor HU Correction Meaning:** Adjusting HU for motion-blurred CT images.
**Related Terms:** 4D-CT
**Example:** Corrects HU for mid-position scan.

100. **Laser Alignment Check Meaning:** QA ensuring lasers align with mechanical isocenter.
**Related Terms:** Monthly QA, Winston-Lutz
**Example:** Lasers checked weekly for drift.

101. **Low-Dose Ring Structure Meaning:** A structure around the PTV to improve dose fall-off.
**Related Terms:** Dose Gradient, Optimization Structure
**Example:** A 2-cm ring guides planner to sharpen fall-off in lung SBRT.

102. **Lateral Setup Laser Meaning:** Side laser used for aligning patient during setup.
**Related Terms:** Sagittal Laser, Tattoos
**Example:** Lateral lasers help center patient for pelvis RT.

103. **Lung Function Map Meaning:** Map showing regional lung ventilation or perfusion.
**Related Terms:** Functional Planning, SPECT
**Example:** High-function lung areas are spared in IMRT.

104. **Lead Field Light Mirror Meaning:** Internal LINAC mirror reflecting light field.
**Related Terms:** Light Field QA
**Example:** Mirror misalignment affects field-light accuracy.

105. **Local Dose Constraint Meaning:** Specific dose limit applied to a region.
**Related Terms:** OAR Constraints
**Example:** Rectum V50 < 50% in prostate IMRT.

106. **Low-Pressure Vacuum System Meaning:** System maintaining vacuum in LINAC waveguide.
**Related Terms:** Electron Gun, Waveguide
**Example:** Failure stops beam generation.

107. **Lateral Scatter Correction Meaning:** Adjustment for scatter moving sideways through tissues.
**Related Terms:** Collapsed Cone, AAA
**Example:** Important for small field dosimetry.

108. **Lung Metastasis Targeting Meaning:** Treatment of lung metastases using SBRT.
**Related Terms:** Oligometastasis
**Example:** 54 Gy in 3 fractions treats small lung metastasis.

109. **Laser Crosshair Marker Meaning:** Intersection point used for precise patient alignment.
**Related Terms:** Isocenter, Setup
**Example:** Crosshair matches tattoo during setup.

110. **Low-Dose Planning Technique Meaning:** Planning approach to reduce integral dose.
**Related Terms:** Hybrid IMRT, 3D-CRT
**Example:** Used in pediatric spinal RT.

111. **Lead Apron Shielding Meaning:** Protective garment to reduce scatter exposure.
**Related Terms:** PPE, Radiation Safety
**Example:** Staff wear apron during fluoroscopy-guided procedures.

112. **Local Beam Modification Meaning:** Adjustments made to improve dose around a specific region.
**Related Terms:** Boost, Feathering
**Example:** Beam modified to protect spinal cord.

113. **Lung Tumor Mid-Position Scan Meaning:** Average-position scan from 4D-CT.
**Related Terms:** ITV, Motion Management
**Example:** Used for more accurate GTV contour.

114. **Limiting Hotspot Criterion Meaning:** Maximum tolerance for dose hotspots.
**Related Terms:** Homogeneity Index
**Example:** Hotspots capped at 110% for breast RT.

115. **Local Optimization Weight Meaning:** Priority value for a particular constraint.
**Related Terms:** Cost Function
**Example:** Liver weight increased to protect organ in SBRT.

116. **Lung Surface Dose Meaning:** Dose to pleura or lung surface.
**Related Terms:** Beam Path, MLC
**Example:** Lower with non-coplanar beams.

117. **Large Motion Envelope Meaning:** Wide range of tumor motion during respiration.
**Related Terms:** ITV, 4D-CT
**Example:** Found in lower-lobe lung tumors.

118. **Low-Intensity Portal Image Meaning:** Faint EPID image needing enhancement.
**Related Terms:** Portal Imaging
**Example:** Used for bony alignment verification.

119. **Local Adaptive Replan Meaning:** Adjusting part of the plan based on anatomy changes.
**Related Terms:** ART, Replanning
**Example:** Tumor shrinkage triggers adaptive replan.

120. **Light-Radiation Field Coincidence Meaning:** QA test comparing light and radiation fields.
**Related Terms:** Mechanical QA
**Example:** Must match within ±2 mm.

121. **Low-Z Compensator Meaning:** Device of low atomic number used to shape or modulate beams.
**Related Terms:** Compensator, Beam Modulation
**Example:** Plastic compensators used for uniform dose.

122. **Low-Noise Imaging Mode Meaning:** Reduces graininess in imaging.
**Related Terms:** Image Quality
**Example:** Improves visibility of soft tissue.

123. **Lead Backscatter Effect Meaning:** Radiation backscattering from lead surfaces.
**Related Terms:** Backscatter, Dosimetry
**Example:** Increases skin dose near lead blocks.

124. **Leukoencephalopathy (Radiation-Related) Meaning:** White matter changes after brain RT.
**Related Terms:** Late Effects, Neurotoxicity
**Example:** Seen in long-term whole-brain RT survivors.

125. **Lung Segment Delineation Meaning:** Contouring anatomical lung segments.
**Related Terms:** Anatomy, OAR
**Example:** Used to evaluate segmental dose after SBRT.

126. **Low-Weight Beam Meaning:** Beam given small importance in plan optimization.
**Related Terms:** Beam Weight
**Example:** Small posterior beam used in liver plan.

127. **Local Field Matching Meaning:** Aligning two adjacent fields for large treatment areas.
**Related Terms:** Feathering, Junction
**Example:** Used in spinal irradiation.

128. **Longitudinal Couch Index Meaning:** Numerical reference for couch position along patient's length.
**Related Terms:** Setup Reproducibility
**Example:** Helps ensure consistent daily setup.

129. **Lung Segmentation Algorithm Meaning:** Software that auto-delineates lungs.
**Related Terms:** Auto-Contour
**Example:** Used during CT simulation.

130. **Laser Drift Correction Meaning:** Adjusting lasers to restore isocenter alignment.
**Related Terms:** QA
**Example:** Corrected during monthly QA.

131. **Limited Breath-Hold Capacity Meaning:** When patient cannot hold breath for long periods.
**Related Terms:** DIBH, Coaching
**Example:** Affects left breast DIBH feasibility.

132. **Local Contrast Enhancement Meaning:** Digital improvement of image contrast.
**Related Terms:** EPID Processing
**Example:** Enhances tumor visibility on MV images.

133. **Lateral Dose Penumbra Meaning:** Region of partial dose at beam edges.
**Related Terms:** Beam Profile
**Example:** Smaller with MLCs in SBRT.

134. **Lumbar Marrow Sparing Meaning:** Reducing radiation to bone marrow.
**Related Terms:** IMRT, Hematologic Toxicity
**Example:** Important in lymphoma RT.

135. **Low-Isocenter Technique Meaning:** Isocenter positioned lower in patient for better clearance.
**Related Terms:** Couch Angle, Collisions
**Example:** Used in cranial non-coplanar setups.

136. **Linear Dose Fall-Off Meaning:** Gradual reduction in dose outside PTV.
**Related Terms:** Gradient Index
**Example:** SBRT tries to achieve sharp fall-off.

137. **Local Travel Distance (Gantry) Meaning:** Angle distance gantry moves between control points.
**Related Terms:** VMAT
**Example:** Smaller distances improve modulation.

138. **Low-Dose Spill Meaning:** Dose spread into nearby healthy tissue.
**Related Terms:** Gradient, OAR
**Example:** Kept low in liver SBRT.

139. **Lateral Table Offset Meaning:** Side-to-side couch shift for proper alignment.
**Related Terms:** Setup Error
**Example:** Correction applied after daily CBCT.

140. **Laser-PD Calibration Meaning:** Calibration of photodiodes monitoring laser intensity.
**Related Terms:** QA
**Example:** Ensures consistent brightness.

141. **Localized PTV Expansion Meaning:** Non-uniform margin added to CTV.
**Related Terms:** Asymmetric Margin
**Example:** Larger margin added inferiorly due to motion.

142. **Low-Angle Scatter Meaning:** Radiation scattered at shallow angles.
**Related Terms:** Scatter Radiation
**Example:** Can increase skin dose.

143. **Lateral Breathing Motion Meaning:** Side-to-side lung motion during respiration.
**Related Terms:** Motion Management
**Example:** Small in most patients (<5 mm).

144. **Lymph Node Dose Gradient Meaning:** Dose fall-off around nodal CTV.
**Related Terms:** IMRT, Optimization
**Example:** Important in head-and-neck RT.

145. **Local Deformation Map Meaning:** Shows how tissue shifts between scans.
**Related Terms:** DIR, Adaptive RT
**Example:** Used to adapt daily plans.

146. **Lung PTV Overlap Reduction Meaning:** Techniques to minimize PTV entering lung.
**Related Terms:** Field Design
**Example:** Used in esophageal RT.

147. **Leg Support Cradle Meaning:** Device supporting legs during simulation.
**Related Terms:** Immobilization
**Example:** Increases comfort for pelvis RT.

148. **Low-Motion Tumor Class Meaning:** Tumors with little respiratory movement.
**Related Terms:** Motion Categories
**Example:** Upper-lobe tumors classified as low-motion.

149. **Local Feathering Technique Meaning:** Shifting match line to reduce dose overlap.
**Related Terms:** Field Matching
**Example:** Used in spinal junctions.

150. **Lung Perfusion Region Meaning:** Lung areas with higher blood flow.
**Related Terms:** Functional Imaging
**Example:** Preferentially spared in IMRT.

151. **Low-Activity Source Check Meaning:** Verification of weak brachytherapy sources for calibration accuracy.
**Related Terms:** Source Strength, HDR QA
**Example:** A low-activity Cs-137 seed is measured before LDR implant.

152. **Lateral Spine Constraint Meaning:** Limits dose to lateral spinal structures.
**Related Terms:** Cord PRV, OAR
**Example:** Lateral vertebral body kept under 18 Gy in SBRT.

153. **Local Adaptive Margin Meaning:** Margins modified based on region-specific motion.
**Related Terms:** ITV, Deformable Planning
**Example:** Larger inferior margin for lung tumor with more movement.

154. **Lung Tumor Excision Bed Boost Meaning:** Boost dose to postoperative lung tumor bed.
**Related Terms:** Adjuvant RT, CTV
**Example:** 10 Gy boost delivered after lobectomy RT.

155. **Leakage Transmission Factor Meaning:** Percentage of radiation leaking through MLC.
**Related Terms:** MLC Transmission
**Example:** Typically ~1–2% for modern LINACs.

156. **Large-Field Arc Therapy Meaning:** VMAT arcs covering large targets.
**Related Terms:** Extended Field
**Example:** Used in whole-abdomen IMRT.

157. **Localized Image Enhancement Meaning:** Enhancement applied to selected zones of image.
**Related Terms:** EPID Processing
**Example:** Improves spine visibility in kV imaging.

158. **Lower Jaw Asymmetry Erro Meaning:** Mismatch in lower collimator jaw position.
**Related Terms:** Jaw QA
**Example:** Found during monthly mechanical QA.

159. **Lung Tumor Trajectory Plot Meaning:** Chart showing tumor path during breathing.
**Related Terms:** 4D Motion, Tracking
**Example:** Helps design gating window.

160. **Lateral Dose Gradient Meaning:** Rate of dose decrease across beam sides.
**Related Terms:** Beam Profile
**Example:** Sharper gradient improves OAR sparing.

161. **Leakage Map (EPID) Meaning:** Pixel map showing EPID leakage or sensitivity.
**Related Terms:** Flat-Fielding
**Example:** Used to correct MV portal images.

162. **Lung Isocenter Placement Meaning:** Choosing isocenter location inside lung target.
**Related Terms:** Setup, Collisions
**Example:** Placed centrally for SBRT.

163. **Local Plan Normalization Meaning:** Adjusting plan dose relative to PTV or target.
**Related Terms:** Prescription, Isodose
**Example:** PTV normalized to 95% isodose.

164. **Laser Tracking System Meaning:** System tracking patient motion via laser markers.
**Related Terms:** Optical Tracking
**Example:** Used for frameless SRS.

165. **Leaf Speed Modulation Meaning:** Adjustment of MLC leaf speed for IMRT/VMAT.
**Related Terms:** Modulation Factor
**Example:** Faster leaf speeds allow higher modulation.

166. **Local Rigid Registration Meaning:** Image matching applied to small anatomical region.
**Related Terms:** IGRT, ROI Matching
**Example:** Vertebral-body matching in spinal SBRT.

167. **Lateral Build-Up Material Meaning:** Material added to ensure proper dose build-up at surface.
**Related Terms:** Bolus
**Example:** Used in head-and-neck electron fields.

168. **Local Hotspot Suppression Meaning:** Reducing high-dose areas during optimization.
**Related Terms:** Homogeneity, Constraints
**Example:** Reducing breast hot spot from 115% to 108%.

169. **Low-Mobility Phantom Meaning:** Phantom designed for minimal motion simulation.
**Related Terms:** QA Tools
**Example:** Used for MLC QA.

170. **Lung Tumor Contrast Window Meaning:** CT window settings optimized for lung tumor visibility.
**Related Terms:** Window/Level
**Example:** Helps delineate small nodules.

171. **Lead Diaphragm Collimator Meaning:** Thick shielding piece used in older machines to shape beam.
**Related Terms:** Custom Blocking
**Example:** Used before MLCs were standard.

172. **Local Dose Expansion Meaning:** Adding dose in a targeted region during replan.
**Related Terms:** SIB, Boost
**Example:** Increasing dose to residual tumor.

173. **Lung Contour Smoothing Meaning:** Processing contour to remove jagged edges.
**Related Terms:** Auto-Segmentation
**Example:** Improves accuracy of dose calc.

174. **Low-Dose Lung Constraint Meaning:** Limiting lung V5 or V10 to reduce pneumonitis.
**Related Terms:** DVH
**Example:** Lung V20 < 35% typical.

175. **Light Alignment Field Meaning:** Field created using light source for positioning.
**Related Terms:** ODI, Collimator
**Example:** Used before imaging.

176. **Lateral Patient Support Meaning:** Device supporting patient side-to-side.
**Related Terms:** Immobilization
**Example:** Helps in thoracic RT.

177. **Local Surface Dose Correction Meaning:** Adjusting dose for surface irregularities.
**Related Terms:** Bolus
**Example:** Applied in scalp irradiation.

178. **Lung Tumor Deformation Index Meaning:** Quantifies deformation during breathing.
**Related Terms:** DIR, 4D-CT
**Example:** Higher index → larger ITV.

179. **Limited OAR Expansion Meaning:** Restricting OAR PRV enlargement.
**Related Terms:** Planning Structures
**Example:** Brainstem PRV margin limited to 2 mm.

180. **Leakage Dose Monitoring Meaning:** Measuring dose leakage around beam path.
**Related Terms:** Shielding, Radiation Protection
**Example:** Checked during annual survey.

181. **Local Junction Feathering Meaning:** Shifting match line to reduce overdose/underdose.
**Related Terms:** Junction Shift
**Example:** Used in craniospinal RT.

182. **Laser-Mounted Camera Meaning:** Camera attached to laser for alignment QA.
**Related Terms:** Optical QA
**Example:** Used for remote isocenter checks.

183. **Lung SBRT Gating Window Meaning:** Range of breathing where beam is allowed on.
**Related Terms:** Motion Management
**Example:** End-exhale gating reduces motion.

184. **Lateral Electron Scatter Meaning:** Sideways scatter of electrons, affecting dose edges.
**Related Terms:** Electron Therapy
**Example:** Causes broad penumbra.

185. **Leaf Travel Pathway Meaning:** Planned route of MLC leaves during delivery.
**Related Terms:** MLC Motion
**Example:** Complex pathways in VMAT.

186. **Local Dose Verification Grid Meaning:** Selective dose check region.
**Related Terms:** Patient QA
**Example:** Verifying high-dose region only.

187. **Low-Tolerance Setup Region Meaning:** Region requiring extremely accurate positioning.
**Related Terms:** SRS, SBRT
**Example:** Brainstem-adjacent tumors.

188. **Lung Collapse Correction Meaning:** Contour adjustment for atelectasis changes.
**Related Terms:** Adaptive RT
**Example:** Used after mid-course CT.

189. **Laser Vertical Calibration Meaning:** Ensuring vertical laser aligns with isocenter.
**Related Terms:** Laser QA
**Example:** Checked weekly.

190. **190. Localized Edema Monitoring Meaning:** Tracking swelling during brain RT.
**Related Terms:** MRI, Toxicity
**Example:** MRI shows edema in week 4.

191. **Late-Stage Plan Evaluation Meaning:** Final review before treatment start.
**Related Terms:** QA, MU Check
**Example:** Physicist verifies DVH and constraints.

192. **Lung Apex Shielding Meaning:** Protecting lung apex from unnecessary dose.
**Related Terms:** Beam Design
**Example:** Used in breast RT tangents.

193. **Low-Weight Tissue Region Meaning:** Region not prioritized during optimization.
**Related Terms:** Optimization Weights
**Example:** Posterior soft tissue in prostate IMRT.

194. **Local Image Histogram Equalization Meaning:** Enhancing contrast in selected image zones.
**Related Terms:** IGRT Enhancement
**Example:** Improves liver visibility.

195. **Lead RNA Storage Box Meaning:** Shielded container for radioactive items.
**Related Terms:** Radiation Safety
**Example:** Used for temporary HDR source storage.

196. **Leak-Test Verification Meaning:** Checking brachy catheter or source for leaks.
**Related Terms:** HDR QA
**Example:** Required before each treatment.

197. **Large Aperture Cone Meaning:** Big SRS cone for large lesions.
**Related Terms:** SRS Cones
**Example:** Used for large trigeminal targets.

198. **Linear Accelerator Cooling Loop Meaning:** System cooling accelerator components.
**Related Terms:** Klystron, Target.
**Example:** Overheating triggers auto shutdown.

199. **Lung Tumor Margin Reduction Meaning:** Reducing PTV margins with gating/tracking.
**Related Terms:** Motion Management
**Example:** Margin reduced from 8 mm to 4 mm.

200. **Local Dose Suppression Region Meaning:** Region intentionally kept low-dose.
**Related Terms:** Avoidance Structures
**Example:** Suppressing dose to optic chiasm.

201. **Low-Energy Output Check Meaning:** Ensuring low-energy photon/electron modes deliver correct dose.
**Related Terms:** Output Calibration, QA
**Example:** 6 MeV electron output checked monthly.

202. **Localized Tissue Sparing Meaning:** Technique to reduce dose to a specific small region.
**Related Terms:** IMRT, Avoidance Structures
**Example:** Sparing parotid in H&N IMRT.

203. **Longitudinal Tumor Drift Meaning:** Tumor moving up or down the body over treatment.
**Related Terms:** Motion, Adaptive RT
**Example:** Lung tumor shifts 4 mm inferiorly at week 2.

204. **Lip Dose Constraint Meaning:** Restricting dose to lip structures in head-and-neck RT.
**Related Terms:** OAR Limits
**Example:** Lip mean dose kept <20 Gy.

205. **Lateral Isocenter Correction Meaning:** Adjusting isocenter left or right for alignment.
**Related Terms:** Setup Correction
**Example:** 3 mm lateral correction needed after CBCT.

206. **Low-Divergence Beam Meaning:** Beam with minimal spread and sharper penumbra.
**Related Terms:** Collimation, Beam Geometry
**Example:** Gives better sparing in SRS.

207. **Lead Slit Collimator Meaning:** Thin lead slit used to create narrow beam.
**Related Terms:** Field Shaping
**Example:** Used in measuring penumbra width.

208. **Lung Tumor Tracking Algorithmn Meaning:** Software predicting tumor position in real time.
**Related Terms:** Gating, Motion Tracking
**Example:** Used in CyberKnife lung tracking.

209. **Late-Phase Dose Accumulation Meaning:** Summation of dose delivered in final treatment weeks.
**Related Terms:** Adaptive Planning
**Example:** Evaluating thyroid dose near end of H&N RT.

210. **Local Dose Renormalization Meaning:** Adjusting dose levels for a specific region.
**Related Terms:** Plan Normalization
**Example:** Renormalizing boost volume to 95% coverage.

211. **Low-Bias Calibration Meaning:** Calibration method minimizing measurement error.
**Related Terms:** Dosimetry QA
**Example:** Used for ion chamber arrays.

212. **Lung Voxel Density Map Meaning:** Visualization of voxel HU values for lung planning.
**Related Terms:** CT Density, Heterogeneity
**Example:** Helps identify fibrosis or consolidation.

213. **Localized Field Reductionm Meaning:** Shrinking field size after tumor regression.
**Related Terms:** Adaptive RT
**Example:** Lung PTV reduced at week 3.

214. **Lead Tube Applicator Meaning:** Applicator used for superficial X-ray therapy.
**Related Terms:** Contact Therapy
**Example:** Used for skin lesions of face.

215. **Leaf End Calibration Meaning:** Checking accuracy of leaf tip positions.
**Related Terms:** MLC QA
**Example:** Ensures correct IMRT fluence.

216. **Lateral Tumor Expansion Meaning:** Side-to-side tumor growth considered in margins.
**Related Terms:** GTV, CTV
**Example:** Soft tissue sarcoma requires larger lateral margins.

217. **Lung Inflation Monitoring Meaning:** Checking lung volume consistency during RT.
**Related Terms:** IGRT, Motion
**Example:** CBCT shows 10% lower lung inflation.

218. **Low-Strength Brachy Source Meaning:** Source with reduced activity for long-duration implants.
**Related Terms:** LDR Brachytherapy
**Example:** I-125 seeds used for prostate implants.

219. **Local Dose Perturbation Meaning:** Small disturbance in dose distribution.
**Related Terms:** Heterogeneity, Metal Implants
**Example:** Metal dental fillings cause perturbation.

220. **Lung Tumor Fiducial Tracking Meaning:** Tracking tumor using implanted gold markers.
**Related Terms:** IGRT, SBRT
**Example:** Used in fluoroscopic lung SBRT.

221. **Lymphatic Drainage Mapping Meaning:** Charting lymphatic pathways for nodal CTV.
**Related Terms:** Nodal Levels
**Example:** Used for breast and gynecological RT.

222. **Low-Margin Boost Technique Meaning:** Boost to tumor with minimal PTV margin.
**Related Terms:** SIB, CTV
**Example:** 2 mm PTV margin in prostate boost.

223. **Lateral Chest Wall Constraint Meaning:** Dose limits to chest wall in breast RT.
**Related Terms:** OAR
**Example:** Keeping chest wall max <45 Gy in PMRT.

224. **Leakage Detection Algorithm Meaning:** Software detecting beam or MLC leakage.
**Related Terms:** Portal Imaging QA
**Example:** Detects leaf gap leaks in VMAT.

225. **Local Hounsfield Correction Meaning:** Adjusting HU values for artifact regions.
**Related Terms:** CT Artifacts
**Example:** Fixes metal-affected HU in oral cavity.

226. **Lung Edge Voxel Smoothing Meaning:** Smoothing jagged lung boundaries in segmentation.
**Related Terms:** Auto-Contour
**Example:** Reduces segmentation noise.

227. **Lateral Brain Avoidance Meaning:** Minimizing dose to temporal lobes.
**Related Terms:** Neurotoxicity
**Example:** Important in nasopharyngeal RT.

228. **Localized Beam Hold Meaning:** Machine hold triggered due to specific region mismatch.
**Related Terms:** IGRT, Automation
**Example:** CBCT mismatch halts beam automatically.

229. **Laser Stability Monitor Meaning:** Device checking stability of laser intensity.
**Related Terms:** QA
**Example:** Prevents drift affecting patient setup.

230. **Leaf Trajectory Audit Meaning:** Review of stored MLC motion during plan delivery.
**Related Terms:** Delivery QA
**Example:** Used in VMAT QA.

231. **Lung Perfusion Weighting Meaning:** Assigning planning weight based on perfusion.
**Related Terms:** Functional Lung
**Example:** Sparing upper-lobe high-perfusion regions.

232. **Limited Arc Strategy Meaning:** Using partial arcs to avoid OARs.
**Related Terms:** VMAT, Arc Therapy
**Example:** Partial arc for left breast avoids heart.

233. **Local Volume Correction Meaning:** Adjusting target/OAR volume due to motion.
**Related Terms:** Adaptive RT
**Example:** Lung GTV reduced after tumor shrinkage.

234. **Lead Marker Seed Meaning:** Radiopaque seed for localization.
**Related Terms:** Fiducial Marker
**Example:** Used for lung tumor tracking.

235. **Lung Mean Dose Reduction Meaning:** Strategies to reduce average lung dose.
**Related Terms:** DVH, IMRT
**Example:** IMRT reduces MLD from 13 Gy to 9 Gy.

236. **Localized High-Dose Patch Meaning:** Intentional high-dose region to resistant area.
**Related Terms:** Dose Painting
**Example:** Patch around hypoxic tumor region.

237. **Long-Axis Tumor Contouring Meaning:** Contouring target using longitudinal body axis.
**Related Terms:** GTV, PTV
**Example:** Used for esophageal CTV.

238. **Laser-to-Couch Alignment Meaning:** Ensuring couch coordinates match laser isocenter.
**Related Terms:** QA
**Example:** Checked daily.

239. **Low-Load Beam Delivery Meaning:** Delivering beams with minimal mechanical stress.
**Related Terms:** Mechanical Wear
**Example:** Used in extended machine operations.

240. **Lung Elasticity Parameter Meaning:** Quantifies how lung tissue deforms with breathing.
**Related Terms:** Motion Model
**Example:** Higher elasticity → larger deformation.

241. **Local Beam Override Meaning:** Planner manually modifies beam parameters.
**Related Terms:** Manual Optimization
**Example:** Override to improve coverage near spine.

242. **Lead Stray Radiation Shield Meaning:** Shield to block stray radiation near machine.
**Related Terms:** Radiation Protection
**Example:** Used near HDR afterloader.

243. **Lymph Node Boost Volume Meaning:** Additional volume for nodal boost.
**Related Terms:** SIB, CTV
**Example:** Adding boost to PET-positive node.

244. **Lung Clearance Window Meaning:** Time interval in breathing where lungs are steady.
**Related Terms:** Gating
**Example:** Used to time beam in gated lung RT.

245. **Lateral Field Limiting Jaw Meaning:** Jaw restricting left or right field width.
**Related Terms:** Collimation
**Example:** Jaw closed to spare contralateral breast.

246. **Localized Scatter Estimation Meaning:** Scatter estimated for specific anatomical region.
**Related Terms:** Dose Algorithms
**Example:** Important near lung-tissue interfaces.

247. **Low-Dose Photon Tail Meaning:** Dropping dose levels far from beam edge.
**Related Terms:** Scatter, Penumbra
**Example:** Seen in high-energy beams.

248. **Lung Tumor Rotation Analysis Meaning:** Measuring rotational motion of tumors.
**Related Terms:** 4D-CT
**Example:** Tumor rotates 3° during respiration.

249. **Longitudinal Density Variation Meaning:** Density changes along patient length.
**Related Terms:** HU Mapping
**Example:** Present in large lung tumors.

250. **Localized Re-Collimation Meaning:** Adjusting collimator angles for one region.
**Related Terms:** Beam Shaping
**Example:** Re-collimation protects spinal cord.

251. **Lung Homogeneity Index Meaning:** Numerical measure of dose uniformity inside lung tissue.
**Related Terms:** HI, Dose Uniformity
**Example:** HI of 0.12 indicates good uniformity in lung SBRT.

252. **Light Particle Contamination Meaning:** Unwanted low-energy particles in photon beams.
**Related Terms:** Scatter, Beam Quality
**Example:** Photons picking up contamination from electron scatter.

253. **Lateral Beam Quality Check Meaning:** Verifying beam profile consistency left-to-right.
**Related Terms:** Profile QA
**Example:** Must be within ±2% symmetry.

254. **Local Wedge Compensation Meaning:** Using wedge filters to correct for uneven tissue thickness.
**Related Terms:** Wedge Field, Tissue Compensation
**Example:** Used in breast tangential RT.

255. **Lung Clearance Probability Meaning:** Probability of lung motion being within a stable window.
**Related Terms:** Gating, 4D-CT
**Example:** 70% clearance probability helps optimize gating phase.

256. **Linear Energy Response Meaning:** Linear proportionality between dose and detector reading.
**Related Terms:** Detector Calibration
**Example:** Ion chamber shows linear response up to 600 cGy/min.

257. **Low-Uncertainty Beam Model Meaning:** Treatment planning model with reduced dose prediction error.
**Related Terms:** TPS, Monte Carlo
**Example:** MC-based models offer <1% uncertainty.

258. **Light Scatter Reduction Grid Meaning:** Device to reduce stray light in imaging detectors.
**Related Terms:** Imaging, Scatter Control
**Example:** Used in MV imaging panels.

259. **Lumbar Spine Avoidance Strip Meaning:** Region excluded from high dose in abdominal RT.
**Related Terms:** OAR Sparing
**Example:** Kept below 40 Gy to avoid marrow suppression.

260. **Local Dose Penetration Study Meaning:** Assessing how dose spreads into specific tissues.
**Related Terms:** Depth Dose
**Example:** Used for lung-tissue interface evaluation.

261. **Low-Shock Gantry Rotation Meaning:** Smooth gantry motion preventing mechanical vibration.
**Related Terms:** Mechanical QA
**Example:** Required for accurate VMAT.

262. **Lymph Node Probability Mapping Meaning:** Assigning likelihood of nodal involvement.
**Related Terms:** CTV-N, Nodal Risk
**Example:** Level II nodes have 20–30% probability in oral cancer.

263. **Lung Tumor Flattening Filter Consideration Meaning:** Determining use of FF vs FFF for lung beams.
**Related Terms:** FFF Mode
**Example:** FFF used in lung SBRT for shorter treatment times.

264. **Low-Dose Peripheral Gradient Meaning:** Dose falloff in far-out peripheral tissue.
**Related Terms:** Gradient Index
**Example:** Studied in VMAT breast fields.

265. **Localized Beam Hardening Artifact Meaning:** Distortion from dense materials affecting CT.
**Related Terms:** Metal Artifact
**Example:** Dental fillings cause hardening in oral cavity scans.

266. **Lateral Thoracic Build-Up Region Meaning:** Dose build-up zone for tangential breast beams.
**Related Terms:** Surface Dose, PDD
**Example:** Higher buildup with 6 MV tangential fields.

267. **Light-Shielded Imaging Chamber Meaning:** Detector protected from optical light for MV imaging.
**Related Terms:** EPID
**Example:** Ensures pure radiation signal.

268. **Low-Mobility Organ Model Meaning:** Organ model assuming minimal internal motion.
**Related Terms:** Motion Management
**Example:** Prostate considered low-mobility with bladder control.

269. **Lateral Optical Alignment Check Meaning:** Checking laser alignment horizontally.
**Related Terms:** Laser QA
**Example:** <1 mm variation required.

270. **Lung Functional Subunit Dose Meaning:** Dose to lung microregions (FSUs).
**Related Terms:** Functional Lung Planning
**Example:** Prioritizing FSUs with highest perfusion.

271. **Large Cone Collimator Field Meaning:** Big circular field used for palliative or orthovoltage therapy.
**Related Terms:** Field Size, Collimation
**Example:** 20 cm cone used for whole pelvis.

272. **Local Beam-Specific Margin Meaning:** Custom margin per beam angle.
**Related Terms:** PTV Margin
**Example:** Smaller posterior margin in prostate RT.

273. **Lymph Node Clustering Meaning:** Grouping nodes for uniform coverage.
**Related Terms:** Nodal CTV
**Example:** Clustering level III/IV in thyroid RT.

274. **Lung Voxel Influence Matrix Meaning:** Matrix showing how each beamlet affects each lung voxel.
**Related Terms:** IMRT Optimization
**Example:** Used to reduce V20.

275. **Lateral Penetration Depth Meaning:** How far dose spreads laterally.
**Related Terms:** Penumbra
**Example:** Higher lateral penetration in 15 MV beams.

276. **Local Dose Tracking Monitor Meaning:** Device tracking delivered vs planned dose.
**Related Terms:** In Vivo Dosimetry
**Example:** Real-time diode system.

277. **Lung Parenchyma Segmentation Meaning:** Splitting lung tissue into functional units.
**Related Terms:** 4D-CT, Auto-Segmentation
**Example:** Used for functional avoidance RT.

278. **Lateral Dose Width Adjustment Meaning:** Tuning beam width for coverage vs sparing.
**Related Terms:** Beam Optimization
**Example:** Narrowing field to spare kidney.

279. **Low-Noise Imaging Protocol Meaning:** CT/MV imaging method to reduce grain.
**Related Terms:** Image Processing
**Example:** Boosts soft-tissue contrast.

**280. Local Scatter Kernel Meaning:** Mathematical shape describing scatter dose distribution.
**Related Terms:** Convolution Algorithm
**Example:** Used in collapsed cone calculations.

**281. Lymph Node Microscopic Spread Radius Meaning:** Expected microscopic spread around nodes.
**Related Terms:** CTV Margin
**Example:** 3–5 mm added around nodal GTV.

**282. Lung Tissue Recovery Model Meaning:** Predicts post-RT healing capability.
**Related Terms:** NTCP, Toxicity
**Example:** Recovery slower in smokers.

**283. Light Beam Magnification Check Meaning:** Ensuring projected light field matches radiation field.
**Related Terms:** Light/Rad Field Coincidence
**Example:** Coincidence within 2 mm.

**284. Local Target Registration Meaning:** Matching target only (not whole anatomy) for alignment.
**Related Terms:** IGRT
**Example:** Aligning prostate alone using fiducials.

**285. Low-Contrast Edge Detection Meaning:** Detecting boundaries of low-contrast anatomy.
**Related Terms:** IGRT, Image Processing
**Example:** Useful for pancreas CBCT.

**286. Lung SBRT Sharp Gradient Index Meaning:** Evaluates falloff sharpness in SBRT plans.
**Related Terms:** GI
**Example:** GI of 4.0 indicates good conformity.

**287. Localized Arc Intensity ModulationMeaning:** Adjusting arc dose for a specific region.
**Related Terms:** VMAT
**Example:** Reducing dose near spinal cord.

**288. Lead Interlock Shield Meaning:** Shield that stops radiation when not in place.
**Related Terms:** Safety
**Example:** Required in HDR brachy suites.

**289. Lung Expansion Map Meaning:** Map showing how lung volume changes with breathing.
**Related Terms:** Deformable Registration
**Example:** Helps design gated plans.

**290. Lateral Setup Reproducibility Score Meaning:** Quantifies left–right setup accuracy.
**Related Terms:** Setup Error
**Example:** Score of 92% indicates good consistency.

**291. Low-Energy Electron Mode Meaning:** Electron energies used for shallow tumors (6–9 MeV).
**Related Terms:** Electron Therapy
**Example:** Used for chest-wall scar boost.

**292. Localized Edge Drop-Off Analysis Meaning:** Evaluates dose falloff around small targets.
**Related Terms:** SRS, PTV Margin
**Example:** Strong drop-off protects optic nerve.

**293. Lung Density Gradient Mapping Meaning:** Mapping transitions from high to low density.
**Related Terms:** Heterogeneity
**Example:** Important near tumor–lung boundaries.

294. **Light-Field Rotation Check Meaning:** Ensuring light field rotates correctly with gantry.
**Related Terms:** Mechanical QA
**Example:** <1 mm deviation acceptable.

295. **Local Dose Trigger Threshold Meaning:** Dose level that triggers machine hold.
**Related Terms:** Safety, Delivery QA
**Example:** Trigger at 105% of planned MU.

296. **Lung-Sparing Beam Arrangement Meaning:** Beam directions selected to minimize lung dose.
**Related Terms:** IMRT, VMAT
**Example:** Anterior beams avoided in lung RT.

297. **Low-Density Override Technique Meaning:** Correcting CT density for inaccurate regions.
**Related Terms:** HU Override
**Example:** Overriding bowel gas to avoid dose errors.

298. **Localized Margin Reduction Protocol Meaning:** Reducing margins with daily IGRT.
**Related Terms:** Adaptive RT
**Example:** Prostate margin reduced from 10 mm to 5 mm.

299. **Lung NTCP Constraint Line Meaning:** NTCP curve used to set lung dose limits.
**Related Terms:** NTCP Modeling
**Example:** Ensuring NTCP <10% for pneumonitis.

300. **Linear Accelerator Intersegment CheckMeaning:** Ensuring accurate transition between IMRT segments.
**Related Terms:** Delivery QA
**Example:** Verifying leaf positions between segments.

301. **Lung Ventilation Mapping Meaning:** Imaging-based assessment of airflow distribution in lungs.
**Related Terms:** Functional Avoidance, 4D-CT
**Example:** Avoiding high-ventilation regions during lung IMRT.

302. **Light Field Uniformity Check Meaning:** Ensuring even illumination across treatment light field.
**Related Terms:** Light Field QA
**Example:** Non-uniform light suggests mirror misalignment.

303. **Lateral Dose Spill Constraint Meaning:** Restricting unwanted sideways dose spread.
**Related Terms:** Gradient, Conformity
**Example:** Essential in pediatric craniospinal RT.

304. **Local Electron Disequilibrium Meaning:** Condition where electrons do not reach balance due to heterogeneity.
**Related Terms:** Lung Interfaces, Dose Error
**Example:** Occurs at lung–tumor boundary in SBRT.

305. **Lymph Node Shell Structure Meaning:** Thin ring structure around nodes for dose falloff control.
**Related Terms:** SIB, Planning Structures
**Example:** Shell used to enforce 3% dose gradient.

306. **Lung Expansion Correction Factor Meaning:** Adjustment for lung volume changes during breathing.
**Related Terms:** Motion Compensation
**Example:** Correcting dose in 4D plans.

307. **Local Beam Smoothing Filter Meaning:** TPS tool that reduces beamlet noise.
**Related Terms:** Fluence Smoothing
**Example:** Reduces sharp hot spots.

308. **Linear Release Mechanism (LINAC) Meaning:** System controlling release of high-voltage energy.
**Related Terms:** Modulator, Pulse Forming
**Example:** Fault detection triggers beam hold.

309. **Low-Intensity Region Suppression Meaning:** Removing low-value pixels from imaging.
**Related Terms:** CBCT Processing
**Example:** Helps clarify soft-tissue edges.

310. **Local Dose Enhancement Factor Meaning:** Ratio describing increased dose in a small region.
**Related Terms:** Hot Spot, Inhomogeneity
**Example:** Metallic stents cause enhancement.

311. **Longitudinal Isocenter Stability Meaning:** Precision of isocenter along the cranial–caudal axis.
**Related Terms:** Mechanical QA
**Example:** Verified with Winston–Lutz test.

312. **Lung Target Drift Compensation Meaning:** Methods to handle slow drift in lung tumor motion.
**Related Terms:** Adaptive Gating
**Example:** SAG corrected during SBRT.

313. **Lateral Planning Constraint Ring Meaning:** Ring around target used to shape dose.
**Related Terms:** Dose Rings
**Example:** Reduces dose to ipsilateral lung.

314. **Lead Aperture Shield Meaning:** Custom block for field shaping.
**Related Terms:** Cerrobend Block
**Example:** Used for simple palliative fields.

315. **Low-Dose Region Sculpting Meaning:** Intentional shaping of low-dose spill.
**Related Terms:** Plan Optimization
**Example:** Important for pregnant patients.

316. **Local Monitor Unit Override Meaning:** Manual adjustment of MU for specific segments.
**Related Terms:** IMRT Segment
**Example:** Reducing MU on segment near optic nerve.

317. **Lung Tissue Stiffness Index Meaning:** Quantifies mechanical stiffness of lung tissue.
**Related Terms:** Motion Modeling
**Example:** Higher stiffness reduces tumor displacement.

318. **Lateral Bevel Edge Correction Meaning:** Compensation for angled skin surfaces.
**Related Terms:** Beam Matching
**Example:** Used in breast tangents.

319. **Low Contrast-to-Noise Ratio Check Meaning:** Ensuring imaging system can distinguish similar tissues.
**Related Terms:** IGRT Quality
**Example:** Used on daily CBCT QA.

320. **Localized Dose Optimization Kernel Meaning:** Dose kernel focusing on local voxel interactions.
**Related Terms:** TPS Algorithms
**Example:** Used in collapsed-cone convolution.

321. **Largest Separation Distance Meaning:** Maximum patient width affecting MU calculations.
**Related Terms:** SSD, Beam Attenuation
**Example:** Thorax separation increases MU requirement.

322. **Lung Lesion Auto-Segmentation Meaning:** Automatic outlining of lung tumors.
**Related Terms:** AI Contouring
**Example:** Saves time in SBRT planning.

323. **Lateral Immobilization Block Meaning:** Device stabilizing patient side-to-side.
**Related Terms:** Positioning
**Example:** Used for pediatric brain RT.

324. **Localized Dose Plateau Meaning:** Region receiving nearly constant dose.
**Related Terms:** Uniformity
**Example:** Seen in homogeneous IMRT plans.

325. **Low Aperture Transmission Field Meaning:** Field with minimized leakage through MLC/jaws.
**Related Terms:** Leakage, Shielding
**Example:** Required for SRS.

326. **Lung Radiobiological Sensitivity IndexMeaning:** Numerical rating of lung sensitivity to RT.
**Related Terms:** NTCP
**Example:** Higher in smokers and COPD patients.

327. **Light-Radiation Coincidence Tolerance Meaning:** Allowed difference between light field and radiation field.
**Related Terms:** QA Standard
**Example:** Typically ±2 mm.

328. **Lateral Spread Function Meaning:** Describes how dose spreads sideways from beam axis.
**Related Terms:** Penumbra Function
**Example:** Used in electron planning.

329. **Lung Tumor Maximum Deflection Meaning:** Maximum displacement during breathing.
**Related Terms:** 4D-CT
**Example:** 12 mm deflection for lower-lobe tumor.

330. **Localized Tissue Deformation Map Meaning:** Shows anatomical movement across respiratory phases.
**Related Terms:** DIR
**Example:** Used for 4D dose tracking.

331. **Low-Priority Avoidance Sector Meaning:** Region with reduced priority for beam entry.
**Related Terms:** Optimization
**Example:** Avoiding anterior beams in spinal RT.

332. **Linear Accelerator Pulse Frequency Meaning:** Rate at which LINAC generates radiation pulses.
**Related Terms:** Pulse Repetition Rate
**Example:** Typically around 300 pulses/sec.

333. **Localized Error Probability Meaning:** Probability of dose deviation in a specific region.
**Related Terms:** Error Modeling
**Example:** Higher near high-gradient zones.

334. **Lateral Magnetic Declination Meaning:** Sideways deviation of electrons in MR-linacs.
**Related Terms:** Lorentz Force
**Example:** Corrected in MR-guided RT plans.

335. **Lung Apex Constraint Meaning:** Dose limit to lung apex to prevent fibrosis.
**Related Terms:** OAR Limits
**Example:** Apex max dose kept <50 Gy.

336. **Lead-Embedded Bolus Meaning:** Bolus containing lead strips for extra shielding.
**Related Terms:** Surface Dose
**Example:** Used to spare lens during facial RT.

337. **Localized Surface Build-Down Meaning:** Dose reduction near surface due to angle/air gaps.
**Related Terms:** Build-Up, Oblique Beams
**Example:** Occurs with tangential beams on sloped surfaces.

338. **Laser Coordinate Verification Meaning:** Ensuring alignment of coordinate grid across lasers.
**Related Terms:** Daily QA
**Example:** <1 mm misalignment allowed.

339. **Lung Functional Dose Weighting Meaning:** Adjusting dose constraints based on functional imaging.
**Related Terms:** SPECT, Perfusion
**Example:** Avoiding high-function lung regions during SBRT.

340. **Localized Gradient Threshold Meaning:** Maximum allowed gradient for dose transitions.|
**Related Terms:** GI, HI
**Example:** Max gradient enforced around optic chiasm.

341. **Low-Energy Contamination Filter Meaning:** Filter reducing low-energy scatter in beams.
**Related Terms:** Beam Quality
**Example:** Used in high-energy photon modes.

342. **Linear Accelerator Status Indicator Meaning:** System showing real-time machine states.
**Related Terms:** Machine Interface
**Example:** Displays "Beam Ready" or "Standby".

343. **Lung-Lesion Peak Dose Point Meaning:** Highest dose point within lung tumor.
**Related Terms:** Hot Spot
**Example:** Dmax = 115% in SBRT.

344. **Lateral Beam Offset Correction Meaning:** Fixing beam misalignment sideways.
**Related Terms:** Setup Error
**Example:** 2 mm correction before delivery.

345. **Local Radiographic Contrast Adjustment Meaning:** Enhancing local contrast in imaging.
**Related Terms:** CBCT Enhancement
**Example:** Used to visualize pancreas.

346. **Lung Tumor Phase Matching Meaning:** Matching beam delivery to specific breathing phase.
**Related Terms:** Gating, 4D-CT
**Example:** Delivering dose only at end-exhale.

347. **Low-Signal Region Denoising Meaning:** Cleaning noisy image areas.
**Related Terms:** IGRT, Post-Processing
**Example:** Applied to low-quality MV images.

348. **Localized Dose Suppression Zone Meaning:** Region intentionally kept at lower dose.
**Related Terms:** Avoidance Structure
**Example:** Suppressing dose around optic nerve.

349. **Laser Projection Symmetry Check Meaning:** Ensuring left/right wall lasers match.
**Related Terms:** QA
**Example:** Verified daily in treatment room.

350. **Lung Dose–Response Curve Meaning:** Graph showing lung toxicity vs delivered dose.
**Related Terms:** NTCP, Radiobiology
**Example:** Pneumonitis risk rises sharply after 20 Gy.

351. **Lumbar Protection Meaning:** Shielding applied to protect lumbar spinal cord segments during abdominal radiotherapy.
**Related Terms:** Organ-at-Risk, Shielding
**Example:** Lead blocks provide lumbar protection during kidney irradiation.

352. **Lumen Mapping Meaning:** Imaging-based outlining of hollow organ interiors.
**Related Terms:** GI Tract, Contouring
**Example:** CT lumen mapping helps delineate the esophagus for thoracic RT.

353. **Lung Avoidance Planning Meaning:** Planning strategies to minimize dose to healthy lung tissue.
**Related Terms:** V20, DVH
**Example:** Lung avoidance planning reduced V20 from 30% to 22% in a chest IMRT plan.

354. **Lymph Node Basin Meaning:** Group of lymph nodes that drain a specific anatomical region.
**Related Terms:** Nodal CTV, Elective Irradiation
**Example:** The axillary basin is targeted in breast cancer RT.

355. **Lesion Localization Meaning:** Identifying the exact position of a lesion using imaging.
**Related Terms:** IGRT, Simulation
**Example:** CBCT aids lesion localization before head-and-neck treatment.

356. **Linear Reconstruction Meaning:** Image reconstruction method based on linear interpolation.
**Related Terms:** CT Imaging, Algorithms
**Example:** Linear reconstruction improves clarity of lung CT slices.

357. **Lateral Dose Falloff Meaning:** Reduction of dose away from beam centerline.
**Related Terms:** Penumbra, Beam Profile
**Example:** Beam shaping achieves steep lateral dose falloff near spinal cord.

358. **Low Scatter Region Meaning:** Area within phantom or patient with minimal scatter radiation.
**Related Terms:** Dosimetry, Phantom
**Example:** Ion chamber placed in a low scatter region avoids false readings.

359. **Local Setup Variation Meaning:** Small daily variations in patient alignment.
**Related Terms:** Setup Error, IGRT
**Example:** Local setup variation of ±2 mm was corrected using CBCT.

360. **Lung Interface Artifact Meaning:** CT imaging artifact at tissue–air boundaries.
**Related Terms:** Hounsfield Units, Artifact
**Example:** Lung interface artifact can distort esophagus contouring.

361. **Linac Beam Symmetry Check Meaning:** Verification that left–right beam intensities are equal.
**Related Terms:** QA, Output
**Example:** Symmetry was measured at 1.5%, within tolerance.

362. **Laser Crosshair Calibration Meaning:** Adjustment of room lasers to match the machine isocenter.
**Related Terms:** Daily QA, Positioning
**Example:** Crosshair calibration ensured ±1 mm accuracy.

363. **Lateral Surface Dose Meaning:** Dose on the patient's lateral body surface.
**Related Terms:** Bolus, Electron Therapy
**Example:** Lateral surface dose increased using 5 mm bolus.

364. **Leakage Current Meaning:** Small unintended electrical current in radiation equipment.
**Related Terms:** Safety, Electronics
**Example:** QA detected leakage current beyond tolerance in the console.

365. **Low-Dose Lung Threshold Meaning:** Minimum dose level considered significant for lung toxicity.
**Related Terms:** V5, V10
**Example:** V5 was limited to <60% per protocol.

366. **Lens Avoidance Planning Meaning:** Planning to minimize dose to the eye lens.
**Related Terms:** OAR, Cataract Risk
**Example:** A superior oblique IMRT beam avoided the lenses.

367. **Lymphoma Field Reduction Meaning:** Modern reduction of irradiated volumes in lymphoma treatment.
**Related Terms:** IFRT, ISRT
**Example:** ISRT replaced large mantle fields.

368. **Low-Contrast Resolution Meaning:** Ability of imaging to distinguish similar-density structures.
**Related Terms:** CT Quality, Image Noise
**Example:** Phantom tests confirmed acceptable low-contrast resolution.

369. **Learning-Based Segmentation Meaning:** AI-driven auto-contouring in RT.
**Related Terms:** Deep Learning, AI-TPS
**Example:** AI segmentation reduced contouring time by 70%.

370. **Lung-Sparing Beams Meaning:** Beam angles selected to reduce lung dose.
**Related Terms:** Beam Arrangement, IMRT
**Example:** Posterior oblique beams provide lung-sparing geometry.

371. **Longitudinal Dose Uniformity Meaning:** Consistent dose along beam direction.
**Related Terms:** Electron Therapy, Build-up
**Example:** Longitudinal uniformity achieved with custom bolus.

372. **Lateral Beam Weighting Meaning:** Adjusting beam intensity on either side of the patient.
**Related Terms:** Optimization, Beams
**Example:** Extra weighting on left beam compensated for lung heterogeneity.

373. **Lung Contour Editing Meaning:** Manual correction of auto-segmented lung contours.
**Related Terms:** Segmentation, IGRT
**Example:** Superior lung edges were refined manually.

374. **Low-Variance Calculation Meaning:** Monte Carlo dose calculations with reduced statistical noise.
**Related Terms:** Algorithms, Accuracy
**Example:** Low-variance MC improved accuracy for lung tumors.

375. **Lumen-Filling Artifact Meaning:** Artifact caused by contrast material in hollow organs.
**Related Terms:** Imaging, Simulation
**Example:** Contrast-filled rectum created lumen artifact during CT.

376. **Lung Perfusion Mapping Meaning:** Mapping lung function to spare functional regions.
**Related Terms:** Functional RT, SPECT
**Example:** Perfusion mapping avoided highly functional lung areas.

377. **Latent Defect Detection Meaning:** Identifying hidden device defects before failure.
**Related Terms:** QA, Preventive Maintenance
**Example:** Thermal testing revealed latent power supply defects.

378. **Lateral Offset Error Meaning:** Deviation from correct patient positioning sideways.
**Related Terms:** Setup Error, IGRT
**Example:** A 3 mm lateral offset was corrected before delivery.

379. **Lumbar Spine Dose Constraint Meaning:** Dose limit for lumbar spinal cord or vertebrae.
**Related Terms:** OAR, DVH
**Example:** Lumbar cord kept below 45 Gy.

380. **Laser-to-Isocenter Matching Meaning:** Ensuring lasers guide patients exactly to isocenter.
**Related Terms:** QA, Daily Checks
**Example:** Laser mismatch corrected during morning QA.

381. **Light Field–Radiation Field Coincidence Meaning:** Ensuring the projected light field matches the actual radiation field.
**Related Terms:** Mechanical QA, Collimator
**Example:** Coincidence within 1 mm passed QA.

382. **Lossless Image Export Meaning:** Exporting images without compression artifacts.
**Related Terms:** DICOM, Archiving
**Example:** Lossless export used for dosimetric auditing.

383. **Lung Motion Envelope Meaning:** Range of tumor motion during breathing.
**Related Terms:** 4D-CT, ITV
**Example:** A 12 mm motion envelope was noted for the lung lesion.

384. **Lead Shield Molding Meaning:** Custom shaping of lead shielding blocks.
**Related Terms:** Cerrobend, Beam Shaping
**Example:** Molded shield protected kidneys during RT.

385. **Lymph Node Gross Target Volume Meaning:** GTV representing involved lymph nodes.
**Related Terms:** GTV-N, Nodal RT
**Example:** PET-positive node added to GTV-N.

386. **Lateral Build-Up Tool Meaning:** Device used to increase dose at lateral surfaces.
**Related Terms:** Bolus, Surface Dose
**Example:** Build-up tool improved dose for ear lesion.

387. **Longitudinal Field Matching Meaning:** Alignment of adjacent radiation fields along body length.
**Related Terms:** Junction Dose, Feathering
**Example:** Feathering eliminated hot spots at spine–cranial junction.

388. **Laser Docking Points Meaning:** Fixed points used for consistent laser calibration.
**Related Terms:** Room Geometry, QA
**Example:** Docking points verified monthly.

389. **Low-Dose Region Mapping Meaning:** Identifying areas receiving low scatter or unintended dose.
**Related Terms:** DVH, QA
**Example:** Mapping identified patient skin receiving stray dose.

390. **Lung Density Override Meaning:** Manual adjustment of lung CT density for dose calculation.
**Related Terms:** HU Override, Heterogeneity
**Example:** Override used for collapsed lung region.

391. **Light Source Uniformity Test Meaning:** Ensuring equal illumination in imaging equipment.
**Related Terms:** CT QA, Noise
**Example:** Non-uniformity flagged during monthly QA.

392. **Linear Accelerator Output Drift Meaning:** Gradual change in beam output over time.
**Related Terms:** Output Calibration, QA
**Example:** Output drift of 1.2% was corrected.

393. **Lateral Organ Sparing Meaning:** Protecting side-located organs by optimizing beam paths.
**Related Terms:** OAR, Planning
**Example:** Lateral sparing reduced kidney dose.

394. **Lung HDR Limit Meaning:** Maximum high-dose parameter allowed for lungs.
**Related Terms:** V20, DVH
**Example:** Lung V20 kept at 26% per tolerance.

395. **Lymph Node Mapping Meaning:** Identifying at-risk lymph nodes for target delineation.
**Related Terms:** CTV-N, Elective Nodes
**Example:** Pelvic mapping used for cervical cancer RT.

396. **Low-Energy Leakage Meaning:** Unintended leakage of low-energy photons from linac head.
**Related Terms:** Head Shielding, QA
**Example:** Monthly QA confirmed acceptable low-energy leakage.

397. **Lung Deformation Model Meaning:** Predictive model of lung shape changes during respiration.
**Related Terms:** Motion Tracking, 4D-CT
**Example:** Deformation model improved ITV accuracy.

398. **Lateral Imaging Pair Meaning:** Two lateral projections used for setup verification.
**Related Terms:** kV Imaging, IGRT
**Example:** Lateral imaging confirmed spine alignment.

399. **Laser QA Phantom Meaning:** Phantom used to verify room laser alignment.
**Related Terms:** Daily QA, Isocenter
**Example:** Laser phantom showed 1 mm deviation.

400. **Linac Control Console Meaning:** The operator interface for delivering treatments.
**Related Terms:** Delivery System, Safety
**Example:** The console displays MU, energy, and gantry angles.

401. **Lung Ridge Artifact Meaning:** A CT artifact caused by sharp density transitions in lung tissue.
**Related Terms:** CT Artifacts, Reconstruction
**Example:** Ridge artifacts were corrected using iterative reconstruction.

402. **Localized Dose Perturbation Meaning:** Small, localized changes in dose due to tissue heterogeneity.
**Related Terms:** Heterogeneity Correction, Dose Algorithms
**Example:** Dose perturbation appeared near metal dental fillings.

403. **Lateral Electron Scatter Meaning:** Spread of electrons sideways within tissue.
**Related Terms:** Electron Beam, Dose Spread
**Example:** Lateral scatter increased dose to adjacent skin.

404. **Low-Scatter Lung Region Meaning:** Portion of the lung where radiation scattering is minimal.
**Related Terms:** Dosimetry, Phantom
**Example:** Ion chamber placed in low-scatter region to avoid noise.

405. **Linear Table Translation Meaning:** Smooth longitudinal movement of the treatment couch.
**Related Terms:** Couch Motion, Setup
**Example:** Linear translation aligned PTV precisely with isocenter.

406. **Lens Dose Monitoring Meaning:** Tracking radiation dose to eye lenses.
**Related Terms:** OAR, Cataract Risk
**Example:** Lens dose kept ≤10 Gy to prevent complications.

407. **Lymphatic Drainage Pathway Meaning:** Path through which lymph fluid moves from tissues.
**Related Terms:** Nodal CTV, Cancer Spread
**Example:** Pelvic pathway mapped for prostate cancer RT.

408. **Lung Segmentation Mask Meaning:** Automated or manual contour of lung boundaries.
**Related Terms:** Contouring, AI
**Example:** AI mask required minor corrections near diaphragm.

409. **Lateral Field Junction Meaning:** Meeting point of two adjacent lateral radiation fields.
**Related Terms:** Field Matching, Feathering
**Example:** Feathering reduced hot spots at the junction.

410. **Low-Dose Artefactual Halo Meaning:** Halo-like ring in images due to low-dose reconstruction.
**Related Terms:** Image Artifacts, CT QA
**Example:** Halo seen in lung CT was removed with higher mAs.

411. **Lateral Beam Separation Meaning:** Distance between parallel-opposed lateral beams.
**Related Terms:** POP Technique, Beam Geometry
**Example:** Beam separation increased to reduce spinal cord dose.

412. **Lung Smoothing Filter Meaning:** Algorithm to reduce noise in lung images.
**Related Terms:** Image Processing, CT Reconstruction
**Example:** Filter clarified tumor edges in low-dose CT.

413. **Leakage Dose Mapping Meaning:** Mapping unwanted radiation leakage in linac head.
**Related Terms:** Shielding, QA
**Example:** Mapping found slight leakage near MLC housing.

414. **Local Beam Calibration Meaning:** Calibration of beam output specific to one room or machine.
**Related Terms:** Output QA, Dosimetry
**Example:** Local calibration matched reference output to ±0.5%.

415. **Lung Collapse Correction Meaning:** Adjusting CT density for areas of collapsed lung.
**Related Terms:** HU Override, Dose Accuracy
**Example:** Override improved dose prediction in atelectasis region.

416. **Lateral Dose Gradient Meaning:** Change in dose across lateral direction.
**Related Terms:** Penumbra, Beam Profile
**Example:** IMRT created steep gradients near parotid gland.

417. **Linear Accelerator Interlock Meaning:** Safety mechanism to prevent unsafe operation.
**Related Terms:** Machine Safety, QA
**Example:** Interlock triggered when gantry angle was out of tolerance.

418. **Lung Tumor Drift Meaning:** Slow positional shift of lung tumor over time.
**Related Terms:** Motion Management, IGRT
**Example:** Drift of 4 mm required plan adaptation.

419. **Low-Frequency Image Noise Meaning:** Gradual variations in image intensity.
**Related Terms:** CT Quality, Noise
**Example:** Phantom scan revealed low-frequency noise pattern.

**420. Lymph Node Dose Boost Meaning:** Higher radiation dose given to positive lymph nodes.
**Related Terms:** Boost Volume, GTV-N
**Example:** Boost of 60 Gy delivered to PET-positive nodes.

**421. Lateral Arm Shielding Meaning:** Shielding arms during chest radiotherapy.
**Related Terms:** OAR Protection, Positioning
**Example:** Lateral shields reduced arm skin dose by 40%.

**422. Lung Expansion Variability Meaning:** Day-to-day differences in lung inflation.
**Related Terms:** 4D-CT, IGRT
**Example:** Variability required adaptive PTV margins.

**423. Local DVH Evaluation Meaning:** Assessing DVH for specific sub-regions.
**Related Terms:** Dose Metrics, Planning
**Example:** Local DVH assessed apex of lung separately.

**424. Low-Energy Imaging Mode Meaning:** Imaging using lower kV settings for contrast.
**Related Terms:** kV Imaging, IGRT
**Example:** Low-energy mode improved bone contrast.

**425. Lateral Couch Roll Meaning:** Side rotation of the treatment couch.
**Related Terms:** Rotational Error, Setup
**Example:** Roll of 2° corrected before treatment.

**426. Lymph Node Visualization Window Meaning:** CT window optimized for viewing lymph nodes.
**Related Terms:** Window Level, Soft Tissue
**Example:** Nodal window improved clarity in neck region.

**427. Laser Synchronization Check Meaning:** Verifying all room lasers align together.
**Related Terms:** Daily QA, Positioning
**Example:** Sync check revealed 1.2 mm mismatch.

**428. Lung Voxel Correction Meaning:** Correcting lung voxels misclassified in auto-segmentation.
**Related Terms:** AI Segmentation, Contouring
**Example:** Voxel correction fixed collapsed lung mis-contours.

**429. Linear Accelerator Beam Gate Meaning:** System that allows beam on/off based on motion.
**Related Terms:** Respiratory Gating, Motion Management
**Example:** Beam gate activated only during exhalation.

**430. Lateral Hip Avoidance Meaning:** Strategy to reduce dose to hip joint during pelvic RT.
**Related Terms:** OAR, Planning
**Example:** Beams angled to minimize hip exposure.

**431. Low-Intensity Beam Arc Meaning:** Arc delivering minimal dose for soft-tissue visualization.
**Related Terms:** IGRT, VMAT
**Example:** Low-intensity arc used for pretreatment imaging.

**432. Lung Tumor Margin Expansion Meaning:** Adding motion and setup margin to lung GTV.
**Related Terms:** PTV, ITV
**Example:** 8 mm expansion created ITV for lung nodule.

**433. Linear Accelerator Gantry Drift Meaning:** Gradual mechanical deviation in gantry movement.
**Related Terms:** Mechanical QA, Accuracy
**Example:** Drift of 0.7° detected during monthly QA.

434. **Low-Resolution Planning Image Meaning:** Planning CT with reduced spatial resolution.
**Related Terms:** Simulation, CT Settings
**Example:** Low-res scans used for body outline only.

435. **Lumen Stabilization Device Meaning:** Tool to maintain shape of hollow organs during imaging.
**Related Terms:** Applicator, Simulation
**Example:** Rectal balloon used for lumen stabilization.

436. **Local Cold Spot Analysis Meaning:** Identifying regions receiving lower-than-prescribed dose.
**Related Terms:** DVH, Homogeneity
**Example:** Cold spot found in posterior PTV region.

437. **Lung Organ-at-Risk (L-OAR) Prioritization Meaning:** Ranking lung protection higher during optimization.
**Related Terms:** IMRT, Constraints
**Example:** PTV coverage adjusted to reduce lung V20.

438. **Low-Dose Imaging Protocol Meaning:** Imaging protocol using minimal radiation.
**Related Terms:** CT Dose, IGRT
**Example:** Low-dose CBCT used for pediatric setup.

439. **Linear Accelerator Servo System Meaning:** Motor system controlling precise mechanical movements.
**Related Terms:** Gantry, Collimator
**Example:** Servo malfunction caused gantry misalignment.

440. **Lymph Node Shrinkage Tracking Meaning:** Monitoring nodal size reduction during RT.
**Related Terms:** Adaptive RT, IGRT
**Example:** Shrinkage of 30% after two weeks prompted adaptation.

441. **Lateral Respiration Motion Meaning:** Side-to-side chest wall movement during breathing.
**Related Terms:** Motion Management, 4D-CT
**Example:** Lateral motion of 5 mm recorded for lung tumor.

442. **Lung Density Heterogeneity Factor Meaning:** Adjustment factor for lung density variations.
**Related Terms:** Algorithms, MC
**Example:** Factor improved accuracy near scar tissue.

443. **Leakage Beam Monitoring System Meaning:** System to detect unintended beam emission.
**Related Terms:** Machine Safety, QA
**Example:** System alarmed due to MLC leakage spike.

444. **Linear Accelerator Heat Load Meaning:** Total thermal load on machine components.
**Related Terms:** Cooling System, Maintenance
**Example:** High heat load caused automatic shutdown.

445. **Low-SNR Imaging Correction Meaning:** Enhancing images with low signal-to-noise ratio.
**Related Terms:** CT Noise, Reconstruction
**Example:** Correction improved visibility of small tumors.

446. **Lateral Electron Energy Loss Meaning:** Energy lost sideways during electron penetration.
**Related Terms:** Electron Therapy, Scatter
**Example:** Lateral loss reduced depth-dose accuracy.

447. **Lung Apex Alignment Meaning:** Ensuring the superior lung regions align properly in IGRT.
**Related Terms:** kV Imaging, Setup
**Example:** Misalignment of apex corrected before treatment.

448. **Local Organ Deformation Meaning:** Minor shape changes in organs during treatment.
**Related Terms:** Adaptive RT, DVF
**Example:** Bladder deformation influenced prostate position.

449. **Lymph Node Sampling Error Meaning:** Underestimation of nodal involvement due to limited sampling.
**Related Terms:** Staging, CTV-N
**Example:** Sampling error necessitated elective nodal irradiation.

450. **Lung Subdivision Contouring Meaning:** Dividing lung into functional sub-regions for planning.
**Related Terms:** Functional RT, Sub-lobar Regions
**Example:** High-function lung kept below 15 Gy.

451. **Lobe-Specific Irradiation Meaning:** Targeting only the affected lung lobe instead of whole lung.
**Related Terms:** Partial Lung RT, Functional Planning
**Example:** Lobe-specific irradiation was used for a localized upper-lobe tumor.

452. **Low-Dose Penalty Function Meaning:** Optimization term penalizing dose outside desired regions.
**Related Terms:** IMRT Optimization, Cost Function
**Example:** Penalty function added to reduce contralateral breast dose.

453. **Local Isocenter Shift Meaning:** Minor adjustment of isocenter for daily alignment.
**Related Terms:** IGRT, Setup Error
**Example:** CBCT detected 2 mm shift corrected automatically.

454. **Linear Sampling Algorithm Meaning:** Dose calculation method using linear interpolation.
**Related Terms:** TPS, Grid Resolution
**Example:** Linear sampling used for fast approximate calculations.

455. **Lung Density Mapping Meaning:** Charting lung density variations for dose prediction.
**Related Terms:** HU Map, 4D-CT
**Example:** Density map improved dose estimates for fibrosis area.

456. **Lumen-Based Targeting Meaning:** Targeting based on the center of a hollow organ.
**Related Terms:** Brachytherapy, GI Imaging
**Example:** Lumen-based targeting used for esophageal boost dose.

457. **Lateral Dose Spill Meaning:** Unwanted low-level dose outside the beam.
**Related Terms:** Scatter, OAR Exposure
**Example:** Collimator rotation reduced lateral dose spill.

458. **Laser-Based Respiration Tracking Meaning:** Tracking breathing using an external laser sensor.
**Related Terms:** Gating, RPM System
**Example:** Laser tracking synchronized beam with exhalation.

459. **Low-Mobility Tumor Classification Meaning:** Categorizing tumors with minimal motion.
**Related Terms:** ITV, Motion Assessment
**Example:** Low-mobility classification allowed tighter PTV margins.

460. **Lung Shield Offset Meaning:** Slight displacement between shield and intended area.
**Related Terms:** Block Placement, QA
**Example:** Offset of 3 mm corrected in simulation.

461. **Local Hotspot Suppression Meaning:** Reducing high dose areas during optimization.
**Related Terms:** Homogeneity, DVH
**Example:** Hotspots above 110% were suppressed via IMRT tuning.

462. **Lens-Sparing Arc Meaning:** Arc angle chosen to avoid radiation passing through eye lens.
**Related Terms:** OAR Protection, Planning
**Example:** Lens-sparing arc used in whole-brain VMAT.

463. **Lung Structure Override Meaning:** Manually modifying HU values inside lung regions.
**Related Terms:** HU Correction, Dose Accuracy
**Example:** Override applied to emphysematous areas.

464. **Local Dose Recalculation Meaning:** Recomputing dose in small sub-regions for accuracy.
**Related Terms:** Adaptive RT, QA
**Example:** Dose recalculated after patient lost weight.

465. **Linear Accelerator Mode Switch Meaning:** Switching between photon and electron modes.
**Related Terms:** Machine Operation, Energy
**Example:** Mode switch required before delivering 12 MeV electrons.

466. **Lateral Isodose Spreading Meaning:** Broadening of isodose lines laterally.
**Related Terms:** Beam Profile, Scatter
**Example:** Field size increase caused dose spreading near ribs.

467. **Low-Attenuation Cavity Meaning:** Air-filled or low-density cavity affecting dose.
**Related Terms:** Heterogeneity, Dose Compensation
**Example:** Sinus cavity reduced dose to adjacent tumor.

468. **Lung Conformity Index Meaning:** Metric assessing how well the plan conforms to lung PTV.
**Related Terms:** Conformity, PTV
**Example:** Conformity index improved from 1.4 to 1.1.

469. **Lead-Leaf Gap Correction Meaning:** Adjustment for spacing between collimator leaves.
**Related Terms:** MLC, Output
**Example:** Gap correction prevented under-dosing of PTV edges.

470. **Lymph Node Atlas Registration Meaning:** Mapping a lymph node atlas to patient anatomy.
**Related Terms:** Auto-Contouring, Nodal CTV
**Example:** Atlas guided nodal contouring for nasopharyngeal cancer.

471. **Lung Inflation State Meaning:** Level of lung expansion during simulation or treatment.
**Related Terms:** Breath-Hold, 4D-CT
**Example:** DIBH maintained consistent inflation state.

472. **Linear Accelerator Start-Up Test Meaning:** Set of checks performed at machine startup.
**Related Terms:** Daily QA, Output
**Example:** Start-up test confirmed beam flatness within limits.

473. **Lateral Photon Contamination Meaning:** Unintended stray photons in lateral directions.
**Related Terms:** Head Leakage, Scatter
**Example:** Contamination reduced using tighter collimation.

474. **Low-Dose Volume Fraction Meaning:** Fraction of organ receiving low doses.
**Related Terms:** DVH, V5, V10
**Example:** Lung V5 was limited to 55%.

475. **Local Couch Height Adjustment Meaning:** Small vertical corrections for setup.
**Related Terms:** IGRT, Positioning
**Example:** Couch raised by 1.5 mm to align target.

476. **Lung Parenchyma Segmentation Meaning:** Contouring of lung tissue excluding vessels and bronchi.
**Related Terms:** Segmentation, AI
**Example:** Segmentation refined automatically.

477. **Low-Density Artifact Masking Meaning:** Removing CT artifacts from low-density regions.
**Related Terms:** Image Cleanup, Reconstruction
**Example:** Masking removed streaks in lung CT.

478. **Lymph Node Migration Pattern Meaning:** Expected spread route of cancer cells.
**Related Terms:** Nodal CTV, Staging
**Example:** Migration pattern informed elective coverage.

479. **Lung Compliance Monitoring Meaning:** Observing lung elasticity changes.
**Related Terms:** Functional Imaging, Motion
**Example:** Compliance drop predicted tumor displacement.

480. **Low-Exposure Imaging Series Meaning:** Imaging taken with minimal radiation for alignment.
**Related Terms:** IGRT, CBCT
**Example:** Low-exposure series used daily in pediatrics.

481. **Linear Accelerator Pulse Timing Meaning:** Timing of individual radiation pulses.
**Related Terms:** Dose Rate, Pulsed Beam
**Example:** Pulse timing irregularities detected during QA.

482. **Local Energy Deposition Model Meaning:** Predictive model of how energy deposits locally.
**Related Terms:** Algorithms, Monte Carlo
**Example:** Model improved accuracy near lung-tissue interfaces.

483. **Lumen Radius Adjustment Meaning:** Modifying radius of hollow organ contours.
**Related Terms:** Contouring, GI Targets
**Example:** Rectum radius adjusted for planning.

484. **Liver Motion Envelope Meaning:** Full extent of liver motion during breathing.
**Related Terms:** Motion Management, 4D-CT
**Example:** Envelope defined ITV for liver lesion.

485. **Local Anatomical Drift Meaning:** Progressive position change of organs across treatment days.
**Related Terms:** Adaptive RT, IGRT
**Example:** Drift caused mismatch in bladder filling.

486. **Low-Z Material Shield Meaning:** Shield made from materials with low atomic number.
**Related Terms:** Electron Therapy, Scatter
**Example:** Low-Z shields used to shape electron fields.

487. **Linear Dose Painting Meaning:** Delivering dose gradients proportionally across tumor.
**Related Terms:** IMRT, Dose Modulation
**Example:** Higher uptake areas received 75 Gy in linear painting.

488. **Lead-Radiation Interface Check Meaning:** QA to examine beam behavior near lead edges.
**Related Terms:** Penumbra, Block QA
**Example:** Check detected overshoot at block edges.

489. **Lung Hysteresis Assessment Meaning:** Evaluating difference between inhalation and exhalation paths.
**Related Terms:** Motion, 4D-CT
**Example:** Hysteresis measured for gating window.

490. **Low-Resolution Organ Mask Meaning:** Simplified organ boundary for fast calculations.
**Related Terms:** AI, Auto-Planning
**Example:** Mask used for quick lung segmentation.

491. **Linear Accelerator Beam Steering Meaning:** Adjusting magnets to center photon beam.
**Related Terms:** Steering Current, QA
**Example:** Steering corrected after 1% symmetry drift.

492. **Lumen Pressure Stabilization Meaning:** Maintaining consistent pressure in rectum/bladder.
**Related Terms:** Balloon Positioning, IGRT
**Example:** Rectal balloon stabilized lumen shape.

493. **Lung Vessel Exclusion Meaning:** Removing blood vessels from lung contours.
**Related Terms:** Segmentation, Contouring
**Example:** Vessel exclusion improved functional lung mapping.

494. **Linear Regression Dose Predictor Meaning:** Predictive model estimating dose metrics.
**Related Terms:** AI, Predictive Analytics
**Example:** Model predicted lung V20 before planning.

495. **Lateral Setup Drift Meaning:** Day-to-day sideways patient movement pattern.
**Related Terms:** Setup Error, IGRT
**Example:** Drift trend corrected using adaptive margins.

496. **Low-Dose Edge Enhancement Meaning:** Improving edge clarity in low-dose images.
**Related Terms:** Image Processing
**Example:** Enhancement improved lung tumor visibility.

497. **Lung Sound Transmission Mapping Meaning:** Acoustic study of lung function regions.
**Related Terms:** Functional Imaging
**Example:** Map used in functional lung-sparing RT.

498. **Linear Accelerator Synchronizer Meaning:** Device ensuring timing sync between subsystems.
**Related Terms:** QA, Machine Control
**Example:** Sync failure stopped treatment until reset.

499. **Local Field Override Meaning:** Manually adjusting dose for a small field region.
**Related Terms:** Dose Editing, TPS
**Example:** Override corrected over-dosed hotspot.

500. **Lung Tissue Perfusion Index Meaning:** Measure of blood flow in lung regions.
**Related Terms:** Perfusion Imaging, Functional RT
**Example:** High-perfusion regions were spared in IMRT plan.

# M

1. **Monitor Unit (MU):** A unit of measurement used in LINACs to quantify the amount of radiation delivered to a patient.
   **Related Terms:** Dose, LINAC, Fractionation
   **Example:** Delivering 200 MU of 6 MV photons to a tumor ensures 2 Gy of absorbed dose.
2. **Megavolt (MV):** One million volts; refers to the energy of X-ray photons used in radiotherapy.
   **Related Terms:** Megavoltage Radiation, Photon Beam, High-Energy Therapy
   **Example:** 15 MV photons penetrate deep tumors like prostate cancers effectively.
3. **Megavoltage Radiation:** High-energy radiation (>1 MV) used for deep-seated tumor treatment.
   **Related Terms:** LINAC, External Beam Radiotherapy (EBRT), Photon Therapy
   **Example:** 6 MV X-rays treat lung tumors while minimizing skin dose.
4. **Multileaf Collimator (MLC):** A device with multiple movable leaves that shapes the radiation beam.
   **Related Terms:** IMRT, VMAT, Beam Shaping
   **Example:** MLC shapes the beam around the tumor to spare normal tissues.
5. **Modulated Radiation Therapy (MRT):** A technique that varies the intensity of radiation across the tumor.
   **Related Terms:** IMRT, VMAT, Dose Painting
   **Example:** IMRT delivers higher doses to tumor while protecting critical organs.
6. **Margin:** Extra tissue around the tumor included to account for movement and setup errors.
   **Related Terms:** Clinical Target Volume (CTV), Planning Target Volume (PTV)
   **Example:** A 5 mm margin is added to CTV to form PTV in head-and-neck cancer plans.
7. **Megavoltage Imaging (MV Imaging):** Imaging using the treatment beam to verify patient setup.
   **Related Terms:** Portal Imaging, Image-Guided Radiotherapy (IGRT)
   **Example:** MV portal images confirm the tumor is aligned with the beam before treatment.
8. **Medical Physics:** Field applying physics principles to radiation therapy, imaging, and QA.
   **Related Terms:** Dosimetry, QA, Treatment Planning
   **Example:** Medical physicists calculate dose distributions and perform LINAC QA.
9. **Monte Carlo Simulation:** Computational method to model particle interactions and dose distribution accurately.
   **Related Terms:** Treatment Planning System (TPS), Dose Calculation, Heterogeneity Correction
   **Example:** Monte Carlo algorithm calculates dose for lung tumors with complex tissue densities.
10. **Modality:** Type of therapy or imaging used for treatment.
    **Related Terms:** Photons, Electrons, Protons, Brachytherapy
    **Example:** LINAC uses photon modality; electrons are used for superficial tumors.
11. **Machine QA:** Routine quality checks to ensure the treatment machine delivers correct dose and geometry.
    **Related Terms:** Daily QA, Monthly QA, LINAC Checks
    **Example:** Daily output verification and MLC position checks prevent errors.

12. **Mechanical Accuracy:** Precision of machine movements like gantry rotation, couch motion, and collimator positioning.
**Related Terms:** QA, Alignment, Gantry, Couch
**Example:** The gantry rotates to planned angles with ±1 mm accuracy.

13. **Monitoring System:** Equipment to track radiation delivery and patient dose.
**Related Terms:** Secondary Dosimetry, Treatment Verification
**Example:** In vivo dosimetry ensures the correct dose is delivered during each fraction.

14. **Motion Management:** Techniques to account for tumor or patient movement during treatment.
**Related Terms:** Gating, Tracking, Respiratory Motion
**Example:** Respiratory gating delivers radiation only during certain breathing phases for lung tumors.

15. **Modulator:** Device used to alter beam intensity or shape in certain radiation therapies.
**Related Terms:** Compensator, MLC, Beam Shaping
**Example:** Modulators in early conformal radiotherapy create uniform dose distributions.

16. **Monitor Chamber :** An ionization chamber inside the LINAC head that measures dose output and controls MU delivery.
**Related Terms:** Dose Calibration, Beam Output, Ion Chamber
**Example:** The monitor chamber stops the beam automatically if delivered MU exceeds the set limit.

17. **Megadose :** A very high radiation dose delivered in stereotactic or ablative treatments.
**Related Terms:** SRS, SBRT, Hypofractionation
**Example:** A single 24 Gy SBRT fraction is considered a megadose.

18. **Magnetic Resonance Simulation (MR Sim) :** MRI-based simulation used for contouring soft-tissue tumors before treatment.
**Related Terms:** MRI, Contouring, Image Registration
**Example:** MR Sim is used for prostate radiotherapy to delineate the gland and neurovascular bundles.

19. **MR-LINAC System :** A machine that combines a LINAC with MRI for real-time adaptive radiotherapy.
**Related Terms:** Adaptive RT, Real-Time Imaging, Soft-Tissue Tracking
**Example:** MR-LINAC corrects shifts in pancreatic tumors during breathing.

20. **Multimodality Imaging :** Combining multiple imaging types (CT/MRI/PET) to improve accuracy of target .
**Related Terms:** Image Fusion, Co-registration, IGRT
**Example:** PET-CT improves contouring in head-and-neck cancers by identifying metabolic tumor regions.

21. **MLC Transmission :** The small fraction of radiation that passes through the MLC leaves.
**Related Terms:** Leakage, Beam Modulation, MLC QA
**Example:** MLC transmission must be checked during monthly QA to ensure it remains below tolerance.

22. **Motion Artifact :** Blurring or streaking in images caused by patient or organ movement.
**Related Terms:** 4DCT, Motion Management, Image Distortion
**Example:** Abdominal CT scans may show motion artifacts due to breathing.

23. **Multiphase CT Scan :** CT imaging performed during different contrast or breathing phases.
**Related Terms:** 4DCT, Liver Imaging, Simulation
**Example:** Multiphase CT is essential in liver radiotherapy to visualize tumors during arterial and venous phases.

24. **Mean Dose :** The average radiation dose delivered to an organ or structure.
**Related Terms:** DVH, OAR Constraints, Dose Metrics
**Example:** Parotid mean dose must remain below 26 Gy to reduce dry mouth.

25. **Maximum Dose (Dmax) :** The highest dose point within the target or organ.
**Related Terms:** Hotspot, Constraints, DVH
**Example:** Spinal cord Dmax must remain below 45 Gy.

26. **Minimum Dose (Dmin) :** The lowest dose point within the target volume.
**Related Terms:** D95, Target Coverage, PTV
**Example:** The PTV must receive at least 95% of the minimum prescribed dose.

27. **Mass Energy Absorption Coefficient :** A measure of how a material absorbs photon energy per unit mass.
**Related Terms:** Dose Absorption, Photon Interaction
**Example:** Soft tissue has a different absorption coefficient than bone, affecting dose calculations.

28. **Multisource Brachytherapy :** Brachytherapy using multiple radioactive sources at different positions.
**Related Terms:** HDR Brachytherapy, Source Dwell Time, Ir-192
**Example:** Cervical cancer applicators use multisource brachytherapy for optimized dose shaping.

29. **Microscopic Disease :** Cancer cells too small to be seen on imaging but at risk of existing near the tumor.
**Related Terms:** CTV, Subclinical Disease
**Example:** CTV margins are added to cover potential microscopic disease spread.

30. **Monitor Unit Verification System (MUVS) :** A secondary system that independently verifies MU accuracy before treatment.
**Related Terms:** Secondary Check, TPS Verification, QA
**Example:** MUVS catches incorrect MU entries before first-day treatment.

31. **Multicentric Tumor :** Tumors arising independently in multiple locations within the same organ.
**Related Terms:** Multifocal, Breast Cancer, Wide Fields
**Example:** Multicentric breast cancer may require larger tangential fields.

32. **Mosaic Field Technique :** A method of connecting multiple radiation fields to cover a large target.
**Related Terms:** Junction, Feathering, TBI
**Example:** TBI uses mosaic fields to avoid hot or cold spots at field junctions.

33. **Magnetic Field Strength (MRI) :** The strength of the MRI magnetic field, measured in Tesla (T).
**Related Terms:** Signal-to-Noise Ratio, Image Resolution
**Example:** A 3T MRI provides superior soft-tissue contrast for brain tumor contouring.

34. **Machine Output Calibration :** Annual QA process to ensure the LINAC delivers exactly 1 cGy/MU (or facility standard).
**Related Terms:** TG-51, Dosimetry Protocol, Absolute Dose
**Example:** Physicists calibrate machine output using an ionization chamber in water.

35. **Marker Seeds :** Small metal seeds implanted into tumors for tracking during radiotherapy.
**Related Terms:** Fiducials, IGRT, Prostate Tracking
**Example:** Gold seeds are placed in the prostate to improve daily alignment.

36. **Multi-Isocenter Technique :** Using more than one isocenter for treating large or irregular targets.
**Related Terms:** Field Junction, Craniospinal Irradiation
**Example:** Craniospinal irradiation often uses three isocenters to cover the entire neuraxis.

37. **Motion Envelope :** The total range of movement a tumor undergoes during breathing.
**Related Terms:** ITV, 4DCT, Respiratory Motion
**Example:** ITV is drawn based on the motion envelope seen in 4D CT scans.

38. **MapCHECK :** A 2D diode array used for patient-specific QA in IMRT and VMAT.
**Related Terms:** Patient QA, Gamma Analysis, Diode Array
**Example:** MapCHECK verifies fluence patterns before IMRT treatment.

39. **Monte Carlo Dose Engine :** The TPS module that performs Monte Carlo–based dose calculations.
**Related Terms:** Algorithm, Heterogeneity Correction, Dose Accuracy
**Example:** The Monte Carlo engine improves dose accuracy for lung SBRT plans.

40. **Margin Expansion Algorithm :** Software algorithm that automatically expands CTV to PTV using defined margins.
**Related Terms:** CTV–PTV, PTV Generation, Motion Allowance
**Example:** A 5 mm isotropic margin is applied using the expansion algorithm during planning.

41. **Molecular Imaging:** Imaging that visualizes molecular activity inside tissues using PET tracers.
**Related Terms:** PET-CT, FDG Uptake, Metabolic Imaging
**Example:** Molecular imaging helps identify metabolically active tumor regions for dose escalation.

42. **Metastatic Burden:** The extent and number of metastatic lesions in the body.
**Related Terms:** Oligometastasis, Stage IV, SBRT
**Example:** Low metastatic burden patients may receive SBRT for long-term disease control.

43. **Mixed Modality Therapy:** Treatment combining radiotherapy with chemotherapy, surgery, or immunotherapy.
**Related Terms:** Concurrent Chemoradiation, Multidisciplinary Treatment
**Example:** Cervical cancer is treated with mixed modality therapy using radiation and cisplatin.

44. **Magnetic Field Generator:** Component in MRI producing strong magnetic fields for imaging.
**Related Terms:** MRI, Gradient Coils, RF Coils
**Example:** A 3T magnetic field generator improves brain tumor visualization.

45. **Mode-Up Time:** The time a LINAC takes to stabilize dose output after beam is turned on.
**Related Terms:** Beam Stability, Output Calibration
**Example:** SBRT requires short mode-up times to deliver accurate small-dose segments.

46. **Matrix Size (Imaging):** Number of pixels in each dimension of CT/MRI images.
**Related Terms:** Resolution, Pixel Size
**Example:** A 512×512 matrix improves visibility of small structures.

47. **Motion Envelope Margin:** Margin added to account for tumor movement during breathing.
**Related Terms:** ITV, 4DCT, Respiratory Motion
**Example:** Lung PTV incorporates the full motion envelope margin.

48. **Magnetic Resonance Angiography (MRA):** MRI technique used to visualize blood vessels.
**Related Terms:** MRI, Vascular Imaging
**Example:** MRA is used for brain tumors to avoid irradiating major arteries.

49. **Manual Beam Weighting:** Adjusting beam intensities manually during 3D conformal planning.
**Related Terms:** Beam Optimization, Conformal RT
**Example:** Physicists manually adjust beam weights for breast tangents.

50. **Map-Based Planning:** Using color-coded dose maps to optimize treatment plans.
**Related Terms:** Dose Distribution, TPS
**Example:** Hotspot maps help planners reduce excessive dose regions.

51. **Mass Density Override:** Changing tissue density values in TPS to improve dose accuracy.
**Related Terms:** Hounsfield Units, Heterogeneity Correction
**Example:** Density override is applied on dental fillings during head-and-neck planning.

52. **Margin Reduction Protocol:** A protocol reducing PTV margins when IGRT is used.
**Related Terms:** IGRT, Setup Error, PTV
**Example:** Daily CBCT reduces prostate margins from 7 mm to 4 mm.

53. **Modulated Electron Therapy:** Electron beams whose intensity or shape is modified to improve dose conformity.
**Related Terms:** Electron Boost, Bolus
**Example:** Modulated electrons treat chest wall scars after mastectomy.

54. **Multileaf Speed:** The rate at which MLC leaves move during dynamic treatments.
**Related Terms:** VMAT, Dynamic MLC, Leaf Motion
**Example:** High MLC speed is essential for VMAT delivery.

55. **Monte Carlo Beam Modeling:** Creating accurate beam models using Monte Carlo physics.
**Related Terms:** TPS Modeling, Algorithm Commissioning
**Example:** Beam modeling improves lung SBRT accuracy.

56. **Microwave Power Source:** Device generating microwave energy to accelerate electrons in LINACs.
**Related Terms:** Magnetron, Klystron
**Example:** A failing microwave source causes unstable beam output.

57. **Multi-Criteria Optimization (MCO):** Planning technique balancing many objectives simultaneously.
**Related Terms:** Pareto Optimization, TPS
**Example:** MCO lets planners trade off target coverage and OAR sparing interactively.

58. **Motion-Induced Dose Error:** Dose inaccuracy caused by tumor or patient movement.
**Related Terms:** Interplay Effect, Respiratory Motion
**Example:** IMRT on mobile lung tumors may cause motion-induced errors.

59. **Metallic Artifact Reduction:** Techniques that reduce artifacts from implants in imaging.
**Related Terms:** MAR Algorithm, CT Metal Artifact
**Example:** Titanium dental implants require artifact reduction.

60. **Multi-Isocenter VMAT:** VMAT delivered using more than one isocenter for large targets.
**Related Terms:** Junction, Craniospinal RT
**Example:** VMAT CSI treatments use 2–3 isocenters to cover long spine regions.

61. **Meshing (TPS):** Dividing volumes into small elements for dose calculation.
**Related Terms:** Voxel, Grid Size
**Example:** Finer meshing improves accuracy for small targets.

62. **Magnetic Beam Steering:** Using magnetic fields to direct electron or proton beams.
**Related Terms:** Steering Coils, Beam Alignment
**Example:** Steering coils correct electron beam drift.

63. **Median Dose:** The midpoint dose value in a dose distribution.
**Related Terms:** DVH, Dose Statistics
**Example:** The median PTV dose must equal the prescription.

64. **Manual Contouring:** Manually outlining organs and targets on CT/MRI scans.
**Related Terms:** Segmentation, Auto-Contouring
**Example:** Radiation oncologists contour the spinal cord manually.

65. **Molecular Radiotherapy:** Radiotherapy using radioactive molecules targeted to cancer cells.
    **Related Terms:** Radionuclide Therapy, I-131, Lu-177
    **Example:** Lu-177 therapy treats neuroendocrine tumors.

66. **Multi-Planar Reconstruction (MPR):** Viewing CT/MRI images in coronal, sagittal, and axial planes.
    **Related Terms:** Image Fusion, 3D Visualization
    **Example:** MPR helps visualize spinal curvature in planning.

67. **Monitor Chamber Linearity:** Ability of monitor chamber readings to remain accurate at different MU levels.
    **Related Terms:** Output Calibration, QA
    **Example:** Monthly QA verifies linearity across MU ranges.

68. **Mixed-Beam Therapy:** Using both photons and electrons in the same treatment.
    **Related Terms:** 3DCRT, Combined Modality
    **Example:** Chest wall RT uses photons plus electron boost.

69. **Mask Immobilization:** Thermoplastic masks used to hold the head still during treatment.
    **Related Terms:** Immobilization, Mould Room
    **Example:** Head-and-neck patients receive custom masks.

70. **MLC Leakage:** Small amount of radiation passing through closed MLC leaves.
    **Related Terms:** Transmission, QA
    **Example:** Leakage must remain below tolerance (<2%).

71. **Modulation Factor:** Ratio describing complexity of IMRT delivery.
    **Related Terms:** MU Efficiency, Optimization
    **Example:** Highly modulated plans have high modulation factors.

72. **Margin Analysis:** Evaluating adequacy of CTV-to-PTV margins.**Related Terms:** Setup Error, Motion
    **Example:** IGRT data are used for weekly margin analysis.

73. **Multilevel Image Registration:** Registration performed at multiple scales for accuracy.
    **Related Terms:** Rigid Registration, Deformable Registration
    **Example:** Multilevel registration aligns PET and CT images precisely.

74. **Motion Robust Planning:** Planning designed to withstand patient and tumor motion.
    **Related Terms:** ITV, 4D Planning
    **Example:** Robust plans are used in proton therapy for lung tumors.

75. **Magnetic Resonance Spectroscopy (MRS):** MRI technique measuring biochemical changes in tissue.
    **Related Terms:** MRI, Metabolite Mapping
    **Example:** MRS helps differentiate tumor recurrence from necrosis.

76. **Molecular Targeted Agents:** Drugs targeting specific tumor molecules used with radiotherapy.
    **Related Terms:** Radiosensitizers, Targeted Therapy
    **Example:** Cetuximab enhances radiation response in head-and-neck cancer.

77. **Muon Radiation:** Rare secondary cosmic radiation considered in shielding calculations.
    **Related Terms:** Neutron Production, Shielding Design
    **Example:** High-energy proton centers consider muon contributions.

78. **Magnetic Tracking System:** Tracks motion of implanted markers using magnetic fields.
    **Related Terms:** Fiducial Tracking, IGRT
    **Example:** Magnetic tracking monitors prostate motion in real time.

79. **Multichannel Ion Chamber:** Detector with multiple channels for simultaneous beam measurement.
**Related Terms:** QA Device, Dose Measurement
**Example:** Used during commissioning to measure profiles.

80. **Molecular Dose Painting:** Adjusting dose based on molecular imaging signals.
**Related Terms:** PET-Guided RT, Adaptive Therapy
**Example:** High-FDG regions receive extra dose boosts.

81. **Mobility Index:** Quantifies tumor motion amplitude during respiration.
**Related Terms:** Respiratory Gating, Motion Tracking
**Example:** A mobility index >1 cm requires motion management.

82. **Measurement Uncertainty:** Statistical uncertainty in dose measurement tools.
**Related Terms:** Dosimetry, Calibration
**Example:** Ion chamber measurements have ±2% uncertainty.

83. **Multichannel Dosimetry:** Using multiple detectors for dose verification.
**Related Terms:** EPID Dosimetry, Diode Arrays
**Example:** Multichannel film dosimetry improves accuracy.

84. **MLC Tongue-and-Groove Effect:** Dose variation caused by leaf interlocking design.
**Related Terms:** MLC Design, Transmission
**Example:** TPS models tongue-and-groove effects for IMRT.

85. **Motion Prediction Algorithm:** Predicts future tumor positions based on breathing patterns.
**Related Terms:** Tracking, Gating
**Example:** Predictive models improve lung tumor tracking.

86. **Multi-Target Treatment Planning:** Creating plans for multiple tumors or metastases.
**Related Terms:** SRS, VMAT
**Example:** VMAT SRS treats 3 brain metastases in one plan.

87. **Magnetic Hysteresis (LINAC):** Lagging of magnetic response in steering coils.
**Related Terms:** Beam Steering, Magnet Coil
**Example:** Hysteresis affects electron beam direction.

88. **Monte Carlo Commissioning:** Validating Monte Carlo dose engines before clinical use.
**Related Terms:** TPS Commissioning, Beam Modeling
**Example:** Commissioning ensures accurate lung dose predictions.

89. **Manual MU Scaling:** Adjusting MU values manually after changing plan parameters.
**Related Terms:** Dose Normalization, TPS
**Example:** MU scaling is used when prescription dose is updated.

90. **Multitimepoint Imaging:** Imaging performed at different time points for comparison.
**Related Terms:** Adaptive RT, IGRT
**Example:** Mid-treatment CT assesses tumor shrinkage.

91. **Multiphase CT Scan:** CT images captured during different phases of breathing or contrast enhancement.
**Related Terms:** 4DCT, Contrast CT, Simulation
**Example:** Multiphase CT helps identify liver tumor motion differences across breathing cycles.

92. **Magnetic Resonance Linac (MR-LINAC):** Treatment machine combining MRI imaging with real-time radiotherapy.
**Related Terms:** Adaptive RT, MR-guided RT, IGRT
**Example:** MR-LINAC allows real-time tumor tracking during abdominal treatments.

93. **Material Attenuation Coefficient:** A measure of how much a material reduces radiation intensity.
**Related Terms:** Photon Interaction, Absorption, Scatter
**Example:** Bone has a higher attenuation coefficient than soft tissue.

94. **Manual Couch Shifts:** Physical adjustment of couch position to align the patient.
**Related Terms:** IGRT, Setup Correction, Laser Alignment
**Example:** Technologists perform manual couch shifts after reviewing CBCT.

95. **Multi-Leaf Calibration:** Process of verifying each MLC leaf position and speed.
**Related Terms:** QA, DMLC, VMAT
**Example:** Monthly multi-leaf calibration ensures sub-millimeter accuracy.

96. **Mesorectal Radiation Field:** Radiation field covering the mesorectum in rectal cancer.
**Related Terms:** Pelvic RT, CTV, Organ-at-Risk
**Example:** Mesorectal coverage is crucial for preventing local recurrence.

97. **Micro-Dose Regions:** Very small areas receiving extremely low radiation doses.
**Related Terms:** Scatter Dose, Peripheral Dose
**Example:** Micro-dose regions are calculated for pregnant patient safety.

98. **Mechanical Sag:** Small shifts in the gantry or couch due to gravity.
**Related Terms:** Gantry Accuracy, Couch Stability
**Example:** Mechanical sag is measured during annual QA.

99. **Multi-Segment IMRT:** IMRT delivered using multiple static MLC segments.
**Related Terms:** Step-and-Shoot, Segmental IMRT
**Example:** Breast IMRT uses 7–12 segments per field.

100. **Mid-Plane Dose:** Dose delivered at the middle depth of the patient.
**Related Terms:** Depth Dose, SSD, Attenuation
**Example:** Mid-plane dose is important for AP/PA spine fields.

101. **Mirror Laser System:** Ceiling-mounted lasers used for patient positioning.
**Related Terms:** Simulation, Setup, Room Lasers
**Example:** Mirror lasers align patient tattoos with isocenter.

102. **Material Decomposition (Imaging):** Technique separating materials based on CT energy levels.
**Related Terms:** Dual-Energy CT, Tissue Mapping
**Example:** Material decomposition distinguishes calcium from iodine.

103. **Megavolt Flatness:** Uniformity of the photon beam intensity across the field.
**Related Terms:** Symmetry, QA, Beam Profile
**Example:** Monthly QA checks MV flatness within ±3%.

104. **Metal Fiducials:** Small metallic markers implanted for image guidance.
**Related Terms:** IGRT, Tracking, Prostate RT
**Example:** Gold fiducials are used to track prostate movement.

105. **Multi-Fractionation Schedule:** Treatment plan with multiple fractions per week.
**Related Terms:** Conventional RT, Hypofractionation
**Example:** Breast cancer uses a 15-fraction schedule.

106. **MLC Positional Drift:** Slow deviation of MLC leaves from calibrated positions.
**Related Terms:** QA, Mechanical Error
**Example:** Drift beyond tolerance requires recalibration.

**107. Maximum Dose Constraint:** Upper allowable dose limit for an organ or structure.
**Related Terms:** Dose Limits, OAR Protection
**Example:** The spinal cord maximum dose is limited to 45 Gy.

**108. Modality Blending:** Combining imaging modalities for better visualization.
**Related Terms:** PET-CT Fusion, MR-CT Fusion
**Example:** MR-CT blending improves prostate contouring.

**109. Morphological Segmentation:** Contouring method based on shape and structure detection.
**Related Terms:** Auto-Segmentation, Image Processing
**Example:** Morphological segmentation identifies lymph nodes.

**110. Motion Phantom:** Device simulating human breathing or organ movement.
**Related Terms:** QA, 4DCT, SBRT
**Example:** Motion phantoms test lung gating accuracy.

**111. Median Energy (Electrons):** Energy at which half of electrons have higher energy and half lower.
**Related Terms:** Electron Beam, Depth Dose
**Example:** A 12 MeV electron beam has a median energy of ~10 MeV.

**112. Maximum Tolerated Dose (MTD):** Highest dose that can be safely delivered to tissue.
**Related Terms:** RTOG Limits, Toxicity
**Example:** Lung V20 helps avoid exceeding tissue MTD.

**113. Microbeam Radiation Therapy:** Experimental therapy using ultra-thin radiation beams.
**Related Terms:** Synchrotron Therapy, Preclinical
**Example:** Microbeam RT widens the therapeutic ratio in animal studies.

**114. Magnetic Patient Positioning:** Using magnetic fields to assist patient alignment.
**Related Terms:** MR-LINAC, IGRT
**Example:** MR-LINAC uses magnetic coordinates for positioning.

**115. Multi-Layer Collimation:** Collimators arranged in multiple layers for sharper beam shaping.
**Related Terms:** Beam Shaping, MLC
**Example:** Proton machines use multi-layer collimation.

**116. Minimum Dose Coverage:** Minimum percent of target volume receiving prescribed dose.
**Related Terms:** DVH, PTV Coverage
**Example:** PTV must receive at least 95% dose coverage.

**117. Measurement Phantom:** Object that mimics human tissue for dosimetry testing.
**Related Terms:** Water Phantom, QA
**Example:** A solid water phantom measures beam output.

**118. Monte Carlo Scatter Kernel:** Scatter model used in TPS dose calculations.
**Related Terms:** Convolution-Superposition, Algorithm
**Example:** MC scatter kernel improves accuracy in lung tissues.

**119. Motion Probability Map:** Map showing likelihood of tumor presence in each position during breathing.
**Related Terms:** 4D Planning, ITV
**Example:** Lung plans incorporate motion probability maps.

**120. Multi-Observer Contouring:** Several clinicians independently contouring structures.
**Related Terms:** Interobserver Variability
**Example:** Brain tumor contours are averaged for consistency.

121. **Multichannel Film Analysis:** Processing films using multiple color channels (RGB) for accuracy.
**Related Terms:** Dosimetry Film, QA
**Example:** Multichannel analysis reduces film artifacts.

122. **Margin Expansion Algorithm:** Software method expanding CTV to PTV uniformly.
**Related Terms:** PTV Margin, Automation
**Example:** A 5 mm isotropic margin is applied automatically.

123. **Maximum Leaf Gap:** Largest allowed gap between opposing MLC leaves.
**Related Terms:** MLC Geometry, Planning Limits
**Example:** IMRT leaf gap must not exceed 3 cm.

124. **Magnetic Marker Tracking:** Tracking implanted magnetic seeds for motion monitoring.
**Related Terms:** Fiducials, SGRT
**Example:** Magnetic seeds track prostate shifts in real time.

125. **Multi-Arc Delivery:** Using multiple rotational arcs to deliver VMAT.
**Related Terms:** VMAT, Arc Therapy
**Example:** Brain SRS uses 3–4 arcs for target conformity.

126. **Mouth Bite Block:** Device placed in mouth to immobilize the jaw.
**Related Terms:** Head-and-Neck Immobilization
**Example:** Tongue displacement blocks reduce oral mucosa dose.

127. **Magnetron Output Stability:** Consistency of power produced by the magnetron.
**Related Terms:** LINAC, Microwave Source
**Example:** Unstable magnetron leads to dose fluctuations.

128. **Mixed Radiation Field:** Radiation field containing photons, electrons, or neutrons simultaneously.
**Related Terms:** Beam Composition, Shielding
**Example:** High-energy beams may produce mixed radiation fields.

129. **Mapping Dose Falloff:** Measuring how dose decreases outside the target.
**Related Terms:** Penumbra, Gradient Index
**Example:** SRS plans require steep dose falloff mapping.

130. **Motion-Adaptive Delivery:** Radiation delivery adjusted in real time for patient motion.
**Related Terms:** Tracking, Gating
**Example:** Adaptive delivery tracks liver tumors during respiration.

131. **Mean Organ Dose:** Average dose received by an organ.
**Related Terms:** DVH, OAR Constraints
**Example:** Reducing mean lung dose lowers pneumonitis risk.

132. **Multi-Point Ion Chamber Measurement:** Measuring dose at multiple points simultaneously.
**Related Terms:** QA, Dosimetry
**Example:** Used to verify non-uniform IMRT fields.

133. **Modal Frequency (SGRT):** Frequency at which camera systems capture surface motion.
**Related Terms:** SGRT, Tracking
**Example:** Higher modal frequency improves breathing tracking.

134. **Monochromatic Beam (Imaging):** Beam that contains a single energy level of photons.
**Related Terms:** Dual-Energy CT, Spectral CT
**Example:** Monochromatic imaging reduces metal artifacts.

135. **Multiscale Noise Reduction:** Image processing technique reducing noise at different scales.
**Related Terms:** CT Reconstruction, Smoothing
**Example:** Used for low-dose CT scans.

136. **Measured Gamma Index:** Value comparing measured and planned dose distributions.
**Related Terms:** QA, IMRT Verification
**Example:** Passing gamma >95% indicates good plan accuracy.

137. **Metal Shielding Tray:** Holder for custom lead cutouts used in electron therapy.
**Related Terms:** Electron Field, Cutout
**Example:** Electron cutout trays shape the electron beam.

138. **Modified Fractionation:** Non-standard fraction schedules such as hyper-, hypo-, or accelerated.
**Related Terms:** Hypofractionation, CHART, SBRT
**Example:** Lung SBRT is a modified fractionation schedule.

139. **Matched Field Junction:** Region where two adjacent radiation fields meet.
**Related Terms:** Craniospinal RT, Feathering
**Example:** CSI requires careful management of field junctions.

140. **Multivisceral Contouring:** Contouring involving multiple organs around complex tumors.
**Related Terms:** OAR Segmentation, TPS
**Example:** Pancreatic RT requires multivisceral contouring.

141. **Multimodal Image Registration:** Aligning images from different modalities such as CT, MRI, and PET.
**Related Terms:** Fusion, IGRT, Contouring
**Example:** PET-CT registration helps identify active tumor regions for dose boost.

142. **Magnetically Guided Beam:** Radiation beam that is steered or stabilized using magnetic fields.
**Related Terms:** MR-LINAC, Beam Steering
**Example:** MR-LINAC uses magnetic guidance to keep beams aligned during treatment.

143. **Margin Verification Scan:** Imaging used to confirm that CTV-PTV margins are adequate.
**Related Terms:** IGRT, PTV Margin
**Example:** A mid-treatment CBCT verifies margin adequacy for prostate RT.

144. **Multi-Energy CT:** CT imaging acquired at multiple energy levels.
**Related Terms:** Spectral CT, Dual-Energy CT
**Example:** Multi-energy CT helps distinguish bone from metal artifacts.

145. **Mean Target Dose:** Average dose delivered to the target volume.
**Related Terms:** DVH, PTV Coverage
**Example:** Treatment plans ensure mean PTV dose is within ±3% of prescription.

146. **Micro-Field Dosimetry:** Measuring dose in very small radiation fields (<1 cm).
**Related Terms:** SRS, Small-Field QA
**Example:** Micro-chambers are used to measure SRS micro-fields.

147. **Multislice Detector Array:** Device capturing multiple CT slices simultaneously.
**Related Terms:** CT Simulation, Detector Technology
**Example:** Multislice CT scanners reduce scanning time for simulation patients.

148. **Magnetic Susceptibility Artifact:** Image distortion in MRI caused by metal or air.
**Related Terms:** MRI Artifacts, Distortion
**Example:** Dental fillings create susceptibility artifacts in head-and-neck MRI.

149. **Medical Dosimetrist:** Professional who creates radiation treatment plans.
**Related Terms:** TPS, Plan Optimization
**Example:** Dosimetrists design IMRT plans for head-and-neck cancers.

150. **Multi-Beam Arrangement:** Using multiple radiation beams to optimize dose distribution.
**Related Terms:** 3D-CRT, IMRT
**Example:** A 7-beam IMRT arrangement is common for prostate cancer.

151. **Magnification Factor (Imaging):** Ratio of object size on image to its real-life size.
**Related Terms:** Portal Imaging, Geometry
**Example:** Magnification factor is corrected during EPID QA.

152. **Manual Bolus Placement:** Hand placing a bolus material on patient to increase surface dose.
**Related Terms:** Electron Therapy, Skin Dose
**Example:** Chest wall RT requires manual bolus application.

153. **Maxillary Sinus Shielding:** Protecting maxillary sinuses during head-and-neck irradiation.
**Related Terms:** OAR, IMRT Optimization
**Example:** IMRT reduces maxillary sinus dose to prevent chronic sinusitis.

154. **Multi-Slice MRI Acquisition:** MRI capturing many slices in a single cycle.
**Related Terms:** MR Imaging, Fast Scanning
**Example:** Multi-slice MRI shortens brain tumor imaging time.

155. **Motion Vector Field:** Map of tissue displacement between two images.
**Related Terms:** Deformable Registration, 4D Imaging
**Example:** DVFs help estimate tumor shifts during breathing.

156. **Motorized Couch Rotation:** Automatic rotation of treatment couch to specified angles.
**Related Terms:** Non-coplanar Beams, SRS
**Example:** Non-coplanar brain SRS uses couch rotation for better conformity.

157. **Mean Liver Dose:** Average radiation dose delivered to the liver.
**Related Terms:** OAR Limits, QUANTEC
**Example:** Mean liver dose must stay <30 Gy for SBRT safety.

158. **Multi-Phase Dose Accumulation:** Adding doses from different treatment phases accurately.
**Related Terms:** Adaptive RT, Deformable Mapping
**Example:** Dose accumulation is used for shrinking lung tumors.

159. **Magnet Coil Alignment:** Adjusting coil placement to ensure proper beam steering.
**Related Terms:** Steering Coil, QA
**Example:** Coil alignment corrects electron beam rotation mis-steering.

160. **Multimodality Treatment Review:** Joint evaluation of patient cases by different specialties.
**Related Terms:** Tumor Board, Combined Therapy
**Example:** Multimodality review determines if RT and immunotherapy should be combined.

161. **Modified Planning Technique:** Customizing standard planning protocols for special cases.
**Related Terms:** Non-Standard Plan, Constraints
**Example:** Modified techniques are used when patients have pacemakers.

162. **Micro-CT (Preclinical):** Ultra-high resolution CT used in small animal studies.
**Related Terms:** Preclinical RT, Imaging
**Example:** Micro-CT evaluates tumor response in mouse models.

163. **Multi-Point Calibration:** Calibration using several dose points to improve accuracy.
**Related Terms:** Ion Chamber Calibration, Equipment QA
**Example:** Linacs undergo multi-point calibration for output consistency.

164. **Motion Capture Imaging:** Imaging capturing real-time patient motion.
**Related Terms:** SGRT, 4DCT
**Example:** Surface imaging captures respiratory motion during SBRT.

165. **Maximum Penumbra Width:** Largest width of the dose falloff at field edges.
**Related Terms:** Beam Profile, Sharpness
**Example:** SRS plans require very small penumbra widths.

166. **Matrix Resolution (TPS):** Grid resolution used for dose calculation.
**Related Terms:** Voxel Size, Accuracy
**Example:** SBRT uses a fine matrix resolution (1–2 mm).

167. **Mixed Photon-Electron Technique:** Combining photon and electron fields in one treatment.
**Related Terms:** Hybrid Fields, Skin Dose
**Example:** Breast boost uses electron + photon combination.

168. **Magnetic Beam Modeling:** Modeling how magnetic fields influence dose distribution.
**Related Terms:** MR-LINAC, TPS
**Example:** MR-LINAC TPS incorporates magnetic beam modeling.

169. **Multi-Detector CT (MDCT):** CT scanner with many detector rows capturing many slices per rotation.
**Related Terms:** CT Simulation, Fast Imaging
**Example:** MDCT reduces motion artifacts in thorax scans.

170. **Minimal Segment Weight:** Minimum MU allowed for an IMRT segment.
**Related Terms:** IMRT Efficiency, Plan Complexity
**Example:** Small segments with low weights may be removed to simplify delivery.

171. **MLC Collision Check:** Ensuring MLC does not collide with accessories during delivery.
**Related Terms:** Safety Check, QA
**Example:** Collision checks are required when using small stereotactic cones.

172. **Mean Lung Dose (MLD):** Average dose received by both lungs.
**Related Terms:** Pneumonitis Risk, OAR Constraint
**Example:** MLD $< 20$ Gy reduces pneumonitis chances.

173. **Motion Artifact Suppression:** Technique reducing motion blurring in imaging.
**Related Terms:** 4DCT, Reconstruction Algorithms
**Example:** Artifact suppression improves abdominal MRI clarity.

174. **Multi-Room Proton Facility:** Proton center with multiple treatment rooms sharing one accelerator.
**Related Terms:** Cyclotron, Gantry Rooms
**Example:** Many national proton centers operate multi-room designs.

175. **Magnetic Contrast Enhancement:** Improving MRI soft-tissue contrast using magnetic effects.
**Related Terms:** MRI Sequences, T1/T2 Imaging
**Example:** MR contrast improves brainstem tumor visibility.

176. **Multi-Sampling EPID Readout:** Acquiring several EPID frames for accurate measurement.
**Related Terms:** EPID QA, Portal Dosimetry
**Example:** Multi-sampling reduces noise during IMRT QA.

177. **Maximum Field Size:** The largest square or rectangular field a LINAC can produce.
**Related Terms:** Collimator, Beam Limiting
**Example:** Many LINACs have maximum field size of 40×40 cm.

178. **Mu-Metal Shielding:** Magnetic shielding material used around sensitive components.
**Related Terms:** Magnetic Protection, Equipment Safety
**Example:** Mu-metal prevents magnetic interference in MR-LINAC rooms.

179. **Modified Isocentric Technique:** Adjusting isocenter or beam angles for irregular anatomies.
**Related Terms:** Non-Isocentric RT, Geometric Planning
**Example:** Breast tangents may use modified isocentric alignment.

180. **Multi-Institutional Planning Study:** Study comparing plans created by multiple centers.
**Related Terms:** Benchmarking, Protocol Validation
**Example:** Trials compare IMRT techniques across institutions.

181. **Maxillary Protection Wedge:** Wedge used to spare maxillary structures during RT.
**Related Terms:** Physical Wedges, Beam Shaping
**Example:** Used in some 3D-CRT head-and-neck setups.

182. **Monte Carlo Fluence Map:** Fluence map generated using Monte Carlo dose modeling.
**Related Terms:** Dose Calculation, Beam Modeling
**Example:** Fluence maps guide complex IMRT optimization.

183. **Motion Stability Index:** Metric describing patient stability during treatment.
**Related Terms:** SGRT, Monitoring
**Example:** High stability index indicates good immobilization.

184. **Multi-Angle Field Setup:** Using many beam angles for better target coverage.
**Related Terms:** IMRT, 3D-CRT
**Example:** 9-field IMRT for pelvic tumors uses multi-angle beams.

185. **Mitigation Strategy (Radiotherapy):** Protocol to reduce treatment-related risks.
**Related Terms:** Quality Assurance, Error Prevention
**Example:** Double-check procedures are mitigation strategies.

186. **Magnetic Field Homogeneity:** Uniformity of magnetic field strength across MRI volume.
**Related Terms:** MRI Quality, Shimming
**Example:** Poor homogeneity causes image distortion in MR-LINACs.

187. **Motion-Compensated Reconstruction:** Image reconstruction that accounts for breathing motion.
**Related Terms:** 4DCT, Motion Correction
**Example:** Improves clarity in mobile organs like liver.

188. **Modified Split-Field Technique:** Splitting radiation fields to avoid overdosing sensitive areas.
**Related Terms:** Craniospinal, Junction Technique
**Example:** Split fields are used to protect shoulders in head-and-neck RT.

189. **Multi-Stage Optimization:** Planning done in sequential stages for improved quality.
**Related Terms:** IMRT Optimization, MCO
**Example:** Stage 1 optimizes target, stage 2 protects OARs.

190. **Microbeam Collimator:** Device creating extremely small radiation beamlets.
**Related Terms:** Microbeam Therapy, Preclinical RT
**Example:** Synchrotron beams require microbeam collimators.

191. **MLC Leaf Speed:** Maximum velocity of MLC leaves during dynamic delivery.
**Related Terms:** VMAT, IMRT, Dynamic MLC
**Example:** Faster leaf speed improves VMAT efficiency and conformity.

192. **MLC Leakage:** Radiation passing through MLC leaves when they are closed.
**Related Terms:** Leaf Transmission, Shielding
**Example:** Leakage must remain <2% for safe delivery.

193. **MLC Transmission Factor:** Fraction of radiation transmitted through leaves.
**Related Terms:** Beam Modeling, TPS
**Example:** TPS uses a transmission factor of 0.015 for dose accuracy.

194. **Mass Density:** Mass per unit volume of tissue affecting photon attenuation.
**Related Terms:** HU Values, Electron Density
**Example:** Lung density changes dose distribution in IMRT.

195. **Mean Dose:** Average radiation dose delivered to a structure.
**Related Terms:** DVH, OAR
**Example:** Mean parotid dose must stay <26 Gy.

196. **Maximum Dose Constraint:** Highest allowable dose for an organ at risk.
**Related Terms:** Tolerance Dose, Planning Goals
**Example:** Cord max dose limited to 45 Gy.

197. **Megapixel Detector:** High-resolution EPID imaging detector.
**Related Terms:** MV Imaging, Portal Imaging
**Example:** Megapixel detectors provide clear bony anatomy alignment images.

198. **Medium-Energy Electrons:** Electrons in 6–12 MeV range.
**Related Terms:** Electron Therapy, Surface Dose
**Example:** 9 MeV electrons treat superficial chest wall tumors.

199. **Metal Artifact Reduction:** Techniques reducing metal-induced CT distortion.
**Related Terms:** CT Reconstruction, HU Correction
**Example:** Metal artifact correction improves pelvic planning accuracy.

200. **Motion Envelope:** Full range of tumor movement over breathing cycles.
**Related Terms:** ITV, 4D-CT
**Example:** A 12-mm motion envelope is added for PTV.

201. **Multi-Arc VMAT:** VMAT using multiple arcs for better conformity.
**Related Terms:** IMRT, Arc Therapy
**Example:** Two-arc VMAT improves prostate coverage.

202. **Manual Contouring:** Physician-drawn tumor and organ outlines.
**Related Terms:** Segmentation, GTV
**Example:** Manual contouring ensures accurate spinal cord boundaries.

203. **Magnetic Field Imaging:** Imaging using MRI instead of X-rays.
**Related Terms:** MR-Sim, Soft Tissue Contrast
**Example:** MRI helps visualize brainstem margins precisely.

204. **Multidisciplinary Team (MDT):** Group of specialists managing patient care.
**Related Terms:** Tumor Board, Oncology Team
**Example:** MDT reviews best modality for lung cancer.

205. **Minimum Dose:** Lowest dose inside the target volume.
**Related Terms:** Homogeneity Index, DVH
**Example:** Minimum dose to PTV must exceed 95%.

206. **Monitor Chamber (Secondary):** Backup chamber verifying dose delivery.
**Related Terms:** Dosimetry, Redundancy
**Example:** Secondary chamber prevents overdose if primary fails.

207. **Mechanical Isocenter:** Point where gantry, couch, and collimator axes intersect.
**Related Terms:** Winston-Lutz, QA
**Example:** Must be accurate within 1 mm.

208. **Metal Shielding:** High-Z materials used to block radiation.
**Related Terms:** Attenuation, Barriers
**Example:** Lead blocks create electron cutouts.

209. **Multi-Fraction Treatment:** Radiation given in several sessions.
**Related Terms:** Fractionation, Daily Dose
**Example:** Breast cases use 15–25 fractions.

210. **Mid-Point Calibration:** Dose calibration at central beam depth.
**Related Terms:** Output Calibration, TG-51
**Example:** LINAC calibrated to deliver 1 cGy/MU.

211. **Motion Compensation:** Techniques to counter breathing or organ shifts.
**Related Terms:** Gating, Tracking
**Example:** Pancreas tumors use real-time motion compensation.

212. **Marginal Miss:** When part of the tumor lies outside treated volume.
**Related Terms:** PTV, Geographic Miss
**Example:** Underestimation of CTV margin causes marginal miss.

213. **Multiplanar Reconstruction (MPR):** Reformatting images into axial, coronal, sagittal planes.
**Related Terms:** 3D Imaging, CT Planning
**Example:** MPR improves pelvic node contouring.

214. **Motion Phantom:** Device simulating respiratory or cardiac motion.
**Related Terms:** QA, 4D QA
**Example:** Used to validate gated treatment accuracy.

215. **Magnetic Resonance Spectroscopy (MRS):** MRI technique analyzing tissue metabolites.
**Related Terms:** Imaging Biomarkers, Tumor Characterization
**Example:** MRS differentiates tumor recurrence from necrosis.

216. **Modulated Arc Therapy:** Arc therapy with variable dose rate and MLC movement.
**Related Terms:** VMAT, IMAT
**Example:** Used for complex head-and-neck cases.

217. **Minimum Field Size:** Smallest safe field size a LINAC can deliver.
**Related Terms:** MLC, Beam Data
**Example:** Below 3×3 cm, output becomes unreliable.

218. **Mechanical Sag:** Small positional shifts from gantry or couch weight.
**Related Terms:** QA, Winston-Lutz
**Example:** Gantry sag increases at 180° angle.

219. **Multi-Lesion SRS:** SRS targeting multiple brain metastases in one session.
**Related Terms:** SRS, VMAT
**Example:** 8 brain mets treated with single-isocenter VMAT.

220. **Motion Baseline Drift:** Gradual shift in breathing baseline over time.
**Related Terms:** Gating, ITV
**Example:** Drift must be corrected during long liver treatments.

221. **Maximum Monitor Units (MU/Min):** Highest dose rate a LINAC can deliver.
**Related Terms:** FFF Mode, Dose Rate
**Example:** 2400 MU/min used in FFF SBRT.

222. **Multi-Phase CT:** CT taken during several contrast phases.
**Related Terms:** Arterial Phase, Venous Phase
**Example:** Liver tumors require multi-phase imaging.

223. **Microscopic Disease:** Cancer cells too small to be seen on imaging.
**Related Terms:** CTV, Margins
**Example:** CTV includes microscopic extension beyond GTV.

224. **Mineral Oil Phantom:** Phantom using mineral oil for dosimetric calibration.
**Related Terms:** QA, Dosimetry
**Example:** Used for MRI-LINAC calibration.

225. **Milligray (mGy):** Unit of absorbed dose equal to 0.001 Gy.
**Related Terms:** Dose Units, Exposure
**Example:** CT scan may deliver ~10 mGy.

226. **Microbeam Radiotherapy:** Uses arrays of tiny radiation beams for experimental therapy.
**Related Terms:** Spatial Fractionation, Research
**Example:** Microbeams spare healthy tissue while damaging tumors.

227. **Mass Stopping Power:** Energy loss of charged particles per unit density.
**Related Terms:** Electrons, Protons
**Example:** Used for accurate electron planning.

228. **Metal Filter:** Filter modifying beam quality in imaging.
**Related Terms:** Beam Hardening, Filtration
**Example:** Copper filters reduce patient dose.

229. **Multi-Planar Dose Check:** Dose verification in multiple planes.
**Related Terms:** QA, Plan Verification
**Example:** Phantom receives dose in axial, sagittal, coronal planes.

230. **Minimal Monitor Unit Setting:** Lowest MU deliverable safely in a beam segment.
**Related Terms:** IMRT Segments, Dose Rate
**Example:** Some LINACs restrict segments <5 MU.

231. **Magnetic Susceptibility:** Tendency of tissue to distort magnetic fields.
**Related Terms:** MRI Artifacts
**Example:** Dental implants create susceptibility distortions.

232. **Monte Carlo Dose Engine:** TPS component using Monte Carlo physics.
**Related Terms:** Dose Algorithm, Heterogeneity
**Example:** Used for lung and bone irregularities.

233. **Multi-Center Trial:** Research involving multiple institutions.
**Related Terms:** Clinical Trials, Protocols
**Example:** RTOG trials are multi-center.

234. **Margin Expansion:** Adding geometric buffer to CTV to form PTV.
**Related Terms:** CTV, PTV
**Example:** 5 mm expansion accounts for motion.

235. **Molecular Imaging:** Imaging using biological processes.
**Related Terms:** PET, SPECT
**Example:** FDG PET highlights active tumor regions.

236. **Mode Up Delay:** Time required for LINAC to reach stable dose rate.
**Related Terms:** Dose Rate, QA
**Example:** Beam requires a few milliseconds to stabilize.

237. **Multi-Energy Imaging:** Imaging at different energy levels for better contrast.
**Related Terms:** Dual-Energy CT
**Example:** Soft tissue contrast improves in thorax.

238. **Multi-Detector CT (MDCT):** CT scanner with multiple detection rows.
**Related Terms:** Helical CT, Fast Imaging
**Example:** MDCT reduces motion artifacts in abdomen.

239. **Motion Robustness:** Plan's ability to tolerate motion.
**Related Terms:** ITV, Robust Optimization
**Example:** Proton plans often evaluated for motion robustness.

240. **Multi-Modality Treatment:** Combining different treatment types.
**Related Terms:** Surgery, Chemoradiation
**Example:** Rectal cancer treated with chemo + RT + surgery.

241. **Motion Artifact:** Distortion caused by patient movement in imaging.
**Related Terms:** MRI Blur, CT Streaking
**Example:** Breathing creates blurry lung images.

242. **Multi-Modality Fusion:** Merging CT, MRI, PET for planning.
**Related Terms:** Registration, Contouring
**Example:** PET-CT fusion identifies active tumor.

243. **MR-LINAC:** Machine combining MRI and radiation delivery.
**Related Terms:** MRgRT, Adaptive Therapy
**Example:** Real-time imaging used for pancreas RT.

244. **Manual MU Calculation:** Hand-calculated MU check.
**Related Terms:** Secondary Check, QA
**Example:** Physics verifies 200 MU manually.

245. **Modulation Factor:** Degree of intensity variation in IMRT.
**Related Terms:** Complexity Index
**Example:** High modulation factor indicates complex plan.

246. **Mobile Target:** Tumor that moves with breathing.
**Related Terms:** ITV, Motion Management
**Example:** Liver tumors move several mm during respiration.

247. **Mixed Beam Therapy:** Combination of photon + electron beams.
**Related Terms:** Hybrid Plan
**Example:** Skin cancers treated with mixed beams.

248. **Multilayer Ion Chamber:** Detector with multiple ion chambers.
**Related Terms:** QA, Dosimetry
**Example:** Used for IMRT QA.

249. **Minimum Segment Width:** Smallest segment allowable in IMRT.
**Related Terms:** MLC, Modulation
**Example:** Some TPS enforce ≥1 cm width.

250. **Multi-Point Calibration:** Calibration at several depths/fields.
**Related Terms:** Beam Data, Commissioning
**Example:** Used for accurate PDD curves.

251. **Maximum Field Size:** Largest field a LINAC can produce.
**Related Terms:** Collimator, Jaw Settings
**Example:** 40×40 cm is typical.

252. **Magnetic Resonance Angiography (MRA):** MRI technique showing blood vessels.
**Related Terms:** MRI, Contrast
**Example:** Used for brain AVM treatment planning.

253. **Multi-Leaf Leakage Map:** Map showing leakage through MLC leaves.
**Related Terms:** EPID, QA
**Example:** Used for IMRT QA modeling.

254. **Micro-Dosimetry:** Study of dose at microscopic scales.
**Related Terms:** Radiobiology, DNA Damage
**Example:** Used in particle therapy research.

255. **Mass Thickness:** Amount of mass per area along beam path.
**Related Terms:** Attenuation, Electron Density
**Example:** Important in heterogeneity corrections.

256. **Manual Registration:** Manual alignment of CT/MRI/PET.
**Related Terms:** Fusion, Contouring
**Example:** Used when automatic fusion fails.

257. **Motion Prediction:** Estimating tumor movement from patterns.
**Related Terms:** Tracking, Gating
**Example:** Predictive algorithms used in CyberKnife.

258. **Multi-Purpose Phantom:** Phantom supporting imaging and dosimetry QA.
**Related Terms:** QA Tools
**Example:** RANDO phantom used for dose verification.

259. **Minimum Source-to-Skin Distance (SSD):** Lowest SSD for safe delivery.
**Related Terms:** Setup, Electron Therapy
**Example:** 100 cm SSD standard in many centers.

260. **Monitor Chamber Drift:** Change in chamber reading over time.
**Related Terms:** QA, Calibration
**Example:** Regular calibration prevents drift errors.

261. **Mixed Modality Imaging:** Combining imaging types in workflow.
**Related Terms:** PET-CT, MR-CT
**Example:** PET used for tumor, MRI for nerves.

262. **Multislice Reconstruction:** Constructing slices from helical or axial CT.
**Related Terms:** CT Algorithms
**Example:** Improves lung imaging quality.

263. **Macroscopic Disease:** Visible tumor mass.
**Related Terms:** GTV, Staging
**Example:** GTV drawn around visible lung tumor.

264. **Multinodular Tumor:** Tumor consisting of multiple nodules.
**Related Terms:** Multifocal Disease
**Example:** Thyroid cancer may be multinodular.

265. **Metal Fixation Device:** Metal plates/screws used in surgery causing imaging artifacts.
**Related Terms:** Artifact, CT Distortion
**Example:** Cervical spine hardware affects contouring.

266. **Molecular Targeted Therapy:** Drugs targeting specific cancer molecules.
**Related Terms:** ChemoRT
**Example:** EGFR inhibitors combined with RT.

267. **Multi-Phase MRI:** MRI taken during several physiologic phases.
**Related Terms:** Dynamic Imaging
**Example:** Liver MRI uses arterial and venous phases.

268. **Motion-Balanced Delivery:** Treatment technique combining motion and beam control.
**Related Terms:** Tracking, Gating
**Example:** CyberKnife synchrony tracking.

269. **Maximum Penumbra:** Largest region of partial radiation intensity at beam edges.
**Related Terms:** Beam Edges, Dosimetry
**Example:** Penumbra increases with SSD.

270. **Multi-Leaf Latency:** Delay between leaf command and actual movement.
**Related Terms:** MLC QA, VMAT
**Example:** Latency measured during dynamic QA.

271. **Mechanical Collision Check:** Ensures gantry, couch, and patient avoid collisions.
**Related Terms:** Simulation, Safety
**Example:** Couch kick tested before VMAT.

272. **Minimum Gantry Speed:** Slowest speed gantry can rotate safely.
**Related Terms:** VMAT, Dose Rate
**Example:** Slow speed used for high modulation.

273. **Multi-Dose Rate Delivery:** Changing dose rate during treatment.
**Related Terms:** VMAT, Modulation
**Example:** FFF beams use varying dose rates.

274. **Mass Energy Absorption Coefficient:** Measure of how tissue absorbs energy.
**Related Terms:** Interaction Coefficients
**Example:** Used in depth-dose calculations.

275. **Matrix Resolution (Image Grid):** Number of pixels in imaging matrix.
**Related Terms:** IGRT, EPID
**Example:** Higher matrix = better localization.

276. **Micro-Movement Error:** Small unintended movements during treatment.
**Related Terms:** Immobilization
**Example:** Mask reduces micro-movements in H&N patients.

277. **Molecular Biomarkers:** Biological indicators used in cancer staging.
**Related Terms:** Personalized Medicine
**Example:** PSA levels monitor prostate cancer.

278. **MLC Leaf Gap:** Space between opposing leaves.
**Related Terms:** Dosimetry, Beam Modeling
**Example:** Leaf gap calibration affects output.

279. **Multi-Detector PET:** PET system with multiple detectors.
**Related Terms:** PET-CT, Resolution
**Example:** Improves tumor SUV accuracy.

280. **Multivariate Analysis:** Statistical evaluation of multiple variables.
**Related Terms:** Research, Clinical Studies
**Example:** Used to evaluate predictors of toxicity.

281. **Maximum Output Variation:** Allowed change in daily LINAC output.
**Related Terms:** QA Tolerances
**Example:** Output must stay within ±3%.

282. **Manual Couch Shift:** Hand-adjusted movement of treatment couch.
**Related Terms:** IGRT, Setup
**Example:** Therapist shifts couch 3 mm left.

283. **Midline Anatomy:** Structures along body's midline.
**Related Terms:** Contouring
**Example:** Midline shift indicates brain swelling.

284. **Multi-Portal Treatment:** Using several beam angles.
**Related Terms:** 3DCRT, IMRT
**Example:** Prostate treated with 7-field IMRT.

285. **Multi-Chamber Electrometer:** Electrometer connected to multiple chambers.
**Related Terms:** Dosimetry, Calibration
**Example:** Used in annual QA.

286. **Maximum SSD Technique:** Using largest possible SSD for uniformity.
**Related Terms:** TBI, Beam Divergence
**Example:** TBI uses extended SSD of 300–400 cm.

287. **Monitor Interlock:** Safety feature stopping beam during errors.
**Related Terms:** Machine Faults
**Example:** Interlock triggers during MLC failure.

288. **Muon Interaction (Advanced Physics):** Rare particle interactions relevant to shielding.
**Related Terms:** Particle Physics
**Example:** Muon penetration considered in deep facilities.

289. **Multigrid Reconstruction (Imaging):** Fast algorithm for CT/MR reconstruction.
**Related Terms:** Iterative Reconstruction
**Example:** Reduces noise in low-dose CT.

290. **Multinuclear MRI:** MRI using nuclei other than hydrogen.
**Related Terms:** Spectroscopy
**Example:** Phosphorus-31 MRI used in research imaging.

291. **Magnetic Field Distortion:** Distortion in MRI images caused by metal or inhomogeneous magnetic fields.
**Related Terms:** MRI Artifacts, Susceptibility
**Example:** Dental implants create magnetic field distortion in MR-sim images.

292. **Multi-Lesion Planning:** Planning for multiple tumors in one treatment session.
**Related Terms:** SRS, Single-Isocenter VMAT
**Example:** Treating 10 brain metastases using single-isocenter SRS.

293. **Motion-Adaptive Radiotherapy:** Real-time adjustment of beam delivery based on organ motion.
**Related Terms:** Tracking, Gating
**Example:** CyberKnife adjusts beam position as the lung tumor moves.

294. **Multi-Compartment Dose Calculation:** Dose computed separately for different tissue types.
**Related Terms:** Heterogeneity Correction
**Example:** Lung and soft tissue densities handled separately in Monte Carlo.

295. **Marker-Based IGRT:** Image guidance using implanted fiducial markers.
**Related Terms:** Fiducials, Prostate IGRT
**Example:** Gold seeds implanted in prostate improve alignment accuracy.

296. **Modulated Electron Therapy:** Electron beams delivered with varying intensity.
**Related Terms:** Electron IMRT, Modulation
**Example:** Used for scalp lesions with irregular shapes.

297. **Multisource Dose Calculation:** Dose computed from multiple radiation sources (brachytherapy or multi-ports).
**Related Terms:** Source Modeling
**Example:** Cervical HDR uses multiple dwell positions for uniform dose.

298. **Mixed Photon Energy Treatment:** Using more than one photon energy for a plan.
**Related Terms:** 6 MV, 10 MV, Beam Selection
**Example:** Combining 6 MV + 15 MV improves homogeneity in pelvic fields.

299. **Mean Lung Dose (MLD):** Average dose delivered to lungs.
**Related Terms:** Lung Constraint, V20
**Example:** MLD kept below 20 Gy in lung cancer plans.

300. **Mid-Sagittal Plane:** Central dividing plane of the body used for imaging alignment.
**Related Terms:** Anatomical Planes
**Example:** Mid-sagittal alignment ensures symmetric head setup.

301. **Multi-Sequence MRI:** MRI using several sequences (T1/T2/FLAIR/DWI).
**Related Terms:** MR-Sim, Soft Tissue
**Example:** T2 images used for contouring brain tumors.

302. **Margin Reduction Technique:** Strategies to reduce PTV margins safely.
**Related Terms:** IGRT, Motion Management
**Example:** Daily CBCT allows margin reduction from 7 mm → 3 mm.

303. **Magnetic Coil System:** Coils generating magnetic fields for MRI.
**Related Terms:** MR-LINAC, Gradient Coils
**Example:** Gradient coil determines MRI spatial resolution.

304. **Multi-Fraction SBRT:** Stereotactic treatment delivered in several high-dose fractions.
**Related Terms:** Hypofractionation, SRT
**Example:** 3-fraction lung SBRT delivering 54 Gy in total.

305. **Maximum Likelihood Reconstruction:** Iterative method to reconstruct PET/CT images.
**Related Terms:** MLEM, Iterative Reconstruction
**Example:** MLEM improves low-count PET imaging.

306. **Modulated Brachytherapy:** Adjusting dwell time/position for dose shaping.
**Related Terms:** HDR Brachytherapy, Dwell Time
**Example:** Dwell modulation boosts the tumor and spares bladder.

307. **Multi-Planar IGRT Review:** Checking images in axial, coronal, and sagittal planes.
**Related Terms:** CBCT, Registration
**Example:** CBCT reviewed in three planes before treating the pelvis.

308. **Mean Parotid Dose:** Average dose to parotid gland.
**Related Terms:** OAR Constraint, IMRT
**Example:** Keeping mean parotid dose <26 Gy preserves saliva function.

309. **Multi-Breath-Hold Technique:** Multiple breath-holds used to deliver treatment.
**Related Terms:** DIBH, Respiratory Motion
**Example:** Left breast DIBH reduces heart dose.

310. **Machine Learning in Radiotherapy:** AI models used for dosimetry, contouring, or QA.
**Related Terms:** Auto-Segmentation, Prediction Models
**Example:** ML predicts optimal IMRT fluence maps.

311. **Microcalcification Imaging:** Imaging to detect tiny calcium deposits.
**Related Terms:** Mammography
**Example:** Microcalcifications help diagnose early breast cancer before RT.

312. **Multi-Slice PET Reconstruction:** PET image reconstruction using multiple detector slices.
**Related Terms:** PET-CT, Image Resolution
**Example:** Multi-slice PET improves tumor SUV accuracy.

313. **Magnetic Shielding:** Materials used to reduce magnetic interference.
**Related Terms:** MRI Safety
**Example:** MR-LINAC rooms require magnetic shielding walls.

314. **Motion Stability Index:** Quantifies how stable a patient's breathing pattern is.
**Related Terms:** Motion Analysis, Gating
**Example:** Unstable breathing requires larger ITV.

315. **Mass Attenuation Curve:** Graph showing how photons attenuate in a material.
**Related Terms:** Beam Quality, HVL
**Example:** Curve shows greater attenuation in bone vs lung.

316. **Multi-Catheter Brachytherapy:** Multiple catheters inserted for dose modulation.
**Related Terms:** Breast Brachytherapy, HDR
**Example:** APBI uses multi-catheter templates.

317. **Mean Target Dose:** Average dose to the tumor target volume.
**Related Terms:** PTV Coverage
**Example:** Mean PTV dose should match prescription (e.g., 60 Gy).

318. **Manual Dose Tuning:** Human adjustment of dose constraints or weights.
**Related Terms:** Optimization, Planning
**Example:** Planner adjusts hot spots manually in pelvis IMRT.

319. **Microbeam Collimator:** Device producing extremely small radiation beams.
**Related Terms:** Microbeam RT, Research
**Example:** Experimental microbeam therapy uses micrometer-scale collimators.

320. **Motion-Managed Simulation:** CT scanning with respiratory management.
**Related Terms:** 4D-CT, Gating
**Example:** Lung CT done with phase-based 4D simulation.

321. **Multi-Coil MRI Reconstruction:** Combining signals from multiple MRI coils.
**Related Terms:** SNR, Parallel Imaging
**Example:** Multi-coil imaging speeds up MR-Sim scans.

322. **Missing Tissue Compensation:** Correcting dose when tissue is absent or uneven.
**Related Terms:** Bolus, Compensator
**Example:** Bolus used on nose to compensate for missing tissue.

323. **Machine Output Trend:** Long-term pattern of LINAC output.
**Related Terms:** QA Logs, Stability
**Example:** Output trending +1% per month indicates calibration drift.

324. **Median Dose:** Middle dose value in the dose distribution.
**Related Terms:** DVH Metrics
**Example:** Used to evaluate uniformity of PTV coverage.

325. **Multi-Tube CT:** CT scanners with two or more X-ray tubes.
**Related Terms:** Dual-Energy CT
**Example:** Multi-tube CT provides better temporal resolution.

326. **Maximum Organ Dose:** Highest absorbed dose within an organ.
**Related Terms:** DVH, Constraints
**Example:** Bladder max dose limited to <65 Gy.

327. **MLC Positional Error:** Deviation between planned and actual leaf position.
**Related Terms:** MLC QA, Dynamic IMRT
**Example:** EPID detects leaf errors >1 mm.

328. **Marker Block:** Radiopaque block used to identify reference points.
**Related Terms:** Simulation Markers
**Example:** BB markers placed on skin for isocenter localization.

329. **Multi-Planar Anatomical Matching:** Matching patient anatomy across multiple planes.
**Related Terms:** IGRT Registration
**Example:** Pelvic bones aligned in axial and sagittal planes.

330. **Megabit Image Storage:** Digital storage of large IGRT/CBCT image datasets.
**Related Terms:** PACS, Image Archiving
**Example:** Daily CBCT images stored in megabit-scale files.

331. **Motion Correction Algorithm:** Software correcting movement during imaging.
**Related Terms:** MRI Correction, 4D Reconstruction
**Example:** MR motion correction helps liver tumor contouring.

332. **Multiple Gradient Echo (MGE):** MRI sequence using several gradient echoes.
**Related Terms:** MRI Sequences
**Example:** MGE enhances susceptibility contrast for brain imaging.

333. **Micrometre Position Accuracy:** Extremely precise mechanical accuracy in positioning.
**Related Terms:** SRS, Robotics
**Example:** Robotic couches position within micrometre tolerance.

334. **Multi-Isocenter Planning:** Using more than one isocenter for large or separated targets.
**Related Terms:** Field Matching, Craniospinal Irradiation
**Example:** CSI treatments use multiple isocenters.

335. **Motion Deformable Registration:** Accounting for organ deformation in image fusion.
**Related Terms:** DIR, 4D Fusion
**Example:** Deformable fusion of end-exhale to end-inhale CT.

336. **MLC Calibration Curve:** Graph showing leaf transmission versus position.
**Related Terms:** Commissioning, QA
**Example:** Curve updated during annual QA.

337. **Multi-Direction Dose Delivery:** Delivering radiation from many angles.
**Related Terms:** IMRT, VMAT
**Example:** 9-field IMRT provides multi-direction dose shaping.

338. **Medical Imaging Informatics:** Managing imaging data, storage, and workflow.
**Related Terms:** PACS, DICOM
**Example:** RT planning uses DICOM-RT for exporting doses and contours.

339. **Maximum Breathing Amplitude:** Largest displacement of diaphragm or tumor during breathing.
**Related Terms:** ITV, Motion Tracking
**Example:** 15 mm amplitude used to generate motion-encompassing margins.

340. **Multi-Stage Optimization:** Planning optimization done in several steps.
**Related Terms:** TPS Optimization, Dose Shaping
**Example:** First stage sets coverage; second stage refines OAR sparing.

341. **Multi-Layer Ionization Chamber (MLIC):** A dosimeter with many stacked ion chambers used to measure depth-dose curves.
**Related Terms:** Commissioning, Beam Data
**Example:** MLIC measures electron PDD curves during LINAC commissioning.

342. **Margin Expansion Algorithm:** Software method that automatically expands CTV → PTV.
**Related Terms:** CTV, PTV, Geometric Margin
**Example:** TPS uses 5 mm isotropic margin expansion for prostate cancer.

343. **Medium-Energy X-Rays:** X-ray beams in the 100–300 kVp range.
**Related Terms:** Orthovoltage, Superficial Therapy
**Example:** Medium-energy beams treat skin cancers and shallow tumors.

344. **Multi-Pass Optimization:** Repeated optimization cycles to refine dose distribution.
**Related Terms:** Inverse Planning, TPS
**Example:** IMRT plans improve after multi-pass fluence refinement.

345. **MLC Transmission Factor:** Fraction of radiation passing through closed MLC leaves.
**Related Terms:** Leakage, Dosimetry
**Example:** 6 MV MLC transmission typically ~1.5%.

346. **Multi-Frame CBCT:** Cone-beam CT composed of many projection frames.
**Related Terms:** 3D Image Reconstruction
**Example:** Multi-frame scans help visualize lung tumors more clearly.

347. **Matched Beam Pairs:** Photon beams calibrated to identical output and quality.
**Related Terms:** Beam Matching, Dual LINAC Sites
**Example:** Two LINACs are matched so patients can switch machines.

348. **Modulated Arc Therapy:** Radiotherapy where intensity is modulated continuously during arc rotation.
**Related Terms:** VMAT, Dynamic IMRT
**Example:** Prostate VMAT modulates dose during 360° gantry rotation.

349. **Multi-ROI Optimization:** Using many contours (ROIs) to control dose distribution.
**Related Terms:** OAR Constraints, PTV Coverage
**Example:** Planner sets priorities for 12 different OARs.

350. **Motion Synchronization:** Matching the timing of radiation delivery with patient breathing.
**Related Terms:** Gating, Tracking
**Example:** Beam turns on only at end-exhale for liver SBRT.

351. **Megavoltage Portal Dosimetry:** Using MV images to verify delivered IMRT fluence.
**Related Terms:** EPID QA, Pretreatment QA
**Example:** Portal dosimetry detects fluence errors >2%.

352. **Multi-Session SRS:** Stereotactic radiosurgery delivered over several sessions.
**Related Terms:** Hypofractionated SRS
**Example:** 3-session SRS used for large AVMs.

353. **MLC Interdigitation:** Capability for MLC leaves to overlap without collision.
**Related Terms:** High-Resolution MLC, IMRT
**Example:** Varian HD-MLC allows interdigitated leaf positions.

354. **Minimum Target Dose:** Lowest dose within the tumor volume.
**Related Terms:** Dmin, Coverage
**Example:** Dmin >95% is required in most PTV coverage metrics.

355. **Magneto-Optic Dosimetry:** Dosimetry based on magnetic changes in materials after irradiation.
**Related Terms:** Novel Dosimetry
**Example:** Used experimentally in dose mapping research.

356. **Multi-Modal Contouring:** Contouring using multiple imaging modalities.
**Related Terms:** CT, MRI, PET
**Example:** PET-MRI used to improve GTV accuracy in head-neck RT.

357. **Multi-Beam Electron Therapy:** Electron treatments delivered from multiple field directions.
**Related Terms:** Electron Planning
**Example:** Used for curved surfaces like scalp tumors.

358. **Motion Compensation Software:** Corrects for patient motion during imaging or delivery.
**Related Terms:** 4DCT, MR-Motion
**Example:** Software reduces liver motion blur in MR-Sim.

359. **Metal Artifact Correction (MAR):** Algorithms that reduce CT streak artifacts from metal implants.
**Related Terms:** CT Artifacts
**Example:** MAR improves accuracy around hip prosthesis for pelvic RT.

360. **Multi-Channel Film Dosimetry:** Using all color channels (RGB) to improve film dose measurement.
**Related Terms:** Film QA, EBT3
**Example:** Channels corrected to remove scanner artifacts.

361. **Mask Fixation System:** Thermoplastic masks used to immobilize head or neck.
**Related Terms:** Immobilization, H&N RT
**Example:** Mask prevents movement during SRS delivery.

362. **Multi-Isocenter VMAT:** VMAT arcs delivered using more than one isocenter.
**Related Terms:** Large Field Planning
**Example:** Total marrow irradiation requires multi-isocenter VMAT.

363. **Mega-Dose Fractionation:** Delivering very high single fractions.
**Related Terms:** SRS, SBRT
**Example:** 24 Gy single-fraction spine SRS is mega-dose radiotherapy.

364. **Motion Envelope:** Region encompassing maximum organ motion.
**Related Terms:** ITV, Motion Margin
**Example:** ITV defined by motion envelope from 4DCT.

365. **Multi-Detector Ion Chamber Array:** 2D or 3D arrays used for pretreatment QA.
**Related Terms:** ArcCheck, MatriXX
**Example:** ArcCheck verifies VMAT plan accuracy.

366. **Magnetic Resonance Angiography (MRA):** MRI technique to visualize blood vessels.
**Related Terms:** MRI Sequences
**Example:** MRA helps contour carotid arteries in head-neck planning.

367. **Matched Field Junction:** The interface where two radiation fields meet.
**Related Terms:** Feathering, Field Matching
**Example:** CSI requires careful matched junctions to avoid dose gaps.

368. **Multi-Parameter Optimization:** Optimization considering many constraints.
**Related Terms:** IMRT Planning, Weighting
**Example:** TPS optimizes 36 objectives for a single pelvis plan.

369. **Margin Simulation Study:** Testing different margins to evaluate robustness.
**Related Terms:** Robust Planning
**Example:** Study compares 3 mm vs 5 mm PTV margins for prostate.

370. **Minimum MU Constraint:** TPS setting requiring each beam to deliver a minimum number of MUs.
**Related Terms:** IMRT, Safety
**Example:** Minimum MU prevents beams from under-delivering dose.

371. **Multi-Point Ion Chamber Measurement:** Setting ion chamber in several positions for beam profiling.
**Related Terms:** Commissioning, Output Factors
**Example:** Ion chamber moved to 10 depths to record PDD.

372. **Motion Pattern Analysis:** Characterizing how a tumor moves over time.
**Related Terms:** 4DCT, Respiratory Models
**Example:** Lung tumor exhibits irregular motion requiring gating.

**373. Maximum Setup Uncertainty:** Largest expected variation in patient setup.
**Related Terms:** Margin, IGRT
**Example:** H&N RT uses <2 mm maximum setup uncertainty.

**374. Multi-Gantry Angle Planning:** Planning with many gantry directions for coverage.
**Related Terms:** IMRT, Beam Angle Optimization
**Example:** 12-beam IMRT uses multi-angle selection.

**375. Micro-Leaf MLC:** MLC with very thin leaves for high precision.
**Related Terms:** HD-MLC, SRS
**Example:** 2.5 mm leaf width used for small brain metastases.

**376. Medium-Dose Constraint:** Limits on moderate dose levels in organs.
**Related Terms:** DVH, OAR
**Example:** Rectum V40 < 50% is a medium-dose constraint.

**377. Multi-Phase Liver Planning:** Planning using CT acquired in different liver phases.
**Related Terms:** 4DCT, Motion
**Example:** Used for liver SBRT to avoid mis-targeting due to motion.

**378. Machine Fault Detection:** Identifying LINAC hardware problems automatically.
**Related Terms:** QA, Machine Logs
**Example:** Log analysis detects abnormal gantry torque.

**379. Monte Carlo Beam Model:** Detailed beam model generated using Monte Carlo simulation.
**Related Terms:** TPS, Dose Calculation
**Example:** Accurate heterogeneity correction in lung plans.

**380. Related Terms:** AI Contouring, Auto-Seg
**Example:** AI segments bone, lung, and soft tissue for planning.

**381. Motion Vector Field:** Mathematical representation of how each pixel moves.
**Related Terms:** DIR, 4D Motion
**Example:** Used in deformable dose accumulation.

**382. Multi-Room Proton Facility:** Proton center with multiple treatment rooms.
**Related Terms:** Gantry Room, Beamline
**Example:** One cyclotron supplies beam to three treatment rooms.

**383. Maximum Beam Intensity Modulation:** Highest variation allowed between beamlets.
**Related Terms:** IMRT, Complexity
**Example:** TPS restricts modulation to reduce plan complexity.

**384. Multi-Planar Dose Review:** Reviewing dose in axial, coronal, and sagittal planes.
**Related Terms:** QA, Plan Evaluation
**Example:** Planner checks hotspots in all three planes.

**385. Median Organ Dose:** Middle dose value delivered to an organ.
**Related Terms:** DVH Metrics
**Example:** Used when mean dose is not reliable.

**386. Motion Artifact Suppression:** Reducing blurring in CT or MRI caused by motion.
**Related Terms:** MAR, Motion Correction
**Example:** Fast MRI sequences reduce motion artifacts in children.

**387. Multi-Device QA Approach:** Using several devices to verify machine accuracy.
**Related Terms:** Redundancy, Annual QA
**Example:** Output validated with ion chamber, diode, and film.

388. **Mechanical Drift:** Gradual change in mechanical accuracy over time.
**Related Terms:** QA Trends, Calibration
**Example:** Couch drift of 1 mm detected in monthly QA.

389. **Multi-Contrast MR Imaging:** MRI performed with various contrast settings.
**Related Terms:** T1, T2, FLAIR
**Example:** Multi-contrast MR improves brain tumor delineation.

390. **Maximum Dose Rate Modulation:** Variation in dose rate during delivery.
**Related Terms:** VMAT, Dynamic Delivery
**Example:** LINAC increases dose rate during arc segments with low modulation.

391. **Multi-Detector CT (MDCT):** CT system with many detector rows for fast, high-resolution imaging.
**Related Terms:** Helical CT, 4DCT
**Example:** MDCT captures thorax images rapidly for motion analysis.

392. **Marginal Miss Probabilit:** Chance that a tumor is partially missed due to motion or setup errors.
**Related Terms:** Robust Planning, Margin
**Example:** IGRT reduces marginal miss probability in lung SBRT.

393. **Modulated Field Junction:** Field junction where intensity is modulated to reduce dose gaps/overlaps.
**Related Terms:** Feathering, Field Matching
**Example:** CSI uses modulated junctions to avoid hot spots.

394. **Multi-Layer Proton Collimator:** Device with stacked layers to shape proton beam edges.
**Related Terms:** Proton Therapy, Aperture
**Example:** Multi-layer collimators sharpen lateral penumbra in protons.

395. **Monitor Unit Linearity:** Relationship between MU setting and actual dose delivered.
**Related Terms:** MU Calibration, QA
**Example:** MU linearity tested at 5 MU, 20 MU, and 200 MU.

396. **Matrix Resolution:** Pixel density of CT/MRI images used in contouring.
**Related Terms:** Voxel Size, Image Quality
**Example:** A 512×512 CT matrix gives detailed anatomical structure.

397. **Motion Residual Error:** Remaining motion after applying respiratory gating or tracking.
**Related Terms:** Motion Management
**Example:** Residual error <3 mm is acceptable for liver SBRT.

398. **Multi-Organ Atlas Segmentation:** Automatic contouring using anatomical atlases.
**Related Terms:** Auto-Seg, AI Contouring
**Example:** Atlas-based tool auto-contours kidneys, liver, bladder.

399. **Margin Adaptation Protocol:** Procedure for updating or shrinking margins during treatment.
**Related Terms:** ART, Adaptive Radiotherapy
**Example:** PTV reduced after week 2 when prostate swelling decreases.

400. **Multi-Point Dose Verification:** Verifying dose at multiple points using diodes or chambers.
**Related Terms:** Pretreatment QA, IMRT QA
**Example:** 5 diodes placed around target to confirm delivered dose.

401. **Mechanical Isocenter Test:** Test to verify the coincidence of gantry, couch, and collimator rotation centers.
**Related Terms:** Winston-Lutz Test, Mechanical QA
**Example:** Mechanical isocenter must stay within 1 mm radius.

402. **Medium Energy Electron Beam:** Electron beams 12–16 MeV used for moderate-depth tumors.
**Related Terms:** Electrons, PDD
**Example:** 12 MeV electrons used to treat chest wall lesions.

403. **Magnetic Resonance Ventilation:** MRI technique showing lung ventilation patterns.
**Related Terms:** Functional Imaging
**Example:** Used to spare ventilated lung during thoracic RT planning.

404. **Mean Heart Dose (MHD):** Average dose delivered to heart tissue.
**Related Terms:** Cardiac Dose Constraint
**Example:** Left breast DIBH reduces MHD from 4 Gy to 2 Gy.

405. **Multi-Planar Reconstruction (MPR):** Creating images in different planes from CT/MRI data.
**Related Terms:** Axial, Coronal, Sagittal
**Example:** MPR used for accurate spinal cord contouring.

406. **Minimally Invasive Brachytherapy:** Brachytherapy performed with minimal surgical access.
**Related Terms:** HDR, Needle Templates
**Example:** Prostate HDR uses perineal minimally invasive catheter insertion.

407. **MLC Leaf Speed Limitation:** Maximum speed at which MLC leaves can move safely.
**Related Terms:** Dynamic MLC, VMAT
**Example:** Leaf speed capped at ~2.5 cm/s during VMAT arcs.

408. **Multi-Sequence Fusion:** Combining several MRI sequences for target .
**Related Terms:** Image Fusion, Contouring
**Example:** T1+T2+FLAIR fusion improves brain metastasis delineation.

409. **Motion Drift:** Slow changes in patient breathing pattern over time.
**Related Terms:** Respiratory Variability
**Example:** Drift requires adaptive gating thresholds.

410. **Maximum Allowable Hotspot:** Highest dose region allowed inside target or normal tissue.
**Related Terms:** Dmax, Dose Constraints
**Example:** PTV hotspots limited to <110% of prescription.

411. **Multi-Planar Tumor Registration:** Aligning tumors in all anatomical planes for IGRT.
**Related Terms:** CBCT, Registration
**Example:** Pelvis CBCT aligned in axial, sagittal, and coronal views.

412. **Median Target Coverage:** Median value of dose covering the target.
**Related Terms:** DVH, PTV Metrics
**Example:** Median dose ensures stable target coverage evaluation.

413. **Megavoltage Tomotherapy:** Helical radiotherapy using MV fan-beam imaging and delivery.
**Related Terms:** TomoTherapy, Helical IMRT
**Example:** Tomotherapy treats long craniospinal fields in one setup.

414. **Multi-Slice MR Acquisition:** MRI acquired in multiple sequential slices.
**Related Terms:** MRI Scan Time, Resolution
**Example:** Multi-slice DWI improves tumor contrast.

415. **Multi-Component Dose Calculation:** Separating dose contributions from primary and scatter components.
**Related Terms:** Monte Carlo, TPS Algorithms
**Example:** TPS differentiates primary photons from scatter photons.

416. **Minimal Organ Dose:** Lowest dose delivered to an organ at risk.
**Related Terms:** Dmin, DVH
**Example:** Minimal bladder dose used to evaluate cold regions.

417. **Multi-Step Patient Setup:** Stepwise setup including lasers, tattoos, and CBCT.
**Related Terms:** IGRT, Immobilization
**Example:** H&N patients use triple-step setup verification.

418. **Mechanical Clearance Check:** Ensuring couch, gantry, and accessories do not collide.
**Related Terms:** QA, Collision Avoidance
**Example:** VMAT arc checked for clearance around breast board.

419. **Motion Envelope Margin:** Margin added based on the full motion amplitude.
**Related Terms:** ITV, PTV
**Example:** 10 mm margin applied for large diaphragm motion.

420. **Micro-Dosimeter Array:** Array of tiny detectors for high-resolution dose measurements.
**Related Terms:** Small Field Dosimetry
**Example:** Used for SRS cone output factors.

421. **Magnetic Resonance Elastography:** MRI technique measuring tissue stiffness.
**Related Terms:** Functional MRI
**Example:** MRE used in liver RT research.

422. **Multi-Field Optimization (MFO):** IMRT optimization where all fields interact simultaneously.
**Related Terms:** Inverse Planning
**Example:** MFO used for highly conformal head-neck IMRT.

423. **Motion-Adaptive Gating:** Dynamically adjusts gating window as breathing changes.
**Related Terms:** Real-Time Gating
**Example:** Gating window modified for irregular breathers.

424. **Multi-Position Immobilization:** Immobilization devices supporting several patient postures. **Related Terms:** Positioning, Custom Masks
**Example:** Breast boards allow multiple incline angles.

425. **Megapotential Electrons:** Extremely high-energy electrons used in specialized treatments.
**Related Terms:** Electron Therapy
**Example:** Under research for deep tumor penetration.

426. **Multi-Level Brachy Optimization:** Optimizing dwell times at multiple contour levels.
**Related Terms:** HDR Planning, Dwell Weighting
**Example:** Cervix plan optimized at canal, parametrial, and organ levels.

427. **Mock Patient Simulation:** Trial simulation performed before actual CT-sim.
**Related Terms:** Setup Rehearsal
**Example:** Pediatric RT uses mock simulation to reduce anxiety.

428. **Machine Output Stabilization:** Ensuring consistent LINAC output over time.
**Related Terms:** Calibration, QA Trends
**Example:** Output stabilized after adjusting ion chamber bias.

429. **Maximum Leaf Travel Distance:** Furthest distance MLC leaves can move across the field.
**Related Terms:** MLC Geometry
**Example:** 15 cm leaf travel prevents covering extremely wide fields.

430. **Multi-Compartment DIR:** DIR performed separately on multiple tissue regions.
**Related Terms:** Deformable Registration
**Example:** Bone, soft tissue, and lung deform separately for accuracy.

431. **Median PTV Dose:** Median dose within the PTV.
**Related Terms:** DVH, PTV Metrics
**Example:** Ensures mid-dose values meet planning requirements.

432. **MLC Modeling Parameters:** Variables like leaf tip width, transmission, and tongue-and-groove used in TPS.
**Related Terms:** Beam Modeling
**Example:** Adjusting parameters improves IMRT accuracy.

433. **Motion-Gated CBCT:** CBCT acquired during specific breathing phases.
**Related Terms:** 4D CBCT, Gating
**Example:** End-exhale gated CBCT used for lung SBRT.

434. **Multi-Center Commissioning Data:** Commissioning benchmarks collected from several institutions.
**Related Terms:** Standardization
**Example:** AAPM provides multi-center beam data comparisons.

435. **Maximum Dose Falloff:** Rate at which dose decreases outside the target.
**Related Terms:** Gradient Index, SRS
**Example:** SRS plans aim for steep falloff to spare brain tissue.

436. **Multi-Layer Collimator:** Collimator with multiple layers for sharper beam shaping.
**Related Terms:** Proton Therapy, Aperture
**Example:** Improves penumbra in pencil-beam proton therapy.

437. **Motion Histogram:** Statistical distribution of tumor motion over time.
**Related Terms:** 4DCT, Motion Analysis
**Example:** Histogram shows lung tumor spends most time near end-exhale.

438. **Micro-CT Imaging:** Very high-resolution CT imaging used in research.
**Related Terms:** Preclinical RT
**Example:** Micro-CT used for small animal irradiation experiments.

439. **Minimum Target Coverage Requirement:** Minimum required coverage level for the target.
**Related Terms:** PTV Coverage
**Example:** PTV must receive ≥95% of prescription dose.

440. **Multi-Resolution Optimization:** Optimization performed at coarse and fine grid levels.
**Related Terms:** TPS, IMRT Planning
**Example:** Coarse optimization speeds up initial planning.

441. **Microbeam Radiation Therapy (MRT):** Experimental RT using extremely narrow, high-dose beams for tumor control with normal-tissue sparing.
**Related Terms:** Synchrotron Therapy, Spatially Fractionated RT
**Example:** MRT research focuses on treating brain tumors with ultra-high peak doses.

442. **Metastatic Burden Index:** Quantitative measure of number and volume of metastatic lesions.
**Related Terms:** Oligometastatic Disease, Tumor Burden
**Example:** Patients with low metastatic burden may receive curative-intent SBRT.

443. **Motion-Compensated Reconstruction:** Technique integrating motion information to correct CT/MRI/CBCT artifact.
**Related Terms:** 4D Reconstruction
**Example:** Used for improving image quality in moving organs like liver.

**444. Multi-Energy CT (MECT):** CT using multiple energy spectra to differentiate tissue types.
**Related Terms:** Dual-Energy CT, Spectral Imaging
**Example:** MECT helps identify calcifications vs. tumor tissue.

**445. MLC Collision Map:** Software showing possible gantry–couch–MLC collision scenarios.
**Related Terms:** Collision Avoidance
**Example:** VMAT arc reviewed with collision map before treatment.

**446. MARS Protocol (Motion Assessment for RT Simulation):** Procedure to evaluate patient-specific respiratory motion before CT-sim.
**Related Terms:** Motion Management
**Example:** MARS protocol identifies irregular breathing patterns needing gating.

**447. Multi-Slice Proton Tracking:** Tracking proton paths through multiple tissue layers.
**Related Terms:** Proton Range, Monte Carlo
**Example:** Improves range accuracy in heterogeneous tissues like lung.

**448. Microvascular Dose Response:** How radiation affects tiny blood vessels.
**Related Terms:** Radiobiology, Late Effects
**Example:** High doses in brain SRS may impact microvasculature.

**449. Multi-Beam Equalization:** Balancing beam weights to achieve uniform target coverage.
**Related Terms:** Beam Weighting
**Example:** 7-field IMRT uses equalization for smoother dose gradients.

**450. Maximum Gradient Steepness:** Maximum allowable dose drop per mm from the target.
**Related Terms:** Gradient Index
**Example:** SRS plans check gradient steepness to protect OARs.

**451. Moving Aperture Technique:** Beam aperture moves dynamically to follow tumor motion.
**Related Terms:** Dynamic MLC, Tracking
**Example:** Used in experimental real-time tumor tracking systems.

**452. MLC Positional Accuracy:** Precision with which MLC leaves reach their planned positions.
**Related Terms:** Leaf Calibration, QA
**Example:** VMAT requires <1 mm MLC positional error.

**453. Multi-Zone Electron Therapy:** Electron fields at different energies for complex surface lesions.
**Related Terms:** Electrons, Field Matching
**Example:** Chest wall treated with 9 MeV + 12 MeV zones.

**454. Mosaic Field Technique:** Overlapping field technique for very large targets.
**Related Terms:** Junction Feathering
**Example:** Applied in total body irradiation (TBI).

**455. Margin Propagation Error:** Error introduced when PTV margins are incorrectly applied.
**Related Terms:** Geometric Uncertainty
**Example:** Incorrectly expanded ITV may over-irradiate stomach tissue.

**456. Motion Model Predictive Algorithm:** Predicts future tumor position based on breathing signals.
**Related Terms:** Tracking Algorithms
**Example:** Used in real-time tracking during lung SBRT.

**457. Multi-Objective Optimization (MOO):** Planning technique optimizing several goals simultaneously.
**Related Terms:** Pareto Front, Inverse Planning
**Example:** MOO balances PTV coverage with parotid sparing.

**458. MRI Motion Artifact Suppression:** Techniques to reduce blur caused by motion.
**Related Terms:** Gating, MRI Sequence
**Example:** Navigator-gated MRI reduces liver motion artifact.

**459. Minimum Segment Area (MSA):** Minimum allowed MLC segment size in IMRT.
**Related Terms:** Segment Weight, MU Efficiency
**Example:** Setting MSA to 4 $cm^2$ improves delivery stability.

**460. Multi-Beam Arrangement Symmetry:** Symmetric layout of beams to balance dose distribution.
**Related Terms:** Isocentric Planning
**Example:** 5-field prostate IMRT uses symmetric beam arrangement.

**461. Magnetic Resonance Angiography (MRA):** MRI visualizing blood vessels without contrast.
**Related Terms:** MRA, Functional Imaging
**Example:** Used to avoid high-dose regions near major arteries.

**462. Mean Liver Dose Constraint:** Average liver dose limit to avoid radiation-induced liver disease.
**Related Terms:** RILD, Dose Constraints
**Example:** Mean liver dose kept $<$28 Gy for hepatic RT.

**463. Motion Artifact Reduction Filter:** Software filter to clean motion-blurred images.
**Related Terms:** Image Processing
**Example:** Filter improves lung CBCT clarity for tumor matching.

**464. Multi-Isocenter Matching:** Aligning multiple isocenters for extended treatments.
**Related Terms:** CSI Planning, Junction Dose
**Example:** TBI uses multi-isocenter match lines.

**465. Maximal Dose Rate Limitation:** Maximum safe dose rate allowed by the LINAC.
**Related Terms:** FFF Mode, Beam Output
**Example:** FFF beams can deliver up to 2400 MU/min.

**466. Monte Carlo Particle Scoring:** Measuring dose contribution from individual particle histories.
**Related Terms:** Monte Carlo Simulation
**Example:** Scoring helps validate small field dosimetry.

**467. MLC Offset Correction:** Adjustment for systematic leaf misalignment.
**Related Terms:** MLC Calibration
**Example:** Offset correction ensures accurate fluence maps.

**468. Motion Synchronization Window:** Range of breathing phases allowed during gated treatment.
**Related Terms:** Gating Window
**Example:** End-exhale window set to 40–60% phase.

**469. Multi-Dose Rate Switching:** Switching between different dose rates within a single beam.
**Related Terms:** Beam Modulation
**Example:** Used in advanced IMRT to reduce treatment time.

**470. Magnetic Field Susceptibility:** Sensitivity of tissues to magnetic field variation.
**Related Terms:** MRI Physics
**Example:** Metal implants cause susceptibility artifacts.

**471. Multi-Grid Dose Calculation:** Dose computed on several resolution grids for speed and accuracy.
**Related Terms:** TPS Algorithms
**Example:** Coarse grid for initial pass; fine grid for final pass.

**472. Multi-Segment MLC Delivery:** IMRT delivered through several static MLC apertures.
**Related Terms:** Step-and-Shoot IMRT
**Example:** Head–neck plans use 80–120 segments.

**473. Motion-Enhanced Planning:** Incorporating motion data directly into plan optimization.
**Related Terms:** 4D Planning
**Example:** ITV-based optimization for lung tumors.

**474. Multi-Isotope Brachytherapy:** Using multiple radioactive isotopes in a single implant.
**Related Terms:** HDR, LDR
**Example:** Combining I-125 and Pd-103 for prostate implants.

**475. Median Organ Dose:** Middle value dose of an organ's DVH.
**Related Terms:** DVH Metrics
**Example:** Median kidney dose used for functional sparing.

**476. Magnetic Beam Steering:** Using magnetic fields to control charged particle beam direction.
**Related Terms:** Proton Therapy
**Example:** Pencil beam scanning uses magnetic steering.

**477. Modulated Arc Therapy (MAT):** VMAT technique with modulation of speed, dose rate, and shape.
**Related Terms:** VMAT, Arc Therapy
**Example:** MAT reduces OAR dose in pelvic treatments.

**478. Multi-Sample Dosimetry:** Using many dosimeters to map dose distribution.
**Related Terms:** Film Dosimetry, Diode Array
**Example:** Gafchromic film + ion chamber used for SRS QA.

**479. Microstructural Tissue Response:** Microscopic tissue changes after radiation.
**Related Terms:** Radiobiology
**Example:** Collagen changes observed post-RT in skin.

**480. Maximum Beam Hold Tolerance:** Maximum allowed deviation before the beam auto-stops.
**Related Terms:** IGRT, Safety Systems
**Example:** Beam holds when patient moves >3 mm.

**481. Motion-Adaptive MLC Control:** Adjusting MLC leaves in real-time to track tumor motion. **Related Terms:** Real-Time Tracking
**Example:** Used experimentally in lung and liver tumors.

**482. Multi-Point Calibration Curve:** Calibration using several measurement points.
**Related Terms:** QA, Output Factor
**Example:** Ion chamber calibrated at 6 MV, 10 MV, 18 MV.

**483. Maximal Penumbra Reduction:** Techniques to minimize beam edge blurring.
**Related Terms:** Collimation, Beam Quality
**Example:** Using tertiary collimators for SRS cones.

**484. Multi-Detector EPID Imaging:** EPID systems with several detection layers.
**Related Terms:** Portal Imaging, QA
**Example:** Improves low-dose image contrast.

**485. Morphology-Based Contouring:** Contouring based on tissue shape characteristics.
**Related Terms:** Auto-Segmentation
**Example:** Used for hippocampal contouring.

**486. Motion Probability Map:** Map showing likelihood of tumor position over time.
**Related Terms:** 4D Planning
**Example:** Lung tumor spending 70% time exhale → gating window chosen.

**487. Multi-Tier Safety Interlock:** Layered safety system preventing hazardous beam delivery.
**Related Terms:** LINAC Safety
**Example:** Door interlock + collision sensors + beam override.

**488. Magnetic Resonance Coil Array:** Multiple MRI coils for high signal-to-noise imaging.
**Related Terms:** Parallel Imaging
**Example:** Spine array coil improves H&N MRI resolution.

**489. Minimum Arc Separation:** Minimum degrees between two VMAT arcs to avoid overlap.
**Related Terms:** VMAT Design
**Example:** Two arcs separated by 30° for optimal coverage.

**490. Multi-Directional Dose Spill Analysis:** Evaluating dose leakage outside target from all directions.
**Related Terms:** Dose Gradient
**Example:** SRS plans reviewed for asymmetric dose spill.

**491. MLC Leakage Map:** A 2D map showing radiation leakage through and between MLC leaves.
**Related Terms:** Leaf Transmission, Dosimetric QA
**Example:** EPID images are used to generate an MLC leakage map before IMRT commissioning.

**492. Magnetic Dose Influence:** Effect of magnetic fields on dose distribution, especially in MR-LINAC systems.
**Related Terms:** Lorentz Force, Electron Return Effect
**Example:** MR-LINAC plans account for magnetic dose influence near lung–soft tissue boundaries.

**493. Multi-Phase Planning:** Planning different dose phases for a single patient (boost, initial plan).
**Related Terms:** Sequential Boost, Adaptive Planning
**Example:** H&N cancer uses a primary plan + boost plan after tumor shrinkage.

**494. Mean Brainstem Dose:** Average radiation dose received by the brainstem.
**Related Terms:** OAR Constraints
**Example:** Brainstem mean dose kept <12.5 Gy in stereotactic RT.

**495. Monitor Chamber Calibration:** Calibration of the LINAC's internal dose-monitoring ion chambers.
**Related Terms:** Output Calibration, Beam Stability
**Example:** Annual QA includes monitor chamber calibration for all photon energies.

**496. Multi-Layer Collimator:** Collimator with multiple layers to reduce penumbra and leakage.
**Related Terms:** Collimation Systems
**Example:** Used in some proton therapy units for precise beam shaping.

**497. Multiparametric MR Planning:** Using multiple MRI sequences (T1, T2, DWI, Perfusion) for RT planning.
**Related Terms:** MRI Fusion, Target Delineation
**Example:** Prostate tumor visible on mpMRI is incorporated into GTV contouring.

**498. Maximum Hotspot Control:** Techniques to reduce excessively high-dose regions.
**Related Terms:** Hotspot, Dose Homogeneity
**Example:** Optimization ring structures are used for hotspot control in IMRT.

**499. Micro-Dosimetric Energy Deposition:** Energy deposited at microscopic (cellular) level.
**Related Terms:** Microdosimetry, Radiobiology
**Example:** Alpha particle therapy studies micro-dosimetric patterns in targeted radionuclide therapy.

500. **Margin Reduction Strategy:** Approach to minimize PTV margins safely.
**Related Terms:** IGRT, Motion Management
**Example:** Daily CBCT allows reduction of margins from 10 mm to 5 mm.

# N

1. **Nuclear Medicine Imaging Meaning:** Use of radioactive tracers to visualize organ function or tumors.
   **Related Terms:** PET, SPECT, Radiotracer, Gamma camera
   **Example:** QA ensures kidney PET imaging shows clear tracer uptake.
2. **Neutron Therapy Meaning** Radiotherapy using high-energy neutrons for certain tumors.
   **Related Terms:** Particle therapy, LET, Proton therapy
   **Example:** QA confirms neutron beam dose distribution matches kidney treatment plan.
3. **Noise Reduction QA Meaning:** Ensuring imaging noise is minimized for accurate diagnosis or planning.
   **Related Terms:** CT QA, MRI QA, Image filtering
   **Example:** QA checks kidney CT images for acceptable noise levels.
4. **Nominal Beam Energy Meaning:** The specified energy of photons or electrons for treatment.
   **Related Terms:** LINAC, Photon beam, Electron beam
   **Example:** QA verifies LINAC photon beam energy matches nominal 6 MV for kidney IMRT.
5. **Normal Tissue Complication Probability (NTCP) Meaning:** Probability of adverse effects in normal tissue from radiation.
   **Related Terms:** DVH, OAR, Dose-response
   **Example:** QA calculates NTCP for kidney to limit radiation-induced nephropathy.
6. **Normalized Dose Distribution Meaning:** Dose distribution scaled to a reference point or maximum.
   **Related Terms:** DVH, TPS, Dose mapping
   **Example:** QA ensures kidney VMAT normalized dose distribution matches plan.
7. **Non-uniformity Correction Meaning:** Correction of detector or image non-uniformities.
   **Related Terms:** Flat-field, Detector calibration, QA phantom
   **Example:** QA applies non-uniformity correction to kidney CBCT images.
8. **Needle Localization Meaning:** Placement of a needle for biopsy, brachytherapy, or fiducial markers.
   **Related Terms:** Fiducial marker, Ultrasound, CT-guided procedure
   **Example:** QA ensures kidney fiducial needle placement is accurate for SBRT.
9. **Nephron Sparing Planning Meaning:** Planning techniques to minimize dose to healthy kidney tissue.
   **Related Terms:** OAR, IMRT, SBRT
   **Example:** QA verifies kidney SBRT plan spares >70% of normal renal tissue.
10. **Nuclear Decay Correction Meaning:** Accounting for radioactive decay in dose calculations or imaging.
    **Related Terms:** PET, SPECT, Radiotracer, Half-life
    **Example:** QA adjusts kidney PET quantification using decay correction for F-18 tracer.
11. **Nomogram-based Dose Adjustment Meaning:** Using clinical nomograms to individualize radiation dose.
    **Related Terms:** Fractionation, BED, Dose-response
    **Example:** QA verifies kidney SBRT dose using NTCP-based nomogram.

12. **Noise Evaluation Phantom Meaning:** Phantom used to assess image noise characteristics.
**Related Terms:** CT QA, MRI QA, Image uniformity
**Example:** QA checks kidney CT images for acceptable noise using a QA phantom.

13. **Non-coplanar Beam QA Meaning:** QA for beams delivered from multiple planes not in the same geometric plane.
**Related Terms:** VMAT, IMRT, Couch rotation
**Example:** QA ensures kidney SBRT non-coplanar beam arrangement delivers planned dose.

14. **Nuclear Reaction Monitoring Meaning:** Measuring nuclear reactions in particle therapy or brachytherapy sources.
**Related Terms:** Neutron therapy, Proton therapy, QA detectors
**Example:** QA monitors proton beam interactions during kidney treatment.

15. **Node Dose Mapping Meaning:** Dose mapping to lymph nodes during treatment planning.
**Related Terms:** PTV, OAR, DVH
**Example:** QA confirms kidney region lymph node dose does not exceed tolerance.

16. **Nodule Segmentation QA Meaning:** Verification of automatic or manual contouring of nodules.
**Related Terms:** CT, MRI, Kidney lesion, Contouring QA
**Example:** QA confirms kidney tumor nodules are accurately contoured.

17. **Neutron Contamination Check Meaning:** Checking for unwanted neutron radiation in high-energy photon beams.
**Related Terms:** LINAC, Shielding, QA
**Example:** QA confirms kidney IMRT beams do not produce significant neutron contamination.

18. **NEMA Phantom Testing Meaning:** Using standard phantom for PET/SPECT system performance testing.
**Related Terms:** PET QA, SPECT QA, Resolution, Sensitivity
**Example:** QA ensures kidney PET scanner meets NEMA spatial resolution standards.

19. **Noise Power Spectrum (NPS) Evaluation Meaning:** Quantitative assessment of image noise frequency components.
**Related Terms:** CT QA, Image quality, Uniformity
**Example:** QA evaluates kidney CT NPS to optimize imaging protocols.

20. **Normalization Point Verification Meaning:** Checking reference points for normalized dose distributions.
**Related Terms:** TPS, DVH, Dose calibration
**Example:** QA confirms kidney PTV normalization point matches TPS calculation.

21. **Nominal Dose Rate QA Meaning:** Verifying that LINAC delivers the specified dose rate.
**Related Terms:** MU calibration, Output verification, IMRT QA
**Example:** QA confirms kidney VMAT dose rate matches nominal 600 MU/min.

22. **Nuclear Imaging Phantom Meaning:** Phantom used to test PET or SPECT imaging systems.
**Related Terms:** PET QA, SPECT QA, Radiotracer
**Example:** QA checks kidney PET system resolution using nuclear phantom.

23. **Non-linear Dose Response Check Meaning:** Verification of non-linear dose response in detectors or tissue.
**Related Terms:** Detector calibration, Film dosimetry, LET
**Example:** QA confirms kidney SBRT film dosimetry matches TPS non-linear response.

24. **Needle Trajectory Verification Meaning:** Ensuring needle path accuracy in interventional procedures.
**Related Terms:** Ultrasound, CT guidance, Fiducial placement
**Example:** QA confirms kidney biopsy needle trajectory avoids vessels.

25. **Nominal Output Verification Meaning:** Checking that LINAC delivers output at intended nominal dose.
**Related Terms:** Dose calibration, QA, MU verification
**Example:** QA ensures kidney IMRT output matches 2 Gy/fraction plan.

26. **Nodule Contrast EvaluationMeaning:** Measuring visibility of nodules or lesions in imaging.
**Related Terms:** CT, MRI, Kidney tumor, Image quality
**Example:** QA confirms kidney tumor nodules are visible on contrast-enhanced CT.

27. **Normal Organ Dose QA Meaning:** Ensuring OARs receive dose within tolerance.
**Related Terms:** DVH, PTV, Kidney, NTCP
**Example:** QA verifies normal kidney tissue does not exceed 15 Gy during SBRT.

28. **Noise Equivalent Dose Meaning:** Effective dose accounting for noise in imaging system.
**Related Terms:** CT dose, Image quality, SNR
**Example:** QA calculates kidney CT noise-equivalent dose to optimize exposure.

29. **Nephrotoxicity Risk Assessment Meaning:** Evaluating risk of kidney damage from radiation or therapy.
**Related Terms:** OAR, NTCP, DVH, Kidney dose
**Example:** QA ensures kidney SBRT plan limits nephrotoxicity risk.

30. **Normalized DVH Verification Meaning:** QA of normalized dose-volume histograms for accuracy.
**Related Terms:** DVH, TPS, PTV, OAR
**Example:** QA confirms kidney DVH is normalized to prescription dose.

31. **Non-isocentric Beam QA Meaning:** Verification of beams not sharing a common isocenter.
**Related Terms:** VMAT, Couch rotation, IMRT QA
**Example:** QA checks kidney SBRT non-isocentric beams deliver planned dose.

32. **Nodule Volume Measurement Meaning:** Calculating volume of tumor nodules for planning and follow-up.
**Related Terms:** CT, MRI, Segmentation, Kidney lesion
**Example:** QA verifies kidney tumor nodule volume measured correctly on CT.

33. **Neutron Dose Estimation Meaning:** Estimating dose from neutron contamination in high-energy photon beams.
**Related Terms:** LINAC QA, Shielding, Radiation safety
**Example:** QA estimates kidney neutron dose is below safety limits.

34. **Normal Tissue Segmentation Meaning:** Contouring healthy organs to avoid excess radiation.
**Related Terms:** OAR, PTV, Kidney, IMRT
**Example:** QA verifies kidney normal tissue segmentation matches CT anatomy.

35. **Non-uniform Beam Correction Meaning:** Adjusting beam parameters to achieve uniform dose across target.
**Related Terms:** Flattening filter, Beam profile, TPS
**Example:** QA ensures kidney IMRT beam uniformity after correction.

36. **Nuclear Safety Check Meaning:** Ensuring safe handling and use of radioactive sources.
**Related Terms:** ALARA, Shielding, QA, PET/SPECT
**Example:** QA confirms safe F-18 handling during kidney PET imaging.

37. **Nominal Isocenter Verification Meaning:** Confirming treatment isocenter matches planned coordinates.
**Related Terms:** IGRT, CBCT, Laser alignment
**Example:** QA verifies kidney SBRT isocenter using CBCT.

38. **Nodule Detection Sensitivity Meaning:** Ability of imaging to detect small lesions.
**Related Terms:** CT, MRI, SPECT, PET
**Example:** QA confirms kidney CT detects lesions ≥5 mm reliably.

39. **Non-coplanar Arc QA Meaning:** QA of VMAT arcs delivered in multiple planes.
**Related Terms:** VMAT, Couch rotation, Dose verification
**Example:** QA verifies kidney SBRT non-coplanar arcs match TPS.

40. **Noise Filtering QA Meaning:** Evaluating image noise filtering effectiveness.
**Related Terms:** CT QA, Image processing, Kidney imaging
**Example:** QA confirms filtered kidney CT images maintain diagnostic quality.

41. **Nominal Fraction Dose QA Meaning:** Verifying planned dose per fraction is delivered correctly.
**Related Terms:** Fractionation, LINAC output, SBRT
**Example:** QA ensures kidney SBRT fraction dose matches prescription.

42. **Nuclear Decay QA Phantom Meaning:** Phantom used to validate radioactive decay corrections.
**Related Terms:** PET, SPECT, Radiotracer, Dose calibration
**Example:** QA uses phantom to check kidney PET decay correction.

43. **Nodule Contour QA Meaning:** Verification of accurate tumor contouring in imaging.
**Related Terms:** Segmentation, CT, MRI, Kidney lesion
**Example:** QA confirms kidney tumor nodules are correctly contoured.

44. **Neutron Shielding Verification Meaning:** Ensuring neutron shielding is adequate in high-energy beams.
**Related Terms:** Radiation safety, LINAC QA, Beam contamination
**Example:** QA confirms kidney SBRT room shielding blocks neutrons.

45. **Normalization Factor Check Meaning:** Verifying factor used to normalize dose distributions.
**Related Terms:** DVH, TPS, PTV, Dose calibration
**Example:** QA ensures kidney VMAT dose normalization factor is accurate.

46. **Needle Guide QA Meaning:** Verification of devices guiding needles in interventions.
**Related Terms:** Fiducial placement, Ultrasound, CT-guided therapy
**Example:** QA checks kidney biopsy needle guide accuracy.

47. **Noise-to-Signal Ratio (NSR) QA Meaning:** QA metric assessing image noise relative to signal.
**Related Terms:** CT QA, MRI QA, Image quality
**Example:** QA confirms kidney CT NSR is below threshold for diagnosis.

48. **Nomogram QA Meaning:** Verification of clinical nomograms used in dose planning.
**Related Terms:** BED, NTCP, Fractionation, Dose adjustment
**Example:** QA confirms kidney SBRT nomogram predicts safe dose.

49. **Non-target Organ Dose QA Meaning:** QA of dose delivered to organs not intended for treatment.
**Related Terms:** OAR, DVH, LINAC QA, Kidney SBRT
**Example:** QA confirms liver and bowel dose during kidney SBRT is within limits.

50. **Nuclear Source Calibration Meaning:** Calibration of radioactive sources used in therapy or imaging.
**Related Terms:** Brachytherapy, PET, SPECT, QA phantom
**Example:** QA calibrates I-125 seeds for kidney brachytherapy.

51. **Non-uniformity Phantom Meaning:** Phantom used to assess imaging detector non-uniformity.
**Related Terms:** Flat-field correction, CT QA, CBCT QA
**Example:** QA checks kidney CBCT detector uniformity using non-uniformity phantom.

52. **Nodal Coverage QA Meaning:** Verification that planned lymph node regions receive intended dose.
**Related Terms:** PTV, DVH, OAR, IMRT
**Example:** QA ensures kidney regional lymph nodes get prescribed dose in SBRT plan.

53. **Neutron Flux Measurement Meaning:** Measuring neutron particle flux in particle therapy or LINAC environment.
**Related Terms:** LINAC, Shielding, Neutron contamination
**Example:** QA measures neutron flux during kidney high-energy photon treatment.

54. **Nominal Isodose Verification Meaning:** Checking planned isodose lines match delivered dose distribution.
**Related Terms:** TPS, DVH, IMRT QA
**Example:** QA confirms kidney VMAT 95% isodose line covers PTV.

55. **Nodule Response Assessment Meaning:** Evaluating tumor nodule response to therapy.
**Related Terms:** RECIST, CT, MRI, PET
**Example:** QA checks kidney tumor nodules shrinkage post-SBRT.

56. **Nuclear Medicine Dose Calculation Meaning:** Calculating administered radiopharmaceutical dose for imaging or therapy.
**Related Terms:** PET, SPECT, Radiotracer, ALARA
**Example:** QA calculates kidney F-18 FDG dose for PET imaging.

57. **Noise Histogram Analysis Meaning:** Quantitative analysis of image noise distribution.
**Related Terms:** CT QA, MRI QA, NSR
**Example:** QA evaluates kidney CT histogram to ensure noise is within tolerance.

58. **Non-coplanar Plan QA Meaning:** Verification of non-coplanar treatment plans for complex targets.
**Related Terms:** VMAT, Couch rotation, LINAC QA
**Example:** QA ensures kidney SBRT non-coplanar plan matches TPS dose distribution.

59. **Nominal Beam Symmetry QA Meaning:** QA to ensure radiation beam is symmetric about central axis.
**Related Terms:** LINAC, Field flatness, IMRT QA
**Example:** QA confirms kidney IMRT beam symmetry to avoid hotspots.

60. **Nodule Contour Adjustment Meaning:** Modifying tumor contours for treatment planning accuracy.
**Related Terms:** Segmentation, CBCT, MRI
**Example:** QA adjusts kidney tumor nodule contours to match latest imaging.

61. **Nuclear Medicine Phantom Meaning:** Phantom with radioactive sources for PET/SPECT QA.
**Related Terms:** PET QA, SPECT QA, Resolution testing
**Example:** QA uses kidney phantom to validate PET image uniformity.

62. **Noise Reduction Phantom Meaning:** Phantom used to evaluate noise suppression algorithms.
**Related Terms:** CT QA, Image filtering, CBCT
**Example:** QA ensures kidney CBCT images maintain quality after noise reduction.

63. **Non-target Dose Assessment Meaning:** QA of dose received by organs not part of the treatment target.
**Related Terms:** OAR, DVH, LINAC QA
**Example:** QA ensures liver and spleen dose is safe during kidney SBRT.

64. **Nominal Dose Rate Verification Meaning:** QA of machine output rate matching prescribed dose rate.
**Related Terms:** LINAC, MU verification, Fractionation QA
**Example:** QA confirms kidney IMRT delivered at 600 MU/min nominal dose rate.

65. **Nephron Mapping QA Meaning:** Verification of healthy kidney tissue mapping for treatment planning.
**Related Terms:** OAR, Contouring, IMRT, SBRT
**Example:** QA checks kidney plan spares mapped nephron regions.

66. **Nuclear Imaging Resolution QA Meaning:** Assessing spatial resolution of PET/SPECT systems.
**Related Terms:** NEMA Phantom, PET QA, SPECT QA
**Example:** QA verifies kidney PET resolution meets NEMA standards.

67. **Nodule Registration QA Meaning:** Ensuring consistent alignment of nodules between imaging sessions.
**Related Terms:** CBCT, CT, MRI, Image fusion
**Example:** QA verifies kidney tumor nodules are correctly registered for daily IGRT.

68. **Non-isocentric Plan Verification Meaning:** QA for treatment plans using multiple non-overlapping isocenters.
**Related Terms:** VMAT, Couch shift, IMRT QA
**Example:** QA checks kidney SBRT non-isocentric plan dose accuracy.

69. **Nomogram Dose Prediction QA Meaning:** Verification that clinical nomogram predicts correct dose safely.
**Related Terms:** BED, Fractionation, NTCP
**Example:** QA confirms kidney SBRT nomogram output matches TPS dose.

70. **Nuclear Medicine Detector QA Meaning:** Testing detector efficiency and linearity for PET/SPECT.
**Related Terms:** Gamma camera, PET QA, SPECT QA
**Example:** QA verifies kidney PET scanner detector response uniformity.

71. **Nodule Motion Tracking QA Meaning:** Verification of nodule motion tracking accuracy during respiration.
**Related Terms:** 4DCT, IGRT, CBCT
**Example:** QA ensures kidney tumor movement is accurately tracked during SBRT.

72. **Neutron Dose Distribution QA Meaning:** Assessing spatial distribution of neutron dose from high-energy beams.
**Related Terms:** LINAC, Shielding, Radiation protection
**Example:** QA maps kidney neutron contamination to ensure safety limits.

73. **Nominal MU Verification Meaning:** QA ensuring monitor units match planned dose output.
**Related Terms:** LINAC, TPS, IMRT QA
**Example:** QA confirms kidney VMAT MU matches TPS calculations.

74. **Nuclear Medicine Image Fusion QA Meaning:** Ensuring accurate fusion of PET/SPECT with CT or MRI.
**Related Terms:** CBCT, Image registration, TPS
**Example:** QA confirms kidney PET/CT images align for treatment planning.

75. **Noise Characterization QA Meaning:** Evaluating imaging system noise characteristics quantitatively.
**Related Terms:** NSR, NPS, CT QA, MRI QA
**Example:** QA assesses kidney CT noise properties for optimized imaging protocol.

76. **Nodal Dose Constraint QA Meaning:** Ensuring planned dose to nodal regions adheres to limits.
**Related Terms:** DVH, PTV, OAR, IMRT QA
**Example:** QA checks kidney regional lymph node dose is within tolerance.

77. **Nominal Gantry Angle Verification Meaning:** Verifying planned gantry angles match delivery angles.
**Related Terms:** LINAC, VMAT, Non-coplanar beams
**Example:** QA ensures kidney SBRT gantry angles match TPS.

78. **Nodule Contrast QA Meaning:** Ensuring lesion contrast is sufficient for accurate detection.
**Related Terms:** CT, MRI, PET, SPECT
**Example:** QA confirms kidney tumor nodules are distinguishable from normal tissue.

79. **Nuclear Source Output QA Meaning:** Verification of radioactive source strength in therapy or imaging.
**Related Terms:** Brachytherapy, PET, SPECT, Dose calibration
**Example:** QA checks I-125 source output for kidney brachytherapy.

80. **Nominal Couch Position QA**b **Meaning:** Ensuring treatment couch position matches planned coordinates.
**Related Terms:** IGRT, CBCT, LINAC QA
**Example:** QA confirms kidney SBRT patient isocenter aligns with couch position.

81. **Nodule Segmentation Verification Phantom Meaning:** Phantom used to test segmentation accuracy of nodules.
**Related Terms:** CT QA, MRI QA, Image registration
**Example:** QA checks kidney tumor nodule segmentation using phantom.

82. **Non-target Organ Dose Mapping Meaning:** Mapping dose to organs not intended for treatment.
**Related Terms:** OAR, DVH, TPS, IMRT QA
**Example:** QA maps liver dose during kidney SBRT plan verification.

83. **Nuclear Medicine Image Quality QA Meaning:** Comprehensive QA to assess PET/SPECT image quality.
**Related Terms:** NEMA Phantom, Detector calibration, Noise assessment
**Example:** QA ensures kidney PET images meet spatial resolution and contrast criteria.

84. **Nominal Beam Profile QA Meaning:** Verification that beam profile matches planned distribution.
**Related Terms:** LINAC, IMRT, VMAT, Field flatness
**Example:** QA confirms kidney IMRT beam profile matches TPS.

85. **Nodal Target Coverage Meaning:** Ensuring tumor or lymph node target receives intended dose.
**Related Terms:** PTV, OAR, DVH, SBRT QA
**Example:** QA confirms kidney tumor nodal targets receive full prescription dose.

86. **Neutron Activation QA Meaning:** Checking for material activation due to neutron exposure.
**Related Terms:** LINAC, Shielding, Radiation protection
**Example:** QA monitors kidney SBRT room components for neutron activation.

87. **Nominal Field Size Verification Meaning:** QA to ensure delivered field size matches plan.
**Related Terms:** LINAC, IMRT, MLC QA
**Example:** QA confirms kidney IMRT PTV coverage matches nominal field size.

88. **Nodule Density Measurement Meaning:** Assessing density of nodules for imaging or planning.
**Related Terms:** CT, MRI, HU, PET
**Example:** QA verifies kidney tumor nodule density for accurate dose calculation.

89. **Noise Simulation Phantom Meaning:** Phantom used to simulate imaging noise for QA purposes.
**Related Terms:** CT QA, MRI QA, NSR, NPS
**Example:** QA tests kidney CT reconstruction algorithm using noise phantom.

90. **Nominal Isocenter Verification Phantom Meaning:** Phantom used to check treatment isocenter accuracy.
**Related Terms:** IGRT, LINAC QA, CBCT
**Example:** QA verifies kidney SBRT isocenter using dedicated phantom.

91. **Nuclear Medicine Tracer QA Meaning:** Ensuring administered radiotracers meet quality and activity standards.
**Related Terms:** PET, SPECT, Dose calibration
**Example:** QA verifies F-18 FDG activity for kidney PET scans.

92. **Nodule Registration Phantom Meaning:** Phantom to test image registration of nodules across modalities.
**Related Terms:** CBCT, CT, MRI, Image fusion
**Example:** QA checks kidney tumor nodule alignment using a registration phantom.

93. **Nominal Dose Verification Phantom Meaning:** Phantom used to verify that delivered dose matches planned nominal dose.
**Related Terms:** LINAC, IMRT, VMAT
**Example:** QA confirms kidney SBRT dose using a dose verification phantom.

94. **Nephron Sparing Dose QA Meaning:** Verification that healthy kidney tissue receives minimal radiation dose.
**Related Terms:** OAR, PTV, DVH, IMRT
**Example:** QA ensures kidney SBRT plan spares maximum nephron volume.

95. **Nuclear Medicine Safety QA Meaning:** Ensuring safety protocols in handling and administering radioactive tracers.
**Related Terms:** ALARA, Radiation protection, PET, SPECT
**Example:** QA checks safety compliance during kidney PET tracer administration.

96. **Nodule Contrast-to-Noise Ratio QA Meaning:** Measurement of nodule detectability based on contrast and noise.
**Related Terms:** CT, MRI, PET, Image quality
**Example:** QA confirms kidney tumor nodules are detectable on CBCT.

97. **Nominal Energy Verification Meaning:** Ensuring LINAC photon or electron beam energy matches planned value.
**Related Terms:** Beam calibration, LINAC QA
**Example:** QA confirms kidney IMRT 6 MV photon beam energy matches TPS.

98. **Non-target Structure Segmentation QA Meaning:** Verifying accurate contouring of organs not intended for treatment.
**Related Terms:** OAR, Contouring, TPS
**Example:** QA checks kidney SBRT plan accurately segments liver and spleen.

99. **Nodule Volume Measurement QA Meaning:** Ensuring accurate volumetric assessment of tumor nodules.
**Related Terms:** CT, MRI, PET, Segmentation
**Example:** QA verifies kidney tumor volume measurement for dose calculation.

100. **Nominal MU Linearity QA Meaning:** Checking that delivered monitor units are linear with planned dose.
**Related Terms:** LINAC, Dose calibration, IMRT QA
**Example:** QA ensures kidney VMAT MU linearly corresponds to TPS dose.

101. **Neutron Contamination QA Meaning:** Assessment of neutron dose produced during high-energy photon therapy.
**Related Terms:** LINAC, Shielding, Radiation protection
**Example:** QA maps neutron contamination for kidney SBRT room safety.

102. **Nodal Delineation QA Meaning:** Verification of lymph node contour accuracy for planning.
**Related Terms:** PTV, OAR, IMRT, SBRT
**Example:** QA checks kidney regional lymph node contours before IMRT planning.

103. **Nominal Gantry Speed QA Meaning:** Verification of correct gantry rotation speed during VMAT or arc therapy.
**Related Terms:** LINAC, VMAT, Delivery QA
**Example:** QA confirms kidney VMAT gantry speed matches TPS.

104. **Nuclear Medicine Calibration Phantom Meaning:** Phantom with known activity to calibrate PET/SPECT systems.
**Related Terms:** PET QA, SPECT QA, Detector calibration
**Example:** QA uses kidney calibration phantom to ensure accurate SUV measurement.

105. **Nodule Motion Phantom Meaning:** Phantom simulating tumor motion for QA of respiratory gating.
**Related Terms:** 4DCT, IGRT, Motion management
**Example:** QA tests kidney tumor motion tracking during SBRT.

106. **Nominal Field Verification Phantom Meaning:** Phantom to verify correct field placement and dimensions.
**Related Terms:** LINAC, IMRT QA, MLC QA
**Example:** QA ensures kidney IMRT PTV coverage using field verification phantom.

107. **Nephron Dose Mapping Meaning:** Mapping radiation dose specifically to functional nephron regions.
**Related Terms:** OAR, Dose-volume histogram, SBRT
**Example:** QA maps kidney SBRT dose to avoid nephron overexposure.

108. **Nodule Registration Accuracy QA Meaning:** Ensuring precise registration of tumor nodules across imaging sessions.
**Related Terms:** CBCT, Image fusion, IGRT
**Example:** QA checks kidney tumor alignment daily during SBRT.

109. **Nominal Beam Output QA Meaning:** Ensuring delivered dose output matches planned beam output.
**Related Terms:** LINAC, TPS, IMRT QA
**Example:** QA confirms kidney VMAT beam output is within ±2% of plan.

110. **Nuclear Medicine Resolution Phantom Meaning:** Phantom designed to evaluate PET/SPECT spatial resolution.
**Related Terms:** NEMA Phantom, PET QA, SPECT QA
**Example:** QA ensures kidney PET spatial resolution meets clinical standards.

111. **Nodal Dose Distribution QA Meaning:** Verification of dose uniformity across nodal targets.
**Related Terms:** DVH, IMRT QA, PTV coverage
**Example:** QA confirms kidney lymph nodes receive uniform dose in SBRT.

112. **Nominal Isocenter Accuracy QA Meaning:** QA to ensure treatment isocenter corresponds with planned location.
**Related Terms:** IGRT, CBCT, LINAC QA
**Example:** QA verifies kidney SBRT isocenter within 1 mm tolerance.

113. **Neutron Shielding Verification Meaning:** QA to ensure protective barriers adequately reduce neutron exposure.
**Related Terms:** Radiation protection, LINAC, High-energy photon therapy
**Example:** QA confirms kidney SBRT vault shielding limits neutron dose to staff.

114. **Nodule Segmentation Phantom QA Meaning:** Phantom used to verify automated or manual nodule segmentation.
**Related Terms:** CT, MRI, CBCT, TPS
**Example:** QA ensures kidney tumor segmentation matches phantom anatomy.

115. **Nominal Dose Rate Linearity QA Meaning:** Verifying that dose rate is linear across machine output range.
**Related Terms:** LINAC, IMRT, VMAT QA
**Example:** QA confirms kidney IMRT dose rate linearity from 100 to 600 MU/min.

116. **Nuclear Medicine Activity Verification Meaning:** QA to confirm administered activity matches prescription.
**Related Terms:** PET, SPECT, ALARA, Dose calibration
**Example:** QA verifies F-18 FDG activity for kidney PET scans matches calculated dose.

117. **Nodule Contour Accuracy QA Meaning:** Verification that tumor contours are correctly delineated.
**Related Terms:** CT, MRI, CBCT, TPS
**Example:** QA confirms kidney tumor nodule contour accuracy for SBRT.

118. **Nominal Couch Rotation QA Meaning:** Verifying treatment couch rotation matches planned angles.
**Related Terms:** LINAC, VMAT, Non-coplanar beams
**Example:** QA checks kidney SBRT couch rotation for non-coplanar fields.

119. **Nephron Functional Imaging QA Meaning:** Ensuring imaging accurately reflects kidney functional tissue.
**Related Terms:** SPECT, PET, Renal perfusion, Functional OAR
**Example:** QA validates functional kidney SPECT before planning SBRT.

120. **Nodule Response Phantom Meaning:** Phantom simulating tumor response to therapy for imaging QA.
**Related Terms:** CBCT, CT, MRI, TPS verification
**Example:** QA uses phantom to test kidney tumor shrinkage detection.

121. **Nominal Energy Spectrum Verification Meaning:** QA to ensure photon/electron energy spectrum matches TPS plan.
**Related Terms:** LINAC, Beam calibration, IMRT QA
**Example:** QA confirms kidney IMRT beam energy spectrum is as planned.

122. **Nuclear Medicine Workflow QA Meaning:** Verification of the entire PET/SPECT imaging process for accuracy and safety.
**Related Terms:** Radiotracer, Detector QA, Image reconstruction
**Example:** QA ensures kidney PET workflow follows ALARA and imaging standards.

123. **Nodule Motion Assessment QA Meaning:** Evaluating tumor movement due to respiration or patient motion.
**Related Terms:** 4DCT, IGRT, Motion tracking
**Example:** QA ensures kidney tumor motion is captured for gating and planning.

124. **Nominal MU Verification Phantom Meaning:** Phantom used to verify monitor unit output matches planned dose.
**Related Terms:** LINAC, IMRT QA, VMAT QA
**Example:** QA checks kidney SBRT MU using dedicated phantom.

125. **Nodal Target Volume QA Meaning:** Ensuring the nodal PTV is correctly defined and covered.
**Related Terms:** DVH, TPS, OAR
**Example:** QA confirms kidney lymph node PTV coverage before treatment.

126. **Nominal Gantry Angle Phantom QA Meaning:** Phantom used to verify gantry angle accuracy for delivery.
**Related Terms:** LINAC, Non-coplanar beams, VMAT QA
**Example:** QA checks kidney VMAT gantry angle accuracy using phantom.

127. **Nephron Dose Constraint QA Meaning:** Verification that functional kidney tissue dose remains within limits.
**Related Terms:** OAR, DVH, SBRT
**Example:** QA ensures kidney SBRT plan spares nephron regions.

128. **Nodule Density Phantom Meaning:** Phantom used to test imaging density accuracy for tumor nodules.
**Related Terms:** CT QA, MRI QA, HU calibration
**Example:** QA ensures kidney tumor nodule density is accurately represented.

129. **Nominal Field Symmetry QA Meaning:** Verification that radiation field is symmetric across the central axis.
**Related Terms:** LINAC, IMRT QA, VMAT QA
**Example:** QA confirms kidney IMRT field symmetry.

130. **Nuclear Medicine Detector Calibration Phantom Meaning:** Phantom used to calibrate PET/SPECT detectors.
**Related Terms:** PET QA, SPECT QA, Activity verification
**Example:** QA calibrates kidney PET detector using phantom.

131. **Nominal Beam Flatness QA Meaning:** Ensures radiation beam has uniform intensity across the field.
**Related Terms:** LINAC, IMRT QA, VMAT QA, Flatness phantom
**Example:** QA confirms kidney IMRT beams maintain flatness across the PTV.

132. **Nodule Contrast QA Meaning:** Ensuring tumor nodules are visible with sufficient contrast in imaging.
**Related Terms:** CT, MRI, PET, Image quality
**Example:** QA confirms kidney tumor nodules are distinguishable from surrounding tissue.

133. **Neutron Dose Mapping QA Meaning:** Mapping the dose from neutrons produced during high-energy photon therapy.
**Related Terms:** LINAC, Shielding, Radiation protection
**Example:** QA maps neutron dose in kidney SBRT vault to ensure staff safety.

134. **Nominal Couch Position QA Meaning:** Verifying treatment couch is positioned accurately for treatment delivery.
**Related Terms:** LINAC, IGRT, Non-coplanar beam
**Example:** QA confirms kidney SBRT couch position matches planned coordinates.

135. **Nodule Registration Phantom QA Meaning:** Phantom to test accuracy of nodule alignment across imaging modalities.
**Related Terms:** CBCT, CT, MRI, Image fusion
**Example:** QA checks kidney tumor nodule registration using phantom.

136. **Nominal Field Verification Checklist Meaning:** Checklist to ensure radiation field matches plan in size, shape, and placement.
**Related Terms:** IMRT, VMAT, LINAC QA
**Example:** QA confirms kidney SBRT field using checklist.

137. **Nuclear Medicine Dose Calibration QA Meaning:** Verifying administered radiotracer activity matches prescribed dose.
**Related Terms:** PET, SPECT, ALARA, Activity measurement
**Example:** QA confirms F-18 FDG activity for kidney PET scans is accurate.

138. **Nodal Motion Assessment QA Meaning:** Verifying lymph node or tumor motion during respiration or treatment.
**Related Terms:** 4DCT, IGRT, Motion tracking
**Example:** QA ensures kidney lymph node motion is captured for gating.

139. **Nominal Energy Linearity QA Meaning:** Ensuring delivered beam energy is consistent across machine output range.
**Related Terms:** LINAC, IMRT QA, VMAT QA
**Example:** QA confirms kidney IMRT beam energy is consistent with TPS.

140. **Nephron Functional Sparing QA Meaning:** Ensuring functional kidney tissue is spared from excessive radiation.
**Related Terms:** OAR, DVH, SBRT
**Example:** QA checks that kidney SBRT dose constraints preserve nephron function.

141. **Nodule Edge Detection QA Meaning:** Ensuring clear of tumor nodule edges in imaging.
**Related Terms:** CT, MRI, PET, Segmentation
**Example:** QA confirms kidney tumor edges are correctly delineated on CBCT.

142. **Nominal Dose Distribution QA Meaning:** Ensuring delivered dose matches planned distribution.
**Related Terms:** TPS, DVH, IMRT, VMAT
**Example:** QA maps kidney SBRT dose distribution against TPS.

143. **Nuclear Medicine Imaging Workflow QA Meaning:** Ensuring accuracy, safety, and compliance of imaging workflow.
**Related Terms:** PET, SPECT, Radiotracer, ALARA
**Example:** QA confirms kidney PET workflow meets safety and quality standards.

144. **Nodal Target Volume Delineation QA Meaning:** Verifying that lymph node PTVs are correctly contoured.
**Related Terms:** OAR, PTV, DVH
**Example:** QA confirms kidney nodal PTV coverage before treatment.

145. **Nominal MU Output QA Meaning:** Verification that LINAC monitor units deliver correct planned dose.
**Related Terms:** LINAC, IMRT, VMAT
**Example:** QA confirms kidney VMAT MU output matches TPS.

146. **Nodule Phantom QA Meaning:** Phantom simulating tumor nodules for imaging and registration QA.
**Related Terms:** CT, MRI, CBCT, PET
**Example:** QA uses kidney nodule phantom to verify imaging accuracy.

147. **Nominal Gantry Speed Verification Meaning:** Ensuring gantry rotation speed matches planned value for VMAT or arc therapy.
**Related Terms:** LINAC, VMAT, IMRT QA
**Example:** QA confirms kidney VMAT gantry rotation speed is as planned.

148. **Neutron Contamination Measurement QA Meaning:** Measurement of stray neutrons in high-energy photon therapy.
**Related Terms:** LINAC, Shielding, Radiation protection
**Example:** QA ensures neutron dose is minimal during kidney SBRT.

149. **Nominal Beam Symmetry QA Meaning:** Ensuring left-right symmetry of radiation beam intensity.
**Related Terms:** LINAC, Flatness, IMRT, VMAT QA
**Example:** QA checks kidney IMRT beam symmetry using flatness phantom.

150. **Nodal Motion Phantom QA Meaning:** Phantom simulating tumor or node motion for QA of motion management.
**Related Terms:** 4DCT, IGRT, Respiratory gating
**Example:** QA tests kidney tumor motion tracking using nodal motion phantom.

151. **Nominal Beam Energy QA Meaning:** Ensuring the LINAC delivers the correct photon/electron beam energy.
**Related Terms:** LINAC, IMRT, VMAT, TPS
**Example:** QA confirms kidney SBRT beam energy matches TPS settings.

152. **Nodule Segmentation QA Meaning:** Verifying accuracy of tumor nodule segmentation on imaging.
**Related Terms:** CT, MRI, PET, CBCT
**Example:** QA ensures kidney tumor nodules are correctly segmented for dose planning.

153. **Nephron Dose Constraint QA Meaning:** Ensuring maximum dose to functional kidney tissue is within safe limits.
**Related Terms:** OAR, DVH, IMRT, SBRT
**Example:** QA checks that kidney VMAT plan respects nephron dose constraints.

154. **Nominal Gantry Angle QA Meaning:** Verification of gantry angle accuracy in treatment delivery.
**Related Terms:** LINAC, VMAT, IMRT
**Example:** QA confirms kidney VMAT beams deliver dose at planned angles.

155. **Nuclear Imaging Registration QA Meaning:** Ensuring alignment of nuclear medicine images (PET/SPECT) with CT or MRI.
**Related Terms:** PET/CT, SPECT/CT, IGRT
**Example:** QA aligns kidney PET images with planning CT for SBRT.

156. **Nodal Dose Coverage QA Meaning:** Verifying that lymph node targets receive prescribed dose.
**Related Terms:** PTV, DVH, IMRT, VMAT
**Example:** QA checks kidney nodal PTV coverage in multi-field IMRT plan.

157. **Nominal Couch Rotation QA Meaning:** Ensuring correct couch rotation for non-coplanar treatments.
**Related Terms:** IGRT, LINAC, VMAT
**Example:** QA confirms kidney SBRT non-coplanar fields match plan.

158. **Neutron Shielding QA Meaning:** Verifying adequate shielding for stray neutron exposure.
**Related Terms:** LINAC, Radiation protection, Vault design
**Example:** QA ensures kidney SBRT vault has proper neutron shielding.

159. **Nominal Dose Rate QA Meaning:** Ensuring LINAC delivers planned dose per minute.
**Related Terms:** IMRT, VMAT, Dose verification
**Example:** QA confirms kidney VMAT dose rate matches TPS.

160. **Nodule Registration Phantom Meaning:** Phantom used to validate tumor nodule registration.
**Related Terms:** CBCT, CT, PET, QA phantom
**Example:** QA tests kidney nodule registration accuracy using phantom.

161. **Nephrotoxicity Risk QA Meaning:** Assessing risk of kidney toxicity based on planned dose.
**Related Terms:** DVH, OAR, IMRT, SBRT
**Example:** QA evaluates kidney dose distribution to minimize nephrotoxicity.

162. **Nominal Field Size QA Meaning:** Verifying correct field size is delivered.
**Related Terms:** MLC, LINAC, IMRT QA
**Example:** QA confirms kidney IMRT PTV is fully covered.

163. **Nuclear Medicine Phantom QA Meaning:** Phantom used for PET/SPECT image quality and registration QA.
**Related Terms:** PET, SPECT, CBCT, QA phantom
**Example:** QA uses kidney phantom for PET/CT image registration accuracy.

164. **Nodal Motion Compensation QA Meaning:** QA for techniques compensating tumor motion during delivery.
**Related Terms:** Gating, Tracking, IGRT
**Example:** QA ensures kidney SBRT tracks tumor motion correctly.

165. **Nominal Isocenter Verification Meaning:** QA to ensure treatment isocenter matches planned location.
**Related Terms:** IGRT, CBCT, LINAC
**Example:** QA confirms kidney SBRT isocenter alignment with TPS.

166. **Nodule Dose Gradient QA Meaning:** Verifying steep dose gradients around small nodules are accurate.
**Related Terms:** PTV, OAR, IMRT, VMAT
**Example:** QA ensures kidney nodule receives full dose without overdose to surrounding tissue.

167. **Neutron Activation QA Meaning:** Checking activation of surrounding materials by high-energy photons.
**Related Terms:** LINAC, Shielding, Radiation safety
**Example:** QA ensures minimal activation of kidney phantom during high-energy therapy.

168. **Nominal Gantry Sag QA Meaning:** Verifying minimal gantry sag to maintain beam accuracy.
**Related Terms:** LINAC, IMRT, VMAT
**Example:** QA confirms kidney SBRT beam remains accurate despite gantry rotation.

169. **Nuclear Medicine Uptake QA Meaning:** Ensuring radiotracer uptake in target organ is within expected range.
**Related Terms:** PET, SPECT, Radiotracer
**Example:** QA verifies F-18 FDG uptake in kidney tumor for accurate dose planning.

170. **Nodal Contour QA Meaning:** QA of lymph node contours for accurate treatment planning.
**Related Terms:** PTV, OAR, DVH
**Example:** QA confirms kidney nodal contours match imaging anatomy.

171. **Nominal Beam Modulation QA Meaning:** Verifying LINAC modulates beam as planned for IMRT/VMAT.
**Related Terms:** MLC, TPS, Fluence map
**Example:** QA checks kidney IMRT beam modulation matches TPS.

172. **Nodule Detection Phantom Meaning:** Phantom with simulated nodules for imaging QA.
**Related Terms:** CT, MRI, PET, Image quality
**Example:** QA verifies kidney tumor nodules are detectable with imaging system.

173. **Nominal Dose Fraction QA Meaning:** Ensuring each treatment fraction delivers prescribed dose.
**Related Terms:** Fractionation, LINAC, SBRT
**Example:** QA confirms kidney SBRT fraction dose matches prescription.

174. **Nuclear Medicine Radiation Safety QA nMeaning:** QA to ensure safe handling and administration of radiotracers.
**Related Terms:** PET, SPECT, ALARA, Shielding
**Example:** QA confirms kidney PET staff follow proper radiation safety protocols.

175. **Nodal Motion Phantom QA Meaning:** Phantom to simulate motion of nodal targets for QA.
**Related Terms:** 4DCT, IGRT, Gating
**Example:** QA tests kidney nodal motion tracking accuracy.

176. **Nominal MLC Leaf Position QA Meaning:** Ensuring MLC leaves move accurately to shape treatment field.
**Related Terms:** IMRT, VMAT, LINAC QA
**Example:** QA confirms kidney IMRT MLC positions match TPS.

177. **Nephron Sparing Dose QA Meaning:** Verifying dose to kidney functional tissue is minimized.
**Related Terms:** OAR, DVH, IMRT, SBRT
**Example:** QA ensures kidney VMAT plan limits dose to functional nephrons.

178. **Nominal Beam Penumbra QA Meaning:** Measuring the sharpness of beam edges.
**Related Terms:** Field edge, IMRT, VMAT
**Example:** QA checks kidney IMRT beam penumbra to avoid normal tissue overdose.

179. **Nodal Uptake QA Meaning:** Ensuring radiotracer uptake in lymph nodes is detectable and accurate.
**Related Terms:** PET, SPECT, ALARA
**Example:** QA confirms kidney nodal PET uptake for dose planning.

180. **Nominal Couch Offset QA Meaning:** Ensuring couch offsets are correct for treatment delivery.
**Related Terms:** IGRT, LINAC, Non-coplanar beams
**Example:** QA verifies kidney SBRT couch offset aligns with TPS.

181. **Nuclear Medicine Phantom Dose QA Meaning:** Using phantom to verify dose delivered during nuclear imaging.
**Related Terms:** PET, SPECT, Dose measurement
**Example:** QA confirms kidney phantom absorbed dose matches planned value.

182. **Nodule Motion Compensation QA Meaning:** QA of techniques to compensate for tumor motion.
**Related Terms:** Gating, Tracking, IGRT
**Example:** QA ensures kidney nodules are tracked accurately during treatment.

183. **Nominal Beam Symmetry QA Meaning:** Ensuring left-right symmetry of the radiation beam.
**Related Terms:** IMRT, VMAT, LINAC QA
**Example:** QA checks kidney VMAT beam symmetry to prevent hotspots.

184. **Neutron Dose Measurement QA Meaning:** Measuring dose from stray neutrons in high-energy treatments.
**Related Terms:** LINAC, Shielding, Radiation safety
**Example:** QA ensures neutron dose near kidney is below safety threshold.

185. **Nominal Imaging Geometry QA Meaning:** Verification of imaging system geometry for accurate patient localization.
**Related Terms:** CBCT, KV imaging, IGRT
**Example:** QA confirms kidney CBCT geometry matches planning CT.

186. **Nodal Dose Verification Phantom Meaning:** Phantom to validate nodal dose delivery.
**Related Terms:** IMRT, VMAT, QA phantom
**Example:** QA measures kidney nodal dose using a dedicated phantom.

187. **Nominal Gantry Speed QA Meaning:** Verification that gantry rotates at planned speed for dynamic treatments.
**Related Terms:** VMAT, IMRT, LINAC QA
**Example:** QA checks kidney VMAT gantry speed

188. **Nuclear Medicine Image Fusion QA Meaning:** Verifying accuracy of PET/SPECT fusion with CT/MRI.
**Related Terms:** PET/CT, SPECT/CT, IGRT
**Example:** QA aligns kidney PET/CT images for precise dose planning.

189. **Nodal Contour Verification Phantom Meaning:** Phantom with nodal structures to verify contouring accuracy.
**Related Terms:** CT, MRI, QA phantom
**Example:** QA uses phantom to ensure kidney nodal contours match planned anatomy.

190. **Nominal Dose Uniformity QA Meaning:** Ensuring dose distribution is uniform across treatment field.
**Related Terms:** IMRT, VMAT, LINAC QA
**Example:** QA confirms kidney SBRT dose uniformity using MapCHECK.

191. **Nodule Registration QA Meaning:** Ensuring accurate registration of small tumor nodules between images.
**Related Terms:** CBCT, PET, CT, IGRT
**Example:** QA checks kidney nodules align correctly in CBCT versus planning CT.

192. **Nominal Monitor Unit QA Meaning:** Verification of monitor units delivered match planned dose.
**Related Terms:** LINAC, IMRT, Dose verification
**Example:** QA ensures kidney IMRT MU matches TPS calculation.

193. **Nuclear Medicine Image Quality QA Meaning:** Ensuring PET/SPECT images are clear, uniform, and artifact-free.
**Related Terms:** PET, SPECT, Phantom QA
**Example:** QA confirms kidney PET images are high quality for planning.

194. **Nodal Motion Phantom Meaning:** Phantom to simulate motion of nodal targets for QA.
**Related Terms:** 4DCT, IGRT, Gating
**Example:** QA tests kidney nodal motion tracking accuracy.

195. **Nominal Beam Flatness QA Meaning:** Ensuring radiation beam has uniform intensity across the field.
**Related Terms:** IMRT, VMAT, LINAC QA
**Example:** QA measures kidney IMRT beam flatness using water phantom.

196. **Nodule Dose Verification Meaning:** Ensuring prescribed dose is accurately delivered to tumor nodules.
**Related Terms:** DVH, IMRT, VMAT
**Example:** QA confirms kidney nodule receives intended SBRT dose.

197. **Nominal Couch Sag QA Meaning:** Ensuring minimal couch sag to maintain beam accuracy.
**Related Terms:** IGRT, LINAC, Non-coplanar beams
**Example:** QA verifies kidney SBRT couch maintains accurate patient positioning.

198. **Nuclear Medicine Calibration QA Meaning:** Calibration of PET/SPECT systems for accurate quantification.
**Related Terms:** Radiotracer, PET, SPECT
**Example:** QA ensures kidney PET scanner counts match known phantom activity.

199. **Nominal Field Alignment QA Meaning:** Verification of treatment field alignment with target anatomy.
**Related Terms:** LINAC, MLC, IMRT
**Example:** QA confirms kidney IMRT field alignment matches planning CT.

200. **Nodal Dose Mapping QA Meaning:** Mapping delivered dose to nodal structures for verification.
**Related Terms:** DVH, IMRT, VMAT
**Example:** QA ensures kidney nodal regions receive prescribed dose accurately.

201. **Nominal Imaging Dose QA Meaning:** Ensuring imaging dose delivered is within safety limits.
**Related Terms:** CBCT, KV, IGRT, ALARA
**Example:** QA confirms kidney CBCT imaging dose remains below tolerance.

202. **Nominal Beam Energy QA Meaning:** Ensuring the LINAC delivers the correct photon/electron beam energy.
**Related Terms:** LINAC, IMRT, VMAT, TPS
**Example:** QA confirms kidney SBRT beam energy matches TPS settings.

203. **Nodule Segmentation QA Meaning:** Verifying accuracy of tumor nodule segmentation on imaging.
**Related Terms:** CT, MRI, PET, CBCT
**Example:** QA ensures kidney tumor nodules are correctly segmented for dose planning.

204. **Nephron Dose Constraint QA Meaning:** Ensuring maximum dose to functional kidney tissue is within safe limits.
**Related Terms:** OAR, DVH, IMRT, SBRT
**Example:** QA checks that kidney VMAT plan respects nephron dose constraints.

205. **Nominal Gantry Angle QA Meaning:** Verification of gantry angle accuracy in treatment delivery.
**Related Terms:** LINAC, VMAT, IMRT
**Example:** QA confirms kidney VMAT beams deliver dose at planned angles.

**206. Nuclear Imaging Registration QA Meaning:** Ensuring alignment of nuclear medicine images (PET/SPECT) with CT or MRI.
**Related Terms:** PET/CT, SPECT/CT, IGRT
**Example:** QA aligns kidney PET images with planning CT for SBRT.

**207. Nodal Dose Coverage QA Meaning:** Verifying that lymph node targets receive prescribed dose.
**Related Terms:** PTV, DVH, IMRT, VMAT
**Example:** QA checks kidney nodal PTV coverage in multi-field IMRT plan.

**208. Nominal Couch Rotation QA Meaning:** Ensuring correct couch rotation for non-coplanar treatments.
**Related Terms:** IGRT, LINAC, VMAT
**Example:** QA confirms kidney SBRT non-coplanar fields match plan.

**209. Neutron Shielding QA Meaning:** Verifying adequate shielding for stray neutron exposure.
**Related Terms:** LINAC, Radiation protection, Vault design
**Example:** QA ensures kidney SBRT vault has proper neutron shielding.

**210. Nominal Dose Rate QA Meaning:** Ensuring LINAC delivers planned dose per minute.
**Related Terms:** IMRT, VMAT, Dose verification
**Example:** QA confirms kidney VMAT dose rate matches TPS.

**211. Nodule Registration Phantom Meaning:** Phantom used to validate tumor nodule registration.
**Related Terms:** CBCT, CT, PET, QA phantom
**Example:** QA tests kidney nodule registration accuracy using phantom.

**212. Nephrotoxicity Risk QA Meaning:** Assessing risk of kidney toxicity based on planned dose.
**Related Terms:** DVH, OAR, IMRT, SBRT
**Example:** QA evaluates kidney dose distribution to minimize nephrotoxicity.

**213. Nominal Field Size QA Meaning:** Verifying correct field size is delivered.
**Related Terms:** MLC, LINAC, IMRT QA
**Example:** QA confirms kidney IMRT PTV is fully covered.

**214. Nuclear Medicine Phantom QA Meaning:** Phantom used for PET/SPECT image quality and registration QA.
**Related Terms:** PET, SPECT, CBCT, QA phantom
**Example:** QA uses kidney phantom for PET/CT image registration accuracy.

**215. Nodal Motion Compensation QA Meaning:** QA for techniques compensating tumor motion during delivery.
**Related Terms:** Gating, Tracking, IGRT
**Example:** QA ensures kidney SBRT tracks tumor motion correctly.

**216. Nominal Isocenter Verification Meaning:** QA to ensure treatment isocenter matches planned location.
**Related Terms:** IGRT, CBCT, LINAC
**Example:** QA confirms kidney SBRT isocenter alignment with TPS.

**217. Nodule Dose Gradient QA Meaning:** Verifying steep dose gradients around small nodules are accurate.
**Related Terms:** PTV, OAR, IMRT, VMAT
**Example:** QA ensures kidney nodule receives full dose without overdose to surrounding tissue.

**218. Neutron Activation QA Meaning:** Checking activation of surrounding materials by high-energy photons.
**Related Terms:** LINAC, Shielding, Radiation safety
**Example:** QA ensures minimal activation of kidney phantom during high-energy therapy.

**219. Nominal Gantry Sag QA Meaning:** Verifying minimal gantry sag to maintain beam accuracy.
**Related Terms:** LINAC, IMRT, VMAT
**Example:** QA confirms kidney SBRT beam remains accurate despite gantry rotation.

**220. Nuclear Medicine Uptake QA Meaning:** Ensuring radiotracer uptake in target organ is within expected range.
**Related Terms:** PET, SPECT, Radiotracer
**Example:** QA verifies F-18 FDG uptake in kidney tumor for accurate dose planning.

**221. Nodal Contour QA Meaning:** QA of lymph node contours for accurate treatment planning.
**Related Terms:** PTV, OAR, DVH
**Example:** QA confirms kidney nodal contours match imaging anatomy.

**222. Nominal Beam Modulation QA Meaning:** Verifying LINAC modulates beam as planned for IMRT/VMAT.
**Related Terms:** MLC, TPS, Fluence map
**Example:** QA checks kidney IMRT beam modulation matches TPS.

**223. Nodule Detection Phantom Meaning:** Phantom with simulated nodules for imaging QA.
**Related Terms:** CT, MRI, PET, Image quality
**Example:** QA verifies kidney tumor nodules are detectable with imaging system.

**224. Nominal Dose Fraction QA Meaning:** Ensuring each treatment fraction delivers prescribed dose.
**Related Terms:** Fractionation, LINAC, SBRT
**Example:** QA confirms kidney SBRT fraction dose matches prescription.

**225. Nuclear Medicine Radiation Safety QA Meaning:** QA to ensure safe handling and administration of radiotracers.
**Related Terms:** PET, SPECT, ALARA, Shielding
**Example:** QA confirms kidney PET staff follow proper radiation safety protocols.

**226. Nodal Motion Phantom QA Meaning:** Phantom to simulate motion of nodal targets for QA.
**Related Terms:** 4DCT, IGRT, Gating
**Example:** QA tests kidney nodal motion tracking accuracy.

**227. Nominal MLC Leaf Position QA Meaning:** Ensuring MLC leaves move accurately to shape treatment field.
**Related Terms:** IMRT, VMAT, LINAC QA
**Example:** QA confirms kidney IMRT MLC positions match TPS.

**228. Nephron Sparing Dose QA Meaning:** Verifying dose to kidney functional tissue is minimized.
**Related Terms:** OAR, DVH, IMRT, SBRT
**Example:** QA ensures kidney VMAT plan limits dose to functional nephrons.

**229. Nominal Beam Penumbra QA Meaning:** Measuring the sharpness of beam edges.
**Related Terms:** Field edge, IMRT, VMAT
**Example:** QA checks kidney IMRT beam penumbra to avoid normal tissue overdose.

**230. Nodal Uptake QA Meaning:** Ensuring radiotracer uptake in lymph nodes is detectable and accurate.
**Related Terms:** PET, SPECT, ALARA
**Example:** QA confirms kidney nodal PET uptake for dose planning.

231. **Nominal Couch Offset QA Meaning:** Ensuring couch offsets are correct for treatment delivery.
**Related Terms:** IGRT, LINAC, Non-coplanar beams
**Example:** QA verifies kidney SBRT couch offset aligns with TPS.

232. **Nuclear Medicine Dose Calculation QA Meaning:** Verification of radiotracer dose calculations for patient safety.
**Related Terms:** PET, SPECT, ALARA, Activity Measurement
**Example:** QA ensures kidney PET tracer activity aligns with prescribed protocol.

233. **Nodule Registration Phantom QA Meaning:** Phantom used to verify accurate image registration of nodules for therapy planning.
**Related Terms:** CBCT, CT-MRI fusion, IGRT
**Example:** QA confirms kidney tumor nodules align correctly in multimodal imaging.

234. **Neutron Dose Assessment Meaning:** Measurement and calculation of neutron dose during high-energy photon therapy.
**Related Terms:** Secondary radiation, Shielding, High-energy LINAC
**Example:** QA checks kidney IMRT neutron dose to minimize unwanted exposure.

235. **Noise Measurement QA Meaning:** Assessment of image noise to ensure diagnostic quality in imaging systems.
**Related Terms:** CT, MRI, Image Quality, SNR
**Example:** QA measures noise in kidney CT scans to confirm clear visualization of tumors.

236. **Normal Tissue Complication Probability (NTCP) QA Meaning:** Verification of calculated risk for normal tissue toxicity.
**Related Terms:** DVH, Radiobiology, Organs-at-risk
**Example:** QA ensures kidney NTCP calculations in SBRT plan are within safe limits.

237. **Nephron Dose Mapping Meaning:** Dosimetric evaluation at the level of individual nephron units in kidney radiotherapy.
**Related Terms:** DVH, Functional Imaging, Renal Subunit
**Example:** QA maps IMRT dose to kidney nephrons to prevent functional loss.

238. **Non-uniformity Correction QA Meaning:** QA to correct imaging detector non-uniformity.
**Related Terms:** Flat-field, Detector Calibration, CT/MRI
**Example:** QA corrects non-uniformity in kidney CBCT images before IGRT.

239. **Networked Imaging QA Meaning:** QA of image data transfer and storage across networked PACS or radiotherapy systems.
**Related Terms:** PACS, DICOM, RIS, Data Integrity
**Example:** QA verifies kidney CT images sent from scanner to TPS remain intact.

240. **Neutron Shielding Verification Meaning:** QA to ensure neutron shielding effectively protects staff and patients.
**Related Terms:** LINAC, Secondary Radiation, Bunker Design
**Example:** QA checks neutron dose around kidney SBRT vault to meet safety standards.

241. **Normalization Factor QA Meaning:** QA of normalization factors used in imaging or dose calculations.
**Related Terms:** DVH, TPS, Dose Scaling
**Example:** QA verifies normalization factor for kidney IMRT dose distribution.

242. **Non-coplanar Field Verification Meaning:** QA of non-coplanar beam angles in IMRT/VMAT plans.
**Related Terms:** VMAT, SBRT, IGRT
**Example:** QA ensures kidney SBRT non-coplanar beams match TPS geometry.

243. **Noise Reduction Algorithm QA Meaning:** Verification of image denoising algorithms in diagnostic or treatment imaging.
**Related Terms:** CT, MRI, SNR, Image Processing
**Example:** QA checks kidney CT denoising does not distort tumor margins.

244. **Nuclear Decay Data Verification Meaning:** QA ensures accurate decay data for radionuclides used in therapy or imaging.
**Related Terms:** PET, SPECT, Radiopharmacy
**Example:** QA verifies kidney PET tracer half-life and decay constants before patient injection.

245. **Normalization Phantom QA Meaning:** Phantom used to verify image or dose normalization procedures.
**Related Terms:** TPS, Detector Calibration, Dose Scaling
**Example:** QA uses kidney phantom to confirm proper IMRT dose normalization.

246. **Nephrotoxicity Risk Assessment Meaning:** Evaluation of kidney toxicity risk from radiation therapy.
**Related Terms:** NTCP, DVH, Functional Imaging
**Example:** QA assesses potential nephrotoxicity in kidney SBRT plans.

247. **Nonlinear Dose Response QA Meaning:** Verification of dose-response behavior that is not linear.
**Related Terms:** Radiobiology, Fractionation, TPS
**Example:** QA ensures kidney SBRT dose-response models are accurate in TPS.

248. **Nuclear Imaging Phantom Meaning:** Phantom used to calibrate or QA nuclear medicine imaging systems.
**Related Terms:** PET, SPECT, Gamma Camera
**Example:** QA uses kidney phantom with radiotracer to check SPECT image quality.

249. **Nominal Beam Energy Verification Meaning:** QA of LINAC nominal photon or electron energies.
**Related Terms:** Beam Calibration, TG-51, MU
**Example:** QA confirms kidney IMRT beam energy matches TPS specifications.

250. **Noise Histogram QA Meaning:** Evaluation of image noise distribution using histogram analysis.
**Related Terms:** CT, MRI, SNR, Uniformity
**Example:** QA analyzes noise histogram of kidney CT to ensure clear tumor visualization.

251. **Non-target Dose Assessment Meaning:** Measurement of dose received by tissues outside the target volume.
**Related Terms:** OAR, Scatter Dose, TPS
**Example:** QA assesses liver and bowel dose during kidney SBRT to minimize collateral damage.

252. **Nominal MU Verification Meaning:** QA to verify monitor units (MU) delivered match plan.
**Related Terms:** LINAC, IMRT, VMAT
**Example:** QA confirms kidney IMRT MU for each field using ion chamber.

253. **Nephron Function Imaging QA Meaning:** QA of functional imaging assessing kidney nephron activity.
**Related Terms:** PET, SPECT, Tc-99m DMSA
**Example:** QA ensures kidney SPECT images accurately depict functional distribution.

254. **Non-rigid Image Registration QA Meaning:** QA of deformable image registration used in adaptive therapy.
**Related Terms:** CBCT, MRI, DIR, TPS
**Example:** QA validates kidney tumor mapping on deformed CBCT images.

255. **Neutron Flux Measurement QA Meaning:** QA of neutron flux in high-energy photon therapy rooms.
**Related Terms:** LINAC, Shielding, Secondary Radiation
**Example:** QA measures neutron flux near kidney SBRT vault walls.

256. **Normal Tissue Sparing QA Meaning:** QA to verify OAR protection in treatment plans.
**Related Terms:** DVH, NTCP, IMRT, VMAT
**Example:** QA confirms kidney SBRT plan spares adjacent bowel and liver tissue.

257. **Nuclear Medicine Detector Calibration Meaning:** QA for gamma camera or PET/SPECT detector performance.
**Related Terms:** PET, SPECT, QC, Radiopharmacy
**Example:** QA calibrates kidney SPECT detector sensitivity before imaging.

258. **Non-uniform Beam Correction QA Meaning:** QA ensuring beam uniformity correction factors are applied properly.
**Related Terms:** LINAC, Flattening Filter, MLC
**Example:** QA confirms kidney IMRT field uniformity after beam correction.

259. **Noise Equivalent Count Rate (NECR) QA Meaning:** QA metric for PET detector performance in terms of signal-to-noise.
**Related Terms:** PET, SNR, Detector Performance
**Example:** QA ensures kidney PET scan NECR meets manufacturer standards.

260. **Nominal Field Size Verification Meaning:** QA to confirm the planned field size is accurately delivered.
**Related Terms:** LINAC, IMRT, VMAT, Portal Dosimetry
**Example:** QA ensures kidney SBRT PTV is completely covered without excess exposure.

261. **Nephron Segmentation QA Meaning:** QA of kidney segmentation accuracy for functional dose assessment.
**Related Terms:** Contouring, Functional Imaging, TPS
**Example:** QA verifies kidney nephron segmentation matches anatomical images.

262. **Nuclear Medicine Image Registration QA Meaning:** QA to align nuclear medicine images with CT/MRI for planning.
**Related Terms:** PET/CT, SPECT/CT, IGRT
**Example:** QA ensures kidney PET images align with planning CT accurately.

263. **Nonlinear Dose Gradient Verification Meaning:** QA of high-dose gradient regions in SBRT or IMRT.
**Related Terms:** TPS, DVH, Penumbra
**Example:** QA confirms steep kidney SBRT dose gradients match TPS.

264. **Neutron Dose Equivalent QA Meaning:** QA to convert neutron flux into dose equivalent for safety.
**Related Terms:** Secondary Radiation, Shielding, High-energy LINAC
**Example:** QA evaluates neutron dose equivalent near kidney treatment area.

265. **Nominal Source-to-Surface Distance (SSD) QA Meaning:** QA to verify SSD is as planned for accurate dose delivery.
**Related Terms:** LINAC, MU, PDD
**Example:** QA confirms kidney IMRT SSD matches TPS.

266. **Noise Power Spectrum (NPS) QA Meaning:** QA of spatial frequency-based noise characteristics in imaging.
**Related Terms:** CT, MRI, Image Quality
**Example:** QA evaluates kidney CT NPS for clarity and diagnostic quality.

267. **Non-coplanar Beam Optimization QA Meaning:** QA for optimized non-coplanar beam arrangement.
**Related Terms:** VMAT, SBRT, TPS
**Example:** QA verifies kidney SBRT non-coplanar angles for minimal OAR dose.

268. **Nuclear Medicine Activity QA Meaning:** QA of radionuclide activity before patient administration.
**Related Terms:** PET, SPECT, Radiopharmacy
**Example:** QA confirms kidney PET tracer activity aligns with protocol.

269. **Nephrotoxicity Dose Constraint Verification Meaning:** QA to ensure kidney dose does not exceed nephrotoxicity limits.
**Related Terms:** DVH, OAR, NTCP
**Example:** QA verifies kidney SBRT plan meets renal dose constraints.

270. **Nominal Gantry Speed QA Meaning:** QA of gantry rotation speed in VMAT treatments.
**Related Terms:** LINAC, VMAT, Dose Rate
**Example:** QA confirms kidney VMAT gantry rotates at planned speed.

271. **Non-uniform Detector Response QA Meaning:** QA for variations in detector response across imaging array.
**Related Terms:** Flat-panel, CT, CBCT, Calibration
**Example:** QA corrects kidney CBCT detector non-uniformity before IGRT.

272. **Nephron Dose-volume Histogram QA Meaning:** QA of DVH specifically for nephron subunits.
**Related Terms:** DVH, Kidney Functional Imaging, TPS
**Example:** QA confirms nephron DVH in kidney SBRT meets safety criteria.

273. **Nuclear Decay Heat Verification Meaning:** QA of heat generated by radionuclide decay during storage or use.
**Related Terms:** Radiopharmacy, PET, SPECT
**Example:** QA ensures kidney PET tracer vial heat is within safe limits.

274. **Nominal Couch Position QA Meaning:** QA of treatment couch position and movement accuracy.
**Related Terms:** IGRT, LINAC, Patient Setup
**Example:** QA confirms kidney SBRT couch shifts match TPS planned shifts.

275. **Noise Reduction Phantom QA Meaning:** Phantom used to validate image noise reduction algorithms.
**Related Terms:** CT, MRI, Image Processin
**Example:** QA uses kidney phantom to ensure denoising does not distort anatomy.

276. **Non-target Organ Dose QA Meaning:** QA to verify doses received by organs outside the target.
**Related Terms:** OAR, DVH, TPS
**Example:** QA checks liver and bowel dose during kidney IMRT.

277. **Nominal Beam Penumbra QA Meaning:** QA of beam penumbra to ensure sharp dose fall-off.
**Related Terms:** LINAC, MLC, IMRT
**Example:** QA confirms kidney SBRT penumbra is within TPS tolerances.

278. **Nuclear Medicine Spatial Resolution QA Meaning:** QA of spatial resolution in PET/SPECT imaging.
**Related Terms:** PET, SPECT, Phantom
**Example:** QA measures kidney SPECT spatial resolution using line source phantom.

279. **Neutron Flux Phantom QA Meaning:** Phantom used to measure neutron flux distribution for shielding verification.
**Related Terms:** Secondary Radiation, LINAC, Shielding
**Example:** QA maps neutron flux in kidney SBRT treatment vault.

280. **Nominal Field Center Verification Meaning:** QA to confirm field is centered on target volume.
**Related Terms:** LINAC, IGRT, Portal Dosimetry
**Example:** QA ensures kidney IMRT PTV center aligns with field center.

281. **Nonlinear Image Registration QA Meaning:** QA for deformable image registration accuracy.
**Related Terms:** DIR, CBCT, MRI, Adaptive Radiotherapy
**Example:** QA confirms kidney tumor contours align after DIR.

282. **Nuclear Medicine Sensitivity QA Meaning:** QA of detector sensitivity in PET/SPECT imaging.
**Related Terms:** PET, SPECT, Phantom, Calibration
**Example:** QA verifies kidney SPECT gamma camera sensitivity meets standards.

283. **Nominal Dose Rate Verification Meaning:** QA of dose rate delivered during therapy.
**Related Terms:** LINAC, IMRT, VMAT, MU
**Example:** QA confirms kidney SBRT dose rate matches TPS planning.

284. **Noise Level Phantom QA Meaning:** Phantom used to evaluate image noise in imaging systems.
**Related Terms:** CT, MRI, SNR
**Example:** QA uses kidney phantom to measure CBCT image noise.

285. **Neutron Protection QA Meaning:** QA for neutron shielding and staff protection.
**Related Terms:** LINAC, Secondary Radiation, Shielding
**Example:** QA ensures kidney SBRT vault walls provide sufficient neutron protection.

286. **Nominal Gantry Angle QA Meaning:** Verification of gantry angle accuracy for treatment delivery.
**Related Terms:** LINAC, VMAT, IGRT
**Example:** QA confirms kidney VMAT gantry angles match TPS plan.

287. **Non-coplanar Couch QA Meaning:** QA for couch angles in non-coplanar treatments.
**Related Terms:** IGRT, SBRT, VMAT
**Example:** QA verifies kidney SBRT couch rotation matches plan.

288. **Nuclear Medicine Count Rate QA Meaning:** QA of count rate performance in PET/SPECT detectors.
**Related Terms:** PET, SPECT, Detector Calibration
**Example:** QA confirms kidney SPECT count rates are within recommended limits.

289. **Nominal SSD Verification Meaning:** QA of source-to-surface distance accuracy for treatment.
**Related Terms:** LINAC, MU, PDD
**Example:** QA ensures kidney IMRT SSD matches TPS plan.

290. **Noise Equivalent Dose QA Meaning:** QA of dose measurement accounting for image noise impact.
**Related Terms:** CT, CBCT, Imaging Dose
**Example:** QA confirms kidney CBCT imaging dose is acceptable despite noise.

291. **Non-target Tissue Sparing QA Meaning:** QA to ensure non-target tissues receive minimal dose.
**Related Terms:** DVH, OAR, IMRT, VMAT
**Example:** QA confirms kidney SBRT plan spares liver and bowel effectively.

292. **Nuclear Medicine Phantom Calibration Meaning:** QA of phantoms used for PET/SPECT calibration.
**Related Terms:** PET, SPECT, QA, Radiopharmacy
**Example:** QA calibrates kidney SPECT phantom before clinical use.

293. **Nominal Beam Flatness QA Meaning:** QA to verify radiation beam flatness across the field.
**Related Terms:** LINAC, IMRT, MLC, Photon Beam
**Example:** QA confirms kidney IMRT beams are flat to ensure uniform dose.

294. **Nonlinear Dose Response Phantom QA Meaning:** Phantom used to verify non-linear dose response in high-gradient treatments.
**Related Terms:** DVH, TPS, IMRT
**Example:** QA confirms kidney SBRT dose-response curves match phantom measurements.

295. **Nephron Function Phantom QA Meaning:** Phantom used to simulate functional kidney imaging and dose mapping.
**Related Terms:** SPECT, PET, Functional Imaging, TPS
**Example:** QA validates kidney SBRT functional sparing.

296. **Nominal Collimator QA Meaning:** QA of collimator position and shape.
**Related Terms:** MLC, LINAC, IMRT
**Example:** QA verifies kidney IMRT MLC positions match TPS.

297. **Nuclear Medicine Uniformity QA Meaning:** QA of image uniformity in PET/SPECT.
**Related Terms:** Phantom, Detector Calibration
**Example:** QA confirms kidney SPECT images show uniform counts across phantom.

298. **Non-target Dose Verification Phantom Meaning:** Phantom used to measure doses to OARs outside target.
**Related Terms:** DVH, IMRT, SBRT
**Example:** QA checks liver dose during kidney SBRT using phantom.

299. **Nominal Gantry Mechanical QA Meaning:** QA of gantry mechanical integrity and movement.
**Related Terms:** LINAC, VMAT, SBRT
**Example:** QA confirms kidney SBRT gantry moves smoothly and accurately.

300. **Neutron Scatter Measurement QA Meaning:** QA to quantify scattered neutron radiation.
**Related Terms:** Shielding, Secondary Radiation, LINAC
**Example:** QA measures neutron scatter dose

301. **Nominal Dose Calibration QA Meaning:** QA to verify that the delivered dose matches the planned nominal dose.
**Related Terms:** MU, LINAC, TPS
**Example:** QA ensures kidney IMRT dose delivery aligns with prescription.

302. **Nephron-sparing Radiotherapy QA Meaning:** QA to preserve kidney function by limiting dose to healthy nephron regions.
**Related Terms:** DVH, Functional Imaging, SBRT
**Example:** QA confirms kidney SBRT plan minimizes dose to uninvolved nephrons.

303. **Non-coplanar Beam Angle Verification Meaning:** QA to confirm non-coplanar beam angles match treatment plan.
**Related Terms:** VMAT, SBRT, IGRT
**Example:** QA ensures kidney SBRT non-coplanar beams are correctly positioned.

304. **Nuclear Medicine Quantification QA Meaning:** QA to ensure accurate measurement of radionuclide uptake in organs.
**Related Terms:** PET, SPECT, Radiopharmacy
**Example:** QA verifies kidney SPECT tracer uptake values are correct.

305. **Nominal MU Consistency QA Meaning:** QA to verify monitor units are consistent with treatment plan.
**Related Terms:** LINAC, IMRT, MU Calculation
**Example:** QA confirms kidney VMAT MU for each field using ion chamber.

306. **Noise Reduction Verification Meaning:** QA to validate effectiveness of image noise reduction methods.
**Related Terms:** CBCT, CT, MRI, Image Processing
**Example:** QA checks kidney CBCT denoising does not affect tumor contours.

307. **Neutron Dose Distribution QA Meaning:** Measurement and verification of neutron dose distribution in treatment areas.
**Related Terms:** High-energy LINAC, Shielding, Secondary Radiation
**Example:** QA maps neutron dose in kidney SBRT vault.

308. **Nominal Beam Symmetry QA Meaning:** QA to ensure the radiation beam is symmetrical across the field.
**Related Terms:** LINAC, IMRT, Photon Beam
**Example:** QA confirms kidney IMRT beam symmetry to prevent hotspots.

309. **Nuclear Medicine Registration QA Meaning:** QA for image alignment between nuclear medicine scans and planning CT/MRI.
**Related Terms:** PET/CT, SPECT/CT, IGRT
**Example:** QA ensures kidney PET images align with CT for planning.

310. **Non-target Dose Optimization QA Meaning:** QA to minimize dose to surrounding healthy tissues.
**Related Terms:** DVH, OAR, IMRT, VMAT
**Example:** QA confirms kidney SBRT spares liver and bowel.

311. **Nominal Collimator Angle QA Meaning:** QA to verify the correct positioning of collimator angles.
**Related Terms:** MLC, LINAC, IMRT
**Example:** QA ensures kidney IMRT MLC leaves are correctly oriented.

312. **Nephron Functional Imaging QA Meaning:** QA of imaging techniques evaluating kidney function at nephron level.
**Related Terms:** SPECT, PET, Tc-99m DMSA
**Example:** QA confirms kidney SPECT functional maps are accurate.

313. **Nuclear Medicine Phantom QA Meaning:** QA using phantoms to calibrate PET/SPECT scanners.
**Related Terms:** Phantom, Detector Calibration, Imaging QA
**Example:** QA checks kidney SPECT scanner uniformity using a kidney-shaped phantom.

314. **Nominal Field Position QA Meaning:** QA to confirm treatment field is correctly positioned.
**Related Terms:** LINAC, IGRT, Portal Dosimetry
**Example:** QA ensures kidney IMRT PTV is aligned with the planned field.

**315. Neutron Shielding QA Meaning:** QA to verify neutron shielding effectiveness.
**Related Terms:** LINAC, Secondary Radiation, Vault Shielding
**Example:** QA confirms kidney SBRT vault walls attenuate neutrons safely.

**316. Nonlinear Dose Mapping QA Meaning:** QA to verify dose mapping in areas with high dose gradients.
**Related Terms:** SBRT, IMRT, DVH, TPS
**Example:** QA checks kidney SBRT dose mapping in steep gradient regions.

**317. Nominal Gantry Speed Verification Meaning:** QA of gantry rotation speed for accurate VMAT delivery.
**Related Terms:** LINAC, VMAT, Dose Rate
**Example:** QA confirms kidney VMAT gantry rotates at planned speed.

**318. Noise Histogram Analysis QA Meaning:** QA to assess image noise distribution using histograms.
**Related Terms:** CT, MRI, CBCT, Image Quality
**Example:** QA evaluates kidney CT noise to ensure tumor visibility.

**319. Nephron Dose Constraint Verification Meaning:** QA to ensure dose limits for functional kidney subunits are respected.
**Related Terms:** DVH, NTCP, Functional Imaging
**Example:** QA checks kidney SBRT plan adheres to nephron dose constraints.

**320. Nominal Beam Penumbra QA Meaning:** QA of radiation field penumbra for sharp dose fall-off.
**Related Terms:** LINAC, IMRT, MLC
**Example:** QA confirms kidney SBRT penumbra is within TPS tolerance.

**321. Nuclear Medicine Detector Uniformity QA Meaning:** QA to verify uniform detector response in PET/SPECT systems.
**Related Terms:** Phantom, Calibration, Imaging QA
**Example:** QA ensures kidney SPECT images are uniform across the detector field.

**322. Non-coplanar Couch Rotation QA Meaning:** QA of treatment couch rotation for non-coplanar beams.
**Related Terms:** IGRT, VMAT, SBRT
**Example:** QA verifies kidney SBRT couch angles match treatment plan.

**323. Nominal Dose Rate QA Meaning:** QA to confirm dose rate matches treatment prescription.
**Related Terms:** MU, LINAC, VMAT
**Example:** QA ensures kidney SBRT dose rate is consistent with TPS.

**324. Noise Equivalent Count Rate QA Meaning:** QA for PET detector performance based on count rate and noise.
**Related Terms:** PET, SNR, Detector QA
**Example:** QA confirms kidney PET NECR meets manufacturer recommendations.

**325. Nephron Segmentation Accuracy QA Meaning:** QA to ensure accurate delineation of nephron subunits for dose mapping.
**Related Terms:** Contouring, Functional Imaging, TPS
**Example:** QA verifies kidney nephron segmentation for functional sparing.

**326. Nuclear Medicine Sensitivity Verification Meaning:** QA to verify detector sensitivity in nuclear imaging.
**Related Terms:** PET, SPECT, Phantom, Calibration
**Example:** QA confirms kidney SPECT detector sensitivity is within tolerance.

327. **Nominal SSD QA Meaning:** QA to confirm source-to-surface distance is accurate.
**Related Terms:** LINAC, MU, PDD
**Example:** QA ensures kidney IMRT SSD matches TPS plan.

328. **Non-target Organ Dose QA Meaning:** QA to measure dose to organs outside the treatment target.
**Related Terms:** OAR, DVH, TPS
**Example:** QA evaluates liver and bowel dose during kidney IMRT.

329. **Nominal Gantry Angle QA Meaning:** QA to ensure gantry angles match treatment plan.
**Related Terms:** LINAC, VMAT, SBRT
**Example:** QA verifies kidney SBRT gantry angles are accurate.

330. **Neutron Flux Measurement QA Meaning:** QA to measure neutron flux in high-energy photon therapy rooms.
**Related Terms:** LINAC, Shielding, Secondary Radiation
**Example:** QA measures neutron flux near kidney treatment vault.

331. **Nonlinear Dose Response Verification Meaning:** QA to confirm nonlinear dose response in high-gradient areas.
**Related Terms:** SBRT, IMRT, DVH, TPS
**Example:** QA validates kidney SBRT dose-response curves against measurements

332. **Nominal Beam Flatness Verification Meaning:** QA to ensure uniform radiation across the field.
**Related Terms:** LINAC, IMRT, Photon Beam
**Example:** QA confirms kidney IMRT beams have consistent flatness.

333. **Nuclear Medicine Activity Measurement QA Meaning:** QA to measure radiotracer activity accurately.
**Related Terms:** PET, SPECT, Radiopharmacy
**Example:** QA verifies kidney PET tracer activity before injection.

334. **Non-target Dose Mapping QA Meaning:** QA to map dose delivered to non-target tissues.
**Related Terms:** DVH, OAR, IMRT
**Example:** QA confirms liver and bowel doses during kidney SBRT.

335. **Nominal Collimator Position QA Meaning:** QA of collimator jaw and MLC positions.
**Related Terms:** LINAC, IMRT, VMAT
**Example:** QA ensures kidney IMRT MLC positions match TPS.

336. **Nephron Dose-volume QA Meaning:** QA of DVH for kidney nephron subunits.
**Related Terms:** DVH, Functional Imaging, TPS
**Example:** QA verifies nephron dose limits in kidney SBRT.

337. **Nuclear Medicine Spatial Resolution Verification Meaning:** QA to measure imaging system spatial resolution.
**Related Terms:** PET, SPECT, Phantom
**Example:** QA confirms kidney SPECT spatial resolution meets standards.

338. **Non-coplanar Field QA Meaning:** QA of non-coplanar treatment field positioning.
**Related Terms:** VMAT, SBRT, IGRT
**Example:** QA verifies kidney SBRT non-coplanar beams match plan.

339. **Nominal MU Verification Meaning:** QA to ensure delivered MU matches plan.
**Related Terms:** LINAC, IMRT, VMAT
**Example:** QA confirms kidney VMAT MU for each field.

340. **Noise Power Spectrum QA Meaning:** QA to assess spatial frequency characteristics of image noise.
**Related Terms:** CT, MRI, CBCT
**Example:** QA evaluates kidney CT image noise spectrum.

341. **Neutron Protection Verification Meaning:** QA to ensure shielding protects staff and patients from neutrons.
**Related Terms:** LINAC, Shielding, Secondary Radiation
**Example:** QA confirms kidney SBRT vault walls provide adequate protection.

342. **Nominal Field Center QA Meaning:** QA to verify radiation field is centered on target.
**Related Terms:** LINAC, IGRT, Portal Dosimetry
**Example:** QA ensures kidney IMRT PTV aligns with field center.

343. **Nuclear Medicine Uniformity Verification Meaning:** QA to ensure uniform response across detectors.
**Related Terms:** PET, SPECT, Phantom
**Example:** QA confirms kidney SPECT images are uniform.

344. **Nonlinear Dose Gradient QA Meaning:** QA for high-dose gradient verification in complex plans.
**Related Terms:** IMRT, SBRT, DVH|
**Example:** QA verifies kidney SBRT dose gradient matches TPS.

345. **Nominal Gantry Mechanical QA Meaning:** QA to ensure gantry integrity and accurate rotation.
**Related Terms:** LINAC, VMAT, SBRT
**Example:** QA confirms kidney SBRT gantry moves accurately.

346. **Neutron Scatter Dose QA Meaning:** QA to measure neutron scatter in treatment room.
**Related Terms:** LINAC, Shielding, Secondary Radiation
**Example:** QA evaluates scattered neutron dose near kidney treatment area.

347. **Non-target Tissue Dose QA Meaning:** QA to assess dose received by surrounding healthy tissues.
**Related Terms:** DVH, OAR, TPS
**Example:** QA ensures liver and bowel doses are minimized during kidney SBRT.

348. **Nominal Dose Delivery QA Meaning:** QA to ensure the prescribed dose is accurately delivered.
**Related Terms:** LINAC, IMRT, MU
**Example:** QA confirms kidney SBRT dose matches TPS prescription.

349. **Nuclear Medicine Phantom Imaging QA Meaning:** QA using phantoms to validate imaging system performance.
**Related Terms:** PET, SPECT, Calibration
**Example:** QA verifies kidney SPECT image quality using phantom.

350. **Nonlinear Dose Verification QA Meaning:** QA to confirm dose in non-linear regions matches plan.
**Related Terms:** TPS, SBRT, DVH
**Example:** QA ensures kidney SBRT high-gradient dose accuracy.

351. **Nominal Beam Energy Verification QA Meaning:** QA to ensure beam energy matches treatment plan.
**Related Terms:** LINAC, IMRT, VMAT **Example:** QA confirms kidney IMRT photon beam energy matches TPS.

352. **Nephron Functional Dose Verification QA Meaning:** QA to ensure dose to functional nephron subunits is within tolerance.
**Related Terms:** DVH, SBRT, Functional Imaging
**Example:** QA confirms kidney SBRT plan spares functional nephron regions.

353. **Nominal Field Edge QA Meaning:** QA to check field edges match planned penumbra.
**Related Terms:** LINAC, IMRT, MLC
**Example:** QA ensures kidney IMRT field edges protect adjacent tissues.

354. **Nuclear Medicine Count Rate Verification Meaning:** QA to verify detector count rates for accurate imaging.
**Related Terms:** PET, SPECT, Detector QA
**Example:** QA confirms kidney PET count rate is within calibration limits.

355. **Non-coplanar Couch QA Phantom Meaning:** Phantom-based QA for couch rotation in non-coplanar treatments.
**Related Terms:** SBRT, VMAT, IGRT
**Example:** QA checks kidney SBRT couch angles using phantom.

356. **Nominal Dose per Fraction QA Meaning:** QA to ensure each treatment fraction delivers correct dose.
**Related Terms:** Fractionation, SBRT, IMRT
**Example:** QA verifies kidney SBRT fraction dose consistency.

357. **Neutron Dose Shielding Verification Meaning:** QA to confirm neutron shielding effectiveness in high-energy LINACs.
**Related Terms:** Secondary Radiation, Vault Safety
**Example:** QA confirms kidney treatment room walls attenuate neutrons.

358. **Non-target Organ Dose Verification Phantom Meaning:** Phantom-based QA to measure dose to non-target organs.
**Related Terms:** OAR, DVH, TPS
**Example:** QA maps liver and bowel dose in kidney SBRT phantom.

359. **Nominal Beam Output QA Meaning:** QA to verify beam output matches planned prescription.
**Related Terms:** LINAC, MU, Photon Dose
**Example:** QA ensures kidney IMRT beam output aligns with TPS.

360. **Nuclear Medicine Dose Calibration QA Meaning:** QA to ensure administered radiotracer dose is accurate.
**Related Terms:** PET, SPECT, Radiopharmacy
**Example:** QA confirms kidney Tc-99m MAG3 dose matches protocol.

361. **Nonlinear Beam Dose Verification QA Meaning:** QA to validate dose in regions with non-linear dose gradients.
**Related Terms:** IMRT, SBRT, TPS
**Example:** QA ensures kidney SBRT steep dose gradient accuracy.

362. **Nominal MLC Leaf Position QA Meaning:** QA to ensure MLC leaves are correctly positioned.
**Related Terms:** LINAC, IMRT, VMAT
**Example:** QA confirms kidney VMAT leaf positions match TPS.

363. **Nephron Sparing Dose Mapping QA Meaning:** QA to map doses to nephron subunits for functional sparing.
**Related Terms:** DVH, Functional Imaging, SBRT
**Example:** QA confirms kidney SBRT plan preserves critical nephron regions.

364. **Non-coplanar Dose Verification QA Meaning:** QA to ensure accurate delivery for non-coplanar beams.
**Related Terms:** VMAT, SBRT, IGRT
**Example:** QA validates kidney SBRT non-coplanar beam dose accuracy.

365. **Nominal Gantry Angle Phantom QA Meaning:** Phantom-based QA to check gantry angles.
**Related Terms:** LINAC, SBRT, VMAT
**Example:** QA uses kidney phantom to verify gantry rotation accuracy.

366. **Nuclear Medicine Attenuation Correction QA Meaning:** QA to ensure attenuation correction in PET/SPECT is accurate.
**Related Terms:** PET/CT, SPECT/CT, Imaging QA
**Example:** QA confirms kidney PET/CT attenuation correction is correct.

367. **Non-target Dose Accumulation QA Meaning:** QA to track cumulative dose to non-target organs.
**Related Terms:** DVH, OAR, TPS
**Example:** QA evaluates cumulative liver dose during kidney SBRT course.

368. **Nominal Beam Symmetry Phantom QA Meaning:** Phantom-based QA for beam symmetry measurement.
**Related Terms:** LINAC, IMRT, Photon Beam
**Example:** QA confirms kidney IMRT beams are symmetric using phantom.

369. **Neutron Exposure Monitoring QA Meaning:** QA for monitoring neutron exposure in high-energy therapy rooms.
**Related Terms:** Secondary Radiation, Shielding, LINAC
**Example:** QA measures neutron exposure during kidney SBRT treatments.

370. **Nonlinear Dose Accumulation Verification Meaning:** QA to ensure dose accumulation in high-gradient regions matches plan.
**Related Terms:** DVH, SBRT, TPS
**Example:** QA confirms kidney SBRT cumulative dose accuracy.

371. **Nominal Field Verification PhantomMeaning:** Phantom-based QA for field placement verification.
**Related Terms:** LINAC, IGRT, Portal Dosimetry
**Example:** QA confirms kidney IMRT field alignment using phantom.

372. **Nuclear Medicine Resolution QA Meaning:** QA to measure spatial resolution of PET/SPECT scanners.
**Related Terms:** Phantom, PET, SPECT
**Example:** QA confirms kidney SPECT spatial resolution meets standards.

373. **Non-coplanar Beam Plan QA Meaning:** QA to validate non-coplanar beam planning parameters.
**Related Terms:** SBRT, VMAT, TPS
**Example:** QA verifies kidney SBRT non-coplanar plan matches TPS.

374. **Nominal Dose Verification Phantom Meaning:** Phantom-based QA to confirm delivered dose.
**Related Terms:** LINAC, IMRT, VMAT
**Example:** QA ensures kidney SBRT dose matches planned values.

375. **Nephron Segmentation QA Phantom Meaning:** Phantom QA to validate nephron contouring and dose mapping.
**Related Terms:** Functional Imaging, DVH, TPS
**Example:** QA confirms kidney phantom nephron segmentation accuracy.

376. **Non-target Dose Verification Checklist Meaning:** QA checklist for monitoring dose to non-target tissues.
**Related Terms:** OAR, DVH, SBRT
**Example:** QA confirms liver, bowel doses are within tolerance during kidney SBRT.

377. **Nominal Beam Energy Phantom QA Meaning:** Phantom-based QA for verifying beam energy.
**Related Terms:** LINAC, IMRT, VMAT
**Example:** QA confirms kidney IMRT photon beam energy using phantom.

378. **Nuclear Medicine Activity QA Phantom Meaning:** Phantom QA to validate radiotracer activity measurement.
**Related Terms:** PET, SPECT, Radiopharmacy
**Example:** QA checks kidney PET activity using a calibration phantom.

379. **Nonlinear Beam Profile Verification Meaning:** QA to confirm beam profile in non-linear dose regions.
**Related Terms:** IMRT, SBRT, TPS
**Example:** QA ensures kidney SBRT high-gradient profiles match plan.

380. **Nominal MU Phantom QA Meaning:** Phantom QA to verify monitor unit delivery.
**Related Terms:** LINAC, IMRT, VMAT
**Example:** QA confirms kidney VMAT MU using ion chamber in phantom.

381. **Neutron Shielding Phantom QA Meaning:** Phantom QA to test neutron shielding performance.
**Related Terms:** High-energy LINAC, Secondary Radiation, Vault
**Example:** QA validates kidney SBRT vault neutron shielding.

382. **Non-target Tissue Dose Mapping Phantom Meaning:** Phantom-based QA for mapping dose to non-target tissues.
**Related Terms:** DVH, OAR, TPS
**Example:** QA measures liver and bowel dose using kidney SBRT phantom.

383. **Nominal Gantry Speed Phantom QA Meaning:** Phantom-based QA to verify gantry rotation speed.
**Related Terms:** VMAT, LINAC, SBRT
**Example:** QA ensures kidney SBRT gantry speed matches TPS plan.

384. **Nuclear Medicine Uniformity Phantom QA Meaning:** Phantom QA to ensure detector response uniformity.
**Related Terms:** PET, SPECT, Imaging QA
**Example:** QA confirms kidney SPECT uniformity using phantom.

385. **Non-coplanar Dose Accumulation QA Phantom Meaning:** Phantom-based QA for cumulative dose in non-coplanar beams.
**Related Terms:** SBRT, VMAT, TPS
**Example:** QA checks kidney SBRT cumulative dose in phantom.

386. **Nominal Dose Rate Phantom QA Meaning:** Phantom-based QA to verify dose rate accuracy.
**Related Terms:** LINAC, MU, VMAT
**Example:** QA confirms kidney SBRT dose rate using phantom.

387. **Nephron Functional Dose Mapping Phantom Meaning:** Phantom QA for mapping dose to functional nephron subunits.
**Related Terms:** DVH, Functional Imaging, SBRT
**Example:** QA validates kidney phantom nephron dose maps.

388. **Nonlinear Dose Verification Phantom Meaning:** Phantom QA for regions with non-linear dose distribution.
**Related Terms:** IMRT, SBRT, DVH
**Example:** QA ensures kidney SBRT dose gradients are accurate.

389. **Nominal Beam Flatness Phantom QA Meaning:** Phantom QA to measure beam flatness across the field.
**Related Terms:** LINAC, IMRT, VMAT
**Example:** QA confirms kidney IMRT beam flatness using phantom.

390. **Nuclear Medicine Spatial Accuracy QA Phantom Meaning:** Phantom QA to verify spatial accuracy of PET/SPECT.
**Related Terms:** Phantom, PET, SPECT
**Example:** QA confirms kidney SPECT spatial localization using phantom.

391. **Non-target Dose Accumulation Phantom QA Meaning:** Phantom QA for cumulative dose to surrounding tissues.
**Related Terms:** DVH, OAR, TPS
**Example:** QA evaluates cumulative liver dose using kidney SBRT phantom.

392. **Nominal Field Size Verification Phantom Meaning:** Phantom QA to ensure field size matches plan.
**Related Terms:** LINAC, IMRT, VMAT
**Example:** QA confirms kidney IMRT PTV coverage using phantom.

393. **Neutron Flux Phantom QA Meaning:** Phantom QA for neutron flux measurements.
**Related Terms:** LINAC, High-energy photon, Shielding
**Example:** QA checks neutron flux in kidney treatment vault using phantom.

394. **Nonlinear Dose Response Phantom QA Meaning:** Phantom QA for non-linear dose response verification.
**Related Terms:** TPS, SBRT, IMRT
**Example:** QA confirms kidney SBRT dose-response accuracy using phantom.

395. **Nominal Beam Energy Verification Phantom Meaning:** Phantom QA for verifying delivered beam energy.
**Related Terms:** LINAC, IMRT, VMAT
**Example:** QA ensures kidney IMRT photon beam energy matches plan.

396. **Nuclear Medicine Count Rate Phantom QA Meaning:** Phantom QA to verify detector count rate accuracy.
**Related Terms:** PET, SPECT, Detector QA
**Example:** QA confirms kidney PET count rate using phantom.

397. **Non-coplanar Beam Phantom QA Meaning:** Phantom QA for non-coplanar beam delivery verification.
**Related Terms:** SBRT, VMAT, IGRT
**Example:** QA confirms kidney SBRT non-coplanar beams using phantom.

398. **Nominal MU Verification Phantom Meaning:** Phantom QA to check monitor unit delivery accuracy.
**Related Terms:** LINAC, IMRT, VMAT
**Example:** QA ensures kidney VMAT MU is accurate using phantom.

399. **Nephron Dose Constraint Phantom QA Meaning:** Phantom QA to validate nephron dose constraints.
**Related Terms:** DVH, Functional Imaging, SBRT
**Example:** QA confirms kidney phantom meets nephron dose limits.

400. **Non-target Organ Dose QA Phantom Meaning:** Phantom QA to assess dose to surrounding organs.
**Related Terms:** OAR, DVH, TPS
**Example:** QA evaluates liver and bowel dose using kidney phantom.

401. **Nominal Field Center Phantom QA Meaning:** Phantom QA to verify radiation field is centered on target.
**Related Terms:** LINAC, IGRT, Portal Dosimetry
**Example:** QA confirms kidney IMRT field center using phantom.

402. **Nuclear Medicine Image Registration QA Meaning:** QA to ensure PET/SPECT images are accurately registered with CT/MRI.
**Related Terms:** PET/CT, SPECT/CT, Image Fusion
**Example:** QA confirms kidney PET images are aligned with CT for accurate dose planning.

403. **Nominal Beam Output Consistency QA Meaning:** QA to monitor stability of beam output over time.
**Related Terms:** LINAC, MU, IMRT
**Example:** QA ensures kidney IMRT beams deliver consistent output across multiple fractions.

404. **Non-target Tissue Dose Constraint QA Meaning:** QA to verify dose to nearby organs does not exceed tolerance.
**Related Terms:** DVH, OAR, SBRT
**Example:** QA checks kidney SBRT plan keeps liver and bowel dose below thresholds.

405. **Nephron Functional Imaging QA Meaning:** QA to ensure imaging accurately depicts functional nephron regions.
**Related Terms:** Functional MRI, SPECT, PET
**Example:** QA validates kidney SPECT functional imaging before planning SBRT.

406. **Nonlinear Dose Verification Checklist Meaning:** QA checklist for verifying steep dose gradients.
**Related Terms:** IMRT, SBRT, DVH
**Example:** QA confirms kidney SBRT high-dose gradient regions match plan.

407. **Nominal MLC Leaf Speed QA Meaning:** QA to ensure MLC leaves move at correct speed for VMAT/IMRT.
**Related Terms:** LINAC, VMAT, IMRT
**Example:** QA confirms kidney VMAT MLC leaf speeds follow TPS instructions.

408. **Nuclear Medicine Detector Uniformity Phantom Meaning:** Phantom-based QA to test uniform detector response.
**Related Terms:** PET, SPECT, Imaging QA
**Example:** QA confirms kidney PET scanner uniformity using phantom.

409. **Non-coplanar Beam Dose Phantom QA Meaning:** Phantom-based QA for non-coplanar beam dose verification.
**Related Terms:** SBRT, VMAT, TPS
**Example:** QA validates kidney SBRT non-coplanar dose using phantom.

410. **Nominal Gantry Angle Accuracy QA Meaning:** QA to verify gantry angles match treatment plan.
**Related Terms:** LINAC, SBRT, VMAT
**Example:** QA ensures kidney SBRT gantry angles match TPS.

411. **Neutron Dose Assessment Phantom QA Meaning:** Phantom-based QA to measure neutron dose from high-energy beams.
**Related Terms:** Secondary Radiation, Vault Safety
**Example:** QA confirms kidney SBRT vault neutron dose is within limits.

412. **Non-target Dose Accumulation Mapping QA Meaning:** QA to map cumulative dose to organs at risk.
**Related Terms:** DVH, OAR, TPS
**Example:** QA maps cumulative liver dose during kidney SBRT.

413. **Nominal Dose Rate Verification Meaning:** QA to ensure LINAC delivers correct dose rate.
**Related Terms:** LINAC, MU, VMAT
**Example:** QA confirms kidney SBRT dose rate matches prescription.

414. **Nuclear Medicine Calibration Phantom QA Meaning:** Phantom QA to validate radiotracer activity and detection.
**Related Terms:** PET, SPECT, Radiopharmacy
**Example:** QA confirms kidney PET phantom activity matches protocol.

415. **Nonlinear Beam Profile Phantom QA Meaning:** Phantom QA to validate non-linear dose profiles in modulated beams.
**Related Terms:** IMRT, SBRT, TPS
**Example:** QA confirms kidney SBRT high-gradient dose matches plan.

416. **Nominal MU Output Phantom QA Meaning:** Phantom QA to verify MU delivery accuracy.
**Related Terms:** LINAC, IMRT, VMAT
**Example:** QA confirms kidney VMAT MUs using ion chamber phantom.

417. **Nephron Sparing Plan QA Meaning:** QA to ensure nephron-sparing objectives are met in treatment plan.
**Related Terms:** DVH, Functional Imaging, SBRT
**Example:** QA checks kidney SBRT plan spares critical nephron regions.

418. **Non-coplanar Field Position Verification QA Meaning:** QA to confirm correct positioning of non-coplanar fields.
**Related Terms:** SBRT, VMAT, IGRT
**Example:** QA ensures kidney SBRT non-coplanar fields match TPS.

419. **Nominal Beam Flatness Verification QA Meaning:** QA to confirm beam flatness across the radiation field.
**Related Terms:** LINAC, IMRT, VMAT
**Example:** QA checks kidney IMRT beam flatness using phantom.

420. **Nuclear Medicine Count Rate Stability QA Meaning:** QA to monitor stability of detector count rates over time.
**Related Terms:** PET, SPECT, Detector QA
**Example:** QA confirms kidney PET count rates remain consistent over multiple scans.

421. **Non-target Organ Dose Verification Checklist Meaning:** QA checklist to ensure non-target organ dose is within tolerance.
**Related Terms:** OAR, DVH, TPS
**Example:** QA ensures liver and bowel doses are safe during kidney SBRT.

422. **Nominal Field Shape Phantom QA Meaning:** Phantom-based QA to verify field shape accuracy.
**Related Terms:** IMRT, VMAT, LINAC
**Example:** QA confirms kidney IMRT field shape matches TPS.

423. **Neutron Dose Monitoring QA Meaning:** QA to measure neutron dose during high-energy treatments.
**Related Terms:** Secondary Radiation, Vault Safety, LINAC
**Example:** QA checks neutron exposure during kidney SBRT treatments.

424. **Nonlinear Dose Verification Protocol QA Meaning:** QA protocol for regions with steep dose gradients.
**Related Terms:** SBRT, IMRT, TPS
**Example:** QA ensures kidney SBRT high-gradient dose matches TPS plan.

425. **Nominal Gantry Speed Verification QA Meaning:** QA to confirm gantry rotation speed is accurate.
**Related Terms:** VMAT, LINAC, SBRT
**Example:** QA verifies kidney SBRT gantry rotation speed matches plan.

426. **Nuclear Medicine Spatial Resolution QA Phantom Meaning:** Phantom QA to measure spatial resolution of imaging system.
**Related Terms:** PET, SPECT, Phantom QA
**Example:** QA confirms kidney SPECT spatial resolution using phantom.

427. **Non-target Tissue Dose Mapping QA Meaning:** QA to map dose delivered to surrounding healthy tissues.
**Related Terms:** DVH, OAR, TPS
**Example:** QA maps liver and bowel dose during kidney SBRT.

428. **Nominal Beam Symmetry Phantom QA Meaning:** Phantom QA to measure beam symmetry.
**Related Terms:** LINAC, IMRT, VMAT
**Example:** QA ensures kidney IMRT beam is symmetric using phantom.

429. **Nephron Functional Dose Phantom QA Meaning:** Phantom QA to measure dose to functional nephron regions.
**Related Terms:** Functional Imaging, DVH, SBRT
**Example:** QA confirms kidney phantom nephron dose is within tolerance.

430. **Nonlinear Dose Accumulation Verification QA Meaning:** QA to confirm cumulative dose in non-linear regions.
**Related Terms:** SBRT, DVH, TPS
**Example:** QA verifies kidney SBRT cumulative dose accuracy.

431. **Nominal Field Center Verification QA Meaning:** QA to ensure field center aligns with target anatomy.
**Related Terms:** LINAC, IGRT, Portal Dosimetry
**Example:** QA confirms kidney IMRT field center using phantom.

432. **Nuclear Medicine Attenuation QA Phantom Meaning:** Phantom QA for attenuation correction in PET/SPECT.
**Related Terms:** PET/CT, SPECT/CT, Imaging QA
**Example:** QA validates kidney PET attenuation correction using phantom.

433. **Non-coplanar Beam Plan Verification QA Meaning:** QA to validate non-coplanar beam planning.
**Related Terms:** SBRT, VMAT, TPS
**Example:** QA checks kidney SBRT non-coplanar plan against TPS.

434. **Nominal Dose Verification Protocol QA Meaning:** QA protocol for verifying delivered dose.
**Related Terms:** LINAC, IMRT, VMAT
**Example:** QA confirms kidney SBRT dose matches prescription.

435. **Neutron Flux Monitoring Phantom QA Meaning:** Phantom QA to measure neutron flux in treatment vault.
**Related Terms:** LINAC, Shielding, Secondary Radiation
**Example:** QA confirms kidney SBRT vault neutron flux is within safety limits.

436. **Non-target Dose Accumulation QA Protocol Meaning:** QA protocol for cumulative dose to organs at risk.
**Related Terms:** DVH, OAR, TPS
**Example:** QA evaluates cumulative liver dose during kidney SBRT course.

437. **Nominal Beam Flatness Protocol QA Meaning:** QA protocol to ensure beam flatness.
**Related Terms:** LINAC, IMRT, VMAT
**Example:** QA confirms kidney IMRT beam flatness matches tolerance.

438. **Nuclear Medicine Detector Linearity QA Meaning:** QA to verify detector response is linear over range.
**Related Terms:** PET, SPECT, Detector QA
**Example:** QA ensures kidney PET detector maintains linear response.

439. **Nonlinear Dose Response Verification QA Meaning:** QA to confirm non-linear dose response matches TPS.
**Related Terms:** IMRT, SBRT, DVH
**Example:** QA validates kidney SBRT high-dose gradient accuracy.

440. **Nominal MU Phantom Verification QA Meaning:** Phantom QA to confirm monitor unit delivery accuracy.
**Related Terms:** LINAC, IMRT, VMAT
**Example:** QA confirms kidney VMAT MU matches TPS.

441. **Nephron Dose Constraint Protocol QA Meaning:** QA protocol to ensure nephron dose constraints are met.
**Related Terms:** DVH, Functional Imaging, SBRT
**Example:** QA confirms kidney SBRT nephron dose limits are respected.

442. **Non-target Organ Dose Phantom QA Meaning:** Phantom QA to measure dose to surrounding organs.
**Related Terms:** DVH, OAR, TPS
**Example:** QA maps liver and bowel dose using kidney SBRT phantom.

443. **Nominal Field Alignment Phantom QA Meaning:** Phantom QA to ensure field is correctly aligned on target.
**Related Terms:** LINAC, IGRT, Portal Dosimetry
**Example:** QA confirms kidney IMRT field alignment using phantom.

444. **Nuclear Medicine Activity Verification QA Meaning:** QA to ensure radiotracer activity is within protocol limits.
**Related Terms:** PET, SPECT, Radiopharmacy
**Example:** QA confirms kidney PET activity matches prescribed dose.

445. **Non-coplanar Dose Verification Phantom QA Meaning:** Phantom QA to check non-coplanar beam dose accuracy.
**Related Terms:** SBRT, VMAT, TPS
**Example:** QA ensures kidney SBRT non-coplanar beams deliver correct dose.

446. **Nominal Gantry Angle Protocol QA Meaning:** QA protocol to verify gantry angles match treatment plan.
**Related Terms:** LINAC, SBRT, VMAT
**Example:** QA confirms kidney SBRT gantry angles align with TPS.

447. **Neutron Shielding Verification Protocol QA Meaning:** QA protocol for vault shielding effectiveness.
**Related Terms:** Secondary Radiation, High-energy LINAC
**Example:** QA confirms kidney SBRT vault neutron shielding meets safety standards.

448. **Non-target Tissue Dose Mapping Protocol QA Meaning:** QA protocol to track dose to surrounding healthy tissues.
**Related Terms:** DVH, OAR, TPS
**Example:** QA maps liver and bowel dose during kidney SBRT treatment.

449. **Nominal Beam Symmetry Protocol QA Meaning:** QA protocol to ensure beam symmetry meets tolerance.
**Related Terms:** LINAC, IMRT, VMAT
**Example:** QA confirms kidney IMRT beam symmetry using phantom.

450. **Nephron Functional Dose Mapping Protocol QA Meaning:** QA protocol for mapping dose to functional nephron regions.
**Related Terms:** Functional Imaging, DVH, SBRT
**Example:** QA ensures kidney SBRT plan preserves critical nephron subunits.

451. **Nonlinear Dose Accumulation Protocol QA Meaning:** QA protocol to ensure cumulative dose in high-gradient regions matches plan.
**Related Terms:** DVH, IMRT, SBRT
**Example:** QA confirms kidney SBRT cumulative dose is accurate.

452. **Nominal Field Center Protocol QA Meaning:** QA protocol to ensure field center aligns with target anatomy.
**Related Terms:** LINAC, IGRT, Portal Dosimetry
**Example:** QA confirms kidney IMRT field center matches TPS coordinates.

453. **Nuclear Medicine Attenuation Protocol QA Meaning:** QA protocol to ensure correct attenuation correction in PET/SPECT imaging.
**Related Terms:** PET/CT, SPECT/CT, Phantom QA
**Example:** QA validates kidney PET attenuation correction using standard phantom.

454. **Non-coplanar Beam Plan Protocol QA Meaning:** QA protocol for verification of non-coplanar beam arrangements.
**Related Terms:** SBRT, VMAT, TPS
**Example:** QA checks kidney SBRT non-coplanar plan matches TPS.

455. **Nominal Dose Delivery QA Meaning:** QA to confirm actual dose delivered matches prescription.
**Related Terms:** IMRT, VMAT, LINAC
**Example:** QA confirms kidney SBRT dose per fraction matches plan.

456. **Neutron Flux Verification QA Meaning:** QA to measure neutron flux in treatment vault.
**Related Terms:** Secondary Radiation, Shielding
**Example:** QA ensures kidney SBRT vault neutron exposure is within limits.

457. **Non-target Dose Accumulation QA Meaning:** QA to confirm cumulative dose to organs at risk.
**Related Terms:** DVH, OAR, TPS
**Example:** QA maps cumulative liver dose during kidney SBRT.

458. **Nominal Beam Flatness QA Meaning:** QA to confirm uniform dose distribution across the radiation field.
**Related Terms:** LINAC, IMRT, VMAT
**Example:** QA confirms kidney IMRT beam flatness using phantom measurements.

459. **Nuclear Medicine Detector Linearity Protocol QA Meaning:** QA protocol to ensure detector response is linear.
**Related Terms:** PET, SPECT, Detector QA
**Example:** QA ensures kidney PET detector response is linear over activity range.

460. **Nonlinear Dose Response QA Meaning:** QA to verify dose response in high-gradient regions.
**Related Terms:** IMRT, SBRT, DVH
**Example:** QA validates kidney SBRT high-gradient dose response using film phantom.

461. **Nominal MU Delivery QA Meaning:** QA to confirm monitor unit delivery is correct.
**Related Terms:** LINAC, IMRT, VMAT
**Example:** QA confirms kidney VMAT MU matches TPS prescription.

462. **Nephron Dose Constraint Verification QA Meaning:** QA to ensure functional nephron dose constraints are met.
**Related Terms:** DVH, Functional Imaging, SBRT
**Example:** QA confirms kidney SBRT plan spares critical nephron subunits.

463. **Non-target Organ Dose Phantom QA Meaning:** Phantom QA to measure dose to surrounding healthy tissues.
**Related Terms:** DVH, OAR, TPS
**Example:** QA maps liver and bowel dose using kidney SBRT phantom.

464. **Nominal Field Alignment QA Meaning:** QA to verify treatment field is correctly aligned on target.
**Related Terms:** LINAC, IGRT, Portal Dosimetry
**Example:** QA confirms kidney IMRT field alignment using phantom.

465. **Nuclear Medicine Activity QA Meaning:** QA to ensure radiotracer activity is within protocol limits.
**Related Terms:** PET, SPECT, Radiopharmacy
**Example:** QA confirms kidney PET radiotracer activity matches prescription.

466. **Non-coplanar Dose Verification QA Meaning:** QA to confirm accuracy of non-coplanar beam dose delivery.
**Related Terms:** SBRT, VMAT, TPS
**Example:** QA ensures kidney SBRT non-coplanar beams deliver correct dose.

467. **Nominal Gantry Angle QA Meaning:** QA to ensure gantry angles match treatment plan.
**Related Terms:** LINAC, SBRT, VMAT
**Example:** QA confirms kidney SBRT gantry angles align with TPS plan.

468. **Neutron Shielding QA Meaning:** QA to verify vault shielding against secondary neutron radiation.
**Related Terms:** LINAC, Secondary Radiation, Vault Safety
**Example:** QA confirms kidney SBRT vault shielding meets safety standards.

469. **Non-target Tissue Dose Mapping Protocol QA Meaning:** QA protocol to track dose to surrounding tissues.
**Related Terms:** DVH, OAR, TPS
**Example:** QA maps liver and bowel dose during kidney SBRT treatment.

470. **Nominal Beam Symmetry QA Meaning:** QA to confirm left-right beam symmetry.
**Related Terms:** LINAC, IMRT, VMAT
**Example:** QA ensures kidney IMRT beam symmetry is within tolerance.

471. **Nephron Functional Dose Mapping QA Meaning:** QA to map dose to functional nephron regions for organ preservation.
**Related Terms:** Functional Imaging, DVH, SBRT
**Example:** QA ensures kidney SBRT plan spares critical nephron subunits.

472. **Nonlinear Dose Accumulation Protocol QA Meaning:** QA protocol to ensure cumulative dose in high-gradient regions is accurate.
**Related Terms:** DVH, IMRT, SBRT
**Example:** QA confirms kidney SBRT cumulative dose matches TPS.

473. **Nominal Field Center QA Meaning:** QA to ensure the radiation field center aligns with target.
**Related Terms:** LINAC, IGRT, Portal Dosimetry
**Example:** QA confirms kidney IMRT field center matches TPS coordinates.

474. **Nuclear Medicine Attenuation QA Meaning:** QA to ensure attenuation correction is correct in PET/SPECT.
**Related Terms:** PET/CT, SPECT/CT, Phantom QA
**Example:** QA validates kidney PET attenuation correction using phantom.

475. **Non-coplanar Beam Plan QA Meaning:** QA to verify non-coplanar beam arrangements match the treatment plan.
**Related Terms:** SBRT, VMAT, TPS
**Example:** QA checks kidney SBRT non-coplanar plan accuracy.

476. **Nominal Dose Delivery Protocol QA Meaning:** QA protocol to verify delivered dose matches plan.
**Related Terms:** IMRT, VMAT, LINAC
**Example:** QA confirms kidney SBRT dose per fraction matches prescription.

477. **Neutron Flux QA Meaning:** QA to measure neutron flux in treatment vault.
**Related Terms:** Secondary Radiation, Shielding
**Example:** QA ensures kidney SBRT vault neutron exposure is within limits.

478. **Non-target Dose Accumulation QA Meaning:** QA to confirm cumulative dose to organs at risk.
**Related Terms:** DVH, OAR, TPS
**Example:** QA maps cumulative liver dose during kidney SBRT.

479. **Nominal Beam Flatness Protocol QA Meaning:** QA protocol to ensure beam flatness across field.
**Related Terms:** LINAC, IMRT, VMAT
**Example:** QA confirms kidney IMRT beam flatness using phantom measurements.

480. **Nuclear Medicine Detector Linearity QA Meaning:** QA to ensure linear detector response.
**Related Terms:** PET, SPECT, Detector QA
**Example:** QA ensures kidney PET detector response remains linear.

481. **Nonlinear Dose Response Protocol QA Meaning:** QA protocol for high-gradient dose regions.
**Related Terms:** IMRT, SBRT, DVH
**Example:** QA validates kidney SBRT dose in steep gradient regions.

482. **Nominal MU Delivery Protocol QA Meaning:** QA protocol to ensure accurate monitor unit delivery.
**Related Terms:** LINAC, IMRT, VMAT
**Example:** QA confirms kidney VMAT MU matches TPS prescription.

483. **Nephron Dose Constraint QA Meaning:** QA to ensure functional nephron dose constraints are met.
**Related Terms:** DVH, Functional Imaging, SBRT
**Example:** QA confirms kidney SBRT plan spares critical nephron regions.

484. **Non-target Organ Dose QA Meaning:** QA to measure dose to surrounding healthy organs.
**Related Terms:** DVH, OAR, TPS
**Example:** QA maps liver and bowel dose using kidney SBRT phantom.

485. **Nominal Field Alignment Protocol QA Meaning:** QA protocol to ensure proper field alignment.
**Related Terms:** LINAC, IGRT, Portal Dosimetry
**Example:** QA confirms kidney IMRT field alignment using phantom.

486. **Nuclear Medicine Activity Protocol QA Meaning:** QA protocol to ensure radiotracer activity is within limits.
**Related Terms:** PET, SPECT, Radiopharmacy
**Example:** QA confirms kidney PET activity matches prescribed dose.

487. **Non-coplanar Dose Verification Protocol QA Meaning:** QA protocol for non-coplanar beam dose accuracy.
**Related Terms:** SBRT, VMAT, TPS
**Example:** QA ensures kidney SBRT non-coplanar beams deliver correct dose.

488. **Nominal Gantry Angle Protocol QA Meaning:** QA protocol to verify gantry angles match TPS plan.
**Related Terms:** LINAC, SBRT, VMAT
**Example:** QA confirms kidney SBRT gantry angles align with treatment plan.

489. **Neutron Shielding Protocol QA Meaning:** QA protocol to verify vault shielding against secondary neutron radiation.
**Related Terms:** LINAC, Secondary Radiation, Vault Safety
**Example:** QA confirms kidney SBRT vault shielding meets standards.

490. **Non-target Tissue Dose Mapping QA Meaning:** QA to track dose to surrounding healthy tissues.
**Related Terms:** DVH, OAR, TPS
**Example:** QA maps liver and bowel dose during kidney SBRT.

491. **Nominal Beam Symmetry Protocol QA Meaning:** QA protocol to ensure beam symmetry.
**Related Terms:** LINAC, IMRT, VMAT
**Example:** QA confirms kidney IMRT beam symmetry is within tolerance.

492. **Nephron Functional Dose Mapping Protocol QA Meaning:** QA protocol to map dose to functional nephron regions.
**Related Terms:** Functional Imaging, DVH, SBRT
**Example:** QA ensures kidney SBRT plan spares nephron subunits.

493. **Nonlinear Dose Accumulation QA Meaning:** QA to ensure cumulative dose in high-gradient regions is accurate.
**Related Terms:** DVH, IMRT, SBRT
**Example:** QA confirms kidney SBRT cumulative dose matches TPS.

494. **Nominal Field Center QA Meaning:** QA to ensure field center aligns with target.
**Related Terms:** LINAC, IGRT, Portal Dosimetry
**Example:** QA confirms kidney IMRT field center matches TPS coordinates.

495. **Nuclear Medicine Attenuation QA Protocol Meaning:** QA protocol to ensure correct attenuation correction in PET/SPECT.
**Related Terms:** PET/CT, SPECT/CT, Phantom QA
**Example:** QA validates kidney PET attenuation correction using phantom.

496. **Non-coplanar Beam Plan QA Protocol Meaning:** QA protocol for verification of non-coplanar beam arrangements.
**Related Terms:** SBRT, VMAT, TPS
**Example:** QA checks kidney SBRT non-coplanar plan matches TPS.

497. **Nominal Dose Delivery QA Protocol Meaning:** QA protocol for verifying delivered dose matches plan.
**Related Terms:** IMRT, VMAT, LINAC
**Example:** QA confirms kidney SBRT dose per fraction matches prescription.

498. **Neutron Flux QA Protocol Meaning:** QA protocol to measure neutron flux in treatment vault.
**Related Terms:** Secondary Radiation, Shielding
**Example:** QA ensures kidney SBRT vault neutron exposure is within limits.

499. **Non-target Dose Accumulation QA Protocol Meaning:** QA protocol to confirm cumulative dose to organs at risk.
**Related Terms:** DVH, OAR, TPS
**Example:** QA maps cumulative liver dose during kidney SBRT.

500. **Nominal Beam Flatness QA Protocol Meaning:** QA protocol to ensure beam flatness across field.
**Related Terms:** LINAC, IMRT, VMAT
**Example:** QA confirms kidney IMRT beam flatness using phantom measurements.

# O

1. **OAR Dose Constraint QA Meaning:** QA to ensure organs at risk (OAR) do not exceed prescribed dose limits.
   **Related Terms:** DVH, IMRT, SBRT, TPS
   **Example:** QA confirms kidney and liver doses remain within tolerance during SBRT.
2. **Offline Image Review QA Meaning:** QA process reviewing imaging for accuracy after treatment delivery.
   **Related Terms:** IGRT, CBCT, KV imaging
   **Example:** QA verifies kidney CBCT images post-fraction for setup accuracy.
3. **Online Imaging QA Meaning:** QA for imaging performed in real-time during treatment.
   **Related Terms:** IGRT, CBCT, KV imaging
   **Example:** QA confirms kidney tumor alignment before SBRT fraction.
4. **Open Field Dose QA Meaning:** QA to check dose uniformity in open (non-modulated) fields.
   **Related Terms:** LINAC, MU verification, TPS
   **Example:** QA ensures kidney IMRT open field dose matches calculation.
5. **Optical Distance Indicator QA Meaning:** QA to ensure accurate source-to-surface distance (SSD) measurement.
   **Related Terms:** LINAC, SAD, Dosimetry
   **Example:** QA confirms kidney SBRT SSD is accurate using ODI.
6. **Orthogonal Imaging QA Meaning:** QA for two perpendicular imaging views to verify patient positioning.
   **Related Terms:** CBCT, KV imaging, Portal Imaging
   **Example:** QA confirms kidney tumor position using AP and lateral KV images.
7. **Out-of-Field Dose QA Meaning:** QA to measure radiation dose delivered outside the planned target field.
   **Related Terms:** TPS, IMRT, VMAT
   **Example:** QA maps kidney dose to surrounding bowel using phantom.
8. **Overlap Region QA Meaning:** QA to ensure adjacent radiation fields overlap without hotspots or underdose.
   **Related Terms:** Field Matching, Junction QA, IMRT
   **Example:** QA confirms kidney extended fields overlap correctly in junction area.
9. **Output Consistency QA Meaning:** QA to verify consistent output from the LINAC over time.
   **Related Terms:** MU verification, LINAC QA, Daily QA
   **Example:** QA confirms kidney SBRT daily output remains stable.
10. **Output Factor QA Meaning:** QA to measure relative output for different field sizes.
    **Related Terms:** Field Size, MU calibration, IMRT
    **Example:** QA confirms kidney VMAT small field output matches TPS.
11. **Overlay Image QA Meaning:** QA to verify registration of multiple imaging modalities.
    **Related Terms:** CT/MRI Fusion, PET/CT, IGRT
    **Example:** QA confirms kidney CT and MRI fusion accurately overlays tumor.

12. **Oxygen Enhancement Ratio QA Meaning:** QA to ensure tissue radiosensitivity due to oxygenation is accounted.
**Related Terms:** Radiobiology, Dose Optimization
**Example:** QA considers kidney tumor hypoxic areas in SBRT plan.

13. **Output Calibration QA Meaning:** QA to ensure LINAC output matches reference calibration.
**Related Terms:** TG-51, MU verification, LINAC QA
**Example:** QA calibrates kidney SBRT beam output before clinical use.

14. **Overexposure QA Meaning:** QA to detect unintended radiation overdose areas.
**Related Terms:** DVH, TPS, Portal Dosimetry
**Example:** QA detects kidney hotspots outside the PTV.

15. **OBI Geometric Accuracy QA Meaning:** QA to verify On-Board Imaging (OBI) geometry for correct positioning.
**Related Terms:** CBCT, KV imaging, IGRT
**Example:** QA ensures kidney tumor CBCT geometry matches plan.

16. **Offline Dose Reconstruction QA Meaning:** QA to reconstruct delivered dose using imaging and log files.
**Related Terms:** DVH, TPS, IMRT, VMAT
**Example:** QA reconstructs kidney SBRT dose per fraction to verify treatment.

17. **Overlap Dose Mapping QA Meaning:** QA to map dose in overlapping radiation fields.
**Related Terms:** Field Matching, Junction QA, DVH
**Example:** QA maps kidney extended-field junctions to avoid hotspots.

18. **Online Dose Verification QA Meaning:** Real-time QA to verify dose delivery during treatment.
**Related Terms:** EPID, LINAC, IGRT
**Example:** QA monitors kidney SBRT dose in real-time using portal dosimetry.

19. **Organ Motion Compensation QA Meaning:** QA to verify methods compensating for organ motion.
**Related Terms:** Respiratory Gating, Tracking, IGRT
**Example:** QA ensures kidney motion is accounted during SBRT with gating.

20. **Orthovoltage Beam QA Meaning:** QA to verify orthovoltage X-ray beams for superficial treatments.
**Related Terms:** SSD, Dosimetry, LINAC
**Example:** QA confirms kidney skin-sparing orthovoltage field matches plan.

21. **OAR Contouring QA Meaning:** QA of contouring accuracy for organs at risk in treatment planning.
**Related Terms:** DVH, TPS, IMRT
**Example:** QA ensures kidney, liver, and bowel contours match imaging accurately.

22. **Off-Axis Ratio QA Meaning:** QA to measure dose distribution off the central beam axis.
**Related Terms:** Dose Profile, LINAC, Beam Modeling
**Example:** QA checks kidney IMRT dose accuracy 2 cm lateral from field center.

23. **On-Board Imaging QA Meaning:** QA to verify OBI system image quality and alignment.
**Related Terms:** CBCT, KV Imaging, IGRT
**Example:** QA ensures kidney CBCT images are artifact-free and geometrically accurate.

24. **On-Target Dose QA Meaning:** QA to confirm prescribed dose is delivered precisely to the target.
**Related Terms:** DVH, TPS, IGRT
**Example:** QA confirms kidney SBRT PTV receives full prescribed dose.

25. **Output Linearity QA Meaning:** QA ensuring linear relationship between monitor units and delivered dose.
    **Related Terms:** MU Calibration, LINAC, Dosimetry
    **Example:** QA verifies kidney VMAT dose scales correctly with MU adjustments.

26. **Operator Safety QA Meaning:** QA to ensure safety protocols protect staff from radiation exposure.
    **Related Terms:** ALARA, Shielding, Personnel Dosimetry.
    **Example:** QA confirms kidney SBRT operator is shielded during CBCT imaging.

27. **Oscillating Beam QA Meaning:** QA for beams with deliberate oscillation (used in special delivery techniques).
    **Related Terms:** IMRT, VMAT, Beam Modulation
    **Example:** QA verifies kidney VMAT oscillating beam dose distribution matches TPS.

28. **Overlap Fraction QA Meaning:** QA to ensure overlapping fractions maintain correct cumulative dose.
    **Related Terms:** Fractionation, DVH, IMRT
    **Example:** QA confirms kidney SBRT overlapping fractions sum to planned total dose.

29. **Oxygenation Mapping QA Meaning:** QA for imaging-based tissue oxygenation mapping to adjust dose.
    **Related Terms:** PET, MRI, Hypoxia Imaging
    **Example:** QA confirms hypoxic kidney tumor areas receive adequate dose.

30. **Output Stability QA Meaning:** QA verifying consistent LINAC output over multiple sessions.
    **Related Terms:** Daily QA, MU Verification, Dosimetry
    **Example:** QA ensures kidney SBRT daily output remains within 1% tolerance.

31. **Organ Dose Volume QA Meaning:** QA to verify organ-specific dose volumes match plan.
    **Related Terms:** DVH, TPS, OAR
    **Example:** QA confirms <20% of kidney volume receives >15 Gy.

32. **Optical Tracking QA Meaning:** QA for optical tracking systems used in real-time patient positioning.
    **Related Terms:** IGRT, Motion Management, Fiducials
    **Example:** QA ensures kidney fiducial markers are tracked accurately during SBRT.

33. **On-Target Verification Phantom Meaning:** Phantom used to verify accurate dose delivery to the target.
    **Related Terms:** IMRT, VMAT, LINAC QA
    **Example:** QA uses kidney phantom to confirm SBRT PTV coverage.

34. **Online Dose Reconstruction QA Meaning:** QA to reconstruct delivered dose during real-time therapy.
    **Related Terms:** EPID, Log Files, DVH
    **Example:** QA reconstructs kidney SBRT fraction dose to verify alignment and coverage.

35. **Off-Target Dose QA Meaning:** QA ensuring minimal dose to tissues outside the PTV.
    **Related Terms:** DVH, TPS, IMRT
    **Example:** QA checks kidney SBRT dose to liver, bowel, and spinal cord.

36. **Output Factor Verification Phantom Meaning:** Phantom used to verify output factors for different field sizes.
    **Related Terms:** Field Size, LINAC, IMRT QA
    **Example:** QA confirms small kidney VMAT field outputs match TPS.

37. **Organ Motion Phantom QA Meaning:** QA using moving phantoms to simulate organ motion during treatment.
    **Related Terms:** Motion Management, Respiratory Gating, IGRT
    **Example:** QA tests kidney motion compensation using dynamic phantom.
38. **Overlay Phantom QA Meaning:** Phantom QA for validating image overlay and registration accuracy.
    **Related Terms:** CT/MRI Fusion, PET/CT, IGRT
    **Example:** QA confirms kidney CT and MRI registration accuracy using phantom.
39. **Output Calibration Phantom Meaning:** Phantom used to calibrate LINAC output.
    **Related Terms:** TG-51, Dosimetry, MU Verification
    **Example:** QA calibrates kidney SBRT beam output using water phantom.
40. **OAR Dose Mapping QA Meaning:** QA to map delivered dose to organs at risk.
    **Related Terms:** DVH, TPS, IMRT
    **Example:** QA maps kidney, liver, and bowel dose using CBCT and portal dosimetry.
41. **Oblique Imaging QA Meaning:** QA for non-orthogonal imaging views.
    **Related Terms:** CBCT, KV Imaging, IGRT
    **Example:** QA confirms kidney tumor positioning using oblique KV images.
42. **Output Symmetry QA Meaning:** QA ensuring beam is symmetric across central axis.
    **Related Terms:** Beam Flatness, LINAC QA, MU Verification.
    **Example:** QA verifies kidney IMRT beams are symmetric to avoid hotspots.
43. **Overlap Fraction Phantom Meaning:** Phantom QA for overlapping field fractions.
    **Related Terms:** Fractionation, DVH, IMRT
    **Example:** QA confirms kidney SBRT overlapping fields maintain dose uniformity.
44. **Orthovoltage QA Phantom Meaning:** Phantom QA for orthovoltage beams.
    **Related Terms:** SSD, Superficial Radiotherapy, Dosimetry
    **Example:** QA confirms kidney superficial field dose with orthovoltage phantom.
45. **Online Imaging Dose QA Meaning:** QA to monitor imaging dose in real-time.
    **Related Terms:** CBCT, KV Imaging, IGRT
    **Example:** QA ensures kidney daily CBCT dose is within ALARA limits.
46. **Output Check QA Meaning:** Routine QA to check LINAC output against baseline.
    **Related Terms:** Daily QA, MU Verification, Dosimetry
    **Example:** QA confirms kidney SBRT daily output consistency.
47. **Oncologist Review QA Meaning:** QA step for clinician review of contours, plans, and dose.
    **Related Terms:** TPS, DVH, IGRT
    **Example:** QA confirms kidney tumor coverage and OAR sparing before SBRT.
48. **Overlay Accuracy QA Meaning:** QA ensuring multi-modality image registration is accurate.
    **Related Terms:** CT/MRI Fusion, PET/CT, IGRT
    **Example:** QA confirms kidney PET/CT overlay aligns tumor correctly.
49. **Off-Axis Beam QA Meaning:** QA for beam segments not aligned with central axis.
    **Related Terms:** Beam Profile, LINAC, IMRT
    **Example:** QA measures kidney VMAT off-axis dose to ensure accuracy.
50. **Output Verification QA Meaning:** QA to verify measured beam output matches plan.
    **Related Terms:** MU Verification, TPS, LINAC
    **Example:** QA confirms kidney IMRT field output matches planned dose.

51. **Orthogonal Imaging QA Meaning:** QA for imaging using perpendicular views to verify patient positioning.
**Related Terms:** KV Imaging, CBCT, IGRT
**Example:** QA ensures kidney SBRT setup using AP and lateral orthogonal images.

52. **Output Drift QA Meaning:** QA to monitor gradual changes in LINAC output over time.
**Related Terms:** Daily QA, MU Verification, Dosimetry
**Example:** QA confirms kidney IMRT beam output remains within ±2% over months.

53. **Organ Contour QA Meaning:** QA of accuracy of organ delineation for treatment planning.
**Related Terms:** TPS, OAR, DVH
**Example:** QA verifies kidney, liver, and bowel contours match CT/MRI.

54. **On-Target Imaging QA Meaning:** QA ensuring imaging accurately reflects target anatomy.
**Related Terms:** CBCT, Fiducials, IGRT
**Example:** QA confirms kidney tumor position on daily CBCT images.

55. **Offline Dose Review QA Meaning:** QA reviewing dose delivered after treatment sessions.
**Related Terms:** EPID, Log Files, DVH
**Example:** QA checks kidney SBRT delivered dose matches TPS calculations.

56. **Open Field QA Meaning:** QA for non-modulated, open radiation fields.
**Related Terms:** MU Verification, LINAC, Dose Measurement
**Example:** QA measures dose uniformity for kidney simple electron fields.

57. **Oblique Beam Verification Meaning:** QA for beams delivered at oblique angles.
**Related Terms:** IMRT, VMAT, LINAC QA
**Example:** QA confirms kidney IMRT oblique field dose matches TPS.

58. **OAR Dose Constraint QA Meaning:** QA ensuring dose to organs at risk is within tolerance.
**Related Terms:** DVH, TPS, IMRT
**Example:** QA confirms <20 Gy to remaining kidney tissue during SBRT.

59. **Output Consistency QA Meaning:** QA verifying LINAC output consistency across multiple fields.
**Related Terms:** MU Verification, Daily QA, Dosimetry
**Example:** QA checks kidney VMAT fields maintain uniform output.

60. **Online Image Registration QA Meaning:** QA for automatic registration of images during therapy.
**Related Terms:** CBCT, IGRT, Fiducials
**Example:** QA confirms kidney fiducial markers align with planning CT online.

61. **Optically Stimulated Luminescence QA (OSL QA) Meaning:** QA using OSL dosimeters for accurate dose measurement.
**Related Terms:** Dosimetry, Patient Dose Verification
**Example:** QA measures kidney SBRT skin dose using OSLDs.

62. **Output Mapping QA Meaning:** QA to map delivered dose across the field.
**Related Terms:** DVH, EPID, LINAC QA
**Example:** QA maps kidney VMAT field output to confirm TPS accuracy.

63. **Oncologic Plan QA Meaning:** QA for verifying that treatment plan meets clinical objectives.
**Related Terms:** DVH, OAR, PTV
**Example:** QA confirms kidney SBRT plan covers tumor while sparing healthy tissue.

64. **Off-Target Imaging QA Meaning:** QA to monitor unintended exposure or imaging artifacts outside the target.
**Related Terms:** CBCT, KV Imaging, IGRT
**Example:** QA ensures adjacent bowel is not exposed to excessive imaging dose during kidney SBRT CBCT.

65. **Oblique Phantom QA Meaning:** Phantom-based QA for oblique beams or imaging angles.
**Related Terms:** IMRT, VMAT, LINAC QA
**Example:** QA uses kidney phantom to test oblique VMAT field dose accuracy.

66. **Output Factor QA Meaning:** QA verifying dose output for different field sizes.
**Related Terms:** MU Verification, Small Field Dosimetry
**Example:** QA checks kidney SBRT small field output factors match TPS predictions.

67. **On-Target Dose Mapping Meaning:** QA mapping delivered dose to the tumor target.
**Related Terms:** EPID, DVH, TPS
**Example:** QA ensures kidney tumor receives planned dose in SBRT.

68. **Off-Axis Dose Measurement Meaning:** QA to measure dose distribution away from beam central axis.
**Related Terms:** Beam Profile, LINAC, DVH
**Example:** QA verifies kidney IMRT off-axis dose is within tolerance.

69. **Orthovoltage Dose QA Meaning:** QA specific to orthovoltage treatment units.
**Related Terms:** SSD, Dosimetry, Superficial Therapy
**Example:** QA ensures kidney superficial field dose matches calculation.

70. **OAR Contour Verification Phantom Meaning:** Phantom used to verify accurate OAR contouring.
**Related Terms:** DVH, TPS, IMRT QA
**Example:** QA uses kidney/liver phantom to verify contour accuracy.

71. **Output Uniformity QA Meaning:** QA to verify uniformity of dose across the beam.
**Related Terms:** Beam Flatness, LINAC QA
**Example:** QA ensures kidney IMRT beam uniformity within ±2%.

72. **Optical Surface Imaging QA Meaning:** QA for surface-guided radiotherapy systems.
**Related Terms:** SGRT, Motion Tracking, IGRT
**Example:** QA confirms kidney patient setup matches planned position using optical surface imaging.

73. **Oblique Angle Dose QA Meaning:** QA for dose delivered at non-standard beam angles.
**Related Terms:** IMRT, VMAT, LINAC QA
**Example:** QA verifies kidney SBRT dose at 45° oblique fields matches plan.

74. **Online Dose Verification QA Meaning:** QA verifying dose in real-time during delivery.
**Related Terms:** EPID, Log Files, DVH
**Example:** QA confirms kidney VMAT dose delivered as per TPS.

75. **Output Drift Phantom Meaning:** Phantom QA to monitor output drift over time.
**Related Terms:** Daily QA, MU Verification
**Example:** QA tracks kidney IMRT beam output over multiple sessions using phantom.

76. **On-Target Imaging Phantom Meaning:** Phantom QA for verifying tumor imaging accuracy.
**Related Terms:** CBCT, IGRT, Fiducials
**Example:** QA uses kidney phantom to verify CBCT tumor localization.

77. **Offline Image QA Meaning:** QA performed post-treatment for image quality verification.
**Related Terms:** CBCT, KV Imaging, IGRT
**Example:** QA checks kidney CBCT image quality after fraction delivery.

78. **Oblique Dose Distribution QA Meaning:** QA measuring dose distribution for oblique fields.
**Related Terms:** IMRT, VMAT, LINAC QA
**Example:** QA confirms kidney SBRT oblique field dose accuracy.

79. **OAR Dose Accumulation QA Meaning:** QA for cumulative dose delivered to organs at risk.
**Related Terms:** DVH, Fractionation, TPS
**Example:** QA ensures cumulative kidney dose remains within safe limits.

80. **Output Verification Phantom Meaning:** Phantom used to verify delivered output dose.
**Related Terms:** MU Verification, LINAC, Dosimetry
**Example:** QA confirms kidney VMAT field output using phantom.

81. **Oblique Field Phantom QA Meaning:** Phantom QA for verifying oblique radiation fields.
**Related Terms:** IMRT, VMAT, LINAC QA
**Example:** QA tests kidney SBRT oblique field dose distribution.

82. **Online Imaging Dose Mapping Meaning:** QA mapping dose from imaging during treatment.
**Related Terms:** CBCT, KV Imaging, ALARA
**Example:** QA confirms kidney CBCT imaging dose stays within safe limits.

83. **Output Reproducibility QA Meaning:** QA to ensure LINAC output is reproducible over multiple sessions.?
**Related Terms:** MU Verification, Daily QA
**Example:** QA checks kidney IMRT output reproducibility within ±2%.

84. **On-Target Fiducial QA Meaning:** QA verifying fiducials accurately indicate tumor location.
**Related Terms:** IGRT, CBCT, Motion Tracking
**Example:** QA confirms kidney fiducials remain within tumor volume during SBRT.

85. **Orthogonal Beam Alignment QA Meaning:** QA verifying alignment of perpendicular beams.
**Related Terms:** KV Imaging, LINAC, IGRT
**Example:** QA ensures kidney orthogonal IMRT fields are aligned correctly.

86. **OAR Sparing QA Meaning:** QA to ensure organs at risk receive minimal radiation dose.
**Related Terms:** DVH, TPS, IMRT
**Example:** QA verifies kidney SBRT plan spares remaining renal tissue.

87. **Online Image Fusion QA Meaning:** QA for real-time multimodality image registration.
**Related Terms:** CT/MRI, PET/CT, IGRT
**Example:** QA confirms kidney PET/CT fused images align tumor accurately.

88. **Output Factor Phantom QA Meaning:** Phantom QA for verifying output factors for different field sizes.
**Related Terms:** MU Verification, Small Field Dosimetry
**Example:** QA ensures small kidney SBRT field output factors match TPS.

89. **Oblique Image Registration QA Meaning:** QA ensuring accurate registration of oblique images.
**Related Terms:** CBCT, IGRT, Fiducials
**Example:** QA verifies kidney tumor alignment in oblique CBCT images.

90. **On-Target Motion QA Meaning:** QA for verifying tumor motion tracking during treatment.
**Related Terms:** Motion Management, Fiducials, IGRT
**Example:** QA confirms kidney SBRT target remains within PTV during breathing cycles.

91. **Off-Target Monitoring QA Meaning:** QA to track unintended dose outside the target volume.
**Related Terms:** DVH, TPS, IMRT
**Example:** QA monitors liver dose during kidney SBRT delivery.

92. **Online Dose Accumulation QA Meaning:** QA for real-time cumulative dose verification.
**Related Terms:** DVH, TPS, EPID
**Example:** QA accumulates kidney SBRT dose fraction-by-fraction to confirm accuracy.

93. **Oblique Field Dose Verification Meaning:** QA for verifying delivered dose of oblique fields.
**Related Terms:** IMRT, VMAT, LINAC QA
**Example:** QA checks kidney VMAT oblique field dose matches TPS.

94. **Output Consistency Phantom QA Meaning:** Phantom QA for verifying consistent output across multiple fields.
**Related Terms:** MU Verification, LINAC, Daily QA
**Example:** QA confirms kidney IMRT beam output consistency using phantom.

95. **Online Imaging QA Protocol Meaning:** Protocol for routine QA of real-time imaging systems.
**Related Terms:** CBCT, KV Imaging, IGRT
**Example:** QA ensures kidney CBCT images are clear, accurate, and aligned daily.

96. **Off-Axis Phantom QA Meaning:** Phantom QA for off-axis dose verification.
**Related Terms:** Beam Profile, IMRT, LINAC QA
**Example:** QA verifies kidney VMAT off-axis dose accuracy using phantom.

97. **Output Calibration QA Protocol Meaning:** Protocol to ensure accurate LINAC output calibration.
**Related Terms:** MU Verification, TG-51, Dosimetry
**Example:** QA confirms kidney SBRT output calibration aligns with TPS.

98. **Oblique Beam Phantom Meaning:** Phantom used for QA of oblique beam geometry and dose.
**Related Terms:** VMAT, IMRT, LINAC QA
**Example:** QA confirms kidney SBRT oblique field coverage using phantom.

99. **On-Target Alignment QA Meaning:** QA to verify tumor alignment with planned PTV.
**Related Terms:** CBCT, Fiducials, IGRT
**Example:** QA ensures kidney SBRT tumor is aligned to PTV daily.

100. **OAR Dose Verification Phantom Meaning:** Phantom QA to confirm organs at risk dose is within tolerance.
**Related Terms:** DVH, IMRT, TPS
**Example:** QA verifies kidney, liver, and bowel dose using phantom.

101. **Oblique Imaging Phantom QA Meaning:** Phantom used to test image quality and dose accuracy for oblique imaging angles.
**Related Terms:** CBCT, KV Imaging, IGRT
**Example:** QA ensures kidney tumor is correctly visualized in oblique CBCT images.

102. **Offline Dose Reconstruction QA Meaning:** QA to reconstruct delivered dose using treatment logs post-fraction.
**Related Terms:** EPID, Log Files, DVH
**Example:** QA reconstructs kidney SBRT dose after each fraction to confirm accuracy.

103. **On-Target Verification Phantom Meaning:** Phantom QA to verify tumor localization and beam delivery.
**Related Terms:** IGRT, Fiducials, CBCT
**Example:** QA confirms kidney SBRT target alignment using on-target phantom.

104. **Output Linearity QA Meaning:** QA ensuring LINAC output is linear across MU ranges.
**Related Terms:** MU Verification, Dosimetry, Daily QA
**Example:** QA confirms kidney IMRT small and large MU outputs are linear.

105. **Oblique CBCT QA Meaning:** QA for cone-beam CT images acquired at oblique angles.
**Related Terms:** CBCT, IGRT, Fiducials
**Example:** QA checks kidney SBRT oblique CBCT image geometry.

106. **OAR Dose Accumulation Phantom Meaning:** Phantom QA for cumulative dose to organs at risk.
**Related Terms:** DVH, Fractionation, TPS
**Example:** QA ensures kidney dose to healthy tissue is within tolerance using phantom.

107. **Output Verification Protocol Meaning:** Standard protocol to verify LINAC output.
**Related Terms:** MU Verification, TG-51, Dosimetry
**Example:** QA confirms kidney VMAT output aligns with TPS calculations.

108. **Orthogonal Beam Phantom QA Meaning:** Phantom QA for verifying perpendicular beam alignment.
**Related Terms:** IGRT, KV Imaging, LINAC QA
**Example:** QA tests kidney SBRT AP-lateral orthogonal beam setup using phantom.

109. **Online Imaging Dose QA Meaning:** QA for patient dose from imaging during treatment.
**Related Terms:** CBCT, KV Imaging, ALARA
**Example:** QA maps kidney CBCT imaging dose during SBRT to stay below limits.

110. **Oblique Dose Phantom QA Meaning:** Phantom QA to validate dose delivery for oblique beams.
**Related Terms:** IMRT, VMAT, LINAC QA
**Example:** QA verifies kidney SBRT oblique field dose using phantom.

111. **On-Target Fluence QA Meaning:** QA ensuring planned fluence reaches the tumor accurately.
**Related Terms:** EPID, IMRT, VMAT
**Example:** QA measures kidney VMAT fluence with MapCHECK phantom.

112. **Output Constancy QA Meaning:** QA monitoring consistent LINAC output over time.
**Related Terms:** Daily QA, MU Verification, Dosimetry
**Example:** QA ensures kidney IMRT output remains within ±2% daily.

113. **OAR Contour Phantom QA Meaning:** Phantom QA for verifying organ at risk contours.
**Related Terms:** DVH, TPS, IMRT QA
**Example:** QA checks kidney, liver, bowel contours using anthropomorphic phantom.

114. **Off-Axis Output QA Meaning:** QA for dose delivered away from central axis.
**Related Terms:** Beam Profile, LINAC, DVH
**Example:** QA measures kidney IMRT off-axis dose accuracy.

115. **Oblique Beam Dose Verification Protocol Meaning:** Protocol for verifying dose delivered by oblique fields.
**Related Terms:** IMRT, VMAT, LINAC QA
**Example:** QA confirms kidney SBRT oblique beam dose matches TPS.

116. **Online Dose Logging QA Meaning:** QA recording dose delivered in real-time.
**Related Terms:** EPID, DVH, IGRT
**Example:** QA logs kidney VMAT dose per fraction to compare with TPS.

117. **Output Reproducibility Phantom Meaning:** Phantom QA to confirm consistent output across sessions.
**Related Terms:** MU Verification, Daily QA, LINAC
**Example:** QA confirms kidney SBRT VMAT field output reproducibility using phantom.

118. **OAR Dose Limit QA Meaning:** QA verifying maximum allowed dose to organs at risk.
**Related Terms:** DVH, TPS, IMRT
**Example:** QA ensures kidney SBRT dose to contralateral kidney stays below 15 Gy.

119. **Orthovoltage Beam QA Meaning:** QA specific to orthovoltage superficial X-ray beams.
**Related Terms:** SSD, Dosimetry, Superficial Therapy
**Example:** QA verifies kidney superficial field dose matches TPS.

120. **Oblique Field Alignment QA Meaning:** QA verifying accurate alignment of oblique radiation fields.
**Related Terms:** IMRT, VMAT, LINAC QA
**Example:** QA confirms kidney SBRT oblique fields align with PTV.

121. **Online Image Quality QA Meaning:** QA verifying clarity and accuracy of images acquired during treatment.
**Related Terms:** CBCT, KV Imaging, IGRT
**Example:** QA checks kidney SBRT CBCT images for sharpness and contrast.

122. **Output Factor Verification Protocol Meaning:** QA to verify output factors for various field sizes.
**Related Terms:** Small Field Dosimetry, MU Verification
**Example:** QA ensures kidney SBRT small field output factors are accurate.

123. **Oblique Imaging Dose Mapping Meaning:** QA mapping dose delivered during oblique imaging.
**Related Terms:** CBCT, KV Imaging, ALARA
**Example:** QA maps dose to kidney during oblique CBCT imaging.

124. **On-Target Phantom QA Meaning:** Phantom QA for verifying tumor location and beam delivery.
**Related Terms:** IGRT, Fiducials, CBCT
**Example:** QA ensures kidney SBRT tumor is correctly targeted using phantom.

125. **Offline Image Registration QA Meaning:** QA verifying image alignment post-treatment.
**Related Terms:** CBCT, IGRT, Fiducials
**Example:** QA checks kidney CBCT images aligned to planning CT after fraction.

126. **Oblique Beam Flatness QA Meaning:** QA for beam flatness in oblique fields.
**Related Terms:** LINAC, Beam Profile, IMRT
**Example:** QA ensures kidney SBRT oblique fields maintain uniform dose.

127. **Output Drift Monitoring Protocol Meaning:** QA to track long-term output changes.
**Related Terms:** Daily QA, MU Verification, Dosimetry
**Example:** QA monitors kidney IMRT beam output over several months.

128. **OAR Dose Mapping QA Meaning:** QA mapping delivered dose to organs at risk.
**Related Terms:** DVH, TPS, IMRT
**Example:** QA confirms kidney dose to healthy tissue during SBRT is within limits.

129. **Online Imaging Workflow QA Meaning:** QA for ensuring imaging procedures follow standard workflow.
**Related Terms:** CBCT, IGRT, Fiducials
**Example:** QA confirms kidney CBCT imaging steps follow IGRT protocol.

130. **Oblique Field Phantom Verification Meaning:** Phantom QA to verify dose and alignment of oblique fields.
**Related Terms:** IMRT, VMAT, LINAC QA
**Example:** QA confirms kidney SBRT oblique field dose using phantom.

131. **Output Calibration Phantom QA Meaning:** Phantom QA to validate LINAC output calibration.
**Related Terms:** MU Verification, TG-51, Dosimetry
**Example:** QA confirms kidney VMAT output calibration using phantom.

132. **On-Target Fluence Mapping Meaning:** QA mapping delivered fluence to the tumor.
**Related Terms:** EPID, IMRT, VMAT
**Example:** QA maps kidney VMAT fluence to confirm TPS accuracy.

133. **Orthogonal Alignment QA Meaning:** QA ensuring perpendicular beams are correctly aligned.
**Related Terms:** KV Imaging, IGRT, LINAC
**Example:** QA confirms kidney IMRT orthogonal fields match PTV.

134. **Offline Dose QA Meaning:** QA reviewing dose delivery after treatment.
**Related Terms:** EPID, DVH, TPS
**Example:** QA confirms kidney SBRT fraction dose matches plan.

135. **Oblique Dose Mapping Phantom Meaning:** Phantom QA for mapping oblique field dose distribution.
**Related Terms:** IMRT, VMAT, LINAC QA
**Example:** QA maps kidney SBRT oblique field dose using phantom.

136. **Online Dose QA Protocol Meaning:** Protocol for QA of real-time dose verification.
**Related Terms:** EPID, Log Files, DVH
**Example:** QA ensures kidney SBRT dose delivered matches TPS.

137. **Output Constancy Phantom Meaning:** Phantom QA to monitor LINAC output constancy.
**Related Terms:** Daily QA, MU Verification
**Example:** QA checks kidney IMRT beam output consistency using phantom.

138. **Oblique Beam Reproducibility QA Meaning:** QA ensuring oblique beam dose reproducibility.
**Related Terms:** IMRT, VMAT, LINAC QA
**Example:** QA confirms kidney SBRT oblique fields reproduce dose accurately.

139. **OAR Dose Evaluation QA Meaning:** QA to evaluate dose received by organs at risk.
**Related Terms:** DVH, IMRT, TPS
**Example:** QA ensures kidney contralateral dose is below 15 Gy.

140. **Online Image QA Protocol Meaning:** Standard protocol for QA of real-time imaging systems.
**Related Terms:** CBCT, KV Imaging, IGRT
**Example:** QA confirms kidney CBCT image quality and alignment daily.

141. **Oblique Field Dose Reproducibility Phantom Meaning:** Phantom QA to verify dose reproducibility of oblique fields.
**Related Terms:** IMRT, VMAT, LINAC QA
**Example:** QA confirms kidney SBRT oblique fields deliver reproducible dose.

142. **Output Factor Mapping QA Meaning:** QA mapping dose output for various field sizes.
**Related Terms:** Small Field Dosimetry, MU Verification
**Example:** QA maps kidney SBRT small field output factors using phantom.

143. **On-Target Dose Verification Phantom Meaning:** Phantom QA for verifying tumor dose accuracy.
**Related Terms:** EPID, IMRT, VMAT
**Example:** QA confirms kidney SBRT target dose using phantom.

144. **Offline Imaging QA Protocol Meaning:** Protocol for QA of post-treatment imaging.
**Related Terms:** CBCT, KV Imaging, IGRT
**Example:** QA checks kidney CBCT image alignment after treatment.

145. **Oblique Beam Alignment Phantom Meaning:** Phantom QA for oblique beam alignment verification.
**Related Terms:** IMRT, VMAT, LINAC QA
**Example:** QA confirms kidney SBRT oblique field alignment using phantom.

146. **Online Fluence QA Meaning:** QA ensuring delivered fluence matches plan in real-time.
**Related Terms:** EPID, IMRT, VMAT
**Example:** QA measures kidney VMAT fluence using EPID.

147. **Output Uniformity Phantom QA Meaning:** Phantom QA for verifying dose uniformity across beam.
**Related Terms:** Beam Flatness, LINAC QA
**Example:** QA ensures kidney IMRT field uniformity using water phantom.

148. **Oblique CBCT Dose QA Meaning:** QA measuring dose from oblique CBCT imaging.
**Related Terms:** CBCT, ALARA, KV Imaging
**Example:** QA confirms kidney CBCT imaging dose is safe.

149. **On-Target Motion Phantom QA Meaning:** Phantom QA for tumor motion tracking.
**Related Terms:** Fiducials, IGRT, Motion Management
**Example:** QA tests kidney SBRT motion tracking accuracy using phantom.

150. **OAR Dose Accumulation Protocol Meaning:** Protocol to monitor cumulative dose to organs at risk.
**Related Terms:** DVH, IMRT, TPS
**Example:** QA confirms kidney dose to healthy tissue stays below tolerance across fractions.

151. **Output Drift QA Meaning:** QA monitoring long-term variations in LINAC output.
**Related Terms:** Daily QA, MU Verification, Dosimetry
**Example:** QA tracks kidney IMRT beam output over several months to ensure consistency.

152. **Oblique Field Dose Optimization Meaning:** QA ensuring oblique beams deliver optimal dose to the target.
**Related Terms:** IMRT, VMAT, TPS
**Example:** QA confirms kidney SBRT oblique fields achieve PTV coverage while sparing OARs.

153. **Online Imaging Alignment QA Meaning:** QA verifying patient alignment during real-time imaging.
**Related Terms:** CBCT, Fiducials, IGRT
**Example:** QA confirms kidney fiducials align with PTV during SBRT CBCT.

154. **Off-Axis Ratio Verification Meaning:** QA measuring dose distribution away from central axis.
**Related Terms:** Beam Profile, LINAC QA, IMRT
**Example:** QA verifies kidney IMRT off-axis dose matches TPS.

155. **OAR Contour Verification Protocol Meaning:** QA protocol to confirm accuracy of OAR contours.
**Related Terms:** TPS, DVH, IMRT QA
**Example:** QA confirms kidney, liver, and bowel contours are correct on planning CT.

156. **Output Reproducibility QA Meaning:** QA to ensure consistent LINAC output over multiple sessions.
**Related Terms:** Daily QA, MU Verification, EPID
**Example:** QA ensures kidney VMAT output is reproducible daily using phantom.

157. **Oblique Beam Fluence QA Meaning:** QA for delivered fluence in oblique beams.
**Related Terms:** IMRT, VMAT, EPID
**Example:** QA maps kidney SBRT fluence for oblique fields to match TPS.

158. **Online Dose Monitoring Protocol Meaning:** QA procedure for monitoring real-time dose during treatment.
**Related Terms:** EPID, DVH, IGRT
**Example:** QA confirms kidney VMAT dose delivery matches TPS in real time.

159. **Oblique Field Alignment QA Meaning:** QA verifying precise alignment of oblique radiation fields.
**Related Terms:** IMRT, VMAT, LINAC QA
**Example:** QA ensures kidney SBRT oblique fields are correctly positioned relative to PTV.

160. **Output Factor QA Meaning:** QA verifying output factors for different field sizes.
**Related Terms:** Small Field Dosimetry, MU Verification
**Example:** QA ensures kidney SBRT small field output factors match TPS calculations.

161. **Offline Image QA Protocol Meaning:** QA procedure for verifying post-treatment imaging accuracy.
**Related Terms:** CBCT, KV Imaging, IGRT
**Example:** QA checks kidney CBCT images for alignment with planning CT after fraction.

162. **On-Target Motion QA Meaning:** QA to verify tumor tracking and motion compensation.
**Related Terms:** Fiducials, IGRT, Motion Management
**Example:** QA ensures kidney SBRT target motion is accurately tracked with fiducials.

163. **Oblique Dose Verification Phantom Meaning:** Phantom QA for validating oblique beam dose delivery.
**Related Terms:** IMRT, VMAT, LINAC QA
**Example:** QA maps kidney SBRT oblique field dose using phantom.

164. **Online Image Registration QA Meaning:** QA verifying correct registration of real-time images with planning CT.
**Related Terms:** CBCT, Fiducials, IGRT
**Example:** QA confirms kidney CBCT images are properly registered before SBRT delivery.

165. **Output Uniformity QA Meaning:** QA to ensure uniform dose distribution across beam field.
**Related Terms:** Beam Flatness, LINAC QA, Phantom
**Example:** QA checks kidney IMRT fields for uniform dose using water phantom.

166. **Oblique Beam Profile Verification Meaning:** QA measuring beam profile for oblique treatment angles.
**Related Terms:** IMRT, VMAT, LINAC QA
**Example:** QA confirms kidney SBRT oblique beam profiles match TPS.

167. **Online Fluence Mapping QA Meaning:** QA to map delivered fluence in real-time.
**Related Terms:** EPID, IMRT, VMAT
**Example:** QA verifies kidney VMAT fluence matches TPS in real-time.

168. **Output Constancy Phantom QA Meaning:** Phantom QA to monitor long-term consistency of beam output.
**Related Terms:** Daily QA, MU Verification, EPID
**Example:** QA ensures kidney IMRT output remains within tolerance using phantom.

169. **Oblique CBCT Image Quality QA Meaning:** QA ensuring clarity and accuracy of oblique CBCT images.
**Related Terms:** CBCT, KV Imaging, IGRT
**Example:** QA confirms kidney SBRT oblique CBCT images are sharp and artifact-free.

170. **Online Dose Logging QA Meaning:** QA recording and verifying dose delivered per fraction.
**Related Terms:** EPID, DVH, IGRT
**Example:** QA logs kidney VMAT dose per fraction to ensure TPS compliance.

171. **Oblique Field Penumbra QA Meaning:** QA to measure field edge sharpness for oblique beams.
**Related Terms:** IMRT, VMAT, LINAC QA
**Example:** QA confirms kidney SBRT oblique field penumbra within tolerance.

172. **Offline Dose Verification QA Meaning:** QA to verify dose after treatment using logs or phantom measurements.
**Related Terms:** DVH, EPID, TPS
**Example:** QA checks kidney SBRT dose delivered matches planning CT.

173. **Oblique Beam Alignment Protocol Meaning:** QA procedure to confirm correct alignment of oblique beams.
**Related Terms:** IMRT, VMAT, LINAC QA
**Example:** QA ensures kidney SBRT oblique beams are positioned accurately.

174. **Output Reproducibility Protocol Meaning:** QA procedure to ensure reproducible beam output over multiple sessions.
**Related Terms:** Daily QA, MU Verification, Phantom
**Example:** QA ensures kidney IMRT beam output is consistent daily.

175. **Online Imaging Dose Assessment Meaning:** QA mapping dose delivered during real-time imaging.
**Related Terms:** CBCT, KV Imaging, ALARA
**Example:** QA confirms kidney CBCT imaging dose remains below safe limits.

176. **Oblique Beam Flatness Phantom QA Meaning:** Phantom QA for measuring flatness of oblique beams.
**Related Terms:** Beam Profile, LINAC QA, IMRT
**Example:** QA checks kidney SBRT oblique fields for uniformity using phantom.

177. **Offline Registration QA Meaning:** QA verifying alignment of images post-fraction.
**Related Terms:** CBCT, Fiducials, IGRT
**Example:** QA ensures kidney CBCT images are aligned to planning CT after treatment.

178. **Oblique Field Dose Mapping Meaning:** QA mapping dose delivered in oblique beams.
**Related Terms:** IMRT, VMAT, LINAC QA
**Example:** QA maps kidney SBRT oblique beam dose to confirm TPS.

179. **On-Target Phantom Verification Meaning:** Phantom QA for verifying tumor targeting and beam delivery.
**Related Terms:** IGRT, Fiducials, CBCT
**Example:** QA confirms kidney SBRT target alignment using phantom.

180. **Output Linearity Verification Meaning:** QA to ensure linear dose output across different MU settings.
**Related Terms:** MU Verification, TG-51, Daily QA
**Example:** QA confirms kidney IMRT small and large MU outputs are linear.

181. **Oblique Beam Dose Verification QA Meaning:** QA to confirm the dose delivered by oblique beams matches TPS.
**Related Terms:** IMRT, VMAT, EPID
**Example:** QA verifies kidney SBRT oblique beam dose using MapCHECK.

182. **Online Patient Setup QA Meaning:** QA to ensure correct patient positioning during treatment.
**Related Terms:** CBCT, Fiducials, IGRT
**Example:** QA confirms kidney SBRT patient is aligned with planning CT prior to beam-on.

183. **Output Consistency Check Meaning:** QA checking consistency of LINAC output over time.
**Related Terms:** Daily QA, MU Verification, EPID
**Example:** QA confirms kidney IMRT output remains within ±2% tolerance.

184. **Oblique Field Penumbra Measurement Meaning:** QA measuring sharpness and width of field edges for oblique beams.
**Related Terms:** IMRT, VMAT, LINAC QA
**Example:** QA verifies kidney SBRT field edges are sharp and within TPS tolerance.

185. **Offline Fluence QA Meaning:** QA to verify delivered fluence using post-treatment analysis.
**Related Terms:** EPID, MapCHECK, IMRT
**Example:** QA confirms kidney VMAT fluence matches TPS after treatment.

186. **Oblique Beam MLC Verification Meaning:** QA checking MLC positions for oblique beams.
**Related Terms:** IMRT, VMAT, Leaf Position QA
**Example:** QA ensures kidney SBRT MLC leaves match planned positions.

187. **Online Dose Accumulation QA Meaning:** QA to track cumulative dose delivered across multiple fractions.
**Related Terms:** DVH, EPID, IGRT
**Example:** QA ensures kidney SBRT cumulative dose matches treatment plan.

188. **Oblique Field Output Factor QA Meaning:** QA verifying output factors for oblique field sizes.
**Related Terms:** Small Field Dosimetry, MU Verification
**Example:** QA confirms kidney SBRT small oblique field outputs match TPS.

189. **Offline CBCT Image QA Meaning:** QA checking CBCT image quality post-fraction.
**Related Terms:** KV Imaging, IGRT, Artifact QA
**Example:** QA verifies kidney CBCT images have no distortion after treatment.

190. **Oblique Beam Flatness QA Meaning:** QA measuring flatness across oblique beam field.
**Related Terms:** Beam Profile, Phantom QA, LINAC QA
**Example:** QA ensures kidney SBRT oblique field flatness is within tolerance.

191. **Online Registration Verification Meaning:** QA to confirm real-time image registration accuracy.
**Related Terms:** CBCT, Fiducials, IGRT
**Example:** QA aligns kidney CBCT images to planning CT prior to VMAT delivery.

192. **Output Drift Monitoring Meaning:** Continuous QA tracking LINAC output over time.
**Related Terms:** MU Verification, Daily QA, EPID
**Example:** QA monitors kidney IMRT output drift monthly.

193. **Oblique Beam Symmetry QA Meaning:** QA ensuring symmetric dose distribution in oblique fields.
**Related Terms:** Beam Flatness, IMRT QA
**Example:** QA confirms kidney SBRT oblique beam symmetry across PTV.

194. **Offline Motion Analysis QA Meaning:** QA evaluating patient/tumor motion post-treatment.
**Related Terms:** Fiducials, IGRT, CBCT
**Example:** QA analyzes kidney SBRT target motion using CBCT logs.

195. **Oblique Dose Gradient QA Meaning:** QA measuring dose fall-off in oblique fields.
**Related Terms:** IMRT, VMAT, LINAC QA
**Example:** QA ensures kidney SBRT oblique field gradients protect OARs.

196. **Online Verification Phantom Meaning:** Phantom QA for real-time image and dose verification.
**Related Terms:** EPID, IGRT, CBCT
**Example:** QA uses kidney phantom to validate VMAT delivery during treatment.

197. **Output Factor Mapping QA Meaning:** QA mapping output factors for all field sizes.
**Related Terms:** MU Verification, Small Field Dosimetry
**Example:** QA confirms kidney SBRT output factors match TPS predictions.

198. **Oblique Field Registration QA Meaning:** QA verifying proper registration of oblique fields to patient anatomy.
**Related Terms:** IGRT, CBCT, Fiducials
**Example:** QA confirms kidney SBRT oblique fields align with PTV using CBCT.

199. **Offline Dose Mapping Meaning:** QA mapping delivered dose after treatment.
**Related Terms:** DVH, EPID, TPS
**Example:** QA verifies kidney VMAT dose distribution matches plan.

200. **Oblique Beam Verification Protocol Meaning:** QA procedure for all oblique beam checks.
**Related Terms:** IMRT, VMAT, Phantom QA
**Example:** QA protocol confirms kidney SBRT oblique fields match TPS.

201. **Online Motion Tracking QA Meaning:** QA monitoring real-time tumor motion during treatment.
**Related Terms:** Fiducials, IGRT, CBCT
**Example:** QA ensures kidney SBRT fiducials track tumor motion accurately.

202. **Output Reproducibility Assessment Meaning:** QA evaluating consistency of beam output.
**Related Terms:** Daily QA, MU Verification, Phantom
**Example:** QA confirms kidney VMAT output reproducibility weekly.

203. **Oblique Field Dose Analysis Meaning:** QA analyzing delivered dose in oblique fields.
**Related Terms:** IMRT, VMAT, DVH
**Example:** QA confirms kidney SBRT oblique field dose matches TPS predictions.

204. **Offline Phantom QA Meaning:** QA using phantom after treatment to validate dose and imaging.
**Related Terms:** EPID, DVH, LINAC QA
**Example:** QA confirms kidney SBRT dose accuracy using phantom.

205. **Oblique Beam Dose Calibration Meaning:** QA to calibrate dose output for oblique angles.
**Related Terms:** MU Verification, LINAC QA
**Example:** QA calibrates kidney SBRT oblique beam using ion chamber.

206. **Online Image Quality Assessment Meaning:** QA for clarity and accuracy of real-time images.
**Related Terms:** CBCT, KV Imaging, IGRT
**Example:** QA ensures kidney SBRT online images are artifact-free.

207. **Output Stability QA Meaning:** QA measuring output consistency across fractions.
**Related Terms:** MU Verification, Daily QA, Phantom
**Example:** QA monitors kidney VMAT output stability over several weeks.

208. **Oblique Beam Alignment Phantom Meaning:** Phantom used to verify alignment of oblique beams.
**Related Terms:** IMRT, VMAT, LINAC QA
**Example:** QA ensures kidney SBRT oblique beams match planning CT using phantom.

209. **Offline Registration Phantom Meaning:** Phantom QA for verifying image registration post-treatment.
**Related Terms:** CBCT, Fiducials, IGRT
**Example:** QA confirms kidney CBCT post-fraction alignment with phantom.

210. **Oblique Field Output QA Meaning:** QA verifying output for oblique fields.
**Related Terms:** MU Verification, LINAC QA
**Example:** QA confirms kidney SBRT oblique field output matches TPS.

211. **Online Dose QA Checklist Meaning:** Checklist ensuring all aspects of online dose verification are completed.
**Related Terms:** EPID, DVH, IGRT
**Example:** QA confirms kidney VMAT online dose QA is complete before beam-on.

212. **Oblique Beam QA Protocol Meaning:** Standard procedure for QA of oblique beams.
**Related Terms:** IMRT, VMAT, LINAC QA
**Example:** QA protocol ensures kidney SBRT oblique beams are correctly delivered.

213. **Output Calibration Verification Meaning:** QA confirming correct calibration of beam output.
**Related Terms:** MU Verification, TG-51, LINAC QA
**Example:** QA verifies kidney IMRT output calibration using ion chamber.

214. **Oblique Field Fluence Verification Phantom Meaning:** Phantom QA for fluence accuracy in oblique fields.
**Related Terms:** MapCHECK, IMRT, VMAT
**Example:** QA confirms kidney SBRT oblique fluence distribution matches TPS.

215. **Offline Dose Recalculation QA Meaning:** QA recalculating dose from delivered fraction for verification.
**Related Terms:** DVH, EPID, TPS
**Example:** QA recalculates kidney SBRT dose after fraction to ensure TPS accuracy.

216. **Oblique Beam Symmetry Verification Meaning:** QA ensuring beam symmetry in oblique treatment angles.
**Related Terms:** Beam Flatness, IMRT QA
**Example:** QA confirms kidney SBRT oblique beam symmetry matches TPS.

217. **Online Phantom Verification Protocol Meaning:** QA procedure using phantom for real-time verification.
**Related Terms:** EPID, IGRT, CBCT
**Example:** QA protocol confirms kidney SBRT beam delivery and imaging alignment.

218. **Output Mapping QA Meaning:** QA mapping delivered beam output across field sizes.
**Related Terms:** MU Verification, Phantom QA
**Example:** QA maps kidney VMAT output factors to confirm TPS predictions.

219. **Oblique Field Dose Logging Meaning:** Recording delivered dose for oblique beams.
**Related Terms:** DVH, EPID, TPS
**Example:** QA logs kidney SBRT oblique field dose for verification.

220. **Offline Dose Comparison QA Meaning:** QA comparing delivered dose to planned dose post-fraction.
**Related Terms:** DVH, EPID, TPS
**Example:** QA confirms kidney VMAT delivered dose matches TPS.

221. **Oblique Beam Phantom QA Meaning:** Phantom QA specifically for oblique beams.
**Related Terms:** IMRT, VMAT, LINAC QA
**Example:** QA confirms kidney SBRT oblique beam fluence and dose using phantom.

222. **Online Dose Reporting QA Meaning:** QA reporting real-time delivered dose to verify treatment.
**Related Terms:** DVH, EPID, IGRT
**Example:** QA reports kidney VMAT dose for each fraction.

223. **Output Verification Phantom Meaning:** Phantom QA used to verify LINAC output.
**Related Terms:** MU Verification, TG-51, Daily QA
**Example:** QA confirms kidney IMRT output using water phantom.

224. **Oblique Field Penumbra QA Phantom Meaning:** Phantom used to measure penumbra of oblique fields.
**Related Terms:** IMRT, VMAT, LINAC QA
**Example:** QA confirms kidney SBRT oblique field penumbra using phantom.

225. **Offline Imaging QA Protocol Meaning:** QA procedure for verifying imaging post-treatment.
**Related Terms:** CBCT, KV Imaging, Artifact QA
**Example:** QA confirms kidney CBCT image quality post-fraction.

226. **Oblique Beam Dose QA Phantom Meaning:** Phantom QA for dose verification of oblique beams.
**Related Terms:** IMRT, VMAT, LINAC QA
**Example:** QA confirms kidney SBRT oblique dose distribution with phantom.

227. **Online Dose Verification Phantom Meaning:** Phantom used for real-time dose verification.
**Related Terms:** EPID, IGRT, DVH
**Example:** QA ensures kidney VMAT dose delivery matches TPS during treatment.

228. **Output QA Protocol Meaning:** Comprehensive QA procedure for verifying LINAC output.
**Related Terms:** MU Verification, TG-51, Daily QA
**Example:** QA ensures kidney IMRT beam output remains within tolerance.

229. **Oblique Field Alignment QA Phantom Meaning:** Phantom used to verify alignment of oblique fields.
**Related Terms:** IMRT, VMAT, LINAC QA
**Example:** QA confirms kidney SBRT oblique field alignment with phantom.

230. **Offline Fluence Verification QA Meaning:** QA to verify delivered fluence after treatment.
**Related Terms:** EPID, MapCHECK, IMRT
**Example:** QA confirms kidney VMAT oblique fluence matches TPS.

231. **Oblique Beam Output Verification Meaning:** QA confirming output of oblique beams matches plan.
**Related Terms:** MU Verification, IMRT, VMAT
**Example:** QA ensures kidney SBRT oblique field output matches TPS.

232. **Online Fluence QA Phantom Meaning:** Phantom for real-time verification of fluence delivery.
**Related Terms:** EPID, IMRT, VMAT
**Example:** QA confirms kidney VMAT fluence matches TPS during treatment.

233. **Output Linearity QA Phantom Meaning:** Phantom QA to verify linear output across MU range.
**Related Terms:** MU Verification, TG-51
**Example:** QA ensures kidney IMRT output linearity across low and high MU settings.

234. **Oblique Field QA Checklist Meaning:** QA checklist for oblique beam verification.
**Related Terms:** IMRT, VMAT, LINAC QA
**Example:** QA confirms kidney SBRT oblique fields meet all QA criteria.

235. **Offline Dose Verification Phantom Meaning:** Phantom QA to confirm dose delivery post-treatment.
**Related Terms:** DVH, EPID, TPS
**Example:** QA confirms kidney VMAT dose matches plan using phantom.

236. **Oblique Beam Dose Recalculation QA Meaning:** QA recalculating delivered dose for oblique beams.
**Related Terms:** DVH, TPS, IMRT QA
**Example:** QA recalculates kidney SBRT oblique field dose for verification.

237. **Online Dose QA Protocol Meaning:** QA procedure for verifying real-time dose.
**Related Terms:** EPID, DVH, IGRT
**Example:** QA ensures kidney VMAT online dose verification is completed before delivery.

238. **Oblique Beam Dose Mapping Phantom Meaning:** Phantom used to map dose for oblique beams.
**Related Terms:** IMRT, VMAT, LINAC QA
**Example:** QA confirms kidney SBRT oblique dose distribution using phantom.

239. **Output QA Phantom Meaning:** Phantom QA to verify LINAC beam output.
**Related Terms:** MU Verification, Daily QA, TG-51
**Example:** QA confirms kidney IMRT output is within tolerance using phantom.

240. **Oblique Field Symmetry QA Phantom Meaning:** Phantom to verify dose symmetry in oblique fields.
**Related Terms:** Beam Flatness, IMRT QA, VMAT QA
**Example:** QA confirms kidney SBRT oblique field symmetry using phantom.

241. **Offline Dose QA Protocol Meaning:** QA procedure for post-treatment dose verification.
**Related Terms:** DVH, EPID, TPS
**Example:** QA confirms kidney VMAT delivered dose matches plan.

242. **Oblique Beam Fluence Mapping Meaning:** QA mapping fluence of oblique beams.
**Related Terms:** IMRT, VMAT, EPID
**Example:** QA verifies kidney SBRT oblique fluence matches TPS.

243. **Online Beam Alignment QA Meaning:** QA verifying real-time beam alignment.
**Related Terms:** EPID, IGRT, Fiducials
**Example:** QA confirms kidney VMAT beam is correctly aligned to PTV during treatment.

244. **Oblique Field Output Mapping QA Meaning:** QA mapping output across oblique field sizes.
**Related Terms:** MU Verification, IMRT QA, VMAT QA
**Example:** QA ensures kidney SBRT oblique output factors match TPS.

245. **Offline Phantom Dose QA Meaning:** Phantom QA for verifying dose post-treatment.
**Related Terms:** EPID, DVH, IMRT QA
**Example:** QA confirms kidney SBRT dose using phantom analysis.

246. **Oblique Beam Flatness Verification Phantom Meaning:** Phantom QA to confirm flatness of oblique beams.
**Related Terms:** Beam Profile, LINAC QA, IMRT QA
**Example:** QA checks kidney SBRT oblique beam flatness using water phantom.

247. **Online Imaging Dose Logging Meaning:** QA recording delivered dose from imaging during treatment.
**Related Terms:** CBCT, KV Imaging, ALARA**Example:** QA logs kidney CBCT dose during SBRT fraction.

248. **Oblique Field QA Phantom Meaning:** Phantom QA for comprehensive oblique field verification.
**Related Terms:** IMRT, VMAT, LINAC QA
**Example:** QA confirms kidney SBRT oblique field alignment, output, and dose using phantom.

249. **Output Verification QA Protocol Meaning:** QA procedure to verify beam output across energies and fields.
**Related Terms:** MU Verification, Daily QA, TG-51
**Example:** QA confirms kidney IMRT output across multiple field sizes.

250. **Oblique Beam Dose QA Protocol Meaning:** Standard QA procedure for oblique beam dose verification.
**Related Terms:** IMRT, VMAT, LINAC QA, EPID
**Example:** QA ensures kidney SBRT oblique beam dose matches TPS predictions.

251. **Oblique Beam MLC QA Protocol Meaning:** QA procedure to verify MLC positions for oblique beams.
**Related Terms:** IMRT, VMAT, Leaf Position QA
**Example:** QA ensures kidney SBRT MLC leaves are positioned accurately.

252. **Online Fiducial QA Meaning:** QA verifying real-time visibility and tracking of fiducial markers.
**Related Terms:** IGRT, CBCT, Marker Tracking
**Example:** QA confirms kidney SBRT fiducials are tracked accurately during treatment.

253. **Output Calibration QA Phantom Meaning:** Phantom used to verify output calibration of LINAC beams.
**Related Terms:** TG-51, MU Verification, Daily QA
**Example:** QA confirms kidney IMRT output calibration using water phantom.

254. **Oblique Field Dose Uniformity QA Meaning:** QA ensuring uniform dose distribution in oblique fields.
**Related Terms:** IMRT, VMAT, Beam Flatness
**Example:** QA verifies kidney SBRT oblique field dose uniformity using phantom.

255. **Offline MLC Position Verification Meaning:** QA checking MLC leaf positions after treatment.
**Related Terms:** IMRT, VMAT, EPID
**Example:** QA confirms kidney VMAT MLC positions match planned TPS positions.

256. **Oblique Beam Profile QA Meaning:** QA measuring dose distribution across oblique beam profile.
**Related Terms:** LINAC QA, IMRT, VMAT
**Example:** QA confirms kidney SBRT oblique beam profile matches TPS.

257. **Online Dose Accumulation Verification Meaning:** QA ensuring cumulative dose delivered matches plan in real-time.
**Related Terms:** DVH, EPID, IGRT
**Example:** QA confirms kidney VMAT accumulated dose aligns with plan.

258. **Oblique Field Flatness Measurement Meaning:** QA measuring flatness of radiation dose across oblique fields.
**Related Terms:** Beam Profile, IMRT, Phantom QA
**Example:** QA ensures kidney SBRT oblique beam flatness is within tolerance.

259. **Offline Dose Gradient QA Meaning:** QA measuring dose fall-off across the treatment field.
**Related Terms:** DVH, IMRT, VMAT
**Example:** QA confirms kidney SBRT oblique field gradients protect organs at risk.

260. **Oblique Beam Dose Logging Meaning:** QA recording delivered dose of oblique beams for verification.
**Related Terms:** DVH, EPID, IMRT QA
**Example:** QA logs kidney SBRT oblique beam dose for review.

261. **Online Dose Mapping QA Meaning:** QA mapping real-time dose delivery to ensure plan accuracy.
**Related Terms:** DVH, EPID, IGRT
**Example:** QA confirms kidney VMAT dose distribution during treatment.

262. **Oblique Field Dose QA Phantom Meaning:** Phantom used to verify oblique field dose distribution.
**Related Terms:** IMRT, VMAT, LINAC QA
**Example:** QA ensures kidney SBRT oblique dose distribution matches TPS using phantom.

263. **Output Verification Phantom QA Meaning:** Phantom QA to verify LINAC output across all energies.
**Related Terms:** TG-51, MU Verification, Daily QA
**Example:** QA confirms kidney IMRT output using water phantom.

264. **Oblique Beam Dose Verification Protocol Meaning:** QA procedure ensuring accurate oblique beam dose delivery.
**Related Terms:** IMRT, VMAT, LINAC QA
**Example:** QA ensures kidney SBRT oblique beam dose matches TPS.

265. **Offline Fluence Analysis QA Meaning:** QA evaluating delivered fluence patterns after treatment.
**Related Terms:** EPID, MapCHECK, IMRT
**Example:** QA confirms kidney VMAT fluence accuracy post-treatment.

266. **Oblique Field Symmetry Verification Meaning:** QA ensuring symmetric dose distribution in oblique fields.
**Related Terms:** Beam Flatness, IMRT, VMAT
**Example:** QA confirms kidney SBRT oblique beam symmetry across PTV.

267. **Online Beam Flatness QA Meaning:** QA measuring beam flatness in real-time.
**Related Terms:** EPID, IGRT, LINAC QA
**Example:** QA ensures kidney VMAT beam flatness meets TPS specifications.

268. **Oblique Beam Penumbra QA Meaning:** QA measuring beam edge sharpness for oblique angles.
**Related Terms:** IMRT, VMAT, LINAC QA
**Example:** QA confirms kidney SBRT oblique field penumbra is within tolerance.

269. **Offline Image Registration QA Meaning:** QA verifying post-treatment image registration accuracy.
**Related Terms:** CBCT, Fiducials, IGRT
**Example:** QA confirms kidney CBCT post-fraction alignment with planning CT.

270. **Oblique Field Dose Recalculation QA Meaning:** QA recalculating dose for oblique fields to verify delivery.
**Related Terms:** DVH, IMRT, VMAT
**Example:** QA recalculates kidney SBRT oblique dose to ensure accuracy.

271. **Online Fluence Verification QA Meaning:** QA verifying delivered fluence in real-time.
**Related Terms:** EPID, IGRT, MapCHECK
**Example:** QA confirms kidney VMAT fluence matches TPS during treatment.

272. **Oblique Beam Alignment QA Meaning:** QA ensuring oblique beams are aligned with patient anatomy.
**Related Terms:** IGRT, CBCT, Fiducials
**Example:** QA ensures kidney SBRT oblique beams align with PTV.

273. **Offline Dose Logging QA Meaning:** QA documenting dose delivered for each fraction post-treatment.
**Related Terms:** DVH, EPID, TPS
**Example:** QA logs kidney VMAT delivered dose for verification.

274. **Oblique Field QA Checklist Protocol Meaning:** QA checklist for verifying oblique field delivery.
**Related Terms:** IMRT, VMAT, LINAC QA
**Example:** QA confirms kidney SBRT oblique fields meet all QA requirements.

275. **Output Reproducibility QA Meaning:** QA ensuring consistent LINAC output across multiple fractions.
**Related Terms:** MU Verification, TG-51, Daily QA
**Example:** QA confirms kidney IMRT output reproducibility weekly.

276. **Oblique Beam Fluence QA Phantom Meaning:** Phantom used to verify fluence in oblique beams.
**Related Terms:** IMRT, VMAT, EPID
**Example:** QA confirms kidney SBRT oblique fluence matches TPS.

277. **Online Dose Accumulation QA Protocol Meaning:** QA procedure for monitoring cumulative dose in real-time.
**Related Terms:** DVH, EPID, IGRT
**Example:** QA ensures kidney VMAT cumulative dose matches TPS plan.

278. **Oblique Field Output QA Meaning:** QA verifying output of oblique fields.
**Related Terms:** MU Verification, LINAC QA
**Example:** QA confirms kidney SBRT oblique field output matches plan.

279. **Offline Beam Profile QA Meaning:** QA checking beam profile accuracy post-treatment.
**Related Terms:** LINAC QA, IMRT, VMAT
**Example:** QA ensures kidney VMAT beam profile matches TPS.

280. **Oblique Beam Dose Mapping QA Meaning:** QA mapping dose delivered by oblique beams.
**Related Terms:** DVH, IMRT, VMAT
**Example:** QA confirms kidney SBRT oblique field dose distribution matches TPS.

281. **Online Beam Alignment Verification Meaning:** QA confirming real-time beam alignment with patient anatomy.
**Related Terms:** IGRT, EPID, Fiducials
**Example:** QA ensures kidney VMAT beam is aligned during delivery.

282. **Oblique Field Dose Logging Phantom Meaning:** Phantom QA recording dose delivery for oblique fields.
**Related Terms:** IMRT, VMAT, DVH
**Example:** QA confirms kidney SBRT oblique dose using phantom logs.

283. **Offline Fluence Mapping QA Meaning:** QA mapping fluence post-treatment for verification.
**Related Terms:** EPID, MapCHECK, IMRT?
**Example:** QA ensures kidney VMAT fluence matches TPS after fraction.

284. **Oblique Beam Dose Verification Phantom Meaning:** Phantom QA for verifying oblique beam dose.
**Related Terms:** IMRT, VMAT, LINAC QA
**Example:** QA confirms kidney SBRT oblique dose distribution matches TPS.

285. **Online Dose Verification Protocol Meaning:** QA procedure to verify real-time dose delivery.
**Related Terms:** EPID, DVH, IGRT
**Example:** QA ensures kidney VMAT dose verification is completed prior to beam-on.

286. **Oblique Field Dose QA Protocol Meaning:** Standard QA procedure for oblique field verification.
**Related Terms:** IMRT, VMAT, LINAC QA
**Example:** QA ensures kidney SBRT oblique field dose matches TPS.

287. **Output QA Verification Phantom Meaning:** Phantom QA confirming LINAC output verification.
**Related Terms:** TG-51, MU Verification, Daily QA
**Example:** QA confirms kidney IMRT output using verification phantom.

288. **Oblique Beam Symmetry QA Protocol Meaning:** QA procedure for verifying oblique beam symmetry.
**Related Terms:** Beam Flatness, IMRT, VMAT
**Example:** QA confirms kidney SBRT oblique beam symmetry matches plan.

289. **Offline Dose Comparison Protocol Meaning:** QA comparing delivered dose to planned dose post-treatment.
**Related Terms:** DVH, EPID, TPS
**Example:** QA ensures kidney VMAT delivered dose aligns with TPS.

290. **Oblique Field Output Mapping Phantom Meaning:** Phantom used to map output for oblique fields.
**Related Terms:** MU Verification, IMRT QA, VMAT QA
**Example:** QA confirms kidney SBRT oblique output matches TPS.

291. **Online Fluence QA Protocol Meaning:** QA procedure for real-time fluence verification.
**Related Terms:** EPID, MapCHECK, IGRT
**Example:** QA ensures kidney VMAT fluence delivery matches TPS.

292. **Oblique Beam Dose Logging QA Meaning:** QA recording delivered dose of oblique beams.
**Related Terms:** DVH, EPID, IMRT QA
**Example:** QA logs kidney SBRT oblique beam dose for verification.

293. **Offline Beam Alignment QA Meaning:** QA verifying beam alignment after treatment.
**Related Terms:** IGRT, CBCT, Fiducials
**Example:** QA confirms kidney SBRT beam alignment post-fraction.

294. **Oblique Field Dose Gradient Phantom Meaning:** Phantom used to measure dose gradient for oblique fields.
**Related Terms:** IMRT, VMAT, LINAC QA
**Example:** QA confirms kidney SBRT oblique field gradients protect OARs.

295. **Online Beam Output Verification Meaning:** QA confirming real-time LINAC output accuracy.
**Related Terms:** MU Verification, EPID, IGRT
**Example:** QA ensures kidney VMAT output matches TPS during delivery.

296. **Oblique Beam Dose QA Checklist Meaning:** QA checklist for verifying oblique beam dose delivery.
**Related Terms:** IMRT, VMAT, LINAC QA
**Example:** QA confirms kidney SBRT oblique beams meet all QA criteria.

297. **Offline Dose Recalculation Protocol Meaning:** QA procedure recalculating delivered dose post-treatment.
**Related Terms:** DVH, TPS, IMRT QA
**Example:** QA recalculates kidney VMAT dose to confirm plan accuracy.

298. **Oblique Field Fluence Mapping QA Meaning:** QA mapping fluence for oblique fields.
**Related Terms:** EPID, MapCHECK, IMRT QA
**Example:** QA confirms kidney SBRT oblique fluence matches TPS.

299. **Online Dose Reporting Protocol Meaning:** QA procedure reporting real-time delivered dose.
**Related Terms:** DVH, EPID, IGRT
**Example:** QA reports kidney VMAT dose for each fraction.

300. **Oblique Beam Output Mapping QA Meaning:** QA mapping delivered output across oblique beams.
**Related Terms:** MU Verification, LINAC QA, IMRT QA
**Example:** QA confirms kidney SBRT oblique field output matches TPS.

301. **Online Beam Profile QA Meaning:** QA procedure to verify beam profile in real-time.
**Related Terms:** LINAC QA, EPID, IMRT QA
**Example:** QA ensures kidney VMAT beam profile matches TPS during delivery.

302. **Oblique Field Dose Logging QA Protocol Meaning:** QA procedure for recording dose delivered by oblique fields.
**Related Terms:** DVH, EPID, IMRT QA
**Example:** QA logs kidney SBRT oblique beam dose for verification.

303. **Offline Fluence Verification Phantom Meaning:** Phantom QA to verify delivered fluence after treatment.
**Related Terms:** MapCHECK, EPID, IMRT QA
**Example:** QA confirms kidney VMAT fluence matches TPS post-treatment.

304. **Oblique Beam Dose Gradient QA Meaning:** QA measuring dose gradient for oblique beams to protect OARs.
**Related Terms:** DVH, IMRT, VMAT
**Example:** QA confirms kidney SBRT oblique field gradient is within tolerance.

305. **Online Dose Accumulation Phantom QA Meaning:** Phantom QA to monitor cumulative dose in real-time.
**Related Terms:** DVH, EPID, IGRT
**Example:** QA confirms kidney VMAT cumulative dose matches TPS using phantom.

306. **Oblique Field Output Verification Protocol Meaning:** QA procedure to verify output of oblique fields.
**Related Terms:** MU Verification, LINAC QA
**Example:** QA confirms kidney SBRT oblique field output matches TPS.

307. **Offline Beam Penumbra QA Meaning:** QA measuring sharpness of beam edges post-treatment.
**Related Terms:** IMRT, VMAT, LINAC QA
**Example:** QA ensures kidney SBRT beam penumbra matches planned value.

308. **Oblique Beam Symmetry QA Phantom Meaning:** Phantom QA to measure symmetry of oblique beams.
**Related Terms:** Beam Flatness, IMRT, VMAT
**Example:** QA confirms kidney SBRT oblique beam symmetry using phantom.

309. **Online Fluence Logging QA Meaning:** QA recording real-time fluence delivery for verification.
**Related Terms:** EPID, MapCHECK, IGRT
**Example:** QA logs kidney VMAT fluence delivery in real-time.

310. **Oblique Field Dose Verification Checklist Meaning:** QA checklist to verify dose delivery of oblique fields.
**Related Terms:** IMRT, VMAT, LINAC QA
**Example:** QA ensures kidney SBRT oblique fields meet all QA criteria.

311. **Offline Dose Accumulation Verification Meaning:** QA comparing cumulative delivered dose to planned dose.
**Related Terms:** DVH, TPS, IMRT QA
**Example:** QA confirms kidney VMAT accumulated dose aligns with TPS.

312. **Oblique Beam Flatness Phantom QA Meaning:** Phantom QA to measure beam flatness of oblique beams.
**Related Terms:** IMRT, VMAT, LINAC QA
**Example:** QA ensures kidney SBRT oblique beam flatness is uniform using phantom.

313. **Online Dose Gradient Verification Meaning:** QA to verify dose fall-off across the field in real-time.
**Related Terms:** DVH, IMRT, VMAT
**Example:** QA ensures kidney SBRT dose gradient protects adjacent organs.

314. **Oblique Field Dose Recalculation Phantom Meaning:** Phantom QA to recalculate dose for oblique fields.
**Related Terms:** DVH, IMRT, VMAT
**Example:** QA confirms kidney SBRT oblique field dose matches TPS.

315. **Offline Beam Alignment Phantom Meaning:** Phantom QA to check beam alignment post-treatment.
**Related Terms:** IGRT, CBCT, Fiducials
**Example:** QA verifies kidney SBRT beam alignment using phantom.

316. **Oblique Beam Dose Reporting QA Meaning:** QA procedure for documenting delivered oblique beam dose.
**Related Terms:** DVH, EPID, IMRT QA
**Example:** QA reports kidney SBRT oblique beam dose for each fraction.

317. **Online Output Mapping QA Meaning:** QA to map LINAC output across field in real-time.
**Related Terms:** MU Verification, EPID, IGRT
**Example:** QA ensures kidney VMAT output distribution matches TPS.

318. **Oblique Field Fluence Phantom QA Meaning:** Phantom used to verify fluence delivery in oblique fields.
**Related Terms:** IMRT, VMAT, EPID
**Example:** QA confirms kidney SBRT oblique fluence using phantom.

319. **Offline Dose Logging Phantom Meaning:** Phantom QA for recording dose delivered in each fraction.
**Related Terms:** DVH, EPID, IMRT QA
**Example:** QA logs kidney VMAT fraction dose using phantom.

320. **Oblique Beam Dose Verification QA Protocol Meaning:** QA procedure to verify dose delivery of oblique beams.
**Related Terms:** IMRT, VMAT, LINAC QA
**Example:** QA confirms kidney SBRT oblique beam dose matches TPS.

321. **Online Beam Output Phantom QA Meaning:** Phantom QA to verify LINAC output in real-time.
**Related Terms:** MU Verification, EPID, IGRT
**Example:** QA ensures kidney VMAT beam output using phantom verification.

322. **Oblique Field Symmetry Phantom Verification Meaning:** Phantom QA to verify left-right symmetry in oblique fields.
**Related Terms:** Beam Flatness, IMRT, VMAT
**Example:** QA confirms kidney SBRT oblique beam symmetry using phantom.

323. **Offline Fluence Mapping Phantom Meaning:** Phantom QA to map fluence post-treatment.
**Related Terms:** EPID, MapCHECK, IMRT QA
**Example:** QA confirms kidney VMAT delivered fluence using phantom.

324. **Oblique Beam Output QA Checklist Meaning:** QA checklist for verifying output of oblique beams.
**Related Terms:** MU Verification, LINAC QA
**Example:** QA ensures kidney SBRT oblique beam output meets plan.

325. **Online Dose Mapping Phantom Meaning:** Phantom QA to verify real-time dose mapping.
**Related Terms:** DVH, EPID, IGRT
**Example:** QA confirms kidney VMAT dose mapping using phantom.

326. **Oblique Field Dose Gradient Verification Phantom Meaning:** Phantom QA for verifying dose fall-off of oblique fields.
**Related Terms:** DVH, IMRT, VMAT
**Example:** QA ensures kidney SBRT dose gradient meets tolerance.

327. **Offline Beam Flatness Verification Meaning:** QA to check beam flatness post-treatment.
**Related Terms:** IMRT, VMAT, LINAC QA
**Example:** QA ensures kidney VMAT beam flatness matches TPS.

328. **Oblique Beam Dose Logging Phantom Meaning:** Phantom QA to record dose delivered by oblique beams.
**Related Terms:** DVH, EPID, IMRT QA
**Example:** QA logs kidney SBRT oblique beam dose using phantom.

329. **Online Fluence Recalculation QA Meaning:** QA recalculating fluence in real-time to verify delivery.
**Related Terms:** EPID, MapCHECK, IGRT
**Example:** QA confirms kidney VMAT delivered fluence matches TPS.

330. **Oblique Field Dose Recalculation Verification Meaning:** QA verifying recalculated dose of oblique fields post-treatment.
**Related Terms:** DVH, IMRT, VMAT
**Example:** QA confirms kidney SBRT oblique dose accuracy.

331. **Offline Beam Output QA**
**Meaning:** QA checking LINAC output after treatment.
**Related Terms:** MU Verification, TG-51, IMRT QA
**Example:** QA confirms kidney VMAT output matches plan.

332. **Oblique Beam Dose Phantom QA Meaning:** Phantom QA to verify dose delivered by oblique beams.
**Related Terms:** IMRT, VMAT, LINAC QA
**Example:** QA ensures kidney SBRT oblique beam dose using phantom.

333. **Online Dose Gradient Phantom QA Meaning:** Phantom QA measuring dose gradient in real-time.
**Related Terms:** DVH, IMRT, VMAT
**Example:** QA confirms kidney VMAT dose gradient using phantom.

334. **Oblique Field Fluence Logging QA Meaning:** QA recording fluence delivered in oblique fields.
**Related Terms:** EPID, MapCHECK, IMRT QA
**Example:** QA logs kidney SBRT oblique fluence.

335. **Offline Dose Verification Checklist Meaning:** QA checklist verifying delivered dose after treatment.
**Related Terms:** DVH, EPID, TPS
**Example:** QA confirms kidney VMAT delivered dose matches TPS.

336. **Oblique Beam Output Mapping Phantom Meaning:** Phantom QA mapping output across oblique beams.
**Related Terms:** MU Verification, LINAC QA, IMRT QA
**Example:** QA confirms kidney SBRT oblique output using phantom.

337. **Online Dose Logging QA Phantom Meaning:** Phantom QA for real-time dose logging.
**Related Terms:** DVH, EPID, IGRT
**Example:** QA logs kidney VMAT dose delivery using phantom.

338. **Oblique Field Symmetry Logging QA Meaning:** QA recording symmetry of oblique fields.
**Related Terms:** Beam Flatness, IMRT, VMAT
**Example:** QA logs kidney SBRT oblique beam symmetry.

339. **Offline Fluence Output Verification Meaning:** QA verifying fluence output post-treatment.
**Related Terms:** EPID, MapCHECK, IMRT QA
**Example:** QA ensures kidney VMAT delivered fluence matches TPS.

340. **Oblique Beam Dose Recalculation QA Phantom Meaning:** Phantom QA to recalculate oblique beam dose.
**Related Terms:** DVH, IMRT, VMAT
**Example:** QA confirms kidney SBRT oblique dose using phantom.

341. **Online Beam Penumbra QA Phantom Meaning:** Phantom QA to verify beam edge sharpness in real-time.
**Related Terms:** IMRT, VMAT, LINAC QA
**Example:** QA ensures kidney VMAT beam penumbra is within tolerance.

342. **Oblique Field Dose Mapping QA Phantom Meaning:** Phantom QA mapping dose delivered by oblique fields.
**Related Terms:** DVH, IMRT, VMAT
**Example:** QA confirms kidney SBRT oblique field dose distribution using phantom.

343. **Offline Dose Gradient Logging QA Meaning:** QA recording dose gradient post-treatment.
**Related Terms:** DVH, IMRT, VMAT
**Example:** QA logs kidney VMAT dose gradient for verification.

344. **Oblique Beam Output Logging QA Meaning:** QA recording output of oblique beams.
**Related Terms:** MU Verification, LINAC QA, IMRT QA
**Example:** QA logs kidney SBRT oblique output using EPID.

345. **Online Dose Mapping QA Protocol Meaning:** QA procedure to map delivered dose in real-time.
**Related Terms:** DVH, EPID, IGRT
**Example:** QA ensures kidney VMAT dose mapping matches TPS.

346. **Oblique Field Dose Gradient Logging Phantom Meaning:** Phantom QA to log dose gradient of oblique fields.
**Related Terms:** DVH, IMRT, VMAT
**Example:** QA confirms kidney SBRT oblique field gradient using phantom.

347. **Offline Fluence Mapping QA Protocol Meaning:** QA procedure mapping fluence after treatment.
**Related Terms:** EPID, MapCHECK, IMRT QA
**Example:** QA confirms kidney VMAT delivered fluence post-treatment.

348. **Oblique Beam Dose Logging Protocol Meaning:** QA procedure for recording delivered oblique beam dose.
**Related Terms:** DVH, EPID, IMRT QA
**Example:** QA logs kidney SBRT oblique dose for fraction verification.

349. **Online Beam Output Logging QA Phantom Meaning:** Phantom QA for real-time LINAC output logging.
**Related Terms:** MU Verification, EPID, IGRT
**Example:** QA logs kidney VMAT beam output using phantom.

350. **Oblique Field Dose Mapping QA Protocol Meaning:** QA procedure for mapping delivered dose of oblique fields.
**Related Terms:** DVH, IMRT, VMAT **Example:** QA confirms kidney SBRT oblique dose distribution matches TPS.

351. **Online Field Aperture Verification Meaning:** QA to ensure MLC and jaw apertures match the planned field in real-time.
**Related Terms:** IMRT, VMAT, LINAC QA
**Example:** QA confirms kidney SBRT MLC leaf positions during treatment.

352. **Oblique Beam Alignment QA Protocol Meaning:** QA procedure to check alignment of oblique beams.
**Related Terms:** EPID, CBCT, IGRT
**Example:** QA ensures kidney SBRT oblique beam alignment matches TPS.

353. **Offline Dose Accumulation Logging Phantom Meaning:** Phantom QA for recording cumulative dose post-treatment.
**Related Terms:** DVH, EPID, IMRT QA
**Example:** QA logs kidney VMAT accumulated dose using phantom.

354. **Oblique Field Flatness Verification Meaning:** QA checking flatness of oblique fields post-treatment.
**Related Terms:** IMRT, VMAT, Beam Profile QA
**Example:** QA ensures kidney SBRT oblique field flatness matches TPS.

355. **Online Fiducial Tracking QA Meaning:** QA for real-time tracking of fiducial markers during treatment.
**Related Terms:** IGRT, CBCT, Fluoroscopy QA
**Example:** QA confirms kidney SBRT fiducials are accurately tracked.

356. **Oblique Beam Output Phantom QA Meaning:** Phantom QA for measuring output of oblique beams.
**Related Terms:** MU Verification, EPID, IMRT QA
**Example:** QA ensures kidney SBRT oblique beam output using phantom.

357. **Offline Fluence Logging Protocol Meaning:** QA procedure for post-treatment recording of fluence.
**Related Terms:** EPID, MapCHECK, IMRT QA
**Example:** QA logs kidney VMAT fluence after treatment.

358. **Oblique Field Dose Verification Checklist Meaning:** QA checklist to verify dose delivery for oblique fields.
**Related Terms:** IMRT, VMAT, LINAC QA
**Example:** QA confirms kidney SBRT oblique fields meet all QA criteria.

359. **Online Beam Profile Logging Meaning:** QA procedure to record beam profile in real-time.
**Related Terms:** EPID, IMRT QA, VMAT
**Example:** QA ensures kidney VMAT beam profile matches TPS during delivery.

360. **Oblique Beam Symmetry Logging Phantom Meaning:** Phantom QA for recording left-right symmetry in oblique beams.
**Related Terms:** Beam Flatness, IMRT, VMAT
**Example:** QA logs kidney SBRT oblique beam symmetry using phantom.

361. **Offline Dose Gradient Logging Phantom Meaning:** Phantom QA to record dose gradient after treatment.
**Related Terms:** DVH, IMRT, VMAT
**Example:** QA logs kidney VMAT dose gradient using phantom.

362. **Oblique Field Output Verification Phantom Meaning:** Phantom QA to measure output of oblique fields.
**Related Terms:** MU Verification, LINAC QA
**Example:** QA ensures kidney SBRT oblique field output using phantom.

363. **Online Fluence Mapping QA Phantom Meaning:** Phantom QA for real-time fluence mapping.
**Related Terms:** EPID, MapCHECK, IMRT QA
**Example:** QA confirms kidney VMAT fluence delivery using phantom.

364. **Oblique Beam Dose Logging QA Phantom Meaning:** Phantom QA for recording delivered oblique beam dose.
**Related Terms:** DVH, EPID, IMRT QA
**Example:** QA logs kidney SBRT oblique beam dose using phantom.

365. **Offline Beam Profile Logging Meaning:** QA for recording LINAC beam profile post-treatment.
**Related Terms:** IMRT, VMAT, LINAC QA
**Example:** QA logs kidney VMAT beam profile using film or phantom.

366. **Oblique Field Dose Mapping QA Protocol Meaning:** QA procedure for mapping dose of oblique fields.
**Related Terms:** DVH, IMRT, VMAT
**Example:** QA confirms kidney SBRT oblique dose distribution matches TPS.

367. **Online Dose Logging QA Protocol Meaning:** QA procedure for real-time dose recording.
**Related Terms:** DVH, EPID, IGRT
**Example:** QA ensures kidney VMAT dose logging matches TPS in real-time.

368. **Oblique Beam Flatness Logging Phantom Meaning:** Phantom QA for recording flatness of oblique beams.
**Related Terms:** IMRT, VMAT, Beam Profile QA
**Example:** QA logs kidney SBRT oblique beam flatness using phantom.

369. **Offline Fluence Output Logging Meaning:** QA procedure to record fluence output after treatment.
**Related Terms:** EPID, MapCHECK, IMRT QA
**Example:** QA logs kidney VMAT delivered fluence post-treatment.

370. **Oblique Field Dose Accumulation Phantom Meaning:** Phantom QA to track cumulative dose for oblique fields.
**Related Terms:** DVH, IMRT, VMAT
**Example:** QA confirms kidney SBRT oblique field cumulative dose using phantom.

371. **Online Beam Symmetry QA Meaning:** QA procedure for real-time beam symmetry verification.
**Related Terms:** IMRT, VMAT, LINAC QA
**Example:** QA ensures kidney VMAT beam symmetry during treatment delivery.

372. **Oblique Beam Dose Recalculation Logging Phantom Meaning:** Phantom QA for recalculated dose logging in oblique beams.
**Related Terms:** DVH, IMRT, VMAT
**Example:** QA confirms kidney SBRT oblique dose using phantom logging.

373. **Offline Dose Mapping Phantom Meaning:** Phantom QA for post-treatment dose mapping.
**Related Terms:** DVH, EPID, IMRT QA
**Example:** QA maps kidney VMAT delivered dose using phantom.

374. **Oblique Field Output Logging QA Meaning:** QA procedure for recording output of oblique fields.
**Related Terms:** MU Verification, LINAC QA
**Example:** QA logs kidney SBRT oblique field output using EPID.

375. **Online Fluence Recalculation Phantom Meaning:** Phantom QA for real-time recalculation of fluence.
**Related Terms:** EPID, MapCHECK, IGRT
**Example:** QA confirms kidney VMAT delivered fluence using phantom recalculation.

376. **Oblique Beam Dose Logging QA Protocol Meaning:** QA procedure to record dose delivery for oblique beams.
**Related Terms:** DVH, EPID, IMRT QA
**Example:** QA logs kidney SBRT oblique beam dose per fraction.

377. **Offline Beam Output Logging Phantom Meaning:** Phantom QA for recording LINAC output post-treatment.
**Related Terms:** MU Verification, EPID, IMRT QA
**Example:** QA confirms kidney VMAT output using phantom logging.

378. **Oblique Field Dose Gradient Logging QA Meaning:** QA procedure for logging dose gradient in oblique fields.
**Related Terms:** DVH, IMRT, VMAT
**Example:** QA logs kidney SBRT oblique field dose gradient.

379. **Online Beam Output Logging QA Protocol Meaning:** QA procedure for real-time beam output recording.
**Related Terms:** MU Verification, EPID, IGRT
**Example:** QA ensures kidney VMAT output matches TPS in real-time.

380. **Oblique Beam Dose Mapping QA Phantom Meaning:** Phantom QA for mapping oblique beam dose.
**Related Terms:** DVH, IMRT, VMAT
**Example:** QA maps kidney SBRT oblique beam dose using phantom.

381. **Offline Dose Gradient Logging QA Protocol Meaning:** QA procedure for recording dose gradient after treatment.
**Related Terms:** DVH, IMRT, VMAT
**Example:** QA logs kidney VMAT dose gradient using phantom.

382. **Oblique Field Dose Accumulation Logging QA Meaning:** QA for recording cumulative dose of oblique fields.
**Related Terms:** DVH, IMRT, VMAT
**Example:** QA confirms kidney SBRT oblique cumulative dose using phantom.

383. **Online Dose Gradient Logging Phantom Meaning:** Phantom QA for recording dose gradient in real-time.
**Related Terms:** DVH, IMRT, VMAT
**Example:** QA logs kidney VMAT dose gradient using phantom.

384. **Oblique Beam Output Recalculation QA Phantom Meaning:** Phantom QA to recalculate oblique beam output.
**Related Terms:** MU Verification, EPID, IMRT QA
**Example:** QA confirms kidney SBRT oblique beam output using phantom.

385. **Offline Fluence Mapping Logging QA Phantom Meaning:** Phantom QA to log post-treatment fluence mapping.
**Related Terms:** EPID, MapCHECK, IMRT QA
**Example:** QA confirms kidney VMAT delivered fluence using phantom logging.

386. **Oblique Field Beam Alignment QA Phantom Meaning:** Phantom QA to verify alignment of oblique fields.
**Related Terms:** IGRT, CBCT, Fiducials
**Example:** QA ensures kidney SBRT oblique field alignment using phantom.

387. **Online Beam Flatness QA Protocol Meaning:** QA procedure for real-time verification of beam flatness.
**Related Terms:** IMRT, VMAT, LINAC QA
**Example:** QA ensures kidney VMAT beams are flat across PTV during delivery.

388. **Oblique Beam Dose Recalculation Logging Protocol Meaning:** QA procedure to log recalculated oblique beam dose.
**Related Terms:** DVH, IMRT, VMAT
**Example:** QA logs kidney SBRT oblique dose recalculation per fraction.

389. **Offline Dose Logging QA Phantom Meaning:** Phantom QA for recording delivered dose after treatment.
**Related Terms:** DVH, EPID, IMRT QA
**Example:** QA logs kidney VMAT fraction dose using phantom.

390. **Oblique Field Fluence Output Logging Phantom Meaning:** Phantom QA for logging fluence output in oblique fields.
**Related Terms:** EPID, MapCHECK, IMRT QA
**Example:** QA confirms kidney SBRT oblique fluence using phantom.

391. **Online Dose Accumulation Logging QA Phantom Meaning:** Phantom QA for recording cumulative dose in real-time.
**Related Terms:** DVH, EPID, IGRT
**Example:** QA logs kidney VMAT cumulative dose using phantom.

392. **Oblique Beam Dose Gradient Recalculation QA Phantom Meaning:** Phantom QA for recalculating dose gradient of oblique beams.
**Related Terms:** DVH, IMRT, VMAT
**Example:** QA confirms kidney SBRT oblique dose gradient using phantom.

393. **Offline Beam Symmetry Logging QA Meaning:** QA procedure for recording beam symmetry post-treatment.
**Related Terms:** IMRT, VMAT, LINAC QA
**Example:** QA logs kidney VMAT beam symmetry using film or phantom.

394. **Oblique Field Dose Recalculation Logging Phantom Meaning:** Phantom QA for logging recalculated oblique field dose.
**Related Terms:** DVH, IMRT, VMAT
**Example:** QA confirms kidney SBRT oblique field dose using phantom.

395. **Online Beam Dose Logging QA Phantom Meaning:** Phantom QA for real-time beam dose recording.
**Related Terms:** DVH, EPID, IGRT
**Example:** QA logs kidney VMAT dose delivery using phantom.

396. **Oblique Beam Output Recalculation Logging QA Meaning:** QA procedure to log recalculated oblique beam output.
**Related Terms:** MU Verification, EPID, IMRT QA
**Example:** QA confirms kidney SBRT oblique beam output using phantom.

397. **Offline Fluence Dose Mapping QA Phantom Meaning:** Phantom QA to map delivered fluence post-treatment.
**Related Terms:** EPID, MapCHECK, IMRT QA
**Example:** QA maps kidney VMAT delivered fluence using phantom.

398. **Oblique Field Beam Profile Logging QA Phantom Meaning:** Phantom QA for logging beam profile of oblique fields.
**Related Terms:** IMRT, VMAT, LINAC QA
**Example:** QA logs kidney SBRT oblique beam profile using phantom.

399. **Online Dose Recalculation QA Phantom Meaning:** Phantom QA for real-time recalculation of delivered dose.
**Related Terms:** DVH, EPID, IGRT
**Example:** QA confirms kidney VMAT delivered dose matches TPS in real-time.

400. **Oblique Beam Flatness QA Phantom Meaning:** Phantom QA for verifying flatness of oblique beams.
**Related Terms:** IMRT, VMAT, LINAC QA
**Example:** QA ensures kidney SBRT oblique beam flatness matches plan using phantom.

401. **Offline Beam Flatness Logging Phantom Meaning:** Phantom QA to record LINAC beam flatness post-treatment.
**Related Terms:** IMRT, VMAT, LINAC QA
**Example:** QA logs kidney SBRT beam flatness using water or film phantom.

402. **Oblique Field Dose Verification QA Protocol Meaning:** QA procedure to verify dose delivery for oblique fields.
**Related Terms:** DVH, IMRT, VMAT
**Example:** QA ensures kidney SBRT oblique dose matches TPS.

403. **Online Beam Dose Mapping QA Meaning:** QA procedure to map delivered dose in real-time.
**Related Terms:** DVH, EPID, IGRT
**Example:** QA maps kidney VMAT dose during treatment using phantom.

404. **Oblique Beam Dose Logging Phantom QA Meaning:** Phantom QA for logging delivered dose of oblique beams.
**Related Terms:** DVH, IMRT, VMAT
**Example:** QA logs kidney SBRT oblique beam dose using phantom.

405. **Offline Dose Verification Logging Phantom Meaning:** Phantom QA to verify dose delivery post-treatment.
**Related Terms:** DVH, IMRT, VMAT
**Example:** QA confirms kidney VMAT delivered dose using phantom.

406. **Oblique Field Beam Output QA Meaning:** QA procedure to verify output of oblique fields.
**Related Terms:** MU Verification, LINAC QA
**Example:** QA ensures kidney SBRT oblique beam output using EPID.

407. **Online Fluence Logging QA Phantom Meaning:** Phantom QA to record delivered fluence in real-time.
**Related Terms:** EPID, MapCHECK, IMRT QA
**Example:** QA logs kidney VMAT fluence during treatment using phantom.

408. **Oblique Beam Dose Accumulation QA Protocol Meaning:** QA procedure for recording cumulative dose of oblique beams.
**Related Terms:** DVH, IMRT, VMAT
**Example:** QA ensures kidney SBRT cumulative dose using phantom.

409. **Offline Beam Dose Mapping Phantom Meaning:** Phantom QA to map dose delivered post-treatment.
**Related Terms:** DVH, EPID, IMRT QA
**Example:** QA maps kidney VMAT delivered dose using phantom.

410. **Oblique Field Fluence Mapping QA Phantom Meaning:** Phantom QA for mapping fluence of oblique fields.
**Related Terms:** EPID, MapCHECK, IMRT QA
**Example:** QA confirms kidney SBRT oblique fluence using phantom.

411. **Online Beam Output Logging Phantom Meaning:** Phantom QA to log LINAC beam output in real-time.
**Related Terms:** MU Verification, EPID, IGRT
**Example:** QA logs kidney VMAT beam output during treatment.

412. **Oblique Beam Dose Verification Logging Phantom Meaning:** Phantom QA to log dose verification for oblique beams.
**Related Terms:** DVH, IMRT, VMAT
**Example:** QA logs kidney SBRT oblique dose verification using phantom.

413. **Offline Fluence Recalculation QA Phantom Meaning:** Phantom QA for post-treatment recalculation of fluence.
**Related Terms:** EPID, MapCHECK, IMRT QA
**Example:** QA confirms kidney VMAT delivered fluence using recalculation phantom.

414. **Oblique Field Beam Profile QA Phantom Meaning:** Phantom QA to check beam profile of oblique fields.
**Related Terms:** IMRT, VMAT, LINAC QA
**Example:** QA checks kidney SBRT oblique beam profile using phantom.

415. **Online Dose Gradient Logging QA Protocol Meaning:** QA procedure to log dose gradients in real-time.
**Related Terms:** DVH, IMRT, VMAT
**Example:** QA logs kidney VMAT dose gradient per fraction using phantom.

416. **Oblique Beam Dose Mapping QA Protocol**
**Meaning:** QA procedure for mapping dose in oblique beams.
**Related Terms:** DVH, IMRT, VMAT
**Example:** QA ensures kidney SBRT oblique dose distribution matches TPS.

417. **Offline Beam Output Recalculation Logging QA Meaning:** QA procedure to log recalculated beam output post-treatment.
**Related Terms:** MU Verification, EPID, IMRT QA
**Example:** QA confirms kidney VMAT beam output using phantom recalculation.

418. **Oblique Field Flatness QA Phantom Meaning:** Phantom QA to measure flatness of oblique fields.
**Related Terms:** IMRT, VMAT, LINAC QA
**Example:** QA ensures kidney SBRT oblique field flatness matches plan.

419. **Online Beam Dose Logging QA Protocol Meaning:** QA procedure for recording delivered beam dose in real-time.
**Related Terms:** DVH, EPID, IGRT
**Example:** QA logs kidney VMAT beam dose using phantom during delivery.

420. **Oblique Beam Dose Recalculation QA Protocol Meaning:** QA procedure to recalculate and log oblique beam dose.
**Related Terms:** DVH, IMRT, VMAT
**Example:** QA confirms kidney SBRT oblique beam dose using phantom.

421. **Offline Beam Symmetry Logging Phantom Meaning:** Phantom QA to log LINAC beam symmetry post-treatment.
**Related Terms:** IMRT, VMAT, LINAC QA
**Example:** QA logs kidney VMAT beam symmetry using phantom.

422. **Oblique Field Dose Mapping Logging Phantom Meaning:** Phantom QA to log dose mapping of oblique fields.
**Related Terms:** DVH, IMRT, VMAT
**Example:** QA maps kidney SBRT oblique dose using phantom.

423. **Online Fluence Output Logging QA Protocol Meaning:** QA procedure for recording fluence output in real-time.
**Related Terms:** EPID, MapCHECK, IMRT QA
**Example:** QA logs kidney VMAT delivered fluence using phantom.

424. **Oblique Beam Dose Gradient Logging QA Phantom Meaning:** Phantom QA to record dose gradient in oblique beams.
**Related Terms:** DVH, IMRT, VMAT
**Example:** QA logs kidney SBRT oblique dose gradient using phantom.

425. **Offline Dose Accumulation Logging QA Phantom Meaning:** Phantom QA to log cumulative dose post-treatment.
**Related Terms:** DVH, EPID, IMRT QA
**Example:** QA logs kidney VMAT cumulative dose using phantom.

426. **Oblique Field Dose Recalculation QA Protocol Meaning:** QA procedure to recalculate oblique field dose post-treatment.
**Related Terms:** DVH, IMRT, VMAT
**Example:** QA confirms kidney SBRT oblique field dose using phantom.

427. **Online Beam Flatness Logging QA Phantom Meaning:** Phantom QA for recording real-time beam flatness.
**Related Terms:** IMRT, VMAT, LINAC QA
**Example:** QA logs kidney VMAT beam flatness during delivery.

428. **Oblique Beam Fluence Logging QA Phantom Meaning:** Phantom QA to log delivered fluence in oblique beams.
**Related Terms:** EPID, MapCHECK, IMRT QA
**Example:** QA logs kidney SBRT oblique beam fluence using phantom.

429. **Offline Dose Gradient Logging QA Phantom Meaning:** Phantom QA to log dose gradient post-treatment.
**Related Terms:** DVH, IMRT, VMAT
**Example:** QA logs kidney VMAT dose gradient using phantom.

430. **Oblique Field Beam Dose Logging QA Phantom Meaning:** Phantom QA to log dose delivery in oblique fields.
**Related Terms:** DVH, IMRT, VMAT
**Example:** QA logs kidney SBRT oblique beam dose using phantom.

431. **Online Beam Dose Recalculation QA Protocol Meaning:** QA procedure to recalculate delivered dose in real-time.
**Related Terms:** DVH, EPID, IGRT
**Example:** QA confirms kidney VMAT dose matches TPS in real-time.

432. **Oblique Beam Output Logging QA Phantom Meaning:** Phantom QA to log oblique beam output.
**Related Terms:** MU Verification, EPID, IMRT QA
**Example:** QA logs kidney SBRT oblique beam output using phantom.

433. **Offline Fluence Mapping Logging QA Phantom Meaning:** Phantom QA for logging post-treatment fluence mapping.
**Related Terms:** EPID, MapCHECK, IMRT QA
**Example:** QA maps kidney VMAT delivered fluence using phantom.

434. **Oblique Field Dose Accumulation QA Phantom Meaning:** Phantom QA to record cumulative dose of oblique fields.
**Related Terms:** DVH, IMRT, VMAT
**Example:** QA ensures kidney SBRT cumulative dose using phantom.

435. **Online Beam Dose Mapping Logging Phantom Meaning:** Phantom QA to log delivered beam dose in real-time.
**Related Terms:** DVH, EPID, IGRT
**Example:** QA logs kidney VMAT dose per fraction using phantom.

436. **Oblique Beam Dose Verification QA Phantom Meaning:** Phantom QA to verify delivered dose in oblique beams.
**Related Terms:** DVH, IMRT, VMAT
**Example:** QA confirms kidney SBRT oblique beam dose using phantom.

437. **Offline Beam Output Logging QA Phantom Meaning:** Phantom QA to record LINAC output post-treatment.
**Related Terms:** MU Verification, EPID, IMRT QA
**Example:** QA logs kidney VMAT beam output using phantom.

438. **Oblique Field Beam Dose Gradient Logging QA Meaning:** QA procedure to record dose gradient of oblique fields.
**Related Terms:** DVH, IMRT, VMAT
**Example:** QA logs kidney SBRT oblique field dose gradient.

439. **Online Fluence Dose Logging QA Phantom Meaning:** Phantom QA to record delivered fluence in real-time.
**Related Terms:** EPID, MapCHECK, IMRT QA
**Example:** QA logs kidney VMAT fluence during delivery.

440. **Oblique Beam Dose Mapping Logging QA Protocol Meaning:** QA procedure for logging oblique beam dose mapping.
**Related Terms:** DVH, IMRT, VMAT
**Example:** QA logs kidney SBRT oblique dose using phantom.

441. **Offline Dose Verification Logging QA Protocol Meaning:** QA procedure to verify dose delivery post-treatment.
**Related Terms:** DVH, IMRT, VMAT
**Example:** QA confirms kidney VMAT delivered dose using phantom.

442. **Oblique Field Beam Output Logging QA Protocol Meaning:** QA procedure to log oblique beam output.
**Related Terms:** MU Verification, LINAC QA
**Example:** QA logs kidney SBRT oblique field output using EPID.

443. **Online Dose Accumulation Logging QA Protocol Meaning:** QA procedure for real-time cumulative dose recording.
**Related Terms:** DVH, EPID, IGRT
**Example:** QA logs kidney VMAT cumulative dose during treatment.

444. **Oblique Beam Dose Recalculation Logging QA Phantom Meaning:** Phantom QA to recalculate and log dose of oblique beams.
**Related Terms:** DVH, IMRT, VMAT
**Example:** QA confirms kidney SBRT oblique beam dose using phantom.

445. **Offline Beam Flatness QA Phantom Meaning:** Phantom QA for recording LINAC beam flatness post-treatment.
**Related Terms:** IMRT, VMAT, LINAC QA
**Example:** QA logs kidney VMAT beam flatness using phantom.

446. **Oblique Field Dose Mapping QA Phantom Meaning:** Phantom QA for mapping oblique field dose.
**Related Terms:** DVH, IMRT, VMAT
**Example:** QA maps kidney SBRT oblique dose using phantom.

447. **Online Beam Output Verification QA Phantom Meaning:** Phantom QA to verify LINAC beam output in real-time.
**Related Terms:** MU Verification, EPID, IGRT
**Example:** QA confirms kidney VMAT beam output during treatment.

448. **Oblique Beam Fluence Output Logging QA Phantom Meaning:** Phantom QA to log fluence output of oblique beams.
**Related Terms:** EPID, MapCHECK, IMRT QA
**Example:** QA logs kidney SBRT oblique beam fluence using phantom.

449. **Offline Dose Gradient Logging QA Protocol Meaning:** QA procedure for logging dose gradient post-treatment.
**Related Terms:** DVH, IMRT, VMAT
**Example:** QA logs kidney VMAT dose gradient using phantom.

450. **Oblique Field Beam Dose Recalculation QA Phantom Meaning:** Phantom QA to recalculate and log oblique field dose.
**Related Terms:** DVH, IMRT, VMAT
**Example:** QA confirms kidney SBRT oblique beam dose using phantom.

451. **Orthogonal Imaging QA:** QA for imaging using two perpendicular angles.
**Related Terms:** IGRT, QA, Patient setup.
**Radiotherapy Example:** Verifying orthogonal X-rays for head-and-neck RT positioning.

452. **Oblique Angle Imaging Correction:** Correcting imaging distortions from non-standard angles.
**Related Terms:** IGRT, QA, Imaging correction.
**Radiotherapy Example:** Correcting oblique CBCT images for spinal tumor alignment.

453. **Organ Dose Mapping Imaging:** Mapping radiation dose distribution to specific organs using imaging.
**Related Terms:** Dosimetry, IGRT, QA.
**Radiotherapy Example:** Mapping liver dose using CT and proton therapy planning.

454. **Onboard Imaging QA:** QA for imaging devices integrated into treatment machines.
**Related Terms:** IGRT, LINAC, CBCT.
**Radiotherapy Example:** Verifying CBCT quality on LINAC before daily patient setup.

455. **Optical Imaging QA:** QA for optical imaging systems used in radiation therapy.
**Related Terms:** Surface imaging, IGRT, QA.
**Radiotherapy Example:** Verifying surface-guided RT system accuracy for breast treatments.

456. **Ocular Dose Assessment:** Measuring radiation dose delivered to the eyes.
**Related Terms:** Dosimetry, Shielding, QA.
**Radiotherapy Example:** Estimating lens dose during head-and-neck proton therapy.

457. **Orientation Verification Imaging:** Imaging to confirm correct patient orientation before treatment.
**Related Terms:** IGRT, QA, Patient setup.
**Radiotherapy Example:** CBCT verification of prostate patient orientation.

458. **Orthogonal Image Dose Correlation:** Comparing orthogonal imaging to verify dose delivery accuracy.
**Related Terms:** IGRT, QA, Imaging.
**Radiotherapy Example:** Correlating AP and lateral images to confirm spinal tumor coverage.

459. **Oblique Angle Dose Verification:** Verifying dose at non-standard imaging angles.
**Related Terms:** QA, Dosimetry, Imaging.
**Radiotherapy Example:** Measuring dose delivered through an oblique beam to avoid critical structures.

460. **Organ Motion Imaging Assessment:** Assessing organ movement during therapy using imaging.
**Related Terms:** Motion management, IGRT, Proton therapy.
**Radiotherapy Example:** Imaging liver motion during respiration to adjust beam delivery.

461. **Onboard Imaging Dose Tracking:** Monitoring dose delivery using imaging integrated into treatment machine.
**Related Terms:** IGRT, QA, Real-time tracking.
**Radiotherapy Example:** Tracking dose to prostate using CBCT during treatment.

462. **Optical Imaging for Dose Verification:** Using optical imaging to assess delivered dose.
**Related Terms:** QA, Imaging, Surface dose.
**Radiotherapy Example:** Measuring skin dose in breast radiotherapy using optical cameras.

463. **Orientation Verification QA:** QA for verifying patient positioning and orientation.
**Related Terms:** IGRT, QA, Alignment.
**Radiotherapy Example:** Checking head-and-neck patient alignment using lasers and CBCT.

464. **Ocular Dose Imaging Assessment:** Imaging-based assessment of dose to eyes.
**Related Terms:** QA, Dosimetry, Proton therapy.
**Radiotherapy Example:** Verifying eye dose during cranial proton therapy.

465. **Overlap Imaging Correction:** Correcting dose or image overlap in multi-angle imaging.
**Related Terms:** QA, Imaging, Dosimetry.
**Radiotherapy Example:** Adjusting overlapping portal images in pelvic treatments.

466. **Optical Coherence Imaging QA:** QA for optical coherence imaging used in surface or tissue imaging.
**Related Terms:** QA, Imaging, Optical imaging.
**Radiotherapy Example:** Verifying skin surface maps in superficial radiation therapy.

467. **Organ-Specific Dose Imaging:** Imaging to evaluate dose delivered to specific organs.
**Related Terms:** Dosimetry, QA, Imaging.
**Radiotherapy Example:** Mapping liver dose during stereotactic body radiotherapy (SBRT).

468. **Objective function (noun):** Mathematical expression defining goals and constraints in optimization.
**Related Terms:** Inverse planning, Cost function.
**Example in Radiotherapy:** Objective functions guide IMRT dose optimization.

469. **Observer variability (noun):** Differences in results between observers performing the same task.
**Related Terms:** Inter-observer variation, contouring uncertainty.
**Example in Radiotherapy:** Seen in target delineation studies.

470. **Occlusion effect (noun):** Blocking of radiation or signal by intervening structures.
**Related Terms:** Attenuation, Shadowing.
**Example in Radiotherapy:** Occurs near dense implants.

471. **Offline adaptive planning (noun):** Plan modification performed between treatment fractions.
**Related Terms:** Adaptive RT, Replanning.
**Example in Radiotherapy:** Used when anatomy changes significantly.

472. **Offline correction (noun):** Adjustment applied after data acquisition or delivery.
**Related Terms:** Post-processing, QA.
**Example in Radiotherapy:** Used for setup trend corrections.

473. **Offset correction (noun):** Adjustment compensating for baseline displacement.
**Related Terms:** Zero shift, Calibration.
**Example in Radiotherapy:** Applied in detector readouts.

474. **On-axis dose (noun):** Dose measured along the central beam axis.
**Related Terms:** Central axis dose, Depth dose.
**Example in Radiotherapy:** Used for beam commissioning.

475. **Online adaptive radiotherapy (noun):** Real-time treatment plan adaptation during delivery.
**Related Terms:** MR-guided RT, Adaptive workflow.
**Example in Radiotherapy:** Adjusts for daily anatomy changes.

476. **Online imaging verification (noun):** Imaging performed immediately before or during treatment.
**Related Terms:** IGRT, CBCT.
**Example in Radiotherapy:** Used for daily patient positioning.

477. **On-treatment imaging dose (noun):** Radiation dose from verification imaging.
**Related Terms:** Imaging dose, CBCT dose.
**Example in Radiotherapy:** Considered in cumulative dose assessment.

478. **Open beam configuration (noun):** Beam delivered without modifiers or shaping devices.
**Related Terms:** Reference field, Calibration setup.
**Example in Radiotherapy:** Used for baseline output checks.

479. **Operational tolerance (noun):** Acceptable deviation during system operation.
**Related Terms:** QA limits, Action level.
**Example in Radiotherapy:** Defined in machine QA protocols.

480. **Optical distance indicator (noun):** Device indicating source-to-surface distance.
**Related Terms:** ODI, SSD.
**Example in Radiotherapy:** Used during patient setup.

481. **Optical imaging guidance (noun):** Use of cameras for patient positioning.
**Related Terms:** Surface imaging, SGRT.
**Example in Radiotherapy:** Assists with motion monitoring.

482. **Optical tracking accuracy (noun):** Precision of position measured using optical systems.
**Related Terms:** Surface guidance, Setup accuracy.
**Example in Radiotherapy:** Important for frameless SRS.

483. **Optimization convergence (noun):** State where further iterations yield minimal improvement.
**Related Terms:** Solver stability, Planning efficiency.
**Example in Radiotherapy:** Indicates completion of IMRT optimization.

484. **Optimization priority (noun):** Relative importance assigned to objectives.
**Related Terms:** Weighting factor, Trade-off.
**Example in Radiotherapy:** Higher priority given to spinal cord sparing.

485. **Optimization robustness (noun):** Plan stability against uncertainties.
**Related Terms:** Robust planning, Sensitivity analysis.
**Example in Radiotherapy:** Essential in proton therapy.

486. **Organ-at-risk constraint (noun):** Dose limit applied to normal tissue.
**Related Terms:** OAR limit, Planning objective.
**Example in Radiotherapy:** Parotid mean dose constraint.

487. **Organ motion envelope (noun):** Total range of organ movement.
**Related Terms:** ITV, Motion margin.
**Example in Radiotherapy:** Used in lung planning.

488. **Output calibration (noun):** Process of setting machine dose output.
**Related Terms:** Absolute dosimetry, TG-51.
**Example in Radiotherapy:** Performed annually or after repairs.

489. **Output consistency (noun):** Stability of delivered dose over time.
**Related Terms:** Output constancy, QA.
**Example in Radiotherapy:** Checked during daily QA.

490. **Output correction factor (noun):** Multiplier adjusting measured or planned output.
**Related Terms:** Scatter factor, MU correction.
**Example in Radiotherapy:** Used for wedges or trays.

491. **Over-travel limit (noun):** Maximum allowed motion beyond intended range.
**Related Terms:** Mechanical interlock, Safety system.
**Example in Radiotherapy:** Prevents gantry collision.

492. **Over-irradiation risk (noun):** Potential for delivering excess dose.
**Related Terms:** Hot spot, Safety margin.
**Example in Radiotherapy:** Minimized through QA checks.

493. **Overlap region (noun):** Area where two radiation fields intersect.
**Related Terms:** Junction, Field matching.
**Example in Radiotherapy:** Managed to avoid hot or cold spots.

494. **Overshoot correction (noun):** Adjustment preventing exceeding target values.
**Related Terms:** Control loop, Stability.
**Example in Radiotherapy:** Used in dynamic MLC motion.

495. **Partial organ irradiation (noun):** Treatment where only part of an organ receives dose.
**Related Terms:** Sub-volume dosing, OAR sparing.
**Example in Radiotherapy:** Common in head and neck RT.

496. **Out-of-field dose (noun):** Radiation dose outside the treatment field.
**Related Terms:** Leakage, Scatter dose.
**Example in Radiotherapy:** Relevant for secondary cancer risk.

497. **Outlier rejection (noun):** Removal of abnormal data points.
**Related Terms:** Data filtering, QA analysis.
**Example in Radiotherapy:** Applied to QA trend data.

498. **Overall treatment accuracy (noun):** Combined precision of planning, setup, and delivery.
**Related Terms:** End-to-end accuracy, QA.
**Example in Radiotherapy:** Critical for stereotactic treatments.

499. **Oxygen enhancement ratio (noun):** Increase in radiation effectiveness due to oxygen.
**Related Terms:** Hypoxia, Radiobiology.
**Example in Radiotherapy:** Considered in tumor response modeling.

500. **Organ Motion Compensation (noun):** Techniques used to account for internal organ movement during radiation delivery to maintain target accuracy.
**Related Terms:** Respiratory Gating, Tracking, ITV.
**Example in Radiotherapy:** Organ motion compensation is applied in lung SBRT using respiratory gating or tumor tracking systems.

# P

1. **Palliation Radiotherapy:** Using radiation to relieve symptoms rather than cure disease.
   **Related Terms:** Palliative care, Symptom management, Pain relief.
   **Radiotherapy Example:** Treating painful bone metastasis to reduce pain.
2. **Particle Beam Therapy:** Using protons or heavy ions for high-precision tumor irradiation.
   **Related Terms:** Proton therapy, Heavy ion therapy, Particle therapy planning.
   **Radiotherapy Example:** Treating liver tumors with proton beams to spare surrounding tissue.
3. **Particle Therapy Planning:** Planning the delivery of particle beams to achieve optimal tumor dose and minimal normal tissue exposure.
   **Related Terms:** Treatment planning system (TPS), Dose optimization, Beam shaping.
   **Radiotherapy Example:** Designing a proton therapy plan for lung cancer using TPS.
4. **Particle Therapy Dose Optimization:** Adjusting beam parameters to deliver the prescribed dose accurately while sparing healthy tissue.
   **Related Terms:** Dose painting, LET optimization, IMPT (Intensity-Modulated Proton Therapy).
   **Radiotherapy Example:** Optimizing proton dose to liver tumor while minimizing liver toxicity.
5. **Particle Radiosurgery:** High-precision, single or few fraction particle treatment for small lesions.
   **Related Terms:** Stereotactic radiosurgery, Proton radiosurgery, Gamma Knife.
   **Radiotherapy Example:** Treating a small brain metastasis with proton radiosurgery.
6. **Particle Fractionation Strategy:** Dividing particle therapy dose into multiple fractions to maximize tumor control and minimize toxicity.
   **Related Terms:** Fractionation, Dose per fraction, Treatment schedule.
   **Radiotherapy Example:** Delivering a liver proton treatment over 5 fractions to reduce side effects.
7. **Particle Dose Verification:** Confirming that the delivered particle dose matches the planned dose.
   **Related Terms:** Dose QA, Treatment verification, Dosimetry.
   **Radiotherapy Example:** Using ionization chambers to verify proton dose to a tumor.
8. **Particle Beam Shaping:** Modifying beam geometry to conform precisely to tumor shape.
   **Related Terms:** Collimation, MLC, Beam modulation.
   **Radiotherapy Example:** Shaping proton beam for irregular liver tumor contours.
9. **Particle Range Verification:** Ensuring the particle beam penetrates to the correct depth in tissue.
   **Related Terms:** Bragg peak, Range shifter, Dose deposition.
   **Radiotherapy Example:** Verifying proton range using water phantom measurements.
10. **Particle Beam Modulation:** Adjusting intensity or energy of the particle beam for uniform dose coverage.
    **Related Terms:** IMPT, Energy modulation, Dose painting.
    **Radiotherapy Example:** Modulating proton spots to cover a heterogeneous tumor.
11. **Proton Therapy:** Using proton beams for precise radiation treatment, exploiting the Bragg peak.
    **Related Terms:** Particle therapy, IMPT, Pencil beam scanning.
    **Radiotherapy Example:** Treating pediatric brain tumors with minimal normal tissue exposure.

12. **Proton Therapy Planning:** Designing a proton treatment plan for optimal dose delivery to the tumor.
**Related Terms:** TPS, Beam arrangement, Dose optimization.
**Radiotherapy Example:** Planning proton therapy for a skull base tumor.

13. **Proton Beam Range Measurement:** Measuring the depth protons travel in tissue or phantom to confirm accuracy.
**Related Terms:** Bragg peak verification, Range QA, Dosimetry.
**Radiotherapy Example:** Using a water phantom to measure the proton beam range for lung tumors.

14. **Proton Beam Dose Calculation:** Computing the dose delivered by a proton beam to tumor and surrounding tissues.
**Related Terms:** TPS, Dose grid, Monte Carlo simulation.
**Radiotherapy Example:** Calculating proton dose for head-and-neck cancer using Monte Carlo methods.

15. **Proton Beam Scattering Correction:** Adjusting for beam spread due to interactions in tissue or materials.
**Related Terms:** Multiple Coulomb scattering, Dose broadening, Range correction.
**Radiotherapy Example:** Correcting proton dose in a liver tumor due to beam scattering in ribs.

16. **Proton Radiosensitizer Study:** Investigating drugs that enhance tumor sensitivity to proton therapy.
**Related Terms:** Radiosensitizers, Combined modality therapy, Chemoradiation.
**Radiotherapy Example:** Testing a drug that increases proton therapy efficacy in pancreatic cancer.

17. **Proton Beam Dose Mapping:** Mapping the spatial distribution of proton dose in tissue or phantom.
**Related Terms:** Dose distribution, TPS verification, Dosimetry.
**Radiotherapy Example:** Creating a 3D proton dose map for prostate cancer.

18. **Proton Beam Bragg Peak Verification:** Ensuring the Bragg peak occurs at the planned tumor depth.
**Related Terms:** Range verification, Proton therapy QA, Dosimetry.
**Radiotherapy Example:** Using a water phantom to confirm Bragg peak location for head-and-neck proton therapy.

19. **Proton Beam Motion Compensation:** Correcting for tumor motion to ensure accurate dose delivery.
**Related Terms:** Motion management, Respiratory gating, Image-guided therapy.
**Radiotherapy Example:** Gating proton therapy to lung tumor motion during breathing cycles.

20. **Proton Beam Adaptive Therapy:** Modifying treatment plans based on anatomical changes during therapy.
**Related Terms:** Adaptive therapy, Daily imaging, Dose recalculation.
**Radiotherapy Example:** Adjusting liver proton therapy plan as tumor shrinks mid-treatment.

21. **Photon Beam Dosimetry:** Measuring dose delivered by photon beams for treatment verification.
**Related Terms:** LINAC QA, Dosimeter, Ion chamber.
**Radiotherapy Example:** Verifying IMRT photon dose using a 2D ion chamber array.

22. **Photon Dose Calculation Algorithms:** Computational methods for determining photon dose in tissue.
**Related Terms:** TPS, Monte Carlo, Convolution-superposition.
**Radiotherapy Example:** Using Monte Carlo to calculate dose in heterogeneous lung tissue.

23. **Photon Dose Mapping:** Creating spatial distribution of photon dose in target volume.
**Related Terms:** Dose distribution, 3D dose verification, DVH analysis.
**Radiotherapy Example:** Mapping photon dose for a breast IMRT plan.

24. **Photon Beam Quality Assurance:** QA procedures to ensure photon beams meet clinical specifications.
**Related Terms:** LINAC QA, Beam calibration, Flatness and symmetry.
**Radiotherapy Example:** Performing monthly QA on a linear accelerator for photon beams.

25. **Photon Energy Calibration:** Adjusting photon beam energy to match treatment specifications.
**Related Terms:** LINAC calibration, Energy verification, Dosimetry QA.
**Radiotherapy Example:** Calibrating 6 MV photon beam before patient treatments.

26. **Photon Output Verification:** Confirming consistent dose output from photon beams.
**Related Terms:** Daily QA, Dose constancy, LINAC monitoring.
**Radiotherapy Example:** Measuring photon output with ion chamber before IMRT delivery.

27. **Photon Beam Profile Assessment:** Evaluating uniformity of photon beam across treatment field.
**Related Terms:** Beam flatness, Symmetry, QA phantom.
**Radiotherapy Example:** Assessing beam profile with water phantom for head-and-neck IMRT.

28. **Photon Attenuation Measurement:** Measuring reduction in photon intensity passing through materials.
**Related Terms:** Tissue attenuation, LINAC QA, Depth dose.
**Radiotherapy Example:** Measuring photon attenuation through lung tissue for planning.

29. **Photon Scatter Correction:** Correcting dose calculations for scatter effects.
**Related Terms:** Scatter factor, TPS correction, Monte Carlo.
**Radiotherapy Example:** Applying scatter correction in photon dose calculation for pelvis.

30. **Photon Therapy Dose Verification:** Confirming delivered photon dose matches planned dose.
**Related Terms:** QA, Dosimetry, Portal dosimetry.
**Radiotherapy Example:** Using electronic portal imaging to verify photon dose for prostate IMRT.

31. **Photomultiplier Tube Calibration:** Calibrating PMTs used in dosimetry or imaging systems.
**Related Terms:** Detector calibration, QA, Radiation measurement.
**Radiotherapy Example:** Calibrating PMTs in a scintillation dosimeter for photon measurements.

32. **Photographic Film Dosimetry:** Measuring dose distribution using radiation-sensitive film.
**Related Terms:** Film QA, 2D dosimetry, Dose mapping.
**Radiotherapy Example:** Checking IMRT photon dose using radiochromic film.

33. **Photopeak Identification in Spectroscopy:** Detecting the main photon energy peak in a spectrum.
**Related Terms:** Gamma spectroscopy, Energy calibration, PET imaging.
**Radiotherapy Example:** Identifying Tc-99m photopeak during nuclear medicine QA.

34. **Photoelectron Emission Dosimetry:** Measuring dose based on emitted photoelectrons from irradiated materials.
**Related Terms:** Electron emission, Dosimetry, Detector calibration.
**Radiotherapy Example:** Using photoelectron emission to verify superficial photon dose.

35. **Photonic Radiation Quality Index:** Index representing photon beam quality and energy spectrum.
**Related Terms:** Beam quality, QA, Photon spectrum.
**Radiotherapy Example:** Calculating quality index for 6 MV photon beam before treatments.

36. **Photoneutron Contamination Assessment:** Measuring unwanted neutrons produced during high-energy photon therapy.
**Related Terms:** Neutron dose, Photonuclear reactions, LINAC QA.
**Radiotherapy Example:** Assessing neutron contamination from 18 MV photon beam.

37. **Photon Flux Measurement:** Measuring the number of photons per unit area per unit time.
**Related Terms:** Beam intensity, Dosimetry, QA.
**Radiotherapy Example:** Measuring photon flux in LINAC beam for treatment verification.

38. **Photon Beam Penumbra Analysis:** Evaluating the dose gradient at the edge of a photon beam.
**Related Terms:** Penumbra, Field edge, Dose gradient.
**Radiotherapy Example:** Measuring penumbra for head-and-neck IMRT fields.

39. **Photon Beam Flatness Verification:** Ensuring uniform dose across the photon beam field.
**Related Terms:** Beam uniformity, QA, LINAC verification.
**Radiotherapy Example:** Checking flatness of 10x10 cm photon field using a water phantom.

40. **Photon Energy Spectrum Analysis:** Determining energy distribution of photons in a beam.
**Related Terms:** Beam quality, Spectroscopy, Dosimetry.
**Radiotherapy Example:** Analyzing energy spectrum of a 6 MV LINAC beam.

41. **PET Imaging:** Positron Emission Tomography to image metabolic activity.
**Related Terms:** PET/CT, Radiotracer, Nuclear medicine.
**Radiotherapy Example:** Using PET to delineate metabolically active tumor regions.

42. **PET/CT Fusion Imaging:** Combining PET metabolic images with CT anatomical images.
**Related Terms:** Image registration, PET, CT, Target delineation.
**Radiotherapy Example:** Fusing PET/CT to plan lung tumor radiotherapy.

43. **PET/CT Dose Optimization:** Minimizing radiation dose during PET/CT imaging.
**Related Terms:** ALARA, CT dose, PET dose.
**Radiotherapy Example:** Reducing CT exposure in PET/CT simulation for a pediatric patient.

44. **PET/CT Quantitative Analysis:** Measuring tracer uptake for tumor assessment.
**Related Terms:** SUV, PET quantification, Dose planning.
**Radiotherapy Example:** Using SUV values to define PET-based target volumes.

45. **PET Radiotracer Kinetics:** Studying how PET tracers distribute and clear in tissues.
**Related Terms:** Pharmacokinetics, SUV, Dynamic PET.
**Radiotherapy Example:** Assessing tumor tracer uptake over time for therapy planning.

46. **PET Scanner Calibration:** Adjusting PET scanner to ensure accurate imaging and quantification.
**Related Terms:** QA, Dose calibration, Image accuracy.
**Radiotherapy Example:** Calibrating PET scanner before tumor volume delineation.

47. **PET Imaging Quality Assurance:** QA procedures to ensure PET imaging accuracy and consistency.
**Related Terms:** Scanner QA, Image uniformity, Calibration.
**Radiotherapy Example:** Performing daily PET QA to ensure reliable tumor imaging.

48. **PET Radiotracer Dose Calculation:** Calculating the appropriate PET tracer dose for imaging.
**Related Terms:** Activity, ALARA, Radiopharmacy.
**Radiotherapy Example:** Administering correct FDG dose for PET simulation in head-and-neck cancer.

49. **PET Motion Correction:** Correcting for patient or organ motion during PET acquisition.
**Related Terms:** Gating, Image registration, Respiratory motion.
**Radiotherapy Example:** Correcting lung tumor motion during PET imaging for planning.

50. **PET Phantom Studies:** Using phantoms to validate PET imaging performance.
**Related Terms:** QA, Calibration, Image uniformity.
**Radiotherapy Example:** Performing PET phantom study to verify SUV accuracy before clinical scans.

51. **Phase-Contrast X-ray Imaging:** X-ray imaging that uses phase shifts of X-rays to enhance soft tissue contrast.
**Related Terms:** X-ray imaging, Contrast enhancement, Soft tissue visualization.
**Radiotherapy Example:** Imaging small lung lesions before radiation planning.

52. **Pixel-Level Dose Mapping:** Mapping radiation dose at the level of individual detector pixels.
**Related Terms:** Dosimetry, 2D/3D dose distribution, QA.
**Radiotherapy Example:** Using pixel-level maps to verify IMRT photon dose distribution.

53. **Planar Scintigraphy:** 2D imaging using gamma-emitting radiotracers captured by a scintillation camera.
**Related Terms:** Nuclear medicine, Gamma imaging, SPECT.
**Radiotherapy Example:** Using planar bone scans to assess metastasis before radiation.

54. **Portal Imaging:** Imaging the treatment field using the treatment beam to verify patient setup.
**Related Terms:** IGRT, Portal dosimetry, Field verification.
**Radiotherapy Example:** Taking portal images for prostate IMRT verification.

55. **Portal Dosimetry:** Measuring dose delivered using portal imaging systems.
**Related Terms:** Dose verification, Portal imaging, IMRT QA.
**Radiotherapy Example:** Checking photon dose delivery for head-and-neck IMRT.

56. **Pre-Treatment Imaging Verification:** Imaging patient setup before treatment to ensure accurate positioning.
**Related Terms:** IGRT, CBCT, Setup verification.
**Radiotherapy Example:** Using cone-beam CT before lung SBRT.

57. **Projection Radiography:** Standard 2D X-ray imaging using transmitted X-rays to form an image.
**Related Terms:** X-ray, Imaging, Radiography.
**Radiotherapy Example:** Using chest X-ray to check tumor position before treatment.

58. **Proton CT Imaging:** Imaging using protons instead of X-rays to reconstruct tissue density maps.
**Related Terms:** Proton therapy, Imaging, Dose calculation.
**Radiotherapy Example:** Using proton CT for treatment planning in pediatric tumors.

59. **Pulmonary Perfusion Imaging:** Imaging to assess blood flow in the lungs.
**Related Terms:** SPECT, PET, Lung function.
**Radiotherapy Example:** Evaluating lung perfusion before thoracic radiation therapy.

60. **Perfusion Radiotracer Mapping:** Mapping tissue perfusion using injected radiotracers.
**Related Terms:** SPECT, PET, Perfusion imaging.
**Radiotherapy Example:** Mapping myocardial perfusion to avoid cardiac dose during breast RT.

61. **Positron Emission:** Emission of a positron from a radioactive nucleus.
**Related Terms:** PET, $\beta^+$ decay, Radiotracer.
**Radiotherapy Example:** FDG tracer emits positrons for PET imaging in tumor planning.

62. **Positron Annihilation Detection:** Detecting photons from positron-electron annihilation.
**Related Terms:** PET, Coincidence detection, Imaging.
**Radiotherapy Example:** Using PET to visualize brain tumor metabolism.

63. **Positron Range Correction:** Correcting PET imaging for the distance positrons travel before annihilation.
**Related Terms:** PET, Resolution, Dose planning.
**Radiotherapy Example:** Adjusting PET images for accurate tumor delineation in lung.

64. **Proton-Induced Nuclear Reaction:** Nuclear reactions triggered by proton beams interacting with nuclei.
**Related Terms:** Proton therapy, Activation, Nuclear physics.
**Radiotherapy Example:** Assessing secondary activation in proton therapy for safety planning.

65. **Proton Capture Reaction:** Nucleus absorbs a proton, leading to nuclear transformation.
**Related Terms:** Nuclear reaction, Activation, Proton therapy.
**Radiotherapy Example:** Producing short-lived isotopes in tissue during proton therapy.

66. **Proton Emission Probability:** Likelihood of a proton being emitted from a nucleus during decay.
**Related Terms:** Radioactive decay, Nuclear physics, Proton therapy.
**Radiotherapy Example:** Studying proton emission from therapy isotopes.

67. **Proton Lifetime Measurement:** Determining half-life or decay characteristics of a proton-rich nucleus.
**Related Terms:** Nuclear physics, Radioisotope, Decay measurement.
**Radiotherapy Example:** Measuring decay properties of isotopes used in proton therapy QA.

68. **Proton Beam-Induced Activation:** Activation of materials or tissues by proton beams.
**Related Terms:** Secondary radiation, Activation, Safety.
**Radiotherapy Example:** Monitoring induced radioactivity in beamline components.

69. **Proton Therapy Radioisotope Production:** Producing isotopes via proton beams for imaging or therapy.
**Related Terms:** Cyclotron, Radiopharmacy, PET.
**Radiotherapy Example:** Creating F-18 for PET imaging in oncology planning.

70. **Proton Therapy Radiochemistry:** Chemistry of isotopes generated or used in proton therapy.
**Related Terms:** Radiopharmaceuticals, PET tracers, Activation.
**Radiotherapy Example:** Preparing labeled compounds for combined proton-PET therapy.

71. **Photoneutron Reaction:** Neutron production induced by high-energy photon interactions.
**Related Terms:** Photonuclear reaction, LINAC, Secondary neutron.
**Radiotherapy Example:** Assessing neutron dose from 18 MV photon therapy.

72. **Photofission:** Fission of nuclei caused by photon absorption.
**Related Terms:** Photonuclear reaction, Nuclear physics, High-energy photons.
**Radiotherapy Example:** Studying fission in lead shielding during high-energy photon therapy.

73. **Photonuclear Reaction:** Nuclear reaction initiated by photon interaction with a nucleus.
**Related Terms:** Photon, Neutron production, LINAC.
**Radiotherapy Example:** Measuring photonuclear neutron dose in high-energy radiotherapy.

74. **Proton-Proton Chain Reaction:** Fusion process in stars converting hydrogen into helium.
**Related Terms:** Nuclear fusion, Stellar physics, Energy generation.
**Radiotherapy Example:** Conceptual physics, not directly used in clinical RT.

75. **Proton-Rich Nuclei Decay:** Decay of nuclei with excess protons via positron emission or proton emission.
**Related Terms:** Radioactive decay, PET, Nuclear physics.
**Radiotherapy Example:** Studying proton decay for radiotracer development.

76. **Proton Therapy Radioactive Contamination:** Unintended radioactivity generated during proton therapy.
**Related Terms:** Safety, Activation, Secondary radiation.
**Radiotherapy Example:** Measuring contamination levels in proton therapy rooms.

77. **Proton Therapy Secondary Neutrons:** Neutrons produced as by-products of proton therapy interactions.
    **Related Terms:** Secondary radiation, Dose assessment, Shielding.
    **Radiotherapy Example:** Calculating neutron dose for staff safety in proton therapy centers.

78. **Proton Therapy Shielding Calculation:** Determining protective material thickness to attenuate radiation.
    **Related Terms:** Radiation safety, Barrier design, Dose limits.
    **Radiotherapy Example:** Designing concrete walls to shield proton therapy vaults.

79. **Proton Therapy Beamline Optimization:** Designing beamline components for efficient and accurate proton delivery.
    **Related Terms:** Beam optics, Collimation, Energy modulation.
    **Radiotherapy Example:** Optimizing proton nozzle design for pediatric brain tumors.

80. **Proton Therapy Beam Modulation:** Adjusting proton beam energy and intensity to achieve desired dose distribution.
    **Related Terms:** IMPT, Pencil beam scanning, Dose painting.
    **Radiotherapy Example:** Modulating proton beam for heterogeneous liver tumor.

81. **Personal Dosimeter:** Device worn by staff to monitor accumulated radiation exposure.
    **Related Terms:** Radiation safety, TLD, OSL.
    **Radiotherapy Example:** Wearing dosimeters during LINAC operation.

82. **Personal Protective Equipment (PPE):** Safety gear used to protect against radiation exposure.
    **Related Terms:** Lead apron, Thyroid shield, Radiation gloves.
    **Radiotherapy Example:** Wearing lead aprons during diagnostic X-ray procedures.

83. **Personnel Radiation Monitoring:** Tracking cumulative radiation exposure of staff.
    **Related Terms:** Dosimetry, Radiation safety, Occupational exposure.
    **Radiotherapy Example:** Monthly review of staff dosimeter readings.

84. **Protective Shielding Design:** Designing barriers to minimize radiation exposure to staff and public.
    **Related Terms:** Lead, Concrete, Shielding calculation.
    **Radiotherapy Example:** Designing treatment room walls for high-energy photon beams.

85. **Protective Apron Usage:** Using lead aprons to shield staff from scatter radiation.
    **Related Terms:** PPE, Radiation protection, Scatter dose.
    **Radiotherapy Example:** Wearing lead aprons during mobile X-ray procedures.

86. **Protective Barrier Assessment:** Evaluating effectiveness of radiation barriers in a treatment facility.
    **Related Terms:** Shielding, Safety, Dose measurement.
    **Radiotherapy Example:** Measuring dose outside proton therapy vault.

87. **Protective Room Shielding:** Concrete or lead shielding designed for radiation treatment rooms.
    **Related Terms:** Barrier design, Radiation safety, Vault shielding.
    **Radiotherapy Example:** Ensuring walls of LINAC vault meet required thickness.

88. **Public Dose Assessment:** Estimating radiation exposure to the general public near therapy facilities.
    **Related Terms:** Dose limit, Shielding, Safety assessment.
    **Radiotherapy Example:** Calculating exposure at the hospital entrance during proton therapy.

89. **Public Radiation Safety Protocol:** Safety procedures to minimize radiation exposure to the public.
    **Related Terms:** Dose limits, Access restriction, Radiation protection.
    **Radiotherapy Example:** Limiting access to areas adjacent to LINAC vaults.

90. **Pollution Control in Radiotherapy:** Measures to prevent radioactive contamination in therapy environments.
**Related Terms:** Waste management, Decontamination, Safety protocols.
**Radiotherapy Example:** Handling and disposing of radioactive tracers safely.

91. **Post-Irradiation Safety Monitoring:** Monitoring areas and staff after radiation exposure.
**Related Terms:** Radiation survey, Residual dose, Safety check.
**Radiotherapy Example:** Surveying proton therapy room after patient treatment.

92. **Post-Accident Radiation Survey:** Measuring radiation levels after an accidental exposure.
**Related Terms:** Incident response, Radiation monitoring, Decontamination.
**Radiotherapy Example:** Surveying LINAC room after unintended beam activation.

93. **Pulse Radiation Detection:** Detecting short bursts of radiation using fast-response detectors.
**Related Terms:** Dosimetry, Ion chamber, Radiation pulse.
**Radiotherapy Example:** Measuring dose per pulse in a pulsed proton therapy system.

94. **Point Source Shielding Calculation:** Calculating shielding needed to protect from a localized radiation source.
**Related Terms:** Inverse square law, Shielding, Safety assessment.
**Radiotherapy Example:** Determining lead thickness for a brachytherapy source.

95. **Precautionary Dose Limits:** Recommended limits to prevent overexposure in staff or public.
**Related Terms:** ALARA, Regulatory limits, Radiation protection.
**Radiotherapy Example:** Limiting staff exposure to <20 mSv/year in proton therapy centers.

96. **Protective Distance Determination:** Calculating safe distance from radiation sources to reduce exposure.
**Related Terms:** Inverse square law, Shielding, Safety.
**Radiotherapy Example:** Ensuring control room is adequately distant from LINAC vault.

97. **Protective Material Selection:** Choosing appropriate materials to attenuate radiation effectively.
**Related Terms:** Lead, Concrete, Shielding design.
**Radiotherapy Example:** Selecting lead vs. concrete for photon vs. proton therapy barriers.

98. **Procedure-Specific Radiation Safety:** Tailored safety measures for specific radiotherapy procedures.
**Related Terms:** PPE, Protocol, Safety checklists.
**Radiotherapy Example:** Safety protocol for HDR brachytherapy procedure.

99. **Patient Radiation Protection:** Measures to minimize unnecessary radiation exposure to patients.
**Related Terms:** Dose optimization, Shielding, ALARA.
**Radiotherapy Example:** Using bolus to reduce skin dose in breast radiotherapy.

100. **Personal Radiation Exposure Log:** Recording cumulative radiation dose for staff over time.
**Related Terms:** Dosimeter, QA, Occupational safety.
**Radiotherapy Example:** Logging monthly TLD readings for all radiotherapy staff.

101. **Phase-Shift Modulated Therapy:** Radiation therapy where beam phase is modulated to enhance dose precision.
**Related Terms:** IMRT, Modulated therapy, Beam shaping.
**Radiotherapy Example:** Using phase modulation for prostate IMRT to spare the rectum.

102. **Plan Verification Imaging:** Imaging performed to confirm accuracy of a treatment plan before delivery.
**Related Terms:** IGRT, QA, Portal imaging.
**Radiotherapy Example:** Verifying cranial tumor alignment before LINAC delivery.

103. **Planning Target Volume (PTV):** Tumor volume plus margin to account for movement and setup errors.
**Related Terms:** CTV, GTV, Dose planning.
**Radiotherapy Example:** Expanding clinical target volume for lung tumor to create PTV.

104. **Particle Range Verification Imaging:** Imaging to confirm penetration depth of particle beams in tissue.
**Related Terms:** Proton therapy, Dosimetry, Imaging QA.
**Radiotherapy Example:** Using proton CT to verify proton beam stopping point in liver tumor.

105. **Particle Beam Scanning:** Moving a particle beam across the tumor to deliver precise dose distribution.
**Related Terms:** Pencil beam scanning, IMPT, Dose painting.
**Radiotherapy Example:** Scanning proton beams to cover irregularly shaped head-and-neck tumor.

106. **Photon Beam Scanning:** Moving a photon beam across the target to ensure uniform dose.
**Related Terms:** IMRT, Dose modulation, QA.
**Radiotherapy Example:** Using scanned photon beams in SBRT for lung lesions.

107. **Photon Intensity Modulation:** Adjusting photon beam intensity to shape the dose distribution.
**Related Terms:** IMRT, Dose shaping, Beam modulation.
**Radiotherapy Example:** Delivering non-uniform photon intensity for prostate sparing.

108. **Photon Therapy Optimization:** Adjusting photon therapy parameters for maximal tumor coverage and minimal normal tissue dose.
**Related Terms:** IMRT, Dose planning, QA.
**Radiotherapy Example:** Optimizing lung photon fields to reduce heart exposure.

109. **Pulsed Radiation Therapy:** Radiation delivered in short, high-intensity pulses rather than continuously.
**Related Terms:** Dose fractionation, LINAC, Safety.
**Radiotherapy Example:** Using pulsed proton beams in research trials for head-and-neck cancers.

110. **Partial Tumor Irradiation:** Treating only a portion of a tumor to spare normal tissue.
**Related Terms:** Dose painting, SBRT, Conformal therapy.
**Radiotherapy Example:** Boosting dose to hypoxic region within a lung tumor.

111. **Patterned Radiation Therapy:** Delivering radiation using spatial patterns for precision and sparing.
**Related Terms:** Microbeam therapy, IMRT, Dose painting.
**Radiotherapy Example:** Using patterned microbeams for preclinical brain tumor studies.

112. **Proton Arc Therapy:** Proton therapy delivered in an arc around the patient to improve dose conformity.
**Related Terms:** Proton therapy, IMPT, Dose optimization.
**Radiotherapy Example:** Arc proton therapy for complex head-and-neck tumors.

113. **Proton Pencil Beam Scanning:** Scanning a narrow proton beam spot-by-spot across the tumor.
**Related Terms:** IMPT, Beam scanning, Dose painting.
**Radiotherapy Example:** Spot scanning for a pediatric brain tumor to spare healthy tissue.

114. **Proton Dose Painting:** Delivering different doses to specific tumor sub-regions based on biology.
**Related Terms:** IMPT, Biological optimization, Targeted therapy.
**Radiotherapy Example:** Increasing dose to hypoxic tumor regions using proton therapy.

**115. Proton Therapy Adaptive Planning:** Adjusting proton therapy plan during treatment based on imaging and response.
**Related Terms:** IGPT, Plan adaptation, Dose recalculation.
**Radiotherapy Example:** Replanning liver proton therapy after tumor shrinkage.

**116. Proton Re-Irradiation Technique:** Delivering a second course of proton therapy to previously irradiated tissue.
**Related Terms:** Reirradiation, Proton therapy, Safety planning.
**Radiotherapy Example:** Re-treating spinal metastasis with proton therapy.

**117. Proton Spot Scanning:** Delivering proton dose via discrete spots to build a conformal dose distribution.
**Related Terms:** Pencil beam, IMPT, Dose painting.
**Radiotherapy Example:** Spot scanning a pediatric medulloblastoma target.

**118. Proton Therapy Multi-Field Optimization:** Optimizing dose distribution using multiple proton beam angles.
**Related Terms:** IMPT, Beam arrangement, Dose optimization.
**Radiotherapy Example:** Multi-field proton plan for complex head-and-neck tumors.

**119. Proton Therapy Motion Management:** Techniques to account for tumor motion during proton therapy delivery.
**Related Terms:** Breath-hold, Gating, Adaptive therapy.
**Radiotherapy Example:** Using respiratory gating for lung proton therapy.

**120. Proton Therapy Range Shifter:** Device used to adjust proton beam range for shallow tumors.
**Related Terms:** Beam modulation, Proton therapy, Dose shaping.
**Radiotherapy Example:** Using range shifter for superficial breast tumor proton therapy.

**121. Parallel-Plate Ionization Chamber:** Ionization chamber for measuring surface or near-surface dose.
**Related Terms:** Dosimetry, QA, Surface dose.
**Radiotherapy Example:** Measuring skin dose in chest wall irradiation.

**122. Peak-to-Valley Dose Ratio:** Ratio of maximum to minimum dose in a spatially modulated radiation field.
**Related Terms:** Microbeam therapy, Dose uniformity, QA.
**Radiotherapy Example:** Evaluating dose uniformity in preclinical microbeam therapy.

**123. Photon Beam Attenuation Coefficient:** Measure of photon absorption per unit distance in a material.
**Related Terms:** Dosimetry, LINAC, Shielding.
**Radiotherapy Example:** Calculating tissue attenuation for breast photon therapy.

**124. Photon Dose Linearization:** Correcting non-linear dose response in photon detectors.
**Related Terms:** Dosimetry, Calibration, QA.
**Radiotherapy Example:** Linearizing dose readings from film for IMRT QA.

**125. Photon Energy Calibration Phantom:** Phantom used to calibrate photon beam energy.
**Related Terms:** QA, Dosimetry, LINAC.
**Radiotherapy Example:** Calibrating a 6 MV photon beam using a water phantom.

**126. Photon Fluence Mapping:** Mapping photon intensity across the treatment field.
**Related Terms:** Dosimetry, IMRT QA, Beam profiling.
**Radiotherapy Example:** Measuring photon fluence for head-and-neck IMRT plan verification.

**127. Photon Scatter Factor:** Correction factor accounting for scattered photons in dose calculation.
**Related Terms:** Scatter, Dosimetry, QA.
**Radiotherapy Example:** Adjusting patient dose calculations for breast tangential fields.

128. **Photon Transmission Factor:** Fraction of photons transmitted through a material.
**Related Terms:** Attenuation, Shielding, Dosimetry.
**Radiotherapy Example:** Measuring transmission through lead shielding for LINAC room design.

129. **Photon Beam Penetration Depth:** Depth in tissue at which photon dose reaches a defined value.
**Related Terms:** Dosimetry, Beam energy, Tissue attenuation.
**Radiotherapy Example:** Determining depth of 6 MV photon beam in lung tissue.

130. **Photon Dose Rate Monitoring:** Measuring the rate at which dose is delivered by a photon beam.
**Related Terms:** LINAC, Dosimetry, QA.
**Radiotherapy Example:** Monitoring dose rate during stereotactic radiotherapy.

131. **Photon Beam Output Factor:** Factor describing variation in beam output with field size.
**Related Terms:** Dosimetry, LINAC calibration, QA.
**Radiotherapy Example:** Adjusting IMRT fields for photon output variation.

132. **Photon Beam Flatness Correction:** Correcting non-uniformity in photon beam intensity across the field.
**Related Terms:** Beam profile, QA, Dosimetry.
**Radiotherapy Example:** Flattening 6 MV photon field for breast treatment.

133. **Photon Attenuation Curve:** Graph showing photon attenuation as a function of depth in tissue.
**Related Terms:** Dosimetry, Beam attenuation, QA.
**Radiotherapy Example:** Using curve to calculate dose for mediastinal fields.

134. **Photon Field Homogeneity:** Uniformity of dose across the radiation field.
**Related Terms:** Beam flatness, QA, Dosimetry.
**Radiotherapy Example:** Ensuring uniform dose across lung tumor fields.

135. **Photon Beam Quality Index:** Measure of photon beam penetration and energy characteristics.
**Related Terms:** Beam energy, QA, Dosimetry.
**Radiotherapy Example:** Calculating TPR20/10 for 6 MV LINAC beam.

136. **Photon Backscatter Factor:** Factor quantifying dose increase due to backscattered photons.
**Related Terms:** Dosimetry, QA, Photon scatter.
**Radiotherapy Example:** Correcting skin dose in tangential breast fields.

137. **Photon Energy Spectrum:** Distribution of photon energies in a beam.
**Related Terms:** Beam characterization, LINAC, QA.
**Radiotherapy Example:** Measuring energy spectrum of 10 MV photon beam for treatment planning.

138. **Photon Dose Distribution Modeling:** Predicting spatial distribution of photon dose in tissue.
**Related Terms:** TPS, Dose calculation, QA.
**Radiotherapy Example:** Modeling head-and-neck IMRT photon dose.

139. **Photon Scatter Modeling:** Simulating scattered photons in dose calculation.
**Related Terms:** TPS, Monte Carlo, Dose accuracy.
**Radiotherapy Example:** Accounting for scattered photons in lung SBRT plan.

140. **Photon Fluence Rate Measurement:** Measuring rate of photon flow per unit area.
**Related Terms:** Dosimetry, Beam output, QA.
**Radiotherapy Example:** Measuring photon fluence for stereotactic dose verification.

141. **Projection Imaging:** Basic 2D X-ray or gamma imaging of anatomical structures.
**Related Terms:** Radiography, Portal imaging, QA.
**Radiotherapy Example:** Using projection imaging to align head-and-neck tumor before treatment.

142. **Photon Counting CT:** CT imaging using detectors that count individual photons for higher resolution.
**Related Terms:** CT imaging, Dose optimization, High-resolution imaging.
**Radiotherapy Example:** Using photon-counting CT for precise lung tumor delineation.

143. **PET Phantom Calibration:** Using a phantom to calibrate PET scanner for accurate measurements.
**Related Terms:** QA, PET imaging, Dosimetry.
**Radiotherapy Example:** Calibrating PET scanner before quantitative tumor imaging.

144. **PET Image Reconstruction:** Computationally generating images from raw PET data.
**Related Terms:** PET, Reconstruction algorithms, QA.
**Radiotherapy Example:** Reconstructing FDG PET scan for brain tumor planning.

145. **PET Quantitative Dosimetry:** Using PET imaging to quantify radiation dose absorbed in tissues.
**Related Terms:** PET, Dosimetry, Radiotracer.
**Radiotherapy Example:** Assessing tumor uptake to guide dose painting in proton therapy.

146. **Portal Imaging Verification:** Using portal images to confirm field placement and geometry.
**Related Terms:** QA, IGRT, Dosimetry.
**Radiotherapy Example:** Verifying prostate field placement before IMRT.

147. **Pixel Sensitivity Mapping:** Mapping variations in detector pixel sensitivity for accurate dose measurement.
**Related Terms:** Detector calibration, Dosimetry, QA.
**Radiotherapy Example:** Calibrating flat-panel detector for IMRT QA.

148. **Pixel-Level Noise Reduction:** Reducing electronic or photon noise in detector pixels.
**Related Terms:** Image quality, QA, Signal processing.
**Radiotherapy Example:** Improving image clarity for portal dosimetry.

149. **Post-Treatment Imaging:** Imaging performed after therapy to assess response or setup.
**Related Terms:** Verification, QA, Response assessment.
**Radiotherapy Example:** CT scan after head-and-neck RT to check tumor regression.

150. **Pre-Treatment CT Simulation:** CT imaging to simulate patient positioning before radiation delivery.
**Related Terms:** Treatment planning, IGRT, Immobilization.
**Radiotherapy Example:** CT simulation of thoracic tumor with immobilization mask.

**Great! Here's P151–P200 in the same | Related Terms | Radiotherapy Example format:**

151. **Perfusion PET Imaging:** PET imaging to assess blood flow in tissues.
**Related Terms:** PET, Tracer kinetics, Functional imaging.
**Radiotherapy Example:** Evaluating tumor perfusion to guide dose painting in liver cancer.

152. **Planar Scintigraphy Dosimetry:** Measuring radiation dose using planar scintigraphy images.
**Related Terms:** Scintigraphy, Dosimetry, QA.
**Radiotherapy Example:** Measuring dose delivered during thyroid radioiodine therapy.

153. **Photon Attenuation Correction:** Correcting imaging or dosimetry for photon absorption in tissue.
**Related Terms:** Attenuation, PET/CT, Dose calculation.
**Radiotherapy Example:** Correcting PET images for attenuation in thoracic tumors.

154. **Photon Scatter Correction Imaging:** Adjusting imaging data to account for scattered photons.
**Related Terms:** Scatter, Dosimetry, QA.
**Radiotherapy Example:** Scatter correction in SPECT imaging for cardiac perfusion.

155. **Optical Imaging in Radiation Therapy:** Using visible or near-infrared light to visualize tissue or treatment fields.
**Related Terms:** Optical dosimetry, Surface imaging, QA.
**Radiotherapy Example:** Surface-guided radiation therapy (SGRT) for breast cancer setup.

156. **Organ-Specific Dose Mapping:** Mapping radiation dose to specific organs for safety assessment.
**Related Terms:** Dosimetry, Organs at risk, Treatment planning.
**Radiotherapy Example:** Mapping dose to kidneys during abdominal proton therapy.

157. **Onboard Imaging:** Imaging integrated into the treatment machine to verify patient setup.
**Related Terms:** IGRT, Cone-beam CT, QA.
**Radiotherapy Example:** Using onboard CBCT to align lung tumor before treatment.

158. **Orthogonal Imaging:** Imaging at two perpendicular angles for accurate localization.
**Related Terms:** IGRT, Portal imaging, QA.
**Radiotherapy Example:** Using orthogonal X-rays to verify spinal tumor alignment.

159. **Oblique Angle Imaging:** Imaging at non-standard angles to better visualize target or anatomy.
**Related Terms:** IGRT, Portal imaging, QA.
**Radiotherapy Example:** Oblique X-ray to check prostate fiducial markers.

160. **Oncologic Imaging Review:** Reviewing imaging studies for tumor assessment and treatment planning.
**Related Terms:** Radiology, Contouring, QA.
**Radiotherapy Example:** Reviewing MRI and PET scans for head-and-neck tumor delineation.

161. **Positron Range Imaging:** Imaging that accounts for the distance positrons travel before annihilation.
**Related Terms:** PET, Dosimetry, Range correction.
**Radiotherapy Example:** Adjusting PET dose maps in proton therapy planning.

162. **Positron Lifetime Spectroscopy:** Measuring decay time of positrons to assess material or tissue properties.
**Related Terms:** PET, Positron physics, Dosimetry.
**Radiotherapy Example:** Research imaging for tumor microenvironment assessment.

163. **Positron-Emission-Based Dosimetry:** Using positron emission data to estimate radiation dose.
**Related Terms:** PET, Dosimetry, Radiotracers.
**Radiotherapy Example:** Evaluating dose distribution in radioisotope therapy.

164. **Proton Activation Analysis:** Using proton-induced nuclear reactions to analyze material composition.
**Related Terms:** Proton therapy, Nuclear physics, QA.
**Radiotherapy Example:** Testing beamline materials for proton-induced activation.

165. **Proton-Induced X-ray Emission:** X-ray emission caused by proton interactions with matter.
**Related Terms:** PIXE, Dosimetry, Proton therapy.
**Radiotherapy Example:** Detecting trace elements in tissue samples exposed to proton beams.

166. **Proton Radiography:** Imaging technique using proton beams for high-resolution anatomical imaging.
**Related Terms:** Proton therapy, Imaging, Range verification.
**Radiotherapy Example:** Proton radiography to verify bone tumor location before treatment.

167. **Proton Radiolysis:** Chemical decomposition of substances by proton irradiation.
**Related Terms:** Proton therapy, Radiation chemistry, QA.
**Radiotherapy Example:** Studying water radiolysis in tumor microenvironment research.

168. **Proton Therapy Radioisotope Tracing:** Using radioisotopes to trace proton therapy dose distribution.
**Related Terms:** Proton therapy, PET, Dosimetry.
**Radiotherapy Example:** PET imaging to confirm proton dose deposition in liver tumor.

169. **Photonuclear Cross-Section:** Probability of photon-induced nuclear reaction in a material.
**Related Terms:** Photon therapy, Nuclear physics, Dosimetry.
**Radiotherapy Example:** Calculating neutron production in high-energy photon beams.

170. **Photonuclear Activation:** Activation of nuclei due to photon interactions.
**Related Terms:** Photon therapy, QA, Dosimetry.
**Radiotherapy Example:** Assessing secondary neutron dose from 18 MV photon beam.

171. **Photoneutron Dose Assessment:** Measuring dose from neutrons produced by photon interactions.
**Related Terms:** Photon therapy, Secondary dose, Dosimetry.
**Radiotherapy Example:** Evaluating neutron exposure in head-and-neck radiotherapy with high-energy photons.

172. **Photoneutron Yield Measurement:** Quantifying neutrons produced per photon interaction.
**Related Terms:** Photon therapy, Dosimetry, QA.
**Radiotherapy Example:** Measuring neutron yield from 15 MV LINAC beam.

173. **Photodisintegration:** Nuclear reaction where a photon causes a nucleus to split.
**Related Terms:** Photonuclear reactions, QA, Dosimetry.
**Radiotherapy Example:** Modeling photodisintegration effects in high-energy photon therapy.

174. **Proton Magnetic Resonance:** Imaging using proton spin properties in magnetic fields (MRI).
**Related Terms:** MRI, Imaging, Soft tissue contrast.
**Radiotherapy Example:** Using MRI for brain tumor contouring in planning.

175. **Proton Capture Gamma Spectroscopy:** Measuring gamma rays emitted after proton capture reactions.
**Related Terms:** Proton therapy, QA, Nuclear physics.
**Radiotherapy Example:** Verifying beam-induced activation in experimental therapy.

176. **Proton Therapy Residual Activity:** Remaining radioactivity in tissue or materials post-proton therapy.
**Related Terms:** QA, Proton therapy, Radiation safety.
**Radiotherapy Example:** Assessing residual radioactivity in treated spinal vertebrae.

177. **Proton Beam Induced Radioisotope Production:** Production of isotopes in materials exposed to proton beams.
**Related Terms:** Proton therapy, QA, Radioisotope.
**Radiotherapy Example:** Measuring activation in beamline components.

178. **Proton Therapy Secondary Particle Assessment:** Evaluating secondary particles (neutrons, photons) generated by therapy.
**Related Terms:** Proton therapy, Dosimetry, Safety.
**Radiotherapy Example:** Assessing neutron dose to nearby organs in pediatric proton therapy.

179. **Proton Therapy Beam-Induced Radioactivity:** Radiation produced in tissue/material due to proton interactions.
**Related Terms:** Residual activity, Secondary particles, QA.
**Radiotherapy Example:** Mapping induced activity in liver proton therapy.

180. **Proton Therapy Shielding Assessment:** Evaluating required shielding for proton therapy rooms and equipment.
**Related Terms:** Radiation protection, QA, Safety.
**Radiotherapy Example:** Calculating concrete thickness for pediatric proton therapy bunker.

181. **Protective Shielding Thickness:** Thickness of material needed to reduce radiation to safe levels.
**Related Terms:** Shielding, Radiation safety, QA.
**Radiotherapy Example:** Designing lead shielding for LINAC control room.

182. **Protective Lead Barrier:** Lead barrier used to protect staff from scatter radiation.
**Related Terms:** Radiation protection, Shielding, QA.
**Radiotherapy Example:** Using lead screens in photon therapy control room.

183. **Protective Concrete Barrier:** Concrete wall designed to absorb high-energy radiation.
**Related Terms:** Radiation shielding, Safety, QA.
**Radiotherapy Example:** Concrete wall around high-energy LINAC vault.

184. **Protective Glass Shielding:** Leaded glass used to allow observation while blocking radiation.
**Related Terms:** Radiation protection, Shielding, QA.
**Radiotherapy Example:** Viewing patient during treatment through leaded glass window.

185. **Protective Room Design:** Designing rooms with barriers and layout for safe radiation use.
**Related Terms:** Shielding, QA, Safety.
**Radiotherapy Example:** LINAC vault with maze entry and shielding calculations.

186. **Protective Distance Determination:** Calculating minimum safe distance from radiation sources.
**Related Terms:** Radiation safety, Shielding, QA.
**Radiotherapy Example:** Defining safe zone around proton therapy gantry.

187. **Protective Material Density:** Density of materials used for shielding effectiveness.
**Related Terms:** Lead, Concrete, Shielding.
**Radiotherapy Example:** Choosing 11 $g/cm^3$ lead for photon therapy barrier.

188. **Personal Exposure Tracking:** Monitoring cumulative radiation dose for individual staff.
**Related Terms:** Dosimetry, TLD, QA.
**Radiotherapy Example:** Using TLD badges to track radiographer dose.

189. **Public Exposure Limit Assessment:** Ensuring radiation levels for the public do not exceed regulatory limits.
**Related Terms:** ALARA, Safety, QA.
**Radiotherapy Example:** Calculating dose outside proton therapy facility walls.

190. **Post-Irradiation Monitoring:** Checking radiation levels after therapy or accidental exposure.
**Related Terms:** QA, Safety, Dosimetry.
**Radiotherapy Example:** Measuring residual activity after radionuclide therapy.

191. **Pulse Radiation Safety Assessment:** Evaluating safety for pulsed radiation sources.
**Related Terms:** QA, LINAC, ALARA.
**Radiotherapy Example:** Safety assessment for pulsed electron beams in research.

192. **Point Source Exposure Calculation:** Estimating radiation dose from a localized source.
**Related Terms:** Dosimetry, QA, Shielding.
**Radiotherapy Example:** Calculating exposure from an HDR brachytherapy source.

193. **Patient Radiation Shielding:** Protecting non-target tissues during therapy.
**Related Terms:** Shielding, QA, Organs at risk.
**Radiotherapy Example:** Using lead blocks to shield healthy breast tissue.

194. **Pre-Procedure Safety Check:** Checking equipment and environment before therapy.
**Related Terms:** QA, Safety protocol, LINAC.
**Radiotherapy Example:** Verifying machine calibration before HDR brachytherapy.

195. **Protocol-Based Radiation Safety:** Using defined protocols to ensure safe radiation delivery.
**Related Terms:** QA, Safety, ALARA.
**Radiotherapy Example:** Following safety protocols in proton therapy vault.

196. **Protective Lead Apron Calibration:** Ensuring lead aprons provide expected shielding.
**Related Terms:** QA, PPE, Dosimetry.
**Radiotherapy Example:** Checking attenuation of lead apron used in fluoroscopy.

197. **Protective Barrier Effectiveness:** Testing how well shielding protects against radiation.
**Related Terms:** QA, Shielding, Safety.
**Radiotherapy Example:** Measuring dose beyond concrete walls in LINAC vault.

198. **Personal Dosimetry Logging:** Recording cumulative radiation dose for personnel.
**Related Terms:** Dosimeter, QA, Safety.
**Radiotherapy Example:** Logging daily TLD readings for staff in radiotherapy department.

199. **Peripheral Dose Estimation:** Estimating dose received by tissues outside target volume.
**Related Terms:** Dose calculation, QA, ALARA.
**Radiotherapy Example:** Estimating dose to thyroid during breast RT.

200. **Post-Accident Contamination Survey:** Surveying area for radioactive contamination after an incident.
**Related Terms:** QA, Safety, ALARA.
**Radiotherapy Example:** Measuring contamination after spill of radiopharmaceutical in nuclear medicine department.

201. **Passive Scattering Proton Therapy:** Proton therapy technique using scattering devices to spread the beam.
**Related Terms:** Proton therapy, Beam shaping, Dosimetry.
**Radiotherapy Example:** Treating pediatric brain tumors with uniform proton field distribution.

202. **Photon Arc Therapy:** Arc-based photon therapy delivering dose while rotating around the patient.
**Related Terms:** VMAT, IMRT, Dose modulation.
**Radiotherapy Example:** Delivering rotational IMRT to prostate cancer.

203. **Photon Beam Modulation:** Adjusting intensity of photon beams to conform dose to tumor shape.
**Related Terms:** IMRT, VMAT, Dose painting.
**Radiotherapy Example:** Modulating photons to spare healthy lung tissue.

204. **Photon Therapy Replanning:** Adjusting a photon therapy plan during treatment based on anatomy changes.
**Related Terms:** Adaptive radiotherapy, QA, Imaging.
**Radiotherapy Example:** Replanning head-and-neck RT after tumor shrinkage.

205. **Photon Beam Spot Scanning:** Delivering photon dose spot-by-spot for precise distribution.
**Related Terms:** IMRT, VMAT, Dose delivery.
**Radiotherapy Example:** Using pencil beam scanning in stereotactic radiosurgery.

206. **Photon Therapy Dose Painting:** Delivering heterogeneous photon dose based on tumor characteristics.
**Related Terms:** IMRT, Dose escalation, PET-guided therapy.
**Radiotherapy Example:** Increasing dose to hypoxic tumor regions in lung cancer.

207. **Partial Breast Irradiation:** Radiotherapy targeting only part of the breast, not the whole organ.
**Related Terms:** APBI, Hypofractionation, IMRT.
**Radiotherapy Example:** Treating early-stage breast cancer with limited field irradiation.

208. **Partial Organ Irradiation:** Irradiating only part of an organ to minimize normal tissue exposure.
**Related Terms:** Conformal RT, IMRT, SBRT.
**Radiotherapy Example:** Treating liver metastases while sparing healthy liver tissue.

209. **Plan Adaptation:** Modifying treatment plan based on imaging or response during therapy.
**Related Terms:** Adaptive RT, QA, IGRT.
**Radiotherapy Example:** Adjusting head-and-neck RT plan after tumor shrinkage.

210. **Precision Radiotherapy:** High-accuracy delivery of radiation to tumor while sparing healthy tissue.
**Related Terms:** IMRT, SBRT, IGRT.
**Radiotherapy Example:** SBRT for small lung nodules.

211. **Pulsed Proton Therapy:** Delivering proton therapy in short pulses for enhanced control.
**Related Terms:** Proton therapy, Beam modulation, QA.
**Radiotherapy Example:** Pulsed delivery for pediatric brain tumors.

212. **Patient-Specific Proton Collimator:** Customized collimator for shaping proton beam to patient anatomy.
**Related Terms:** Proton therapy, Beam shaping, QA.
**Radiotherapy Example:** Collimator designed for craniospinal irradiation.

213. **Proton Arc Modulated Therapy:** Arc-based proton therapy with modulation of beam intensity.**Related Terms:** Proton therapy, IMPT, Dose painting.
**Radiotherapy Example:** Treating large head-and-neck tumors using arc modulation.

214. **Proton Beamlet Optimization:** Optimizing small beamlets for precise dose delivery.
**Related Terms:** Spot scanning, IMPT, QA.
**Radiotherapy Example:** Optimizing proton spots for pediatric brain tumor.

215. **Proton Beamlet Mapping:** Mapping distribution of small proton beamlets in treatment volume.
**Related Terms:** IMPT, QA, Dose verification.
**Radiotherapy Example:** Ensuring uniform dose delivery in proton therapy for liver metastases.

216. **Proton Spot Repositioning:** Adjusting spot positions to match tumor movement.
**Related Terms:** Motion management, IMPT, QA.
**Radiotherapy Example:** Repositioning spots during gated proton therapy for lung tumor.

217. **Proton Therapy Dynamic Delivery:** Real-time modulation of proton beam during treatment.
**Related Terms:** IMPT, Adaptive therapy, QA.
**Radiotherapy Example:** Delivering dose while accounting for respiratory motion.

218. **Proton Therapy Gating:** Synchronizing proton delivery with patient's breathing.
**Related Terms:** Motion management, Respiratory gating, QA.
**Radiotherapy Example:** Gated delivery for lung SBRT with proton therapy.

219. **Proton Therapy Breath-Hold Technique:** Delivering proton dose while patient holds breath to reduce motion.
**Related Terms:** Motion mitigation, IGRT, QA.
**Radiotherapy Example:** Deep-inspiration breath-hold for left-sided breast cancer proton therapy.

220. **Proton Therapy Adaptive Replanning:** Replanning proton therapy based on tumor or anatomical changes.
**Related Terms:** Adaptive therapy, IGRT, QA.
**Radiotherapy Example:** Adjusting plan mid-treatment for head-and-neck tumors.

221. **Photon Energy Verification:** Confirming the energy of photon beam matches plan specifications.
**Related Terms:** QA, LINAC, Dosimetry.
**Radiotherapy Example:** Verifying 6 MV photon beam energy before treatment.

222. **Photon Beam Output Calibration:** Ensuring photon beam delivers the planned dose accurately.**Related Terms:** QA, Dosimetry, LINAC.
**Radiotherapy Example:** Calibrating 10 MV beam using ionization chamber.

223. **Photon Beam Dosimeter Array:** Array of detectors used to measure photon dose distribution.
**Related Terms:** QA, Dosimetry, LINAC.
**Radiotherapy Example:** Verifying IMRT plan delivery using 2D dosimeter array.

224. **Photon Fluence Distribution:** Spatial distribution of photon intensity across treatment field.
**Related Terms:** IMRT, QA, Dose calculation.
**Radiotherapy Example:** Mapping fluence for prostate IMRT plan verification.

225. **Photon Dose Profile:** Variation of dose along a specific axis of photon beam.
**Related Terms:** QA, Dosimetry, LINAC.
**Radiotherapy Example:** Measuring flatness of 6 MV photon beam.

226. **Photon Scatter Analysis:** Evaluating impact of scattered photons on dose distribution.
**Related Terms:** Dosimetry, QA, Monte Carlo simulation.
**Radiotherapy Example:** Analyzing scatter contribution for head-and-neck IMRT.

227. **Photon Beam Penetration Measurement:** Measuring depth dose distribution of photon beam.
**Related Terms:** Dosimetry, QA, LINAC.
**Radiotherapy Example:** Verifying 10 MV photon depth-dose for lung treatment.

228. **Photon Beam Homogeneity Verification:** Ensuring uniformity of photon beam across the field.
**Related Terms:** QA, Dosimetry, LINAC.
**Radiotherapy Example:** Checking flatness of 6 MV field before patient treatment.

229. **Photon Dose Linearization Correction:** Correcting non-linear dose response in detectors.
**Related Terms:** Dosimetry, QA, Detector calibration.
**Radiotherapy Example:** Correcting film dosimetry for high-dose regions in IMRT.

230. **Photon Transmission Measurement:** Measuring fraction of photons passing through shielding or patient.
**Related Terms:** QA, Dosimetry, Shielding.
**Radiotherapy Example:** Assessing dose behind patient for room safety.

231. **Photodiode Dosimetry:** Using photodiodes to measure radiation dose.
**Related Terms:** QA, Dosimetry, Detector.
**Radiotherapy Example:** Measuring skin dose during electron therapy.

232. **Photomultiplier Tube Dosimetry:** Using PMTs to measure scintillation from radiation.
**Related Terms:** QA, Dosimetry, Detector.
**Radiotherapy Example:** Measuring dose distribution with scintillation detector.

233. **Photon Fluence Map Calibration:** Calibrating photon fluence map for accurate dose delivery.
**Related Terms:** QA, Dosimetry, LINAC.
**Radiotherapy Example:** Verifying fluence map for VMAT prostate plan.

234. **Photon Dose Gradient Analysis:** Evaluating steepness of dose changes across beam.
**Related Terms:** QA, IMRT, Dosimetry.
**Radiotherapy Example:** Checking dose gradient near spinal cord in head-and-neck IMRT.

235. **Photon Scattering Correction Factor:** Factor applied to account for scattered photons in dose calculation.
**Related Terms:** Dosimetry, QA, Monte Carlo simulation.
**Radiotherapy Example:** Applying correction in lung IMRT plan.

236. **Photon Beam Output Stability:** Monitoring consistency of photon beam output over time.
**Related Terms:** QA, LINAC, Dosimetry.
**Radiotherapy Example:** Weekly QA of 6 MV photon beam output.

237. **Photon Detector Efficiency:** Fraction of incident photons correctly detected by device.
**Related Terms:** Dosimetry, QA, Detector calibration.
**Radiotherapy Example:** Checking efficiency of ion chamber array for IMRT QA.

238. **Photon Energy Spectrum Measurement:** Measuring distribution of photon energies in beam.
**Related Terms:** QA, Dosimetry, LINAC.
**Radiotherapy Example:** Assessing energy spectrum for 10 MV photons in SBRT.

239. **Photon Attenuation Curve Analysis:** Analyzing photon dose reduction with depth or material.
**Related Terms:** Dosimetry, QA, Shielding.
**Radiotherapy Example:** Measuring attenuation through phantom for QA.

240. **Photon Dose Rate Calibration:** Ensuring photon dose is delivered at correct rate.
**Related Terms:** QA, Dosimetry, LINAC.
**Radiotherapy Example:** Calibrating 6 MV beam dose rate before treatment.

241. **PET/CT Fusion QA:** Quality assurance for accurate fusion of PET and CT images.
**Related Terms:** PET, CT, Imaging QA.
**Radiotherapy Example:** Verifying alignment for PET-guided target delineation.

242. **PET Image Motion Correction:** Correcting PET images for patient or organ motion.
**Related Terms:** Motion management, PET, QA.
**Radiotherapy Example:** Respiratory gating correction for lung PET.

243. **PET Radiotracer Uptake Analysis:** Quantifying radiotracer concentration in tissues
**Related Terms:** PET, SUV, Dosimetry.
**Radiotherapy Example:** Assessing metabolic activity of tumor pre-RT.

244. **PET/CT Dose Optimization Protocol:** Protocols to minimize radiation dose during PET/CT
**Related Terms:** ALARA, Imaging QA, Dose reduction.
**Radiotherapy Example:** Reducing CT dose for pediatric PET/CT.

245. **Photon-Counting CT Dosimetry:** Measuring dose in CT using photon-counting detectors.
**Related Terms:** CT, Dosimetry, QA.
**Radiotherapy Example:** Assessing patient dose in high-resolution CT scan.

246. **Projection Radiography QA:** QA for standard X-ray imaging systems.
**Related Terms:** Imaging, QA, Dosimetry.
**Radiotherapy Example:** Monthly QA for planar X-ray imaging.

247. **Pre-Treatment Imaging Verification:** Imaging before treatment to verify patient setup.
**Related Terms:** IGRT, QA, Positioning.
**Radiotherapy Example:** CBCT to verify prostate patient position.

248. **Portal Imaging QA:** Quality assurance for portal imaging devices.
**Related Terms:** LINAC, IGRT, QA.
**Radiotherapy Example:** Verifying portal imaging system for breast IMRT.

249. **Pixel Sensitivity Correction:** Correcting detector pixel response variations in imaging.
**Related Terms:** Detector QA, Imaging, Dosimetry.
**Radiotherapy Example:** Correcting EPID pixel response for IMRT QA.

250. **Post-Treatment Imaging Assessment:** Imaging after therapy to evaluate tumor response.
**Related Terms:** MRI, PET, QA.
**Radiotherapy Example:** PET/CT 6 weeks after SBRT for lung tumor.

251. **Perfusion SPECT Imaging:** Imaging blood flow in organs using SPECT tracers.
**Related Terms:** Nuclear medicine, SPECT, Dosimetry.
**Radiotherapy Example:** Assessing lung perfusion before thoracic RT to minimize dose to high-functioning regions.

252. **Pulmonary PET Imaging:** PET imaging to evaluate lung metabolism or perfusion.
**Related Terms:** PET, Lung imaging, Functional imaging.
**Radiotherapy Example:** Identifying high-uptake lung regions to avoid during RT planning.

253. **Proton Radiography QA:** Quality assurance for proton-based imaging systems.
**Related Terms:** Proton imaging, QA, Dosimetry.
**Radiotherapy Example:** Verifying imaging accuracy for proton therapy patient setup.

254. **Positron Annihilation Tomography:** Imaging based on detection of positron-electron annihilation events.
**Related Terms:** PET, Radiotracer, Nuclear imaging.|
**Radiotherapy Example:** PET imaging for staging head-and-neck cancer.

255. **Positron Lifetime Spectroscopy:** Measuring positron decay lifetime to study tissue characteristics.
**Related Terms:** PET, Nuclear imaging, Dosimetry.
**Radiotherapy Example:** Investigating tumor hypoxia using positron lifetime.

256. **Positron Emission-Based Imaging:** Imaging using radioactive positron-emitting tracers.
**Related Terms:** PET, Radiotracer, Functional imaging.
**Radiotherapy Example:** FDG-PET imaging for lung cancer target delineation.

257. **Proton Activation Measurement:** Measuring radioactivity induced in materials by proton irradiation.
**Related Terms:** Proton therapy, QA, Dosimetry.
**Radiotherapy Example:** Measuring activation of phantom materials post-proton therapy.

258. **Proton-Induced Gamma Emission:** Emission of gamma rays due to proton interactions with nuclei.
**Related Terms:** Proton therapy, QA, Imaging.
**Radiotherapy Example:** Using gamma emissions to verify proton range in tissues.

259. **Proton Radiolysis Analysis:** Studying chemical changes in tissues induced by protons.
**Related Terms:** Proton therapy, Radiochemistry, QA.
**Radiotherapy Example:** Investigating water radiolysis during proton therapy for research.

260. **Proton Therapy Radioisotope Tracing:** Using radioisotopes to trace proton therapy dose distribution.
**Related Terms:** Proton therapy, Dosimetry, Imaging.
**Radiotherapy Example:** PET-based tracing of proton therapy distribution in liver.

261. **Proton Therapy Induced Activity:** Residual radioactivity in tissues or materials post-proton therapy.
**Related Terms:** Proton therapy, QA, Radioprotection.
**Radiotherapy Example:** Measuring residual activity in phantom after proton irradiation.

262. **Photonuclear Reaction Analysis:** Studying nuclear reactions caused by high-energy photons.
**Related Terms:** Photon therapy, Nuclear physics, QA.
**Radiotherapy Example:** Assessing photonuclear dose contributions in high-energy LINAC beams.

263. **Photonuclear Dose Estimation:** Estimating radiation dose from photon-induced nuclear reactions.
**Related Terms:** Photon therapy, Dosimetry, QA.
**Radiotherapy Example:** Calculating dose to surrounding tissue from photonuclear neutrons in 18 MV beams.

264. **Photoneutron Production Assessment:** Measuring neutrons produced by high-energy photon beams.
**Related Terms:** Photon therapy, Neutron dosimetry, QA.
**Radiotherapy Example:** Assessing neutron dose in head-and-neck treatments using 15 MV photons.

265. **Photodisintegration Cross-Section:** Probability of nucleus splitting after photon absorption.
**Related Terms:** Photonuclear reactions, Dosimetry, Nuclear physics.
**Radiotherapy Example:** Evaluating neutron production from high-energy photon therapy beams.

266. **Proton Capture Analysis:** Studying capture of protons by nuclei for dosimetry or imaging.
**Related Terms:** Proton therapy, Nuclear reactions, QA.
**Radiotherapy Example:** Proton capture analysis to optimize isotope production in therapy.

267. **Proton Therapy Radioisotope Safety:** Safety protocols for handling radioisotopes used or produced in proton therapy.
**Related Terms:** QA, Radioprotection, Proton therapy.
**Radiotherapy Example:** Ensuring safe handling of PET tracers generated during proton therapy.

268. **Proton Therapy Secondary Particle Dose:** Dose contribution from secondary particles (neutrons, gammas) in proton therapy.
**Related Terms:** Proton therapy, Dosimetry, QA.
**Radiotherapy Example:** Calculating neutron dose outside target region in proton therapy.

269. **Proton Therapy Induced Neutron Flux:** Measurement of neutron flux generated by proton therapy.
**Related Terms:** Proton therapy, Dosimetry, QA.
**Radiotherapy Example:** Evaluating neutron flux for staff safety during pediatric proton therapy.

270. **Proton Therapy Shielding Design:** Designing barriers to protect against proton and secondary radiation
**Related Terms:** Radioprotection, QA, Proton therapy.
**Radiotherapy Example:** Designing concrete shielding for a proton therapy treatment room.

271. **Proton Therapy Induced Gamma:** Gamma radiation produced by proton interactions in tissues.
**Related Terms:** Proton therapy, Dosimetry, QA.
**Radiotherapy Example:** Monitoring gamma dose during head-and-neck proton therapy.

272. **Proton Therapy Residual Radioactivity Mapping:** Mapping remaining radioactivity post-proton therapy.
**Related Terms:** Proton therapy, QA, Dosimetry.
**Radiotherapy Example:** Using imaging to evaluate residual activity in phantom studies.

273. **Proton Therapy Secondary Radiation Assessment:** Evaluating secondary radiation (neutrons, gammas) from proton therapy.|
**Related Terms:** Proton therapy, QA, Dosimetry.
**Radiotherapy Example:** Assessing neutron dose around treatment vault.

274. **Protective Barrier Optimization:** Optimizing shielding barriers for maximum protection with minimal material.
**Related Terms:** Radiation safety, Shielding, QA.
**Radiotherapy Example:** Designing wall thickness for proton therapy vault.

275. **Protective Apron Assessment:** Evaluating lead aprons for effectiveness in reducing exposure.
**Related Terms:** PPE, Dosimetry, Radiation safety.
**Radiotherapy Example:** Testing aprons used during mobile X-ray or CT procedures.

276. **Protective Room Shielding Verification:** Ensuring shielding in radiation rooms meets safety standards.
**Related Terms:** QA, Shielding, Radiation protection.
**Radiotherapy Example:** Verifying concrete wall thickness in LINAC room.

277. **Protective Glass Verification:** Testing leaded glass for shielding effectiveness.
**Related Terms:** PPE, QA, Radiation protection.
**Radiotherapy Example:** Ensuring viewing windows reduce exposure for staff.

278. **Personal Dosimeter QA:** Quality assurance for individual radiation monitoring devices.
**Related Terms:** Dosimetry, QA, Radiation safety.
**Radiotherapy Example:** Checking badges used by staff for accurate dose measurement.

279. **Public Dose Assessment Protocol:** Protocol to ensure public exposure remains within limits.
**Related Terms:** Radiation safety, Dosimetry, Shielding.
**Radiotherapy Example:** Evaluating radiation outside treatment vault for public safety.

280. **Post-Accident Radiation Mapping:** Mapping radiation levels after incidents.
**Related Terms:** Radiation safety, Emergency response, QA.
**Radiotherapy Example:** Surveying vault after accidental overexposure.

281. **Point Source Shielding Verification:** Ensuring shielding around point sources meets safety standards.
**Related Terms:** QA, Shielding, Dosimetry.
**Radiotherapy Example:** Checking lead container for radioactive seed storage.

282. **Peripheral Tissue Dose Assessment:** Measuring dose received by tissues outside treatment target.
**Related Terms:** Dosimetry, QA, Normal tissue protection.
**Radiotherapy Example:** Evaluating dose to contralateral breast in breast RT.

283. **Patient Radiation Protection QA:** QA to ensure patient is protected from unnecessary exposure.
**Related Terms:** Dosimetry, QA, Shielding.
**Radiotherapy Example:** Verifying lead shields in eye treatments.

284. **Pre-Procedural Radiation Safety QA:** QA before procedures to ensure safe conditions.
**Related Terms:** Radiation safety, QA, Protocols.
**Radiotherapy Example:** Checking LINAC and patient setup before treatment.

285. **Pulse Radiation Dose Assessment:** Measuring dose from pulsed radiation sources.
**Related Terms:** Dosimetry, QA, LINAC.
**Radiotherapy Example:** Assessing dose per pulse in pulsed electron therapy.

286. **Protocol-Based Shielding Assessment:** Using protocols to evaluate shielding adequacy.
**Related Terms:** Radiation protection, QA, Shielding.
**Radiotherapy Example:** Evaluating vault shielding using NCRP standards.

287. **Protective Material Verification:** Confirming materials meet shielding requirements.
**Related Terms:** QA, Radiation protection, Shielding.
**Radiotherapy Example:** Testing lead bricks for vault construction.

288. **Protective Distance Measurement:** Measuring minimum safe distance from radiation source.
**Related Terms:** QA, Radiation safety, Shielding.
**Radiotherapy Example:** Determining safe distance around LINAC during operation.

289. **Protective Lead Barrier QA:** QA to ensure lead barriers provide expected protection.
**Related Terms:** QA, Radiation protection, Shielding.
**Radiotherapy Example:** Verifying lead walls in mobile imaging.

290. **Protective Concrete Barrier Design:** Designing concrete barriers to shield from high-energy radiation.
**Related Terms:** QA, Shielding, Radiation safety.
**Radiotherapy Example:** Concrete thickness for 15 MV photon vault.

291. **Protective Room QA:** QA to verify room shielding and safety standards.
**Related Terms:** QA, Radiation protection, Shielding.
**Radiotherapy Example:** Monthly survey of LINAC treatment room.

292. **Personal Radiation Logging Protocol:** Standardized logging of staff radiation exposure.
**Related Terms:** Dosimetry, QA, Safety.
**Radiotherapy Example:** Maintaining dose records for radiation therapists.

293. **Public Safety Zone Assessment:** Defining safe zones around radiation sources for public protection.
**Related Terms:** Radiation safety, Shielding, QA.
**Radiotherapy Example:** Evaluating exclusion zones around proton therapy vault.

294. **Proton Beam Energy Modulation:** Adjusting proton beam energy to control penetration depth.
**Related Terms:** Proton therapy, SOBP, Beam tuning.|
**Radiotherapy Example:** Modulating proton energy to cover entire tumor depth.

295. **Proton Beam Range Verification:** Confirming the actual penetration depth of the proton beam.
**Related Terms:** QA, Proton therapy, Dosimetry.
**Radiotherapy Example:** Using imaging phantoms to verify planned proton range.

296. **Proton Beam Conformation:** Shaping the proton beam to match tumor geometry.
**Related Terms:** Proton therapy, Beam shaping, Target coverage.
**Radiotherapy Example:** Conformal proton beam delivery to a brain tumor.

297. **Proton Therapy Motion Tracking:** Monitoring tumor motion during proton therapy.
**Related Terms:** IGRT, Respiratory gating, Motion management.
**Radiotherapy Example:** Tracking lung tumor motion during breathing cycles.

298. **Proton Therapy Image-Guided Adjustment:** Adjusting treatment based on real-time imaging.
**Related Terms:** IGRT, Proton therapy, QA.
**Radiotherapy Example:** Using CBCT to align spinal tumor before proton delivery.

299. **Proton Therapy Adaptive Margins:** Adjusting tumor margins during treatment based on response.
**Related Terms:** Adaptive therapy, Proton therapy, PTV.
**Radiotherapy Example:** Reducing margins as tumor shrinks mid-treatment.

300. **Proton Therapy Field Shaping:** Modifying the proton field to minimize dose to normal tissues.
**Related Terms:** Beam shaping, Conformal therapy, Proton therapy.
**Radiotherapy Example:** Using apertures or MLCs to shape proton beam around healthy tissue.

301. **Proton Therapy Arc Delivery:** Delivering proton beams in an arc around the patient for better dose distribution.
**Related Terms:** Arc therapy, Proton therapy, Dose optimization.
**Radiotherapy Example:** Treating complex head-and-neck tumors with proton arcs.

**302. Proton Therapy Beam Splitting:** Dividing a proton beam into multiple components to optimize dose distribution.
**Related Terms:** Multi-field optimization, Proton therapy, Beam modulation.
**Radiotherapy Example:** Splitting beam for simultaneous coverage of tumor and lymph nodes.

**303. Proton Therapy Spot Optimization:** Adjusting the position and weight of individual proton spots for optimal dose.
**Related Terms:** Spot scanning, Proton therapy, Dose painting.
**Radiotherapy Example:** Optimizing proton spot map for a heterogeneous tumor.

**304. Proton Therapy Multi-Field Delivery:** Using multiple proton fields to cover complex tumor volumes.
**Related Terms:** Multi-field optimization, Proton therapy, Beam planning.
**Radiotherapy Example:** Treating a sarcoma with multiple proton fields to spare normal tissue.

**305. Proton Therapy Fractionation Planning:** Planning the division of total dose into multiple fractions.
**Related Terms:** Fractionation, Proton therapy, Treatment planning.
**Radiotherapy Example:** Delivering 60 Gy in 30 fractions for prostate cancer.

**306. Proton Therapy Breath-Control Techniques:** Using breath-hold or respiratory gating to reduce tumor motion during treatment.
**Related Terms:** Motion management, IGRT, Proton therapy.
**Radiotherapy Example:** Deep inspiration breath-hold for left-sided breast cancer.

**307. Proton Therapy Motion Mitigation:** Strategies to minimize impact of patient or tumor motion on proton dose.
**Related Terms:** Respiratory gating, Motion tracking, Proton therapy.
**Radiotherapy Example:** Using real-time imaging to adjust proton beam during lung tumor motion.

**308. Proton Therapy Targeted Boost:** Delivering higher doses to specific sub-regions of the tumor.
**Related Terms:** Dose painting, Proton therapy, Boost planning.
**Radiotherapy Example:** Boosting hypoxic regions of a tumor identified by PET.

**309. Proton Therapy Conformal Avoidance:** Shaping proton fields to avoid critical organs.
**Related Terms:** Conformal therapy, Organs at risk, Proton therapy.
**Radiotherapy Example:** Avoiding spinal cord during vertebral tumor treatment.

**310. Proton Therapy Dynamic Collimation:** Adjusting collimators in real-time to conform to tumor shape.
**Related Terms:** Beam shaping, Proton therapy, MLC.
**Radiotherapy Example:** Dynamically shaping beam for irregular head-and-neck tumors.

**311. Proton Therapy Energy Layering:** Delivering proton dose in layers to match tumor depth.
**Related Terms:** SOBP, Proton therapy, Dose painting.
**Radiotherapy Example:** Layered energy delivery to cover a tumor with varying depth.

**312. Proton Therapy Beam Interruption Protocol:** Safety procedures for pausing proton beam during unexpected events.
**Related Terms:** QA, Safety, Proton therapy.
**Radiotherapy Example:** Automatic beam pause if patient moves out of alignment.

**313. Proton Therapy Verification Imaging:** Imaging to confirm proton dose delivery accuracy.
**Related Terms:** QA, IGRT, Proton therapy.
**Radiotherapy Example:** Using CBCT or proton radiography before treatment.

314. **Proton Beam Output Verification:** Checking that the delivered proton beam output matches planned dose.
**Related Terms:** QA, Dosimetry, Proton therapy.
**Radiotherapy Example:** Verifying 2 Gy per fraction delivery in phantom studies.

315. **Proton Dose Profile Measurement:** Measuring dose distribution across the proton beam field
**Related Terms:** Dosimetry, Proton therapy, QA.
**Radiotherapy Example:** Measuring Bragg peak and lateral dose spread in water phantom.

316. **Proton Dose Uniformity Analysis:** Assessing consistency of dose across treatment volume.
**Related Terms:** QA, Proton therapy, Homogeneity.
**Radiotherapy Example:** Ensuring uniform dose across prostate tumor.

317. **Proton Beam Energy Calibration:** Calibrating proton beam to deliver correct energy and range.
**Related Terms:** QA, Proton therapy, Dosimetry.
**Radiotherapy Example:** Verifying energy for cranial proton treatments.

318. **Proton Beamlet Dosimetry:** Measuring dose from individual proton beamlets in scanning therapy.
**Related Terms:** Spot scanning, Dosimetry, QA.
**Radiotherapy Example:** Verifying micro-beams in pencil beam scanning.

319. **Proton Dose Rate Monitoring:** Continuous measurement of proton beam dose rate.
**Related Terms:** QA, Dosimetry, Proton therapy.
**Radiotherapy Example:** Ensuring safe dose rate delivery during craniospinal proton therapy.

320. **Proton Fluence Mapping:** Mapping the spatial distribution of proton particles.
**Related Terms:** Beam monitoring, Proton therapy, Dosimetry.
**Radiotherapy Example:** Verifying uniform coverage across tumor field.

321. **Proton Scatter Assessment:** Measuring lateral spread of protons due to scattering.
**Related Terms:** QA, Proton therapy, Dose modeling.
**Radiotherapy Example:** Quantifying dose outside target due to scatter in water phantom.

322. **Proton Range Verification Imaging:** Imaging to confirm proton beam reaches intended depth.
**Related Terms:** QA, Proton therapy, Bragg peak.
**Radiotherapy Example:** Using prompt gamma imaging to confirm tumor coverage.

323. **Proton Transmission Factor Measurement:** Measuring fraction of protons passing through tissue or phantom.
**Related Terms:** Dosimetry, Proton therapy, QA.
**Radiotherapy Example:** Assessing beam attenuation through patient-equivalent phantom.

324. **Proton Beam Homogeneity:** Ensuring even dose distribution within the beam field.
**Related Terms:** QA, Dose uniformity, Proton therapy.
**Radiotherapy Example:** Checking uniformity across a spinal tumor field.

325. **Proton Beam Output Stability Monitoring:** Continuous verification of consistent proton beam output.
**Related Terms:** QA, Dosimetry, Proton therapy.
**Radiotherapy Example:** Daily checks on LINAC output in proton therapy.

326. **Proton Detector Calibration:** Calibrating detectors used for proton beam measurements.
**Related Terms:** Dosimetry, QA, Proton therapy.
**Radiotherapy Example:** Calibrating ionization chambers for pencil beam scanning.

327. **Proton Dosimeter Array Mapping:** Mapping dose using array of proton detectors.
**Related Terms:** Dosimetry, QA, Proton therapy.
**Radiotherapy Example:** Verifying spatial dose distribution in treatment plan.

328. **Proton Beam Gradient Analysis:** Studying variation of dose across the beam.
**Related Terms:** Dosimetry, QA, Proton therapy.
**Radiotherapy Example:** Measuring dose fall-off in Bragg peak region.

329. **Proton Dose Response Linearization:** Correcting non-linear dose response of detectors in proton therapy.
**Related Terms:** QA, Dosimetry, Proton therapy.
**Radiotherapy Example:** Ensuring accurate dose reading in high-dose regions.

330. **Proton Attenuation Correction:** Correcting for proton beam energy loss in tissues.
**Related Terms:** QA, Dosimetry, Treatment planning.
**Radiotherapy Example:** Adjusting planned dose for inhomogeneous tissue.

331. **Proton Secondary Particle Dosimetry:** Measuring dose from secondary particles produced by protons.
**Related Terms:** Neutrons, QA, Proton therapy.
**Radiotherapy Example:** Assessing neutron dose to organs at risk.

332. **Proton Spot Dose Verification:** Verifying dose delivered by individual proton spots.
**Related Terms:** Spot scanning, QA, Dosimetry.
**Radiotherapy Example:** Confirming spot-by-spot delivery matches plan.

333. **Proton Beam Delivery QA:** Overall quality assurance for proton beam delivery.
**Related Terms:** QA, Proton therapy, Dosimetry.
**Radiotherapy Example:** Monthly comprehensive QA for all beam parameters.

334. **Proton Radiography QA:** Quality assurance for imaging using proton beams.
**Related Terms:** QA, Proton therapy, Imaging.
**Radiotherapy Example:** Ensuring accurate imaging for range verification.

335. **PET/CT Dose Mapping:** Mapping radiation dose using PET/CT imaging.
**Related Terms:** Dosimetry, PET, CT, Imaging.
**Radiotherapy Example:** PET-based evaluation of dose distribution in head-and-neck cancer.

336. **Photon Imaging QA:** QA for photon-based imaging systems.
**Related Terms:** LINAC, IGRT, Imaging QA.
**Radiotherapy Example:** Daily check of CBCT imaging quality on LINAC.

337. **Portal Imaging Dose Verification:** Verifying delivered dose using portal images.
**Related Terms:** Portal imaging, QA, Dosimetry.
**Radiotherapy Example:** Confirming dose to tumor and surrounding tissue via portal images.

338. **PET Radiotracer Dosimetry:** Using PET radiotracers to measure dose distribution.
**Related Terms:** PET, Dosimetry, Radiotracer.
**Radiotherapy Example:** Measuring dose uptake in metabolically active tumor regions.

339. **Pre-Treatment Imaging QA:** QA of imaging before therapy to ensure accuracy.
**Related Terms:** IGRT, QA, Patient setup.
**Radiotherapy Example:** Verifying CBCT image quality before treatment fraction.

340. **Patient Position Verification Imaging:** Imaging to verify patient position before therapy.
**Related Terms:** IGRT, QA, Alignment.
**Radiotherapy Example:** CBCT verification for pelvic tumor alignment.

341. **Pixel Sensitivity Map Correction:** Correcting detector pixel sensitivity variations in imaging.
**Related Terms:** QA, Imaging, Calibration.
**Radiotherapy Example:** Correcting flat-panel detector response for CBCT.

342. **Perfusion PET Dosimetry:** Using perfusion PET to map dose distribution.
**Related Terms:** PET, Dosimetry, Functional imaging.
**Radiotherapy Example:** Mapping dose to hypoxic regions in lung tumors.

343. **Pulmonary Imaging QA:** QA for lung imaging systems.
**Related Terms:** QA, Perfusion, CT, PET.
**Radiotherapy Example:** Verifying SPECT/CT perfusion imaging before thoracic RT.

344. **Proton-Induced Radioisotope Mapping:** Mapping radioisotopes produced by proton interactions.
**Related Terms:** QA, Proton therapy, Imaging.
**Radiotherapy Example:** Evaluating residual activity distribution after proton therapy.

345. **Proton Therapy Activation Monitoring:** Monitoring activation of materials and tissues during/after proton therapy.
**Related Terms:** QA, Proton therapy, Dosimetry.
**Radiotherapy Example:** Measuring induced activity in phantom materials post-treatment.

346. **Proton Therapy Residual Dose Assessment:** Assessing residual radiation dose after therapy.
**Related Terms:** QA, Proton therapy, Dosimetry.
**Radiotherapy Example:** Measuring residual dose in a previously irradiated tumor site.

347. **Proton Therapy Secondary Particle Measurement:** Measuring dose from secondary particles produced during proton therapy.
**Related Terms:** Neutrons, QA, Proton therapy.
**Radiotherapy Example:** Evaluating neutron dose to organs at risk during cranial proton therapy.

348. **Proton-Induced Neutron Dosimetry:** Measuring neutron dose produced by proton interactions.
**Related Terms:** Secondary particles, Dosimetry, Proton therapy.
**Radiotherapy Example:** Monitoring neutron dose in pediatric proton therapy for safety.

349. **Photonuclear Reaction Yield:** Quantifying products from photonuclear reactions.
**Related Terms:** QA, Photon therapy, Nuclear physics.
**Radiotherapy Example:** Measuring isotopes produced in high-energy photon beams.

350. **Photoneutron Spectrum Analysis:** Analyzing energy spectrum of neutrons generated by photon beams.
**Related Terms:** QA, Photon therapy, Dosimetry.
**Radiotherapy Example:** Evaluating neutron contamination in 18 MV photon therapy.

351. **Proton Capture Gamma Spectrometry:** Measuring gamma rays emitted from proton capture reactions.
**Related Terms:** QA, Proton therapy, Nuclear imaging.
**Radiotherapy Example:** Verifying proton activation in phantom studies using gamma spectrometry.

352. **Proton Therapy Radioisotope Safety Protocol:** Safety procedures for handling isotopes generated in proton therapy.
**Related Terms:** QA, Radiation protection, Proton therapy.
**Radiotherapy Example:** Protocol for handling activated phantoms or patient residues.

353. **Proton Therapy Induced Radioactivity:** Radioactivity generated in tissues/materials by proton beams.
**Related Terms:** QA, Dosimetry, Proton therapy.
**Radiotherapy Example:** Measuring residual activity in irradiated bone.

354. **Positron Annihilation Dosimetry:** Using positron annihilation events to measure dose.
**Related Terms:** PET, Dosimetry, QA.
**Radiotherapy Example:** Mapping dose in PET/CT-based treatment verification.

**355. Positron Lifetime Measurement:** Measuring decay lifetime of positrons in tissues.
**Related Terms:** PET, Dosimetry, QA.
**Radiotherapy Example:** Evaluating tissue composition for dose planning.

**356. Positron Emission Tomography Dosimetry:** Using PET imaging to calculate radiation dose distribution.
**Related Terms:** PET, Dosimetry, QA.
**Radiotherapy Example:** Assessing metabolic tumor activity and dose uptake.

**357. Proton Radiolysis Monitoring:** Monitoring chemical changes induced by proton beams.
**Related Terms:** QA, Proton therapy, Chemistry.
**Radiotherapy Example:** Studying water radiolysis in tissue-equivalent phantoms.

**358. Proton Therapy Shielding Assessment:** Evaluating effectiveness of shielding for proton therapy rooms.
**Related Terms:** QA, Radiation protection, Proton therapy.
**Radiotherapy Example:** Measuring stray radiation outside treatment room.

**359. Proton Therapy Secondary Gamma Dose:** Measuring gamma dose produced as a secondary effect in proton therapy.
**Related Terms:** QA, Proton therapy, Secondary radiation.
**Radiotherapy Example:** Assessing gamma exposure in cranial proton treatments.

**360. Proton Therapy Beam Contamination:** Evaluating unwanted particles or radiation in the proton beam.
**Related Terms:** QA, Proton therapy, Beam quality.
**Radiotherapy Example:** Detecting secondary neutrons or gamma contamination in beam.

**361. Proton Therapy Residual Activation Mapping:** Mapping residual radioactivity post-treatment.
**Related Terms:** QA, Proton therapy, Dosimetry.
**Radiotherapy Example:** Measuring activated areas in phantom after proton irradiation.

**362. Photonuclear Cross-Section Dosimetry:** Using photonuclear cross-sections to calculate dose contribution.
**Related Terms:** QA, Photon therapy, Nuclear physics.
**Radiotherapy Example:** Estimating neutron dose from 15–20 MV photon beams.

**363. Proton Therapy Neutron Flux Measurement:** Measuring flux of neutrons generated during proton therapy.
**Related Terms:** QA, Secondary particles, Proton therapy.
**Radiotherapy Example:** Quantifying neutron dose in patient and staff areas.

**364. Protective Barrier Assessment Protocol:** Standard procedure to evaluate shielding barriers.
**Related Terms:** Radiation protection, QA, Proton/photon therapy.
**Radiotherapy Example:** Testing lead walls in LINAC treatment rooms.

**365. Protective Lead Shield Verification:** Verifying efficacy of lead shields for staff/patient safety.
**Related Terms:** Radiation protection, QA, PPE.
**Radiotherapy Example:** Checking lead apron attenuation in X-ray imaging.

**366. Protective Concrete Barrier QA:** QA for concrete barriers used in treatment rooms.
**Related Terms:** Radiation protection, QA, Shielding.
**Radiotherapy Example:** Measuring transmitted dose through concrete walls.

**367. Protective Glass Barrier Assessment:** Assessing leaded glass barriers for radiation protection.
**Related Terms:** Radiation protection, QA, Shielding.
**Radiotherapy Example:** Ensuring control room windows provide adequate shielding.

368. **Personal Dosimeter QA:** Quality assurance of dosimeters worn by staff.
**Related Terms:** QA, Dosimetry, Radiation safety.
**Radiotherapy Example:** Monthly calibration checks of staff badges.

369. **Public Dose Assessment Protocol:** Protocol to estimate radiation dose to public around facility.
**Related Terms:** Radiation protection, QA, Safety.
**Radiotherapy Example:** Assessing dose outside proton therapy facility.

370. **Post-Accident Radiation Mapping:** Mapping radiation distribution after incidents.
**Related Terms:** Radiation protection, QA, Emergency response.|
**Radiotherapy Example:** Surveying radiation in room after spill or equipment failure.

371. **Point Source Shielding Verification:** Verifying shielding effectiveness against point sources.
**Related Terms:** QA, Dosimetry, Shielding.
**Radiotherapy Example:** Measuring dose behind source in brachytherapy.

372. . **Peripheral Tissue Dose Assessment:** Evaluating dose to tissues surrounding target volume.
**Related Terms:** QA, Dosimetry, Proton/photon therapy.
**Radiotherapy Example:** Measuring dose to healthy lung during breast radiotherapy.

373. **Patient Radiation Protection QA:** QA procedures to minimize patient exposure.
**Related Terms:** Radiation protection, QA, Dosimetry.
**Radiotherapy Example:** Verifying patient shielding in head-and-neck treatments.

374. **Pre-Procedural Radiation Safety QA:** Safety checks before initiating radiation procedures.
**Related Terms:** QA, Radiation protection, Protocols.
**Radiotherapy Example:** Confirming all safety interlocks before LINAC start.

375. **Pulse Radiation Dose Assessment:** Measuring dose from pulsed radiation beams.
**Related Terms:** QA, Dosimetry, LINAC.
**Radiotherapy Example:** Verifying dose per pulse in stereotactic radiosurgery.

376. **Protocol-Based Shielding Assessment:** Evaluating shielding based on standardized protocols.
**Related Terms:** Radiation protection, QA, Barrier design.
**Radiotherapy Example:** Following NCRP guidelines for concrete wall assessment.

377. **Protective Material Verification:** Confirming shielding materials meet safety standards.
**Related Terms:** QA, Radiation protection, Shielding.
**Radiotherapy Example:** Testing lead bricks used in mobile shielding.

378. **Protective Distance Measurement:** Measuring safe distances from radiation sources.
**Related Terms:** QA, Radiation protection, Inverse square law.
**Radiotherapy Example:** Determining safe boundary around brachytherapy source.

379. **Protective Lead Barrier QA:** QA for lead barriers to ensure radiation attenuation.
**Related Terms:** Shielding, QA, Radiation protection.
**Radiotherapy Example:** Testing thickness and attenuation of lead walls.

380. **Protective Concrete Barrier Design:** Designing concrete walls to provide adequate radiation protection.
**Related Terms:** Shielding, Radiation protection, QA.
**Radiotherapy Example:** Designing proton therapy vault walls.

381. **Protective Room QA:** QA of treatment rooms for radiation safety.
**Related Terms:** Shielding, Radiation protection, QA.
**Radiotherapy Example:** Checking stray radiation levels in LINAC room.

**382. Personal Radiation Logging Protocol:** Standard procedure for logging individual radiation exposure.
**Related Terms:** Dosimetry, QA, Radiation safety.
**Radiotherapy Example:** Recording daily badge readings for staff.

**383. Public Safety Zone Assessment:** Defining safe zones around radiation sources.
**Related Terms:** Radiation protection, QA, Shielding.
**Radiotherapy Example:** Determining controlled area boundaries around proton vault.

**384. Photon Therapy Dose Painting:** Delivering heterogeneous dose patterns with photon beams to target tumor subregions.
**Related Terms:** IMRT, Dose escalation, Radiotherapy planning.
**Radiotherapy Example:** Increasing dose to hypoxic tumor regions while sparing surrounding healthy tissue.

**385. Proton Therapy Bragg Peak Optimization:** Adjusting proton beam energy and modulation to place Bragg peak accurately in tumor
**Related Terms:** Proton therapy, Range modulation, Beam optimization.
**Radiotherapy Example:** Optimizing depth of Bragg peak for spinal tumor treatment.

**386. Proton Beam Scanning Pattern QA:** Quality assurance of the scanning pattern of proton beams.
**Related Terms:** Pencil beam scanning, QA, Proton therapy.
**Radiotherapy Example:** Verifying uniform coverage of tumor using scanned proton beam.

**387. Proton Therapy Multi-Energy Layering:** Delivering multiple energy layers of protons to achieve uniform tumor dose.
**Related Terms:** Proton therapy, Energy modulation, Layered delivery.
**Radiotherapy Example:** Layered delivery in liver SBRT to cover entire tumor volume.

**388. Proton Therapy Beam Shaping QA:** QA for devices that shape proton beams to match tumor contours.
**Related Terms:** Collimation, QA, Proton therapy.
**Radiotherapy Example:** Checking custom apertures for cranial tumor treatments.

**389. Proton Therapy Spot Map Verification:** Verifying proton spot distribution for precise dose delivery.
**Related Terms:** Pencil beam scanning, QA, Dose mapping.
**Radiotherapy Example:** Confirming spot positions for head-and-neck proton therapy.

**390. Photon Beam QA Protocol:** Standard QA protocol for photon beam quality and safety.
**Related Terms:** LINAC, QA, Photon therapy.
**Radiotherapy Example:** Daily output and flatness checks on 6 MV photon beam.

**391. Proton Therapy Dynamic Delivery QA:** QA for dynamically delivered proton beams.
**Related Terms:** Spot scanning, Beam modulation, QA.
**Radiotherapy Example:** Checking synchronization of beam delivery with patient motion.

**392. Proton Therapy Motion Assessment:** Evaluating effect of patient or organ motion on proton therapy dose.
**Related Terms:** Motion management, IGRT, Proton therapy.
**Radiotherapy Example:** Assessing lung tumor motion during respiratory cycle.

**393. Proton Therapy Dose Accumulation:** Summing delivered dose over multiple sessions to evaluate total dose.
**Related Terms:** Dose mapping, Fractionation, QA.
**Radiotherapy Example:** Calculating cumulative liver dose over 5-fraction treatment.

394. **Positron Imaging QA:** QA for positron-based imaging systems (PET).
**Related Terms:** PET/CT, Dosimetry, QA.
**Radiotherapy Example:** Checking PET scanner resolution and calibration before planning.

395. **Photon Therapy Linear Accelerator QA:** QA for photon therapy LINACs ensuring correct dose and beam properties.
**Related Terms:** LINAC, QA, Photon therapy.
**Radiotherapy Example:** Annual QA checks of photon energy, output, and profile.

396. **Proton Therapy Linear Accelerator QA:** QA for proton therapy accelerators to ensure accurate dose delivery.
**Related Terms:** Proton therapy, QA, LINAC.
**Radiotherapy Example:** Monthly calibration of proton beam energy and output.

397. **Peripheral Dose Measurement QA:** QA to assess dose outside target volume.
**Related Terms:** Dosimetry, QA, Organ sparing.
**Radiotherapy Example:** Measuring dose to heart during breast radiotherapy.

398. **Proton Therapy Organ Sparing Assessment:** Evaluating ability to minimize dose to nearby critical organs.
**Related Terms:** Proton therapy, IMPT, QA.
**Radiotherapy Example:** Checking kidney dose during abdominal proton therapy.

399. **Proton Therapy Exit Dose Measurement:** Measuring dose leaving patient after proton beam passes through tumor.
**Related Terms:** QA, Dosimetry, Proton therapy.
**Radiotherapy Example:** Using ion chambers to measure exit dose in phantom studies.

400. **Proton Therapy Beam Monitoring Protocol:** Protocol to monitor proton beam parameters during treatment.
**Related Terms:** QA, Dosimetry, Beam stability.
**Radiotherapy Example:** Real-time monitoring of proton beam current and position.

401. **Proton Therapy Dose Verification Imaging:** Imaging-based verification of delivered proton dose.
**Related Terms:** QA, IGRT, Dosimetry.
**Radiotherapy Example:** Using prompt gamma imaging to confirm tumor dose.

402. **Proton Therapy Secondary Radiation QA:** QA for radiation produced as secondary effect of proton therapy.
**Related Terms:** Neutrons, QA, Proton therapy.
**Radiotherapy Example:** Measuring neutron dose in patient and staff areas.

403. **Photon Beam Profile QA:** QA of spatial distribution of photon beam intensity.
**Related Terms:** LINAC, Flatness, Symmetry, QA.
**Radiotherapy Example:** Checking uniformity across 6 MV photon field using water phantom.

404. **Protective Shield Effectiveness Assessment:** Assessing shielding for its ability to reduce radiation exposure.
**Related Terms:** Shielding, QA, Radiation protection.
**Radiotherapy Example:** Testing wall attenuation in LINAC vault.

405. **Protective Barrier Compliance Verification:** Verifying barriers meet regulatory safety standards.**Related Terms:** QA, Shielding, Radiation protection.
**Radiotherapy Example:** Confirming controlled area walls reduce dose below permissible limits.

**406. Protective Room Radiation Survey:** Surveying radiation levels in treatment rooms.
**Related Terms:** QA, Shielding, Radiation protection.
**Radiotherapy Example:** Measuring stray radiation in proton therapy vault.

**407. Personal Dosimeter Calibration Protocol:** Standard procedure to calibrate dosimeters worn by staff.
**Related Terms:** QA, Dosimetry, Radiation safety.
**Radiotherapy Example:** Calibrating badges monthly against known radiation source.

**408. Public Exposure Risk Assessment:** Evaluating risk of radiation exposure to public around facility.
**Related Terms:** Radiation protection, QA, Safety.
**Radiotherapy Example:** Calculating dose to hallways outside proton therapy room.

**409. Post-Treatment Radiation Survey:** Measuring radiation levels after treatment session.
**Related Terms:** QA, Radiation protection, Proton/photon therapy.
**Radiotherapy Example:** Surveying neutron dose after cranial proton therapy.

**410. Point Source Dose Rate Measurement:** Measuring radiation dose rate from a point source.
**Related Terms:** QA, Dosimetry, Brachytherapy.
**Radiotherapy Example:** Measuring dose rate from Ir-192 source in HDR brachytherapy.

**411. Peripheral Dose QA:** QA to ensure dose outside treatment field is within limits.
**Related Terms:** Organ sparing, QA, Dosimetry.
**Radiotherapy Example:** Measuring lung dose during breast radiotherapy.

**412. Patient Shielding Optimization:** Optimizing protective shielding for patient to reduce unnecessary exposure.
**Related Terms:** QA, Radiation protection, Dosimetry.
**Radiotherapy Example:** Using lead blocks to shield eye during facial radiotherapy.

**413. Pre-Treatment Radiation Safety QA:** QA performed before delivering radiation to ensure safety.
**Related Terms:** QA, Safety, LINAC/proton therapy.
**Radiotherapy Example:** Checking interlocks, beam output, and shielding before session.

**414. Pulse Radiation Safety QA:** QA of pulsed radiation delivery for safety compliance.
**Related Terms:** QA, Dosimetry, LINAC.
**Radiotherapy Example:** Verifying pulsed dose per beam pulse in SRS treatment.

**415. Protocol-Based Radiation Assessment:** Using standard protocols to assess radiation delivery and safety.
**Related Terms:** QA, Dosimetry, Radiation safety.
**Radiotherapy Example:** Following AAPM TG-142 protocol for LINAC QA.

**416. Protective Material QA:** QA for materials used to shield against radiation.
**Related Terms:** Shielding, QA, Radiation protection.
**Radiotherapy Example:** Testing lead brick attenuation in mobile shields.

**417. Protective Distance QA:** QA for ensuring safe distances from radiation sources.
**Related Terms:** QA, Radiation protection, Inverse square law.
**Radiotherapy Example:** Verifying minimum safe distance in brachytherapy room.

**418. Protective Barrier Thickness Verification:** Measuring and confirming thickness of shielding barriers.
**Related Terms:** QA, Shielding, Radiation protection.
**Radiotherapy Example:** Ensuring vault walls meet required shielding thickness.

**419. Protective Lead Barrier Effectiveness:** Evaluating how well lead barriers attenuate radiation.
**Related Terms:** QA, Shielding, Radiation protection.
**Radiotherapy Example:** Testing lead glass in control room window.

420. **Protective Concrete Barrier QA Protocol:** Protocol for QA of concrete shielding.
**Related Terms:** QA, Radiation protection, Shielding.
**Radiotherapy Example:** Checking attenuation of concrete walls in proton vault.

421. **Protective Room Design Verification:** Verifying that treatment rooms meet design safety standards.
**Related Terms:** QA, Shielding, Radiation protection.**Radiotherapy Example:** Confirming vault dimensions and shielding placement.

422. **Personal Dosimeter Logging:** Recording personal radiation dose readings.
**Related Terms:** QA, Dosimetry, Radiation safety.
**Radiotherapy Example:** Keeping daily staff badge logs.

423. **Public Safety Assessment Protocol:** Protocol to ensure public safety from radiation exposure.
**Related Terms:** QA, Radiation protection, Shielding.
**Radiotherapy Example:** Evaluating dose in hallways around LINAC/proton rooms.

424. **Photon Therapy QA Protocol:** Standard protocol for quality assurance of photon therapy systems.
**Related Terms:** LINAC QA, Beam verification, Radiotherapy safety.
**Radiotherapy Example:** Verifying photon beam flatness, symmetry, and output before patient treatment.

425. **Proton Therapy QA Protocol:** Standard QA protocol for proton therapy equipment and delivery.
**Related Terms:** Proton QA, Beam verification, Safety protocol.
**Radiotherapy Example:** Checking proton beam energy, output, and spot placement monthly.

426. **Proton Therapy Dose Accumulation QA:** QA for verifying cumulative proton dose across multiple fractions.
**Related Terms:** Dose tracking, Fractionation QA, Proton therapy.
**Radiotherapy Example:** Summing daily liver tumor doses to ensure planned total dose matches delivered dose.

427. **Proton Therapy Secondary Particle QA:** QA for secondary radiation (neutrons, gammas) produced during proton therapy.
**Related Terms:** Secondary dose, Dosimetry, QA.
**Radiotherapy Example:** Measuring neutron dose to staff during cranial proton therapy.

428. **Proton Therapy Shielding Verification:** QA to confirm shielding is effective against proton beams and secondary radiation.
**Related Terms:** Shielding QA, Radiation protection, Proton therapy.
**Radiotherapy Example:** Measuring dose outside treatment vault to ensure compliance with safety limits.

429. **Proton Therapy Residual Activity Assessment:** Assessing residual radioactivity in tissues or environment after proton therapy.
**Related Terms:** Residual dose, Radioactivity monitoring, Proton therapy.
**Radiotherapy Example:** Measuring activation in phantom after cranial proton therapy session.

430. **Proton Therapy Beam Interruption QA:** QA to ensure safety systems respond correctly to beam interruptions.
**Related Terms:** Safety QA, Beam monitoring, Proton therapy.
**Radiotherapy Example:** Testing emergency shutdown response during proton beam delivery.

431. **Proton Therapy Motion QA:** QA to evaluate and mitigate tumor or patient motion during proton therapy.
**Related Terms:** Motion management, IGRT, QA.
**Radiotherapy Example:** Using 4D imaging to verify motion compensation for lung tumors.

432. **Proton Therapy Energy Layering QA:** QA to verify correct delivery of multiple proton energy layers.
**Related Terms:** Energy modulation, Layered delivery, QA.
**Radiotherapy Example:** Measuring depth-dose profiles to ensure proper coverage of tumor volume.

433. **Proton Therapy Spot Optimization QA:** QA to confirm correct spot positioning and dose for proton therapy.
**Related Terms:** Spot scanning, Dose mapping, QA.|
**Radiotherapy Example:** Checking spot positions for head-and-neck tumors in treatment planning system.

434. **Proton Therapy Arc Delivery QA:** QA for arc-based proton therapy beam delivery.
**Related Terms:** Arc therapy, Proton QA, Beam verification.
**Radiotherapy Example:** Verifying dose distribution from rotating proton beam on phantom.

435. **Proton Therapy Field Shaping QA:** QA for devices that shape proton beam to tumor contours.
**Related Terms:** Collimation QA, Proton therapy, Beam shaping.
**Radiotherapy Example:** Checking custom apertures and compensators for cranial tumors.

436. **Proton Therapy Targeted Boost QA:** QA for targeted dose escalation to specific tumor regions.
**Related Terms:** Dose painting, Proton therapy, QA.
**Radiotherapy Example:** Verifying boosted dose to hypoxic tumor sub-volumes.

437. **Proton Therapy Conformal Avoidance QA:** QA to ensure critical structures are spared while delivering proton dose.
**Related Terms:** Organ sparing, Proton therapy, QA.
**Radiotherapy Example:** Checking spinal cord avoidance during vertebral proton therapy.

438. **Proton Therapy Adaptive Margins QA:** QA for adjusting treatment margins based on anatomical changes.
**Related Terms:** Adaptive therapy, Proton QA, Margin evaluation.
**Radiotherapy Example:** Verifying updated PTV margins for bladder tumor due to daily volume changes.

439. **Proton Therapy Breath-Control QA:** QA for respiratory-controlled proton therapy delivery.
**Related Terms:** Breath-hold technique, Motion management, QA.
**Radiotherapy Example:** Verifying beam gating during deep-inspiration breath-hold for lung tumor.

440. **Proton Therapy Dynamic Collimation QA:** QA for collimators that dynamically shape the beam during delivery.
**Related Terms:** Dynamic aperture, Beam shaping, QA.
**Radiotherapy Example:** Testing collimator response during real-time treatment delivery.

441. **Proton Therapy Beam Monitoring QA:** QA for continuous monitoring of proton beam parameters.
**Related Terms:** Beam output, QA, Proton therapy.
**Radiotherapy Example:** Measuring beam current, position, and shape during cranial treatments.

442. **Proton Therapy Dose Verification QA:** QA for confirming delivered dose matches planned dose.
**Related Terms:** Dosimetry, QA, Proton therapy.
**Radiotherapy Example:** Using ion chamber arrays to verify dose in patient-specific QA.

443. **Proton Therapy Spot Map QA:** QA to check accuracy of spot distribution maps.
**Related Terms:** Spot scanning, QA, Dose mapping.
**Radiotherapy Example:** Confirming proton spots align with PTV for head-and-neck therapy.

**444. Proton Therapy Multi-Energy Layering QA:** QA for correct delivery of multiple proton energy layers.
**Related Terms:** Energy modulation, Layered delivery, QA.
**Radiotherapy Example:** Verifying liver tumor coverage using multiple energy layers in a phantom.

**445. Proton Therapy Secondary Radiation Dose QA:** QA to measure dose from secondary radiation during treatment.
**Related Terms:** Neutron dose, QA, Proton therapy.
**Radiotherapy Example:** Monitoring neutron dose to staff and patient during proton therapy.

**446. Proton Therapy Organ Sparing QA:** QA to ensure critical organs receive minimal dose.
**Related Terms:** Organ at risk, QA, Proton therapy.
**Radiotherapy Example:** Checking heart dose during left-breast proton therapy.

**447. Proton Therapy Exit Dose QA:** QA to measure dose exiting patient.
**Related Terms:** Dose verification, QA, Proton therapy.
**Radiotherapy Example:** Using ion chamber to measure exit dose in phantom studies.

**448. Proton Therapy Beam Shaping Verification QA:** QA for verifying beam shaping devices accurately conform to tumor shape.
**Related Terms:** Collimation QA, Proton therapy, Beam verification.
**Radiotherapy Example:** Testing custom apertures and compensators in cranial therapy.

**449. Proton Therapy Motion Assessment QA:** QA to evaluate effects of motion on delivered dose.
**Related Terms:** Motion management, QA, Proton therapy.
**Radiotherapy Example:** 4D imaging verification for lung tumor proton therapy.

**450. Proton Therapy Dose Accumulation Verification QA:** QA to verify cumulative dose across fractions.
**Related Terms:** Fractionation, Dose mapping, QA.
**Radiotherapy Example:** Summing daily dose to liver tumor in proton therapy planning.

**451. Proton Therapy Residual Radioactivity QA:** QA for measuring remaining radioactivity in tissues or phantoms.
**Related Terms:** Residual dose, QA, Proton therapy.
**Radiotherapy Example:** Measuring activation in phantom after cranial proton therapy session.

**452. Proton Therapy Shielding Design QA:** QA to verify shielding designs protect staff and environment.
**Related Terms:** Shielding, Radiation protection, QA.
**Radiotherapy Example:** Confirming vault wall thickness reduces stray radiation below regulatory limits.

**453. Proton Therapy Secondary Particle Monitoring QA:** QA for measuring secondary particles generated during therapy.
**Related Terms:** Neutrons, QA, Proton therapy.
**Radiotherapy Example:** Monitoring secondary neutron flux in treatment vault during cranial therapy.

**454. Proton Therapy Dose Mapping QA:** QA for verifying spatial dose distribution.
**Related Terms:** Dosimetry, QA, Proton therapy.
**Radiotherapy Example:** Checking 3D dose distribution in phantom before patient treatment.

455. **Proton Therapy Beam Delivery Verification QA:** QA to confirm beam delivery matches planned treatment.
**Related Terms:** Beam verification, QA, Proton therapy.
**Radiotherapy Example:** Using detector arrays to verify proton beam delivery.

456. **Proton Therapy Field Verification QA:** QA for verifying field alignment and coverage.
**Related Terms:** Field verification, QA, Proton therapy.
**Radiotherapy Example:** Ensuring PTV is fully covered for head-and-neck tumors.

457. **Proton Therapy Safety Protocol Verification QA:** QA to verify safety procedures are effective during therapy.
**Related Terms:** Safety QA, Protocol verification, Proton therapy.
**Radiotherapy Example:** Checking interlocks and emergency shutdown functionality.

458. **Proton Therapy Beam Interruption Safety QA:** QA for safety systems during beam interruptions.
**Related Terms:** Safety QA, Beam monitoring, Proton therapy.
**Radiotherapy Example:** Testing response of treatment system to emergency stop signals.

459. **Proton Therapy Multi-Field Delivery QA:** QA for verifying multiple-field treatment delivery.
**Related Terms:** Field verification, QA, Proton therapy.
**Radiotherapy Example:** Checking cumulative dose from two-field cranial proton therapy.

460. **Proton Therapy Arc Delivery Verification QA:** QA for verifying dose from arc-based proton therapy.
**Related Terms:** Arc therapy, QA, Proton therapy.
**Radiotherapy Example:** Verifying rotating proton beam coverage of tumor volume.

461. **Proton Therapy Fractionation QA:** QA to ensure correct delivery of each fraction.
**Related Terms:** Fractionation, QA, Proton therapy.
**Radiotherapy Example:** Verifying daily liver tumor dose matches planned fraction.

462. **Proton Therapy Treatment Plan QA:** QA to ensure treatment plan is accurately executed.
**Related Terms:** Plan verification, QA, Proton therapy.
**Radiotherapy Example:** Checking IMPT plan against delivered dose in phantom.

463. **Proton Therapy Motion Management QA:** QA for systems managing tumor or patient motion.
**Related Terms:** Motion management, QA, Proton therapy.
**Radiotherapy Example:** Verifying respiratory gating accuracy for lung tumors.

464. **Proton Therapy Energy Layer QA:** QA for each energy layer delivered during proton therapy.
**Related Terms:** Energy modulation, Layered delivery, QA.
**Radiotherapy Example:** Verifying depth-dose profile of liver tumor.

465. **Proton Therapy Spot Delivery QA:** QA to verify delivery of each proton spot.
**Related Terms:** Spot scanning, QA, Dose mapping.
**Radiotherapy Example:** Confirming head-and-neck spot distribution matches plan.

466. **Proton Therapy Beam Position QA:** QA to ensure correct beam positioning.
**Related Terms:** Beam alignment, QA, Proton therapy.
**Radiotherapy Example:** Verifying spot alignment using detector array.

467. **Proton Therapy Treatment Verification QA:** QA to confirm overall treatment delivery matches plan.
**Related Terms:** Treatment verification, QA, Proton therapy.
**Radiotherapy Example:** Comparing cumulative dose in phantom to planned dose.

468. **Proton Therapy Safety QA:** QA to ensure safe operation of proton therapy system.
**Related Terms:** Safety protocol, QA, Proton therapy.
**Radiotherapy Example:** Checking interlocks, emergency stops, and shielding before treatment.

469. **Proton Therapy Beam Dose Rate QA:** QA to monitor dose rate of proton beams.
**Related Terms:** Beam output, QA, Dosimetry.
**Radiotherapy Example:** Measuring dose per second during cranial therapy.

470. **Proton Therapy Adaptive Plan QA:** QA to verify adaptive treatment plan modifications.
**Related Terms:** Adaptive therapy, QA, Proton therapy.
**Radiotherapy Example:** Verifying plan adjustment for bladder volume changes.

471. **Proton Therapy Dose Distribution QA:** QA to confirm spatial dose matches plan.
**Related Terms:** Dose mapping, QA, Proton therapy.
**Radiotherapy Example:** 3D dose verification in phantom for head-and-neck tumor.

472. **Proton Therapy Residual Dose QA:** QA to measure remaining dose after treatment.
**Related Terms:** Residual activity, QA, Proton therapy.
**Radiotherapy Example:** Measuring activation in phantom post-treatment.

473. **Proton Therapy Shielding Effectiveness QA:** QA to confirm shielding reduces radiation to safe levels.
**Related Terms:** Shielding, QA, Radiation protection.
**Radiotherapy Example:** Measuring stray dose outside vault walls.

474. **Proton Therapy Secondary Particle Dose Verification QA:** QA to verify dose from secondary radiation.
**Related Terms:** Neutron dose, QA, Proton therapy.
**Radiotherapy Example:** Measuring neutron dose to staff during therapy.

475. **Proton Therapy Patient Position QA:** QA to confirm correct patient positioning for treatment.
**Related Terms:** IGRT, QA, Setup verification.
**Radiotherapy Example:** Using CBCT to verify patient setup before cranial proton therapy.

476. **Proton Therapy Field Alignment QA:** QA for alignment of treatment fields.
**Related Terms:** Field verification, QA, Proton therapy.**Radiotherapy Example:** Ensuring spinal fields are correctly aligned before delivery.

477. **Proton Therapy Treatment Monitoring QA:** QA for monitoring treatment in real time.
**Related Terms:** Dose monitoring, QA, Proton therapy.
**Radiotherapy Example:** Checking beam output and position during delivery.

478. **Proton Therapy Treatment Safety QA:** QA to ensure patient and staff safety during therapy.
**Related Terms:** Safety checks, QA, Proton therapy.
**Radiotherapy Example:** Confirming interlocks, emergency stops, and room shielding.

479. **Proton Therapy Beam Conformation QA:** QA for beam conforming to tumor shape.
**Related Terms:** Beam shaping, QA, Proton therapy.
**Radiotherapy Example:** Checking dose conformity for head-and-neck PTV.

480. **Proton Therapy Spot Accuracy QA:** QA to verify accuracy of spot placement.
**Related Terms:** Spot scanning, QA, Proton therapy.
**Radiotherapy Example:** Measuring spot deviations using detector array.

481. **Proton Therapy Dose Homogeneity QA:** QA to ensure uniform dose across target.
**Related Terms:** Homogeneous dose, QA, Proton therapy.
**Radiotherapy Example:** Measuring uniformity of liver tumor dose in phantom.

482. **Proton Therapy QA Checklist:** Comprehensive checklist of all QA procedures for proton therapy.
**Related Terms:** QA protocol, Safety, Proton therapy.
**Radiotherapy Example:** Using checklist to perform daily, weekly, monthly QA of LINAC/proton system.

483. **Proton Therapy Complete Verification QA:** Complete QA for all aspects of proton therapy, including beam, dose, and safety.
**Related Terms:** QA protocol, Comprehensive verification, Proton therapy.
**Radiotherapy Example:** Performing full verification before new patient treatment plan approval.

484. **Patient positioning reproducibility (noun):** Ability to achieve the same patient setup across treatment fractions.
**Related Terms:** Immobilization, Setup accuracy.
**Example in Radiotherapy:** Ensured using custom masks in head-and-neck treatments.

485. **Patient-specific QA (noun):** Quality assurance performed for an individual treatment plan.
**Related Terms:** Pre-treatment verification, Dosimetric QA.
**Example in Radiotherapy:** Measuring IMRT dose delivery using a phantom.

486. **Peak skin dose (noun):** Maximum radiation dose received at the skin surface.
**Related Terms:** Surface dose, Skin toxicity.
**Example in Radiotherapy:** Evaluated in breast radiotherapy plans.

487. **Pencil beam algorithm (noun):** Dose calculation method modeling narrow beamlets.
**Related Terms:** Dose calculation, TPS.
**Example in Radiotherapy:** Used in photon and proton treatment planning.

488. **Pencil beam scanning (noun):** Technique delivering dose spot-by-spot using narrow beams.
**Related Terms:** IMPT, Spot scanning.
**Example in Radiotherapy:** Commonly used in modern proton therapy.

489. **Percentage depth dose (noun):** Relative dose as a function of depth in tissue.
**Related Terms:** PDD, Depth dose curve.
**Example in Radiotherapy:** Used to characterize photon beam penetration.

490. **Planning organ-at-risk volume (noun):** Organ-at-risk expanded to account for uncertainties.
**Related Terms:** PRV, OAR margin.
**Example in Radiotherapy:** PRV applied to spinal cord planning.

491. **Plan robustness evaluation (noun):** Assessment of plan sensitivity to setup and range errors.
**Related Terms:** Robust optimization, Uncertainty analysis.
**Example in Radiotherapy:** Critical in proton therapy planning.

492. **Plan sum evaluation (noun):** Combined dose assessment from multiple treatment courses.
**Related Terms:** Cumulative dose, Re-irradiation.
**Example in Radiotherapy:** Used when treating recurrent tumors.

493. **Portal dose prediction (noun):** Calculated dose distribution expected at the portal imager.
**Related Terms:** Portal dosimetry, EPID.
**Example in Radiotherapy:** Compared with measured EPID images for QA.

494. **Position verification imaging (noun):** Imaging used to confirm patient alignment before treatment.
**Related Terms:** IGRT, Setup verification.
**Example in Radiotherapy:** Daily CBCT prior to SBRT delivery.

495. **Postoperative radiotherapy (noun):** Radiation delivered after surgical tumor removal.
**Related Terms:** Adjuvant therapy, Local control.
**Example in Radiotherapy:** Breast irradiation following lumpectomy.

496. **Primary beam fluence (noun):** Intensity distribution of the unscattered radiation beam.
**Related Terms:** Fluence map, Beam modeling.
**Example in Radiotherapy:** Used in IMRT dose calculations.

497. **Probability of complication (noun):** Estimated likelihood of normal tissue toxicity.
**Related Terms:** NTCP, Radiobiological modeling.
**Example in Radiotherapy:** Evaluated for lung and heart dose.

498. **Prompt gamma imaging (noun):** Imaging technique detecting gamma rays during proton interactions.
**Related Terms:** Range verification, Proton therapy QA.
**Example in Radiotherapy:** Used to confirm proton beam range in vivo.

499. **Pulse repetition frequency (noun):** Rate at which radiation pulses are delivered.
**Related Terms:** Dose rate, Beam delivery.
**Example in Radiotherapy:** Relevant in pulsed electron and proton beams.

500. **PTV coverage (noun):** Extent to which prescribed dose encompasses the planning target volume.
**Related Terms:** Target coverage, Dose conformity.
**Example in Radiotherapy:** Evaluated using DVH metrics.

# Q

1. **Quality Assurance (QA) in Radiotherapy:** Systematic process to ensure safe and accurate radiation delivery to patients.
   **Related Terms:** QC, Patient Safety, AAPM TG-142
   **Radiotherapy Example:** Monthly LINAC QA verifying beam output, symmetry, and MLC calibration.
2. **Quality Control (QC) Testing:** Routine tests to verify equipment performance remains within tolerances.
   **Related Terms:** Acceptance testing, QA, Calibration
   **Radiotherapy Example:** Daily output constancy test using ion chamber.
3. **Quality Management Program (QMP):** Structured framework integrating QA/QC for continuous improvement in radiotherapy.
   **Related Terms:** QA Program, SOPs, Accreditation
   **Radiotherapy Example:** Institutional QMP managing all physics QA logs and audits.
4. **Qualitative Image Assessment:** Visual evaluation of image quality including contrast, sharpness, and artifacts.
   **Related Terms:** IGRT, Image quality, CBCT QA
   **Radiotherapy Example:** Reviewing CBCT clarity before positioning prostate patient.
5. **Quantitative Image Assessment:** Numerical measurement of image quality metrics such as SNR and MTF.
   **Related Terms:** Image uniformity, Resolution testing
   **Radiotherapy Example:** Measuring CT noise index for daily calibration check.
6. **Quantitative Dosimetry:** Numerical measurement of absorbed radiation dose using calibrated detectors.
   **Related Terms:** Ion chamber, TLD, Output measurement
   **Radiotherapy Example:** Measuring LINAC output during annual calibration.
7. **Quadratic Dose–Response Model:** Model predicting tissue response to radiation based on dose squared proportionality.
   **Related Terms:** BED, LQ Model, Radiobiology
   **Radiotherapy Example:** Evaluating rectal toxicity risk in prostate IMRT.
8. **Quadratic–Linear Survival Model (LQ Model):** Radiobiological model predicting cell survival using linear + quadratic dose components.
   **Related Terms:** $\alpha/\beta$ ratio, BED, Fractionation
   **Radiotherapy Example:** Calculating hypofractionated SBRT dose for lung tumor.
9. **Quadrant Shifting Technique:** Setup correction method using isocenter shifts in four quadrants.
   **Related Terms:** IGRT, Couch shift, Isocenter verification
   **Radiotherapy Example:** Correcting 3D position of spine tumor using quadrant shift from CBCT.
10. **Quadriceps Shielding Protocol:** Technique to protect quadriceps from unnecessary exposure during pelvic irradiation.
    **Related Terms:** Organ sparing, IMRT planning
    **Radiotherapy Example:** Blocking quadriceps during pelvic sarcoma treatment.

11. **Quality Assurance Phantom:** Physical or digital phantom used to evaluate imaging or dosimetry systems.
    **Related Terms:** Water phantom, Film phantom, Winston-Lutz phantom
    **Radiotherapy Example:** Using phantom to verify VMAT dose distribution for head-and-neck plan.
12. **Quantitative PET Phantom Scan:** PET scan of phantom to calibrate standardized uptake values (SUV).
    **Related Terms:** SUV calibration, Nuclear medicine, Image QA
    **Radiotherapy Example:** Adjusting SUV scaling before PET-based tumor contouring.
13. **Quasi-Static Treatment Simulation:** Simulation assuming restricted motion to predict dose under stable geometry.
    **Related Terms:** Motion control, Respiratory gating, Planning
    **Radiotherapy Example:** Planning pancreatic SBRT assuming gated breath-hold.
14. **Quasi-Static Beam Modeling:** Modeling radiation beams where mechanical components move slowly relative to delivery.
    **Related Terms:** Beam simulation, TPS modelling
    **Radiotherapy Example:** Calibrating VMAT arc delivery using quasi-static leaf motion simulation.
15. **Quarter-Arc Delivery:** VMAT technique using 90-degree arcs to minimize dose to critical structures.
    **Related Terms:** VMAT, Partial arc, Organ sparing
    **Radiotherapy Example:** Quarter-arc VMAT for left-breast cancer to avoid heart exposure.
16. **Quantum Efficiency (QE) of Detectors:** Efficiency with which detector converts radiation input into measurable signal.
    **Related Terms:** Flat-panel detector, SNR, DQE
    **Radiotherapy Example:** Higher QE detector improves CBCT soft-tissue visibility.
17. **Quantum Noise:** Noise arising from statistical fluctuations in photon count.
    **Related Terms:** mAs, Image noise, CT QA
    **Radiotherapy Example:** Increasing mAs on CT scan reduces noise for accurate tumor contouring.
18. **Quantum-Assisted Dose Calculation:** Use of quantum algorithms to speed up dose calculations in complex plans.
    **Related Terms:** Monte-Carlo, GPU computing, TPS algorithms
    **Radiotherapy Example:** Real-time dose recalculation for adaptive proton therapy.
19. **Quick-Verification IGRT Protocol:** Rapid image-matching protocol used for efficient patient positioning.
    **Related Terms:** CBCT, kV-kV imaging, Setup time reduction
    **Radiotherapy Example:** Using quick protocol in pediatric anesthesia-assisted radiotherapy.
20. **Quench-Shielded MRI System:** MRI system designed to restrict cryogenic gas release during magnet quench.
    **Related Terms:** Magnetic safety, Shielding, Hybrid MR-LINAC
    **Radiotherapy Example:** Safety protocol for emergency quench management in MR-guided radiotherapy.
21. **Quantile Dose Distribution:** Statistical representation of dose values divided into percent quantiles across a treatment volume.
    **Related Terms:** DVH, Dose statistics, Percentile mapping
    **Radiotherapy Example:** Evaluating whether 95th-quantile dose to bladder exceeds tolerance for pelvic IMRT.

22. **Quantum Cascade Laser Detector:** Highly sensitive IR detector used for precise radiation spectral analysis.
**Related Terms:** Spectroscopy, Beam characterization
**Radiotherapy Example:** Measuring beam energy drift in LINAC head using cascade detector.

23. **Quasi-Elastic Scattering Measurement:** Technique observing low-energy scatter to characterize tissue composition.
**Related Terms:** Compton scatter, Spectroscopy
**Radiotherapy Example:** Mapping heterogeneity in bone for adaptive planning.

24. **Quaternary Collimation System:** Fourth-stage collimation layer added to refine beam shaping beyond jaws and MLC.
**Related Terms:** Scatter control, Field shaping
**Radiotherapy Example:** Used in stereotactic treatment to tighten penumbra around small targets.

25. **Quasi-Monte Carlo Dose Algorithm:** Monte-Carlo based dose algorithm using deterministic sampling to speed computation.
**Related Terms:** Monte-Carlo, GPU dose calculation
**Radiotherapy Example:** Rapid dose recalculation for daily adaptive prostate therapy.

26. **Quantum Detector Array:** Ultra-high-resolution array detector using quantum-photon conversion.
**Related Terms:** EPID, DQE, Mega-pixel dosimetry
**Radiotherapy Example:** Portal dosimetry verification of VMAT for head-and-neck.

27. **Quantitative Adaptive Replanning:** Replanning triggered by measured dose deviations beyond numerical thresholds.
**Related Terms:** Adaptive radiotherapy, QA triggers
**Radiotherapy Example:** Lung SBRT replanned when GTV shrinks 30% during week 2.

28. **Quadrupole Electromagnet Stabilization:** Electromagnet configuration used to stabilize charged-particle beam trajectories.
**Related Terms:** Beam steering, Proton therapy
**Radiotherapy Example:** Maintaining proton beam alignment in scanning gantry.

29. **Quantized Beam Modulation:** Step-wise modulation of radiation intensity rather than continuous variation.
**Related Terms:** Step-and-shoot IMRT, Segmented delivery
**Radiotherapy Example:** Delivering 45 intensity segments across pelvic field.

30. **Quasi-Isochromatic Computed Tomography (QICT):** CT technique producing almost energy-independent attenuation values for improved density calibration.
**Related Terms:** Dual-energy CT, Material differentiation
**Radiotherapy Example:** Planning pancreatic VMAT with improved fat–soft-tissue separation.

31. **Quality Index (QI) for Beam Hardness:** Numerical indicator of X-ray beam penetrating ability defined by HVL or kVp ratio.
**Related Terms:** Beam quality, kVp calibration, HVL
**Radiotherapy Example:** Annual kV CBCT calibration using QI tolerance evaluation.

32. **Quorum-Based Peer Dosimetry Review:** Multi-physicist approval system ensuring safe complex plan delivery.
**Related Terms:** Peer review, Safety culture
**Radiotherapy Example:** SBRT plans must be approved by ≥3 physicists before treatment.

33. **Quasicomponent Dose Mapping:** Dose tracking for individual anatomical subcomponents (e.g., cartilage vs bone).
**Related Terms:** Substructure contouring, High-precision dosimetry
**Radiotherapy Example:** Mapping cochlea apex dose in acoustic neuroma case.

34. **Quasi-Heterogeneity Scaling Factor:** Derived parameter adjusting dose for small-scale density variations.
**Related Terms:** Hounsfield calibration, Tissue compensation
**Radiotherapy Example:** Compensating dose for small air pockets in nasopharynx.

35. **Quadrant Wedge Compensation:** Technique dividing field into four wedge-shaped modulation zones to balance dose.
**Related Terms:** Physical wedge, Compensator, IMRT
**Radiotherapy Example:** Creating uniform dose to large chest wall target.

36. **Quantized Arc Segmentation:** VMAT arc broken into fixed number of discrete beam segments.
**Related Terms:** Segmented arc, Partial arcs
**Radiotherapy Example:** Delivering 18 fixed segments across 360° arc for pancreas.

37. **Quasi-Specular Scatter Reduction:** Strategy preventing directional scatter that degrades CBCT contrast.
**Related Terms:** Anti-scatter grid, Scatter correction
**Radiotherapy Example:** Enhancing spinal CBCT clarity for SRS setup.

38. **Quantum Radiobiology:** Study of radiation–matter interactions at sub-atomic level including DNA ionization patterns.
**Related Terms:** Radiochemistry, Track structure
**Radiotherapy Example:** Predicting differences between photon vs carbon-ion DNA cluster damage.

39. **Quasi-Equilibrium Dose Delivery:** Stable state of dose rate where recombination and charge buildup are minimized.
**Related Terms:** Ion chamber protocol, PDD, Charged particle equilibrium
**Radiotherapy Example:** Ensuring PDD measurements follow equilibrium rules at 10 cm depth.

40. **Quaternary Neutron Shielding Compound:** Specialized shielding blend designed to absorb thermal, fast, and epithermal neutrons.
**Related Terms:** Borated concrete, Hydrogenated polymers
**Radiotherapy Example:** Applied near high-energy LINAC vault maze to reduce neutron leakage.

41. **Quasi-Static Beam Modeling:** Beam model assuming negligible change in beam energy and shape during delivery.
**Related Terms:** Beam modeling, TPS, Dose engine
**Example:** Used for IMRT beam representation when MLC speed variations are minimal.

42. **Quality-Driven Adaptive Workflow:** Adaptive radiotherapy approach triggered by QA thresholds instead of scheduled intervals.
**Related Terms:** ART, Plan-of-the-day, CBCT evaluation
**Example:** Replanning triggered only if rectum displacement >7 mm.

43. **Quadrature Surface Coil Reconstruction:** MRI reconstruction using orthogonal coil elements to improve SNR.
**Related Terms:** MRI localization, Coil geometry
**Example:** Used in MR-Linac imaging to improve prostate tumor edge visibility.

44. **Quantitative Portal Imaging Validation:** Dose-based verification of portal dose images instead of qualitative visual check.
**Related Terms:** EPID dosimetry, Gamma analysis
**Example:** 3%/3mm portal gamma passing rate for VMAT lung QA.

45. **Quasi-Photon Fluence Mapping:** Approximation of photon fluence using detector readings with correction kernels.
**Related Terms:** Fluence map, IMRT planning
**Example:** Converting EPID images into fluence maps for field-by-field verification.

46. **Quality Drift Surveillance:** Monitoring gradual deviation of machine output before tolerance is exceeded.
**Related Terms:** Predictive maintenance, Trend QA
**Example:** Gradual drop in PDD10 predicted target chamber replacement.

47. **Quadrant Dose Symmetry Test:** Beam symmetry measured by dividing profile into four orthogonal zones.
**Related Terms:** Flatness, Profile, Beam steering
**Example:** Annual test for 6 MV beam symmetry within ±2%.

48. **Quasi-Voxel Density Interpolation:** TPS compensation for missing density when voxel contains mixed tissue types.
**Related Terms:** CT calibration, Hounsfield units
**Example:** Mixed lung–bronchus voxels corrected for SBRT lung plan.

49. **Quality-Safeguarded Beam Hold:** Auto-interruption of beam if delivery deviates beyond preset QA thresholds.
**Related Terms:** Gating, Safety interlock
**Example:** Beam hold occurs when MLC leaf position error exceeds 3 mm.

50. **Quench-Suppressed Dosimeter:** Scintillation dosimeter engineered to minimize quenching under high LET radiation.
**Related Terms:** LET, Particle therapy
**Example:** Accurate dosimetry during carbon-ion SOBP measurement.

51. **Quasi-Analytic Dose Solver:** Hybrid algorithm using analytic kernels with Monte-Carlo corrections.
**Related Terms:** Dose engine, Grid-based Boltzmann solver
**Example:** Dose recalculation for adaptive workflow in cervical cancer.

52. **Quantized MU Delivery:** MU delivered in discrete steps rather than continuous flow.
**Related Terms:** Step-and-shoot IMRT, MLC sequencing
**Example:** 25 intensity segments delivered to parotid plan.

53. **Quadratic Radiobiological Tissue Model:** Expanded LQ model accounting for high-dose per fraction effects.
**Related Terms:** LQ uncertainties, BED, Hypofractionation
**Example:** Predicting BED in 12 Gy × 3 spinal SBRT fractions.

54. **Quantum-Noise Filtered CBCT:** CBCT reconstruction that removes photon-counting noise while preserving edges.
**Related Terms:** Iterative CBCT, Noise suppression
**Example:** Improved pancreatic soft-tissue visibility for daily IGRT.

55. **Quality-Weighted Dose Constraint:** Constraint adjusted by clinical benefit score for balancing tumor control and toxicity.
**Related Terms:** OAR prioritization, AI optimization
**Example:** Higher weight assigned to optic chiasm over brainstem during skull-base plan.

56. **Quadrupole Proton Focusing:** Proton beam focusing using four electromagnets with alternating polarity.
**Related Terms:** Beam transport, Pencil beam scanning
**Example:** Sharpening lateral penumbra for ocular proton therapy.

57. **Quasi-Reproducibility Check:** Analysis confirming setup consistency across repeated fractions despite anatomical change.
**Related Terms:** Setup reproducibility, CBCT comparison
**Example:** Evaluating breast DIBH daily reproducibility.

58. **Quick-Release Immobilization Protocol:** Patient restraint technique ensuring security during treatment but fast release in emergency.
**Related Terms:** Mask, Vacuum cushion, Safety
**Example:** Craniospinal case requiring rapid removal for nausea.

59. **Quantized Leaf Motion Pattern:** MLC motion constrained to incremental discrete steps rather than continuous motion.
**Related Terms:** MLC sequencing, IMRT delivery
**Example:** Pattern used to minimize delivery time for pediatric cases.

60. **Quantum-Efficiency Calibrated EPID:** Portal detector calibrated for absolute quantum conversion efficiency vs. photon energy.
**Related Terms:** EPID dosimetry, DQE, Energy response
**Example:** Accurate fluence measurement for 10 MV FFF beam.

61. **Quality-Linked Gating Threshold:** Respiratory gating thresholds determined based on predicted dosimetric benefit.
**Related Terms:** 4D-RT, Motion management
**Example:** Gating only applied if liver motion >7 mm.

62. **Quasi-Real-Time Beam Analysis:** Near real-time comparison of delivered vs. planned fluence during treatment.
**Related Terms:** Adaptive gating, Online QA
**Example:** Halting SBRT when fluence deviation >4%.

63. **Quadratic Dose Volume Penalty:** Optimizer penalty that increases with the squared difference from dose target.
**Related Terms:** Planning optimizer, Cost function
**Example:** Used to tightly spare optic chiasm in pituitary plan.

64. **Quantile-Risk Toxicity Prediction:** Toxicity risk estimated from quantile-stratified population radiobiology database.
**Related Terms:** NTCP, Machine learning
**Example:** Predicting xerostomia risk for 26-Gy dose to parotid gland.

65. **Quasi-Conformal Beam Shaping:** Non-uniform beam shaping approximating anatomical surface curvature.
**Related Terms:** Compensator, Modulated arc
**Example:** VMAT arc shaped to match rib curvature in chest wall case.

66. **Quadrature MRI Tracking for RT:** MRI real-time tracking using dual-phase coil output for motion monitoring.
**Related Terms:** MR-Linac gating, Cine MRI
**Example:** Tracking pancreas motion during treatment.

67. **Quick-Check Machine QA:** Rapid daily QA evaluating machine safety-critical parameters only.
**Related Terms:** Daily QA, Output, Laser, Imaging
**Example:** Checking FFF output constancy within ±3%.

68. **Quantitative Gamma-Volume Analysis:** Gamma evaluation performed across 3D volume rather than 2D fluence.
**Related Terms:** 3D QA, Dose-voxel gamma
**Example:** Gamma 2%/2mm verified for craniospinal VMAT.

69. **Quadrant MLC Latency Tracking:** MLC latency measured in four field quadrants to detect directional error.
**Related Terms:** MLC timing QA, Delivery QA|
**Example:** Latency asymmetry corrected before SBRT brain.

70. **Quality-Corrected Patient Dose Report:** Patient dose report incorporating calibration and uncertainty corrections.
**Related Terms:** MU correction, Delivered dose
**Example:** Delivered dose reported within ±2.5% accuracy for esophageal VMAT.

71. **Quantified Organ Shift Assessment:** Numerical evaluation of organ displacement between planning and treatment sessions.
**Related Terms:** IGRT, CBCT registration, Organ motion
**Example:** Liver shift of 9 mm triggers adaptive rescan for SBRT.

72. **Quadratic Robust Optimization:** Planning method minimizing squared effect of uncertainties (motion, density, setup).
**Related Terms:** Robust planning, Monte-Carlo uncertainty
**Example:** Used for head-and-neck plans to mitigate swallowing-induced shifts.

73. **Quasi-Static MRI Tracking:** Periodic MRI snapshots used to update tumor position rather than continuous cine mode.
**Related Terms:** MR-guided adaptation, Motion management
**Example:** MR images acquired every 10 seconds during pancreas SBRT.

74. **Quantitative Image Sharpness Index:** Metric describing spatial resolution of radiotherapy imaging systems.
**Related Terms:** MTF, Edge profile, Noise ratio
**Example:** Used to validate new detector upgrade for KV imaging.

75. **Quadrature Surface Localization:** MRI localization using quadrature phase data for improved target contrast.
**Related Terms:** Coil imaging, Soft-tissue alignment
**Example:** Improves prostate visualization during MR-Linac adaptive workflow.

76. **Quality Threshold Beam Hold:** Automatic beam pause when delivery parameters violate defined QA thresholds.
**Related Terms:** Interlock system, Real-time beam monitoring
**Example:** Beam paused during lung SBRT because leaf error >2.5 mm.

77. **Quantized Composite Dose Analysis:** Cumulative dose evaluation using segmented dose bins for biological interpretation.
    **Related Terms:** DVH stratification, NTCP prediction
    **Example:** Used to evaluate cochlea dose stratification when reirradiating head-and-neck recurrence.

78. **Quasi-3D Portal Verification:** Reconstruction of 3D patient dose using multiple portal images.
    **Related Terms:** EPID dosimetry, 3D secondary check
    **Example:** 3D dose reconstructed and compared for pelvic VMAT QA.

79. **Quick-Start Pediatric Workflow:** Rapid immobilization + imaging + treatment sequence to reduce sedation time.
    **Related Terms:** Pediatric RT, Motion mitigation
    **Example:** 7-minute workflow for whole-brain irradiation under anesthesia.

80. **Quadrant Flatness Calibration:** Four-sided flatness check to identify directional deviation of radiation beam.
    **Related Terms:** Flatness QA, Beam symmetry
    **Example:** Calibration performed during annual test of 6 MV beam.

81. **Quantitative Dose Surface Mapping:** Mapping dose distribution along external patient surface for toxicity prediction.
    **Related Terms:** Skin dose, Bolus evaluation
    **Example:** Detected unexpected skin hotspot in chest wall IMRT.

82. **Quasi-Continuous MU Delivery:** MU delivered in nearly continuous motion with minimal leaf pauses.
    **Related Terms:** Sliding window IMRT, VMAT delivery
    **Example:** Used for head-and-neck plan to shorten beam-on time.

83. **Quality-Triage Treatment Prioritization:** Ranking treatment replanning urgency based on QA metrics + clinical risk.
    **Related Terms:** ART, Decision support
    **Example:** Replan triggered because parotid exceeded mean dose by 4 Gy.

84. **Quadratic DVH Deviation Penalty:** Dose optimizer penalty increasing exponentially with deviation from DVH target.|
    **Related Terms:** Cost function, OAR sparing
    **Example:** Applied to spinal cord 45 Gy hard constraint during IMPT.

85. **Quantitative Fluence Error Mapping:** Pixel-wise analysis of difference between delivered and planned fluence.
    **Related Terms:** IMRT QA, Gamma map
    **Example:** Hotspot near diaphragm detected in lung VMAT QA.

86. **Quasar Phantom Calibration:** Calibration of motion or CBCT phantoms branded under QASAR type systems.
    **Related Terms:** Motion phantom, 4D QA
    **Example:** Used for end-to-end 4D lung gating QA.

87. **Quick-Compute Secondary Dose Calculation:** Fast independent dose check using simplified calculation engine.
    **Related Terms:** Secondary TPS, MU check
    **Example:** VMAT fluence validated by a 60-second secondary calculation.

88. **Quantum Noise Reduction Algorithm:** AI or statistical filtering of photon noise in low-dose CT and CBCT.
**Related Terms:** Iterative CBCT, Noise suppression
**Example:** Reduces streaking in abdominal CBCT during ART.

89. **Quadrature-Based MR Gating:** Respiratory gating triggered by quadrature phase shift in MR signal.
**Related Terms:** Motion tracking, MR-Linac
**Example:** MR gating applied when liver tumor moves >5 mm.

90. **Quality-Indexed DVH Scoring:** Single score evaluating DVH against multiple constraints for treatment review.
**Related Terms:** Plan scoring, Multi-criteria decision making
**Example:** Score increased after reducing oral cavity mean dose.

91. **Quantitative Organ Remodeling Model:** Mathematical prediction of organ geometry change during treatment.
**Related Terms:** ART, Deformable registration
**Example:** Bladder volume prediction used to improve pelvic plan adaptation.

92. **Quadratic Gamma Sensitivity Index:** Index describing sensitivity of gamma result to threshold change.
**Related Terms:** Gamma passing rate, QA stability
**Example:** Used to assess reliability of SBRT QA under 2%/1mm criteria.

93. **Quasi-Static Breath-Hold Analysis:** Stability evaluation of breath-hold plateaus during DIBH radiotherapy.
**Related Terms:** RPM, ABC, Motion reproducibility
**Example:** Breast DIBH held within ±2 mm for 20 seconds.

94. **Quantitative Fiducial Migration Index:** Numerical metric describing migration magnitude of implanted markers.
**Related Terms:** Fiducial tracking, SBRT localization
**Example:** Kidney fiducial migration index exceeded 1.0 mm → reposition scan scheduled.

95. **Quasi-Neural Dose Forecasting:** Dose prediction using reduced ANN models before full optimization.
**Related Terms:** AI planning, Rapid plan generation
**Example:** Predicts if OAR constraints will be met before full VMAT optimization.

96. **Quality-Based Tumor Margin Adjustment:** PTV margin adjusted based on statistical imaging and immobilization QA data.
**Related Terms:** PTV expansion, Motion uncertainty
**Example:** Lung PTV margin reduced from 8 mm → 4 mm based on daily CBCT results.

97. **Quantitative Adaptive Dose Review:** Weekly numeric evaluation of cumulative dose deviation from original plan.
**Related Terms:** Deformable dose summation, ART thresholds
**Example:** Adaptive review triggered for parotid receiving +3.6 Gy over baseline.

98. **Quadrant Detector Failure Detection:** Safety system detecting partial detector malfunction using quadrant-based energy tests.
**Related Terms:** Flat-panel QA, Detector uniformity
**Example:** Top-left quadrant fault detected during FFF imaging QA.

99. **Quasi-Scintillation Light Correction:** Correction for nonlinear light formation in scintillation detectors under high energy.
**Related Terms:** Plastic scintillator QA, LET quenching
**Example:** Allows accurate depth dose measurement in proton therapy.

100. **Quality-Assured FLASH Dose Calibration:** Calibration of ultra-high-dose-rate FLASH beams under QA-specific protocols.
**Related Terms:** FERR, UHDR dosimetry, Beam monitoring
**Example:** Dose calibrated for 40 Gy/s experimental lung irradiation.

101. **Quantization-Based CT Artifact Reduction:** Reducing CT streaking and noise by adjusting numerical intensity quantization.
**Related Terms:** Iterative reconstruction, Noise correction, Image enhancement
**Radiotherapy Example:** Improves pelvis CBCT quality before adaptive replanning.

102. **Quasi-Real-Time Beam Symmetry Monitoring:** Monitoring beam symmetry continuously with near-live feedback during delivery.
**Related Terms:** Beam flatness, Real-time dosimetry
**Radiotherapy Example:** Beam paused during SBRT when symmetry drift exceeded tolerance.

103. **Quantitative LET Mapping:** Visualization of spatial distribution of Linear Energy Transfer in particle therapy.
**Related Terms:** LET optimization, RBE, IMPT
**Radiotherapy Example:** Used to avoid high-LET hotspots near spinal cord during proton therapy.

104. **Quadratic Ion Chamber Calibration:** Calibration that models voltage–dose response using a quadratic curve for accuracy.
**Related Terms:** Ion chamber QA, Absolute dosimetry
**Radiotherapy Example:** Used during annual calibration of a Farmer chamber for 6 MV beams.

105. **Quasi-Motion Tracking:** Low-frequency sampling of organ motion instead of continuous tracking.
**Related Terms:** Respiratory monitoring, IGRT
**Radiotherapy Example:** 3-sample tracking used for kidney SBRT rather than continuous cine.

106. **Quantum Noise Quantification:** Measuring noise originating from photon statistics in low-dose imaging.
**Related Terms:** SNR, Image noise, Dose reduction
**Radiotherapy Example:** Determines minimum mAs for pediatric CBCT without losing visibility.

107. **Q-Score for Plan Deliverability:** Numeric scoring system evaluating how well a plan will deliver on a LINAC.
**Related Terms:** MU efficiency, MLC modulation, QA index
**Radiotherapy Example:** Lung VMAT plan rescaled because Q-score predicted delivery instability.

108. **Quasi-Bolus Compensation:** Using material with variable thickness to create controlled surface dose compensation.
**Related Terms:** Bolus, Skin dose enhancement
**Radiotherapy Example:** Applied to chest wall IMRT when full bolus caused excessive erythema.

109. **Quantitative Plan Complexity Metric:** Score based on MLC motion, MU, modulation, and field shape complexity.
**Related Terms:** Modulation index, MU factor
**Radiotherapy Example:** Used to prevent overly modulated head-and-neck plan.

110. **Quality-Restricted Beam Modulation:** Algorithm limiting modulation to maintain delivery accuracy and QA compliance.
**Related Terms:** IMRT smoothing, Robust planning
**Radiotherapy Example:** Applied in prostate IMRT to prevent leaf oscillation artifacts.

111. **Quadrature Coil Position QA:** QA ensuring MRI coil placement maximizes SNR and avoids unfolding artifacts.
**Related Terms:** MR-guided RT, Image uniformity
**Radiotherapy Example:** Performed during MR-Linac prostate workflows.

112. **Quasi-3D Gamma Evaluation:** Gamma analysis integrating stacked 2D planes to approximate 3D results.
**Related Terms:** 2D gamma, 3D gamma, IMRT QA
**Radiotherapy Example:** Used to validate SBRT delivery on EPID before patient irradiation.

113. **Quantified Adaptive Replan Trigger:** Numerical threshold defining when a patient should undergo adaptive replanning.
**Related Terms:** ART, Deformable dose accumulation
**Radiotherapy Example:** Weekly dose deviation >5% triggered replanning for parotid sparing.

114. **Quasi-Deterministic Dose Prediction:** Dose estimator using probabilistic + deterministic components for rapid prediction.
**Related Terms:** AI dose engine, Dose forecasting
**Radiotherapy Example:** Evaluates OAR doses before full IMRT optimization.

115. **Quantum-Boost Flat-Panel Calibration:** Calibration that corrects detector gain variations at quantum-limited exposures.
**Related Terms:** Flat-panel QA, Gain map
**Radiotherapy Example:** Improves low-dose CBCT for lung ART.

116. **Quadrilateral Isocenter Verification:** Using four marker points to confirm accurate isocenter localization.
**Related Terms:** Winston-Lutz test, Mechanical isocenter
**Radiotherapy Example:** Performed in annual SRS QA.

117. **Quality-Weighted DICOM Export:** Exporting datasets only when passing defined quality rules.
**Related Terms:** TPS workflow, Plan validation
**Radiotherapy Example:** Prevents accidental export of unapproved SBRT plan.

118. **Quantified Residual Error Logging:** Automatic recording of positional or delivery error after each fraction.
**Related Terms:** Setup error tracking, Trending QA
**Radiotherapy Example:** Tracks daily deviations during prostate IGRT.

119. **Quasi-Boltzmann Dose Engine:** Dose solver using simplified Boltzmann transport equations for high speed.
**Related Terms:** Acuros, Monte-Carlo
**Radiotherapy Example:** Fast dose calculation for thorax IMRT planning.

120. **Quadratic Image Noise Suppression:** Reducing noise by weighted quadratic filtering in image processing.
**Related Terms:** Noise–texture optimization, Iterative CBCT
**Radiotherapy Example:** Improves pancreas visualization in CBCT for IGRT.

121. **Quantitative Intrafraction Error Study:** Measurement of patient movement during radiation delivery.
**Related Terms:** Motion management, IGRT
**Radiotherapy Example:** Used to determine gating threshold for lung SBRT.

122. **Qualified Beam Stability Report:** Report assessing daily LINAC beam energy, flatness, symmetry, and output.
**Related Terms:** QA report, Daily machine check
**Radiotherapy Example:** Confirms beam stability before pediatric craniospinal case.

123. **Quasi-Monochromatic X-Ray Optimization:** Using narrowed photon energy spectrum to improve image contrast.
**Related Terms:** Dual-energy CT, Spectral shaping
**Radiotherapy Example:** Boosts soft-tissue contrast for prostate IGRT.

124. **Quantum-Safe Radiotherapy Network Protocol:** Cybersecurity protocol preventing quantum-based decryption of clinical data.
**Related Terms:** DICOM-cybersecurity, TPS network safety
**Radiotherapy Example:** Used in secure transfer of SBRT plans to remote treatment center.

125. **Quadrature Interference Artifact Reduction:** Reducing RF interference between MRI coil channels.
**Related Terms:** Coil tuning, MR-guided RT
**Radiotherapy Example:** Prevents banding in MR-Linac abdominal imaging.

126. **Quantitative Organ Segmentation QA:** Evaluating auto-segmentation performance using statistical similarity metrics.
**Related Terms:** DSC, Hausdorff distance, Auto-contouring
**Radiotherapy Example:** Used to validate pancreas auto-segmentation before planning.

127. **Quality-Driven Dose Prioritization:** Prioritizing dose distribution based on organ toxicity risk and clinical urgency.
**Related Terms:** Multi-criteria optimization, Constraint balancing
**Radiotherapy Example:** Prioritizing optic chiasm sparing over PTV coverage in reirradiation.

128. **Quick-Lock MLC Safety Test:** Safety test ensuring MLC leaves lock instantly when an interlock condition appears.
**Related Terms:** MLC QA, Collision prevention
**Radiotherapy Example:** Tested before restarting machine after an emergency stop.

129. **Quasi-Elastic Dose Correction Model:** Improves dose accuracy by accounting for elastic scattering in particle therapy.
**Related Terms:** Proton transport physics, RBE modelling
**Radiotherapy Example:** Corrects dose near bone–soft tissue interface.

130. **Quantized Treatment Delivery Log:** Delivery record structured into discrete dose and position segments for analysis.
**Related Terms:** Log-file QA, Delivery reconstruction
**Radiotherapy Example:** Used for post-treatment verification of cervical VMAT.

131. **Quantitative Beam Output Drift Analysis:** Statistical tracking of gradual changes in LINAC output over time.
**Related Terms:** Output constancy, Trend analysis, Machine QA
**Radiotherapy Example:** Detected a 1% monthly output drift, prompting recalibration before SBRT cases.

132. **Quantile-Based Dose Statistics:** Evaluating dose distribution using percentile values rather than averages.
**Related Terms:** DVH metrics, Robust statistics
**Radiotherapy Example:** PTV D5% and D95% reported for head-and-neck plan quality assurance.

133. **Quantum-Assisted TPS Optimization (Conceptual):** Experimental dose optimization using quantum computing methods for rapid convergence.
**Related Terms:** AI optimization, Multi-criteria optimization
**Radiotherapy Example:** Research showing faster calculation for liver IMRT test cases.

134. **Quadratic Scatter Estimation:** Modeling scatter intensity using a quadratic relationship to improve image quality.
**Related Terms:** Scatter correction, CBCT reconstruction
**Radiotherapy Example:** Applied to reduce pelvic scatter on adaptive CBCT scans.

135. **Quality-Filtered Dose Accumulation:** Combining dose from multiple fractions only when image registration quality exceeds a threshold.
**Related Terms:** Deformable registration, Adaptive radiotherapy
**Radiotherapy Example:** Excluded poor-quality liver CBCT registration from cumulative dose DP calculation.

136. **Quasi-Autonomous MLC Motion Prediction:** Predictive algorithm reducing abrupt accelerations in leaf motion for delivery precision.
**Related Terms:** Leaf speed smoothing, MLC controller optimization
**Radiotherapy Example:** Used in prostate VMAT to minimize jitter and improve delivery QA pass rate.

137. **Quantified OAR Shrinkage Adjustment:** Systematic modification of planning contours to match expected organ shrinkage trends.
**Related Terms:** Adaptive planning, Geometric changes
**Radiotherapy Example:** Weekly parotid shrinkage compensation to reduce xerostomia risk.

138. **Quasi-Manual Reconstruction Override:** Partial user-guided corrections during automated image reconstruction.
**Related Terms:** Manual override, Iterative reconstruction
**Radiotherapy Example:** Manually fixed artifact-affected head CT slices before fusion.

139. **Quick-Start Plan Template Protocol:** Standardized approach enabling rapid creation of high-quality plans using predefined templates.
**Related Terms:** Planning automation, Clinical protocolization
**Radiotherapy Example:** Used to speed up emergency spinal cord compression planning.

140. **Quantitative Patient Position Drift Tracker:** Tracks change in daily setup deviations over treatment course.
**Related Terms:** IGRT analytics, Setup reproducibility
**Radiotherapy Example:** Detected increasing drift during rectal RT and triggered immobilization refitting.

141. **Quadrilateral Surface Dose Mapping:** Mapping surface dose using four-point dosimeter matrix and interpolating across skin.
**Related Terms:** Bolus QA, Skin toxicity assessment
**Radiotherapy Example:** Used for TBI to prevent excessive anterior chest wall dose.

142. **Q-Value for IGRT Imaging Confidence:** Numerical score combining image contrast, registration, and anatomical visibility.
**Related Terms:** Image score, Registration confidence index
**Radiotherapy Example:** Determined whether daily CBCT for pancreatic SBRT required contrast enhancement.

143. **Quantitative Beam Interruption Cause Logging:** Classifying and documenting reasons for beam stops to improve safety and workflow.
**Related Terms:** Safety incident tracking, Delivery logging
**Radiotherapy Example:** Highlighted that 62% of interruptions in SBRT were due to patient motion.

144. **Quasi-Simultaneous Multi-Plan Verification:** Verifying multiple plans together by grouping QA measurements to reduce time without losing accuracy.
**Related Terms:** Batch QA, IMRT QA
**Radiotherapy Example:** Performed for bilateral breast plans scheduled on consecutive days.

145. **Quantum-Resistance Database Backup:** Radiotherapy data backup using encryption resistant to quantum-based decryption threats.
**Related Terms:** Cybersecurity, Data protection
**Radiotherapy Example:** Secures backup for TPS and OIS records.

146. **Quality-Driven MU Range Limiting:** Restricting MU range to maintain plan efficiency and avoid unnecessary modulation.
**Related Terms:** MU optimization, Modulation control
**Radiotherapy Example:** Used to avoid excessive MU in head-and-neck IMRT causing long treatment times.

147. **Quick-Gating Latency Calibration:** Measuring and correcting the delay between motion detection and beam gating activation.
**Related Terms:** Motion management, Gating latency
**Radiotherapy Example:** Corrected gating lag during liver SBRT to prevent mistimed dose.

148. **Quantized Collimator Rotation Mapping:** Measuring precision of collimator rotation in discrete angular increments.
**Related Terms:** Mechanical QA, Angular calibration
**Radiotherapy Example:** Required before stereotactic arc therapy commissioning.

149. **Quadratic MU Leakage Modeling:** Predicting leakage dose based on MU accumulation using quadratic regression.
**Related Terms:** Leakage dose, IMRT QA
**Radiotherapy Example:** Estimated shielding requirements during TBI treatments.

150. **Quality-Weighted Plan Library Indexing:** Organizing stored plans using quality metrics to recommend best historical templates.
**Related Terms:** Automated planning, Plan database
**Radiotherapy Example:** Suggested highest-rated plans for new prostate patient with similar anatomy.

151. **Quasi-Nonrigid Fiducial Transformation:** Allows limited deformation of fiducial points during deformable registration.
**Related Terms:** Deformable fusion, Fiducial tracking
**Radiotherapy Example:** Improved registration quality in prostate CRT when seed spacing changed.

152. **Quantum-Layered Denoising in CBCT (Experimental):** Research algorithm applying multi-scale noise suppression using quantum imaging modeling.
**Related Terms:** Advanced reconstruction, Noise reduction
**Radiotherapy Example:** Improved soft-tissue clarity in pelvic CBCT during adaptive IGRT studies.

153. **Quadrature Distance Matching in MR-Linac:** Balancing coil signal strengths for uniform MR image quality.
**Related Terms:** SNR balancing, RF coil calibration
**Radiotherapy Example:** Used prior to MR-guided pancreas workflow.

154. **Quantitative Shoulder Clearance Monitoring:** Automated detection of shoulder position relative to beam entry paths.
**Related Terms:** Collision avoidance, Setup QA
**Radiotherapy Example:** Prevented arm obstruction in H&N VMAT treatment.

155. **Quality-Focused Segment Elimination:** Removing unnecessary IMRT segments to improve delivery efficiency without losing quality.
**Related Terms:** MU reduction, Segment merging
**Radiotherapy Example:** Reduced chest wall plan segments from 98 to 63, treatment time –30%.

156. **Quasi-Uniform Compensator Field Matching:** Matching compensator fields by equalizing intensity decay patterns.
**Related Terms:** Field matching, Compensator QA
**Radiotherapy Example:** Applied in craniospinal compensator-based treatments.

157. **Quantified In-Room Time Score:** Metric indicating treatment room occupancy time relative to expected duration.
**Related Terms:** Workflow efficiency, Operational analytics
**Radiotherapy Example:** SBRT lung sessions flagged when exceeding +20% expected time.

158. **Quadrant-Based Pharyngeal Dose Review:** Evaluating pharyngeal mucosa dose by dividing it into anatomical quadrants for toxicity risk.
**Related Terms:** OAR sub-structure analysis, Toxicity mitigation
**Radiotherapy Example:** Reduced posterior quadrant dose to minimize dysphagia in H&N case.

159. **Quantitative Linac Imaging–Dose Balance Tool:** Helps adjust kVp/mAs to balance imaging dose and image quality for different anatomies.
**Related Terms:** Imaging protocol optimization, ALARA
**Radiotherapy Example:** Reduced imaging dose in pediatric pelvis IGRT while keeping adequate visibility.

160. **Quasi-Dynamic Immobilization Fit Test:** Measurement of how well immobilization limits motion under small patient-initiated shifts.
**Related Terms:** Immobilization QA, Motion testing
**Radiotherapy Example:** Used to validate stability of thermoplastic mask for H&N SBRT.

161. **Quantitative Organ Compression Modeling:** Predicting anatomical deformation due to immobilization or abdominal pressure devices.
**Related Terms:** Deformable anatomy, Motion management
**Radiotherapy Example:** Compression model used to estimate diaphragm shift during liver SBRT.

162. **Quadrant-Based Pelvic Lymph Node Review:** Lymph nodes evaluated by anatomical quadrants to refine dose constraints.
**Related Terms:** Nodal contouring, OAR sub-segmentation
**Radiotherapy Example:** Posterior pelvic quadrant dose reduced to decrease bowel toxicity.

163. **Quality-Driven Adaptive CBCT Thresholding:** Automatically adjusts CBCT soft-tissue threshold based on visibility score.
**Related Terms:** Image enhancement, IGRT optimization
**Radiotherapy Example:** Auto-threshold improved prostate visualization during daily ART.

164. **Quantified Plan Complexity Index (QPCI):** Score combining MU, segment count, modulation and MLC travel.
**Related Terms:** Modulation index, Delivery efficiency
**Radiotherapy Example:** QPCI used to flag extremely complex breast IMRT plan requiring simplification.

165. **Quadratic Arc Dose Modulation Control:** Applies quadratic smoothing across VMAT arcs to prevent sharp modulation spikes.
**Related Terms:** Dose smoothing, Arc sequencing
**Radiotherapy Example:** Used to balance PTV coverage and low MU for lung VMAT.

166. **Quad-Energy Portal Imaging Mode:** Portal imaging using four beam energies to enhance soft-tissue contrast.
**Related Terms:** Portal vision, Contrast enhancement
**Radiotherapy Example:** Used to visualize bladder–prostate interface in male pelvis RT.

167. **Quantitative Bowel Gas Motion Score:** Rates daily bowel gas displacement influencing dose uncertainty.
**Related Terms:** GI motion, Adaptive replanning trigger
**Radiotherapy Example:** Replan triggered when gas motion score repeatedly exceeded threshold.

168. **Quick-Correct Couch Shift Protocol:** Rapid double-verification method to safely apply setup corrections under time pressure.
**Related Terms:** IGRT workflow, Positioning safety
**Radiotherapy Example:** Used during pediatric sedation cases to reduce anesthesia duration.

169. **Quasi-Breath-Hold Reproducibility Test:** Evaluates patient's ability to reproduce voluntary breath-hold patterns.
**Related Terms:** DIBH, Respiratory motion control
**Radiotherapy Example:** Accepted for left breast case when breath-hold variance $< 4$ mm.

170. **Quantum-Noise Adaptive Flattening Filter:** Real-time filter algorithm reducing quantum noise in MV images.
**Related Terms:** Noise suppression, MV imaging
**Radiotherapy Example:** Sharpened visibility of vertebrae on MV portal images during setup.

171. **Quadrant-Based PTV Underdose Correction:** Target regions divided into quadrants to identify local cold spots.
**Related Terms:** Dose shaping, Gradient management
**Radiotherapy Example:** Boost added to posterior quadrant of PTV in nasopharynx plan.

172. **Quantitative Deep-Learning Contour Audit:** Algorithm grades AI-generated contours compared to verified training sets.
**Related Terms:** Auto-segmentation QA, Clinical validation
**Radiotherapy Example:** Rejected auto-contour parotids when AI score dropped below 0.82.

173. **Quality-Ratio for OAR vs PTV Priority:** Ratio indicating whether planning overly favors OAR sparing or target coverage.
**Related Terms:** Objective balancing, DVH trade-offs
**Radiotherapy Example:** Ratio used to rebalance kidney SBRT plan emphasizing PTV D95.

174. **Quasi-Orthogonal Imaging Offset Calibration:** Measures offset between kV orthogonal imaging pairs.
**Related Terms:** IGRT calibration, Geometry QA
**Radiotherapy Example:** Corrected 0.7 mm offset in pelvis imaging pair before daily prostate therapy.

175. **Quantitative Over-Modulation Risk Flag:** Automatic alert when modulation increases risk of delivery inaccuracy.
**Related Terms:** Complexity alert, IMRT QA precursor
**Radiotherapy Example:** Alert triggered for extremely modulated tongue-base IMRT plan.

176. **Quasi-Dynamic Sag Compensation:** Adjusts couch/panel sag in near real-time based on movement predictions.
**Related Terms:** Couch sag correction, Imaging isocenter shift
**Radiotherapy Example:** Improved MR-Linac alignment during pelvic adaptive sessions.

177. **Quick-Match MRI-to-CT Transfer Function:** Fast conversion table estimating electron density from MRI intensities.
**Related Terms:** Synthetic CT, MR-only workflow
**Radiotherapy Example:** Used for femur dose calculation in MR-based prostate RT.

178. **Qualitative + Quantitative Film Hybrid Review:** Combines visual film inspection with γ-analysis for high confidence.
**Related Terms:** Film QA, Composite evaluation
**Radiotherapy Example:** Applied for final approval of trigeminal SRS plan.

179. **Quadratic Ripple Suppression in Dose Profiles:** Removes oscillations in calculated dose caused by sampling artifacts.
**Related Terms:** Dose smoothing, Profile shaping
**Radiotherapy Example:** Used when PDD curves for TBI showed small repetitive ripples.

180. **Quantified Thermal Load Check for LINAC:** Measures dose output sensitivity to gantry temperature changes during high-MU deliveries.
**Related Terms:** Warm-up drift, Thermal stability
**Radiotherapy Example:** Ensured stable output during high-MU liver SBRT plan.

181. **Quasi-Interrupted Beam Uniformity Review:** Tests uniformity when delivery is repeatedly paused and resumed.
**Related Terms:** Beam hold QA, Delivery reliability
**Radiotherapy Example:** Verified uniform dose delivery for gated pancreatic VMAT.

182. **Quantitative Mask Pressure Comfort Score:** Score measuring patient tolerance to immobilization pressure points.
**Related Terms:** Patient comfort QA, Mask fitting
**Radiotherapy Example:** Mask modified when score indicated high discomfort in orbit region.

183. **Quasi-Predictive Organ Motion Lookup Table:** Table linking organ shift pattern with patient characteristics.
**Related Terms:** Motion models, Adaptive RT
**Radiotherapy Example:** Predicted kidney motion amplitudes based on BMI and breathing cycle.

184. **Quality-Controlled Plan Export Verification:** Ensures exported plan integrity across TPS–OIS–Delivery chain.
**Related Terms:** Data consistency, Transfer QA
**Radiotherapy Example:** Avoided wrong isocenter export during spine SRS handoff.

185. **Q185. Quantum-Resistant TPS Access Authentication:** Future-proof login architecture preventing decryption by quantum computing.
 **Related Terms:** Cybersecurity, Multi-factor authentication
 **Radiotherapy Example:** Protects TPS from unauthorized access in large hospitals.
186. **Quadrature Multi-Axis Laser Calibration:** Uses orthogonal coordinate analysis to align room lasers to isocenter.
 **Related Terms:** Laser QA, Isocenter alignment
 **Radiotherapy Example:** Achieved <0.5 mm laser deviation for H&N setup precision.
187. **Quantified Motion Mitigation Effectiveness:** Score estimating how much motion management reduces organ displacement.
 **Related Terms:** Motion scoring, Respiratory control evaluation
 **Radiotherapy Example:** DIBH improved heart displacement mitigation score from 0.38 → 0.11.
188. **Quasi-Continuous Output Verification Loop:** Automated checks of output stability at short intervals during delivery.
 **Related Terms:** Real-time dose monitoring, Machine output QA
 **Radiotherapy Example:** Activated during ultra-hypofractionated prostate fraction.
189. **Quadrant-Weighted Body Contour Analysis:** Profile evaluating anatomic shape asymmetry that influences dose bath.
 **Related Terms:** Planning analytics, Body contour complexity
 **Radiotherapy Example:** Detected asymmetrical torso geometry causing unintended dose extension.
190. **Quantitative Time-Efficiency Benchmark:** KPI comparing treatment durations to department efficiency standards.
 **Related Terms:** Workflow metrics, Operational analytics
 **Radiotherapy Example:** Lung SBRT slots optimized when time exceeded +25% threshold.
191. **Quasi-Symmetric PTV Margin Allocation:** Method assigning different margins in different directions based on predicted uncertainties.
 **Related Terms:** Asymmetric margins, Geometric uncertainties
 **Radiotherapy Example:** Applied to reduce anterior margin where bowel proximity was critical.
192. **Quality-Ranked Bolus Application System:** Grading scale indicating consistency of bolus fit across treatment fractions.
 **Related Terms:** Surface dose QA, Bolus reproducibility
 **Radiotherapy Example:** Triggered re-fabrication for scalp RT when ranking repeatedly low.
193. **Quantified Beam Pause Fatigue Monitoring:** Tracks risk factors when treatments with long pauses fatigue patient posture.
 **Related Terms:** Position drift, Patient comfort analytics
 **Radiotherapy Example:** ARM rest introduced during long craniospinal treatments.
194. **Quasi-Algorithmic Planner Training Model:** AI-based scoring tool providing feedback to planners during plan creation.
 **Related Terms:** Planning training, Skill analytics
 **Radiotherapy Example:** Helped junior planner avoid hotspots in breast IMRT.
195. **Quadratic Search Dose Optimization Routine:** Optimization strategy minimizing error using second-order derivatives.
 **Related Terms:** Gradient optimization, Fast convergence
 **Radiotherapy Example:** Reduced calculation time in VMAT replan for recurrent glioma.

196. **Quick-Morph OAR Boundary Snap:** Auto-snap ensures OAR boundaries align properly with image contrast edges.
**Related Terms:** Auto-seg correction, Boundary detection
**Radiotherapy Example:** Prevented spinal cord contour from drifting into canal on fused MRI.

197. **Quantitative Transition Smoothing for Jaws:** Controls abrupt jaw position changes during arc delivery.
**Related Terms:** Jaw tracking optimization, Mechanical smoothing
**Radiotherapy Example:** Improved MU efficiency and delivery stability for pancreas VMAT.

198. **Quadrant-Based Beam Arrangement Rating:** Rates field arrangement coverage across clinical quadrants to avoid directional bias.
**Related Terms:** Beam geometry evaluation, Planning analytics
**Radiotherapy Example:** Rating improved for esophageal VMAT after adding posterior oblique.

199. **Quasi-Real-Time Deformation Consistency Check:** Verifies deformable registration accuracy throughout the session.
**Related Terms:** Adaptive QA, Registration safety
**Radiotherapy Example:** Detected incorrect mapping for parotid gland during adaptive H&N treatment.

200. **Quality-Triggered Automatic Re-Prescription Alert:** Alert system recommending physician review when cumulative dose trends deviate from intent.
**Related Terms:** Dose tracking, Clinical safety alert
**Radiotherapy Example:** Triggered re-evaluation when bladder adaptive doses exceeded tolerance early.

201. **Quantitative Dose Steering Model:** Computational model that adjusts optimization to steer dose toward under-covered target regions.
**Related Terms:** Hotspot suppression, PTV cold spot correction
**Radiotherapy Example:** Dose steering improved PTV D98 in cervical plan without increasing bowel dose.

202. **Quick Gamma Normalization Protocol:** Fast standardization of gamma index settings to ensure uniform IMRT QA evaluation.
**Related Terms:** Gamma analysis, QA reproducibility
**Radiotherapy Example:** Normalization automatically set to global max before evaluating lung IMRT QA.

203. **Quantified Portal Dose Transformation:** Converts EPID signals to water-equivalent dose maps for verification.
**Related Terms:** EPID dosimetry, Dose reconstruction
**Radiotherapy Example:** Portal dose transformation validated pancreatic VMAT delivery accuracy.

204. **Quadrant-Based Surface Registration:** Patient alignment based on four independent regions of surface scan.
**Related Terms:** SGRT, Surface matching
**Radiotherapy Example:** Posterior quadrant weighting helped align spine SBRT despite chest motion.

205. **Quasi-Static Target Margin Model:** Margin estimation assuming minimal motion but not true immobilization.
**Related Terms:** Internal margin, Residual motion
**Radiotherapy Example:** Used for shoulder sarcoma where motion was small but not zero.

206. **Quality Normalized Dose Gradient Metric:** Measures how fast dose falls off while maintaining PTV coverage.
**Related Terms:** Gradient index, Conformity
**Radiotherapy Example:** Gradient optimized to spare optic chiasm in pituitary SRS.

207. **Quantitative Anatomy Change Threshold:** Trigger threshold indicating anatomy has changed enough to require replan.
**Related Terms:** ART trigger, Adaptive workflow
**Radiotherapy Example:** Bladder volume change >130% triggered ART in prostate case.

208. **Quick-Check Imaging Isocenter Validation:** Rapid verification that imaging isocenter matches treatment isocenter before delivery.
**Related Terms:** Isocenter QA, Couch shift validation
**Radiotherapy Example:** Performed before every brain SRS fraction.

209. **Quasi-Linear MU Efficiency Rating:** Rate describing MU efficiency relative to modulation complexity.
**Related Terms:** Delivery efficiency, MU optimization
**Radiotherapy Example:** Breast plan revised after MU efficiency rating was below 0.70.

210. **Quantum-Safe Treatment Record Archive:** High-security protocol for lifetime storage of radiotherapy treatment records.
**Related Terms:** Data encryption, Digital compliance
**Radiotherapy Example:** Ensures pediatric RT data remains accessible for follow-up decades later.

211. **Quadratic Leaf Speed Modeling:** Predictive model accounting for nonlinear MLC speed during modulation.
**Related Terms:** Leaf motion constraint, Delivery timing
**Radiotherapy Example:** Used to avoid MLC overshoot during head-and-neck VMAT.

212. **Quantifiable Immobilization Reproducibility Index:** Measures how consistently the immobilization device reproduces patient setup.
**Related Terms:** Setup precision, Mask QA
**Radiotherapy Example:** Spine SRS mask remade after reproducibility score fell below 0.85.

213. **Quick-Sync CBCT Registration Algorithm:** Accelerated image registration to reduce on-couch time.
**Related Terms:** IGRT speed optimization, Registration QA
**Radiotherapy Example:** Reduced prostate CBCT registration from 50 to 15 seconds.

214. **Quality-Assured Shell Expansion Method:** Controlled expansion used to form PTV or PRV from baseline contour.
**Related Terms:** Margin recipe, Planning safety buffer
**Radiotherapy Example:** PRV margin applied to optic nerve in chordoma IMRT.

215. **Quantitative OAR Impact Forecasting:** Predicts effects of small plan adjustments on OAR doses before recalculation.
**Related Terms:** Sensitivity analysis, Plan prediction model
**Radiotherapy Example:** Forecasting enabled safe dose reduction to parotid without full reopt.

216. **Quasi-Surface Bolus Check:** Algorithm detects air gaps and wrinkles in bolus surface.
**Related Terms:** Bolus QA, Skin dose correction
**Radiotherapy Example:** Air gap flagged near ear during scalp RT.

217. **Quantitative Beam Hold Stability Test:** Confirms beam output consistency before and after hold events.
**Related Terms:** Interruption stability, Gating QA
**Radiotherapy Example:** Verified for gated liver VMAT with repeated beam stops.

218. **Quick Feedback Plan Evaluation Tool:** Displays predicted consequences when plan objectives are changed.
**Related Terms:** Optimization preview, DVH predictor
**Radiotherapy Example:** Used to tune brain plan to spare hippocampus while protecting PTV.

219. **Quasi-Adaptive Skin Dose Control:** Adapts plan to maintain minimum skin dose for superficial tumors.
**Related Terms:** Surface optimization, Bolus management
**Radiotherapy Example:** Boost applied automatically for chest wall post-mastectomy plan.

220. **Quantification of Couch Angle Interplay:** Measures dose deviation due to couch rotation interacting with MLC modulation.
**Related Terms:** Couch modeling, IMRT interplay
**Radiotherapy Example:** Lower couch angle used after high interplay predicted for tonsil IMRT.

221. **Quadrant-Based Lung Expansion Score:** Rates lung expansion asymmetry to estimate diaphragm and tumor motion.
**Related Terms:** Motion probability index, Respiratory metric
**Radiotherapy Example:** Used to determine suitability for free-breathing liver RT.

222. **Quasi-Uniform Dose Window Evaluation:** Tests whether most of PTV dose lies within the clinically acceptable band.
**Related Terms:** Homogeneity index, PTV dose conformity
**Radiotherapy Example:** Adjusted hotspots in esophageal plan after failing window test.

223. **Quality-Based Multi-Plan Selection Engine:** Compares candidate plans automatically using weighted clinical criteria.
**Related Terms:** Plan ranking, Automated evaluation
**Radiotherapy Example:** Selected best pancreas VMAT plan from five candidates.

224. **Quick Acquisition Respiratory Sampling:** Short respiratory recording to estimate typical cycle and amplitude.
**Related Terms:** 4D CT preparation, Motion baseline
**Radiotherapy Example:** Used to choose optimal breathing control for lung SBRT.

225. **Quantitative Setup Fatigue Alert:** Tracks patient discomfort risk associated with long immobilization times.
**Related Terms:** Patient tolerance, Safety alerts
**Radiotherapy Example:** Fraction time shortened for spine SRS because fatigue score high.

226. **Quadratic Dose Spill Suppression:** Optimization tool applying squared penalty when low-dose bath exceeds threshold.
**Related Terms:** OAR low-dose control, Dose bath suppression
**Radiotherapy Example:** Reduced low-dose exposure to lung in mediastinal lymphoma plan.

227. **Quasi-Real-Time In-Vivo Calibration Shift:** Detects deviation in detector signal during in-vivo dosimetry.
**Related Terms:** Entrance dose, Diode drift
**Radiotherapy Example:** Calibration shift detected for tongue output diode mid-fraction.

228. **Quantitative Shoulder Tension Index:** Metric detecting patient muscle tension influencing setup reliability.
**Related Terms:** Postural drift risk, Immobilization comfort
**Radiotherapy Example:** Neck support pad added when index exceeded limit in H&N IMRT.

229. **Quick Projected Isodose Inspection:** Fast planar review of key isodose lines without full dose analysis.
**Related Terms:** Visual QA, Planner rapid screening
**Radiotherapy Example:** Verified 50% isodose fall-off around spine cord before final QA.

230. **Quality-Controlled Plan Library Matching:** Auto selection of best-matching adaptive plan for today's anatomy.
**Related Terms:** Plan-of-day, ART
**Radiotherapy Example:** Selected full bladder plan for prostate when volume increased.

231. **Quantitative VMAT Field Sequencing Review:** Evaluates arc segmentation to avoid unnecessary pauses or speed constraints.
**Related Terms:** Arc smoothness, Delivery timing QA
**Radiotherapy Example:** Eliminated small unnecessary segments in rectal VMAT.

232. **Quasi-Static Brain Shift Evaluation:** Estimation of intracranial motion from swelling or CSF redistribution.
**Related Terms:** Brain deformation, Adaptive SRS
**Radiotherapy Example:** Brain shift prompted repeat MRI before large AVM SRS.

233. **Quantitative Neutron Dose Estimation:** Calculates secondary neutron exposure from high-energy photon beams.
**Related Terms:** Secondary cancer risk, Out-of-field dose
**Radiotherapy Example:** Neutron dose calculated for pediatric spine field using 18 MV beam.

234. **Quad-Point Bite Block Stability Test:** Verifies stability at four mouth contact points in H&N immobilization.
**Related Terms:** Dental registration, Setup reproducibility
**Radiotherapy Example:** Bite block remade for base-of-tongue patient after failing test.

235. **Quick GTV Boundary Confidence Rating:** Scoring system reflecting certainty of tumor border visibility.
**Related Terms:** Margin decision tool, GTV contour reliability
**Radiotherapy Example:** High uncertainty near lung–liver interface → expanded ITV margin.

236. **Quantitative Plan Revision Alert System:** AI predicts whether a submitted plan likely requires physician changes.
**Related Terms:** Plan prediction analytics, Review minimization
**Radiotherapy Example:** Notified planner that further optic nerve sparing likely needed.

237. **Quasi-Predictive MU Overflow Assessment:** Forecasts excessive MU risk before optimization completes.
**Related Terms:** Efficiency prediction, Modulation control
**Radiotherapy Example:** Allowed planner to adjust objectives before MU exceeded limits.

238. **Quality-Weighted Composite DVH Score:** Condenses multiple DVH evaluations into one clinically weighted score.
**Related Terms:** Plan scoring, Objective consolidation
**Radiotherapy Example:** Highest DVH score plan selected for bladder IMRT.

**239. Quadrant-Specific Skin Dose Monitor:** Tracks skin dose independently in four anatomical quadrants.
**Related Terms:** Toxicity monitoring, Skin tolerance
**Radiotherapy Example:** Detects higher posterior skin dose during breast boost.

**240. Quantified MLC Tongue-and-Groove Impact:** Estimates dose artifacts caused by T-and-G MLC structure.
**Related Terms:** Leaf overlap modeling, Modulation artifacts
**Radiotherapy Example:** Reduced tongue-and-groove effect in highly modulated brain IMRT.

**241. Quick Optical Surface Engagement Confirmation:** Verifies SGRT camera has good lock on surface before beam enable.
**Related Terms:** SGRT interlock, Patient tracking
**Radiotherapy Example:** Prevented beam-on when hair obscured scalp optical capture.

**242. Quantitative Fractional Dose Drift Log:** Trend log tracking small dose output differences over fractions.
**Related Terms:** Output consistency, PDI
**Radiotherapy Example:** Predicted recalibration need before major drift occurred.

**243. Quadratic Target Overlap Protocol:** Penalizes overlapping boost and base PTVs in optimization.
**Related Terms:** Nested targets, Dose layering
**Radiotherapy Example:** Helped manage sequential boosts in oropharyngeal IMRT.

**244. Quality-Assured Imaging Dose Reduction Strategy:** Systematic method reducing imaging dose while maintaining accuracy.
**Related Terms:** ALARA, IGRT optimization
**Radiotherapy Example:** Pediatric cases switched from daily CBCT to weekly + daily kV.

**245. Quantitative Risk Projection for Dose Accumulation:** Predicts cumulative toxicity based on ART dose accumulation.
**Related Terms:** Dose tracking, OAR risk forecasting
**Radiotherapy Example:** Alert raised when accumulated brainstem dose trending high in re-irradiation.

**246. Quick Adaptive Beam Weight Balancing:** Rapid update of beam weight to correct mild underdose without full reopt.
**Related Terms:** Fast replan, Weight tweaker
**Radiotherapy Example:** Used to compensate for prostate PTV cold region after anatomy change.

**247. Quantified Comfort-vs-Accuracy Trade Index:** Shows whether accessory changes that improve comfort reduce immobilization precision.
**Related Terms:** Setup quality, Patient comfort algorithm
**Radiotherapy Example:** Allowed soft mask padding while maintaining H&N SRS precision.

**248. Quadrant-Controlled Gantry Collision Simulation:** Collision prediction system dividing risk checks by gantry quadrants.
**Related Terms:** Collision avoidance, Safety simulation
**Radiotherapy Example:** Prevented collision with breast/prone board at 90° gantry.

**249. Quasi-Isotropic CBCT Rebinning:** Converts CBCT into nearly isotropic voxel spacing to improve registration.
**Related Terms:** Image processing, Deformable registration
**Radiotherapy Example:** Increased contour accuracy for pancreas ART.

250. **Quantitative Toxicity Expectation Report:** Predicts probabilities of acute and late toxicities from planned dose.
**Related Terms:** NTCP modeling, Predictive analytics
**Radiotherapy Example:** Helped physician decide between IMRT and proton therapy for lung cancer.

251. **Quantitative Organ Surface Dose Mapping:** Method that displays dose on 3D organ surface rather than interior volume.
**Related Terms:** Dose painting on surface, Toxicity prediction
**Radiotherapy Example:** Used to correlate esophageal surface dose with dysphagia after lung RT.

252. **Quick Adaptive Deformable Alignment:** Fast deformable registration method used during online ART.
**Related Terms:** Deformable fusion, Adaptive workflow
**Radiotherapy Example:** Enabled same-session replan for pancreas SBRT after bowel shift.

253. **Quadratic PTV Underdose Penalty Curve:** Penalty increases exponentially as PTV receives lower-than-prescribed dose.
**Related Terms:** Cold spot suppression, Optimization constraints
**Radiotherapy Example:** Eliminated a cold region behind hip prosthesis in pelvic IMRT.

254. **Quasi-Real-Time Lung Motion Detector:** Tracks respiratory motion during treatment using fast image/optical data.
**Related Terms:** Gating monitoring, ITV validation
**Radiotherapy Example:** Beam paused automatically when amplitude exceeded baseline.

255. **Quick Immobilization Pressure Map:** Records pressure distribution between patient and immobilization device.
**Related Terms:** Mask fit QA, Reproducibility prediction
**Radiotherapy Example:** Pressure variance detected mask loosening in H&N boost fractions.

256. **Quantified Machine Performance Trendline:** Statistical trajectory of linac performance parameters across QA tests.
**Related Terms:** Predictive maintenance, QA analytics
**Radiotherapy Example:** Predicted target current drift weeks before failure.

257. **Quality-Indexed PTV Overlap Correction:** Adjusts dose goals when multiple PTVs overlap to prevent overdose.
**Related Terms:** Boost interplay, Nested targets
**Radiotherapy Example:** Maintained safety at junction of prostate PTV + seminal vesicle boost.

258. **Quadrant-Based SGRT Drift Monitor:** Separates surface drift by anatomical quadrants to pinpoint trouble areas.
**Related Terms:** Real-time motion monitoring, SGRT variability
**Radiotherapy Example:** Detected asymmetric shoulder relaxation during clavicle RT.

259. **Quantified Couch Sag Compensation:** Automatic dose correction for couch bending under patient weight.
**Related Terms:** Mechanical modeling, Isocenter shift
**Radiotherapy Example:** Prevented underdose in posterior liver field for high-BMI patient.

260. **Quasi-Biological Energy Weighting Model:** Assigns different biological weight to different photon energies.
**Related Terms:** RBE surrogate, Mixed energy modelling
**Radiotherapy Example:** Evaluated tissue effects when mixing 10 MV and 6 MV for breast IMRT.

261. **Quadratic Dose Deviation Normalization:** Scoring system giving larger penalty for bigger dose error rather than linear.
**Related Terms:** Plan scoring, Weighted deviation
**Radiotherapy Example:** Helped evaluate large deviations in optic nerve dose more critically.

262. **Quantitative Spot Precision Log:** Accuracy record for individual proton spots or photon mini-segments.
**Related Terms:** Beam targeting history, Delivery verification
**Radiotherapy Example:** Flagged gantry bearing wear when spot precision drifted.

263. **Quick OAR Dose Re-Balancing Tool:** Redistribution of dose between multiple OARs to meet combined constraints.
**Related Terms:** Trade-off control, Multi-OAR tuning
**Radiotherapy Example:** Balanced parotid doses without compromising brainstem limit.

264. **Quasi-Static Bolus Reproducibility Score:** Measures consistency of bolus placement across fractions.
**Related Terms:** Bolus QA, Surface dose monitoring
**Radiotherapy Example:** Triggered photography protocol for facial bolus alignment.

265. **Quadratic Beam Orientation Selector:** Optimization that scores gantry/couch combinations using squared penalties.
**Related Terms:** Beam angle optimization, Plan improvement
**Radiotherapy Example:** Identified highly effective noncoplanar angles for brain metastasis.

266. **Quantitative OAR–PTV Competition Index:** Numerical value reflecting how difficult it is to meet competing OAR/PTV goals.
**Related Terms:** Plan complexity prediction, Priority balancing
**Radiotherapy Example:** High index warned physician that optic chiasm dose would be limiting.

267. **Quick GTV Margin Sensitivity Test:** Rapid evaluation of how much dose or OAR impact will change if GTV margin is altered.
**Related Terms:** ITV/GTV expansion prediction, Sensitivity scoring
**Radiotherapy Example:** Supported decision to reduce edge margin for laryngeal preservation.

268. **Quality-Assured Auto-Matching Protocol:** Pre-approved rules for when automatic match is acceptable vs. manual correction needed.
**Related Terms:** IGRT safety policy, Registration validation
**Radiotherapy Example:** In brain SRS, any auto-match shift >1 mm required manual review.

269. **Quantitative Radiodermatitis Likelihood Model:** Risk model predicting skin reaction severity based on surface dose + patient factors.
**Related Terms:** NTCP, Toxicity prediction
**Radiotherapy Example:** Predicted high-grade skin risk for obese breast patient with large field.

270. **Quad-Point Prostate Landmark Verification:** Use of four anatomical landmarks to check prostate alignment.
**Related Terms:** Fiducial-free IGRT, Soft-tissue alignment
**Radiotherapy Example:** Four-point check caught rotation missed by single-plane IGRT.

271. **Quantitative Beam-Hold Latency Report:** Measures delay between motion trigger and actual beam shutdown.
**Related Terms:** Gating latency, Motion-safety QA
**Radiotherapy Example:** System passed liver SBRT threshold (<100 ms shutdown latency).

272. **Quality-Normalized Delivery Complexity Rating:** Scores plan complexity relative to achieved OAR/PTV quality.
**Related Terms:** Efficiency vs. benefit, Plan value metric
**Radiotherapy Example:** Avoided unnecessary modulated plan for simple palliative pelvis.

273. **Quick Simulation Reproducibility Check:** First-fraction test evaluating whether position reproduces simulation without deviation.
**Related Terms:** Baseline validation, Initial setup QA
**Radiotherapy Example:** First brain fraction required no mask adjustment — passed quick check.

274. **Quantified Patient Breathing Regularity Index:** Numerical measure of respiratory consistency.
**Related Terms:** Gating suitability, 4D variance
**Radiotherapy Example:** Low regularity index indicated patient needed abdominal compression.

275. **Quasi-Deformable CBCT Dose Mapping:** Approximate dose warping using low-complexity deformable mapping.
**Related Terms:** Online dose accumulation, Adaptive dose
**Radiotherapy Example:** Detected rising small bowel dose mid-pelvis treatment.

276. **Quality-Filtered Plan Library System:** Plan-of-day library restricted to only clinically high-scoring plans.
**Related Terms:** ART plan selection, Daily adaptation
**Radiotherapy Example:** Excluded bladder plan variant with poor rectum sparing.

277. **Quantitative Shoulder-Roll Compensation:** Position correction to counter shoulder rotation affecting upper thorax alignment.
**Related Terms:** Postural correction, SGRT compensation
**Radiotherapy Example:** Reduced CTV shift in supraclavicular breast RT.

278. **Quadratic Low-Dose Volume Penalty:** Penalizes volume receiving low-dose bath with increasing weight at higher volumes.
**Related Terms:** Lung low-dose sparing, Dose bath control
**Radiotherapy Example:** Reduced V5 in mediastinal lymphoma IMRT.

279. **Quasi-Instantaneous MLC Error Recovery:** Automatic correction/resume after small MLC positioning error without restarting plan.
**Related Terms:** Delivery resiliency, Interruption control
**Radiotherapy Example:** Avoided repeating entire VMAT arc after minor leaf fault.

280. **Quick Symmetry Validation for Opposed Fields:** Fast evaluation of left-right dose symmetry in opposed parallel plans.
**Related Terms:** Midline alignment check, Traditional field QA
**Radiotherapy Example:** Thoracic AP/PA plan validated before patient first fraction.

281. **Quantitative Predictive Dose Aging:** Cumulative dose decay forecast for reirradiation or lifetime toxicity risk.
**Related Terms:** Tissue repair modeling, Long-term NTCP
**Radiotherapy Example:** Evaluated safety of re-irradiating brain after 9-year interval.

282. **Quasi-Robust CTV Edge Compensation:** Boosts dose near edges more sensitive to uncertainties (motion, contouring).
**Related Terms:** Edge robustness, ITV strengthening
**Radiotherapy Example:** Used for lung SBRT tumor adjacent to diaphragm.

**283. Quadrant-Based Body Clearance Check:** Predicts patient-gantry collisions by checking clearance quadrant by quadrant.
**Related Terms:** Collision avoidance simulation
**Radiotherapy Example:** Avoided gantry–shoulder collision in lateral brain plan.

**284. Quick Digital Phantom Dose Validation:** Performs virtual measurement to confirm dose distribution before physical QA.
**Related Terms:** Pre-QA simulation, Virtual QA
**Radiotherapy Example:** Caught optimizer defect before wasting array QA time.

**285. Quantitative Small-Field Output Correction:** Applies output correction factors for small fields to ensure correct dose.
**Related Terms:** DLG tuning, Output factors
**Radiotherapy Example:** Corrected mini-MLC tongue-and-groove effect in trigeminal neuralgia SRS.

**286. Quad-Criterion RTOG Compliance Verification:** Automatic confirmation of conformity, homogeneity, coverage, and fall-off vs. RTOG.
**Related Terms:** Protocol compliance checking
**Radiotherapy Example:** Verified brain SRS parameters for clinical trial enrollment.

**287. Quantified Gating Duty Cycle Projection:** Predicts actual treatment time based on expected beam-on fraction during gating.
**Related Terms:** Treatment duration prediction
**Radiotherapy Example:** Predicted 55% duty cycle led to abdominal compression to shorten session.

**288. Quick Composite Imaging Dose Monitor:** Running total of patient imaging dose across planning and treatment.
**Related Terms:** IGRT dose tracking, ALARA
**Radiotherapy Example:** Pediatric case switched to weekly CBCT after dose threshold.

**289. Quasi-Biological Multi-Objective Ranking:** Weighted scoring combining physical metrics with expected biological effects.
**Related Terms:** NTCP/plan hybrid metric
**Radiotherapy Example:** Chosen IMRT vs proton therapy based on lowest composite score.

**290. Quality-Flagged Hotspot Redistribution:** Redistributes hotspots only if redistribution improves OAR outcome rather than just smoothing.
**Related Terms:** Smart hotspot control, Optimization decision logic
**Radiotherapy Example:** Reduced breast ridge hotspot only if not increasing lung V20.

**291. Quantitative Arm Position Stability Score:** Tracks arm drift during breast/chest RT to avoid setup deviations.
**Related Terms:** Shoulder stabilization, SGRT monitoring
**Radiotherapy Example:** Left arm needed extra support for axillary IMRT.

**292. Quadratic Dose–Volume Trade Metric:** Converts multiple DVH trade-offs into a single optimized curve.
**Related Terms:** Pareto analytics, Plan frontier
**Radiotherapy Example:** Selected dose compromise between rectum vs. bladder in prostate RT.

**293. Quick CT-To-CBCT Air Cavity Matching:** Recognizes changes in bowel/stomach air cavities that may affect dose.
**Related Terms:** Anatomy variation alert, ART trigger
**Radiotherapy Example:** Triggered adaptive workflow when bowel gas entered PTV region.

**294. Quantified Paused-Time Heat Map:** Map showing where treatment time paused most frequently during gated delivery.
**Related Terms:** Gating inefficiency visualization
**Radiotherapy Example:** Beam pauses clustered at end-inspiration → gating window adjusted.

**295. Quad-Model Arc Complexity Estimation:** Uses four parameters (MU, aperture change, speed, segment variation) to estimate VMAT complexity.
**Related Terms:** Modulation score, Delivery efficiency predictor
**Radiotherapy Example:** H&N plan adjusted to reduce segment fluctuation.

**296. Quasi-Static Proton Range Drift Detection:** Monitors range change over time caused by density/weight variation.
**Related Terms:** Proton range uncertainty, ART trigger
**Radiotherapy Example:** Weight loss shifted proton range in esophagus — re-scan ordered.

**297. Quantitative Treatment Break Recovery Protocol:** Calculates additional dose or fractionation adjustment after unplanned break.
**Related Terms:** Proliferation compensation, Treatment delay management
**Radiotherapy Example:** Compensatory boost calculated after 10-day interruption in H&N RT.

**298. Quick In-Room Optical Marker Confirmation:** Validates visibility and correct placement of optical tracking markers before surface tracking.
**Related Terms:** SGRT calibration safety
**Radiotherapy Example:** Marker misalignment detected on arm for DIBH breast case.

**299. Quality-Driven Adaptive Plan Eligibility Score:** Determines whether a patient benefits from ART based on change magnitude and dosimetric impact.
**Related Terms:** ART decision support, Dose–change prioritization
**Radiotherapy Example:** Flagged rectal cancer patient as high priority for ART after significant shrinkage.

**300. Quantitative Real-Time Delivery Verification Index:** Composite score summarizing agreement between planned and delivered delivery metrics in real time.
**Related Terms:** Treatment surveillance, Live QA
**Radiotherapy Example:** Score drop during liver SBRT immediately identified MLC mis-tracking.

**301. Quantitative Pelvic Rotation Index:** Numerical score measuring pelvic rotational variation between fractions.
**Related Terms:** Setup reproducibility, IGRT alignment
**Radiotherapy Example:** High index triggered adaptive repositioning during prostate RT.

**302. Quadratic Nerve-Sparing Dose Model:** Dose model that increases sparing priority exponentially near nerve bundles.
**Related Terms:** OAR gradient boost, Functional avoidance
**Radiotherapy Example:** Protected brachial plexus during head & neck IMRT without compromising PTV.

**303. Quick Missing-Tissue Compensator Estimation:** Auto-prediction of bolus/compensator thickness when external contour changes.
**Related Terms:** ART bolus correction, Surface adaptation
**Radiotherapy Example:** New rib separation required 0.5 cm bolus update in breast plan.

**304. Quantified Organ Filling Change Score:** Measures daily bladder/bowel volume variability to predict dosimetric impact.
**Related Terms:** Hydration protocol compliance, ART trigger
**Radiotherapy Example:** Bladder score drop warned of increased rectum dose.

**305. Quality-Capped Dose Paint Region:** Limits escalation only where model confidence is high to avoid unsafe dose paint.
**Related Terms:** Radiomics-driven planning, Boost regulation
**Radiotherapy Example:** Prevented escalation in uncertain PET-MRI border for brain GBM.

**306. Quantitative Hotspot Displacement Map:** Visual display tracking hotspot migration across adaptive replans.
**Related Terms:** Hotspot stability, Adaptive dose follow-up
**Radiotherapy Example:** Hotspot drift toward duodenum flagged in liver ART.

**307. Quick NTCP Parameter Refit:** Adjusts NTCP curve using patient-specific biomarkers.
**Related Terms:** Precision toxicity prediction, Personalized medicine
**Radiotherapy Example:** NTCP adjusted for smoker in lung IMRT toxicity prediction.

**308. Quadrant-Level IGRT Trust Matrix:** Weights reliability of IGRT match differently for anatomical quadrants.
**Related Terms:** Region-priority matching, Confidence map
**Radiotherapy Example:** Soft-tissue match prioritized anterior prostate region over gas-filled posterior.

**309. Quasi-Proton Equivalent Index:** Score estimating how much photon plan mimics proton dose distribution.
**Related Terms:** Proton benefit prediction, Low-dose bath reduction
**Radiotherapy Example:** Pediatric medulloblastoma IMRT scored low — proton referral advised.

**310. Quality-Based Bolus Necessity Algorithm:** Determines if bolus improves PTV coverage without increasing skin toxicity.
**Related Terms:** Surface dose evaluation, Optimization rule
**Radiotherapy Example:** Eliminated unnecessary bolus for chest wall boost.

**311. Quantitative SGRT Lag Characterization:** Measures delay between real motion and SGRT tracking display.
**Related Terms:** Tracking latency, Gating synchronization
**Radiotherapy Example:** Lag corrected before starting DIBH left breast.

**312. Quad-Beam Exit Dose Validator:** Uses exit-dose logs from four beam directions to estimate internal dose error.
**Related Terms:** Transit dosimetry, Portal verification
**Radiotherapy Example:** Detected spine curvature shift during thoracic IMRT.

**313. Quick Comfort-Driven Immobilization Review:** Checks if discomfort causes posture drift that degrades reproducibility.
**Related Terms:** Patient tolerance QA, Motion prevention
**Radiotherapy Example:** Mask pressure redesigned after facial pain increased drift.

**314. Quantified Treatment Anxiety–Motion Score:** Correlates patient anxiety with measurable intrafraction motion trends.
**Related Terms:** Behavioral radiotherapy, Motion risk model
**Radiotherapy Example:** Music intervention reduced motion score in pediatric RT.

**315. Quadratic Field Junction Stability Model:** Predicts risk of over- or under-dose at field junctions using quadratic penalty.
**Related Terms:** Junction hot/cold avoidance, Field matching
**Radiotherapy Example:** Craniospinal plan passed junction stability model before QA.

316. **Quick Proton Range-GAN Estimator:** AI that predicts proton range shifts based on daily CBCT.
**Related Terms:** Adaptive proton therapy, Range uncertainty
**Radiotherapy Example:** Corrected 3 mm shift in anterior skull base tumor.

317. **Quantitative 4D Lung Cycle Similarity Index:** Measures similarity between historical and current breathing cycles.
**Related Terms:** Motion model reliability, Gating fidelity
**Radiotherapy Example:** Index drop triggered new 4DCT for lung SBRT.

318. **Quasi-Toroidal Dose Cloud Model:** Model describing donut-shaped dose clouds around concave targets.
**Related Terms:** Concave geometry handling, Avoidance ring shaping
**Radiotherapy Example:** Improved coverage around horseshoe-shaped PTV around spinal cord.

319. **Quick Multi-Structure Priority Balancer:** Automatically redistributes planning priorities between multiple competing OARs.
**Related Terms:** Multi-OAR negotiation, Optimization automation
**Radiotherapy Example:** Balanced dose between parotids and cochlea in H&N IMRT.

320. **Quantified BMI-Driven Table Shift Predictor:** Anticipates couch sag/shift based on body habitus and limb positioning.
**Related Terms:** Mechanical prediction model, IGRT correction
**Radiotherapy Example:** Triggered manual verification for high-BMI lung patient.

321. **Quality-Weighted Tumor Control Probability:** TCP estimate adjusted by plan quality and dose conformity rather than only BED.
**Related Terms:** TCP hybrid model, Outcome prediction
**Radiotherapy Example:** Higher score favored VMAT boost over static beams.

322. **Quadrant-Shaped Dose Halo Classification:** Categorizes low-dose halos by orientation around PTV.
**Related Terms:** Scatter mapping, Secondary dose pattern
**Radiotherapy Example:** Right-posterior halo minimized to protect spinal cord.

323. **Quick Anterior–Posterior Shift Alarm:** Real-time alert if AP displacement exceeds preset threshold.
**Related Terms:** Tracking alarm, Motion safety
**Radiotherapy Example:** Prevented pelvic displacement during bladder emptying.

324. **Quantitative Neural Network Plan Auditor:** AI system that checks RT plans for protocol and physics compliance.
**Related Terms:** Automated plan QA, Error prevention
**Radiotherapy Example:** Detected incorrect prescription isocenter shift in pediatric proton case.

325. **Quasi-Continuous Thermal Camera Monitoring:** Thermal sensors verify skin temperature for early radiodermatitis detection.
**Related Terms:** Skin toxicity predictor, Treatment support
**Radiotherapy Example:** Breast RT patient referred for topical care before Grade-2 toxicity.

326. **Quick Fraction-to-Fraction Dose Drift Alarm:** Triggers alert when accumulated dose deviates from expected projection.
**Related Terms:** Dose accumulation QA, Adaptive threshold|
**Radiotherapy Example:** Detected unexpected hip rotation affecting gonadal dose.

327. **Quantitative Deep-Tissue Expansion Score:** Measures internal organ shift from weight change or tumor shrinkage.
**Related Terms:** ART need detection, Soft tissue shift scoring
**Radiotherapy Example:** Score predicted bladder ART requirement by week 3.

328. **Quadratic Fall-Off Efficiency Rating:** Rates steepness and uniformity of dose drop-off beyond target.
**Related Terms:** Dose gradient index, SRS quality
**Radiotherapy Example:** Confirmed superior gradient for Gamma Knife vs LINAC SRS.

329. **Quick-Predict OAR Recovery Estimator:** Estimates long-term recovery based on organ tolerance and dose timing.
**Related Terms:** Toxicity compensation, Long-term NTCP
**Radiotherapy Example:** Supported safe re-irradiation of spinal metastasis after 7 years.

330. **Quantified Hybrid Tracking Confidence:** Confidence score combining SGRT + kV + CBCT alignment.
**Related Terms:** Sensor fusion, Redundancy safety
**Radiotherapy Example:** Required manual match when confidence dropped during neck RT.

331. **Quantitative Proton Range Validation:** Confirms proton stopping range accuracy using imaging or detectors before treatment.
**Related Terms:** Range uncertainty, Prompt-gamma monitoring
**Radiotherapy Example:** Range check ensured no overshoot into spinal cord during pediatric proton craniospinal RT.

332. **Quasi-Real-Time Dose Reconstruction:** Rebuilds delivered dose during treatment using log files and motion tracking signals.
**Related Terms:** Log-file QA, Delivered dose verification
**Radiotherapy Example:** Detected underdosing of lung PTV during VMAT due to breathing variation.

333. **Quality-Based Energy Layer Selection:** Chooses optimal energy layers to balance LET distribution and range uncertainty in proton/ion therapy.
**Related Terms:** Layered energy optimization, LET balancing
**Radiotherapy Example:** Reduced LET hotspots in brainstem during proton boost.

334. **Quantitative Radiomics-Guided Adaptation:** Uses radiomic biomarker trends to decide whether plan adaptation is needed mid-treatment.
**Related Terms:** Response-based ART, AI response evaluation
**Radiotherapy Example:** Radiomics shrinkage pattern triggered adaptive replan on H&N week 4.

335. **Quad-Structure Plan Validation Index:** Scores plan quality based on PTV, high-priority OARs, secondary OARs, and healthy tissue sparing.
**Related Terms:** Composite plan scoring, Multi-criteria evaluation
**Radiotherapy Example:** Index ranked pancreas VMAT plan #3 as optimal among 6 auto-generated plans.

336. **Quasi-Static Tracking Window:** Tracking mode assuming slow/limited motion rather than real-time fast motion, common in pelvic targets.
**Related Terms:** Pelvic IGRT stability, Drift-based tracking
**Radiotherapy Example:** Maintained prostate PTV accuracy without full gating.

337. **Quantified Gradient Fall-Speed Metric:** Measures how rapidly dose falls from PTV edge to surrounding tissue in 3D.
**Related Terms:** High-dose gradient control, OAR proximity safety
**Radiotherapy Example:** Confirmed safe spinal cord fall-off in stereotactic spine RT.

338. **Quick Adaptive Optimization Trigger:** Automatic decision rule for activating re-optimization when deviation surpasses threshold.
**Related Terms:** Adaptive criteria, Smart replanning
**Radiotherapy Example:** Triggered ART when parotid migration exceeded 3 mm laterally.

339. **Quality-Weighted Fraction Priority Table:** Assigns importance to specific fractions depending on biological effect or tumor response window.
**Related Terms:** Radiosensitivity timing, Dose–effect scheduling
**Radiotherapy Example:** Prioritized first 3 fractions in SBRT liver case for highest BED impact.

340. **Quantitative Organ Expansion Model:** Predicts internal organ swelling/shrinkage patterns affecting dose delivery.
**Related Terms:** Organ deformation forecasting, Time-dependent ART
**Radiotherapy Example:** Predicted esophageal dilation during chemoradiation → generated pre-planned adaptive strategy.

341. **Quantitative Electron Contour Deviation Score:** Tracks how much patient surface contour deviates from planned for electron fields.
**Related Terms:** Bolus correction, Electron cutout verification
**Radiotherapy Example:** Triggered custom bolus update for chest wall boost after edema reduction.

342. **Quick Anatomical Deformation Warning:** Instant alert when deformable registration detects significant tissue distortion.
**Related Terms:** ART trigger, DIR consistency
**Radiotherapy Example:** Detected parotid shrinkage requiring replanning during H&N RT.

343. **Quadratic Cranio-Caudal Gradient Preserver:** Algorithm stabilizing dose fall-off along cranio-caudal direction in long targets.
**Related Terms:** Field matching integrity, Gradient uniformity
**Radiotherapy Example:** Used in craniospinal RT to prevent junction mismatch.

344. **Quantified Lung Ventilation Match Score:** Measures agreement between planned and actual ventilation distribution.
**Related Terms:** Functional avoidance, Functional lung RT
**Radiotherapy Example:** Prevented dose increase to high-function lobe during ART.

345. **Quad-Source Imaging Registration Validator:** Verifies IGRT alignment consistency across four imaging sources.
**Related Terms:** Registration redundancy, Verification loop
**Radiotherapy Example:** Detected mismatched kV/kV vs CBCT in prostate positioning.

346. **Quick Dose Hot-Rim Alert:** Warns when ring-shaped hotspots form around high-dose boost borders.
**Related Terms:** Gradient ring control, IMRT quality check
**Radiotherapy Example:** Resolved halo around SRS boost for brain metastasis.

347. **Query-Driven Dose Recovery Predictor:** Estimates if suboptimal early fractions can be compensated later safely.
**Related Terms:** Compensatory dose, BED recovery
**Radiotherapy Example:** Allowed safe boost of week-4 underdosed PTV in bladder RT.

348. **Quad-Spoke Beam Interaction Model:** Predicts hotspot formation when four beams intersect around a concave target.
**Related Terms:** Beam interplay risk, Hotspot prevention
**Radiotherapy Example:** Prevented dose spike at rectum-prostate junction.

349. **Quick Surface-to-Isocenter Vector Check:** Confirms correct relationship between SGRT external contour and internal isocenter.
**Related Terms:** External-internal correlation, Position safety
**Radiotherapy Example:** Detected mask shift in brain RT despite matched lasers.

350. **Quantitative Thermoplastic Memory Assessment:** Measures mask expansion or relaxation due to temperature and time.
**Related Terms:** Immobilization drift, Setup reproducibility
**Radiotherapy Example:** Replaced mask when looseness increased >3 mm.

351. **Quality-Weighted Composite DVH Score:** DVH summarizing PTV/OAR quality in a single numeric result.
**Related Terms:** Plan quality scoring, Automated plan ranking
**Radiotherapy Example:** Score selected best plan among five auto-generated VMAT plans.

352. **Quadratic Low-Dose Bath Suppression:** Exponential penalty for excess low-dose spread to healthy tissue.
**Related Terms:** Healthy tissue protection, Photon scatter minimization
**Radiotherapy Example:** Reduced contralateral breast dose during left breast VMAT.

353. **Quick Fiducial Drift Localization:** Identifies direction and magnitude of gold seed migration.
**Related Terms:** Fiducial stability, IGRT reliability
**Radiotherapy Example:** Detected posterior seed migration in prostate patient.

354. **Quadrant-Priority Intrafraction Tracking:** Prioritizes monitoring of the most motion-sensitive anatomical quadrant.
**Related Terms:** Region-based gating, Adaptive vigilance
**Radiotherapy Example:** Focused tracking on diaphragm-adjacent liver region.

355. **Quantitative Biological Fractionation Score:** Ranks fractionation schemes based on biological advantage for that tumor.
**Related Terms:** BED personalization, Radiosensitivity weighing
**Radiotherapy Example:** Score favored hypofractionation for prostate SBRT case.

356. **Quick Detector Panel Thermal Drift Correction:** Automatic recalibration to correct MV/kV panel heat-induced sag.
**Related Terms:** Imaging QA, Geometric correction
**Radiotherapy Example:** Corrected 1.4 mm EPID shift on long IMRT delivery.

357. **Quadratic Neural Tissue Avoidance Function:** Aggressively increases dose penalty when dose approaches neural tissue tolerance.
**Related Terms:** Neuro-protection, High-risk OAR
**Radiotherapy Example:** Prevented optic chiasm dose spike during skull base RT.

358. **Quick Auto-Beam-Collapse Check:** Ensures beam paths remain clear of collision with couch, headrest, or patient.
**Related Terms:** Collision avoidance, Mechanical safety
**Radiotherapy Example:** Avoided planned couch collision during VMAT spine RT.

**359. Quasi-Isotropic Respiratory Gating Window:** Gating window based on 3-axis motion uniformity rather than single axis.
**Related Terms:** 3D gating, Multi-vector motion
**Radiotherapy Example:** More stable gating for pancreatic SBRT.

**360. Quantified MLC End-Leaf Convergence Score:** Measures efficiency and stability of end-leaf overlap for small fields.
**Related Terms:** Leaf interplay reliability, Small-field accuracy
**Radiotherapy Example:** Improved conformity in SRS 5-mm target.

**361. Quick High-Dose Arc Pause Logic:** Pauses beam automatically when arc enters high-risk OAR zone if motion detected.
**Related Terms:** Motion-aware VMAT, Safety pausing
**Radiotherapy Example:** Prevented bowel overdose during liver VMAT.

**362. Quantitative SBRT Target-Rigidness Check:** Confirms target biomechanics match assumptions for high-precision SBRT.
**Related Terms:** Motion robustness, Target consistency
**Radiotherapy Example:** Identified pancreas case unsuitable for non-adaptive SBRT.

**363. Quasi-Predictive Fractional Regression Model:** Predicts dose-response each week using regression over biomarkers + imaging.
**Related Terms:** Longitudinal radiomics, Response forecast
**Radiotherapy Example:** Predicted volumetric shrinkage by week 3 of H&N RT.

**364. Quadratic Re-Irradiation Safety Envelope:** Combines previous and current dose with exponential OAR sensitivity penalty.
**Related Terms:** Re-irradiation planning, Cumulative tolerance?
**Radiotherapy Example:** Approved safe spinal SBRT after old field review.

**365. Quick Mid-Fraction Drift Corrector:** Resets patient position during treatment if gradual drift detected.
**Related Terms:** Intrafraction correction, Tracking feedback
**Radiotherapy Example:** Corrected 2 mm upward chin motion during brain mask RT.

**366. Quantified Bolus-Skin Gap Detector:** Calculates micro-air gaps between bolus and skin from surface imaging.
**Related Terms:** Bolus adherence QA, Surface dose integrity
**Radiotherapy Example:** Air gap increased under clavicle → bolus taped and re-scanned.

**367. Quick OAR-Border Vulnerability Flag:** Flags when build-up region overlaps OAR boundary at steep gradient.?
**Related Terms:** Gradient-risk mapping, Border-sensitivity
**Radiotherapy Example:** Detected risk at esophagus–lung border during mediastinal RT.

**368. Quadratic Dual-Layer Modulator:** Dual penalty system controlling both PTV homogeneity and OAR fall-off.
**Related Terms:** Optimization balancing, Dual-objective
**Radiotherapy Example:** Achieved uniform rectum sparing in prostate VMAT.

**369. Quantitative DIBH Stability Rating:** Scores number of stable breath-holds and duration reliability.
**Related Terms:** SGRT respiratory evaluation, Gating quality
**Radiotherapy Example:** Required training when stability rating <80%.

370. **Quick Inverse-Dose Hotspot Trim:** Auto-creates sub-structures to limit dose in hotspot regions during optimization.
**Related Terms:** Hotspot smoothing, IMRT tuning
**Radiotherapy Example:** Limited lateral PTV hotspot in pelvis VMAT.

371. **Quantified Beam Modulation Complexity Meter:** Evaluates whether MLC modulation is excessive or clinically unnecessary.
**Related Terms:** Plan complexity index, Delivery robustness
**Radiotherapy Example:** Complexity reduced for safer delivery without losing PTV coverage.

372. **Quick Rotational Axis Shift Scan:** Identifies day-to-day changes in patient rotation center.
**Related Terms:** Rotational IGRT, Alignment consistency
**Radiotherapy Example:** Corrected pelvic rotation axis shift due to muscle tightness.

373. **Quadratic Heterogeneity Distribution Monitor:** Tracks internal density distribution changes affecting dose calculation.
**Related Terms:** Hounsfield drift, Density-change ART
**Radiotherapy Example:** Flagged lung consolidation requiring recalculation.

374. **Quantitative Esophagus Inflation Predictor:** Predicts gas-related esophageal expansion impacting dose.
**Related Terms:** GI motion predictor, Swallow variability
**Radiotherapy Example:** Auto-replan prevented hot spot during lung VMAT.

375. **Quick MLC Interdigitation Safety Check:** Ensures leaf-pair configurations remain safe at tight spacing.
**Related Terms:** Collision-free MLC, Leaf geometry safety
**Radiotherapy Example:** Prevented end-leaf conflict in spine SRS.

376. **Quadrant-Based Artifact Suppression:** Removes reconstruction artifacts by quadrant rather than whole image.
**Related Terms:** CBCT artifact reduction, Local correction
**Radiotherapy Example:** Posterior artifact fixed near spine pedicles.

377. **Quick Daily Dose-Shift Recovery Plan:** Instant micro-boost scheduling if target underdose detected early.
**Related Terms:** Dose catch-up, Fraction compensation
**Radiotherapy Example:** Recovered CTV dose loss during week 2 of bladder RT.

378. **Quantified Midline Symmetry Engine:** Measures anatomical midline variations affecting PTV centering.
**Related Terms:** Symmetry-based alignment, Position strategy
**Radiotherapy Example:** Midline shift from edema triggered new setup instructions.

379. **Quick Dual-Energy Registration Check:** Compares DECT-based soft/tissue matches with CBCT matches for consistency.
**Related Terms:** Dual-energy IGRT, Soft-tissue validation
**Radiotherapy Example:** Improved pancreas alignment accuracy.

380. **Quadratic Counter-Rotation Planner:** Applies compensatory rotational corrections when two joints rotate independently.
**Related Terms:** Pelvis–lumbar decoupling, Torsion correction
**Radiotherapy Example:** Prevented mis-registration from pelvic vs lumbar rotation conflict.

381. **Quasi-4D Dose Tracking:** Estimates accumulated dose over time based on breathing motion without full 4D recalculation.
**Related Terms:** Motion-compensated dosing, Accumulated dose tracking
**Radiotherapy Example:** Detected slow PTV underdose across SBRT lung fractions.

382. **Quiet Beam Mode Verification:** QA mode ensuring modified dose rate for reduced acoustic noise operates correctly.
**Related Terms:** Patient comfort mode, Dose-rate control
**Radiotherapy Example:** Used for long H&N VMAT sessions in pediatric cases.

383. **Quad-Detector Portal QA:** Verifies EPID calibration using four independent detector regions.
**Related Terms:** Portal dosimetry QA, Detector uniformity
**Radiotherapy Example:** Improved VMAT gamma passing for pelvic RT.

384. **Quantitative LET Mapping QA:** Validation of LET distribution maps for particle therapy.
**Related Terms:** LET optimization, Proton RBE QA
**Radiotherapy Example:** Checked LET hotspots near optic nerves in chordoma IMPT.

385. **Quality Scoring for Adaptive Replanning:** Ranks necessity of ART based on tumor change, OAR shift, and dose deviation.
**Related Terms:** Adaptation threshold scoring, AI-driven ART
**Radiotherapy Example:** Triggered ART for pancreatic RT at week 3 after significant stomach shift.

386. **Quantile-Based Dose Gradient Index:** Evaluates dose fall-off by comparing dose values across statistical quantiles.
**Related Terms:** Dose gradient index, Hotspot quantification
**Radiotherapy Example:** Validated safe spinal cord fall-off in vertebral SBRT.

387. **Quadrant-Based Surface Tracking QA:** Evaluates SGRT accuracy in each quadrant of visible surface.
**Related Terms:** SGRT quality, Optical tracking calibration
**Radiotherapy Example:** Ensured accurate breast DIBH surface tracking.

388. **Quasi-Isocentric Field Calibration:** Ensures multibeam linac delivery mimics single isocenter in multi-target SRS.
**Related Terms:** Single-isocenter SRS, Couch rotation QA
**Radiotherapy Example:** Phantom results confirmed isocentric alignment for 8 brain mets.

389. **Quick Patient-Specific Plan Validation:** Automated verification of dose metrics, constraints, MU, and fluence before approval.
**Related Terms:** Auto-plan review, TPS QA
**Radiotherapy Example:** Accelerated approval for a simple breast field plan.

390. **Quality-Weighted BED Calculator:** BED calculation integrating biological sensitivity and clinical priority score.
**Related Terms:** TCP/NTCP estimation, Dose–effect modelling
**Radiotherapy Example:** Identified optimal BED range for esophageal SBRT while sparing heart.

391. **Quadratic Dose–Response Modelling:** Predicts tumor response curve using quadratic trend instead of linear or sigmoid.
**Related Terms:** Dose–effect modeling, Radiosensitivity analysis
**Radiotherapy Example:** Used for modeling prostate radiobiology in hypofractionation.

**392. Quality-Driven Beam Weight Optimization:** Assigns importance to beams based on organ risk and PTV coverage during optimization.
**Related Terms:** Beam weighting, Multi-criteria optimization
**Radiotherapy Example:** Increased posterior beam weight to reduce bowel dose in pelvis RT.

**393. Quantitative Anatomical Drift Monitoring:** Tracks gradual organ or target displacement during long fractionation schedules.
**Related Terms:** Interfraction motion, IGRT monitoring
**Radiotherapy Example:** Identified progressive prostate drift → triggered SBRT adaptation.

**394. Quadrature-Based Dose Reconstruction:** Uses integral quadrature calculations to rebuild delivered dose from fluence logs.
**Related Terms:** Log-based dose reconstruction, Delivery verification
**Radiotherapy Example:** Confirmed 2% MU deviation during VMAT pancreas session.

**395. Quasi-Rigid Organ Deformation Model:** Assumes organs deform partially rather than fully elastic or rigid.
**Related Terms:** Hybrid deformation model, Adaptive contouring
**Radiotherapy Example:** Improved stomach auto-contours for gastric RT.

**396. Quantitative PET-Response Triggered Adaptation:** Uses PET metabolic response to indicate mid-treatment plan changes.
**Related Terms:** Functional adaptation, SUV-based response
**Radiotherapy Example:** Dose boost added for persistent lung tumor FDG hotspot.

**397. Quality-Assured Auto-Segmentation:** Segmentation automatically checked for geometry and anatomical plausibility.
**Related Terms:** Auto-contouring QA, AI contour verification
**Radiotherapy Example:** Auto-corrected parotid contour shrinking during H&N therapy.

**398. Quasi-Static Couch Motion QA:** Tests accuracy of slow couch translation during gated or tracked therapies.
**Related Terms:** Couch drift control, Motion tracking
**Radiotherapy Example:** Ensured couch accuracy during liver gated IMRT.

**399. Quantitative Organ Sparing Index:** Scores radiation toxicity risk reduction relative to conventional planning.
**Related Terms:** OAR protection score, Clinical plan ranking
**Radiotherapy Example:** Demonstrated 57% risk reduction for kidney RT using VMAT.

**400. Quality Fusion Accuracy Metric:** Rates CT–MRI/PET fusion based on landmark and soft-tissue precision.
**Related Terms:** Image registration QA, Fusion validation
**Radiotherapy Example:** Verified PET–CT fusion for pancreatic SBRT target.

**401. Quadrant-Based Dose Validation Phantom:** Phantom split into four dose zones for QA symmetry checks.
**Related Terms:** Symmetry QA, Profile QA
**Radiotherapy Example:** Confirmed equal VMAT dose distribution for spinal RT.

**402. Quasi-Monte Carlo Dose Estimation:** Uses deterministic pseudo-random sampling to accelerate Monte Carlo speed.
**Related Terms:** Fast MC, Collapsed cone, GPU dose
**Radiotherapy Example:** Enabled real-time proton dose adaptation.

403. **Quantitative On-Treatment Imaging Score:** Measures IGRT accuracy based on contrast, SNR, edge precision, and spatial alignment.
**Related Terms:** IGRT QA, Adaptive correction
**Radiotherapy Example:** Signaled declining CBCT contrast in abdomen RT → detector recalibration.

404. **Quasi-Online Adaptive Margin Correction:** Applies reduced margins during treatment based on real-time tracking confidence.
**Related Terms:** Margin reduction, Motion-adaptive PTV
**Radiotherapy Example:** Halved PTV margin during DIBH breast RT.

405. **Quantified Micro-Beam Peak–Valley Ratio:** Ratio describing therapeutic contrast in micro-beam radiotherapy.
**Related Terms:** MRT QA, Spatial fractionation
**Radiotherapy Example:** Verified safe valley dose for pre-clinical brain irradiation.

406. **Quality-Assured Proton Aperture Fabrication:** QA of custom apertures for proton collimation and edge shaping.
**Related Terms:** Brass aperture QA, Cutout verification
**Radiotherapy Example:** Confirmed accurate field shape for pediatric abdominal target.

407. **Quadratic NTCP Estimator:** Predicts complication probability using modified quadratic response function.
**Related Terms:** Toxicity modeling, Normal tissue response
**Radiotherapy Example:** Estimated xerostomia risk in H&N IMRT.

408. **Quantitative Head Drift Detection:** Detects slow head motion during brain SRS despite immobilization.
**Related Terms:** SGRT monitoring, Cranial motion
**Radiotherapy Example:** Triggered automated couch correction for 1.3 mm drift.

409. **Quick SRS Field-to-Field Junction QA:** Verifies hotspot control in multi-isocenter cranial SRS junctions.
**Related Terms:** Field matching QA, Junction dosimetry
**Radiotherapy Example:** Eliminated 15% hotspot between 2 overlapped isocenters.

410. **Quadrant-Based MU Sensitivity Scan:** Finds dose sensitivity to MU errors across anatomical quadrants.
**Related Terms:** MU safety modeling, Delivery robustness
**Radiotherapy Example:** Ensured safe pancreas VMAT delivery under ±2% MU noise.

411. **Quantitative Bone Dose–Porosity Correlation:** Correlates bone density weakening with local radiation dose.
**Related Terms:** Bone toxicity modeling, SRS vertebrae risk prediction
**Radiotherapy Example:** Guided SBRT dose constraint for vertebral body.

412. **Quasi-3D Portal Film Reconstruction:** Recreates 3D fluence from stacked 2D portal films or EPID frames.
**Related Terms:** EPID 3D dosimetry, Log-file QA
**Radiotherapy Example:** Verified 3D VMAT dose to liver.

413. **Quantum Noise Modelling for Imaging QA:** Predicts and compensates for quantum mottle/low-photon noise in KV/CBCT.
**Related Terms:** Scatter reduction, Denoising QA
**Radiotherapy Example:** Improved pediatric abdominal CBCT visibility.

414. **Quick-Turnaround Patient QA Pipeline:** High-speed automated workflow for IMRT/VMAT validation and approval.
**Related Terms:** Auto-gamma, AI QA
**Radiotherapy Example:** Enabled same-day start for palliative spine IMRT.

415. **Quality-Weighted Tumor Control Priority:** Numerical weight reflecting clinical urgency and benefit of dose escalation.
**Related Terms:** Dose boost strategy, Prioritized planning
**Radiotherapy Example:** Boosted high-risk prostate lesion identified by PSMA-PET.

416. **Quantified Dose-Toxicity Gradient Score:** Measures how safely dose curves transition from tumor to organs.
**Related Terms:** Gradient index, Toxicity risk prediction
**Radiotherapy Example:** Reduced risk of esophagitis in lung SBRT plan.

417. **Quasi-Sequential Adaptive Planning:** Creates a series of standby plans anticipating anatomical evolution.
**Related Terms:** Predictive ART, Adaptive library
**Radiotherapy Example:** Used for weekly weight loss trend in H&N RT.

418. **Quadratic Gamma Constraint Model:** Adjusts gamma tolerance depending on anatomical risk and dose priority.
**Related Terms:** Weighted gamma index, Patient-specific QA
**Radiotherapy Example:** Lower threshold near optic chiasm, higher threshold near muscle.

419. **Quantitative Beam Steering Drift Monitoring:** Tracks deviation of steering magnets over time to prevent beam misalignment.
**Related Terms:** Beam steering QA, Output uniformity
**Radiotherapy Example:** Detected slight drift before affecting photon SRS precision.

420. **Quality-Driven Aperture Complexity Index:** Score describing MLC shape complexity vs. clinical benefit.
**Related Terms:** MLC modulation index, IMRT deliverability
**Radiotherapy Example:** Reduced complexity to increase pass rate in pancreas IMRT.

421. **Quasi-Autonomous Machine Output Calibration:** Automated self-calibration of LINAC output using reference detectors.
**Related Terms:** Automatic output QA, Machine learning QA
**Radiotherapy Example:** Eliminated drift in daily output before beam start.

422. **Quantile-Based CBCT HU Stability Curve:** Models stability of CBCT HU values using quantile trends over time.
**Related Terms:** HU calibration QA, Daily CBCT QA
**Radiotherapy Example:** Identified HU instability during brain tumor RT caused by detector warm-up.

423. **Quadrant-Based Collimator Angle Sensitivity:** Tests if field quality varies depending on collimator angle region.
**Related Terms:** Angular QA, MLC geometry QA
**Radiotherapy Example:** Verified stable IMRT fluence at all angles for prostate RT.

424. **Quick-Adaptive Field Margin Scaling:** Scales margins automatically based on IGRT confidence score.
**Related Terms:** Margin adaptation, ART margin control
**Radiotherapy Example:** Margin reduced during stable DIBH breast treatment.

**425. Quantitative Sub-Voxel Dose Accumulation:** Accumulates dose with resolution finer than imaging voxel grid.
**Related Terms:** Deformable dose mapping, High-precision dose summation
**Radiotherapy Example:** Improved dose accuracy for tongue tumor showing tissue shrinkage.

**426. Quality-Adjusted Motion Risk Score:** Predicts treatment risk due to motion and adjusts delivery strategy.
**Related Terms:** Motion prediction, Gating threshold selection
**Radiotherapy Example:** Triggered gating for irregular-lung-breathing patient.

**427. Quadrature-Based 3D Surface Tracking:** Uses multi-vector interpolation for precise SGRT surface mapping.
**Related Terms:** Optical tracking, Surface guidance
**Radiotherapy Example:** Improved face mask-free SRS patient tracking.

**428. Quasi-Online RBE Validation:** Monitors effective biological dose during proton or heavy ion therapy.
**Related Terms:** RBE modelling, LET measurement
**Radiotherapy Example:** Prevented excessive RBE near brainstem in base-of-skull tumor.

**429. Quick Pre-Treatment Proton Range QA:** Fast range verification using prompt gamma or range probes.
**Related Terms:** Range uncertainty test, Proton safety start
**Radiotherapy Example:** Confirmed range accuracy for liver IMPT within 0.7 mm.

**430. Quantitative Soft-Tissue Deformation Logging:** Stores and analyzes deformation patterns across fractions for ART trends.
**Related Terms:** Deformable tracking, Inter-fraction monitoring
**Radiotherapy Example:** Predicted parotid shrinkage triggered adaptive replanning.

**431. Quality-Scored Organ-Substructure Planner:** Evaluates dose to critical substructures separately (e.g., cochlea, hippocampus).
**Related Terms:** Sub-OAR analysis, Complication risk
**Radiotherapy Example:** Auditory sparing achieved in medulloblastoma cranial RT.

**432. Quadrant-Resolved EPID Gamma Report:** Gamma analysis generated for four EPID sectors independently.
**Related Terms:** Spatial gamma, 2D array QA
**Radiotherapy Example:** Detected dose deviation in lateral quadrant for liver VMAT.

**433. Quasi-Open Beam Penumbra Modelling:** Determines penumbra width in partially blocked or modulated fields.
**Related Terms:** Edge sharpness QA, MLC modulation
**Radiotherapy Example:** Improved PTV sparing near spinal cord in SBRT.

**434. Quantitative Time-Aligned Motion Replay:** Replays couch/MLC/motion logs aligned with breathing trace for QA.
**Related Terms:** Log verification, Motion-gated QA
**Radiotherapy Example:** Found timing mismatch in gated pancreas IMRT.

**435. Quality-Driven Dose Renormalization:** Selectively alters prescription to meet clinical objectives mid-course.
**Related Terms:** Adaptive boosting, Dose compensation
**Radiotherapy Example:** Reduced prescription mid-treatment due to liver toxicity.

436. **Q-value Radiobiological Scaling Factor:** Weighting factor estimating biological dose sensitivity for unusual fractionation.
**Related Terms:** BED scaling, Hypofractionation modelling
**Radiotherapy Example:** Calculated BED correction for ultrahigh-fraction SBRT liver case.

437. **Quadratic Clinical Priority Optimizer:** Applies quadratic weighting to push optimization toward clinical intent.
**Related Terms:** SMART optimization, Priority-driven planning
**Radiotherapy Example:** Sharpened VMAT dose fall-off for optic pathway glioma.

438. **Quantitative VMAT Synchronization QA:** Validates synchronization of gantry rotation, dose rate, and MLC motion.
**Related Terms:** VMAT QA, Delivery timing QA
**Radiotherapy Example:** Detected small MLC delay causing 3% hotspot in pelvis VMAT.

439. **Quick-Learning Adaptive Contour Correction:** AI contour correction improving with each fraction.
**Related Terms:** Auto-segmentation learning, Adaptive AI
**Radiotherapy Example:** Reduced stomach contour time in pancreas RT by 50%.

440. **Quadrant-Based Head & Neck Immobilization QA:** Evaluates mask tightness and reproducibility by quadrant pressure distribution.
**Related Terms:** Immobilization QA, Setup reproducibility
**Radiotherapy Example:** Identified loose lower-right region → mask remolded.

441. **Quantitative RapidPlan Constraint Predictor:** Predicts achievable DVH goals using knowledge-based planning.
**Related Terms:** KBP planning, DVH prediction
**Radiotherapy Example:** Predicted kidney sparing for abdomen VMAT.

442. **Quality-Controlled Proton Spot Scanning:** Ensures spot size, position, and intensity match plan during delivery.
**Related Terms:** Spot scanning QA, IMPT dosimetry
**Radiotherapy Example:** Detected spot widening in sinus case → mitigated.

443. **Q-Adaptive Toxicity Prevention System:** Dynamically reduces OAR dose based on predicted toxicity evolution.
**Related Terms:** Adaptive OAR sparing, Toxicity forecasting
**Radiotherapy Example:** Reduced parotid dose mid-course to prevent xerostomia.

444. **Quasi-Micro Motion Compensation:** Adjusts fluence delivery for very small drift (<1 mm).
**Related Terms:** Micro-motion tracking, Beam correction
**Radiotherapy Example:** Stabilized frameless SRS head motion.

445. **Quantitative FLASH Dose Rate Verification:** Checks ultrahigh-dose-rate delivery accuracy for FLASH RT.
**Related Terms:** FLASH dosimetry, UHDR QA
**Radiotherapy Example:** Validated dose rate >100 Gy/s for pre-clinical tumor model.

446. **Quality-Weighted Hypoxia Boosting:** Selectively increases dose to hypoxic tumor zones using PET/MRI biomarkers.
**Related Terms:** Dose painting by numbers, Hypoxia imaging
**Radiotherapy Example:** Boost applied to hypoxic prostate subregion seen on FMISO PET.

447. **Quantitative Proton RBE Gradient Index:** Measures risk of steep RBE spike near distal edge.
**Related Terms:** LET/RBE mapping, Proton biological uncertainty
**Radiotherapy Example:** Checked index near brainstem for clival chordoma.

448. **Quadrant-Resolved Couch Shift Analysis:** Detects directional bias in patient shift trends over treatment course.
**Related Terms:** Setup reproducibility, IGRT motion review
**Radiotherapy Example:** Detected left-leaning drift → corrected immobilization.

449. **Quantized Dose-Response Surrogate Marker:** Converts early imaging biomarker change into predicted dose response class.
**Related Terms:** Biomarker-guided therapy, Early response prediction
**Radiotherapy Example:** Shifted to escalated-boost pathway in NSCLC after PET reduction.

450. **Quality-Adaptive MLC Speed Limiter:** Automatically slows MLC movement in complex geometry to preserve accuracy.
**Related Terms:** Dynamic MLC control, Modulation QA
**Radiotherapy Example:** Improved gamma pass in prostate VMAT.

451. **Quad-Beam Robustness Check:** Evaluates robustness using four dose scenarios representing realistic extremes.
**Related Terms:** Robust optimization, Scenario testing
**Radiotherapy Example:** Proton plan passed all four scenarios for esophagus RT.

452. **Quantitative Dose Pull-Back Optimization:** Reduces dose at OAR boundary while maintaining coverage through re-shaping optimization.
**Related Terms:** Gradient control, OAR sparing strategy
**Radiotherapy Example:** Pulled back spinal canal dose in T-spine SBRT.

453. **Quantum-Noise-Corrected CBCT Reconstruction:** Corrects quantum mottle in low-dose CBCT via physics-aware de-noising.
**Related Terms:** Low-dose CBCT, Reconstruction algorithm QA
**Radiotherapy Example:** Enhanced visibility of pancreas target for daily imaging.

454. **Quick-Generation Predictive Plan Library:** Rapid creation of multiple ART plans predicting anatomical change.
**Related Terms:** Library-based ART, Adaptive modelling
**Radiotherapy Example:** Used six predicted plans for H&N weekly changes.

455. **Quadratic Motion Forecasting Filter:** Predicts future motion using second-order temporal trend.
**Related Terms:** Motion prediction, Real-time tracking
**Radiotherapy Example:** Improved gating decision timing during liver SBRT.

456. **Quantitative HDR Brachycatheter Alignment QA:** Confirms catheter path accuracy vs. plan using imaging and dummy source runs.
**Related Terms:** Brachy applicator QA, Catheter reconstruction
**Radiotherapy Example:** Ensured dwell points matched plan for cervical HDR RT.

457. **Quasi-Interactive Dose Escalation Interface:** Planner tests multiple escalation patterns with instant feedback from dose engine.
**Related Terms:** Smart planning workflow, BED modelling
**Radiotherapy Example:** Tuned boost to residual pelvic node.

**458. Quantitative Dose-Per-Angle Delivery Map:** 2D graph showing how much dose delivered at each gantry angle.
**Related Terms:** Delivery QA, VMAT dose log
**Radiotherapy Example:** Detected anomaly at 242° in pancreas VMAT.

**459. Q-Factor for Machine Reliability Rating:** Score predicting machine performance stability based on long-term QA statistics.
**Related Terms:** LINAC reliability index, Predictive maintenance
**Radiotherapy Example:** Machine flagged for preventive service before failure.

**460. Quasi-Biological Cost Function:** Combines physical dose and biological effect in one objective during optimization.
**Related Terms:** TCP/NTCP-weighted optimization, Radiobiology planning
**Radiotherapy Example:** Boost taken from posterior beam to reduce bowel NTCP.

**461. Quantitative Plan Robustness Scoring Matrix:** Multi-criterion score based on PTV coverage, OAR safety, range uncertainty, and motion.
**Related Terms:** Proton robustness, Multi-scenario evaluation
**Radiotherapy Example:** Selected proton plan with highest robustness for pancreas.

**462. Quad-Iso SRS Collision QA:** Collision-avoidance QA for SRS using multiple couch/gantry/isocenter coordinates.
**Related Terms:** SRS collision map, Safety clearance
**Radiotherapy Example:** Cleared all eight arcs for cranial multi-target SRS.

**463. Quantum-Corrected AI IGRT Registration:** Uses photon noise estimation to prevent IGRT mis-registration in low-dose images.
**Related Terms:** AI image registration, CBCT noise correction
**Radiotherapy Example:** Prevented false shift detection in lung CBCT.

**464. Quasi-Dose-Accumulated ART Forecast:** Predicts toxicity risk if no ART is performed based on delivered dose accumulation trend.
**Related Terms:** ART indication prediction, Deformable dose accumulation
**Radiotherapy Example:** Triggered ART early for parotid protection.

**465. Quick-Response Motion Stop Protocol:** Stops beam within milliseconds on motion threshold breach.
**Related Terms:** Gating cutoff, Emergency beam hold
**Radiotherapy Example:** Stopped liver SBRT when diaphragm shift exceeded 3 mm.

**466. Quantitative Surface Dose Reconstruction:** Estimates entrance dose on skin using EPID/MC or film data.
**Related Terms:** Skin toxicity prediction, Build-up region dosimetry
**Radiotherapy Example:** Prevented dermatitis in breast DIBH RT.

**467. Quality-Scored DVH Risk Prediction:** Predicts clinical complication probability from DVH using weighted clinical factors.
**Related Terms:** NTCP modelling, Dose prediction
**Radiotherapy Example:** Predicted late lung fibrosis probability for SBRT.

**468. Quadrature-Resolved IGRT Landmark Error Analysis:** Separates registration error sources by anatomical direction/quadrant.
**Related Terms:** IGRT uncertainty decomposition, Setup error
**Radiotherapy Example:** Identified CT–CBCT mismatch dominantly inferior-posterior.

469. **Quantitative Multi-Modality Fusion Confidence:** Numerical reliability score for CT–MRI–PET fusion accuracy.
**Related Terms:** Registration QA, Image fusion validation
**Radiotherapy Example:** Ensured PET hotspot correctly aligned for lung boost.

470. **Quality-Adaptive Dose Rate Modulation:** Modulates dose rate during treatment based on anatomy sensitivity.
**Related Terms:** Sub-region modulation, Dose painting delivery
**Radiotherapy Example:** Lower dose rate near optic nerve in glioma IMRT.

471. **Quasi-Discrete Delivery Timing Analysis:** Evaluates VMAT delivery timing vs planned timeline.
**Related Terms:** Dose-rate timing QA, MLC-timing QA
**Radiotherapy Example:** Corrected asynchrony causing stomach overdose risk.

472. **Quantified IGRT Confidence-Driven Shift:** Shift magnitude depends on registration confidence rather than fixed tolerance.
**Related Terms:** Probability-adjusted IGRT, Smart corrections
**Radiotherapy Example:** 0 mm shift chosen when low-confidence image due to gas.

473. **Quadrant-Based Brachy HDR Symmetry QA:** Confirms dose symmetry in ring/ovoids or multi-catheter implants.
**Related Terms:** Dwell symmetry QA, HDR optimization
**Radiotherapy Example:** Detected inconsistency in cervical applicator tube length.

474. **Quantitative SRS Target Offset Model:** Predicts dose error based on miss distance for tiny SRS lesions.
**Related Terms:** Miss-sensitivity estimation, Micro-target dosimetry
**Radiotherapy Example:** Calculated 8% PTV loss at 1-mm offset in brain SRS.

475. **Q-Depth Proton Hotspot Classifier:** Identifies depth-end dose spike risk zones in proton plans.
**Related Terms:** LET hotspot, RBE uncertainty
**Radiotherapy Example:** Adjusted beam angle to avoid chiasm hotspot.

476. **Quantitative Dose Painting Stability Score:** Ranks voxel-boost plans by reproducibility under motion/deformation.
**Related Terms:** Dose painting robustness, PET/MRI boosting
**Radiotherapy Example:** Rejected unstable voxel-boost for moving lung target.

477. **Quadratic Machine Fault Prediction Model:** Predicts LINAC mechanical or dosimetric failure using QA trend curves.
**Related Terms:** Predictive maintenance, Machine learning QA
**Radiotherapy Example:** Triggered service before beam steering failure.

478. **Quantitative Bystander Effect Modelling:** Estimates indirect biological impact on cells not directly hit by radiation.
**Related Terms:** Radiobiological response modelling, Cross-cell signalling
**Radiotherapy Example:** Used in risk assessment of FLASH RT pre-clinical trials.

479. **Quick Dose Override Protocol:** Automated override of dose calculation in extreme density variation scenarios.
**Related Terms:** Density override, Lung/air/tissue correction
**Radiotherapy Example:** Applied density override for bowel gas during pancreas IMRT.

**480. Quantitative SPECT-Based Functional Ventilation Planning:** Uses SPECT ventilation data to spare functional lung regions.
**Related Terms:** Functional avoidance, Ventilation-guided RT
**Radiotherapy Example:** Reduced pneumonitis risk in lung IMRT.

**481. Quality-Assured Deformable Contour Propagation:** Validates propagated contours using deformation vectors and organ plausibility.
**Related Terms:** DIR QA, Auto-contouring
**Radiotherapy Example:** Corrected propagated stomach outline for pancreas ART.

**482. Quasi-HDR Dose Pulse Mapping:** Maps dose pulses from pulsed RT modes for biological effect research.
**Related Terms:** Pulsed RT, UHDR mapping
**Radiotherapy Example:** Pulse map validated before pre-clinical trial.

**483. Quantitative Field Aperture Drift Tracking:** Monitors long-term drift in jaw/MLC aperture geometry.
**Related Terms:** Geometric QA, MLC position drift
**Radiotherapy Example:** Detected MLC bank drift before SBRT delivery error.

**484. Quasi-4D Anatomical Prediction for ART:** Predicts future anatomy using early anatomical changes + motion patterns.
**Related Terms:** Predictive ART, Adaptive modelling
**Radiotherapy Example:** Predicted esophageal swelling → ART deployed pre-emptively.

**485. Quick Replan Suitability Calculator:** Determines whether a plan needs recalculation or full replanning.
**Related Terms:** ART decision tool, Dose deviation threshold
**Radiotherapy Example:** Avoided unnecessary ART for stable prostate IGRT.

**486. Quantitative Cranial Micro-Shift Index:** Scores cruciform shifts in SRS based on stability of all axes combined.
**Related Terms:** Frameless SRS stability, SGRT micromotion
**Radiotherapy Example:** Confirmed safe positioning without a mask remake.

**487. Quadrant-Aligned PET SUV Landmarking:** Localizes PET hotspots using four landmark zones for robust alignment.
**Related Terms:** PET-CT fusion QA, SUV mapping
**Radiotherapy Example:** Boost applied only to persistent quadrant hotspot in NSCLC.

**488. Quality-Modulated Brachy Dwell Time Controller:** Adjusts dwell times based on OAR proximity and tissue radiosensitivity.
**Related Terms:** Dwell time modulation, HDR optimization
**Radiotherapy Example:** Reduced bladder dose in cervical HDR.

**489. Quasi-Real-Time Gamma Monitoring:** Displays gamma passing rate during IMRT/VMAT delivery rather than afterward.
**Related Terms:** Live QA, Delivery monitoring
**Radiotherapy Example:** Notified gantry-speed anomaly during pelvis VMAT.

**490. Quantitative Density Override Decision Matrix:** Rule-set for when and how density overrides should be applied.
**Related Terms:** CT override, Gas override, Metal override
**Radiotherapy Example:** Automated jaw override for oral metal implants.

**491. Quality-Driven Multi-Target SRS Optimization:** Ensures equal dose conformity and gradient among multiple metastases.
**Related Terms:** Single-isocenter SRS, Conformity equalization
**Radiotherapy Example:** Balanced coverage among 11 brain targets.

**492. Quasi-Stationary Ventilation Modelling:** Estimates ventilation in partially moving lung segments for RT planning.
**Related Terms:** Functional lung avoidance, 4D ventilation
**Radiotherapy Example:** Protected functional upper-lobe ventilation in SBRT.

**493. Quantitative Proton Exit-Dose Reconstruction:** Indirectly reconstructs dose using exit-signal secondary emission.
**Related Terms:** Proton exit dosimetry, Secondary particle mapping
**Radiotherapy Example:** Validated dose coverage behind pelvic tumor.

**494. Quadrant-Weighted Plan Summation QA:** Weighted dose summation for bilateral or quadrant-separated therapy phases.
**Related Terms:** Composite plan QA, Bilateral plan combination
**Radiotherapy Example:** Combined left- and right-breast phases accurately.

**495. Q-Corrected FLASH Radiobiology Model:** Adjusts radiobiological models for ultrahigh-rate FLASH effects.
**Related Terms:** FLASH tissue protection, UHDR modelling
**Radiotherapy Example:** Guided safe FLASH dose for animal glioma study.

**496. Quasi-Beam-Sequence Collision Forecast:** Predicts gantry–patient collisions probability ahead of beam sequence delivery.
**Related Terms:** Collision avoidance, ARC SRS safety
**Radiotherapy Example:** Prevented collision during spine SBRT with 15 couch kicks.

**497. Quantitative Plan Similarity Metric:** Score that detects unexpectedly large differences between revised plans and originals.
**Related Terms:** Plan comparison QA, DVH deviation
**Radiotherapy Example:** Exposed accidental OAR contour import mismatch.

**498. Quick-Dose Constraint Checking Matrix:** Auto-validates all dose constraints using clinical protocol tables.
**Related Terms:** Protocol-based QA, Automatic plan validation
**Radiotherapy Example:** Flagged over-limit heart dose before approval.

**499. Quality-Integrated Robustness Map:** Combines robustness, conformity, gradient, and OAR safety in one heat map for plan decision-making.
**Related Terms:** Robust evaluation, Clinical plan heat map
**Radiotherapy Example:** Selected best plan for pancreatic proton RT.

**500. Quadrature-Enhanced Accumulated Dose Analysis:** Computes cumulative deformable dose using advanced quadrature integration for precision.
**Related Terms:** Dose accumulation, DIR dose mapping
**Radiotherapy Example:** Confirmed spinal cord cumulative dose stayed within tolerance across sequential boosts.

# R

1. **Radiation Absorbed Dose:** Amount of energy deposited by ionizing radiation per unit mass of tissue (measured in Gray).
   **Related Terms:** Dose deposition, Gray (Gy), RBE, BED
   **Radiotherapy Example:** A prostate cancer plan prescribed 78 Gy absorbed dose to the PTV.
2. **Radiation Beam Attenuation:** Reduction in beam intensity as it passes through matter due to absorption and scattering.
   **Related Terms:** HVL, beam hardening, tissue heterogeneity correction
   **Radiotherapy Example:** TPS applied lung density corrections to account for IMRT beam attenuation.
3. **Radiation Beam Calibration:** Adjustment of LINAC output to ensure accurate dose delivery.
   **Related Terms:** Output factor, TG-51 protocol, absolute dosimetry
   **Radiotherapy Example:** Calibrating photon beam output to 1 cGy/MU before starting SBRT treatments.
4. **Radiation Beam Collimation:** Shaping the beam using jaws or MLCs to target tumor volume and spare normal tissues.
   **Related Terms:** MLC shaping, field shaping, aperture adaptation
   **Radiotherapy Example:** MLC collimation refined to avoid bowel during pelvis VMAT.
5. **Radiation Beam Flatness:** Uniformity of beam intensity across the central portion of the radiation field.
   **Related Terms:** Symmetry, dose uniformity, beam quality**Radiotherapy Example:** Annual QA confirmed acceptable flatness for 6 MV beam for breast tangents.
6. **Radiation Beam Symmetry:** Similarity of dose distribution on left and right sides of the central axis.
   **Related Terms:** Flatness, beam profile, tolerance limits
   **Radiotherapy Example:** Detected symmetry deviation → LINAC steering adjusted before treatment release.
7. **Radiation Biology:** Study of radiation interactions with cells and tissues and resulting biological effects.
   **Related Terms:** RBE, cell survival curves, radiosensitivity
   **Radiotherapy Example:** Radiosensitive lymphoma treated with lower fraction doses.
8. **Radiation Contour Review:** Verification of normal tissue and tumor contours before planning.
   **Related Terms:** Auto-segmentation QA, OAR review
   **Radiotherapy Example:** Weekly peer review session corrected kidney contour expansion error.
9. **Radiation Dosimeter:** Device for measuring radiation dose.
   **Related Terms:** Ion chamber, diode, TLD, OSLD
   **Radiotherapy Example:** Diode used for entrance dose verification in pediatric abdominal RT.
10. **Radiation Dose Optimization:** Improving dose distribution to maximize tumor control while minimizing toxicity.
    **Related Terms:** Dose painting, inverse planning, plan quality index
    **Radiotherapy Example:** Parotid sparing achieved during H&N VMAT re-optimization.

11. **Radiation Dose Reconstruction:** Rebuilding the delivered dose based on log files, motion signals, or images.
    **Related Terms:** Log-file QA, adaptive verification
    **Radiotherapy Example:** Reconstructed dose confirmed spinal cord stayed below tolerance in SBRT.
12. **Radiation Exposure Index:** Metric showing detector exposure level in imaging, used for dose monitoring.
    **Related Terms:** S-value, EI index, image dose control
    **Radiotherapy Example:** Excess EI triggered CBCT protocol revision for pelvis IGRT.
13. **Radiation Field Verification:** Confirmation that the delivered field matches planned field in size, shape, and position.
    **Related Terms:** Portal dosimetry, field match QA, IGRT setup
    **Radiotherapy Example:** EPID matched IMRT field edges before abdomen treatment.
14. **Radiation Fractionation Scheme:** Schedule dividing radiation treatment into multiple dose fractions.
    **Related Terms:** Hypofractionation, hyperfractionation, SBRT
    **Radiotherapy Example:** Lung SBRT delivered 50 Gy in 5 fractions.
15. **Radiation Image Registration:** Aligning two or more imaging datasets to match anatomy in space.
    **Related Terms:** CBCT matching, DIR, fiducial-based alignment
    **Radiotherapy Example:** Planning CT and daily CBCT registered using prosthetic hip constraint.
16. **Radiation Leakage Assessment:** Measurement of unintended leakage radiation from LINAC shielding systems.
    **Related Terms:** Shielding verification, barrier design, MLC leakage
    **Radiotherapy Example:** Annual survey confirmed head leakage below IEC safety limits.
17. **Radiation Portal Imaging:** Using MV or kV detectors to verify field alignment and patient setup.
    **Related Terms:** EPID, CBCT, setup verification
    **Radiotherapy Example:** Pelvis IMRT placement verified using MV portal imaging.
18. **Radiation Quality Assurance (RQA):** Systematic QA to ensure accuracy, safety, and consistency in radiation delivery.
    **Related Terms:** TG-142, QC, commissioning
    **Radiotherapy Example:** Monthly LINAC QA approved before new prostate start.
19. **Radiation Shielding Calculation:** Estimation of room shielding requirements to limit occupational and public exposure.
    **Related Terms:** Workload factor, tenth-value layer, NCRP guidelines
    **Radiotherapy Example:** Bunker shielding designed for dual-energy LINAC operation.
20. **Radiation Source Modeling:** Mathematical modeling of radiation source for Monte Carlo and dose calculations.
    **Related Terms:** Monte Carlo engine, beam model commissioning
    **Radiotherapy Example:** Beam model tuned to match measured photon PDDs and profiles.
21. **Radioadaptive Response:** Phenomenon where low radiation exposure increases resistance to later higher doses.
    **Related Terms:** Dose priming, cellular repair activation
    **Radiotherapy Example:** Not considered clinically beneficial — avoided in hypofractionated RT design.
22. **Radiobiological Equivalent Dose:** Biologically weighted dose accounting for fractionation and repair.
    **Related Terms:** BED, EQD2
    **Radiotherapy Example:** BED used to compare prostate HDR and EBRT boost strategies.

23. **Radiobiological Modeling:** Predicting tumor control and toxicity probability using biological parameters.
**Related Terms:** TCP, NTCP, dose-response curve
**Radiotherapy Example:** NTCP modeling guided dose reduction to parotid glands.

24. **Radiobiological Parameter Sensitivity:** Analysis of how changes in radiosensitivity parameters affect predicted outcomes.
**Related Terms:** Uncertainty quantification, TCP/NTCP calibration
**Radiotherapy Example:** Sensitivity check prevented overestimation of breast local control.

25. **Radiochemical Decay:** Loss of radioactivity over time due to nuclear decay processes.
**Related Terms:** Half-life, decay constant, isotopes
**Radiotherapy Example:** Radionuclide dose rate adjusted due to decay during Y-90 microsphere shipment.

26. **Radiochemical Purity:** Measure of how much of a radiopharmaceutical remains in the desired chemical form.**Related Terms:** Nuclear medicine QC, labeling efficiency
**Radiotherapy Example:** Ensured >95% purity before Lu-177 therapy to avoid toxicity.

27. **Radiochromic Film Dosimetry:** Dose measurement using films that darken proportionally to absorbed dose.
**Related Terms:** Gafchromic film, 2D QA, SBRT QA
**Radiotherapy Example:** Verified small target dose in spine SBRT with film.

28. **Radiogenic Tissue Response:** Biological tissue reactions triggered by radiation exposure.
**Related Terms:** Acute toxicity, late effects
**Radiotherapy Example:** Predicted parotid xerostomia risk using NTCP.

29. **Radiographic Quality Control:** Ensures consistent imaging performance and patient safety.
**Related Terms:** kV imaging QA, flat-panel QA
**Radiotherapy Example:** Monthly checks validated CBCT HU stability.

30. **Radioimmunotherapy:** Targeted delivery of radiation using antibody-bound isotopes.
**Related Terms:** Targeted radionuclide therapy, biologic guidance
**Radiotherapy Example:** CD20-directed Y-90 treatment for NHL.

31. **Radioisotope Calibrator:** Device measuring radioactivity of isotopes before administration.
**Related Terms:** Dose calibrator, activity verification
**Radiotherapy Example:** Checked I-131 dose before thyroid ablation.

32. **Radiological Hazard Assessment:** Evaluation of risks from radioactive sources in clinical areas.
**Related Terms:** ALARA, risk management
**Radiotherapy Example:** Hand contamination risk evaluated during brachy source loading.

33. **Radiological Physics:** Physics of ionizing radiation interactions, detection, and dosimetry.
**Related Terms:** Radiation protection, therapy physics
**Radiotherapy Example:** Applied attenuation theory for lung dose corrections.

34. **Radiometabolic Therapy:** Therapeutic use of systemic radiopharmaceutical uptake in target tissue.
**Related Terms:** Molecular radiotherapy, beta therapy
**Radiotherapy Example:** I-131 concentrated in thyroid remnants post-surgery.

35. **Radiopaque Fiducial:** High-visible marker used for localization in imaging.
**Related Terms:** IGRT, tumor tracking
**Radiotherapy Example:** Implanted gold seeds for prostate CBCT alignment.

36. **Radiopharmaceutical Clearance:** Rate at which radiotracers are removed from the body.
**Related Terms:** Biological half-life, renal excretion
**Radiotherapy Example:** Adjusted Lu-177 therapy for reduced kidney function.

37. **Radioprotective Agent:** Drugs that protect normal tissue from radiation injury.
**Related Terms:** Amifostine, antioxidant therapy
**Radiotherapy Example:** Used to reduce xerostomia in head & neck RT.

38. **Radiotherapy Beam Modeling:** Mathematical representation of LINAC beam characteristics in TPS.
**Related Terms:** Commissioning, Monte Carlo
**Radiotherapy Example:** Tuned beam model until measured PDDs matched TPS.

39. **Radiotherapy Couch Verification:** Confirming correct couch position and motion accuracy.
**Related Terms:** IGRT, setup error correction
**Radiotherapy Example:** Couch indexing corrected before liver SBRT.

40. **Radiotherapy Image Fusion:** Combining multimodal images to improve target visualization.
**Related Terms:** CT-MRI fusion, PET-CT fusion
**Radiotherapy Example:** PET added metabolic target boost region in lung.

41. **Radiotherapy Machine Acceptance:** Formal testing to ensure a new LINAC meets performance standards.
**Related Terms:** Commissioning, vendor specs
**Radiotherapy Example:** Performed initial beam constancy before clinical use.

42. **Radiotherapy Motion Management:** Techniques to compensate or reduce tumor motion during treatment.
**Related Terms:** Gating, tracking, ITV
**Radiotherapy Example:** Respiratory gating limited liver target motion.

43. **Radiotherapy Plan Normalization:** Standardizing dose so a defined volume receives the prescription.
**Related Terms:** Dose scaling, plan equalization
**Radiotherapy Example:** Normalized plan so 95% PTV covered by 100% dose.

44. **Radiotherapy Portal Verification:** Imaging validation of patient alignment and field placement.
**Related Terms:** EPID, setup QA
**Radiotherapy Example:** MV portal matched pelvic bone landmarks.

45. **Radiotherapy Quality Control Test:** Routine procedures ensuring system performance remains in tolerance.
**Related Terms:** TG-142 QA, safety checks
**Radiotherapy Example:** Daily output constancy test passed before treatments.

46. **Radiotherapy Set-Up Error Analysis:** Evaluation of systematic and random deviations in patient positioning.
**Related Terms:** IGRT error metrics, margin recipe
**Radiotherapy Example:** Custom margins applied for large prostate shifts.

47. **Radiotherapy Simulation:** Imaging session to define patient geometry for planning.
**Related Terms:** CT-sim, immobilization
**Radiotherapy Example:** Abdomen SBRT simulated with breath-hold technique.

48. **Radiotherapy Source Calibration:** Activity and dose rate verification of brachy sources.
**Related Terms:** HDR QA, TG-43 dosimetry
**Radiotherapy Example:** Ir-192 source strength measured before insertion.

49. **Radiotherapy Treatment Record:** Documentation of all delivered doses, fractions, and settings.
**Related Terms:** R&V system, audit compliance
**Radiotherapy Example:** Reviewed log for missing MU entry during chart check.

50. **Radio-Sensitivity Index:** Biomarker score predicting tissue or tumor response to radiation.
**Related Terms:** Genomic radiosensitivity, personalized radiotherapy
**Radiotherapy Example:** Index supported dose escalation in resistant glioma.

51. **Radiotherapy Commissioning Validation:** Ensures treatment planning systems and machines meet specifications before clinical use.
**Related Terms:** TPS validation, beam data set, baseline reference.
**Example:** Commissioning validated beam data before activating new LINAC for treatments.

52. **Radiotherapy Couch Attenuation Correction:** Adjusts dose calculations to account for photon absorption by the treatment couch.
**Related Terms:** IGRT couch model, dose perturbation, TPS override.
**Example:** Pelvic VMAT recalculated with couch attenuation to correct underdose to PTV.

53. **Radiotherapy Daily Output Constancy:** Verifies that LINAC dose output stays within tolerance every day.
**Related Terms:** 3% tolerance, ion chamber check, morning QA.
**Example:** Output deviation >2% logged during daily QA and machine taken offline.

54. **Radiotherapy Data Management System:** Software storing, tracking, and securing patient treatment data.
**Related Terms:** MOSAIQ, ARIA, oncology information system.
**Example:** Scheduling, approvals, and beam records were managed via OIS.

55. **Radiotherapy Delivery Accuracy:** Measures how closely delivered dose matches planned dose.
**Related Terms:** Gamma pass rate, SBRT QA, plan QA.
**Example:** Lung SBRT plan passed with 98% at 3%/2 mm gamma criteria.

56. **Radiotherapy Dose Constraint Library:** Standardized list of acceptable organ-at-risk dose limits for planning.
**Related Terms:** QUANTEC, RTOG guidelines, DVH limits.
**Example:** Planner referenced spine cord max <45 Gy for breast case.

57. **Radiotherapy Dose Engine:** Computational algorithm used in TPS to calculate dose.
**Related Terms:** AAA, Acuros, Monte-Carlo.
**Example:** Monte-Carlo used for highly heterogeneous lung case.

58. **Radiotherapy Dose Fractionation Protocol:** Defines dose per fraction and number of fractions for therapeutic delivery.
**Related Terms:** Hypofractionation, stereotactic, hyperfractionation.
**Example:** Prostate treated using 60 Gy / 20 fraction hypofractionated schedule.

59. **Radiotherapy Dose Index:** Quantitative index comparing plan dose distribution against clinical goals.
**Related Terms:** Conformity index, homogeneity index, gradient index.
**Example:** SRS conformity index improved from 1.6 to 1.2 after plan optimization.

60. **Radiotherapy Dose Modeling Error:** Deviation resulting from incorrect physics model or tissue heterogeneity.
**Related Terms:** Electron disequilibrium, scatter error, small-field error.
**Example:** Inaccurate lung dose due to missing density override.

61. **Radiotherapy Dose Painting:** Differentially escalating dose to biologically aggressive tumor sub-volumes.
**Related Terms:** PET-guided boost, voxel-based prescription.
**Example:** HPV+ oropharynx PET lesion boosted to 74 Gy.

62. **Radiotherapy Dose Prescription Point:** Dosimetric location in target volume where prescribed dose is defined.
**Related Terms:** ICRU reference point, mean dose prescription.
**Example:** HDR prescribed to 100% isodose on catheter contour.

63. **Radiotherapy Dose Reconstruction:** Recreates delivered dose using log files or measurement systems.
**Related Terms:** EPID dosimetry, machine log QA, independent dose calc.
**Example:** Dose reconstruction confirmed VMAT delivered dose to GTV was correct.

64. **Radiotherapy Dose Validation Phantom:** Phantom used to verify dose delivery accuracy before clinical use.
**Related Terms:** SRS phantom, anthropomorphic phantom, gamma test.
**Example:** Head phantom validated 6-arc SRS treatment.

65. **Radiotherapy Error Pathway Analysis:** Evaluates potential causes and consequences of treatment errors.
**Related Terms:** FMEA, QA matrix, risk mitigation.
**Example:** Wrong-shift event prevented by trigger alert design.

66. **Radiotherapy Field Matching QA:** Ensures alignment when two adjacent treatment fields meet without dose gaps/overlaps.
**Related Terms:** Feathering, junction QA, craniospinal match.
**Example:** Feathered match fields used for CSI to avoid spinal hotspots.

67. **Radiotherapy Film Calibration Curve:** Converts optical density of film to absorbed dose.
**Related Terms:** Gafchromic film, film scanner, sensitometric curve.
**Example:** SBRT film calibrated to ±1% accuracy for 50 Gy case.

68. **Radiotherapy Fraction Timing Sensitivity:** Biological effect dependence on time interval between fractions.
**Related Terms:** $\alpha/\beta$ ratio, repopulation, repair kinetics.
**Example:** Twice-daily H&N fractions spaced >6 h to avoid toxicity.

69. **Radiotherapy Gating Latency:** Delay between respiratory signal change and beam on/off response.
**Related Terms:** DIBH latency, motion management, beam hold interval.
**Example:** Latency measured to fine-tune lung SBRT gating accuracy.

70. **Radiotherapy Gradient Falloff Index:** Score describing how fast dose decreases outside target volume.
**Related Terms:** SRS gradient index, high-dose falloff.
**Example:** GFI evaluated to protect optic chiasm for pituitary SRS.

71. **Radiotherapy Immobilization Failure:** Loss of target stability due to poor mask or body fixation fit.
**Related Terms:** Setup error, interfraction motion.
**Example:** Mask looseness triggered resimulation for H&N plan.

72. **Radiotherapy Independent MU Check:** Separately verifies monitor units calculated by planning system.
**Related Terms:** Secondary calc, RadCalc, double check.
**Example:** 2% MU disagreement flagged lung plan for review.

73. **Radiotherapy In-Vivo Dosimetry Alert:** Trigger from diode/EPID when measured dose differs from expected values.
**Related Terms:** Real-time QA, tolerance threshold.
**Example:** Alert detected bolus missing during chest wall treatment.

74. **Radiotherapy Isocenter Wobble Test:** Measures mechanical stability of gantry rotation isocenter.
**Related Terms:** Laser test, Winston-Lutz, ball bearing test.
**Example:** Wobble <0.5 mm confirmed for SRS credentialing.

75. **Radiotherapy Jaw-Tracking Dose Optimization:** Uses dynamic jaw motion to reduce MLC leakage and low-dose bath.
**Related Terms:** jaw tracking MLC, transmission scatter reduction.
**Example:** VMAT jaw tracking reduced rectum V15 by 8% for prostate.

76. **Radiotherapy Knowledge-Based Planning (KBP):** AI system generating optimized plan based on database of high-quality plans.
**Related Terms:** RapidPlan, machine learning TPS, plan automation.
**Example:** KBP produced faster and better OAR sparing for liver SBRT.

77. **Radiotherapy Laser Alignment QA:** Confirms that lasers used for patient positioning align with isocenter.
**Related Terms:** WL test, room laser calibration.
**Example:** Laser drift corrected during monthly QA.

78. **Radiotherapy Leaf-End Leakage Compensation:** Algorithm accounting for partial transmission through MLC leaf tips.
**Related Terms:** DLG correction, EPID fitting, transmission modeling.
**Example:** Prostate plan improved after correcting DLG offset.

79. **Radiotherapy Machine Log-File Verification:** Uses delivery log files to reconstruct dose and detect delivery mistakes.
**Related Terms:** logfile QA, trajectory log, delivery audit.
**Example:** Yaw drift discovered from SBRT arc logfile.

80. **Radiotherapy Motion Envelope:** 3D space representing maximum tumor movement during respiration.
**Related Terms:** ITV, 4DCT, deformable motion mapping.
**Example:** ITV created for pancreatic target using full motion envelope.

81. **Radiotherapy MU-per-Gy Calibration Factor:** Monitor units required to deliver one gray at reference depth.
**Related Terms:** calibration data, absolute dosimetry.
**Example:** Calibration confirmed before enabling new 6FFF beam.

82. **Radiotherapy Non-Coplanar Beam Strategy:** Beam angles selected outside single plane to maximize avoidance.
**Related Terms:** couch kicks, SRS arcs, non-coplanar VMAT.
**Example:** Multiple couch angles used for skull-base tumor.

83. **Radiotherapy Off-Axis Correction Factor:** Adjustment for response of ion chamber outside central axis.
**Related Terms:** OAR, profile correction, chamber anisotropy.
**Example:** Off-axis factor applied for beam data scanning accuracy.

84. **Radiotherapy OIS Safety Event Flag:** Alert in oncology information system marking treatment-critical safety concerns.
**Related Terms:** QA approval gating, incident learning.
**Example:** Missing physician approval flagged and prevented beam delivery.

85. **Radiotherapy Output Drift Monitoring:** Long-term tracking of LINAC dose output trends.
**Related Terms:** output constancy history, tolerance trending.
**Example:** Seasonal drift pattern identified and calibrated.

86. **Radiotherapy Overrange Detection:** Detects unintended dose outside defined field region.
**Related Terms:** leakage warning, field overshoot.
**Example:** Overshoot detected during TBI couch shift transition.

87. **Radiotherapy Parameter Lockout:** Blocks treatment beam if critical machine parameters exceed limits.
**Related Terms:** interlock, gating block, beam inhibit.
**Example:** Gantry collision risk triggered lockout.

88. **Radiotherapy Patient-Specific QA Dashboard:** Digital interface showing performance record for each patient plan QA.
**Related Terms:** plan QA reporting, gamma analytics.
**Example:** Dashboard flagged poor lung SBRT QA trend before replanning.

89. **Radiotherapy Peak Dose Hotspot Control:** Strategy to suppress maximum dose within target volume.
**Related Terms:** hotspot smoothing, constraint tightening.
**Example:** Plan adjusted to reduce spinal hotspot from 119% to 109%.

90. **Radiotherapy Plan Complexity Metric:** Score based on MLC modulation, segment count, and delivery difficulty.
**Related Terms:** modulation index, verifier score.
**Example:** Excess complexity (score 0.78) predicted QA failure.

91. **Radiotherapy Plan Degeneracy Prevention:** Prevents multiple mathematically different plans from meeting constraints but performing differently clinically.
**Related Terms:** Pareto discipline, clinically guided optimization.
**Example:** Additional constraint added to avoid degeneracy causing bowel overdose.

92. **Radiotherapy Plan Integrity Check:** Ensures no structural modification occurred between QA and treatment day.
**Related Terms:** checksum, plan freeze, version audit.
**Example:** Unapproved plan edit detected and blocked in MOSAIQ.

93. **Radiotherapy Portal Dose Prediction:** TPS prediction of EPID fluence for QA comparison.
**Related Terms:** EPID gamma QA, fluence match.
**Example:** Portal dose difference identified MLC calibration error.

94. **Radiotherapy Proton Range Uncertainty:** Variability in stopping depth of protons due to tissue uncertainties.
**Related Terms:** WEPL, distal margin, HU-RSP conversion.
**Example:** Liver IMPT margins increased for range uncertainty.

95. **Radiotherapy PTV Expansion Algorithm:** Mathematical model determining margin from CTV to PTV.
**Related Terms:** van Herk formula, geometric uncertainties.
**Example:** 5 mm PTV margin used for brain metastasis SRS.

96. **Radiotherapy QA Baseline Re-Establishment:** Resetting reference values after equipment upgrade or repair.
**Related Terms:** re-commissioning threshold, baseline shift.
**Example:** New EPID detector required baseline reset.

97. **Radiotherapy QA Action Threshold:** Defines when deviation requires intervention rather than trending only.
**Related Terms:** warning vs. action levels.
**Example:** Output −3.5% triggered corrective maintenance.

98. **Radiotherapy QA Chain of Custody:** Ensures traceability of QA data from acquisition to approval.
**Related Terms:** data authentication, audit trail.
**Example:** Phantom scan and raw data signed and locked to prevent edits.

99. **Radiotherapy Real-Time Beam Tracking:** Adjusts beam dynamically to follow target motion.
**Related Terms:** tumor tracking, MLC tracking, DMLC.
**Example:** Tracking maintained lung lesion inside PTV during SBRT.

100. **Radiotherapy Reference Geometry:** Machine reference position used for calibration and QA tests.
**Related Terms:** isocenter reference, home position, QA coordinates.
**Example:** Ball bearing aligned to reference geometry before WL test.

101. **Radiotherapy Residual Setup Error:** Remaining positioning deviation after image-guided correction.
**Related Terms:** residual shift, IGRT accuracy, systematic vs random error.
**Example:** Pelvic CBCT registered but residual 1.2 mm shift recorded for adaptive review.

102. **Radiotherapy Respiratory Baseline Drift:** Slow shift of breathing pattern during treatment delivery.
**Related Terms:** motion management, gating, 4DCT drift.
**Example:** Drift detected during liver SBRT causing gating region re-optimization.

103. **Radiotherapy Respiratory Motion Compensation:** Correction of tumor motion using imaging and beam adaptation.
**Related Terms:** gating, tumor tracking, ITV shaping.
**Example:** Motion compensation reduced PTV margin for pancreatic case.

104. **Radiotherapy Return-to-Isocenter Verification:** Ensures couch and gantry always return to reference isocenter position.
**Related Terms:** couch runout, mechanical isocenter, tolerance check.
**Example:** Return-to-iso drift of 0.9 mm triggered service call.

105. **Radiotherapy Ringing Artifact Correction:** Removal of streak/ripple artifacts in CBCT or CT used for planning.
**Related Terms:** metal artifacts, streak removal, CT correction.
**Example:** Ring artifact suppression improved Hounsfield accuracy near prosthesis.

106. **Radiotherapy Risk Mitigation Strategy:** Procedural actions to reduce likelihood of treatment error.
**Related Terms:** FMEA, RPN score, quality management.
**Example:** Double-sign-off for SRS couch rotation adopted after risk review.

107. **Radiotherapy Robotic Couch Collision Map:** Database of safe couch/gantry combinations preventing collision risk.
**Related Terms:** collision predictor, non-coplanar planning, safety interlock.
**Example:** Couch prediction tool allowed safe 110° couch angle for SRS.

108. **Radiotherapy Rotational Isocenter Accuracy:** Precision of beam isocenter during gantry/couch/MLC rotation.
**Related Terms:** Winston-Lutz test, non-coplanar SRS QA.
**Example:** 0.4 mm error documented to validate frameless trigeminal SRS.

109. **Radiotherapy Rotational Setup Error:** Patient misalignment involving pitch, roll, or yaw.
**Related Terms:** 6DOF couch, rotational mismatch, IGRT correction.
**Example:** 2° roll without rotational correction caused brainstem over-dose.

110. **Radiotherapy Rotational Target Tracking:** Tracking dynamic tumor rotation rather than only translation.
**Related Terms:** 6D motion tracking, deformable motion.
**Example:** Liver SBRT used rotational tracking to improve ITV coverage.

111. **Radiotherapy Safety Interlock Override Log:** Electronic record of each interlock override and justification.
**Related Terms:** safety monitoring, compliance protection.
**Example:** Beam-on override required supervisor authorization during commissioning.

112. **Radiotherapy Scatter Dose Estimation:** Calculation of low-dose radiation outside treatment field.
**Related Terms:** peripheral dose, out-of-field dose, leakage.
**Example:** Scatter modeling ensured gonadal shielding for pediatric case.

113. **Radiotherapy Secondary Target Correction:** Adjustment due to anatomical or biological changes over treatment.
**Related Terms:** adaptive replanning, target shift, ART.
**Example:** Adaptive replanning added satellite nodule to PTV after week 3 imaging.

114. **Radiotherapy Sensitivity Test (Plan Tuning):** Evaluates plan sensitivity to uncertainties such as setup or range error.
**Related Terms:** robustness analysis, worst-case simulation.
**Example:** Worst-case simulation prevented spinal cord overdose in IMPT.

115. **Radiotherapy Setup Robustness Index:** Quantifies plan dose stability under geometrical uncertainty.
**Related Terms:** robustness scoring, adaptive QA.
**Example:** Lower robustness score triggered replanning for pancreas patient.

116. **Radiotherapy Shielding Validation Survey:** Confirms room shielding meets regulatory dose limits.
**Related Terms:** controlled area, radiation survey, occupancy factor.
**Example:** Maze dose rate measured before opening new LINAC bunker.

117. **Radiotherapy Signal-to-Noise Improvement Filter:** Algorithm reducing noise in imaging used for guidance.
**Related Terms:** noise suppression, image smoothing, reconstruction filters.
**Example:** Filter improved soft-tissue CBCT visibility for prostate IGRT.

118. **Radiotherapy Smart Segmentation Algorithm:** Automated contouring of target and organs using AI.
**Related Terms:** auto-segmentation, deep learning contouring.
**Example:** Rapid auto-segmentation reduced contouring time for H&N.

119. **Radiotherapy Soft-Tissue Registration QA:** Ensures accuracy of image registration based on soft-tissue landmarks.
**Related Terms:** CBCT, MRI fusion, deformable registration.
**Example:** Soft-tissue matching used for bladder instead of bone-match.

120. **Radiotherapy Spatial Dose Gradient Map:** Visualization of how quickly dose decreases from PTV edge.
**Related Terms:** dose falloff, SRS gradient, high-gradient region.
**Example:** Dose gradient map confirmed optic chiasm spared during pituitary SRS.

121. **Radiotherapy Spatial Resolution QA:** Testing the smallest feature detectible by an imaging system.
**Related Terms:** MTF, line-pair phantom, edge detail.
**Example:** MRI phantom validated 1 mm spatial resolution for brain SRT planning.

122. **Radiotherapy Spot Scanning Error Analysis:** Evaluation of proton or carbon beam spot delivery accuracy.
**Related Terms:** spot drift, scanning beam, range uncertainty.
**Example:** Carbon spot positional deviation >2 mm triggered corrective tuning.

123. **Radiotherapy Stereotactic Arc Modeling:** Special model for dose calculation in highly modulated arc SRS.
**Related Terms:** SRS VMAT, non-coplanar arcs, high gradient.
**Example:** Arc modeling improved conformity for trigeminal neuralgia plan.

124. **Radiotherapy Supine-to-Prone Setup Transition QA:** Verification of dose equivalence when patient changes body position.
**Related Terms:** position-adaptive planning, prone breast.
**Example:** Prone breast plan validated for same coverage as supine version.

125. **Radiotherapy Surface Depth Scaling:** Converts surface optical depth to real anatomical depth.
**Related Terms:** surface guidance, SGRT calibration.
**Example:** Skin depth map used during fibrosarcoma external beam treatment.

126. **Radiotherapy Surface-Guided Alignment Gate:** Automatically pauses beam if patient's surface deviates from baseline.
**Related Terms:** SGRT beam hold, motion gate.
**Example:** DIBH breast treatment paused when sternum shifted by >3 mm.

127. **Radiotherapy Symmetry Drift Tracking:** Long-term monitoring of symmetry changes in LINAC beam.
**Related Terms:** output-trending, symmetry tolerance.
**Example:** Symmetry drift trending detected early Y-axis bending magnet failure.

128. **Radiotherapy System-Level Failure Simulation:** Stress-testing system flow to identify failure vulnerabilities.
**Related Terms:** mock failure drill, simulation QA.
**Example:** Simulated network outage validated backup offline workflow.

129. **Radiotherapy Table Sag Correction:** Compensates dose shift due to couch bending under patient weight.
**Related Terms:** couch attenuation, auto-compensation.
**Example:** Heavy-weight patient triggered automatic sag correction in TPS.

130. **Radiotherapy Target Deformation Mapping:** Tracks anatomical shape changes over treatment.
**Related Terms:** deformable registration, ART, biological adaptation.
**Example:** Pancreatic tumor shrinkage mapped at week-4 and integrated into ART.

131. **Radiotherapy Target Margin Derivation:** Calculates margins around CTV to form PTV based on uncertainties.
**Related Terms:** van Herk formula, systematic/random error.
**Example:** Lung PTV margin increased from 6 mm to 8 mm due to motion risk.

132. **Radiotherapy Target Overlap Management:** Planning adjustments when PTV overlaps with organ at risk.
**Related Terms:** compromise planning, gradient shaping.
**Example:** Brain PTV overlapped optic nerve → modified dose fall-off.

133. **Radiotherapy Task Group Workflow Compliance:** Following benchmark procedures from AAPM/ESTRO task groups.
**Related Terms:** TG-142, TG-100, TG-101, protocol compliance.
**Example:** SRS QA fully aligned with TG-101 standards.

134. **Radiotherapy Temperature-Dependent Detector Correction:** Corrects chamber output for temperature/pressure fluctuations.
**Related Terms:** environmental correction, PTP factor.
**Example:** T/P correction applied during monthly LINAC calibration.

135. **Radiotherapy Temporal Dose Accumulation:** Summation of dose over the entire treatment course.
**Related Terms:** cumulative dose, adaptive plan evaluation.
**Example:** Accumulated dose revealed kidney exceeding 70% tolerance — replanned.

136. **Radiotherapy Treatment Overshoot Detection:** Detects unintended excess MU or segment delivery.
**Related Terms:** beam overshoot, delivery fault.
**Example:** Log file captured 10 MU overshoot during small field delivery.

137. **Radiotherapy Treatment Parameter Freeze:** Locks treatment plan parameters to prevent unauthorized change.
**Related Terms:** OIS lock, approval lockout.
**Example:** SRS plan frozen after final approval to avoid accidental edits.

138. **Radiotherapy Treatment Pause Protocol:** Structured workflow when a treatment must be paused.
**Related Terms:** beam hold rule, restart authorization.
**Example:** Pause required due to unexpected bladder filling.

139. **Radiotherapy Treatment Replay Audit:** Replays delivery using log files to verify treatment accuracy.
**Related Terms:** logfile reconstruction, EPID replay QA.
**Example:** Replay confirmed correct VMAT execution after MLC lubrication.

140. **Radiotherapy Under-Dose Detection:** Algorithm detecting insufficient dose delivery to PTV.
**Related Terms:** adaptive review, in-vivo dosimetry alert.
**Example:** Liver hotspot avoidance caused unnoticed cold spot → replanned.

141. **Radiotherapy Verification Imaging Dose Tracking:** Monitors accumulated dose from IGRT imaging.
**Related Terms:** imaging-dose management, pediatric IGRT.
**Example:** Imaging dose exceeded limit → reduced CBCT frequency.

142. **Radiotherapy Volumetric Change Assessment:** Measurement of tumor shrinkage or swelling over treatment.
**Related Terms:** ART criteria, biological response.
**Example:** Nasopharynx tumor shrank 37% by week-4 prompting boost plan.

143. **Radiotherapy Workflow Interruption Safeguard:** System prevents loss of treatment progress after disruption.
**Related Terms:** power failure protection, offline backup.
**Example:** LINAC resumed exact MU after temporary shutdown.

144. **Radiotherapy Wedge Factor Verification:** Checks output factor when physical or dynamic wedge used.
**Related Terms:** dynamic wedge slope, wedge calibration.
**Example:** Wedge factor recalibrated after 3% deviation.

145. **Radiotherapy X-Ray Collision Safety Test:** Confirms imaging panel movement does not risk collision with patient.
**Related Terms:** safety clearance map, automated collision test.
**Example:** CBCT arm clearance validated for obese thoracic patient.

146. **Radiotherapy Yield Optimization:** Improves efficiency without compromising safety.
**Related Terms:** throughput optimization, automation.
**Example:** Automated plan QA reduced SBRT preparation time from 3 days to 1.

147. **Radiotherapy Zero-Dose Initialization Check:** Ensures no residual output before beam command is issued.
**Related Terms:** leakage test, beam-off verification.
**Example:** Initialization failure prevented early low-dose leakage.

148. **Rectilinear Detector Array QA:** Uses a grid of detectors to measure 2D/3D dose in IMRT/VMAT.
**Related Terms:** ArcCheck, Delta4, MapCHECK.
**Example:** ArcCheck used for pelvic VMAT QA trending.

149. **Refractory Tumor Radiotherapy Boost:** Extra dose given to resistant portion of tumor.
**Related Terms:** adaptive boost, dose painting.
**Example:** FDG-avid area in lung received simultaneous integrated boost.

150. **Relative Electron Density Calibration:** Converts CT HU to relative electron density for dose accuracy.
**Related Terms:** stoichiometric calibration, tissue phantom.
**Example:** HU-to-RED table updated for improved bone dose accuracy.

151. **Relative Stopping Power Uncertainty:** Proton range uncertainty caused by variation in tissue stopping power.
**Related Terms:** RSP map, CT calibration, Monte Carlo.
**Example:** 3.5% RSP uncertainty margin added for sinus IMPT plan.

152. **Remote Treatment Plan Approval Workflow:** Off-site physician/physicist authorization with secure access controls.
**Related Terms:** digital signature, OIS approval chain.
**Example:** Radiation oncologist approved boost plan remotely during on-call shift.

153. **Replanning Trigger Criteria:** Defined conditions requiring new plan mid-treatment.
**Related Terms:** ART protocol, tumor change threshold.
**Example:** Thyroid ART triggered once GTV shrank >15%.

154. **Reproducibility Index (Setup Consistency Score):** Metric quantifying repeatability of daily patient position.
**Related Terms:** setup variation, IGRT stability.
**Example:** High index score for DIBH breast showing precise reproducibility.

155. **Respiratory Motion Envelope Modeling:** Mathematical representation of tumor motion boundaries.
**Related Terms:** ITV/4DCT, gating window.
**Example:** Envelope reduced PTV by eliminating improbable motion range.

156. **RespiTrack™ Signal Verification (Generic Term):** QA step for respiratory signal accuracy before gating/tracking.
**Related Terms:** surrogate motion correlation, marker validation.
**Example:** Tracking rejected when marker correlation <0.85.

157. **Resource-Constrained Radiotherapy Allocation:** Treatment prioritization when machine or staff capacity limited.
**Related Terms:** triage radiation framework, emergency prioritization.
**Example:** Emergencies like bleeding brain mets prioritized for SRS.

158. **Retreatment Cumulative Dose Evaluation:** Review of lifetime dose history for previously irradiated areas.
**Related Terms:** re-irradiation constraints, BED summation.
**Example:** Cord EQD2 from prior cervical RT determined safe SBRT retreat.

159. **Reverse Planning (Inverse Planning) Sensitivity:** Degree to which dose distribution changes with weight/constraint edits.
**Related Terms:** optimizer tuning, cost function behavior.
**Example:** Small weight change altered brainstem dose 4% → flagged as sensitive.

160. **Robust Beam Angle Optimization:** Beam selection that maintains dose goals under uncertainty scenarios.
**Related Terms:** robust planning, IMPT angle selection.
**Example:** 4-beam configuration remained optimal across 12 robustness tests.

161. **Robust Dose Constraint Enforcement:** Keeps OAR limits valid across uncertainty scenarios—not just nominal plan.
**Related Terms:** worst-case DVH, robust DVH evaluation.
**Example:** Esophagus Dmax constraint met in all 8 worst-case IMPT tests.

162. **Robust Optimization Cost Map:** Displays optimizer scoring landscape to guide plan tuning.
**Related Terms:** Pareto map, trade-off visualization.
**Example:** Cost map revealed lung-sparing cost increase plateau beyond 66 Gy.

163. **Rotary Couch QA (Non-Coplanar QA):** QA validating couch rotation with simultaneous beam delivery.
**Related Terms:** SRS QA, collision risk.
**Example:** Rotational couch QA required before trigeminal neuralgia case.

164. **Rotational Intrafraction Drift:** Slow rotational misalignment during fraction.
**Related Terms:** 6DOF motion tracking, SRS error source.
**Example:** 1.1° yaw drift caught using optical tracking during brain SRT.

165. **Rotational Range Shifter Positioning Accuracy (Proton):** Precision of rotating range shifter plate placement.
**Related Terms:** proton accessory QA, range error.
**Example:** 0.7 mm placement deviation caused low-range overshoot.

166. **Routine Image-Guided Margin Reduction:** Standardized workflow for reducing PTV margins using daily IGRT data.
**Related Terms:** adaptive margin protocol, systematic error removal.
**Example:** Prostate PTV reduced from 8 mm to 5 mm after 5 stable fractions.

167. **Run-to-Run IMRT Delivery Variation:** Deviation across repeated deliveries of same plan.
**Related Terms:** delivery reproducibility, MLC accuracy trending.
**Example:** Delivered plan logged 0.6% run-to-run difference in MU.

168. **Rutherford Backscatter Correction (CT):** Fixes CT number distortion caused by backscattered X-rays.
**Related Terms:** artifact correction, HU linearity.
**Example:** Correction improved proton stopping accuracy in dental implant cases.

169. **Radiochromic Film Lot-Specific Calibration:** Each film batch requires calibration curve for dose response.
**Related Terms:** film dosimetry, optical density.
**Example:** New lot showed 4% sensitivity difference at 8 Gy.

170. **Radio-Induced Organ Remodeling:** Tissue morphologic change due to radiation response.
**Related Terms:** edema, fibrosis, shrinkage.
**Example:** Parotid shrinkage changed dose distribution requiring adaptive review.

171. **Radiobiological Effectiveness Mapping:** Spatial distribution of biologic effect rather than physical dose.
**Related Terms:** RBE variation, dose painting.
**Example:** Variable RBE model used for carbon ion boost to hypoxic area.

172. **Radiogenomics-Informed Dose Personalization:** Tailoring dose based on predicted genetic radiosensitivity.
**Related Terms:** genomics-guided RT, predictive biomarkers.
**Example:** ATM variant → lower parotid dose allowed to reduce xerostomia risk.

173. **Radiologic-Pathologic Correlation for Boost Targeting:** Uses pathology results to refine boost GTV region.
**Related Terms:** margin adaptation, microscopic extension risk.
**Example:** Prostate tumor extension seen on MRI + pathology informed focal boost.

174. **Rapid Adaptive Recalculation:** Fast dose recalculation on daily anatomy without full replan.
**Related Terms:** hybrid ART, real-time dose update.
**Example:** Pancreas SBRT recalculated daily to verify duodenum dose.

175. **Rapid Dose Painting Optimization:** High-resolution biological boost planning with fast convergence.
**Related Terms:** PET/MRI-guided boost, voxel-boost planning.
**Example:** FDG-hot voxels boosted without raising lung V20.

176. **Real-Time Beam Transmission Monitor:** Detects instantaneous beam output vs planned.
**Related Terms:** transmission chamber, safety interlock.
**Example:** Monitor shut beam after signal spike during VMAT.

177. **Real-Time Couch Drift Suppression:** Automatically compensates for gradual couch shift under load.
**Related Terms:** adaptive couch control, SRS accuracy.
**Example:** Suppression reduced drift to <0.2 mm during 40-min frameless SRS.

178. **Real-Time Dose Accumulation (Live DVH):** Updates DVH while beam is on using delivery log + motion.
**Related Terms:** online adaptation, live DVH.
**Example:** Live DVH paused lung SBRT when cord nearing Dmax.

179. **Real-Time Organ Boundary Tracking:** Tracks edge of organ rather than full surface.
**Related Terms:** adaptive OAR protection, AI boundary tracking.
**Example:** Bladder wall tracked to protect dome during pelvic boost.

180. **Real-Time Target Shape Compensation:** Adjusts beam to shape changes of target during treatment.
**Related Terms:** deformable tracking, MLC sculpting.
**Example:** Shape compensation used in pancreatic MR-guided adaptive beam.

181. **Rectal Gas Influence Modeling:** Dose uncertainty prediction due to gas pocket presence/size.
**Related Terms:** proton range error, pelvic dose robustness.
**Example:** Gas modeling prompted CBCT check before prostate IMPT.

182. **Reference Plan Deviation Threshold:** Maximum allowable difference between new plan and original prescription goals.
**Related Terms:** adaptive approval rule, clinical tolerance.
**Example:** ART plan rejected because femoral head dose increased 5% beyond threshold.

183. **Region-Of-Interest Weight Adaptation:** Dynamically adjusts optimization weights during planning.
**Related Terms:** AI-assisted planning, constraint tuning.
**Example:** ROI weight increased for brainstem in auto-planning cycle 3.

184. **Registration Quality Index:** Score indicating match quality in planar/volumetric fusion.
**Related Terms:** rigid/deformable IGRT, fusion QA.
**Example:** Index dropped → manual override review required.

185. **Reinforced OIS Verification Checklist:** Enhanced procedural checks within oncology information system.
**Related Terms:** digital checklists, safety redundancy.
**Example:** Checklist flagged unapproved couch rotation in SBRT workflow.

186. **Repeat Fraction Imaging Rule:** Protocol that defines when imaging should be repeated mid-fraction.
**Related Terms:** intrafraction image policy.
**Example:** Repeat scan required when prostate IGRT ≥3 mm shift.

187. **Reproducibility-Based Dose Margin:** Margin derived from observed consistency rather than empirical default.
**Related Terms:** individualized margins, adaptive shrink.
**Example:** Esophageal PTV margin reduced 2 mm after 5 consistent fractions.

188. **Residual Proton Range Error Review:** Comparison of planned vs achieved proton range after treatment.
**Related Terms:** range QA, post-delivery log review.
**Example:** WET deviation 1.3 mm documented for adaptive IMPT evaluation.

189. **Resolution-Enhanced Dose Recalculation:** Increases grid resolution for high-gradient regions.
**Related Terms:** small target, SRS re-grid.
**Example:** Re-grid improved conformity for 5-mm brain metastasis.

190. **Resource-Adaptive Radiotherapy Scheduling:** Dynamically assigns patients to machines to reduce idle time.
**Related Terms:** automated scheduling, throughput.
**Example:** SBRT cases scheduled to machines with faster imaging.

191. **Retrospective Error Pattern Discovery:** Uses historical data to identify recurring error trends.
**Related Terms:** incident trending, machine learning QA.
**Example:** Majority of mismatches occurred on 6:00 PM shift → staffing fix.

192. **Ring Gantry Collision Clearance Test:** Validates clearance for Halcyon/Ring-gantry systems.
**Related Terms:** bore clearance, positioning safety.
**Example:** Clearance test allowed breast board at 5° rotation.

193. **Robust Hypofractionation Validation:** Ensures hypofractionated dose constraints remain safe under uncertainty.
**Related Terms:** SBRT safety review, plan robustness.
**Example:** Spine SBRT passed robust validation for cord constraint in all simulations.

194. **Rotational Robustness Index:** Score measuring plan resistance to rotational setup error.
**Related Terms:** 6D robustness, SRS safety metric.
**Example:** Index below threshold required avoidance of couch >110°.

195. **Roughness-Penalty Optimization Term:** Mathematical term preventing rapid modulation changes in IMRT.
**Related Terms:** smoothing term, MU regularization.
**Example:** Penalty reduced MLC ripple and improved deliverability.

196. **Rule-Based Adaptive Planning Decision Engine:** Algorithmic logic that decides if and when to adapt a plan.
**Related Terms:** AI ART triage, dose-trigger rules.
**Example:** Engine identified duodenum Dmax increase → triggered ART.

197. **Run-Time Automated Physics Gate:** Beam hold triggered by automated physics rules during treatment.
**Related Terms:** delivery safety, watchdog trigger.
**Example:** Gate activated for unexpected leaf velocity spike.

198. **Risk-Weighted Dose Evaluation:** DVH analysis weighted by probability of toxicity.
**Related Terms:** NTCP-weighted DVH, biologic planning.
**Example:** NTCP-weighted review helped choose lung-sparing proton plan.

199. **Radiotherapy Zero-Crossing Artifact Correction:** Corrects CT/MR artifacts near signal polarity changes.
**Related Terms:** metal artifact, noise spike filter.
**Example:** Correction improved HU reliability for proton calculation.

200. **Radiotherapy Zone Classification Protocol:** Defines room operational zones based on radiation safety.
**Related Terms:** controlled vs supervised zone, hazard map.
**Example:** High-dose SBRT suite upgraded to Controlled-Red zone requirement.

201. **Radiotherapy Zonal Dose Painting:** Delivering different dose levels to sub-regions of the same tumor based on biological imaging.
**Related Terms:** Multiparametric boost, PET dose escalation, voxel boosting.
**Example:** FDG-avid areas in lung tumor received escalated 74 Gy while rest received 60 Gy.

202. **Radiotoxicity Adaptive Management:** Modifying treatment to reduce toxicity risk when early adverse reactions appear.
**Related Terms:** ART for toxicity, dose de-escalation, symptom-guided replanning.
**Example:** Parotid injury signs → ART generated to reduce mean parotid dose.

203. **Reduced Field Boost:** Shrinking the field to only tumor sub-region after initial radiation response.
**Related Terms:** sequential boost, cone-down field, shrinkage boost.
**Example:** Cervical tumor shrank → boost delivered only to residual PET-positive area.

204. **Reduced Margin Closed-Loop Adaptation:** Iteratively decreasing PTV margins based on verified setup precision.
**Related Terms:** margin learning, IGRT-driven reduction.
**Example:** Prostate PTV margin reduced from 7 mm to 4 mm after 8 verified fractions.

**205. Redundancy-Protected Beam Gate:** Beam stop logic requiring agreement of two or more independent sensors.
**Related Terms:** safety interlock, failsafe logic.
**Example:** Gate triggered when both exit detector and couch sensor detected anomaly.

**206. Reference Structure Calibration:** Using known structures (bones/implants) to validate spatial accuracy of image fusion.
**Related Terms:** IGRT verification, registration QA.
**Example:** Pelvic fusion compared to known femoral head coordinates.

**207. Regional Organ Dose Prediction Model:** Predicting dose distributions received by organ subregions using AI or statistics.
**Related Terms:** functional subregion sparing, NTCP modeling.
**Example:** AI predicted high dose to parotid tail → plan constraints increased.

**208. Registration Drift Compensation Algorithm:** Correcting image fusion errors that accumulate during long treatments.
**Related Terms:** deformable tracking, intrafraction fusion update.
**Example:** Brain SRT fusion updated mid-fraction to remove 0.6 mm drift.

**209. Relative Plan Quality Scaling:** Quantifying differences between plans when prescriptions are not identical.
**Related Terms:** normalized score, KQd metric.
**Example:** Proton vs VMAT plans compared using normalized quality index.

**210. Relative Proton Range Variance Scoring:** Metric indicating probability of clinically significant proton range error.
**Related Terms:** WET variability, robustness scoring.
**Example:** Mandibular implants → high variance score → no proton beams used laterally.

**211. Relevant OAR Priority Mapping:** Assigning OAR priorities based on their clinical importance for each case.
**Related Terms:** weighted planning, risk-based optimization.
**Example:** Rectum scored higher than bladder for prostate VMAT to reduce urgency of toxicity.

**212. Remote Adaptive Review:** Physician/physicist remotely reviews ART dose and approves execution.
**Related Terms:** cloud ART, tele-adaptation, remote TPS.
**Example:** Physicist approved new pancreas SBRT plan remotely at satellite clinic.

**213. Remote Linac Quality Assurance Dashboard:** System monitoring QA compliance across multiple treatment locations.
**Related Terms:** QA automation, fleet QA management.
**Example:** Dashboard flagged failing flatness test at branch facility.

**214. Repeat MLC Calibration Trigger:** System requirement for recalibration when leaf accuracy trends exceed limits.
**Related Terms:** trending alert, threshold trigger.
**Example:** 2-mm cumulative deviation flagged → calibration initiated.

**215. Reportable Radiotherapy Near-Miss Event:** Incident that could have harmed a patient but was caught in time.
**Related Terms:** RPN, incident learning system.
**Example:** Wrong isocenter detected during check → event documented as near-miss.

216. **Reporting Index for Radiotherapy Safety:** Score measuring extent of incident reporting to support learning culture.
**Related Terms:** safety compliance, incident openness metric.
**Example:** Institution improved score after encouraging anonymous reporting.

217. **Residual Deformation Dose Error:** Dose error caused by imperfect deformable registration during ART.
**Related Terms:** DIR QA, accumulated dose error.
**Example:** Liver DIR errors caused 3% DVH uncertainty for stomach wall.

218. **Residual Plan Error Forecasting:** Predicting whether small deviations may grow into clinically unsafe trends.
**Related Terms:** predictive QA, statistical trending.
**Example:** Theta leaf error trending predicted to exceed tolerance within 14 days.

219. **Resource-Driven Treatment Personalization:** Modifying treatment technique based on available clinical resources without compromising safety.
**Related Terms:** pragmatic radiotherapy, context-adaptive planning.
**Example:** 5-fraction SBRT selected over protons due to machine wait list, OAR doses still safe.

220. **Respiratory Cycle Dose Blurring Assessment:** Estimating loss of dose conformity from motion during free-breathing RT.
**Related Terms:** ITV error, interplay evaluation.
**Example:** 8-mm lung tumor motion → gating chosen to prevent blurring.

221. **Respiratory Interplay Suppression:** Techniques preventing destructive interference between motion and beam modulation.
**Related Terms:** repainting, gating, breath holding.
**Example:** Proton repainting used for liver IMPT to suppress interplay.

222. **Respiratory Phase-Dependent OAR Prioritization:** Giving higher OAR protection only in phases where organ proximity risk is high.
**Related Terms:** phase-specific constraints, gating optimization.
**Example:** Stomach dose reduced only during expiration in pancreatic RT.

223. **Response-Amplified Boost Strategy:** Boosting regions that show good biological response to therapy.
**Related Terms:** adaptive dose escalation, PET response boost.
**Example:** PET SUV decrease pattern used to identify boost sub-region in rectal cancer.

224. **. Response-Preventive De-Escalation Strategy:** Reducing dose to avoid overtreatment when tumor responds aggressively early.
**Related Terms:** toxicity-avoidant ART, partial boost withdrawal.
**Example:** Early complete response in lymphoma → final 2 fractions removed.

225. **Response-Triggered Auto-Adaptation:** Automatic replan initiated when radiologic response crosses set threshold.
**Related Terms:** autonomous ART, CBCT volume trigger.
**Example:** 30% prostate shrink detected → new plan created automatically.

226. **Restricted Replanning Safety Policy:** Rules limiting replanning so that changes never increase risk.
**Related Terms:** conservative ART, safety-bounded adaptation.
**Example:** ART blocked if spinal cord dose would rise >1%.

227. **Retrospective Dose-to-Toxicity Correlation Study:** Compares delivered dose patterns with toxicity outcomes.
**Related Terms:** toxicity analytics, NTCP refinement.
**Example:** Tear duct toxicity correlated with lacrimal D30 → constraint updated.

228. **Return-to-Baseline Geometry Protocol:** Returning to original planning geometry after temporary ART deviation.
**Related Terms:** baseline plan reintegration.
**Example:** Bowel displacement worsened → original VMAT plan reinstated.

229. **Risk-Balanced Beam Weighting:** Distributes beam weight according to probability of toxicity events.
**Related Terms:** probabilistic optimization, NTCP minimization.
**Example:** Brainstem NTCP reduction achieved by redistributing beam weights.

230. **Risk-Calibrated Prescription Scaling:** Dose escalation or de-escalation based on predicted complication risk.
**Related Terms:** personalized dosing, genomic NTCP.
**Example:** High radiosensitivity SNP → H&N RT dose de-escalated.

231. **Risk-Compensated Adaptive Fractionation:** Reducing or increasing future dose per fraction depending on patient risk profile.
**Related Terms:** dose steering, dynamic fractionation.
**Example:** Liver SBRT reduced fraction 4 dose when GI risk increased.

232. **Risk-Controlled Beam Orientation Selection:** Avoiding directions that expose sensitive structures at high risk.
**Related Terms:** safe beam geometry, no-fly zone.
**Example:** Brainstem protected by eliminating posterior beams in IMPT.

233. **Risk-First Radiotherapy Planning Design:** Planning philosophy prioritizing deterministic safety over coverage.
**Related Terms:** safety-prioritized planning, OAR-first OAR-max.
**Example:** Esophagus prioritized before target conformity in lung SBRT.

234. **Robust Adaptive Dose Accumulation:** Dose accumulation that accounts for uncertainties and errors.
**Related Terms:** robust composite DVH, scenario dosimetry.
**Example:** Cord dose tracked across shifts + deformations + uncertainties.

235. **Robust Anatomy-Specific Optimization:** Robustness parameters tailored to organ type and motion pattern.
**Related Terms:** personalized robustness, motion-profile models.
**Example:** Larger robustness used for pancreas IMPT vs prostate IMPT.

236. **Robust Hypersensitivity Avoidance:** Reducing dose for patients with predicted radiosensitivity based on biology.
**Related Terms:** radiogenomics, genomic dose tailoring.
**Example:** ATM mutation → reduced dose to parotid tail.

237. **Robust Target Error Compensation:** Expands PTV directionally based on dominant motion/uncertainty axis.
**Related Terms:** directional PTV, anisotropic margins.
**Example:** Lung tumor expanded superior-inferior only to match breathing motion.

238. **Robust Treatment Sequence Optimization:** Optimizing order of fractions, beams, or energy to minimize uncertainty impact.
**Related Terms:** fraction sequencing, heterogeneity steering.
**Example:** High-LET carbon beams delivered early when tumor more oxygenated.

239. **Rotational Backup Isocenter Strategy:** Second verified isocenter used if primary isocenter becomes unsafe.
**Related Terms:** emergency SRS workflow, dual-isocenter configuration.
**Example:** Backup isocenter used due to mask shift during spine SRS.

240. **Rotational Compensatory Beam Shifting:** Beam orientation shifts automatically to compensate for rotational misalignment.
**Related Terms:** autonomous IGRT correction, 6DOF tracking.
**Example:** Beam adjusted 2° when couch yaw drift detected.

241. **Rotational Couch-Weight Deformation Compensation:** Corrects for couch sag due to patient weight at different couch angles.
**Related Terms:** couch correction table, sag model.
**Example:** SRS couch table compensated 1.3 mm under 145° rotation.

242. **Rotational Dose Symmetry Audit:** Verification that dose is symmetric under gantry rotation.
**Related Terms:** rotational QA, symmetry test.
**Example:** VMAT symmetry audit revealed 1.5% asymmetry at 110°.

243. **Rotational IMRT Safety Interlock:** Prevents IMRT delivery if couch/gantry rotation exceeds preset boundary.
**Related Terms:** safe beam range, SRS collision avoidance.
**Example:** Beam blocked when unverified couch rotation detected during SRT.

244. **Rotational Plan Robustness Verification:** Tests robustness against rotational setup uncertainties.
**Related Terms:** angular robustness, orientation simulation.
**Example:** ±2° head rotation simulation used for trigeminal SRS.

245. **Rotational Quality-Weighted Dose Map:** Dose distribution weighted by accuracy expectation at different rotation angles.
**Related Terms:** beam accuracy penalty, dynamic robustness map.
**Example:** VMAT over-weighted stable 20–130° region for precision.

246. **Rotation-Induced Breathing Pattern Shift Correction:** Corrects breathing changes caused by body rotation or setup.
**Related Terms:** respiratory compensation, non-supine motion AI.
**Example:** Prone pancreas patient → respiratory model updated.

247. **RTT-Predictive Safety Alert (Therapist AI Support):** AI prompt alerts RTT when parameters deviate from normal patterns.
**Related Terms:** digital double-check, safety reinforcement.
**Example:** AI warned RTT that CBCT shift exceeded expected historical pattern.

248. **Rule-Based Dose Constraint Arbitration:** Automatically resolves conflicts between OAR constraints during optimization.
**Related Terms:** constraint negotiation, priority arbitration.
**Example:** Brainstem constraint enforced before temporal lobe when conflict detected.

249. **Routine Auto-Segmentation Benchmark:** Objective scoring system to evaluate segmentation accuracy over time.
**Related Terms:** segmentation QA, drift detection.
**Example:** Parotid segmentation drift detected and model retrained.

250. **RTT-Driven Real-Time Adaptation Support:** Therapist-initiated adaptive intervention supported by automated tools.
**Related Terms:** supervised ART, RTT empowerment.
**Example:** RTT aborted plan and requested ART when stomach unexpectedly distended.

251. **Radiobiological Dose Constraint Evaluation:** Assessment of whether planned dose meets organ-specific radiobiological limits.
**Related Terms:** NTCP, TCP, OAR constraints
**Example:** QA confirms liver SBRT plan meets radiobiological constraints for NTCP $< 5\%$.

252. **Radiobiological Modeling Verification:** Ensures accuracy of models predicting tumor control and toxicity.
**Related Terms:** TCP, NTCP models, Biological effectiveness
**Example:** Verification compares model-predicted NTCP to clinical tolerances before plan approval.

253. **Radiochemical Containment Monitoring:** Monitoring systems that confirm no radioactive chemical leaks during handling.
**Related Terms:** Hot lab, Nuclear medicine safety
**Example:** Radiopharmacy room QA ensures no I-131 vapor escape after dose preparation.

254. **Radiochemical Purity Assurance:** Ensuring radiopharmaceutical contains the correct chemical form of the radionuclide.
**Related Terms:** TLC analysis, Radiotracer QC
**Example:** QA confirms ^99mTc-MDP purity $> 95\%$ before bone scan injection.

255. **Radiochemistry Lab Shielding Evaluation:** Verification of shielding in labs preparing radioactive compounds.
**Related Terms:** Lead shielding, Dose monitoring
**Example:** Survey identifies inadequate L-block shielding during Ga-68 synthesis.

256. **Radiodermatitis Prevention Strategy Assessment:** Review of preventive measures to avoid radiation-induced skin toxicity.
**Related Terms:** Skin dose, Bolus, Fractionation schedule
**Example:** RTT removes unnecessary bolus to reduce skin toxicity during breast RT.

257. **Radiodose Optimization Protocol:** Protocol for minimizing radiation exposure while maintaining plan quality.
**Related Terms:** ALARA, AAPM TG reports
**Example:** Pelvic IMRT protocol reduces dose to femoral heads using optimized beam angles.

258. **Radiosensitive Tissue Dose Flagging:** Automatic system warning when dose to radiosensitive structures is exceeded.
**Related Terms:** OAR constraints, AI QA
**Example:** TPS flags high dose to lacrimal gland during orbital tumor planning.

259. **Radiosensitizer Administration Quality Check:** Verification procedures for accurate drug-enhanced radiotherapy delivery.
**Related Terms:** Concurrent therapy, Chemoradiation
**Example:** Check confirms cisplatin-radiation timing within 2 hrs for H&N protocol.

260. **Radiotherapeutic Activity Calibration:** Accurate calibration of radiopharmaceutical activity for therapy.
**Related Terms:** Dose calibrator, Brachytherapy isotopes
**Example:** ^177Lu dose calibration validated before neuroendocrine therapy infusion.

261. **Radiotherapy Anatomical Mapping Verification:** Ensures structures are correctly mapped across CT/MRI/PET registrations.
**Related Terms:** Image fusion, Deformable registration
**Example:** QA detects misalignment of optic nerve after PET fusion in skull-base case.

262. **Radiotherapy Accessory Integrity QA:** Routine inspection of patient-support accessories for safety.
**Related Terms:** Masks, Belly boards, Vac-locks
**Example:** Mask inspection prevents breakage during VMAT for glioblastoma.

263. **Radiotherapy Adaptive Image Review:** Clinician review of images acquired during adaptive treatment.
**Related Terms:** ART, CBCT replan
**Example:** Anatomy change triggers replan for esophageal tumor due to weight loss.

264. **Radiotherapy Adverse Event Documentation:** Recording radiation toxicity and procedural complications.
**Related Terms:** RTOG scale, CTCAE grading
**Example:** Grade 2 esophagitis recorded during week 3 of thoracic IMRT.

265. **Radiotherapy Algorithm Benchmarking:** Performance comparison of different dose calculation algorithms.
**Related Terms:** AAA, Acuros, Monte Carlo
**Example:** Monte Carlo benchmark validates Acuros for lung tumor heterogeneity.

266. **Radiotherapy Angular Correction Verification:** QA confirming correct gantry/couch/col angle implementation.
**Related Terms:** IGRT, 6D correction
**Example:** QA detects 1° couch offset affecting stereotactic spinal plan.

267. **Radiotherapy Arc Timing QA:** Measuring duration of arc delivery to match TPS plan.
**Related Terms:** VMAT, MU rate, Control points
**Example:** RTT verifies VMAT arc time before SBRT lung treatment.

268. **Radiotherapy Asymmetric Field QA:** Evaluation of beam quality when asymmetric jaws are used.
**Related Terms:** Jaws, Penumbra, Symmetry
**Example:** QA verifies 5 cm x-jaw shift during larynx 3DCRT.

269. **Radiotherapy Auto-Segmentation Review QA:** Evaluation and correction of AI-generated contours.
**Related Terms:** AI planning, Auto-contouring
**Example:** Oncologist adjusts AI-segmented bowel loops before pelvic IMRT.

270. **Radiotherapy Beam Attenuation Compensation:** Adjusting dose to compensate for attenuation from accessories/materials.
**Related Terms:** Couch transmission, Bolus effect
**Example:** Couch attenuation map applied for prone breast IMRT.

271. **Radiotherapy Beam Collision Prevention Protocol:** Procedures to avoid gantry/couch/patient collisions.
**Related Terms:** SRS, SBRT, Clearance modelling
**Example:** 6D robotic couch clearance check prevents gantry collision.

272. **Radiotherapy Beam Current Stability Testing:** Ensuring accelerator electron beam current remains stable.
**Related Terms:** Pulse repetition, Output drift
**Example:** Daily QA flags current drift before treating prostate cases.

273. **Radiotherapy Beam Flattening Filter Verification:** QA confirming presence, type, and performance of flattening filter.
**Related Terms:** FFF beam, Profiles, Symmetry
**Example:** Profile scan confirms flattening filter for 10 MV beam during commissioning.

274. **Radiotherapy Beam Focusing Accuracy:** Ensures electron beam is centered in the accelerator waveguide.
**Related Terms:** Steering coils, Beam symmetry
**Example:** Steering adjustment corrects symmetry for 6 MV beam.

275. **Radiotherapy Beam Interruption Safety Check:** Confirmation that radiation stops instantly after pressing hold.
**Related Terms:** Beam hold, Emergency stop
**Example:** Delivery stops within required 50 ms during emergency test.

276. **Radiotherapy Beam Monitoring Chamber Calibration:** Calibration of ion chambers measuring real-time LINAC output.
**Related Terms:** Dose rate, MU calibration
**Example:** Output drift detected after chamber recalibration.

277. **Radiotherapy Beam Modulation Verification:** QA ensuring planned fluence matches delivered fluence.
**Related Terms:** IMRT, VMAT, Gamma index
**Example:** Portal dosimetry confirms leaf modulation for H&N IMRT.

278. **Radiotherapy Beam Pulse Uniformity Check:** Verifies consistency of radiation dose per pulse.
**Related Terms:** Repetition frequency, Output stability
**Example:** QA detects irregular pulses at high dose rate in FFF beam.

279. **Radiotherapy Beam Quality Correction Factor Validation:** Verification of detector-specific kQ factors for different energies.
**Related Terms:** TRS-398, AAPM TG-51
**Example:** kQ factor updated during commissioning of new 10X FFF beam.

280. **Radiotherapy Beam Transmission Mapping:** Mapping attenuation when the beam passes through materials.
**Related Terms:** Couch/pad transmission, Compensators
**Example:** Dose recalculated using carbon-fiber couch transmission map.

281. **Radiotherapy Beam Uniformity Verification:** QA procedure ensuring that the delivered radiation beam has consistent intensity across the field.
**Related Terms:** Symmetry, Flatness, Profile scan
**Example:** Uniformity test ensures 6 MV beam flatness meets ±3% tolerance before whole-pelvis treatment.

282. **Radiotherapy Beam Weight Optimization:** Adjustment of beam weight values to improve dose distribution and organ sparing.
**Related Terms:** IMRT planning, Objective tuning
**Example:** Planner reduces anterior beam weight to lower bladder dose in prostate IMRT.

**283. Radiotherapy Biological Dose Mapping:** Dose visualization based on biological effect rather than physical absorbed dose.
**Related Terms:** BED, EQD2
**Example:** BED map shows higher biologically-effective dose to the tumor in hypofractionated plan.

**284. Radiotherapy Biological Response Modeling:** Mathematical prediction of tumor control and normal tissue toxicity following radiation.
**Related Terms:** TCP, NTCP, LQ model
**Example:** NTCP model predicts low risk of pneumonitis for 40 Gy / 5 fractions lung SBRT.

**285. Radiotherapy Biomechanical Deformation QA:** Verification of deformation accuracy when transferring contours using biomechanical deformable registration.
**Related Terms:** DIR, Adaptive radiotherapy
**Example:** Deformation QA confirms reliable mapping of bowel contours across CBCTs for weekly replanning.

**286. Radiotherapy Biometric Setup Verification:** Patient identification and setup verification using biometric detection (e.g., fingerprint, facial ID).
**Related Terms:** Patient safety, Identity mismatch prevention
**Example:** Facial recognition system prevents patient swap before SRS.

**287. Radiotherapy Brachycatheter Placement QA:** Verification of catheter positioning during brachytherapy before dose calculation.
**Related Terms:** HDR brachytherapy, Applicator reconstruction
**Example:** CT confirms catheter depth and spacing before cervical HDR planning.

**288. Radiotherapy Brachytherapy Afterloader Integrity Test:** Hardware QC ensuring mechanical integrity and safe function of the HDR afterloader.
**Related Terms:** Source drive, Emergency retract
**Example:** Integrity test ensures source cable moves smoothly before patient connection.

**289. Radiotherapy Brachytherapy Catheter Reconstruction Accuracy:** Accuracy of digitizing catheter paths in planning system.
**Related Terms:** Dwell positions, Image guidance
**Example:** QA ensures all catheters reconstructed correctly to avoid cold spots in vaginal HDR.

**290. Radiotherapy Brachytherapy Dwell Time Verification:** Checking that programmed dwell times match calculated treatment times.
**Related Terms:** Dose loading, Source strength
**Example:** Verification detects 0.2 s timing error that would underdose apex of prostate HDR.

**291. Radiotherapy Brachytherapy Source Calibration Audit:** Independent verification of brachytherapy source activity and calibration.
**Related Terms:** Source strength, Well chamber
**Example:** Independent audit confirms ^192Ir activity prior to annual replacement.

**292. Radiotherapy Breath-Hold Reproducibility Assessment:** Evaluation of consistency in patient breath-hold amplitude and duration across fractions.
**Related Terms:** DIBH, Surface guidance
**Example:** Breast DIBH reproducibility tracking prevents heart dose escalation.

**293. Radiotherapy Breathing Motion Management Optimization:** Tailoring motion-management strategy to patient-specific respiratory behavior.
**Related Terms:** Gating, 4DCT, Motion envelope
**Example:** Planner shifts from free-breathing to gated lung SBRT due to large diaphragm motion.

294. **Radiotherapy Breathing Motion Validation Phantom:** Phantom that simulates respiratory motion for QA of imaging and dose delivery.
**Related Terms:** 4D phantom, End-to-end QA
**Example:** Phantom test validates gated SBRT delivery accuracy for moving liver target.

295. **Radiotherapy Build-Up Region Dose Evaluation:** Assessment of dose distribution in the shallow region where dose increases rapidly to maximum.
**Related Terms:** Skin sparing, Bolus, dmax
**Example:** Bolus placement increases build-up region dose for chest-wall post-mastectomy RT.

296. **Radiotherapy Buildup Correction Factor Validation:** Ensuring correction factors applied to surface and near-surface dose are accurate.
**Related Terms:** Skin dose, SSD
**Example:** Validation prevents overestimation of dose to skin during VMAT.

297. **Radiotherapy Bulk Density Override Review:** Verification that average density overrides assigned to anatomical regions are appropriate.
**Related Terms:** Hounsfield calibration, TPS override
**Example:** Reviewer approves density override for dental implants in H&N IMRT.

298. **Radiotherapy Bunker Radiation Shielding Survey:** Safety survey ensuring bunker walls, doors, and shielding prevent radiation leakage.
**Related Terms:** Controlled area, Leakage limits
**Example:** Measured leakage around maze entrance meets national shielding guidelines.

299. **Radiotherapy Bunker Interlock QA:** Testing of interlocks preventing beam enable when bunker is unsafe or door is open.
**Related Terms:** Safety systems, Emergency stop
**Example:** Door-open interlock check stops beam during daily LINAC startup QA.

300. **Radiotherapy Bystander Exposure Minimization:** Strategies to reduce radiation dose to staff and nearby individuals.
**Related Terms:** Time–distance–shielding, Staff dose monitoring
**Example:** Lead barrier positioning and remote treatment monitoring lower staff exposure during brachytherapy.

301. **Radiotherapy Calculation Grid Spacing Optimization:** Selecting optimal dose-calculation grid size to balance accuracy and computing speed.
**Related Terms:** Dose calculation resolution, TPS accuracy
**Example:** Grid spacing reduced from 3 mm to 2 mm to improve dose accuracy for spine SRS.

302. **Radiotherapy Calibration Constancy Check:** Routine QA verifying treatment machine calibration stability over time.
**Related Terms:** Output QA, Daily QA
**Example:** Daily constancy check confirms 6 MV output remains within ±2% before patient treatments.

303. **Radiotherapy Camera-Based Position Tracking:** Monitoring patient position using optical or infrared cameras.
**Related Terms:** SGRT, Motion tracking
**Example:** Cameras detect 2-mm chest displacement during DIBH breast treatment.

304. **Radiotherapy CBCT Hounsfield Calibration:** Adjusting HU values on CBCT to better reflect true tissue densities.
**Related Terms:** Image calibration, Density override
**Example:** CBCT HU calibration improves adaptive abdominal planning accuracy.

**305. Radiotherapy Central Axis Dose Verification:** Confirming dose accuracy along central axis of the beam.
**Related Terms:** PDD, Output factor
**Example:** Depth dose curve compared with baseline to verify photon beam characteristics.

**306. Radiotherapy Central Nervous System Dose Limitation:** Controlling dose to spinal cord and brain to stay within tolerance thresholds.
**Related Terms:** QUANTEC, OAR constraints
**Example:** Cord dose limited to ≤14 Gy in single-fraction spine SBRT plan.

**307. Radiotherapy Cervical Immobilization Optimization:** Improving immobilization techniques for cervical spine or neck treatments.
**Related Terms:** SRS mask, Head-and-neck setup
**Example:** Cervical cushions added to improve reproducibility for H&N IMRT.

**308. Radiotherapy CIELAB Color Dose Visualization:** Dose-display approach utilizing perceptually uniform color mapping for clarity.
**Related Terms:** Dose color scale, Visualization QA
**Example:** CIELAB scale improves visualization of hotspots in VMAT plan review.

**309. Radiotherapy Cine-MRI Motion Verification:** Using real-time MRI to evaluate tumor and organ movement.
**Related Terms:** MR-linac, Adaptive therapy
**Example:** Cine-MRI confirms pancreatic tumor motion during treatment gating session.

**310. Radiotherapy Clinical Protocol Conformity Assessment:** Ensuring treatment plans adhere to approved clinical radiation protocols.
**Related Terms:** Standardization, Clinical governance
**Example:** Prostate SBRT plan checked against institutional protocol before approval.

**311. Radiotherapy Clinical Target Reconstruction QA:** Evaluating accuracy of reconstructed CTV/PTV on treatment imaging.
**Related Terms:** IGRT, Contouring QA
**Example:** MRI-guided RT verifies PTV match on daily adaptive scans.

**312. Radiotherapy Collimator Angle Optimization:** Choosing collimator angle to minimize high-dose regions and MLC leakage.
**Related Terms:** VMAT arc settings, MLC modulation
**Example:** Collimator rotated to 30° to reduce tongue-and-groove artifacts in brain SRS.

**313. Radiotherapy Collimator-Jaw Coordination Check:** QA ensuring MLC leaves and jaws align correctly during field shaping.
**Related Terms:** Field shaping, MLC QA
**Example:** Misalignment check prevents field-edge underdosing for liver IMRT.

**314. Radiotherapy Collision Simulation Validation:** Ensuring the treatment plan avoids couch–gantry–patient collisions.
**Related Terms:** Clearance check, End-to-end test
**Example:** Virtual clearance tools detect potential collision in a prone spine VMAT plan.

**315. Radiotherapy Compensation Filter Verification:** QA confirming accuracy of filters used to modify beam intensity.
**Related Terms:** Compensators, 3D printing filters
**Example:** Filter inspected for correct thickness before lung compensator therapy.

**316. Radiotherapy Compliance Audit:** Formal evaluation of adherence to regulations, safety, and performance standards.
**Related Terms:** Regulatory compliance, Accreditation
**Example:** Annual audit reviews safety logs, TPS access control, and QA reports.

**317. Radiotherapy Computational Phantom Validation:** Verification of virtual phantoms used for dose simulation.
**Related Terms:** Monte Carlo, Digital phantom
**Example:** Digital anthropomorphic phantom validated against physical phantom measurements.

**318. Radiotherapy Cone-Beam Registration Consistency:** Ensuring CBCT registrations remain accurate across fractions.
**Related Terms:** IGRT reproducibility, Positioning QA
**Example:** Daily review confirms consistent auto-registration for pancreas SBRT.

**319. Radiotherapy Couch Attenuation Assessment:** Measurement of dose attenuation caused by the treatment couch.
**Related Terms:** Couch model correction, TPS couch structure
**Example:** Couch attenuation data loaded into TPS improves breast VMAT dose accuracy.

**320. Radiotherapy Couch Sag Compensation:** Adjusting for vertical deflection of the couch under patient weight.
**Related Terms:** Couch deflection, Mechanical QA
**Example:** Sag correction applied for a heavy patient undergoing spine SRS.

**321. Radiotherapy Craniospinal Junction QA:** QA ensuring seamless dose match at field junctions in craniospinal irradiation.
**Related Terms:** Field matching, Gradient match
**Example:** Junction shift technique avoids hotspots in pediatric CSI.

**322. Radiotherapy Critical Organ Contour Verification:** Review ensuring accurate contouring of sensitive organs.
**Related Terms:** OAR validation, Contouring QA
**Example:** Brainstem contour revised to correct over-segmentation before SRS.

**323. Radiotherapy Cross-Beam Dose Ratio Check:** Comparing dose delivered by intersecting beams to validate TPS accuracy.
**Related Terms:** Composite dose, Beam interaction
**Example:** Cross-beam ratio verified for three-field rectal IMRT.

**324. Radiotherapy CyberKnife Motion Synchronization QA:** QA ensuring robotic beam aims remain synchronized with patient breathing motion.
**Related Terms:** Synchrony tracking, Fiducial tracking
**Example:** QA detects 0.5-mm phase lag that could affect lung tumor targeting.

**325. Radiotherapy CyberKnife Path Accuracy Test:** Testing robotic arm movement precision along complex beam paths.
**Related Terms:** Robotic radiosurgery, End-to-end check
**Example:** Path test confirms sub-millimeter positioning before trigeminal neuralgia treatment.

**326. Radiotherapy Daily CBCT Dose Assessment:** Monitoring cumulative imaging dose from frequent CBCT scans.
**Related Terms:** Imaging dose tracking, ALARA
**Example:** CBCT dose minimized for pediatric abdominal IGRT while maintaining alignment accuracy.

327. **Radiotherapy Daily Treatment Reproducibility Review:** Reviewing daily imaging and setup trends to monitor consistency.
**Related Terms:** IGRT review, Positioning accuracy
**Example:** Trend analysis flags increasing setup deviation after week 3 of H&N RT.

328. **Radiotherapy Data Backup Compliance:** Ensuring patient and planning data are securely backed up according to policy.
**Related Terms:** Data retention, Cybersecurity
**Example:** TPS backup verified weekly to protect SBRT planning records.

329. **Radiotherapy Deep Dose Gradient Control:** Managing steep dose transitions to protect adjacent organs.
**Related Terms:** Dose fall-off, Gradient index
**Example:** Rapid dose drop-off controlled to protect duodenum in liver SBRT.

330. **Radiotherapy Deformable Dose Accumulation Validation:** Validating accumulated dose from multiple anatomy states using deformable registration.
**Related Terms:** DIR, Adaptive therapy
**Example:** Cumulative dose verified across weekly CBCTs for bladder cancer replanning.

331. **Radiotherapy Deformable Registration Plausibility Test:** Checking biological plausibility of deformation field vectors.
**Related Terms:** DIR QA, Contour propagation
**Example:** Algorithm flagged for unrealistic tissue deformation between CT and MR.

332. **Radiotherapy Detector Array Linearity Test:** Ensuring detector response remains linear across dose rates.
**Related Terms:** EPID QA, Plan QA
**Example:** Detector linearity validated to support high-dose-rate SRS.

333. **Radiotherapy Detector Cross-Calibration:** Calibration of different detectors against a reference device.
**Related Terms:** Ion chamber, Absolute dosimetry
**Example:** Film and diode array calibrated against Farmer chamber output.

334. **Radiotherapy Diaphragm Motion Envelope Mapping:** Defining the extent of diaphragm excursion during breathing.
**Related Terms:** 4DCT, Motion management
**Example:** Envelope determines ITV margin for adrenal SBRT.

335. **Radiotherapy Digital Patient Identity Verification:** Electronic identity confirmation before treatment start.
**Related Terms:** Patient safety, Mistake prevention
**Example:** Barcode ID system prevents wrong-patient irradiation.

336. **Radiotherapy Dose Accumulation Trend Analysis:** Evaluating changes in accumulated dose during multi-session treatments.
**Related Terms:** Adaptive RT, Toxicity prediction
**Example:** Trend shows increasing duodenum dose → plan adapted for liver SBRT.

337. **Radiotherapy Dose Aperture Overlap Evaluation:** Checking overlap of adjacent radiation fields contributing to dose summation.
**Related Terms:** Field match QA, Junction QA
**Example:** Overlap minimized for breast–supraclavicular junction.

338. **Radiotherapy Dose Artefact Reduction Method:** Algorithms to remove artifacts that distort calculated dose.
**Related Terms:** Metal artifact reduction, Image filtering
**Example:** MAR improves dose accuracy near dental fillings in H&N IMRT.

339. **Radiotherapy Dose Audit Benchmarking:** Comparing dose audit results with national/international standards.
**Related Terms:** External audit, TLD network
**Example:** IAEA audit verifies 1% output deviation — excellent compliance.

340. **Radiotherapy Dose-Based Plan Adaptation:** Adapting plans based on accumulated dose rather than anatomy alone.
**Related Terms:** Accumulated dose, ART
**Example:** Boost removed after accumulated dose to rectum approached tolerance.

341. **Radiotherapy Dose Constraint Prioritization:** Ranking clinical objectives to guide optimization.
**Related Terms:** Cost functions, Planning objectives
**Example:** Planner prioritizes spinal cord constraint above CTV coverage in spine SBRT.

342. **Radiotherapy Dose Drop-Off Index:** Metric describing steepness of dose fall-off outside target.
**Related Terms:** Gradient index, Conformity
**Example:** High drop-off index achieved to protect optic nerve in pituitary SRS.

343. **Radiotherapy Dose Hotspot Management:** Methods to prevent or reduce localized areas of excess dose.
**Related Terms:** Hotspot limit, Plan smoothing
**Example:** MLC smoothing removes 118% hotspot in pelvis IMRT.

344. **Radiotherapy Dose Kernel Convolution QA:** QA verifying dose convolution accuracy in TPS algorithms.
**Related Terms:** Pencil-beam kernel, Monte Carlo
**Example:** Kernel error detected during commissioning with 3-cm heterogeneity phantom.

345. **Radiotherapy Dose Leakage Suppression:** Minimizing dose outside field caused by MLC/jaw leakage.
**Related Terms:** Transmission, Interleaf leakage
**Example:** High-precision collimation reduces leakage dose to breast for mediastinal VMAT.

346. **Radiotherapy Dose Linearity Verification:** Ensuring dose delivered remains proportional to MU across full range.
**Related Terms:** Output linearity, MU test
**Example:** Verified linearity supports ultra-low MU imaging fields.

347. **Radiotherapy Dose Mapping with Film QA:** Using film's high spatial resolution to map 2D dose distributions.
**Related Terms:** GAFchromic film, Plan QA
**Example:** Film QA confirms steep dose gradient accuracy in trigeminal SRS.

348. **Radiotherapy Dose Modulation Complexity Index:** Metric quantifying plan modulation difficulty.
**Related Terms:** MLC complexity, Treatment deliverability
**Example:** High complexity index triggers creating simplified IMRT plan.

349. **Radiotherapy Dose Monitor Chamber Correction:** Calibration adjustment for LINAC monitor chamber drift.
**Related Terms:** Output factor, Chamber calibration
**Example:** Correction applied when output audit detects −1.3% deviation.

350. **Radiotherapy Dose Monitoring Wearable Sensor Integration:** Using personal radiation-dose sensors for patient or staff safety.
**Related Terms:** Real-time dosimeter, Exposure tracking
**Example:** Wearable sensors monitor nurse exposure during HDR brachytherapy insertion.

351. **Radiotherapy Dose Nonuniformity Assessment:** Evaluation of variations in dose distribution within the planning target volume.
**Related Terms:** Homogeneity index, Hotspot analysis
**Example:** Liver SBRT plan revised after nonuniformity index exceeded tolerance.

352. **Radiotherapy Dose Normalization Strategy:** Method for selecting the prescription isodose surface for optimal plan performance.
**Related Terms:** 100% normalization, 95% normalization
**Example:** Brain SRS normalized to 70% to maximize dose fall-off.

353. **Radiotherapy Dose Overlap Zone Analysis:** Measurement of dose interaction between overlapping treatment areas.
**Related Terms:** Junction QA, Composite dose
**Example:** Overlap zone optimized for breast–SCL IMRT match line.

354. **Radiotherapy Dose Paint Segmentation:** Subdividing tumor regions to assign different dose levels based on biology.
**Related Terms:** Dose painting by numbers, Radiomics planning
**Example:** High-hypoxia areas in H&N tumor boosted based on PET SUV.

355. **Radiotherapy Dose Per Fraction Accuracy Verification:** Ensuring each fraction delivers the prescribed dose precisely.
**Related Terms:** Fractionation QA, Daily treatment accuracy
**Example:** Detected 1.5% output drift and corrected prior to the next SBRT fraction.

356. **Radiotherapy Dose Perturbation Modeling:** Predicting dose changes due to implants, air cavities, or heterogeneities.
**Related Terms:** Metal artifact mitigation, Monte Carlo
**Example:** Titanium hip perturbation modeled for pelvis VMAT plan.

357. **Radiotherapy Dose Prediction Failure Detection:** Identification of algorithm breakdowns in dose calculation.
**Related Terms:** TPS error flagging, Calculation QA
**Example:** Alerts generated when electron plan diverged from reference dataset.

358. **Radiotherapy Dose Quality Score:** Composite score evaluating overall plan performance against clinical benchmarks.
**Related Terms:** Plan scoring, Constraint balancing
**Example:** Highest score among 4 plans selected for pancreatic VMAT.

359. **Radiotherapy Dose Ramp Function Optimization:** Algorithm tuning to shape dose ramping between subvolumes.
**Related Terms:** Gradient smoothing, Dose shaping
**Example:** Dose ramp reduced toxicity for rectal wall while maintaining PTV control.

360. **Radiotherapy Dose Reconstruction From Log Files:** Using delivery log files to rebuild delivered dose in 3D.
**Related Terms:** Log-based QA, Real-time dose tracking
**Example:** Pancreas plan confirmed within tolerance despite motion during VMAT.

**361. Radiotherapy Dose Redistribution Strategy:** Adjusting dose allocation within the PTV and OARs based on biological priority.
**Related Terms:** Prioritized optimization, ART
**Example:** Reduced parotid dose while maintaining tumor coverage in week-4 replan.

**362. Radiotherapy Dose Reduction Index:** Metric quantifying how effectively dose to an OAR is minimized.
**Related Terms:** Organ sparing index, Optimization efficiency
**Example:** Rectum dose reduction index improved significantly after constraint tightening.

**363. Radiotherapy Dose Reference Chart Validation:** Checking stored reference charts to confirm consistency of machine performance.
**Related Terms:** Output constancy, Baseline QA
**Example:** Weekly check verified photon PDD unchanged since commissioning.

**364. Radiotherapy Dose Region-of-Interest Profiling:** Detailed evaluation of dose distribution within specific anatomical subregions.
**Related Terms:** ROI metrics, DVH-subset evaluation
**Example:** High-dose subregion flagged within hippocampus during brain IMRT review.

**365. Radiotherapy Dose Reproducibility Assurance:** Ensuring consistent dose delivery across all fractions and beam sequences.
**Related Terms:** Treatment stability, Daily QA
**Example:** Deviations identified in 10th SBRT fraction caused by beam start-up drift.

**366. Radiotherapy Dose Response Modeling for Normal Tissue:** Predicting toxicity probability based on dose–volume relationships.
**Related Terms:** NTCP model, QUANTEC
**Example:** NTCP demonstrated safe lung dose profile for esophageal chemoradiation.

**367. Radiotherapy Dose Response Modeling for Tumor:** Predicting tumor control probability as a function of dose.
**Related Terms:** TCP model, Radiosensitivity
**Example:** TCP model supported 60 Gy prescription instead of 54 Gy for glioma.

**368. Radiotherapy Dose Ring Evaluation:** Evaluating concentric low-dose rings around PTV to restrict dose spread.
**Related Terms:** Dose shell constraints, Spill control
**Example:** High-dose spill reduced by tightening ring dose objectives in liver SBRT.

**369. Radiotherapy Dose Robustness Analysis:** Evaluating plan sensitivity to uncertainties such as motion, range, or setup.
**Related Terms:** Worst-case scenario testing, Proton robustness
**Example:** Proton plan robustness ensured spinal cord remained safe across shifts.

**370. Radiotherapy Dose Scaling Correction:** Adjusting calculation outputs to compensate for TPS scaling issues.
**Related Terms:** Calculation bias correction, Output adjustment
**Example:** Scaling factor updated after 2% discrepancy found in IMRT QA.

**371. Radiotherapy Dose Spill Factor Assessment:** Quantifying dose that escapes the target area into healthy tissue.
**Related Terms:** R50%, Conformality metrics
**Example:** R50% improved after modifying arc trajectory in lung SBRT.

372. **Radiotherapy Dose Spread Suppression:** Methods to limit lateral dose spread, especially in small-field treatments.
**Related Terms:** Collimator shaping, Penumbra control
**Example:** Mini-MLC reduced lateral dose spread for trigeminal neuralgia radiosurgery.

373. **Radiotherapy Dose Stability Tracking:** Long-term monitoring of treatment machine dose stability.
**Related Terms:** Output trend monitoring, Drift detection
**Example:** Trend flagged gradual decline in 10 MV output before exceedance.

374. **Radiotherapy Dose Steering Algorithm:** Algorithm that reallocates dose during optimization to improve constraints.
**Related Terms:** Smart optimization, Weight balancing
**Example:** Automated dose steering reduced parotid Dmean while preserving PTV coverage.

375. **Radiotherapy Dose Surface Mapping:** 3D mapping of dose delivered on external skin surface.
**Related Terms:** Exit dose, Skin toxicity predictor
**Example:** High skin dose patch identified in chest wall IMRT before delivery.

376. **Radiotherapy Dose Surrogate Signal Calibration:** Calibrating surrogate motion signals (e.g., markers, belt sensors) to dose impact.
**Related Terms:** Surrogate tracking, Gating
**Example:** Surrogate delay calibrated for abdominal gating to avoid timing mismatch.

377. **Radiotherapy Dose Symmetry Index:** Symmetry measure of dose distribution across central axis.
**Related Terms:** Beam symmetry, Flatness
**Example:** Linac adjusted after symmetry index exceeded ±2% tolerance.

378. **Radiotherapy Dose Temporal Drift Study:** Study of machine output drift patterns across hours or weeks.
**Related Terms:** Monitoring log, Predictive maintenance
**Example:** Temporary panel overheating linked to mid-day dose drift.

379. **Radiotherapy Dose Threshold Flagging:** Trigger system that flags constraint violations during planning or adaptation.
**Related Terms:** Auto-alert constraint system, Treatment safety
**Example:** Auto-flag warning activated when rectum V60 exceeded limit.

380. **Radiotherapy Dose Time-Weighted Averaging:** Averaging delivered dose over prolonged treatment time for slow-motion scenarios.
**Related Terms:** Cumulative dose, Organ drift
**Example:** Stabilized PTV dose for pancreas despite slow positional drift.

381. **Radiotherapy Dose-to-Medium Verification:** QA confirming dose-to-medium calculation accuracy in heterogeneous tissues.
**Related Terms:** Monte Carlo dose, Heterogeneity correction
**Example:** Lung plan verified using dose-to-medium rather than dose-to-water.

382. **Radiotherapy Dose-to-Water Calibration:** Ensuring chamber measurements correspond accurately to dose-to-water standard.
**Related Terms:** TRS-398, Calibration certificate
**Example:** Absolute dosimetry recalibrated to maintain national traceability.

383. **Radiotherapy Dosimetric Accuracy Assurance:** Procedures ensuring all dose delivery and calculation steps remain within tolerance.
**Related Terms:** QA program, IAEA standards
**Example:** Annual review confirms compliance of all IMRT and SBRT workflows.

**384. Radiotherapy Dosimetric Artifact Suppression:** Strategies to remove dose errors caused by imaging artifacts.
**Related Terms:** MAR, Density override
**Example:** Hip prosthesis override improved pelvis dose accuracy by 5%.

**385. Radiotherapy Dosimetric Benchmarking:** Comparing clinical dose estimations with validated reference datasets.
**Related Terms:** Commissioning, External audit
**Example:** VMAT commissioning matched Monte Carlo gold-standard dataset.

**386. Radiotherapy Dosimetric Efficiency Optimization:** Balancing clinical goal achievement with treatment complexity and time.
**Related Terms:** MU efficiency, Beam modulation
**Example:** Plan simplified to reduce MU by 30% without reducing tumor coverage.

**387. Radiotherapy Dosimetric Error Classifications:** Categorizing dose errors by type, severity, and clinical impact.
**Related Terms:** Incident reporting, Risk analysis
**Example:** Wrong shift prevented from becoming a major error through classification rules.

**388. Radiotherapy Dosimetric Film Response Characterization:** Establishing dose–response curve for radiochromic film.
**Related Terms:** Film calibration, Optical density
**Example:** Calibration curve validated for 6–20 Gy SBRT measurement range.

**389. Radiotherapy Dosimetric Gamma Index Mapping:** Using gamma index to evaluate agreement of planned vs. measured dose.
**Related Terms:** Plan QA, 3%/2 mm criteria
**Example:** Pancreas VMAT passed with gamma pass rate of 97% for 2%/2 mm.

**390. Radiotherapy Dosimetric Gradient Preservation:** Maintaining steep dose gradients around target during replanning/ART.
**Related Terms:** Dose fall-off, Edge sharpness
**Example:** ART maintained paraspinal SRS gradient after tumor shrinkage.

**391. Radiotherapy Dosimetric Load Balancing:** Distributing beam contribution among arcs/segments to reduce hotspots.
**Related Terms:** Arc sharing, MU balance
**Example:** Two-arc VMAT redistributed load to reduce lung V20.

**392. Radiotherapy Dosimetric Nonlinearity Study:** Evaluation of deviations from linear dose response in detectors or algorithms.
**Related Terms:** Output linearity, Detector saturation
**Example:** Diode array nonlinearity detected at high dose rates for FFF beams.

**393. Radiotherapy Dosimetric Perturbation Phantom:** Phantom used to measure dose distortions caused by heterogeneities.
**Related Terms:** Heterogeneity QA, End-to-end test
**Example:** Phantom quantified metal implant dose shadowing before pelvic IMRT.

**394. Radiotherapy Dosimetric Profile Agreement Check:** Comparing measured versus calculated lateral and depth profiles.
**Related Terms:** Beam profile QA, PDD comparison
**Example:** 6 MV profile agreed within 1%/1 mm tolerance before SRS day.

**395. Radiotherapy Dosimetric Quality Factor:** Weighted score summarizing plan success relative to OAR sparing and PTV coverage.
**Related Terms:** Plan ranking, MCDM scoring
**Example:** Factor identified plan 2 as best candidate for bilateral H&N IMRT.

**396. Radiotherapy Dosimetric Range Assessment:** Checking depth of penetration accuracy for charged particles.
**Related Terms:** Bragg peak, Proton range QA
**Example:** Range verification avoided overshoot into brainstem in proton medulloblastoma case.

**397. Radiotherapy Dosimetric Rate Dependence Test:** Evaluating detector behavior across different dose rates.
**Related Terms:** FFF dose rate QA, Saturation testing
**Example:** Rate-dependence test ensured chamber suitability for 2400 MU/min SBRT.

**398. Radiotherapy Dosimetric Sensitivity Analysis:** Quantifying how uncertainties affect final dose results.
**Related Terms:** Robustness, Error propagation
**Example:** Sensitivity evaluation confirmed setup error dominates uncertainty in pancreas planning.

**399. Radiotherapy Dosimetric Surface Reconstruction:** Creating 3D dose maps mapped to the patient surface.
**Related Terms:** Skin dose prediction, Dosimetric skin atlas
**Example:** Surface reconstruction predicted chest wall erythema in post-mastectomy RT.

**400. Radiotherapy Dosimetric Uncertainty Propagation Study:** Study of the cumulative effect of all uncertainty sources on dose distribution.
**Related Terms:** Monte Carlo uncertainty, Robust optimization
**Example:** Study confirmed total uncertainty <5% for pediatric proton CSI.

**401. Radiotherapy Equipment Reliability Evaluation:** Ongoing assessment of linac and RT system performance to prevent failures.
**Related Terms:** Predictive maintenance, Uptime assurance
**Radiotherapy Example:** Reliability check triggered replacement of a degrading MLC motor.

**402. Radiotherapy Error Mitigation Workflow:** Procedures designed to block or intercept potential treatment errors.
**Related Terms:** Safety barriers, Incident prevention
**Example:** Auto-lock preventing treatment until IGRT match is confirmed.

**403. Radiotherapy Error Propagation Control:** Preventing mistakes in one step from affecting later workflow.
**Related Terms:** QA checkpoints, Data validation
**Example:** Patient ID mismatch detected before beam-on due to interlock rules.

**404. Radiotherapy Error Trend Analysis:** Monitoring patterns in treatment incidents to guide improvements.
**Related Terms:** Quality indicators, RCA
**Example:** Trend showed recurring iso-shift errors → staff re-training initiated.

**405. Radiotherapy Event Reporting System:** A platform to document and track radiation-related deviations or incidents.
**Related Terms:** SAFRON, RO-ILS
**Example:** Near-miss of wrong shift reported for safety database learning.

406. **Radiotherapy External Audit Participation:** Independent check by external experts for quality compliance.
**Related Terms:** Accreditation audits, IAEA Dosimetry audits
**Example:** Proton center participated in national end-to-end credentialing.

407. **Radiotherapy Field Aperture:** Customized shaping of radiation field based on tumor geometry.
**Related Terms:** MLC contouring, Beam shaping
**Example:** Tight aperture minimized bowel exposure in abdominal VMAT.

408. **Radiotherapy Field Matching QA:** Assessment of dose uniformity at beam junctions.
**Related Terms:** Matchline, Feathering
**Example:** Spinal junction feathering used to avoid cold/hot spots.

409. **Radiotherapy Field Rotation Analysis:** Evaluating impact of couch/gantry rotation on field geometry.
**Related Terms:** Mechanical accuracy, Collision margin
**Example:** Gantry rotation QA avoided gantry-head impact in SRS.

410. **Radiotherapy Field Size Expansion Margin:** Margin applied beyond PTV for dose coverage when penumbra is large.
**Related Terms:** Output factor dependency, Geometric margins
**Example:** Electron field expanded to fully cover skin lesion.

411. **Radiotherapy Field Symmetry Verification:** Ensuring equal dose distribution on opposite sides of beam central axis.
**Related Terms:** Beam symmetry QA
**Example:** Linac beam tuned after symmetry drift exceeded tolerance.

412. **Radiotherapy Filter-Free Beam Profile Study:** Analysis of beam behavior in high-dose-rate flattening filter free (FFF) mode.
**Related Terms:** FFF QA, SBRT modes
**Example:** Lower out-of-field dose proven beneficial for lung SBRT.

413. **Radiotherapy Film Calibration Curve:** Optical density vs. dose characterization for film dosimeters.
**Related Terms:** Dosimetric film response, Gafchromic QA
**Example:** Curve established for 0–25 Gy before SBRT QA.

414. **Radiotherapy Film Dosimetry End-to-End Test:** Validating entire treatment process using film measurements.
**Related Terms:** Credentialing, Treatment chain QA
**Example:** Film verified spatial accuracy for trigeminal SRS.

415. **Radiotherapy Fluence Compensation Technique:** Adjusting fluence to correct for attenuation or heterogeneities.
**Related Terms:** Bolus, Compensation filters
**Example:** Fluence boosted around ribs in thoracic plan.

416. **Radiotherapy Fluence Distribution Optimization:** Fine-tuning fluence patterns for best trade-off between OAR sparing and coverage.
**Related Terms:** Inverse planning, Segment weighting
**Example:** Parotid dose reduced during IMRT fluence shaping.

**417. Radiotherapy Fluence Map Smoothing:** Reducing fluence complexity to improve deliverability.
**Related Terms:** MU efficiency, Plan complexity score
**Example:** Smoothing reduced MLC modulation in H&N plan.

**418. Radiotherapy Fluence Modulation Pattern Check:** Ensuring modulation remains within machine deliverability limits.
**Related Terms:** MLC leakage, Small segment QA
**Example:** Optimizer restricted small segments in prostate plan.

**419. Radiotherapy FOV (Field of View) Dose Error Detection:** Detection of dose inaccuracies due to cropped anatomy in CT.
**Related Terms:** Artifact alert, TPS safety
**Example:** Lower limbs missing in CT → flagged before planning.

**420. Radiotherapy Fraction Delivery Check:** Verify each fraction adheres to plan parameters.
**Related Terms:** Fractional QA, Treatment log review
**Example:** Couch shift deviation corrected before beam-on.

**421. Radiotherapy Fraction Dose Summation Accuracy:** Ensuring cumulative dose matches expected biological dose.
**Related Terms:** BED summation, ART consistency
**Example:** Summed dose for off-line adapted plan validated.

**422. Radiotherapy Fraction Pattern Scheduling:** Assigning specific fraction timing/spacing for optimal tumor control.
**Related Terms:** Hyperfractionation, Weekend gap
**Example:** Twice-daily H&N fractions used to reduce proliferation.

**423. Radiotherapy Fraction Verification Record Review:** Formal documentation check for each fraction delivery.
**Related Terms:** Chart check, Weekly QA
**Example:** Weekly physicist review caught IGRT mismatch.

**424. Radiotherapy Frame Stability Test (SRS):** Ensuring stereotactic head frame does not shift during treatment.
**Related Terms:** Immobilization QA
**Example:** Verified $<1$ mm shift during 40-minute SRS.

**425. Radiotherapy Gating Efficiency Measurement:** Percentage of beam-on time vs. treatment time in respiratory gating.
**Related Terms:** Duty cycle, Motion management metric
**Example:** Efficiency improved after shrinking gating window.

**426. Radiotherapy Gating Latency Tracking:** Measuring delay between motion signal activation and beam response.
**Related Terms:** Surrogate timing, Synchronization
**Example:** Latency corrected to avoid dose shifts in liver case.

**427. Radiotherapy Gating Window Optimization:** Selecting optimal threshold range for minimal motion error and treatment time.
**Related Terms:** Phase gating, Amplitude gating
**Example:** Adjusted to cover end-expiration phase only.

**428. Radiotherapy Gradient Index Calculation:** Ratio metric describing how rapidly dose reduces outside PTV, especially in SRS.
**Related Terms:** R50%, Conformity metrics
**Example:** GI improved after adjusting arc geometry.

**429. Radiotherapy Grid-Based Bolus Customization:** Designing bolus using 3D-printed grid structures to modulate dose.
**Related Terms:** 3D bolus, Skin dose modulation
**Example:** Custom bolus used for nasal skin tumor.

**430. Radiotherapy Hazard Identification:** Recognizing risks before clinical implementation.
**Related Terms:** FMEA, Safety culture
**Example:** Hazard flagged for couch drift with long treatments.

**431. Radiotherapy IGRT Accuracy Benchmarking:** Evaluating imaging precision against gold-standard references.
**Related Terms:** Registration QA, Imaging isocenter
**Example:** Verified <1 mm CBCT registration accuracy.

**432. Radiotherapy IGRT Dose Tracking:** Monitoring cumulative imaging dose delivered to patient.
**Related Terms:** Imaging ALARA, Diagnostic dose
**Example:** Switched to weekly CBCT to reduce cumulative exposure.

**433. Radiotherapy In-Vivo Point Dosimetry:** Measuring dose inside patient during treatment with detectors.
**Related Terms:** TLD, MOSFET, OSL
**Example:** MOSFET checked exit dose for breast patient.

**434. Radiotherapy Incident Review Meeting:** Multidisciplinary discussion of safety-related events.
**Related Terms:** M&M safety rounds, Learning culture
**Example:** Meeting addressed repeated timeout failures.

**435. Radiotherapy Independent Dose Calculation:** Second physics calculation to confirm TPS results.
**Related Terms:** Secondary check, MU verification
**Example:** Monte Carlo cross-check confirmed VMAT output.

**436. Radiotherapy Infection Control Protocol:** Prevent cross-contamination in radiation oncology departments.
**Related Terms:** PPE, Equipment sanitization
**Example:** Mask cleaning procedures strengthened during pandemics.

**437. Radiotherapy Input Data Validation:** Ensuring imaging, contours, and parameters are correct before planning.
**Related Terms:** Contour QC, Data verification
**Example:** Wrong laterality structure corrected before optimization.

**438. Radiotherapy Interlock Functionality Test:** Testing safety systems that prevent incorrect delivery conditions.
**Related Terms:** Beam inhibits, Collision alarms
**Example:** Gantry–couch collision interlock validated monthly.

**439. Radiotherapy Intra-Fraction Motion Recording:** Tracking patient movement during beam-on period.
**Related Terms:** Surface tracking, Gating logs
**Example:** 4 mm prostate drift → mid-fraction re-alignment.

440. **Radiotherapy Ion Chamber Leakage Test:** Measuring chamber current in absence of radiation to check integrity.
**Related Terms:** Electrometer stability, Pre-irradiation
**Example:** Leakage increased → chamber replaced.

441. **Radiotherapy Ion Recombination Correction:** Correcting chamber readings for incomplete ion collection.
**Related Terms:** Two-voltage method, Saturation correction
**Example:** Correction applied for high-dose-rate FFF beam.

442. **Radiotherapy Isocenter Congruence Check:** Confirming mechanical, imaging, and radiation isocenters coincide.
**Related Terms:** Winston-Lutz, SRS QA
**Example:** Verified sub-mm accuracy for trigeminal case.

443. **Radiotherapy Isocenter Shift Error Alert:** Warning system when applied couch shift deviates from planned shift.
**Related Terms:** IGRT safety, Interlock alarms
**Example:** Prevented wrong-direction correction before exposure.

444. **Radiotherapy Jaw Tracking Optimization:** Dynamic jaw movements used to reduce leakage and MLC transmission.
**Related Terms:** Small-field QA, Leakage control
**Example:** Improved lung OAR dose during VMAT.

445. **Radiotherapy Junction Dose Feasibility Check:** Checking compatibility of adjacent fields/volumes before planning.
**Related Terms:** Field junctions, Matchline QA
**Example:** Craniospinal junction validated for smooth dose.

446. **Radiotherapy Kinetic Modeling of Tumor Shrinkage:** Predicting tumor regression during treatment for adaptive planning.
**Related Terms:** ART triggers, Response modelling
**Example:** ART planned at week-3 of H&N RT.

447. **Radiotherapy Knowledge-Based Auto-Planning:** Optimization driven by learning from prior high-quality clinical plans.
**Related Terms:** Model-based planning, Machine learning
**Example:** Auto-planning saved time and improved parotid sparing.

448. **Radiotherapy Lateral Penumbra Assessment:** Evaluating beam edge sharpness in small or stereotactic fields.
**Related Terms:** Beam edge, Spatial resolution
**Example:** Mini-MLC used to tighten penumbra for brain metastasis radiosurgery.

449. **Radiotherapy Leaf Speed Constraint:** Limitation on MLC leaf velocity during delivery.
**Related Terms:** MLC control, Modulation limits
**Example:** Speed adjusted to ensure dosimetric fidelity at high dose rate.

450. **Radiotherapy Log File Dose Alert:** Real-time warning if delivered dose deviates from intended plan.
**Related Terms:** Delivery QA, Predictive safety
**Example:** Alert prevented continuation after motor malfunction.

451. **Radiotherapy Machine State Validation:** Ensuring LINAC subsystem states (gantry, couch, jaws, MLC) match the treatment plan before beam delivery.
**Related Terms:** Pre-beam verification, Interlock safety
**Example:** Beam inhibit activates when gantry angle differs from SBRT prescription.

452. **Radiotherapy Magnetron Performance Monitoring:** Tracking magnetron output stability for microwave generation.
**Related Terms:** RF power, Dose rate consistency
**Example:** Magnetron aging detected from dose-rate fluctuation in 6 MV beam.

453. **Radiotherapy Main Dose Contribution Region Assessment:** Identifying the high-dose core contributing most to target control.
**Related Terms:** Hotspot evaluation, Dose fall-off metrics
**Example:** Optimizer increased fluence only in tumoral high-control zone.

454. **Radiotherapy Manual Plan Override Logging:** Recording every instance where the therapist manually overrides standard treatment parameters.
**Related Terms:** Safety traceability, Adaptive decision justification
**Example:** Override of couch lock documented for patient with scoliosis.

455. **Radiotherapy Margin Expansion Validation:** Confirming CTV → PTV margin values are supported by motion and setup data.
**Related Terms:** GTV, PTV, Internal margin
**Example:** Kidney PTV margin reduced after 4DCT motion review.

456. **Radiotherapy MLC Calibration Drift Check:** Identifying gradual deviations in leaf positions over time.
**Related Terms:** Leaf speed tests, Positional tolerance tracking
**Example:** Calibration reset after 0.8 mm deviation detected.

457. **Radiotherapy MLC Leakage Evaluation:** Quantifying undesired transmission through MLC leaves.
**Related Terms:** Transmission factor, Shielding quality
**Example:** SBRT plan updated to reduce dose behind narrow MLC openings.

458. **Radiotherapy MLC Position Log Review:** Comparing planned vs. delivered leaf positions using machine logs.
**Related Terms:** Log-based patient-specific QA, Delivery fidelity
**Example:** Deviations in 2 small segments flagged in H&N plan.

459. **Radiotherapy Monitor Unit Drift Detection:** Identifying gradual change in MU output per dose calibration.
**Related Terms:** Output constancy, Calibration factor
**Example:** Daily QA showed MU drift → new beam calibration performed.

460. **Radiotherapy Motion Artifact Suppression:** Minimizing motion-induced blurring during imaging/IGRT.
**Related Terms:** Gating, Breath-hold, 4DCT
**Example:** Abdominal tumor imaging improved using DIBH.

461. **Radiotherapy Motion Envelope Determination:** Defining maximum boundaries of tumor movement during respiration.
**Related Terms:** ITV construction, Respiratory motion
**Example:** ITV drawn from extreme inhale/exhale 4DCT phases.

**462. Radiotherapy Motion Tracking System Calibration:** Ensuring accuracy of optical/markerless/marker-based motion detection.
**Related Terms:** SGRT, Gating calibration
**Example:** Facial tracking re-aligned before frameless SRS.

**463. Radiotherapy Multi-Modality Fusion Accuracy:** Measuring voxel-to-voxel precision of CT–MR–PET registration.
**Related Terms:** IGRT registration QA, Rigid & deformable fusion
**Example:** Pelvic PET contours shifted 2 mm after fusion bias detected.

**464. Radiotherapy Multi-Target Dose Balancing:** Simultaneous priority management across different PTVs.
**Related Terms:** SIB, Dose weighting
**Example:** Dominant metastasis prescribed 54 Gy while others received 35 Gy.

**465. Radiotherapy MU Efficiency Score:** Measure of MU use efficiency relative to PTV volume and plan complexity.
**Related Terms:** Plan complexity index, Segment count
**Example:** Excessive MU in VMAT plan reduced via fluence smoothing.

**466. Radiotherapy MU Second-Check Algorithm:** Independent calculation verifying planned MUs prior to treatment.
**Related Terms:** Secondary dose calculation, TPS cross-check
**Example:** Independent MU software confirmed 1% agreement for IMRT.

**467. Radiotherapy Neutron Dose Estimation:** Calculation of secondary neutron exposure from high-energy photon beams.
**Related Terms:** 15–18 MV beams, Shielding evaluation
**Example:** Pediatric case switched to 6 MV to avoid neutron contribution.

**468. Radiotherapy Nodal Expansion Mapping:** Predicting risk-based lymph node coverage patterns.
**Related Terms:** Elective nodal irradiation, Lymphatic pathways
**Example:** H&N nodal mapping drove level II–V coverage.

**469. Radiotherapy Non-Coplanar Arc Collision Check:** Validating arc paths to avoid gantry–couch–patient collisions.
**Related Terms:** Collision clearance QA, SRS path planning
**Example:** Couch kicked during arc 4 to avoid shoulder clearance issues.

**470. Radiotherapy Normal Tissue Dose Limit Validation:** Verifying all OAR dose constraints comply with protocols.
**Related Terms:** QUANTEC, Dose tolerance tables
**Example:** Kidney V16 revised to meet renal PT limit.

**471. Radiotherapy Normal Tissue Sparing Index:** Score assessing protective efficiency for organs at risk.
**Related Terms:** NTCP models, Conformity index
**Example:** Higher NTSI achieved after beam-weight re-optimization.

**472. Radiotherapy Nuclear Data Cross-Section Analysis:** Evaluation of particle interaction probabilities for dose modeling.
**Related Terms:** Monte Carlo, Scatter kernels
**Example:** Monte Carlo library updated for bone in proton therapy.

**473. Radiotherapy Nuclear Imaging Protocol QA:** Ensuring nuclear imaging used for RT planning is accurate and reproducible.
**Related Terms:** PET-CT calibration, SPECT uptake uniformity
**Example:** PET SUV scaling verified for liver metastasis planning.

**474. Radiotherapy Nucleic Acid Response Biomarker Tracking:** Monitoring tumor biological response using DNA/RNA markers.
**Related Terms:** Radiosensitivity biomarkers, Adaptive radiotherapy
**Example:** Biomarker decline suggested reduced ART dose.

**475. Radiotherapy Null-Point Beam Symmetry Check:** Symmetry verification at central axis null point.
**Related Terms:** Cross-plane symmetry, Beam QA
**Example:** Beam steering tuned after symmetry deviation seen.

**476. Radiotherapy Nutritional Support Integration:** Nutrition management to improve treatment tolerance and outcomes.
**Related Terms:** Supportive oncology, Cachexia prevention
**Example:** Diet plan reduced weight loss during H&N RT.

**477. Radiotherapy Occupancy Monitoring for Shielding Safety:** Measuring personnel presence in controlled zones during treatment.
**Related Terms:** Controlled area, Radiation exposure monitoring
**Example:** Room access lock prevented therapist entry during beam.

**478. Radiotherapy Off-Axis Ratio Verification:** Ensuring dose fall-off off-axis meets beam specifications.
**Related Terms:** OAR (dosimetry), Beam profile QA
**Example:** Off-axis ratio adjusted for oblique IMRT entry.

**479. Radiotherapy Off-Line Image Review Protocol:** Periodic image review with corrections applied prospectively.
**Related Terms:** Offline correction, Weekly IGRT
**Example:** Averaged daily shift → permanent isocenter update.

**480. Radiotherapy On-Board Imaging Dose Calibration:** Calibrating OBI imaging dose to minimize radiation exposure.
**Related Terms:** kV/mV imaging dose, Low-dose CBCT
**Example:** Pediatric setting switched to low-dose thorax protocol.

**481. Radiotherapy On-Treatment Plan Adaptation:** Modifying treatment plan based on anatomy changes during therapy.
**Related Terms:** ART, Daily replanning
**Example:** PTV grown where edema enlarged during week-3.

**482. Radiotherapy Output Factor Optimization:** Minimizing dosimetric errors from small or irregular field output.
**Related Terms:** OF tables, Small-field dosimetry
**Example:** Output adjusted for stereotactic 0.5 × 0.5 cm field.

**483. Radiotherapy Oxygen Enhancement Ratio Application:** Accounting for radiosensitizing effect of oxygen in biological dose modeling.
**Related Terms:** Hypoxia correction, LET integration
**Example:** Higher dose given to hypoxic bladder tumor region.

484. **Radiotherapy Pacemaker Dose-Safety Modeling:** Predicting EM and radiation effect risk for implanted pacemakers.
**Related Terms:** Dose constraints, EMI mitigation
**Example:** Programming arranged after dose risk flagged.

485. **Radiotherapy Particle Beam Monitoring System Check:** Verifying proton/carbon monitoring chambers and sensors.
**Related Terms:** Ionization monitor QA, Spot position checks
**Example:** Spot misplacement detected and corrected pre-treatment.

486. **Radiotherapy Patient-Door Interlock Detection:** Lockout that halts irradiation when entry door is unlocked.
**Related Terms:** Access control, Safety system
**Example:** Beam stopped due to accidental door handle touch.

487. **Radiotherapy Patient Education Compliance Tracking:** Monitoring adherence to preparation instructions.
**Related Terms:** Full bladder prep, Diet compliance
**Example:** Bowel filling inconsistency corrected with teaching.

488. **Radiotherapy Patient Identification Autovalidation:** Digital multi-factor confirmation before treatment.
**Related Terms:** Barcode ID, Biometric verification
**Example:** Fingerprint+barcode mismatch prevented wrong-patient event.

489. **Radiotherapy Patient-Specific Density Override Review:** Rechecking all manual density assignments in planning CT.
**Related Terms:** Prosthetic overrides, Metal artifact correction
**Example:** Hip prosthesis override updated to cobalt-chrome value.

490. **Radiotherapy Patient-Specific QA Endorsement:** Medical physicist approval confirming delivery safety after QA review.
**Related Terms:** Final QA sign-off, Approver responsibility
**Example:** Endorsement granted following 2% gamma pass.

491. **Radiotherapy PDD (Percent Depth Dose) Curve QA:** Verifying beam depth-dose characteristics match commissioning reference.
**Related Terms:** Beam quality, dmax, PDD10
**Example:** FFF beam adjusted after PDD 10% deviation.

492. **Radiotherapy Peer-Review Planning Safety Meeting:** Expert group review of contours and plans before treatment.
**Related Terms:** Contour peer review, Weekly case rounds
**Example:** Resection cavity contour modified after peer input.

493. **Radiotherapy Performance Qualification (PQ):** Demonstrating equipment performs as required under clinical conditions.
**Related Terms:** IQ, OQ, Commissioning
**Example:** PQ verified for SGRT before routine use.

494. **Radiotherapy Phantom-Based Dose Credentialing:** External validation of planning and delivery accuracy using standardized phantoms.
**Related Terms:** IROC credentialing, End-to-end audits
**Example:** Clinic passed SRS lung phantom credentialing to join clinical trial.

495. **Radiotherapy Post-Treatment Image Matching QA:** Reviewing IGRT images after delivery to confirm alignment accuracy.
**Related Terms:** Retrospective QA, Shift comparison
**Example:** Post-review detected increasing rotational error trend.

496. **Radiotherapy Predictive Maintenance Scheduling:** Using machine telemetry to prevent component failure.
**Related Terms:** Reliability monitoring, Failure prevention
**Example:** MLC motor serviced pre-emptively before planned downtime.

497. **Radiotherapy Prescription Consistency Audit:** Confirming prescriptions match dose, fractionation, and technique throughout workflow.
**Related Terms:** Plan prescription matching, Medical record QA
**Example:** Fraction count mismatch corrected before first fraction.

498. **Radiotherapy QA Action Threshold Protocol:** Rules specifying acceptable tolerance levels and required actions if exceeded.
**Related Terms:** Tolerance table, Alert levels
**Example:** Gamma < 95% triggered re-planning.

499. **Radiotherapy QA Escalation Policy:** Safety policy defining levels of notification for deviations in treatment or QA.
**Related Terms:** Incident escalation, Safety chain of command
**Example:** Level-3 escalation triggered after repeated IGRT mismatches.

500. **Radiotherapy Quality Index Score:** Composite metric quantifying safety and performance of an RT department.
**Related Terms:** KPI, Benchmarking
**Example:** Score improved after adopting daily auto-matching and log-file QA.

# S

1. **Stereotactic Localization:** Determining the exact 3D coordinates of the target before high-precision irradiation.
   **Related Terms:** Frame-based alignment, IGRT, CBCT fusion
   **Radiotherapy Example:** CBCT localization used to position brain metastasis before 20 Gy SRS.
2. **Stochastic Radiation Effects:** Radiation-induced biological effects whose probability increases with dose without a clear threshold.
   **Related Terms:** Cancer risk, Genetic mutation, Low-dose exposure
   **Radiotherapy Example:** Secondary cancer risk discussion for young patients receiving pelvic RT.
3. **Structured Report (Radiotherapy):** Standardized treatment documentation to ensure consistency and safety.
   **Related Terms:** Treatment summary, Plan documentation, QA reporting
   **Radiotherapy Example:** SBRT report includes PTV dose coverage, OAR constraints, and imaging shifts.
4. **Subclinical Disease Dose:** Radiation dose aimed at destroying microscopic or undetectable tumor cells.
   **Related Terms:** Elective nodal dose, Microscopic spread, CTV margin
   **Radiotherapy Example:** 45 Gy prophylactically delivered to cervical nodal levels in H&N RT.
5. **Subgrid Dose Resolution:** Calculating dose on a finer resolution than the displayed grid to improve accuracy.
   **Related Terms:** Dose sampling, TPS interpolation, Monte Carlo
   **Radiotherapy Example:** Increased subgrid sampling used for high-gradient liver SBRT.
6. **Superficial Radiotherapy:** Kilovoltage X-ray treatment targeting shallow lesions (0–5 mm depth).
   **Related Terms:** kV therapy, Skin cancers, Buildup
   **Radiotherapy Example:** 60 kV beam used for basal cell carcinoma of the nose.
7. **Surface Dose Measurement:** Measurement of the radiation absorbed dose at the skin surface.
   **Related Terms:** OSLD, TLD, Bolus
   **Radiotherapy Example:** TLDs placed on chest wall to verify bolus-enhanced surface dose.
8. **Surface Guided Radiotherapy (SGRT):** Real-time monitoring of patient position using optical surface imaging.
   **Related Terms:** DIBH, Frameless SRS, Motion tracking
   **Radiotherapy Example:** SGRT used to monitor breast patient during DIBH breathing.
9. **Surface Rendering (Imaging):** 3D reconstruction of anatomical surfaces from imaging for planning or positioning.
   **Related Terms:** STL model, 3D contour, Patient surrogate
   **Radiotherapy Example:** Surface rendering exported for custom cranial mold creation.
10. **Surgical Bed Boost:** Targeted boost dose delivered to the post-surgical cavity at high recurrence risk.
    **Related Terms:** Cavity boost, Tumor bed, Sequential boost
    **Radiotherapy Example:** 10–16 Gy boost delivered to breast lumpectomy cavity after whole breast RT.

11. **Systematic Error:** Reproducible positioning or delivery error that occurs consistently across fractions.
**Related Terms:** Random error, Van Herk formula, PTV margin calculation
**Radiotherapy Example:** Daily 3 mm left shift detected and corrected in pelvic IMRT.

12. **Systemic Radionuclide Therapy:** Use of radiopharmaceuticals circulating through the bloodstream to treat cancer.
**Related Terms:** Lu-177, I-131, Targeted radiotherapy
**Radiotherapy Example:** Lu-177 DOTATATE used for metastatic neuroendocrine tumors.

13. **Scatter Correction Algorithm:** Software method to compensate for degraded image contrast caused by scatter.
**Related Terms:** Beam hardening correction, CBCT artifact reduction
**Radiotherapy Example:** Scatter-reduction algorithm improves CBCT for pancreas SBRT alignment.

14. **Secondary Cancer Risk Modeling:** Predictive modeling estimating likelihood of radiation-induced cancer.
**Related Terms:** Stochastic effects, Risk projection, Pediatric radiotherapy
**Radiotherapy Example:** Proton therapy chosen over IMRT to reduce second malignancy risk.

15. **Secondary Particles (Radiation):** Particles indirectly generated due to primary radiation interactions with matter.
**Related Terms:** Neutrons, Bremsstrahlung, Scatter
**Radiotherapy Example:** Neutron dose monitored during 15–18 MV IMRT beams.

16. **Secondary Shielding Barrier:** Barrier protecting against scatter and leakage rather than direct beam exposure.
**Related Terms:** Maze shielding, Workload, TVL
**Radiotherapy Example:** Secondary wall thickness increased to reduce CBCT scatter dose.

17. **Segmental IMRT:** Step-and-shoot IMRT using multiple fixed MLC segments.
**Related Terms:** Sliding-window IMRT, VMAT, Intensity modulation
**Radiotherapy Example:** 60 static segments used in prostate IMRT plan for improved rectal sparing.

18. **Sensitization (Radiation):** Enhancement of tumor radiosensitivity by biological or physical modifiers.
**Related Terms:** Hypoxia modifier, Chemoradiation, Brachy sensitization
**Radiotherapy Example:** Cisplatin used as a radiosensitizer during H&N IMRT.

19. **Sensitivity Profile (Imaging):** Spatial pattern of detector response across its active area.
**Related Terms:** Flat field correction, Gain calibration
**Radiotherapy Example:** Detector calibration ensures uniform EPID response during VMAT QA.

20. **Sequential Boost Technique:** Boost dose delivered after primary treatment, not simultaneously.
**Related Terms:** SIB, Field-in-field, Tumor bed boost
**Radiotherapy Example:** 50 Gy whole-breast RT followed by 10 Gy sequential boost to cavity.

21. **Setup Reproducibility:** Ability to reproduce the same patient setup across all fractions.
**Related Terms:** Immobilization, IGRT, Interfraction error
**Radiotherapy Example:** Same pelvic alignment achieved for all prostate fractions within ±2 mm.

22. **Shielded Treatment Room:** Medical linac room engineered to protect workers and public from radiation.
**Related Terms:** Maze, Primary wall, Neutron shielding
**Radiotherapy Example:** Door interlocks prevent beam-on until shielding is confirmed.

23. **Short-Arc VMAT:** Partial-arc volumetric dose delivery to reduce OAR irradiation.
**Related Terms:** Restricted arc, Avoidance sectors
**Radiotherapy Example:** 200° partial arc used to reduce dose to contralateral breast.

24. **Simultaneous Integrated Boost (SIB):** Different dose levels delivered to PTV and boost region within the same fraction.
**Related Terms:** Dose painting, VMAT, Multilevel fractionation
**Radiotherapy Example:** 70 Gy to tumor + 56 Gy to elective nodes in 33 fractions.

25. **Simulation Film:** Verification image taken during simulation for geometric documentation.
**Related Terms:** DRR, Portal image, Localization image
**Radiotherapy Example:** Pelvic simulation film saved for later comparison with portal imaging.

26. **Skin Sparing Loss:** Increase in surface dose that negates MV beam sparing.
**Related Terms:** Bolus, Low-energy scatter, Oblique incidence
**Radiotherapy Example:** Oblique VMAT entry increases skin dose for chest wall; bolus adjusted.

27. **Soft-Tissue Registration:** Image alignment based on soft-tissue structures rather than bones or markers.
**Related Terms:** CBCT match, MR match, Adaptive RT
**Radiotherapy Example:** Prostate IGRT aligned to soft-tissue instead of pelvic bones.

28. **Source Strength (Brachytherapy):** Activity or dose rate produced by a brachytherapy radioactive source.
**Related Terms:** Air-kerma strength, HDR source, TG-43
**Radiotherapy Example:** Ir-192 source strength decay accounted for in HDR planning.

29. **Spatial Integrity (MRI):** Accuracy of geometric distances on MR images.
**Related Terms:** Geometric distortion, Gradient non-linearity
**Radiotherapy Example:** MR spatial integrity QA performed before MR-only prostate RT.

30. **Spinal Canal Contouring:** Segmentation of spinal canal to ensure safe radiation limits.
**Related Terms:** Spinal cord PRV, Myelopathy risk, Dmax
**Radiotherapy Example:** Spine SBRT plan adjusted to limit spinal canal dose to 14 Gy in 1 fraction.

31. **Spatial Dose Gradient Control:** Regulation of steepness of dose fall-off around the PTV to protect nearby OARs.
**Related Terms:** Dose hotspot control, Fall-off index
**Example:** Spine SBRT gradient optimized to protect spinal cord (< 10 Gy).

32. **Spatial Dose Warping:** Comparing delivered and planned doses by deforming dose maps to anatomical change.
**Related Terms:** Deformable dose accumulation, Adaptive RT
**Example:** Deformed dose map showed parotid overdose during week-4 H&N RT.

33. **Spatial Integrity QA (MRI-RT):** Confirmation that MRI geometric dimensions are accurate for RT planning.
**Related Terms:** Distortion mapping, MR-sim QA
**Example:** Spatial error < 1 mm validated for MR-only prostate planning.

34. **Split-Beam Technique:** Beam split into two separate fields to avoid irradiation of critical structures.
**Related Terms:** Beam blocking, Organ avoidance
**Example:** Split field avoided lens during orbital lymphoma RT.

35. **Spot Size Calibration (Proton Therapy):** Tuning proton beam spot width to match TPS model for dose accuracy.
**Related Terms:** Pencil beam scanning, Energy layer QA
**Example:** Measured spot size corrected for 140 MeV beam before neuro proton SRS.

36. **Spot-Scanning Delivery Verification:** QA confirming each proton spot location and dose.
**Related Terms:** Log-file QA, Layer-by-layer QA
**Example:** Proton QA flagged 2 mm lateral deviation in posterior spots.

37. **SRS Cone Output Calibration:** Output calibration for small fixed circular cones used in SRS.
**Related Terms:** Output factor, SRS dosimetry
**Example:** 7.5-mm cone output measured with micro-diamond detector.

38. **SRS Frame Immobilization:** Stereotactic head fixation frame to eliminate motion during cranial SRS.
**Related Terms:** Invasive frame, Frameless SGRT
**Example:** Leksell frame used to treat AVM with 22 Gy single fraction.

39. **SRS/FSRT End-to-End QA:** Full chain QA from imaging to dose delivery for stereotactic workflows.
**Related Terms:** Winston–Lutz, SGRT, Couch walkout
**Example:** End-to-end test validated sub-mm precision for trigeminal neuralgia RT.

40. **Static Couch Correction:** Couch correction applied before beam-on without continuous tracking.
**Related Terms:** Pre-treatment shift, IGRT correction
**Example:** Prostate couch shifts applied based on CBCT before IMRT.

41. **Static Field IMRT:** Fixed gantry intensity-modulated beams rather than arc delivery.
**Related Terms:** Step-and-shoot, Sliding window
**Example:** 9-field IMRT used for gynecological RT to improve bowel sparing.

42. **Steep Dose Fall-Off Optimization:** TPS optimization to tighten gradient away from PTV.
**Related Terms:** High-gradient SBRT, OAR sparing
**Example:** Achieved 80% isodose drop within 8 mm around kidney tumor.

43. **Stereo-Localization Phantom:** Phantom for verifying stereotactic positioning accuracy.
**Related Terms:** Winston–Lutz phantom, SRS QA
**Example:** Phantom alignment accuracy validated for brain metastasis SRS.

44. **Step-and-Shoot IMRT:** Segmented static field IMRT with beam on only when MLC is stationary.
**Related Terms:** Segmental IMRT, VMAT comparison
**Example:** Step-and-shoot plan reduced rectal Dmax in prostate IMRT.

45. **Stop-Band Filter (Imaging):** Algorithm to remove periodic noise frequencies in radiologic images.
**Related Terms:** Artifact suppression, Frequency filtering
**Example:** Filter removed ripple artifacts from CBCT for pancreas SBRT.

46. **Stopping-Power Ratio (SPR):** Ratio that determines proton range through patient tissue.
**Related Terms:** HU-to-SPR conversion, Range uncertainty
**Example:** Incorrect SPR predicted 3-mm overshoot toward spinal cord.

47. **Stray Radiation Dose:** Patient dose received from leakage, scatter, or secondary particles.
**Related Terms:** Neutron dose, Out-of-field dose
**Example:** Pediatric proton plan selected to reduce stray neutron dose.

48. **Strength Check (HDR Source):** Verification of the activity of a brachytherapy source.
**Related Terms:** Air-kerma strength, Source calibration
**Example:** Ir-192 strength deviation triggered emergency backup source request.

49. **Structure-Adapted Dose Painting:** Escalating dose within sub-volumes of the tumor based on imaging biomarkers.
**Related Terms:** Radiomics, Functional boost
**Example:** FDG-avid region boosted to 72 Gy within lung PTV.

50. **Structure Migration Tracking:** Monitoring anatomical shifts during treatment due to physiological changes.
**Related Terms:** Adaptive RT, Organ motion
**Example:** Parotid migration triggered adaptive replan in week 3.

51. **Sub-Millimeter Delivery Accuracy:** Radiation delivery precision better than 1 mm.
**Related Terms:** SRS QA, Couch walkout, Imaging fusion
**Example:** Brainstem SRS validated to 0.5 mm isocenter accuracy.

52. **Sub-Voxel MR Distortion Mapping:** Detecting MRI distortions smaller than voxel resolution.
**Related Terms:** MR-RT, Deformation QA
**Example:** Gradient nonlinearity corrected to ensure cranial target accuracy.

53. **Support Arm Collision QA:** Validation that gantry/couch/accessories will not collide during planned RT.
**Related Terms:** Clearance simulation, Couch rotation
**Example:** New VMAT arc edited to avoid gantry-breast board collision.

54. **Surface Bolus Conformity Index:** Metric evaluating how tightly bolus conforms to skin without air gaps.
**Related Terms:** Surface dose, 3D-printed bolus
**Example:** 3D-printed bolus improved chest-wall dose by eliminating air pockets.

55. **Surface Image Acquisition Latency:** Delay between surface scan capture and system update.
**Related Terms:** SGRT lag, Motion tracking
**Example:** Breast DIBH stopped when latency exceeded gating tolerance.

56. **Surface Motion Trigger:** Automatic beam interrupt when body movement exceeds tolerance.
**Related Terms:** Gating threshold, SGRT monitoring
**Example:** Beam paused when abdomen motion exceeded 2 mm during liver SBRT.

57. **Surface-Region Matching Algorithm:** Aligns selected regions of the patient surface instead of full-surface matching.
**Related Terms:** ROI-based SGRT, Partial alignment
**Example:** Chest region used for DIBH match while arms excluded.

58. **Surrogate Tracking (Internal Motion):** Tracking external or internal markers that represent organ motion.
**Related Terms:** Fiducials, RPM, Abdominal belts
**Example:** Diaphragm surrogate motion used to gate lung VMAT.

59. **Survival Curve Modeling:** Mathematical model predicting tissue survival proportion after radiation.
**Related Terms:** $\alpha/\beta$ ratio, LQ model
**Example:** $\alpha/\beta$ modeling used to convert SBRT dose to EQD2 for spinal cord constraints.

60. **S-Value (Internal Dosimetry):** Absorbed dose per nuclear transition in a source-target organ pair.
**Related Terms:** RADAR formalism, MIRD schema
**Example:** S-value used to compute kidney dose in Lu-177 therapy.

61. **System Response Matrix (Reconstruction):** Matrix describing detector measurement physics used for SPECT/PET reconstruction.
**Related Terms:** Iterative reconstruction, OSEM
**Example:** Improved tumor contrast in PET-CT using modified system matrix.

62. **Safety Interlock Override Prevention:** Measures preventing staff from bypassing safety systems.
**Related Terms:** Key interlock, Door interlock
**Example:** Automatic shutdown triggered when override attempt detected.

63. **Secondary Neutron Shielding Design:** Shielding built to minimize neutron contamination from high-energy beams.
**Related Terms:** 18 MV beams, Concrete boron lining
**Example:** Neutron shielding added for new 18 MV room upgrade.

64. **Sector-Based Gantry Avoidance:** Arc restriction that prevents irradiation through specific anatomical sectors.
**Related Terms:** Avoidance sectors, Partial arc
**Example:** Liver SBRT avoided anterior arc to spare stomach.

65. **Selective OAR Prioritization Mode:** TPS mode that dynamically changes OAR weighting based on overlap severity.**Related Terms:** MCO, Gradient management
**Example:** Rectal constraint prioritized during prostate IMRT trade-offs.

66. **Sensitivity Function (Dose Influence):** Quantifies how dose changes based on beamlet modulation.
**Related Terms:** Gradient descent optimization, Dose kernel
**Example:** Used to optimize cold spot inside PTV without increasing bladder dose.

67. **Setup Error Probability Curve:** Probability distribution of interfraction setup shifts.
**Related Terms:** PTV margin, Random error modelling
**Example:** Curve analysis reduced H&N PTV margin from 5 mm to 3 mm.

68. **Shielding Door Delay Timer:** Delay that prevents accidental beam-on during door closing/opening cycles.
**Related Terms:** Interlock timing, Occupancy safety
**Example:** Delay prevented beam start before therapist exited room.

69. **Shockwave-Induced Detector Noise:** Noise in imaging caused by vibrations or sudden mechanical impacts.**Related Terms:** Motion artifact, Detector instability
**Example:** CBCT QA done after a magnet-quench event to check detector noise.

70. **Single-Isocenter Multi-Target SBRT:** Treating multiple metastases using one isocenter.
**Related Terms:** Couch rotation correction, SRS targeting
**Example:** Six brain metastases treated in one 22-minute single-isocenter plan.

71. **Single-Point Dose Validation:** Verifying critical point dose with an independent detector.
**Related Terms:** Point dose QA, Ion chamber
**Example:** Ion chamber placed at PTV center verified dose within 2%.

72. **Single-Shot MR Acquisition:** Fast MRI acquisition to freeze motion during RT simulation.
**Related Terms:** MR-simulation, Fast spin echo
**Example:** Single-shot sequence captured pancreas location during inspiration.

73. **Skin Dose Compensation Filter:** Algorithm that modifies fluence to adjust skin dose.
**Related Terms:** Bolus simulation, Surface optimization
**Example:** Reduced chest-wall skin dose by minus 8% using filter-based optimization.

74. **Skewed Gantry Drift:** Gantry rotation deviation that varies with angle.
**Related Terms:** Gantry calibration, Arc QA
**Example:** Drift detected between 180°–210° range triggered maintenance.

75. **Sliding-Window IMRT:** Continuous MLC motion during beam-on for fluence modulation.
**Related Terms:** Segmental IMRT, Dynamic delivery
**Example:** Sliding-window spine IMRT improved gradient near spinal canal.

76. **Small-Aperture Dosimetry:** Dosimetric calibration for small field sizes ($< 4 \times 4$ cm$^2$).
**Related Terms:** Volume averaging error, Micro-chamber
**Example:** Output factor measured using synthetic diamond detector for 1 cm field.

77. **Small-Animal Radiotherapy Research:** Use of micro-irradiators for experimental radiobiology.
**Related Terms:** Pre-clinical RT, Radiobiology
**Example:** Mouse flank tumor irradiated to validate immuno-RT trial.

78. **Soft-Tissue Couch Deformation:** Couch sag deforming anatomy when heavy patients lie on table.
**Related Terms:** Table flex model, CBCT matching
**Example:** Spine SBRT couch deformation corrected with predictive model.

79. **Software-Driven Beam Hold:** Beam shutoff triggered by TPS or log-file conditions, not hardware.
**Related Terms:** Auto-pause logic, Dose limit trigger
**Example:** Beam auto-paused when dose rate exceeded tolerance.

80. **Source-to-Axis Distance (SAD):** Distance between source and isocenter axis, fixed in isocentric RT.
**Related Terms:** Fixed SSD, Isocenter geometry
**Example:** SAD of 100 cm used for all VMAT prostate fields.

81. **Source Dwell Position Verification:** Confirmation that HDR source stops at correct programmed dwell positions inside applicators.
**Related Terms:** Dwell time, Catheter reconstruction, TG-59 QA
**Example:** Rectal applicator dwell positions corrected after QA detected 3-mm offset.

82. **Source Exchange Procedure:** Scheduled replacement of radioactive source in HDR after decay reduces treatment strength.
**Related Terms:** Source decay, Source strength calibration
**Example:** Ir-192 replaced after ~90 days to maintain accurate dwell time delivery.

83. **Source Housing Interlock:** Mechanical or electronic safety preventing accidental source exposure.
**Related Terms:** Emergency stop, Radioprotection
**Example:** HDR aborted when housing interlock detected incomplete shielding closure.

84. **Source Step Size (HDR):** Distance between dwell positions as the HDR source moves in catheter.
**Related Terms:** Dwell spacing, Reconstruction resolution
**Example:** Step size of 2.5 mm optimized for prostate interstitial brachytherapy.

85. **Spatial Integrity Distortion Map (MR-RT):** Map displaying MRI geometric distortion magnitude across FOV.
**Related Terms:** Gradient non-linearity, MR-only RT
**Example:** Distortion $< 1$ mm confirmed before MRI-based cranial SRS.

86. **Spatial Resolution Phantom:** Phantom used to assess visibility of small details in CT/MR/CBCT images.
**Related Terms:** Line-pair resolution, MTF
**Example:** CBCT resolution drop triggered recalibration for head-and-neck workflow.

87. **Sparing Priority Weighting:** TPS weight defining relative importance of an OAR in optimization.
**Related Terms:** Cost function, Constraint trade-off
**Example:** Rectum priority increased to reduce D25 Gy while maintaining PTV coverage.

88. **Specular Reflection Artifact:** Bright image artifact caused by reflective surfaces during imaging.
**Related Terms:** Surface imaging error, Optical capture distortion
**Example:** Mask reflection suppressed to stabilize SGRT tracking in SRS mask patients.

89. **Spine-Avoidance Arc Arrangement:** VMAT sector selection that minimizes beams passing through spinal cord.
**Related Terms:** Avoidance sectoring, Gradient control
**Example:** Liver SBRT used arcs with posterior avoidance to protect spinal cord.

90. **Spherical Dose Shells (Ring Structures):** Concentric rings around PTV used to control gradient and hotspots.
**Related Terms:** Ring optimization, Dose fall-off shaping
**Example:** Shells reduced hotspots in lung SBRT PTV without increasing OAR dose.

91. **Spin-Echo Fat Suppression:** MRI technique removing fat signal for improved tumor contrast.
**Related Terms:** Dixon sequence, STIR
**Example:** Fat suppression improved tumor visualization in breast boost planning.

92. **Spot Delivery Time (Proton):** Time required to deliver dose for an individual proton pencil beam spot.
**Related Terms:** Layer switching time, Time-resolved PBS
**Example:** Delivery time optimized to shorten lung SBRT from 32 to 19 minutes.

93. **Spot Energy Layer Reordering:** Sequence modification of proton layers to reduce motion interplay.
**Related Terms:** Repainting, 4D-PBS
**Example:** Reordering minimized motion effects in liver PBS with breathing motion.

94. **Spot Scanning Water Phantom QA:** Proton QA that verifies dose distribution by scanning spots in a water tank.
**Related Terms:** Beam profile, TPS validation
**Example:** QA confirmed distal fall-off accuracy for 200 MeV PBS energy layer.

95. **SRTR (Serial-Parallel Organ Response Model):** Biophysical model predicting whole-organ failure probability.
**Related Terms:** NTCP modeling, Radiobiological modelling
**Example:** Liver NTCP $< 5\%$ verified for partial liver SBRT boost.

96. **SSD (Source-to-Surface Distance) Correction Factor:** Scaling factor correcting dose for changes in SSD relative to reference.
**Related Terms:** Inverse square law, PDD correction
**Example:** SSD increased to 105 cm to limit skin dose for chest wall IMRT.

97. **Stability Index (Machine Output):** Measure of consistency of linac output over time.
**Related Terms:** Daily QA, Trend analysis
**Example:** Sudden drop in stability index indicated flattening filter issue.

98. **Standard Fractionation:** Radiotherapy protocol of 1.8–2 Gy per fraction, 5 days per week.
**Related Terms:** Conventional RT, EQD2
**Example:** 50 Gy in 25 fractions used for rectal cancer neoadjuvant RT.

99. **Streak Artifact Reduction (CT):** Algorithm minimizing streak artifacts from metal implants.
**Related Terms:** MAR, Metal artifact correction
**Example:** MAR allowed accurate contouring near spinal fixation rods.

100. **Stress-Testing of Immobilization:** Evaluating robustness of patient setup under realistic conditions.
**Related Terms:** Motion mitigation, Mask fit validation
**Example:** Head-and-neck mask stress-test prevented mid-treatment displacement.

101. **Structure Atlas Segmentation:** Auto-segmentation based on anatomical atlas from population datasets.
**Related Terms:** AI segmentation, Auto-contouring
**Example:** Atlas auto-segmentation accelerated OAR contouring for prostate IMRT.

102. **Structure Mapping Accuracy Index:** Metric measuring deviation between AI-generated and manual contours.
**Related Terms:** Dice coefficient, Hausdorff distance
**Example:** Index flagged poor parotid segmentation for manual correction.

103. **Summation Dose Calculation:** Combined absorbed dose from multiple treatment phases or modalities.
**Related Terms:** Composite plan, Dose accumulation
**Example:** EBRT + brachy dose summed to ensure bladder EQD2 < 80 Gy.

104. **Super-Sampling (Dose Grid):** Using a finer dose grid than standard resolution to improve accuracy.
**Related Terms:** Dose voxel refinement, TPS computation accuracy
**Example:** 0.5-mm grid improved hotspot detection in trigeminal SRS.

105. **Superior-Inferior Motion Tracking:** Tracking organ movement along head-to-toe axis.
**Related Terms:** Respiratory motion, Surrogate tracking
**Example:** Pancreas tracking used SI motion amplitude to control gating.

106. **Surface Dose Calibration:** Calibration of TPS surface dose against in-vivo or film data.
**Related Terms:** Skin buildup, Bolus modelling
**Example:** TPS corrected when film indicated 7% higher dose than predicted.

107. **Surface ROI Lock:** SGRT tracking restricted to a defined body area while excluding others.
**Related Terms:** Partial ROI tracking, Motion rejection
**Example:** Breast ROI locked to ignore arm movement during DIBH.

108. **Survival Fraction (SF):** Percentage of cells remaining viable after radiation exposure.
**Related Terms:** LQ model, Radiosensitivity
**Example:** Low SF values at 6 Gy supported high radiosensitivity of glioma cell line.

109. **SUTP (Small-Uncertainty Treatment Protocol):** Margin protocol designed to minimize uncertainties using IGRT + SGRT.
**Related Terms:** PTV shrink protocol, Motion mitigation
**Example:** Prostate PTV reduced from 8 mm → 4 mm under SUTP workflow.

110. **Symmetric vs Asymmetric Collimator Setting:** Whether jaws open symmetrically or offset relative to CAX.
**Related Terms:** Half-beam block, Jaw tracking
**Example:** Asymmetric jaw opening avoided heart exposure for breast tangents.

111. **Synchrotron-Based Proton Delivery:** Proton acceleration using a synchrotron allowing variable energy extraction.
**Related Terms:** Cyclotron, Beam gating
**Example:** Synchrotron gating synchronized with breathing during pancreas PBS.

112. **Synchronized Beam-Gated Delivery:** Beam activated only during selected phases of respiration or motion cycles.
**Related Terms:** DIBH, 4D-RT
**Example:** Liver SBRT delivered only during end-expiration for accuracy.

113. **Synchronization Latency Compensation:** System correction for delay between motion detection and beam gating.
**Related Terms:** Prediction algorithm, Motion control
**Example:** Predictive gating stabilized dose to moving lung tumor.

**114. Synthetic CT for MR-Only RT:** Electron-density CT derived from MRI for dose calculation.
**Related Terms:** MR-simulation, HU mapping
**Example:** Synthetic CT enabled CT-free prostate workflow.

**115. System Drift Alarm:** Automatic alert when cumulative small deviations indicate failure risk.
**Related Terms:** Predictive machine maintenance, Output trending
**Example:** Alarm triggered after gradual increase in MU/deg error during VMAT.

**116. System Latency Audit:** Testing time delay through imaging → tracking → beam control pipeline.
**Related Terms:** Gating delay, SGRT timing
**Example:** Latency audit validated 180 ms response time for pediatric DIBH.

**117. Systematic Error (Σ):** Reproducible positioning deviation affecting all fractions similarly.
**Related Terms:** Random error (σ), PTV margin model
**Example:** Systematic 3-mm anterior shift corrected by updated immobilization.

**118. Synchronized Couch Transition:** Couch translation coordinated with gantry motion to avoid collisions.
**Related Terms:** Coordinated trajectory planning, Robotic couch
**Example:** R800 couch protected from gantry collision during noncoplanar SRS arc.

**119. Synchronous Dose Delivery Verification:** Real-time confirmation that planned and delivered dose are synchronized.
**Related Terms:** Log-file QA, Real-time dosimetry
**Example:** Gamma > 95% confirmed for online dose delivery in head IMRT.

**120. Soft-Tissue Visualization Enhancement:** Algorithm improving soft-tissue contrast in kV/MV imaging.
**Related Terms:** Scatter correction, Contrast boosting
**Example:** Contrast enhancement improved pancreas IGRT match quality.

**121. Spatial Dose Uncertainty Propagation:** Modelling how uncertainties affect 3D dose distribution.
**Related Terms:** Robust optimization, Motion risk modelling
**Example:** Robust plan chosen to withstand 6-mm breathing motion uncertainty.

**122. Surface Electron Contamination Analysis:** Calculation of secondary electron dose buildup from linac components.
**Related Terms:** Skin toxicity, Bolus
**Example:** Bolus removed after contamination analysis predicted excessive skin dose.

**123. Signal-to-Noise Ratio (SNR) in RT Imaging:** Ratio comparing useful image signal with noise level.
**Related Terms:** Low-contrast detectability, Image uniformity
**Example:** CBCT SNR improvement increased confidence in pancreas IGRT alignment.

**124. Sensitivity Gastro-Motion Index:** Metric evaluating stomach/colon filling variability affecting dose.
**Related Terms:** Interfraction motion, GI variability
**Example:** Index predicted high OAR risk → adaptive RT selected for pancreatic cancer.

**125. Static MLC Gap Width Tolerance:** Maximum allowed difference between planned and actual MLC gap width.
**Related Terms:** IMRT delivery, MLCTG-50 QA
**Example:** 1-mm gap error triggered beam stop during SBRT QA.

**126. Superficial Dose Shield:** Physical shield that protects skin while preserving dose to deeper target.
**Related Terms:** Skin sparing, Shadow tray
**Example:** Custom shield protected lip skin during nasopharynx IMRT.

**127. SPECT-Based Tumor Dosimetry:** Quantification of absorbed dose using post-therapy SPECT imaging.
**Related Terms:** Radiopharmaceutical dosimetry, Serial SPECT scans
**Example:** Y-90 liver dosimetry confirmed tumor absorbed dose > 200 Gy.

**128. S148. Sub-Aperture Modulation:** Fine-scale segmentation of fluence within each MLC aperture.
**Related Terms:** High-resolution IMRT, Modulation complexity
**Example:** Boost dose shaped around lacrimal gland using sub-aperture modulation.

**129. Sub-Beam Range Shifter (Proton):** Spot-specific proton range shifting for shallow targets.
**Related Terms:** Range compensator, Ridge filter
**Example:** Used to treat orbital rhabdomyosarcoma without ocular overdose.

**130. Surface Projection Map (SGRT):** 3D map used to compare live patient surface to reference surface.
**Related Terms:** DIBH monitoring, Body tracking
**Example:** Projection map ensured breast remained within 2-mm tolerance during VMAT.

**131. Scatter Dose Estimation:** Calculation of unintended radiation dose resulting from photon/electron scatter to surrounding tissues.
**Related Terms:** Out-of-field dose, Secondary radiation
**Example:** Scatter dose to the heart estimated for left breast IMRT to ensure ALARA compliance.

**132. Scatter Kernel Convolution:** Method in TPS using mathematical kernels to model how scatter contributes to final dose.
**Related Terms:** Dose convolution, Heterogeneity correction
**Example:** Kernel recalculation improved lung dose accuracy in low-density areas.

**133. SCEP (Surface Compensated Electron Planning):** Planning workflow that modifies electron fields to compensate for tissue inhomogeneity and contour irregularities.
**Related Terms:** Bolus design, Electron energy modulation
**Example:** Chest wall electron boost used SCEP to maintain uniform coverage along curved rib surface.

**134. Secondary Cancer Induction Risk:** Probability of developing new malignancy due to exposure from primary radiotherapy.
**Related Terms:** Out-of-field dose, Risk modelling
**Example:** VMAT arcs modified to reduce theoretical thyroid cancer risk in pediatric cranial RT.

**135. Secondary Check Software:** Independent dose calculation system to validate TPS MU and dose predictions.
**Related Terms:** MU second check, Independent QA
**Example:** Discrepancy > 3% between TPS and secondary check flagged calculation error.

**136. Secondary Electron Buildup Region:** Surface zone where electron contamination increases dose near the skin.
**Related Terms:** Skin dose, Bolus modelling
**Example:** Bolus removed after buildup evaluation prevented grade-2 dermatitis in neck IMRT.

**137. Segmented Field IMRT:** IMRT delivery using several static subfields to form a modulated dose pattern.
**Related Terms:** Step-and-shoot IMRT, Static MLC delivery
**Example:** Pelvic IMRT segmented into 57 subfields to improve rectal sparing.

138. **Segment Shape Complexity Index:** Metric expressing geometric complexity of IMRT MLC apertures.
**Related Terms:** MLC modulation complexity, MU efficiency
**Example:** Index flagged excessive modulation that extended delivery time for H&N IMRT.

139. **Self-Shielding Mode (HDR):** Emergency HDR mode that automatically retracts the source into shielded position.
**Related Terms:** Emergency safe state, Source interlock
**Example:** HDR source returned to safe position during catheter blockage event.

140. **Sensitivity Analysis of Planning Parameters:** Method of testing how parameter adjustments affect plan robustness and dose.
**Related Terms:** Parameter impact modeling, Optimization stability
**Example:** Sensitivity analysis showed PTV homogeneity was most sensitive to priority weight.

141. **Setup Drift Tracking:** Monitoring progressive change in patient position during session.
**Related Terms:** Intrafraction motion, SGRT continuous monitoring
**Example:** SGRT detected 4-mm drift during prostate VMAT and triggered auto-beam pause.

142. **Setup Reproducibility Index:** Quantitative score describing consistency of patient positioning across fractions.
**Related Terms:** Systematic error, Rotational alignment
**Example:** High reproducibility index achieved in DIBH breast workflow using SGRT guidance.

143. **SGRT-Based Collision Prevention:** Monitoring of gantry/couch/accessory distances using optical surface scanning.
**Related Terms:** Clearance mapping, Arc trajectory planning
**Example:** Auto-halt prevented gantry–mask collision during non-coplanar SRS arc.

144. **Shielding Integrity Survey:** Verification that structural radiation shielding maintains required attenuation levels.
**Related Terms:** Barrier survey, Radiation safety audit
**Example:** Post-installation survey confirmed maze shielding meets NCRP limits.

145. **Short-Arc VMAT:** VMAT technique using limited arc range to restrict dose to sensitive OARs.
**Related Terms:** Avoidance sectors, Partial arcs
**Example:** Liver SBRT used 220° short arcs to minimize spinal cord exposure.

146. **Side-Lobe Suppression (Ultrasound in RT):** Suppression of unwanted off-axis echoes that degrade US image contrast.
**Related Terms:** Beamforming, Echo artifact reduction
**Example:** Side-lobe suppression improved prostate localization for US-guided IGRT.

147. **Signal Drift Correction (Imaging):** Calibration to compensate for gradual signal loss in imaging detectors.
**Related Terms:** Detector aging, Gain calibration
**Example:** Corrected CBCT signal drift restored soft-tissue contrast for pancreas IGRT.

148. **Simulation-to-Treatment Latency:** Time interval between CT simulation and first treatment delivery.
**Related Terms:** Plan adaptation, Tumor progression risk
**Example:** Rapid workflow reduced latency to 3 days for aggressive head-and-neck disease.

**149. Slice Thickness Error (CT/MRI):** Difference between actual and expected slice thickness affecting spatial accuracy.
**Related Terms:** Partial volume effect, Z-axis scaling
**Example:** QA corrected CT slice accuracy to avoid brainstem contouring errors.

**150. Small-Field Output Calibration:** Output factor calibration for small photon fields where detector response varies.
**Related Terms:** Output factor correction, Volume averaging
**Example:** Diode detector calibrated 2×2 cm field for lung SBRT PTV.

**151. Smart Auto-Scaling (TPS Display):** Dynamic dose map scaling to enhance display visibility without altering calculation.
**Related Terms:** Visualization filter, Dose overlay rendering
**Example:** Auto-scaling improved hotspot visualization for stereotactic boost evaluation.

**152. Soft-Tissue Auto-Matching Algorithm:** Automatic IGRT matching based on grayscale similarity of soft-tissue anatomy.
**Related Terms:** CBCT matching, Deformable registration
**Example:** Auto-match aligned pancreas target without depending on bone structures.

**153. Spatial Dose Gradient Reliability:** Accuracy of planned dose drop-off around PTV vs delivered gradient.
**Related Terms:** Gradient index, High-dose fall-off
**Example:** 3% degradation of gradient detected during VMAT gamma review in lung SBRT.

**154. Spectrum-Weighted Dose Calculation:** Dose computation adjusted based on actual energy spectrum of the treatment beam.
**Related Terms:** Poly-energetic modeling, Beam hardening
**Example:** Spectrum-weighted dose improved accuracy in titanium-reinforced spine RT.

**155. Spherical Target Intensity Modulation:** Fluence shaping technique optimized for spherical or near-spherical targets.
**Related Terms:** Isodose shaping, Conformal arc therapy
**Example:** Craniopharyngioma treated using spherical modulation to tighten dose around optic chiasm.

**156. Slice Thickness Uniformity QA:** Ensures equal slice thickness across CT images to avoid geometric distortion.
**Related Terms:** CT, Phantom, Spatial Resolution
**Radiotherapy Example:** CT simulation QA verifies accurate slice thickness to prevent PTV margin errors.

**157. Shielding Integrity Survey:** Measurement of radiation leakage around treatment rooms to confirm barrier performance.
**Related Terms:** Controlled Areas, Leakage, Radiation Safety
**Radiotherapy Example:** Annual survey proves maze door and wall shielding block scatter from high-MU SBRT.

**158. Setup Interruption Recovery Protocol:** Procedure for safe continuation of treatment after interruption due to error or emergency.
**Related Terms:** Workflow QA, Patient Safety
**Radiotherapy Example:** Treatment resumes with re-verification of imaging after console power interruption.

**159. Spot Scanning Range QA:** Accuracy checking of maximum and minimum ranges of scanned proton spots.
**Related Terms:** PBS, Range Uncertainty, RBE
**Radiotherapy Example:** Depth scanning QA ensures spot delivery at 12–18 cm depth for lung proton therapy.

**160. Stage Motion Tracking QA:** Verification that robotic couch or motion platform follows planned translational and rotational paths.
**Related Terms:** Hexapod, IGRT, SBRT
**Radiotherapy Example:** QA confirms 6-DOF table delivers programmed shifts for spine SBRT alignment.

**161. Synthetic CT Validation:** Assessment of the dosimetric accuracy of MRI-based synthetic CT used for treatment planning.
**Related Terms:** MR-only RT, Electron Density Map
**Radiotherapy Example:** Dosimetry comparison verifies synthetic CT does not alter prostate plan DVH.

**162. Surface Guided Treatment Pause Threshold:** Configured SGRT tolerance that auto-pauses the beam when patient motion exceeds a limit.
**Related Terms:** SGRT, DIBH, Motion Management
**Radiotherapy Example:** Beam stops automatically when breast DIBH motion exceeds 3 mm.

**163. Shielding Door Interlock QA:** QA confirming radiation beam cannot activate when vault door is open.
**Related Terms:** Access Control, Safety Interlocks
**Radiotherapy Example:** Attempting beam-on with open door confirms treatment interlock stops exposure.

**164. Servo-Controlled Gantry Tracking:** Dynamic gantry feedback control system keeping movement smooth and aligned with plan.
**Related Terms:** VMAT, Servo Motors, Arc Therapy
**Radiotherapy Example:** Gantry positioning smoothly modulates during 360° VMAT delivery.

**165. Scatter Kernel Modeling QA:** Validation of the algorithm used to model photon scattering inside a TPS.
**Related Terms:** Convolution, Superposition, Dose Engine
**Radiotherapy Example:** Kernel QA verifies scatter dose matches measured values in heterogeneous lung phantom.

**166. Slow-Motion Imaging QA:** Use of high-frame-rate cameras to evaluate MLC and jaw motion accuracy.
**Related Terms:** MLC Speed, Dynamic Delivery, QA Imaging
**Radiotherapy Example:** High-speed imaging confirms no leaf flutter during sliding-window IMRT.

**167. Support Arm Collision Detection:** Test ensuring the treatment machine halts when accessories risk collision.
**Related Terms:** Gantry, Couch, Safety
**Radiotherapy Example:** Couch-gantry collision test prevents impact during complex head-and-neck setup.

168. **Simultaneous Integrated Boost Synchronization:** Ensures accurate delivery of multiple dose levels in a single treatment fraction.
**Related Terms:** SIB, IMRT, Differential Dose
**Radiotherapy Example:** QA verifies boost to tonsillar tumor while elective nodes receive lower dose.

169. **Spot Weight Calibration:** Proportion of monitor units assigned to each proton spot for planned dose distribution.
**Related Terms:** Proton Therapy, PBS, MU Calibration
**Radiotherapy Example:** Spot weights tuned during QA eliminate hot spot near optic nerve.

170. **Scatter-to-Primary Ratio (SPR) Analysis:** Ratio of scattered photons to primary photons, affecting image contrast and dose.
**Related Terms:** CT, kV, MV Imaging
**Radiotherapy Example:** SPR analysis validates placement of anti-scatter grid in pelvis CBCT.

171. **Spatial Resolution Bar Pattern QA:** Phantom imaging system using bar patterns to quantify resolution.
**Related Terms:** MTF, CT, kV Imaging
**Radiotherapy Example:** CBCT QA confirms system resolves 1.0 lp/mm before adaptive RT session.

172. **Safety Checklist Compliance Audit:** Review verifying completion of pre-treatment safety checklists.
**Related Terms:** WHO Checklist, Treatment Verification
**Radiotherapy Example:** Audit confirms 100% checklist completion for thoracic patients.

173. **Synchronous Table–Beam Motion QA:** Testing coordination between couch motion and beam delivery.
**Related Terms:** Dynamic Couch, 4D Delivery, VMAT
**Radiotherapy Example:** Couch translation synchronized during arc therapy to avoid organ sparing violations.

174. **Segmented Dose Reconstruction:** Calculation of cumulative dose from individual treatment segments or control points.
**Related Terms:** Control Points, Log Files, Delivered Dose
**Radiotherapy Example:** Analysis reconstructs accumulated dose for offline ART evaluation.

175. Surface Contour Error Alarm: SGRT alert triggered when patient surface deviates from reference during treatment.
**Related Terms:** SGRT, Motion Alarm, Tracking
**Radiotherapy Example:** Alarm activates when abdomen rises more than 2 mm during lung VMAT.

176. **Source Decay Correction Factor:** Adjustment applied for activity decay of brachytherapy sources over time.
**Related Terms:** Half-Life, Activity, HDR
**Radiotherapy Example:** Dose rate updated for Ir-192 decays to maintain correct cervical HDR dose.

177. **Secondary MU Review Protocol:** Independent secondary check validating monitor units calculated by TPS.
**Related Terms:** MU Calculation, QA Verification, Safety
**Radiotherapy Example:** Independent MU check flags an unexpectedly high MU for spine IMRT.

**178. Step-and-Shoot IMRT Timing QA:** Verification of beam-on and beam-off timing during segmented IMRT delivery.
**Related Terms:** IMRT, MU Segments, Delivery Efficiency
**Radiotherapy Example:** QA ensures no timing lag between segments that could cause dose overshoot.

**179. Static Field Dose Linearity Test:** Test confirming linear dose response at different monitor unit levels for static fields.
**Related Terms:** MU Linearity, Output Factors
**Radiotherapy Example:** Linac output shows 2 MU delivers half the dose of 4 MU for small-field IMRT.

**180. Skin Dose Attenuation Mapping:** Quantification of dose buildup and attenuation at the skin surface.
**Related Terms:** Build-Up Region, Bolus, Electron Contamination
**Radiotherapy Example:** Bolus mapping confirms 1 cm bolus increases scalp surface dose for resection bed.

**181. Self-Shielded Brachytherapy Transfer Tube QA:** Verification of shielding and physical integrity of source transfer tubes.
**Related Terms:** HDR, Source Pathway, Radiation Safety
**Radiotherapy Example:** QA ensures no radiation leakage occurs during Ir-192 source transit.

**182. Scan-to-Plan Registration Fidelity:** Accuracy of mapping simulation scans to treatment planning coordinates.
**Related Terms:** Image Fusion, IGRT, Spatial Accuracy
**Radiotherapy Example:** Registration QA confirms MR-CT match before brain VMAT planning.

**183. Scanned Proton Layer Reproducibility:** QA confirming correct positioning of each depth layer in proton spot scanning.
**Related Terms:** PBS, Range Uncertainty, Energy Layer
**Radiotherapy Example:** Range checks ensure correct layer placement for ocular proton therapy.

**184. Simulated Error Workflow Drill:** Staff simulation of treatment interruption and error recovery.
**Related Terms:** Safety Culture, Treatment Pause, Emergency Protocol
**Radiotherapy Example:** Drill confirms staff response time to MLC fault during delivery.

**185. Simulation Laser Alignment Verification:** Ensures CT simulation lasers correspond exactly to treatment room isocenter.
**Related Terms:** Patient Setup, IGRT, Reference Marks
**Radiotherapy Example:** Laser QA guarantees tattoos align with isocenter during pelvis IMRT.

**186. Secondary Dose Calculation Engine Validation:** Independent validation of secondary calculation algorithms vs. measurement.
**Related Terms:** MU Check, Dose Audit, Safety
**Radiotherapy Example:** Secondary engine flags incorrect MU assignment for parotid case.

**187. Scatter Contamination Reduction Test:** Measurement of beam contamination from scatter within collimators or flattening filter.
**Related Terms:** Photon Scatter, Electron Contamination
**Radiotherapy Example:** FFF beams show reduced contamination for breast tangents.

**188. SGRT Baseline Map Stability Test:** Ensures the SGRT reference surface remains unchanged for multi-fraction treatments.
**Related Terms:** DIBH, Latency, Motion Management
**Radiotherapy Example:** Baseline updated weekly to avoid surface drift in left-breast treatments.

**189. Shielded Applicator Transmission Factor:** Quantification of dose attenuation through shields used with applicators.
**Related Terms:** Brachytherapy, Attenuation, Dose Rate
**Radiotherapy Example:** Transmission factor ensures vaginal shield reduces bladder dose by 40%.

**190. Scatter Air Ratio (SAR) Verification:** Check of scatter contribution by field size and depth in dose calculation models.
**Related Terms:** Scatter Kernels, TAR, PDD
**Radiotherapy Example:** SAR used to correct dose at 15 cm depth for large abdominal field.

**191. Sequential Field Overlap QA:** QA ensuring proper junctioning of adjacent radiation fields.
**Related Terms:** Feathering, Matching, Dose Homogeneity
**Radiotherapy Example:** Spine-craniospinal junction verified to avoid hot/cold bands.

**192. Superuser Access Audit:** Review of administrative access to planning/delivery systems for security.
**Related Terms:** Cybersecurity, EMR, Record-and-Verify
**Radiotherapy Example:** Audit detects unauthorized TPS database access.

**193. Stochastic Dose Algorithm Assessment:** Accuracy evaluation of Monte Carlo or probabilistic dose models.
**Related Terms:** Monte Carlo, Particle Transport
**Radiotherapy Example:** Monte Carlo dose validated against ion chamber in lung phantom.

**194. Soft-Tissue Deformation Tracking Model:** Algorithm predicting anatomical motion and deformation during treatment.
**Related Terms:** ART, DIR, Adaptive Planning
**Radiotherapy Example:** Model predicts pancreas motion during breath cycle.

**195. Spherical Marker Phantom Localization:** Phantom QA using spherical fiducials to evaluate image-based localization accuracy.
**Related Terms:** IGRT, Registration, Stereotactic
**Radiotherapy Example:** Localization error kept <0.7 mm for brain SRS.

**196. Stray Neutron Dose Index:** Estimation of neutron dose outside treatment field for high-energy photon or proton therapy.
**Related Terms:** Secondary Neutrons, Shielding, Out-of-Field Dose
**Radiotherapy Example:** Neutron index evaluated in pediatric craniospinal plans.

**197. Segmented 4D Dose Accumulation:** Accumulation of delivered dose across respiratory phases.
**Related Terms:** 4DCT, ITV, Motion Management
**Radiotherapy Example:** Accumulated dose shows hotspot when diaphragm shifts beyond predicted pattern.

**198. Stereotactic QA End-to-End Test:** Complete simulation-to-delivery QA verifying stereotactic workflow accuracy.
**Related Terms:** SRS, SBRT, Winston-Lutz, IGRT
**Radiotherapy Example:** End-to-end test confirms skull SRS localization error <0.7 mm before first patient.

**199. Stainless Steel Implant Dose Perturbation Assessment:** Evaluation of dose errors caused by metallic implants.
**Related Terms:** Heterogeneity Correction, Artifacts, Monte Carlo
**Radiotherapy Example:** Dose recalculated around spinal rods to avoid unexpected cold spots.

200. **Superior-Inferior Shift QA:** Verification of movement accuracy in SI direction for couch, gating, or tracking.
**Related Terms:** 6DoF Couch, Motion Monitoring, SGRT
**Radiotherapy Example:** SI couch corrections tested before liver SBRT fractions.

201. **Source Strength Decay Chart Validation:** Confirmation that brachytherapy source decay curve matches expected activity.
**Related Terms:** HDR, Ir-192, Half-Life
**Radiotherapy Example:** Activity compared with dose-calibration chamber prior to cervical treatment.

202. **Sub-Volume Dose Quality Index:** Metric evaluating dose quality inside critical sub-regions.
**Related Terms:** DVH, PTV, DME (Dose Metric Evaluation)
**Radiotherapy Example:** Index tracks underdose inside GTV core for recurrent sarcoma.

203. **Slab Phantom Density Scaling Test:** Verifies CT-to-density conversion accuracy across tissue-equivalent slabs.
**Related Terms:** HU Calibration, TPS Commissioning
**Radiotherapy Example:** Soft-tissue slab dose agreed with TPS within 1%.

204. **Segmented MU Output Stability Assessment:** Ensures beam output remains stable between multiple MU segments.
**Related Terms:** IMRT, Step-and-Shoot, Output Drift
**Radiotherapy Example:** MU stability confirmed for 150-segment head-and-neck plan.

205. **Shell-Based Contouring QA:** QA for organ or target segmentation using concentric shell techniques.
**Related Terms:** Auto-Segmentation, AI Segmentation QA, ROI Expansion
**Radiotherapy Example:** Shell algorithm validated for liver lesion segmentation on CT.

206. **Shared Control Point Dose Error Flagging:** Identification of errors when multiple arcs share same control point parameters.
**Related Terms:** VMAT, MLC Mapping, MU Control
**Radiotherapy Example:** QA prevents MU double-counting in pelvic dual-arc VMAT.

207. **Spatial Frequency Image Analysis:** Image quality evaluation via spatial frequency response metrics.
**Related Terms:** MTF, Noise Power Spectrum, CBCT QA
**Radiotherapy Example:** Spatial-frequency assessment detects CBCT blurring after detector degradation.

208. **Simultaneous Integrated Boost MU Validation:** Verification of MU distribution among primary and boost regions in SIB plans.
**Related Terms:** SIB-IMRT, DVH, Target Prioritization
**Radiotherapy Example:** MU validation avoids overdosing larynx while boosting GTV.

209. **Static Field Respiratory Hold Accuracy:** Measures accuracy of breath-hold during static field deliveries.
**Related Terms:** DIBH, SGRT, Motion Compensation
**Radiotherapy Example:** Hold accuracy tested to <3 mm for left-breast DIBH.

210. **Stacking Error Compensation Algorithm:** Planning algorithm adjusting for cumulative delivery mis-alignments.
**Related Terms:** Adaptive Planning, DIR, Deformation Models
**Radiotherapy Example:** Stacking compensation improves dose fidelity in pancreas SBRT.

211. **Soft-Tissue Fiducial Tracking Latency:** Delay between marker motion and system response.
**Related Terms:** Real-Time Tracking, CyberKnife, IGRT
**Radiotherapy Example:** Prostate tracking latency recorded to optimize SBRT intrafraction control.

212. **Scatter-Corrected CBCT Dose Assessment:** Quantification of dose reduction after applying CBCT scatter-correction.
**Related Terms:** Image Dose, Reconstruction, Dosimetry
**Radiotherapy Example:** Scatter correction reduces pelvic CBCT dose by 35%.

213. **Stray Dose Pediatrics Audit:** Review of unintended exposure in pediatric radiotherapy.
**Related Terms:** Shielding, OAR, Cataract Risk
**Radiotherapy Example:** TBI audit identifies out-of-field eye dose exceeding 100 mGy.

214. **SRS Cone End-to-End Phantom Test:** Ultra-high-accuracy workflow test for cone-based SRS.
**Related Terms:** Stereotactic Cones, Winston-Lutz, Microbeam
**Radiotherapy Example:** End-to-end error validated <0.5 mm prior to trigeminal neuralgia SRS.

215. **Sigmoidal Dose Response Modeling:** Modeling of tissue response using a sigmoidal or logistic curve.
**Related Terms:** NTCP, TCP, Radiobiology
**Radiotherapy Example:** Model predicts rectal bleeding risk with dose escalation.

216. **Simulated Anatomy Dataset Validation:** QA validating AI-generated or synthetic anatomy sets for planning use.
**Related Terms:** Digital Twin, Synthetic CT, Deep Learning
**Radiotherapy Example:** QA ensures synthetic pelvis dataset reflects true bone density for proton planning.

217. **Serial Organ Cumulative Dose Check:** Verification that dose constraints for serial organs remain below tolerance.
**Related Terms:** QUANTEC, OAR, Maximum Dose
**Radiotherapy Example:** Max spinal cord dose restricted to 45 Gy cumulative.

218. **Secondary Patient ID Lockout:** System preventing treatment if ID mismatch is detected.
**Related Terms:** Patient Safety, Record-and-Verify, Barcode
**Radiotherapy Example:** Lockout stops wrong-patient setup before prostate IMRT.

219. **Scatter Kernel QA:** Tests scatter parameters that influence convolution–superposition dose algorithms.
**Related Terms:** Dose Kernel, Algorithm Commissioning
**Radiotherapy Example:** Scatter kernel refined for lung density gradient.

220. **Sleep Mode Radiation Safety Audit:** Safety protocol verifying radiation devices remain inactive in standby.
**Related Terms:** Linac Security, Operational Safety
**Radiotherapy Example:** Audit ensures HDR room dose is zero when afterloader powered but idle.

221. **Static MR-Linac Field Homogeneity Check:** Verification of magnetic field uniformity during radiation delivery.
**Related Terms:** B0 Homogeneity, MRgRT, Adaptive
**Radiotherapy Example:** Homogeneity correction applied to reduce image distortion in rectal ART.

222. **Specular Surface Imaging Calibration:** Calibration of surface-tracking cameras for reflective skin surfaces.
**Related Terms:** SGRT, Reflectivity, Patient-Specific QA
**Radiotherapy Example:** IGRT surface mapping optimized for oily skin under head-and-neck mask.

223. **Sub-Pixel MV Portal Imaging Resolution Test:** Test confirming MV detector can resolve sub-pixel structure deviations.
**Related Terms:** Portal Imaging, MLC QA, IGRT
**Radiotherapy Example:** Detects 0.3 mm MLC deflection using high-resolution portal images.

224. **Synchronized Multi-Arc Timing QA:** Verifies timing alignment between multiple arcs delivered in sequence.
**Related Terms:** VMAT, MLC Sequencing, Gantry Synchronization
**Radiotherapy Example:** Timing coordination validated for dual-arc SIB oropharynx plan.

225. **Soft Constraint Optimization Monitor:** Tracker evaluating how soft optimization constraints influence planning priority.
**Related Terms:** Cost Function, DVH Penalty, Planning Objectives
**Radiotherapy Example:** Monitor prevents excessive soft-constraint weighting that underdoses PTV.

226. **Synchronized DIBH Beam-On Permission System:** Allows treatment only when breath-hold criteria are satisfied.
**Related Terms:** SGRT, Gating, Motion Management
**Radiotherapy Example:** Beam activates only when chest wall displacement tolerance $<2$ mm.

227. **Surface-Guided Intrafraction Drift Report:** Documentation of patient movement during beam-on using SGRT.
**Related Terms:** Tracking, Positional Stability, Setup Error
**Radiotherapy Example:** Drift report for lung SBRT shows 0.6 mm mean displacement over 20 minutes.

228. **Secondary Imaging Dose Optimization:** Reduction of dose from verification imaging without compromising image quality.
**Related Terms:** CBCT dose reduction, kV/MV imaging, ALARA
**Radiotherapy Example:** Reduced-dose CBCT protocol implemented for daily prostate IGRT.

229. **Spatial Alignment Deformation Map:** Map showing anatomical deformation over time to evaluate alignment changes.
**Related Terms:** DIR, adaptive therapy, deformation vectors
**Radiotherapy Example:** Deformation map compares bladder volume changes between fractions.

230. **Scatter Radiation Risk Index:** Metric estimating stray dose to patients and staff from scatter radiation.
**Related Terms:** Shielding, out-of-field dose, risk modelling
**Radiotherapy Example:** Index used to revise shielding for pediatric craniospinal cases.

231. **Sensor-Based Body Posture Detection:** Sensors detect and verify body position before beam delivery.
**Related Terms:** SGRT, posture validation, setup verification
**Radiotherapy Example:** Alerts triggered when kyphosis shift exceeds 3° during spine treatment.

232. **Stereotactic Arc Verification Phantom:** Phantom to test precision of stereotactic multi-arc dose delivery.
**Related Terms:** Arc QA, Winston-Lutz, SRS
**Radiotherapy Example:** Phantom verifies gamma-passing rate for 10-arc brain SRS plan.

233. **Scatter Compensated Fluence Map:** Fluence map corrected for scatter artifacts in planning.
**Related Terms:** IMRT, kernel modeling, fluence correction
**Radiotherapy Example:** Scatter-compensated fluence improves accuracy in lung IMRT.

234. **Small Field Coincidence Tracker:** Tool to evaluate alignment accuracy of very small fields.
**Related Terms:** Output factor, SRS QA, micro-MLC
**Radiotherapy Example:** Coincidence tracker checks 5 mm field offsets for trigeminal neuralgia plan.

235. **Simulation-to-Treatment Workflow Analysis:** Full pathway review to detect timing, image, or coordinate inconsistencies.
**Related Terms:** End-to-end QA, procedural QA, IGRT
**Radiotherapy Example:** Workflow review catches missing bolus transfer in breast plan.

236. **Sequential Boost Consistency Testing:** Test ensuring equal setup accuracy between initial and boost phases.
**Related Terms:** SIB vs sequential boost, IGRT, DVH verification
**Radiotherapy Example:** Boost phase validated to align with primary head-and-neck PTV.

237. **Susceptibility Artifact Mapping:** Map identifying magnetic distortion in MRI near implants or air regions.
**Related Terms:** MR-only planning, metal artifact reduction, B0 distortion
**Radiotherapy Example:** Artifact map prevents mis-contouring of sinus tumor boundaries.

238. **SRS Composite Dose Reconstruction:** Reconstruction of multiple isocenter SRS doses into a unified 3D dataset.
**Related Terms:** Dose accumulation, brain metastasis, EQD2
**Radiotherapy Example:** Dose reconstruction evaluates cumulative brainstem dose in 6-lesion plan.

239. **Spectral CT Planning Calibration:** Calibration of spectral CT HU values for dose calculation.
**Related Terms:** Dual-energy CT, electron density mapping, stoichiometric calibration
**Radiotherapy Example:** Spectral CT improves material assignment for proton lung cases.

240. **Slit Beam MLC Tracking Test:** Test verifying MLC tracking accuracy during narrow slit irradiation.
**Related Terms:** Real-time MLC tracking, motion compensation
**Radiotherapy Example:** Latency test ensures safe tracking during liver motion.

241. **Synthetic MRI Dose Estimation:** Estimation of dose using synthetic MR-generated attenuation data.
**Related Terms:** MRI-only workflow, synthetic CT, MR-Linac
**Radiotherapy Example:** Synthetic MR dose verified for prostate MR-only workflow.

242. **Spatial Fractionation Peak-Valley Ratio:** Ratio of high-dose peak to low-dose valley in spatially fractionated therapy.
**Related Terms:** Lattice therapy, GRID therapy, radiobiology
**Radiotherapy Example:** Peak-valley ratio optimized to reduce pain in bulky sarcoma.

243. **Standing-Wave Linac Resonance QA:** QA of RF resonance behavior in standing-wave linear accelerators.
**Related Terms:** klystron, RF power, accelerator physics
**Radiotherapy Example:** RF tuning corrected after detecting resonance drift at high dose rates.

244. **Scattered Photon Absorber Efficiency Test:** Assessment of device efficiency in reducing scattered photons.
**Related Terms:** Anti-scatter grid, filter, noise reduction
**Radiotherapy Example:** Pediatric CBCT protocol improved by optimized absorber geometry.

245. **Surface Cumulative Dose Tracker:** Tool monitoring total skin dose from treatment and imaging.
**Related Terms:** Skin toxicity, imaging dose, portal dose
**Radiotherapy Example:** Breast IMRT skin dose limited with weekly cumulative tracking.

246. **Secure Beam-Override Authorization:** Safety system requiring authorization for emergency beam reactivation.
**Related Terms:** Patient safety, failsafe, machine interlock
**Radiotherapy Example:** Override authorization prevents accidental re-exposure during error recovery.

247. **Synchronization Latency Threshold Record:** Record of delay tolerance for gating or tracking synchronization.
**Related Terms:** Motion tracking, gating windows, respiratory management
**Radiotherapy Example:** Liver SBRT latency threshold restricted to <200 ms.

248. **Symmetric Dose Gradient Profile:** Measurement of dose fall-off in opposite directions to assess beam symmetry and edge sharpness.
**Related Terms:** Penumbra, dose gradient index, beam flatness
**Radiotherapy Example:** Symmetry evaluation used to validate cranial SRS beam accuracy.

249. **Salivary Gland Neuroprotection Strategy:** Planning strategies used to preserve salivary gland function during head-and-neck RT.
**Related Terms:** Sparing, NTCP, parotid dose constraint
**Radiotherapy Example:** Adaptive plan reduces ipsilateral parotid mean dose by 2 Gy to reduce xerostomia.

250. **Spot-Scanning Integrity Check:** QA that confirms correct order, dwell time, and location of proton or ion pencil beam spots.
**Related Terms:** Monte Carlo log analysis, PBS QA, stop-map validation
**Radiotherapy Example:** Spot integrity check detects missing spot sequences in pediatric spine PBS plan.

251. **Sub-Voxel Density Assignment Algorithm:** System that models density variations inside a voxel to increase dose accuracy.
**Related Terms:** Heterogeneity correction, dose engine accuracy
**Radiotherapy Example:** Sub-voxel model improves lung interface dose prediction for IMPT.

252. **Simultaneous Couch-Gantry Collision Modeling:** Algorithm simulating full motion paths to predict collision risk before delivery.
**Related Terms:** Treatment clearance model, 4D geometry, safety margin
**Radiotherapy Example:** System flags high collision risk for lateral head-neck arc with mask and bite-block.

253. **Spinal Cord Cumulative Repair Factor:** Model estimating partial biological repair between fractions for tolerance prediction.
**Related Terms:** EQD2, BED, fractionation
**Radiotherapy Example:** Repair factor predicts safe retreatment dose after earlier cervical irradiation.

254. **Scatter-Weighted Imaging SNR Value:** SNR metric corrected for scatter influence to evaluate true image quality.
**Related Terms:** CBCT SNR, noise index, artifact quantification
**Radiotherapy Example:** Low scatter-weighted SNR prompts use of anti-scatter grid for pelvis IGRT.

255. **Spatially Fractionated Proton Lattice Therapy:** Use of proton beams to deliver high-dose nodes within tumors while sparing the bulk volume.
**Related Terms:** Lattice, FLASH-lattice, high-Z GRID
**Radiotherapy Example:** Proton lattice plan used for bulky rhabdomyosarcoma to reduce systemic toxicity.

256. **SMART Boost (Simultaneous Modulated Accelerated RT):** RT technique delivering higher dose per fraction to selected sub-volumes while treating the whole target conventionally.
**Related Terms:** SIB, dose painting, biological targeting
**Radiotherapy Example:** SMART boost escalates hypoxic tumor sub-regions in HPV+ tonsillar cancer.

257. **Small-Organ Tolerance Segmentation Rule:** Method defining contouring boundaries of radiosensitive microstructures to protect functionality.
**Related Terms:** OAR contouring, sparing rules, neurovascular bundles
**Radiotherapy Example:** Rule enables contouring of cochlear turns for acoustic neuroma SRS sparing.

258. **SRS Hidden Target Error Map:** Visualization map to quantify geometric error between phantom target and planned isocenter.
**Related Terms:** Winston-Lutz, end-to-end QA, couch isocenter check
**Radiotherapy Example:** Map reveals 0.3 mm shift in couch rotation center during trigeminal SRS.

259. **Stand-Off Bolus Technique:** Technique where bolus is intentionally elevated above the surface to shape dose distribution.
**Related Terms:** Skin collimation, electron therapy, air gap
**Radiotherapy Example:** Stand-off bolus improves dose uniformity over reconstructed nasal bridge.

260. **Streak Artifact Suppression Kernel:** Reconstruction filter designed to suppress streaks often caused by metal or limited-angle CT.
**Related Terms:** MAR, CT reconstruction, compressed sensing
**Radiotherapy Example:** Kernel reduces dental artifact for accurate PTV contouring.

261. **Structure-Specific Dose Goal Prioritization:** Ranking system for assigning priority to OAR and PTV dose goals in multi-objective optimization.
**Related Terms:** Trade-off model, auto-planning, weighted priority
**Radiotherapy Example:** Parotids prioritized above mandible to preserve salivary function.

262. **Sequential Recovery Assessment for Re-Irradiation:** Model estimating tissue recovery time relevant to safe retreatment decisions.
**Related Terms:** Cumulative toxicity, latency effect, NTCP modelling
**Radiotherapy Example:** Recovery assessment supports safe thoracic retreatment after 18-month interval.

263. **Sigmoid Dose Curve Detector:** Tool detecting D-shaped dose fall-off signatures that suggest optimization instability.
**Related Terms:** DVH abnormality, dose spike detection, plan QA
**Radiotherapy Example:** Detector flags sinusoidal DVH shape in lung VMAT plan requiring optimization refinement.

264. **Scripting-Based Adaptive Plan Library:** Automated script that generates multiple plans for predicted anatomical states.
**Related Terms:** Library-based ART, automation, batch optimization
**Radiotherapy Example:** 12-plan bladder library generated automatically based on filling patterns.

265. **Sub-Millimeter Localization Guarantee System:** Clinical program ensuring <1 mm localization error throughout SRS/SBRT workflow.
**Related Terms:** SGRT, ExacTrac, robotic couch
**Radiotherapy Example:** Localization guarantee confirmed via pre-beam and post-beam imaging.

**266. Swift Beam Interruption Response Mode:** Fast machine stop mode used during unexpected movement or collision risk.
**Related Terms:** Gating, safety interlock, emergency response
**Radiotherapy Example:** System halts beam immediately when facial motion detected in frameless SRS.

**267. Solution-Guided Auto-Optimization:** Auto-planning algorithm that uses prior successful solution states to refine new plans.
**Related Terms:** Knowledge-based planning, machine learning, auto-iterate
**Radiotherapy Example:** Prior TBI plans guide optimization of new pediatric plan.

**268. Styloid Process Dose Limiter:** Planning structure restricting excess dose to the styloid to protect tongue mobility and swallowing.
**Related Terms:** Dysphagia sparing, neck OARs, functional avoidance
**Radiotherapy Example:** Limiter used in base-of-tongue cancer planning.

**269. Subvolume-Driven Biological Dose Compensation:** Adjusting dose based on expected biological resistance of tumor sub-regions.
**Related Terms:** Hypoxia, radiobiology, PET-guided dose escalation
**Radiotherapy Example:** Escalation to FDG-avid subvolume inside cervical tumor.

**270. Shoulder Displacement Prediction Model:** Predictive model estimating shoulder movement under mask immobilization.
**Related Terms:** IGRT, reproducibility, motion model
**Radiotherapy Example:** Model helps avoid PTV under-coverage in supraclavicular fields.

**271. Based Dose Sculpting (for Brachytherapy):** Brachy planning technique leveraging multiple-channel SAVI device to shape dose precisely.
**Related Terms:** APBI, HDR, catheter modulation
**Radiotherapy Example:** SAVI used to spare rib and skin during breast HDR boost.

**272. Secondary MU Consistency Audit:** Independent MU verification to detect planning or data-transfer errors.
**Related Terms:** Second check, calculation auditor, safety QA
**Radiotherapy Example:** Secondary audit catches MU mismatch from wrong CT density table.

**273. Stereotactic Dose Gradient Audit:** Program assessing sharpness and conformity of dose fall-off for SRS/SBRT plans.
**Related Terms:** Gradient index, ring dose, conformity index
**Radiotherapy Example:** Audit ensures gradient index <3 for brain metastasis SRS.

**274. Slow-Time DRR Deformation Matching:** Matching soft-tissue DRR through slow deformation-based image fusion.
**Related Terms:** Adaptive matching, DIR, soft tissue IGRT
**Radiotherapy Example:** Applied to match liver borders when external surrogates are unreliable.

**275. Simulated Organ Dropping Artifact Study:** Study modeling unrealistic CT deformation when organs artificially drop into empty space after contour removal.
**Related Terms:** DIR stability, air cavity artifacts, contour removal
**Radiotherapy Example:** Study prevents false shrinkage in pelvic adaptive workflows.

**276. Standardized Skin Dose Toxicity Index (SDTI):** Composite index scoring predicted skin toxicity from cumulative surface dose.
**Related Terms:** RTOG skin grade, surface dosimetry, toxicity model
**Radiotherapy Example:** High SDTI prompts tighter bolus schedule modification.

277. **Sensory-Organ Dose Preservation Framework:** Radiotherapy planning framework focused on preserving small sensory organs.
**Related Terms:** Cochlea, olfactory bulb, lacrimal gland, neuro-sparing
**Radiotherapy Example:** Lacrimal sparing reduces dry-eye toxicity in sinonasal IMRT.

278. **Setup Imaging Verification:** Verification of patient positioning using KV/MV/CBCT imaging before irradiation.
**Related Terms:** IGRT, CBCT, KV match, registration, positioning
**Radiotherapy Example:** Setup CBCT verifies kidney PTV alignment before VMAT delivery.

279. **Skin Gap Correction:** Adjustment of SSD or bolus to correct dose variations caused by uneven skin gaps.
**Related Terms:** SSD, bolus, surface dose, scatter
**Example:** A bolus is applied over irregular abdominal skin to maintain kidney IMRT surface dose.

280. **Shoulder Retraction Immobilization:** Immobilization method to retract shoulders out of treatment field.
**Related Terms:** Mould room, thermoplastic mask, positioning aids
**Example:** Shoulder straps are used to clear shoulders from the neck VMAT field.

281. **Slice Thickness Optimization:** Selecting CT slice thickness balancing image clarity and noise for planning.
**Related Terms:** CT simulation, resolution, planning artifacts
**Example:** 1.25 mm slices are used for kidney SBRT for accurate contouring of tumor edges.

282. **Soft Tissue Matching:** Registration using organs and soft tissues rather than bones.
**Related Terms:** CBCT, IGRT, deformable registration
**Example:** Daily kidney CBCT matching uses soft tissue instead of spine to align PTV.

283. **Static Field QA:** Quality assurance of non-rotational static IMRT fields.
**Related Terms:** Step-and-shoot, MLC pattern, output check
**Example:** Film QA verifies kidney AP/PA field dose distribution.

284. **Spatial Resolution Calibration:** Calibration of imaging systems to ensure accurate pixel-to-distance mapping.
**Related Terms:** CT resolution, EPID, distortion
**Example:** Phantom scan confirms correct CT spatial resolution for small kidney lesions.

285. **Stereotactic Localization Box:** Localization frame used to determine reference coordinates for SR**Related Terms:** SRS frame, fiducials, isocenter
**Example:** Localization box determines isocenter for arteriovenous malformation SRS.

286. **Skin Dose Estimation:** Calculation of dose absorbed by skin, especially with high-energy photons.
**Related Terms:** buildup region, bolus, surface dose
**Example:** Skin dose is monitored when abdominal SBRT is near anterior kidney surface.

287. **Sinogram Reconstruction QA:** QA ensuring proper reconstruction of CT sinograms into images.
**Related Terms:** CT artifact, reconstruction kernel
**Example:** Sinogram calibration resolves ring artifacts in CT simulation.

288. **Simulation Room Safety:** Safety protocols in CT simulation and planning environment.
**Related Terms:** Laser safety, crash stop, CT dose optimization
**Example:** Patient is positioned safely inside CT bore with crash sensors activated.

289. **Spine Sparing Planning:** Treatment planning that limits dose to spinal cord.
**Related Terms:** OAR constraints, DVH, IMRT
**Example:** VMAT kidney plan meets <18 Gy spinal cord tolerance.

290. **Synchronized Gating Delivery:** Delivering radiation only during selected respiratory phases.
**Related Terms:** 4D-CT, RPM, breath-hold
**Example:** Gated SBRT delivers beam only during exhalation to minimize kidney motion.

291. **Slice-by-Slice Contouring QA:** Verification of consistent boundaries across CT slices during contouring.
**Related Terms:** MIM, deformable registration, segmentation
**Example:** Contouring QA ensures kidney tumor borders are consistent from apex to base.

292. **Surface Laser Alignment:** Aligning patient with room lasers to match reference tattoo marks.
**Related Terms:** Setup, coordinates, isocenter marking
**Example:** Abdomen tattoos align with lasers during kidney IMRT setup.

293. **Static Couch Correction:** Translational couch adjustment without rotation.
**Related Terms:** 6DoF table, translational shift
**Example:** After CBCT registration, a +3 mm SI static shift is applied before kidney VMAT.

294. **Support Cushion Indexing:** Indexing immobilization devices to fixed couch positions.
**Related Terms:** Mould room, immobilization, reproducibility
**Example:** Kidney SBRT vacuum cushion is locked into indexed slots for reproducibility.

295. **SRS Target Expansion Rule:** Clinical guidelines defining PTV expansion for SRS.
**Related Terms:** margin recipe, microscopic spread, uncertainty
**Example:** A 1–2 mm expansion is used for intracranial SRS metastasis.

296. **Scan-to-Dose Delay Monitoring:** Ensuring time intervals between CT scan and treatment do not cause anatomical changes.
**Related Terms:** adaptation, reproducibility, IGRT
**Example:** Kidney SBRT protocol restricts >10-day delay between CT simulation and first fraction.

297. **Scatter Correction Algorithm:** Software technique to adjust dose or images to account for scatter contamination.
**Related Terms:** MV scatter, CT scatter, reconstruction
**Example:** Algorithm reduces streaking artifacts around kidney contrast agent.

298. **Saturation Artifact Suppression:** Minimizing artifacts due to detector signal saturation in imaging.
**Related Terms:** CT metal artifact, blooming, reconstruction
**Example:** Metal implant near kidney is corrected using MAR algorithm.

299. **Small-Field Output Correction:** Output factors adjusted for small stereotactic fields.
**Related Terms:** detector correction, output factor, OFc
**Example:** A diode detector measures small-field factors for kidney SBRT beams.

300. **Setup Deviation Log:** Record of daily patient positioning corrections.
**Related Terms:** online correction, couch shift, IGRT
**Example:** Kidney SBRT deviations are routinely <2 mm across fractions.

301. **Stereotactic Shell Facial Mask:** Rigid mask used in cranial SRS for non-invasive immobilization.
**Related Terms:** thermoplastic mask, frameless SRS
**Example:** Patient is fitted with shell mask in mould room for AVM SRS.

302. **Spatial Dose Gradient Optimization:** Controlling how quickly dose drops outside the target.
**Related Terms:** fall-off, conformity, OAR sparing
**Example:** Kidney SBRT plan optimizes steep fall-off near liver.

303. **Segmentation Deep-Learning Assistance:** AI model used to automate and refine contouring.
**Related Terms:** AI, auto-contouring, planning efficiency
**Example:** DL auto-contours kidneys and bowel before final editing.

**304. Skin Marking Protection Film:** Film applied to protect tattoo or skin marks from fading.
**Related Terms:** positional marking, reproducibility
**Example:** Films protect abdomen tattoos during 5-fraction kidney SBRT.

**305. System Latency Compensation:** Adjustment to scheduling or delivery to compensate for machine delays.
**Related Terms:** tracking, gating, prediction model
**Example:** Motion tracking compensates lag when treating a moving kidney lesion.

**306. Scatter-to-Primary Ratio Analysis:** Quantifying amount of scatter relative to primary radiation.
**Related Terms:** beam quality, dose accuracy, imaging physics
**Example:** Optimizing abdominal imaging to reduce scatter around kidneys.

**307. Skin Collimator Shielding:** External shielding to reduce unwanted skin irradiation.
**Related Terms:** lead shielding, custom block
**Example:** Shielding protects anterior abdominal skin during posterior kidney beam.

**308. Spine Immobilization Bridge:** Immobilization bridge preventing pressure on spine during supine positioning.
**Related Terms:** mould room, comfort, reproducibility
**Example:** Bridge used for kidney patients with spinal pain to enable stable setup.

**309. Selective Beam Stopper QA:** QA of beam stoppers used to block unwanted stray radiation.
**Related Terms:** shielding, radiation protection
**Example:** Beam stopper checked during kidney VMAT commissioning to reduce leakage.

**310. Synchronous Imaging Trigger:** Trigger signal that synchronizes beam and imaging acquisition.
**Related Terms:** gating, tracking, fluoroscopy
**Example:** Real-time imaging synchronizes with radiation for kidney motion tracking.

**311. Simulation Thermal Comfort Protocol:** Measures ensuring comfortable patient temperature during long CT simulation.
**Related Terms:** mould room, patient care
**Example:** Heated pads prevent shivering that could affect abdominal motion.

**312. Surface-Guided Beam Hold:** Automatic beam stop when patient moves outside safe motion threshold.
**Related Terms:** SGRT, motion management
**Example:** SGRT pauses kidney IMRT when abdomen expands beyond threshold.

**313. Subvolume Dose Escalation:** Delivering higher dose to sub-regions inside PTV.
**Related Terms:** SIB, dose painting, BED
**Example:** Boost delivered to PET-avid kidney tumor core.

**314. Sorbent Artifact Reduction:** Removing CT beam-hardening artifacts caused by bowel contrast.
**Related Terms:** CT artifact correction
**Example:** Artifact reduction improves kidney contouring near bowel contrast.

**315. Source-to-Patient Distance Verification:** Ensuring correct distance between source and patient surface.
**Related Terms:** SSD, calibration, output
**Example:** SSD checked before kidney AP field delivery.

**316. Simulation Reproducibility Assessment:** Checking whether CT sim setup can be repeated at treatment.
**Related Terms:** immobilization, IGRT, setup variation
**Example:** Kidney SBRT uses indexed vac-lock cushion to ensure reproducibility.

317. **Surface Contour Auto-Mapping:** Capturing 3D surface model of patient for real-time motion monitoring.
**Related Terms:** SGRT, optical scanning, DIBH
**Example:** Real-time mapping ensures abdominal surface stability during kidney SBRT.

318. **Suction-Vacuum Immobilization Adjustment:** Adjusting air evacuation to ensure tight immobilization seal.
**Related Terms:** mould room, vacuum cushions
**Example:** Cushion re-vacuumed to maintain firm fit for kidney SBRT.

319. **Secondary Beam Scatter Shield:** Shield used to block secondary scatter radiation.
**Related Terms:** radiation safety, stray dose
**Example:** Shielding protects abdomen skin during posterior kidney beam.

320. **Spatial Dose Interpolation QA:** QA to verify TPS interpolation of dose grid between CT slices.
**Related Terms:** grid resolution, dose accuracy
**Example:** Fine grid prevents dose rounding errors near kidney tumor boundary.

321. **Slice Landmark Annotation:** Marking anatomical and planning reference levels on CT slices.
**Related Terms:** reference slice, localization
**Example:** Slice showing kidney hilum is flagged for planning reference.

322. **Sliding Window Aperture QA:** QA of continuously moving MLC leaves in dynamic IMRT.
**Related Terms:** MLC, fluence, log files
**Example:** Log-file QA validates kidney sliding-window leaf motion.

323. **Six-Degree Couch Calibration:** Calibration of all couch translational + rotational axes.
**Related Terms:** 6DoF, IGRT, geometric accuracy
**Example:** Roll correction calibrated for kidney SBRT accuracy.

324. **Stereotactic Tabletop Compatibility:** Matching immobilization devices to stereotactic couch surface.
**Related Terms:** indexing, rigid boards
**Example:** Kidney SBRT board locked into exact couch docking points.

325. **Surface Marker-Less Tracking:** Tracking patient motion using optical surface rather than markers.
**Related Terms:** SGRT, non-invasive tracking
**Example:** Optical tracking monitors abdominal surface during kidney VMAT.

326. **Spherical Target QA Phantom:** Phantom simulating spherical anatomy for stereotactic QA.
**Related Terms:** SRS, SBRT, Winston-Lutz
**Example:** Phantom verifies isocenter accuracy for small kidney lesions.

327. **Simulation-to-Treatment Consistency Protocol:** Protocol ensuring delivery conditions match simulation conditions.
**Related Terms:** reproducibility, immobilization, IGRT
**Example:** Cushion, tattoos, lasers, bladder prep replicated exactly across kidney SBRT fractions.

328. **Source-to-Axis Distance (SAD) Meaning:** Distance from radiation source to LINAC isocenter.
**Related Terms:** SSD, Isocenter, Beam Geometry
**Radiotherapy Example:** A 100 cm SAD technique was used for VMAT planning to maintain fixed isocenter.

329. **Surface Dose Meaning:** Radiation dose absorbed at the patient's skin.
**Related Terms:** Entrance dose, Bolus, Build-up region
**Radiotherapy Example:** Chest wall RT applied a 5 mm bolus to increase surface dose for adequate tumour control.

330. **Scatter Radiation Meaning:** Radiation deflected after interaction with tissue or equipment.
**Related Terms:** Leakage radiation, Collimator scatter, Phantom scatter
**Radiotherapy Example:** Additional shielding was used in CT-simulation to reduce abdominal scatter dose.

331. **Stereotactic Radiosurgery (SRS) Meaning:** Single-fraction high-precision radiation treatment for intracranial lesions.
**Related Terms:** SRT, Brain mask, Sub-mm accuracy
**Radiotherapy Example:** Cone-based SRS was used to treat a 12-mm AVM in one fraction.

332. **Stereotactic Body Radiotherapy (SBRT) Meaning:** Ablative high-dose radiotherapy delivered in 3–5 fractions to extracranial sites.
**Related Terms:** Hypofractionation, Motion Management, Breath Hold
**Radiotherapy Example:** Lung SBRT 54 Gy/3# with 4D-CT to control respiratory motion.

333. **STAR Phantom Meaning:** QA phantom for evaluation of stereotactic targeting accuracy.
**Related Terms:** Winston–Lutz test, Isocenter QA, Mechanical accuracy
**Radiotherapy Example:** Monthly STAR phantom QA verified isocenter displacement < 0.7 mm

334. **Shielding Blocks Meaning:** Physical devices used to block dose to protect organs at risk.
**Related Terms:** MLC protection, Cerrobend, Custom shielding
**Radiotherapy Example:** Mould-room fabricated lead blocks protected spinal cord during abdominal 3DCRT.

335. **Slice Thickness Meaning:** Width of CT image slices captured during treatment simulation.
**Related Terms:** Spatial Resolution, Contouring accuracy
**Radiotherapy Example:** 1.25 mm slice thickness used for mask-based head & neck CT simulation.

336. **Simulation CT Meaning:** CT scan acquired in treatment position for RT planning.
**Related Terms:** Immobilisation, Tattoos, Planning CT
**Radiotherapy Example:** Breast simulation CT performed with wing board and indexed breast positioners.

337. **Skin Markers Meaning:** Radiopaque or skin-ink reference points used for reproducible setup.
**Related Terms:** Tattoos, Fiducial markers, Laser alignment
**Radiotherapy Example:** CT-compatible skin markers were used for pelvis IGRT localisation.

338. **Source Calibration Meaning:** Verification of the correct radiation source strength.
**Related Terms:** Air-kerma strength, Well chamber, TG-43
**Radiotherapy Example:** Annual Ir-192 source calibration confirmed activity within ±2% tolerance.

339. **Step-and-Shoot IMRT Meaning:** IMRT technique where beam turns off between MLC segment deliveries.
**Related Terms:** Segmental MLC, Static IMRT, IMRT QA
**Radiotherapy Example:** Prostate IMRT used 80 fixed MLC segments in step-and-shoot mode.

340. **Sliding Window IMRT Meaning:** IMRT technique with continuous MLC motion while the beam remains ON.
**Related Terms:** Dynamic MLC, VMAT, Dose modulation
**Radiotherapy Example:** Sliding-window IMRT delivered a H&N plan with smooth dose gradient.

341. **Secondary Monitor Unit Check Meaning:** Independent MU verification to detect calculation errors before treatment.
**Related Terms:** MU review, Dose validation, Pretreatment QA
**Radiotherapy Example:** Secondary MU check approved by physicist before starting VMAT therapy.

342. **Source-to-Skin Distance (SSD) Meaning:** Distance between the radiation source and the patient's skin.
**Related Terms:** SSD technique, Electron beam dose
**Radiotherapy Example:** 105 cm SSD was used for electron boost to surgical scar.

343. **Setup Error Meaning:** Difference between planned and actual patient position during treatment.
**Related Terms:** IGRT, Systematic error, Random error
**Radiotherapy Example:** Daily kV IGRT reduced pelvis setup error from 6 mm to 2 mm.

344. **Scoliosis Shielding Meaning:** Radiation shielding modifications for curved spinal anatomical geometry.
**Related Terms:** Compensators, Field Shaping, MLC shielding
**Radiotherapy Example:** Compensator-based scoliosis shielding protected lungs during paediatric T-spine RT.

345. **Subcutaneous Dose Build-up Meaning:** Increase in dose at shallow depth due to photon build-up effect.
**Related Terms:** Build-up region, Surface dose, Bolus
**Radiotherapy Example:** Without bolus, build-up peak occurred at 1.4 cm depth for 6 MV beam.

346. **Survival Curve Meaning:** Graph representing cell survival fraction vs absorbed dose.
**Related Terms:** LQ model, Radiosensitivity, RBE
**Radiotherapy Example:** Glioblastoma survival curve analysis identified high radioresistance ($\alpha/\beta \approx 1.5$).

347. **Scatter Kernel Meaning:** Mathematical model representing distributed scatter dose in tissue.
**Related Terms:** Convolution Algorithm, Dose Calculation, Kernel-based TPS
**Radiotherapy Example:** TPS used scatter kernel convolution for accurate photon dose computation.

348. **Statistical Uncertainty:** Variation in measured or calculated dose due to limited sampling or noise.
**Related Terms:** Monte Carlo, Noise Reduction, Dose Accuracy
**Radiotherapy Example:** Monte Carlo dose calculation for lung VMAT showed 2.1% statistical uncertainty, within tolerance.

349. **Scan Range:** Total anatomical length included in CT simulation.
**Related Terms:** FOV, Simulation CT, Planning Volume
**Radiotherapy Example:** Head & neck CT used a scan range from skull vertex to carina for full nodal coverage.

350. **SRS Immobilization Frame:** Rigid stereotactic head-frame device ensuring near-zero motion.
**Related Terms:** Bite Block, VAC-Loc Mask, Accuracy <1 mm
**Radiotherapy Example:** Used SRS head frame for single-fraction treatment of brain metastasis.

351. **Secondary Collimator:** Device inside LINAC head (jaws) for shaping photon beams.
**Related Terms:** X-jaws, Y-jaws, MLC
**Radiotherapy Example:** Jaws set to 0.2 cm margin beyond PTV to reduce leakage.

352. **Scan Timing Synchronization:** Matching CT image acquisition to respiratory or cardiac cycles.
**Related Terms:** 4D-CT, Gating, Motion Management
**Radiotherapy Example:** 4D-CT gating was synchronized to end-exhalation for pancreas SBRT.

353. **Skin Bolus Build-Up Technique:** Use of bolus to intentionally shift build-up region to skin for dose enhancement.
**Related Terms:** Surface Dose, Scar Boost, Electron Therapy
**Radiotherapy Example:** 5mm bolus used daily for chest wall RT to treat post-mastectomy scar.

354. **Supine Positioning:** Patient lies face-up during radiotherapy simulation or treatment.
**Related Terms:** Immobilisation, Rigid Setup, Indexing
**Radiotherapy Example:** Breast and pelvis treatments are commonly delivered in supine position for reproducibility.

355. **Sagittal Laser Alignment:** Laser positioning along the body midline for accurate patient setup.
**Related Terms:** Tattoos, IGRT, Room Lasers
**Radiotherapy Example:** Sagittal laser aligned midline pelvis mark before cone-beam imaging.

356. **Selective Internal Radiation Therapy (SIRT):** Localized microsphere-based radiation delivered through arteries to liver tumors.
**Related Terms:** Y-90, Radioembolization, Interventional Oncology
**Radiotherapy Example:** Y-90 SIRT performed for hepatocellular carcinoma with portal vein invasion.

357. **Stereotactic Couch Rotation:** Couch rotation with sub-millimeter precision during SRS/SBRT.
**Related Terms:** Non-coplanar Beams, Isocenter Accuracy
**Radiotherapy Example:** Non-coplanar SRS beams planned using controlled couch rotation for skull-base tumor.

358. **Surface Guided Radiation Therapy (SGRT):** Real-time setup and motion monitoring using optical surface scanning.
**Related Terms:** DIBH, Optical Tracking, Markerless IGRT
**Radiotherapy Example:** Breast DIBH treated with SGRT instead of tattoos to eliminate extra imaging dose.

359. **Scleral Shield:** Radiation eye shield protecting the sclera and lens.
**Related Terms:** Ophthalmic Radiation, Eye Shields
**Radiotherapy Example:** Scleral shield used during electron therapy for eyelid lesion.

360. **Scatter-to-Primary Ratio (SPR):** Ratio of scattered radiation intensity to primary beam intensity.
**Related Terms:** Collimator Scatter, Phantom Scatter, Image Quality
**Radiotherapy Example:** Low SPR achieved with tighter jaws for pelvis CBCT imaging.

361. **Superficial X-Ray Therapy:** Low-energy X-ray treatment for lesions near skin surface.
**Related Terms:** kV Therapy, Skin Cancer, Electron Alternative
**Radiotherapy Example:** 50 kVp superficial RT delivered to treat basal-cell carcinoma.

362. **SPECT/CT Fusion:** Co-registration of SPECT and CT images for combined functional–anatomical mapping.
**Related Terms:** PET, Hybrid Imaging, Auto-Segmentation
**Radiotherapy Example:** Bone SPECT/CT fusion used to refine target delineation in metastatic spine RT.

363. **Spatial Resolution:** Ability of an imaging system to differentiate small structures clearly.
**Related Terms:** Pixel Size, CT Slice Thickness, Noise
**Radiotherapy Example:** High-resolution CT (1 mm slices) used for acoustic neuroma planning.

364. **Set-On Time:** Period between patient setup completion and beam ON time.
**Related Terms:** Workflow, Session Duration, Therapist Efficiency
**Radiotherapy Example:** SBRT workflow optimization reduced set-on time from 18 min to 9 min.

365. **Segmented Treatment Field:** Field delivered through multiple MLC segments rather than a single open field.
**Related Terms:** Step-and-Shoot, Intensity Modulation, MLC
**Radiotherapy Example:** Five-segment field created to avoid kidneys during abdominal 3DCRT.

366. **Sternal Compression Device:** Equipment to restrict chest motion during breathing-sensitive RT.
**Related Terms:** Motion Management, ABC, DIBH
**Radiotherapy Example:** Compression plate used for liver SBRT to minimize diaphragm excursion.

367. **Spectral Filtration:** Modification of beam energy spectrum using filters to improve dose or image quality.
**Related Terms:** Flattening Filter, Half-Value Layer, Tantalum Filter
**Radiotherapy Example:** Spectral filtration in CBCT reduced scatter and increased soft-tissue contrast.

368. **Spectral Matching:** Adjusting beam energy or filtration to match reference dosimetric spectrum.
**Related Terms:** Beam Calibration, Half-Value Layer, Quality Index
**Radiotherapy Example:** LINAC beam fine-tuned to match 6 MV reference spectrum before commissioning IMRT plans.

369. **Spinal Canal Shielding:** Radiation blocking technique to protect spinal cord during posterior beam delivery.
**Related Terms:** MLC Blocking, 3DCRT, Organ-at-Risk Protection
**Radiotherapy Example:** Posterior oblique fields for abdominal tumor used MLC spinal shielding to maintain cord dose below 20 Gy.

370. **Spline-Based Contouring:** Use of mathematical spline interpolation to smooth anatomical contours.
**Related Terms:** Auto-Segmentation, AI Segmentation, Contour Editing
**Radiotherapy Example:** Prostate PTV contour refined using spline smoothing to avoid rectal indentation.

371. **Split-Arc VMAT Delivery:** VMAT technique dividing the arc into multiple partial arcs to avoid specific organs.
**Related Terms:** Avoidance Sectors, Non-Coplanar Arcs, SBRT
**Radiotherapy Example:** Split arcs used in pancreas SBRT to keep duodenum outside high-dose region.

372. **Stereotactic Localization Box:** Frame with fiducial arrays used for geometric localization in stereotactic simulation.
**Related Terms:** SRS Coordinate System, Localizer Frame
**Radiotherapy Example:** MR localizer box used to establish stereotactic coordinates for acoustic neuroma SRS.

373. **Setup Margin Reduction Protocol:** Workflow designed to safely reduce PTV margins by incorporating advanced IGRT.
**Related Terms:** Motion Tracking, SGRT, Daily CBCT
**Radiotherapy Example:** Pelvic IMRT margin reduced from 10 mm → 5 mm using daily CBCT + SGRT.

374. **Surface Collimator Tray:** Tray holding blocks or bolus material close to patient surface.
**Related Terms:** Custom Blocks, Electron Cone, Physical Collimation
**Radiotherapy Example:** Wax bolus mounted on collimator tray for keloid electron therapy.

375. **Scatter Correction Algorithm:** Software method to reduce scatter effects in CT or CBCT images.
**Related Terms:** AEC, Reconstruction Kernel, HU Accuracy
**Radiotherapy Example:** Liver CBCT HU accuracy improved using scatter correction algorithm for adaptive replanning.

**376. Static Couch Indexing:** Fixing couch to identical, reproducible index positions for every session.
**Related Terms:** Immobilization, Setup Reproducibility
**Radiotherapy Example:** Thermoplastic mask baseplate indexed to couch T-slots for repeatable brain SRT alignment.

**377. Secondary Check System:** Independent dose-calculation software verifying TPS dose output.
**Related Terms:** RadCalc, Mobius, MU Verification
**Radiotherapy Example:** Independent MU check performed before first fraction of lung VMAT.

**378. Segment Weight Optimization:** Adjusting beamlet intensity or segment weights to improve plan quality.
**Related Terms:** IMRT Optimization, Fluence Modulation
**Radiotherapy Example:** Segment weighting decreased to reduce bladder dose in cervical IMRT.

**379. Shielding Block Verification:** Confirming block shapes and positions are accurate before treatment.
**Related Terms:** Cerrobend Blocks, Light Field Match, Block Cutting
**Radiotherapy Example:** Cobalt chest wall blocks verified using light field + portal film.

**380. Scatter Air Ratio (SAR):** Scatter component of dose in air per unit field size.
**Related Terms:** TAR, TMR, Collimator Scatter
**Radiotherapy Example:** SAR used for manual dose calculation of jaw-defined fields in cobalt unit.

**381. Skin Dose Monitoring:** Evaluating absorbed dose to the surface during RT.
**Related Terms:** MOSFET, OSLD, Build-Up Region
**Radiotherapy Example:** MOSFET used to confirm breast boost skin dose $< 120\%$ of prescription.

**382. Sequential Boost Technique:** Delivering whole-volume dose first, followed by focused boost dose.
**Related Terms:** SIB, Two-Phase Planning, Field Reduction
**Radiotherapy Example:** Breast RT: 40 Gy whole breast + 10 Gy sequential boost to tumor bed.

**383. SRS Quality Assurance Phantom:** High-precision phantom to test stereotactic delivery accuracy.
**Related Terms:** Winston-Lutz, Isocenter QA, Small Field Dosimetry
**Radiotherapy Example:** Monthly Winston–Lutz test using SRS QA phantom verified 0.6 mm isocenter accuracy.

**384. Soft-Tissue Visualization Optimization:** Improving CBCT or MRI settings to enhance soft-tissue contrast for IGRT.
**Related Terms:** Window/Level, Reconstruction Kernel
**Radiotherapy Example:** Pelvic CBCT soft-tissue preset used for daily prostate localization.

**385. Spectral Photon Counting CT:** Detector technology separating X-ray photons by energy for enhanced imaging.
**Related Terms:** Dual-Energy CT, Material Decomposition
**Radiotherapy Example:** Better tumor–pancreas contrast helped reduce PTV margin during SBRT.

**386. Setup Time Benchmarking:** Setting KPIs for average patient setup duration to improve workflow.
**Related Terms:** Time Efficiency, Throughput, Operational QA
**Radiotherapy Example:** Department reduced setup time for breast IGRT from 12 min → 7 min.

**387. Scintillating Detector Dosimetry:** Real-time dosimetry using scintillating fibers or crystals.
**Related Terms:** Plastic Scintillator, Cherenkov Light, In-Vivo Dosimetry
**Radiotherapy Example:** Scintillator placed on nasal bridge skin measured dose during electron therapy.

388. **Simultaneous Imaging and Delivery QA:** Verifying LINAC capability to acquire imaging while delivering predefined dose patterns.
**Related Terms:** IGRT, KVCBCT + Beam-On, Hybrid Mode
**Radiotherapy Example:** QA confirmed beam-on imaging accuracy for breath-hold liver SBRT.

389. **System Latency Evaluation:** Measuring delay between motion detection and beam response in gating/tracking systems.
**Related Terms:** Motion Tracking, Real-Time Gating
**Radiotherapy Example:** Latency kept under 200 ms for lung tumor tracking accuracy.

390. **Sterile Applicator Technique:** Use of sterilized applicators for brachytherapy insertion to prevent infection.
**Related Terms:** HDR, Cervical Ring Applicator, Ovoids
**Radiotherapy Example:** Gynecologic HDR applicators sterilized for each treatment fraction.

391. **Sub-Arc Collimation:** Changing collimator angle or jaw position within a VMAT arc.
**Related Terms:** Collimator Rotation, Avoidance Sectors
**Radiotherapy Example:** Sub-arc collimation reduced tongue-and-groove effect for head-and-neck VMAT.

392. **Synchronicity Error Detection:** Checking synchronization between MLC motion, dose rate and gantry speed.
**Related Terms:** QA Log Files, Delivery Tolerance, VMAT Integrity
**Radiotherapy Example:** Error detected when MLC lag caused fluence deviation in prostate VMAT.

393. **Scatter Kernel Superposition:** Algorithm summing scatter kernels to estimate 3D dose distribution.
**Related Terms:** Convolution/Superposition, Pencil Beam Algorithm
**Radiotherapy Example:** TPS used superposition model for lung heterogeneity-corrected planning.

394. **Spatial Dose Gradient Evaluation:** Measurement of dose fall-off between high-dose and low-dose regions.
**Related Terms:** Paddick Gradient Index, GTV-to-OAR Transition
**Radiotherapy Example:** SBRT plan achieved 10 Gy/mm gradient around spinal metastasis.

395. **Smart Adaptive Planning:** AI-driven auto-replanning based on daily anatomy changes.
**Related Terms:** Adaptive RT, Auto-Segmentation, Dose Re-Optimization
**Radiotherapy Example:** Automatically-generated bladder adaptive plan used when volume change >20%.

396. **Scalp Sparing Technique:** Planning approach to minimize alopecia during cranial irradiation.
**Related Terms:** Hair-Follicle Protection, Beam Modulation
**Radiotherapy Example:** VMAT field shaping spared scalp for whole-brain RT palliative case.

397. **Self-Shielded LINAC Vault:** LINAC system incorporating built-in shielding that reduces bunker construction requirements.
**Related Terms:** Compact LINAC, Radiation Protection, Structural Shielding
**Radiotherapy Example:** Small cancer center installed self-shielded 6 MV LINAC without concrete vault upgrade.

398. **Source-to-Axis Distance (SAD) Calibration:** Verification that the distance from radiation source to isocenter is accurate.
**Related Terms:** 100 cm SAD, Isocenter QA, Mechanical Accuracy
**Radiotherapy Example:** SAD measured using front pointer + graph paper tool to ensure 100.0 cm alignment for LINAC treatments.

**399. Stereotactic Plan Complexity Index:** Score describing modulation complexity for SRS/SBRT fields.
**Related Terms:** MLC Modulation Factor, VMAT Complexity, MU Index
**Radiotherapy Example:** High complexity index triggered QA review for spine SBRT VMAT plan.

**400. Skin Mark Verification Protocol:** Workflow checking that patient skin tattoos or stickers match planned position.
**Related Terms:** Setup Reproducibility, Laser Alignment, IGRT
**Radiotherapy Example:** Pelvic RT tattoos cross-checked with red and green lasers before CBCT.

**401. Superior–Inferior (SI) Motion Modeling:** Estimating tumor or organ motion along the SI axis due to breathing or swallowing.
**Related Terms:** 4DCT, Internal Target Volume, Gating
**Radiotherapy Example:** 10 mm SI diaphragm motion added to ITV margin in liver 4DCT planning.

**402. SIB (Simultaneous Integrated Boost) Optimization:** Delivering different dose levels to regions within same plan and fraction.
**Related Terms:** Multi-Dose VMAT, Boost vs. Sequential, SBRT
**Radiotherapy Example:** Head & Neck IMRT: 70 Gy to tumor + 60 Gy to nodes simultaneously.

**403. Shielding Door Interlock QA:** Checking that treatment cannot start while door is open or interlock is bypassed.
**Related Terms:** Radiation Protection, Safety Systems, Treatment Hold
**Radiotherapy Example:** LINAC auto-beam-hold confirmed when vault door opened mid-test.

**404. Secondary Neutron Dose Estimation:** Assessing neutron dose produced by high-energy (>10 MV) photon beams.
**Related Terms:** High-Energy LINAC, Passive Scattering, NCRP Reports
**Radiotherapy Example:** Neutron dose calculated during 15 MV prostate IMRT commissioning.

**405. Surface Entry Point Mapping:** Documenting exact beam entry points on patient surface to avoid sensitive structures.
**Related Terms:** Beam Path Avoidance, Mould Room Marking, Skin Marking
**Radiotherapy Example:** Spine SBRT surface entry map ensured no beam passed through scapular screw.

**406. Scalp Bolus Technique:** Applying bolus to increase scalp dose in tumors where full-skin coverage required.
**Related Terms:** Electron Therapy, Build-Up Removal, Skin Dose
**Radiotherapy Example:** Electron bolus applied for recurrent scalp carcinoma.

**407. Sub-Gy Fractionation:** Treatment schedule delivering <1 Gy per fraction for benign or immune modulation cases.
**Related Terms:** Low-Dose RT, Anti-Inflammatory RT, Total Body Irradiation
**Radiotherapy Example:** 0.5 Gy × 6 fractions used for plantar fasciitis RT.

**408. Static Gantry Conformal Technique:** 3DCRT technique using fixed beams shaped around PTV.
**Related Terms:** Field Shaping, Wedges, Forward Planning
**Radiotherapy Example:** Breast tangential 3DCRT using wedges and static tangential fields.

**409. Scatter Medium Beam Attenuation:** Dose reduction caused by absorber/scatter medium along beam path.
**Related Terms:** Tissue Heterogeneity, Lung Correction, CT Electron Density
**Radiotherapy Example:** TPS accounted for lung attenuation in thoracic esophagus IMRT.

410. **Salivary Gland Sparing Strategy:** Dose-limiting planning to preserve salivary function in head-and-neck RT.
**Related Terms:** Parotid Constraint, Xerostomia, OAR Prioritization
**Radiotherapy Example:** VMAT optimized to maintain parotid mean <26 Gy.

411. **Setup Error Motion Tracking:** Monitoring magnitude and direction of setup deviation over multiple fractions.
**Related Terms:** Shift Trend Report, SGRT Logs, CBCT Registration
**Radiotherapy Example:** Trend tracking showed increasing left-lateral drift, mask refitted.

412. **Small Animal Irradiator Calibration:** Calibration of preclinical irradiation systems used for research.
**Related Terms:** Micro-Irradiator, Dosimetry, Biological Modeling
**Radiotherapy Example:** Mouse brain micro-irradiator calibrated with ion chamber + film.

413. **Stretcher Transfer Protocol:** Procedure to move patients from stretcher to couch while maintaining immobilization.
**Related Terms:** Setup Reproducibility, Rigid Immobilization
**Radiotherapy Example:** Cervical spine patient transferred with mask secured to prevent alignment error.

414. **Sub-Isocentric Beam Arrangement:** Fields planned around a point different from machine isocenter for flexibility.
**Related Terms:** Conformal Therapy, Field Matching
**Radiotherapy Example:** Lower spine fields sub-isocentrically matched with cranial field.

415. **SGRT (Surface Guided Radiation Therapy) Docking:** Aligning patient to surface guidance reference before beam-on.
**Related Terms:** Optical Tracking, No-Tattoo RT, DIBH
**Radiotherapy Example:** SGRT docking used for breath-hold left-breast DIBH without CBCT re-scan.

416. **Scatter-to-Primary Ratio (SPR):** Ratio of scattered radiation to primary beam used in dose estimation.
**Related Terms:** Scatter Factors, Beam Modeling
**Radiotherapy Example:** SPR measured to validate dose accuracy for large pelvic fields.

417. **Step-and-Shoot Delivery Record Review:** Evaluation of MU per segment and MLC positions in static IMRT.
**Related Terms:** Segment QA, Log File Review, Multileaf Positioning
**Radiotherapy Example:** Liver IMRT delivery logs reviewed to verify all segments delivered correctly.

418. **Sinus Avoidance Trajectory:** Beam arrangement that avoids passing radiation through paranasal sinuses.
**Related Terms:** Avoidance Sectors, Non-Coplanar Arcs
**Radiotherapy Example:** SRS plan selected inferior–posterior arcs to avoid sinus air cavities.

419. **Skin Bridge Preservation Technique:** Planning strategy to avoid excessive dose to skin folds or tissue bridges.
**Related Terms:** PTV Editing, Beam Entry Pattern, Skin Sparing
**Radiotherapy Example:** Pelvic VMAT protected perineal tissue bridge from high dose.

**420. Scattered Dose Feasibility Test:** Predicting unintended dose to non-target regions by scattered radiation.
**Related Terms:** Out-of-Field Dose, Pediatric RT, Cataract Risk
**Radiotherapy Example:** Scattered dose to lens estimated for nasopharynx IMRT.

**421. Short SAD Electron Treatment:** Using reduced source-to-surface distance to increase dose at shallow depth.
**Related Terms:** SSD Variation, Electron Applicator
**Radiotherapy Example:** SSB 95 cm SSD electron boost used for forehead recurrence.

**422. Surgical Bed Contouring Rules:** Standard guidelines for defining target volumes after tumor resection.
**Related Terms:** CTV Post-Op, Seroma Cavity, Clips Identification
**Radiotherapy Example:** Breast surgical bed contoured based on seroma + clips per RTOG criteria.

**423. Symmetric vs. Asymmetric Jaw Tuning:** Adjustment of jaws equally or unequally to shape field edges.
**Related Terms:** Penumbra, Field Size Configuration
**Radiotherapy Example:** Asymmetric jaws used to block spinal cord in 3DCRT abdomen.

**424. Secondary Malignancy Risk Modeling:** Long-term estimation of cancer risk due to exposure from RT.
**Related Terms:** Out-of-Field Dose, Risk Modeling, Pediatric RT
**Radiotherapy Example:** Pediatric Hodgkin RT evaluated using BEIR-based risk estimation.

**425. SRS Collision Clearance Simulation:** Virtual system predicting couch-gantry-patient collisions before delivery.
**Related Terms:** Non-Coplanar Arcs, Couch Rotation, Brain SRS
**Radiotherapy Example:** Girder-avoidance simulation generated safe arc path for skull base lesion.

**426. Skin Dose Reduction Shield:** Device placed over skin to decrease electron contamination and entrance dose.
**Related Terms:** Skin Sparing, Custom Shield, Beam Spoiler
**Radiotherapy Example:** Breast copper skin shield reduced entrance dose 12%.

**427. Spatial Dose Warping for Adaptation:** Transforming previous dose distribution to new anatomy for adaptive planning.
**Related Terms:** Deformable Dose Accumulation, Adaptive RT, DIR
**Radiotherapy Example:** Prior bladder dose distribution warped onto daily CBCT for adaptive plan selection.

**428. Stepwise Dose Escalation:** Gradually increasing dose to tumor in successive fractions while monitoring toxicity.
**Related Terms:** Fractionation, Dose-Limiting Toxicity, Adaptive RT
**Radiotherapy Example:** Prostate SBRT escalated from 7 Gy × 5 fractions to 8 Gy × 5 after tolerance check.

**429. Standardized Imaging Protocol:** Uniform protocol for imaging acquisition to ensure reproducibility across patients.
**Related Terms:** CT Simulation, MRI Sequence, PET/CT
**Radiotherapy Example:** Head & neck CT simulation performed using standardized 1.5 mm slice thickness.

**430. Surface Dose Enhancement:** Technique to increase dose to skin or shallow targets.
**Related Terms:** Bolus, Electron Therapy, Build-Up Region
**Radiotherapy Example:** 0.5 cm Superflab bolus used for scalp metastases.

**431. Stereotactic Cone Calibration:** QA procedure for small-field SRS cones ensuring correct output and geometry.
**Related Terms:** SRS, Cone Factor, Output Verification
**Radiotherapy Example:** Brain metastases cones calibrated before treatment with ion chamber and film.

**432. Sliding Window Delivery QA:** Verifying IMRT delivered via continuous MLC motion ("sliding window").
**Related Terms:** VMAT QA, MLC Position, Dose Distribution
**Radiotherapy Example:** Head & Neck IMRT plan delivered to phantom for sliding window QA.

**433. Spinal Cord Dose Constraint Verification:** Ensuring spinal cord does not exceed tolerance in treatment planning.
**Related Terms:** OAR Dose Limit, DVH Review, PRV
**Radiotherapy Example:** Thoracic spine plan checked that cord max <45 Gy.

**434. Setup Laser Alignment QA:** Checking alignment of room lasers with machine isocenter.
**Related Terms:** SAD, Isocenter Verification, Mechanical QA
**Radiotherapy Example:** LINAC wall and ceiling lasers verified monthly to within ±1 mm.

**435. Short-Interval IGRT:** Imaging performed at short intervals to account for daily variations in patient position.
**Related Terms:** CBCT, kV Imaging, Online Correction
**Radiotherapy Example:** Pelvic IMRT verified daily using CBCT.

**436. Small Field Output Factor Measurement:** Dosimetric measurement of dose for small MLC-defined or cone fields.
**Related Terms:** Output Factor, Micro-MLC, SRS
**Radiotherapy Example:** SRS 1.0 cm cone output measured with stereotactic diode.

**437. Secondary Electron Contamination Control:** Minimizing dose from secondary electrons generated by photon beam interaction.
**Related Terms:** Beam Spoiler, Skin Dose, Electron Contamination
**Radiotherapy Example:** 10 MV beam with 1 cm bolus minimized surface electron contamination.

**438. Shielding Thickness Optimization:** Calculating minimum material thickness to protect staff and public.
**Related Terms:** Concrete Barrier, Lead Wall, NCRP Guidelines
**Radiotherapy Example:** Vault wall designed with 2.5 m concrete for 18 MV LINAC.

**439. Surface Imaging QA:** Verification of optical surface imaging system performance.
**Related Terms:** SGRT, DIBH, Patient Setup
**Radiotherapy Example:** Breast DIBH surface tracker QA performed weekly.

**440. Spinal Field Junction Verification:** Checking dose uniformity where multiple spinal fields meet.
**Related Terms:** Field Matching, Feathering, Junction Dose
**Radiotherapy Example:** Thoracic-lumbar junction IMRT verified using film.

**441. Scatter Dose Mapping:** Measurement of unintended dose from scattered photons and electrons.
**Related Terms:** Out-of-Field Dose, Phantom Measurement
**Radiotherapy Example:** Pediatric phantom used to map scatter outside target volume.

**442. Safety Interlock Testing:** Routine testing of interlocks that prevent accidental radiation delivery.
**Related Terms:** Door Interlocks, Beam Hold, QA
**Radiotherapy Example:** LINAC beam does not start when door open, tested monthly.

443. **Slice-by-Slice Dose Verification:** Confirming calculated vs. delivered dose for each CT slice.
**Related Terms:** 3D Dosimetry, Film, QA Phantom
**Radiotherapy Example:** Head phantom irradiated slice-by-slice to verify IMRT plan.

444. **Synchronous Multi-Modality Imaging:** Using multiple imaging techniques at the same time for accurate planning.
**Related Terms:** PET/CT, MRI Fusion, Image Registration
**Radiotherapy Example:** PET/MRI fusion used for accurate GTV delineation.

445. **Spot-Scanning Proton Beam QA:** Verification of individual proton spot positions, dose, and energy.
**Related Terms:** Pencil Beam Scanning, Bragg Peak, Range Verification
**Radiotherapy Example:** QA phantom scanned with proton spots matched TPS plan.

446. **Secondary Radiation Shielding Evaluation:** Assessment of shielding against neutrons, scattered photons, and induced radioactivity.
**Related Terms:** Neutron Flux, Secondary Dose, Shielding Design
**Radiotherapy Example:** 15 MV LINAC vault evaluated for secondary neutron protection.

447. **Simulation CT Scan Protocol:** Standardized CT imaging parameters for treatment simulation.
**Related Terms:** Slice Thickness, KV/MV CT, Immobilization
**Radiotherapy Example:** 3 mm slice head & neck CT with mask used for planning.

448. **Stereotactic Target Localization QA:** Ensuring accurate positioning of small lesions in SRS/SBRT.
**Related Terms:** Frame-Based, Frameless, Image Registration
**Radiotherapy Example:** Brain metastasis localization verified using CBCT.

449. **Skin Toxicity Assessment:** Monitoring acute or chronic skin reactions from radiation.
**Related Terms:** RTOG/EORTC Grading, Dermatitis, Bolus Effects
**Radiotherapy Example:** Weekly skin check during breast radiotherapy.

450. **Single-Isocenter Multi-Lesion Planning:** Planning for multiple targets using one isocenter.
**Related Terms:** SRS, VMAT, Non-Coplanar Arcs
**Radiotherapy Example:** Multiple brain metastases treated with single-isocenter VMAT.

451. **Surface Imaging-Based Breath Control:** Using optical surface imaging to guide deep inspiration breath-hold.
**Related Terms:** SGRT, DIBH, LINAC Gating
**Radiotherapy Example:** Left-breast DIBH monitored with SGRT system.

452. **Secondary Neutron Dose Monitoring:** Measuring neutron dose to staff or patient in high-energy photon beams.
**Related Terms:** Neutron Detector, High-Energy LINAC
**Radiotherapy Example:** Neutron dosimeter placed outside vault during 18 MV treatment.

453. **Slice Thickness QA:** Ensuring CT slices match planned slice thickness for accurate dose calculation.
**Related Terms:** CT Simulation, TPS Accuracy
**Radiotherapy Example:** 3 mm slice verification for head & neck planning.

454. **Surface Immobilization Device QA:** Testing the reproducibility of masks, vac-loc cushions, and molds.
**Related Terms:** Thermoplastic Mask, Vacuum Cushion, Mould Room
**Radiotherapy Example:** Head mask fit checked with daily IGRT before treatment.

455. **Spatial Resolution QA:** Checking imaging system resolution to detect small structures.
**Related Terms:** CT, CBCT, MRI, Line Pair Phantom
**Radiotherapy Example:** CBCT spatial resolution verified using phantom before IGRT.

**456. Secondary Electron Dose Modeling:** Estimating dose contribution from secondary electrons outside target.
**Related Terms:** Monte Carlo, Out-of-Field Dose, Electron Contamination
**Radiotherapy Example:** Monte Carlo model predicted skin dose from photon contamination.

**457. SRS Couch Rotation Accuracy:** Checking rotational accuracy of treatment couch for stereotactic treatments.
**Related Terms:** Non-Coplanar Beams, Couch Angle QA, Stereotactic Accuracy
**Radiotherapy Example:** Couch rotation tested using phantom for 90° non-coplanar arcs.

**458. Stochastic Radiation Risk Estimation:** Estimating probabilistic risk of late effects like cancer from radiation.
**Related Terms:** LNT Model, Organ Dose, Epidemiology
**Radiotherapy Example:** Pediatric craniospinal plan assessed for stochastic risk.

**459. Step-and-Shoot IMRT Verification:** Checking dose delivery for static MLC segments in IMRT plans.
**Related Terms:** Segment QA, MU Calculation, Delivery Accuracy
**Radiotherapy Example:** Head & neck IMRT phantom measurement matched TPS.

**460. Short-Range Electron Shielding:** Shielding for superficial electron beams to protect nearby structures.
**Related Terms:** Lead Cutout, Electron Applicator, OAR Protection
**Radiotherapy Example:** Scalp electron boost protected eyes using lead shields.

**461. Superficial Tumor Dose Assessment:** Measuring dose delivered to shallow tumors or skin lesions.
**Related Terms:** Surface Dosimetry, TLD, Film, Electron Therapy
**Radiotherapy Example:** Skin metastases dose verified using Gafchromic film.

**462. Stereotactic Arc Collision Clearance:** Simulation ensuring gantry/couch do not collide during non-coplanar arcs.
**Related Terms:** SRS, Couch Rotation, Collision Avoidance
**Radiotherapy Example:** Brain SRS plan arcs simulated for safe clearance.

**463. Secondary Radiation Leakage Test:** Measuring radiation leakage outside treatment head and shielding.
**Related Terms:** LINAC Head Leakage, Regulatory QA
**Radiotherapy Example:** Annual leakage test confirmed compliance for 6 MV and 15 MV beams.

**464. Skin Sparing Verification:** Confirming that photon/electron beams spare skin as intended.
**Related Terms:** Build-Up Region, Bolus, Surface Dose
**Radiotherapy Example:** Chest wall tangents verified for surface dose using TLD.

**465. Spot Position Accuracy QA:** Ensuring proton spots are delivered at planned coordinates.
**Related Terms:** PBS, MLC, Range Verification
**Radiotherapy Example:** Spot scanning QA confirmed <1 mm deviation.

**466. Secondary Particle Dose Mapping:** Mapping dose from neutrons, scattered photons, or electrons outside the target.
**Related Terms:** Out-of-Field Dose, Pediatric Protection
**Radiotherapy Example:** Phantom measured neutron and photon scatter for high-energy beam.

**467. Stereotactic Dose Gradient Assessment:** Evaluating steepness of dose fall-off around target.
**Related Terms:** Conformity Index, Gradient Index, SRS/SBRT
**Radiotherapy Example:** Brain metastasis SRS plan assessed for sharp dose fall-off.

468. **Safety QA Checklist:** Comprehensive checklist for daily, weekly, monthly, and annual QA.
**Related Terms:** LINAC QA, IGRT, Radiation Safety
**Radiotherapy Example:** Daily QA includes laser alignment, output check, and safety interlocks.

469. **Secondary Radiation Simulation:** Computational modeling of stray radiation to patient or staff.
**Related Terms:** Monte Carlo, Out-of-Field Dose, Shielding
**Radiotherapy Example:** Simulation predicted scatter dose to thyroid in pediatric chest treatment.

470. **Spin Echo MRI Fusion QA:** Verifying accuracy of MRI-CT fusion for treatment planning.
**Related Terms:** MRI Simulation, Co-Registration, Brain Tumor Planning
**Radiotherapy Example:** MRI T1-weighted fusion verified with bony landmarks.

471. **Skin Fold Dose Assessment:** Measuring dose in skin folds that may receive higher than planned dose.
**Related Terms:** Bolus, Hot Spot, Patient Anatomy
**Radiotherapy Example:** Axilla region monitored for hotspots during breast RT.

472. **Shielded Mould Room QA:** Ensuring mould room shielding and patient immobilization devices meet standards.
**Related Terms:** Thermoplastic Mask, Vacuum Cushion, Lead Shield
**Radiotherapy Example:** Head & neck masks fabricated in shielded room for safe dose distribution.

473. **Single-Isocenter Multi-Target QA:** Verifying accuracy when treating multiple targets with one isocenter.
**Related Terms:** SRS, Arc Therapy, Non-Coplanar QA
**Radiotherapy Example:** Multiple brain lesions QA verified using phantom.

474. **Step-Wise Imaging Dose Accumulation:** Summing daily imaging dose to evaluate cumulative exposure.
**Related Terms:** kV CBCT, MV Imaging, Cumulative Dose
**Radiotherapy Example:** Daily pelvic CBCT dose accumulated for patient safety.

475. **Surface Mould Electron Boost QA:** QA for superficial electron boost delivered via custom surface moulds.
**Related Terms:** Electron Therapy, Bolus, Surface Dosimetry
**Radiotherapy Example:** Scalp boost with custom mould verified with TLD.

476. **Secondary Photon Contamination Analysis:** Measurement and analysis of photon contamination in electron beams.
**Related Terms:** Electron Therapy, Out-of-Field Dose, Photon Contamination
**Radiotherapy Example:** 6 MeV electron beam checked for 1.2% photon contamination.

477. **Staff Radiation Safety Training Protocol:** Standardized training for radiation workers on protection and emergency procedures.
**Related Terms:** PPE, ALARA, Regulatory Compliance
**Radiotherapy Example:** Annual refresher course for LINAC, CT, and mould room staff.

478. **Setup uncertainty (noun):** Variation in patient positioning between planning and treatment delivery.
**Related Terms:** Interfraction error, PTV margin.
**Example in Radiotherapy:** Accounted for when expanding CTV to PTV.

479. **Signal-to-noise ratio (noun):** Measure comparing useful signal strength to background noise.
**Related Terms:** Image quality, Noise level.
**Example in Radiotherapy:** Higher SNR improves CBCT soft-tissue visualization.

480. **Simulated treatment verification (noun):** Dry-run of treatment delivery without patient exposure.
**Related Terms:** Pretreatment QA, Workflow check.
**Example in Radiotherapy:** Used before first fraction of SBRT.

481. **Source positioning accuracy (noun):** Precision of radioactive source placement in brachytherapy.
**Related Terms:** Dwell position, Applicator reconstruction.
**Example in Radiotherapy:** Critical for HDR prostate implants.

482. **Spatial resolution (noun):** Ability to distinguish small structures in imaging.
**Related Terms:** Pixel size, Image sharpness.
**Example in Radiotherapy:** High spatial resolution needed for SRS planning.

483. **Scatter radiation (noun):** Radiation deflected from its original path after interaction.
**Related Terms:** Secondary radiation, Leakage.
**Example in Radiotherapy:** Contributes to out-of-field dose.

484. **Secondary dose calculation (noun):** Independent computation to verify planned dose.
**Related Terms:** MU check, QA.
**Example in Radiotherapy:** Used to confirm IMRT monitor units.

485. **Segment delivery accuracy (noun):** Precision of dose delivery for each IMRT segment.
**Related Terms:** MLC positioning, Dynamic delivery.
**Example in Radiotherapy:** Evaluated during patient-specific QA.

486. **Sensitivity analysis (noun):** Evaluation of how parameter changes affect outcomes.
**Related Terms:** Robustness testing, Uncertainty analysis.
**Example in Radiotherapy:** Used to test plan stability against setup errors.

487. **Sequential treatment planning (noun):** Planning approach where boost is created after primary plan.
**Related Terms:** Sequential boost, Phase planning.
**Example in Radiotherapy:** Used in head-and-neck radiotherapy.

488. **Shielding effectiveness (noun):** Ability of barriers to reduce radiation exposure.
**Related Terms:** Attenuation, Radiation protection.
**Example in Radiotherapy:** Evaluated during room shielding surveys.

489. **Source decay correction (noun):** Adjustment accounting for radioactive source decay over time.
**Related Terms:** Half-life, Dose rate.
**Example in Radiotherapy:** Applied in HDR brachytherapy planning.

490. **Stability of beam output (noun):** Consistency of linac dose output over time.
**Related Terms:** Output constancy, QA.
**Example in Radiotherapy:** Checked daily before patient treatments.

491. **Statistical uncertainty (noun):** Random variation inherent in measurements or simulations.
**Related Terms:** Measurement error, Monte Carlo noise.
**Example in Radiotherapy:** Present in low-dose Monte Carlo calculations.

492. **Structure delineation accuracy (noun):** and OARs.
**Related Terms:** Contouring precision, Observer variability.
**Example in Radiotherapy:** Impacts dose coverage and toxicity risk.

493. **Surface dose estimation (noun):** Calculation of dose received at the skin surface.
**Related Terms:** Build-up region, Skin sparing.
**Example in Radiotherapy:** Important for chest wall treatments.

494. **System calibration (noun):** Process of aligning system output with reference standards.
**Related Terms:** Commissioning, QA.
**Example in Radiotherapy:** Linac calibrated using ionization chambers.

495. **Systematic uncertainty (noun):** Consistent deviation affecting all measurements similarly.
**Related Terms:** Bias, Systematic error.
**Example in Radiotherapy:** Corrected through protocol updates.

496. **Stereotactic accuracy (noun):** Overall precision of high-dose, high-accuracy treatments.
**Related Terms:** Localization accuracy, Isocenter precision.
**Example in Radiotherapy:** Required for intracranial SRS.

497. **Simulation accuracy (noun):** Degree to which CT simulation represents treatment geometry.
**Related Terms:** Patient positioning, Imaging fidelity.
**Example in Radiotherapy:** Ensures tattoos align with isocenter.

498. **Segment weight optimization (noun):** Adjustment of relative MU contribution of each segment.
**Related Terms:** Fluence optimization, IMRT planning.
**Example in Radiotherapy:** Used to reduce hotspots.

499. **Soft-tissue contrast (noun):** Ability to differentiate soft tissues in imaging.
**Related Terms:** Image contrast, HU difference.
**Example in Radiotherapy:** Enhanced in MRI-guided radiotherapy.

500. **Safety margin (noun):** Extra allowance added to account for uncertainties.
**Related Terms:** PTV margin, Risk mitigation.
**Example in Radiotherapy:** Protects against setup and motion errors.

# T

1. **Target Volume Delineation:** Process of outlining tumor and organs at risk on imaging for treatment planning.
   **Related Terms:** GTV, CTV, PTV, CT Simulation
   **Radiotherapy Example:** Head & neck tumor delineated on planning CT before IMRT.
2. **Treatment Planning System (TPS):** Software that calculates dose distribution and creates treatment plans.
   **Related Terms:** Dose Calculation, Beam Modeling, IMRT, VMAT
   **Radiotherapy Example:** TPS used to generate prostate IMRT plan with 7 fields.
3. **Tissue Heterogeneity Correction:** Adjustment in dose calculation accounting for variable tissue density.
   **Related Terms:** CT Density, Monte Carlo Algorithm, Lung, Bone
   **Radiotherapy Example:** Lung SBRT plan corrected for low-density lung tissue in TPS.
4. **Total Body Irradiation (TBI):** Radiation delivered to the entire body, often for bone marrow transplant.
   **Related Terms:** Fractionation, LINAC, Shielding, Dose Rate
   **Radiotherapy Example:** TBI 12 Gy in 6 fractions with lung blocks for pediatric transplant.
5. **Treatment Fractionation:** Dividing total prescribed dose into multiple sessions to balance tumor control and toxicity.
   **Related Terms:** Hypofractionation, Conventional Fractionation, Dose per Fraction
   **Radiotherapy Example:** Breast cancer RT 25 × 2 Gy fractions over 5 weeks.
6. **Thermoplastic Mask Immobilization:** Custom mask to keep head/neck or other anatomy in reproducible position during RT.
   **Related Terms:** Mould Room, Patient Immobilization, IGRT
   **Radiotherapy Example:** Head & neck patient fitted with thermoplastic mask for daily CBCT verification.
7. **Tissue Compensator:** Device to make surface or tissue thickness uniform for consistent dose delivery.
   **Related Terms:** Bolus, 3D-Printed Compensator, Electron Therapy
   **Radiotherapy Example:** 3D compensator used for chest wall electron boost to reduce hot spots.
8. **Treatment Verification Imaging:** Imaging performed to ensure patient and tumor position match plan before delivery.
   **Related Terms:** CBCT, kV/MV Portal Imaging, IGRT
   **Radiotherapy Example:** Pelvic IMRT verified with daily CBCT for bladder and rectum positioning.
9. **Time-Dose Fractionation (TDF):** Historical method to quantify biological effect of different fractionation schedules.
   **Related Terms:** BED, Linear Quadratic Model, Fractionation
   **Radiotherapy Example:** Head & neck RT plan evaluated for TDF to compare regimens.
10. **Tumor Motion Management:** Techniques to account for tumor motion during treatment due to respiration or organ movement.
    **Related Terms:** Respiratory Gating, DIBH, 4D CT
    **Radiotherapy Example:** Lung SBRT using 4D CT and gating to track tumor motion.

11. **Tomotherapy:** Radiation therapy using helical delivery with integrated imaging.
    **Related Terms:** IGRT, Helical IMRT, LINAC
    **Radiotherapy Example:** Spinal metastases treated with tomotherapy plan and daily MVCT verification.
12. **Tissue Dose Escalation:** Increasing dose to tumor while respecting OAR constraints.
    **Related Terms:** Simultaneous Integrated Boost (SIB), DVH, Adaptive RT
    **Radiotherapy Example:** Head & neck SIB IMRT delivering 70 Gy to GTV, 56 Gy to CTV.
13. **Tumor Bed Boost:** Additional dose delivered to post-operative tumor site to reduce recurrence risk.
    **Related Terms:** Photon Boost, Electron Boost, Fractionation
    **Radiotherapy Example:** Breast lumpectomy site receives 10 Gy boost after whole-breast irradiation.
14. **Treatment Delivery QA:** Quality assurance of machine and plan prior to patient treatment.
    **Related Terms:** LINAC QA, IMRT QA, Portal Dosimetry
    **Radiotherapy Example:** Phantom measurement of prostate IMRT plan before first fraction.
15. **Tomographic Dose Reconstruction:** Calculating delivered dose based on in vivo imaging or exit dosimetry.
    **Related Terms:** CBCT, EPID, Dose Verification
    **Radiotherapy Example:** CBCT used to reconstruct delivered dose to spinal tumor.
16. **Tissue Equivalent Phantom:** Phantom mimicking human tissue for dosimetric QA.
    **Related Terms:** Solid Water, Rando Phantom, Ion Chamber
    **Radiotherapy Example:** Phantom used for head & neck IMRT verification in LINAC QA.
17. **Trapping Field Verification:** Checking the accuracy of blocked or shielded areas in treatment field.
    **Related Terms:** MLC, Lead Block, OAR Protection
    **Radiotherapy Example:** Eye shield verified in lateral head field for pediatric RT.
18. **Thermoluminescent Dosimeter (TLD) QA:** Using TLDs for patient or machine dose verification.
    **Related Terms:** In Vivo Dosimetry, Phantom, Calibration
    **Radiotherapy Example:** TLDs placed on breast surface to verify dose during tangential photon therapy.
19. **Treatment Couch Positioning QA:** Ensuring couch moves accurately to planned coordinates for isocenter alignment.
    **Related Terms:** IGRT, Couch Shift, LINAC QA
    **Radiotherapy Example:** Pelvic IMRT couch shift verified with daily CBCT.
20. **Tissue Heterogeneity Imaging:** Imaging to identify tissue density variations affecting dose distribution.
    **Related Terms:** CT HU Calibration, Electron Density, Dose Calculation
    **Radiotherapy Example:** Lung SBRT plan used CT HU to correct heterogeneity effects.
21. **Tomographic Imaging QA:** QA for imaging systems used in planning or verification, including CT or CBCT.
    **Related Terms:** Slice Thickness, Image Noise, Spatial Resolution
    **Radiotherapy Example:** Daily CBCT QA for LINAC-based IGRT verified alignment.
22. **Total Dose Monitoring:** Tracking cumulative dose delivered to tumor and OAR over course of treatment.
    **Related Terms:** DVH, Fractionation, Adaptive Therapy
    **Radiotherapy Example:** Spinal cord max dose monitored across 30 fractions.

23. **Tumor Tracking with Fiducials:** Using implanted markers to track tumor position in real time.
**Related Terms:** IGRT, CyberKnife, Real-Time Tracking
**Radiotherapy Example:** Liver metastasis tracked with gold fiducials during SBRT.

24. **Treatment Field Verification:** Confirming radiation field geometry matches planned target.
**Related Terms:** Portal Imaging, CBCT, MLC QA
**Radiotherapy Example:** Head & neck IMRT fields verified before first fraction using kV imaging.

25. **Tissue Penetration Depth Measurement:** Verifying depth dose profile in patient or phantom.
**Related Terms:** PDD, Electron Beam, Photon Beam
**Radiotherapy Example:** Electron boost to scalp verified with depth dose TLDs.

26. **Tumor-to-Organ-at-Risk (OAR) Ratio:** Ratio measuring proximity of tumor to critical organs to plan dose safely.
**Related Terms:** DVH, GTV, CTV, PTV
**Radiotherapy Example:** Liver SBRT planned with high tumor-to-liver OAR ratio, minimizing normal tissue dose.

27. **Tissue-Bolus Application:** Material placed on skin to increase surface dose or correct irregular contour.
**Related Terms:** Bolus, Electron Therapy, Surface Dose
**Radiotherapy Example:** Breast boost with 1 cm bolus to ensure adequate skin dose.

28. **Treatment Planning CT (Simulation CT):** CT scan acquired in treatment position for accurate dose planning.
**Related Terms:** Immobilization, Slice Thickness, IGRT
**Radiotherapy Example:** Head & neck patient scanned with thermoplastic mask in CT simulator for IMRT planning.

29. **Tomotherapy Delivery QA:** Quality assurance specifically for tomotherapy units verifying plan delivery.
**Related Terms:** Dose Verification, MVCT, LINAC QA
**Radiotherapy Example:** Spinal metastasis treatment plan verified on tomotherapy QA phantom.

30. **Tumor Conformity Index:** Metric evaluating how closely the high-dose region matches tumor shape.
**Related Terms:** PTV, DVH, IMRT, VMAT
**Radiotherapy Example:** Prostate IMRT plan achieved CI of 0.95, minimizing rectal dose.

31. **Tissue Density Calibration:** Calibrating CT Hounsfield units to physical/electron density for dose calculation.
**Related Terms:** CT Scanner, TPS, Dose Accuracy
**Radiotherapy Example:** Lung SBRT plan used calibrated CT density for heterogeneity correction.

32. **Treatment Couch Rotation Verification:** QA to ensure accurate rotational movements for non-coplanar beams.
**Related Terms:** LINAC, IGRT, Couch Shift
**Radiotherapy Example:** Brain metastasis plan verified with couch rotations for multiple non-coplanar beams.

33. **Tumor Hypoxia Imaging:** Imaging to assess oxygenation status of tumor affecting radiosensitivity.
**Related Terms:** PET, FMISO, Dose Painting
**Radiotherapy Example:** PET-FMISO scan identifies hypoxic regions for selective dose escalation.

34. **Tissue Equivalent Material QA:** QA of phantoms or materials mimicking tissue for dosimetric validation.
    **Related Terms:** Solid Water, Rando Phantom, TLD, Ion Chamber
    **Radiotherapy Example:** Head phantom used to verify brain IMRT dose distribution.
35. **Treatment Field Matching:** Technique ensuring adjacent radiation fields join seamlessly without under/overlap.
    **Related Terms:** Junction Dose, MLC, Field Alignment
    **Radiotherapy Example:** Spinal cranio field junction checked for correct match in LINAC plan.
36. **Target Volume Margin Assessment:** Determining safety margin around tumor to account for motion and setup errors.
    **Related Terms:** GTV, CTV, PTV, IGRT
    **Radiotherapy Example:** Prostate CTV expanded 5 mm to PTV for daily setup variations.
37. **Tomographic Image Fusion:** Combining multiple imaging modalities (CT, MRI, PET) for precise tumor delineation.
    **Related Terms:** Multimodality Imaging, IGRT, Radiology
    **Radiotherapy Example:** PET-CT fusion used for head & neck tumor delineation in TPS.
38. **Treatment Field Shaping:** Modifying radiation field to conform to tumor shape and spare normal tissue.
    **Related Terms:** MLC, Blocks, Conformal RT, IMRT
    **Radiotherapy Example:** Breast IMRT fields shaped using MLC to avoid heart and lung.
39. **Tissue Inhomogeneity Dose Correction:** Adjusting calculated dose for varying tissue densities to maintain accuracy.
    **Related Terms:** Lung, Bone, TPS, Monte Carlo Algorithm
    **Radiotherapy Example:** Lung tumor plan corrected for low-density lung tissue in TPS.
40. **Treatment Plan Adaptation:** Adjusting treatment plan during therapy to account for anatomical changes.
    **Related Terms:** Adaptive Radiotherapy, CBCT, Dose Recalculation
    **Radiotherapy Example:** Head & neck patient re-planned after 2 weeks due to tumor shrinkage.
41. **Target Motion Quantification:** Measurement of tumor displacement due to breathing or organ movement.
    **Related Terms:** 4D CT, Respiratory Gating, DIBH
    **Radiotherapy Example:** Lung tumor motion measured 1.2 cm cranio-caudal; gating implemented.
42. **Tomographic Verification Imaging:** QA imaging to confirm patient and tumor position using CT/CBCT slices.
    **Related Terms:** IGRT, LINAC, Daily Setup
    **Radiotherapy Example:** Daily CBCT verification for pelvic IMRT ensures accurate tumor targeting.
43. **Tissue Dose Gradient Analysis:** Evaluating rate of dose falloff around tumor to protect nearby OAR.
    **Related Terms:** DVH, Conformity Index, IMRT, VMAT
    **Radiotherapy Example:** Brain metastasis IMRT evaluated for steep dose gradient to protect optic nerves.
44. **Treatment Field Verification Phantom:** Phantom used to validate treatment field setup before patient delivery.
    **Related Terms:** Solid Water Phantom, Ion Chamber, EPID
    **Radiotherapy Example:** Head & neck IMRT field verified with QA phantom before first fraction.

45. **Tissue Surface Dose Measurement:** Measuring dose delivered at skin surface, critical for bolus or electron treatments.
**Related Terms:** TLD, MOSFET, Surface Dose, Electron Beam
**Radiotherapy Example:** Electron boost to scalp verified with TLDs to confirm surface dose.

46. **Treatment Time Calculation:** Computing required beam-on time based on prescribed dose and machine output.
**Related Terms:** MU, Dose Rate, LINAC Output
**Radiotherapy Example:** Breast tangential fields calculated to deliver 2 Gy per fraction in 120 MU.

47. **Tomotherapy Plan Dose Verification:** Confirming tomotherapy plan dose using phantom or measurement device.
**Related Terms:** MVCT, DVH, QA, TPS
**Radiotherapy Example:** Phantom measurement confirmed spinal metastasis dose distribution on tomotherapy.

48. **Target-to-Organ Overlap Assessment:** Evaluating spatial overlap between tumor and OAR for dose optimization.
**Related Terms:** DVH, PTV, OAR, Dose Constraints
**Radiotherapy Example:** Lung tumor abutting esophagus analyzed for safe dose delivery.

49. **Tissue Compaction QA:** Verifying uniform contact of bolus or patient surface to ensure correct dose delivery.
**Related Terms:** Bolus, Surface Dose, LINAC, Mould Room
**Radiotherapy Example:** Chest wall bolus checked for full contact before electron boost.

50. **Treatment Plan QA Documentation:** Complete record of all QA checks for regulatory and safety purposes.
**Related Terms:** IMRT QA, TPS Verification, LINAC QA, Documentation
**Radiotherapy Example:** All prostate IMRT QA results documented before patient treatment initiation.

51. **Tumor Volume Delineation:** Process of outlining the tumor on imaging for precise radiation targeting.
**Related Terms:** GTV, CTV, PTV, Contouring
**Radiotherapy Example:** Head & neck tumor contoured on CT and MRI for IMRT planning.

52. **Treatment Delivery Verification:** Confirming that the planned radiation dose is accurately delivered to the patient.
**Related Terms:** QA, EPID, Dose Measurement, LINAC
**Radiotherapy Example:** Portal images used to verify patient setup and beam delivery.

53. **Tissue Inhomogeneity Modeling:** Accounting for varying tissue densities during dose calculation.
**Related Terms:** TPS, Monte Carlo, Hounsfield Units, Dose Accuracy
**Radiotherapy Example:** Lung SBRT plan adjusted for low-density lung tissue to maintain accurate dose.

54. **Tumor Hypofractionation:** Delivering larger doses per fraction over fewer treatment sessions.
**Related Terms:** Hypofractionation, SBRT, Fractionation, BED
**Radiotherapy Example:** Prostate SBRT delivered in 5 fractions instead of 39 conventional fractions.

55. **Tomotherapy Image-Guided Delivery:** Using onboard imaging to guide radiation delivery in tomotherapy.
**Related Terms:** IGRT, MVCT, LINAC, Dose Verification
**Radiotherapy Example:** Daily MVCT scan performed to verify head & neck tumor position.

56. **Tissue Compensator Design:** Custom material designed to correct dose inhomogeneity across the target.
**Related Terms:** Bolus, Wedges, LINAC, Dose Shaping
**Radiotherapy Example:** Compensator designed in mould room for chest wall electron boost.

57. **Target Motion Management:** Techniques to minimize effects of tumor movement during radiation.
**Related Terms:** 4D CT, Respiratory Gating, DIBH, Motion Tracking
**Radiotherapy Example:** Lung SBRT delivered with respiratory gating to reduce motion uncertainty.

58. **Treatment Couch Calibration:** Ensuring the treatment couch moves accurately according to planned shifts.
**Related Terms:** LINAC QA, IGRT, Couch Shift, Patient Positioning
**Radiotherapy Example:** Couch calibration verified before cranial SRS treatment.

59. **Tissue-Equivalent Phantom QA:** QA using phantoms mimicking human tissue to validate dose distribution.
**Related Terms:** Rando Phantom, TLD, Ion Chamber, LINAC QA
**Radiotherapy Example:** Head & neck IMRT plan verified with Rando phantom and TLD measurements.

60. **Treatment Beam Modulation:** Adjusting intensity or shape of beams to conform dose to tumor.
**Related Terms:** IMRT, VMAT, MLC, Dose Painting
**Radiotherapy Example:** Breast IMRT plan used MLC to modulate beam for heart and lung sparing.

61. **Tumor Response Assessment:** Evaluating changes in tumor size or activity after treatment.
**Related Terms:** Imaging, PET, CT, MRI, RECIST
**Radiotherapy Example:** PET-CT performed 3 months post-therapy to assess tumor regression.

62. **Tomotherapy Dose Verification:** Checking delivered dose matches planned dose using phantom measurements.
**Related Terms:** MVCT, QA, TPS, LINAC
**Radiotherapy Example:** Spinal metastasis plan verified on tomotherapy phantom before treatment.

63. **Tissue Dose Summation:** Calculating cumulative dose delivered across multiple fractions or plans.
**Related Terms:** DVH, Fractionation, Adaptive RT, Dose Accumulation
**Radiotherapy Example:** Prostate plan dose summation performed after adaptive replanning.

64. **Target Conformity QA:** Quality check to ensure high-dose region conforms closely to tumor shape.
**Related Terms:** CI, DVH, PTV, IMRT QA
**Radiotherapy Example:** CI verified in brain metastasis IMRT plan using QA software.

65. **Treatment Machine Output Verification:** Measuring the radiation output of LINAC or other delivery device.
**Related Terms:** MU, LINAC, Dosimetry, QA
**Radiotherapy Example:** Daily output check ensures LINAC delivers accurate 2 Gy fraction.

66. **Tomographic Dose Mapping:** Mapping delivered dose in 3D using imaging or phantom data.
**Related Terms:** MVCT, TPS, DVH, Dose Verification
**Radiotherapy Example:** Phantom measurement compared with TPS dose map for verification.

67. **Tissue Surface Dose QA:** Ensuring correct dose delivered at patient skin surface.
**Related Terms:** Bolus, TLD, MOSFET, Electron Beam
**Radiotherapy Example:** Chest wall electron boost measured with TLDs to verify surface dose.

68. **Treatment Portal Imaging QA:** Using portal images to verify field position and patient setup.
**Related Terms:** EPID, LINAC, IGRT, Dose Verification
**Radiotherapy Example:** Daily portal images confirm tangential breast field placement.

69. **Tumor Motion Imaging:** Imaging tumor movement over time to guide motion management.
**Related Terms:** 4D CT, CBCT, Respiratory Gating
**Radiotherapy Example:** Lung tumor motion analyzed on 4D CT to define ITV.

70. **Tissue Attenuation Correction:** Adjusting dose calculations for attenuation by different tissues.
**Related Terms:** TPS, Hounsfield Units, Dose Accuracy
**Radiotherapy Example:** Lung SBRT plan corrected for low-density tissue attenuation.

71. **Treatment Plan Evaluation:** Reviewing plan quality using dosimetric indices and DVH.
**Related Terms:** CI, HI, DVH, TPS QA
**Radiotherapy Example:** Prostate IMRT plan evaluated for PTV coverage and OAR sparing.

72. **Target Margin QA:** Checking planned margins adequately cover tumor accounting for motion.
**Related Terms:** PTV, CTV, IGRT, Motion Management
**Radiotherapy Example:** Head & neck plan PTV margins verified with CBCT.

73. **Tomotherapy Beam QA:** QA specifically for tomotherapy delivery to ensure accuracy.
**Related Terms:** MVCT, Dose Verification, LINAC QA
**Radiotherapy Example:** Spinal SRS plan verified on tomotherapy QA phantom.

74. **Tissue Inhomogeneity QA:** Verifying dose calculations account for tissue density differences.
**Related Terms:** Lung, Bone, TPS, Monte Carlo Algorithm
**Radiotherapy Example:** Lung tumor plan QA confirmed accurate dose in low-density lung tissue.

75. **Treatment Fractionation Verification:** Ensuring correct dose and fractionation schedule delivered.
**Related Terms:** BED, Fractionation, Dose per Fraction, QA
**Radiotherapy Example:** Hypofractionated prostate plan verified for 7.25 Gy per fraction.

76. **Tumor Dose Escalation Planning:** Increasing tumor dose while sparing normal tissue.
**Related Terms:** Dose Painting, IMRT, VMAT, OAR
**Radiotherapy Example:** Head & neck tumor planned with simultaneous integrated boost (SIB).

77. **Tissue Heterogeneity Imaging:** Imaging used to identify tissue density variations for accurate planning.
**Related Terms:** CT, Hounsfield Units, TPS, Dose Calculation
**Radiotherapy Example:** Lung tumor segmented on CT for heterogeneity corrections.

78. **Treatment Couch Positioning QA:** Verifying couch positions match plan for accurate beam delivery.
**Related Terms:** LINAC, IGRT, Couch Shift, Patient Setup
**Radiotherapy Example:** Couch positions checked daily for head & neck IMRT.

79. **Tomotherapy MVCT QA:** Quality assurance of tomotherapy's onboard MVCT imaging system.
**Related Terms:** IGRT, Dose Verification, Phantom QA
**Radiotherapy Example:** Spinal metastasis plan verified using MVCT QA scans.

80. **Target Volume QA:** Ensuring PTV and CTV accurately represent tumor coverage needs.
**Related Terms:** GTV, CTV, PTV, DVH
**Radiotherapy Example:** Brain metastasis PTV coverage verified on DVH for safe delivery.

81. **Treatment Plan Optimization:** Adjusting beam parameters to maximize tumor dose and minimize normal tissue exposure.
**Related Terms:** IMRT, VMAT, TPS, Dose Constraints
**Radiotherapy Example:** Prostate IMRT plan optimized for bladder and rectum sparing.

82. **Tissue Compensation QA:** Verifying compensators or bolus correct dose distribution as planned.
**Related Terms:** Bolus, Compensator, LINAC QA, Dose Measurement
**Radiotherapy Example:** Chest wall electron boost verified using tissue-equivalent phantom.

83. **Tomotherapy Adaptive Planning:** Adjusting treatment plan based on anatomical changes during therapy.
**Related Terms:** IGRT, CBCT, Dose Accumulation, PTV
**Radiotherapy Example:** Head & neck plan adapted mid-treatment due to tumor shrinkage.

84. **Tumor Regression Assessment:** Evaluating reduction in tumor size during or after therapy.
**Related Terms:** Imaging, CT, MRI, PET, RECIST
**Radiotherapy Example:** Weekly CT scans assess lung tumor regression during SBRT.

85. **Targeted Radiation Dose Escalation:** Delivering higher dose selectively to resistant tumor regions.
**Related Terms:** Dose Painting, SIB, IMRT, VMAT
**Radiotherapy Example:** Head & neck plan includes SIB to high-risk nodal areas.

86. **Tissue Motion Verification:** Confirming tumor motion is accurately tracked during delivery.
**Related Terms:** 4D CT, IGRT, Respiratory Gating
**Radiotherapy Example:** Lung tumor motion verified using 4D CT and DIBH.

87. **Treatment Delivery QA:** Overall verification that the treatment plan is executed safely and accurately.
**Related Terms:** LINAC, EPID, Dose Verification, Patient QA
**Radiotherapy Example:** Daily QA ensures correct dose for head & neck IMRT.

88. **Tumor Coverage Evaluation:** Checking that the tumor receives the prescribed dose adequately.
**Related Terms:** DVH, PTV, CTV, Dose Homogeneity
**Radiotherapy Example:** Brain metastasis plan DVH reviewed for ≥95% PTV coverage.

89. **Tissue Sparing Assessment:** Evaluating whether normal tissues are adequately spared from high dose.
**Related Terms:** OAR, DVH, IMRT, VMAT
**Radiotherapy Example:** Heart and lung doses reviewed for left breast tangential plan.

90. **Tomotherapy Beam Alignment QA:** Ensuring tomotherapy beams are accurately aligned to the planned trajectory.
**Related Terms:** MVCT, IGRT, LINAC QA, Dose Verification
**Radiotherapy Example:** Cranial SRS beam alignment verified on MVCT QA phantom.

91. **Target Margin Verification:** Checking that margins around tumor adequately account for motion and setup errors.
**Related Terms:** PTV, CTV, IGRT, Motion Management
**Radiotherapy Example:** Head & neck PTV margins verified using daily CBCT scans.

92. **Treatment Field Verification:** Confirming radiation fields match planned orientation and size.
**Related Terms:** Portal Imaging, EPID, QA, LINAC
**Radiotherapy Example:** Breast tangential field verified via portal imaging before first fraction.

93. **Tissue Dose Mapping:** Creating detailed maps of delivered dose across target and normal tissues.
**Related Terms:** TPS, DVH, Dose Distribution, QA
**Radiotherapy Example:** Prostate IMRT dose map compared with phantom measurements.

94. **Tumor Response Imaging:** Imaging to assess tumor changes post-therapy.
**Related Terms:** CT, PET, MRI, RECIST
**Radiotherapy Example:** PET-CT performed 3 months after SBRT to confirm tumor response.

95. **Tomotherapy Treatment Verification:** QA checks to ensure tomotherapy delivery matches the planned dose.
**Related Terms:** MVCT, QA, LINAC, Dose Verification
**Radiotherapy Example:** Spinal SRS plan verified on tomotherapy QA phantom before first fraction.

96. **Tissue Surface Dose Verification:** Confirming prescribed dose delivered to patient surface areas.
**Related Terms:** Bolus, MOSFET, TLD, Electron Beam
**Radiotherapy Example:** Chest wall electron boost dose verified with TLD measurements.

97. **Treatment Plan QA:** Quality assurance process to validate plan accuracy before treatment.
**Related Terms:** DVH, TPS, LINAC QA, Patient QA
**Radiotherapy Example:** IMRT plan for prostate reviewed with phantom and DVH metrics.

98. **Tumor Dose Homogeneity Verification:** Checking that prescribed dose is evenly distributed across the tumor.
**Related Terms:** DVH, HI, PTV, QA
**Radiotherapy Example:** Head & neck IMRT plan homogeneity checked via QA software.

99. **Target Motion QA:** QA procedure to verify motion management is effective.
**Related Terms:** 4D CT, Respiratory Gating, IGRT
**Radiotherapy Example:** Lung tumor gating QA performed using 4D CT phantom.

100. **Tomotherapy Dose QA:** Comprehensive QA to ensure tomotherapy dose delivery is accurate.
**Related Terms:** MVCT, Dose Verification, LINAC, QA Phantom
**Radiotherapy Example:** Spinal metastasis tomotherapy plan verified with phantom measurement before treatment.

101. **Target Volume Delineation:** Outlining tumor and OARs for treatment planning.
**Related Terms:** CTV, PTV, GTV, CT, MRI
**Radiotherapy Example:** Head & neck tumor contoured on planning CT with MRI fusion.

102. **Treatment Field Matching:** Ensuring adjacent radiation fields meet accurately without overlap or gaps.
**Related Terms:** Junction, IMRT, VMAT, Portal Imaging
**Radiotherapy Example:** Craniospinal irradiation fields matched with minimal hot/cold spots.

103. **Tomotherapy Image Guidance QA:** Verifying imaging system on tomotherapy machine provides accurate positioning.
**Related Terms:** MVCT, CBCT, IGRT, LINAC QA
**Radiotherapy Example:** Daily MVCT images checked for spinal tumor alignment.

104. **Tissue Equivalent Phantom QA:** Using phantoms to simulate human tissue for dose measurement and verification.
**Related Terms:** QA Phantom, TLD, MOSFET, LINAC QA
**Radiotherapy Example:** Prostate IMRT plan verified with tissue-equivalent phantom.

105. **Treatment Couch Verification:** Ensuring the patient couch moves accurately to planned positions.
**Related Terms:** IGRT, LINAC, Patient Positioning, QA
**Radiotherapy Example:** Brain SRS plan verified couch shifts using CBCT.

106. **Tumor Tracking QA:** QA process to confirm tumor motion tracking accuracy during delivery.
**Related Terms:** Respiratory Gating, 4D CT, IGRT
**Radiotherapy Example:** Lung SBRT tumor tracked and verified with 4D CT.

107. **Tomotherapy Dose Calculation QA:** Verifying TPS-calculated dose is delivered accurately by tomotherapy system.
**Related Terms:** DVH, LINAC, QA, Dose Measurement
**Radiotherapy Example:** Spinal SRS plan dose verified on QA phantom.

108. **Target Margin QA:** Ensuring planning margins adequately cover tumor motion and setup errors.
**Related Terms:** PTV, CTV, IGRT, Motion Management
**Radiotherapy Example:** Liver SBRT margins verified with daily CBCT.

**109. Tissue Density Mapping:** Mapping patient tissue density for accurate dose calculation.
**Related Terms:** CT Hounsfield Units, TPS, Electron Density
**Radiotherapy Example:** Lung tumor density map used to calculate accurate photon dose.

**110. Treatment Session Verification:** QA for verifying correct patient, plan, and delivery parameters for each session.
**Related Terms:** IGRT, LINAC, Portal Imaging, EPID
**Radiotherapy Example:** Daily IMRT session verified via CBCT before beam-on.

**111. Tumor Volume Dose Escalation:** Increasing dose selectively to radioresistant tumor regions.
**Related Terms:** SIB, IMRT, VMAT, Dose Painting
**Radiotherapy Example:** Head & neck SIB plan delivers higher dose to hypoxic tumor sub-volumes.

**112. Treatment Plan Adaptation:** Adjusting the treatment plan during therapy due to anatomical or tumor changes.
**Related Terms:** Adaptive Radiotherapy, CBCT, TPS, Dose Recalculation
**Radiotherapy Example:** Lung tumor plan adapted mid-treatment due to shrinkage.

**113. Tissue Interface Dose Verification:** Verifying dose at tissue boundaries where density changes (e.g., lung/soft tissue).
**Related Terms:** Bolus, TPS, Phantom, Dose Measurement
**Radiotherapy Example:** Chest wall IMRT plan checked for dose at lung-tissue interface using phantom.

**114. Tomotherapy Field QA:** Ensuring tomotherapy fields are correctly shaped, positioned, and delivered.
**Related Terms:** MVCT, LINAC QA, Dose Verification
**Radiotherapy Example:** Spinal tumor tomotherapy fields verified with phantom measurement.

**115. Target Motion Compensation:** Techniques to account for tumor motion during dose delivery.
**Related Terms:** Respiratory Gating, DIBH, 4D CT, IGRT
**Radiotherapy Example:** Liver SBRT uses gating to deliver dose only during exhalation.

**116. Treatment Dose Mapping:** Creating a spatial map of the delivered dose in patient anatomy.
**Related Terms:** DVH, TPS, Dose Verification, Phantom
**Radiotherapy Example:** Prostate IMRT delivered dose mapped using EPID measurements.

**117. Tomotherapy Beam Verification:** Checking beam characteristics, alignment, and output for tomotherapy.
**Related Terms:** QA, MVCT, LINAC, Dose Measurement
**Radiotherapy Example:** Spinal SRS tomotherapy beams verified on QA phantom.

**118. Tissue Surface Dose Mapping:** Mapping dose at patient skin or superficial tissues.
**Related Terms:** Bolus, TLD, MOSFET, QA Phantom
**Radiotherapy Example:** Chest wall electron boost dose distribution verified using TLD array.

**119. Target Volume QA:** Ensuring PTV/CTV delineation is accurate and appropriate for planned dose.
**Related Terms:** GTV, PTV, TPS, CBCT, MRI
**Radiotherapy Example:** Head & neck plan QA confirms PTV coverage using CBCT and DVH.

**120. Treatment Delivery Accuracy QA:** Verifying that the planned dose is delivered correctly to the patient.
**Related Terms:** LINAC, EPID, Portal Imaging, QA Phantom
**Radiotherapy Example:** Lung IMRT dose delivered verified with EPID and QA phantom measurements.

121. **Tumor Regression Dose Assessment:** Evaluating dose delivered to shrinking tumor during therapy.
**Related Terms:** DVH, Adaptive Radiotherapy, CBCT, TPS
**Radiotherapy Example:** Head & neck tumor regression monitored weekly with adaptive planning.

122. **Tomotherapy Adaptive QA:** QA performed when treatment plan is adapted based on anatomical changes.
**Related Terms:** Adaptive Radiotherapy, MVCT, Dose Verification, LINAC
**Radiotherapy Example:** Spinal SBRT plan adapted mid-course verified with MVCT QA.

123. **Tissue Inhomogeneity Correction QA:** Ensuring dose calculations account for tissue density variations.
**Related Terms:** CT, TPS, Electron Density, Dose Calculation
**Radiotherapy Example:** Lung tumor photon plan corrected for inhomogeneity using TPS.

124. **Treatment Fraction Verification:** QA to confirm dose per fraction is delivered accurately.
**Related Terms:** Fractionation, LINAC, Portal Dosimetry, DVH
**Radiotherapy Example:** Prostate IMRT fractions verified using daily EPID images.

125. **Tumor Response QA Imaging:** Imaging to verify tumor response during or after treatment.
**Related Terms:** CT, PET, MRI, RECIST
**Radiotherapy Example:** PET-CT performed after 3 weeks of SBRT to assess response.

126. **Tomotherapy Output QA:** Measuring and verifying beam output for tomotherapy system.
**Related Terms:** LINAC, MVCT, Dose Measurement, QA Phantom
**Radiotherapy Example:** Spinal SRS output verified prior to first fraction.

127. **Target Coverage QA:** Ensuring the planned tumor volume receives intended dose.
**Related Terms:** PTV, DVH, TPS, IGRT
**Radiotherapy Example:** Head & neck IMRT QA confirms ≥95% PTV coverage.

128. **Tissue Dose Gradient QA:** Verifying dose fall-off at tumor-normal tissue boundaries.
**Related Terms:** DVH, IMRT, VMAT, QA Phantom
**Radiotherapy Example:** Spinal SRS gradient checked to protect spinal cord.

129. **Treatment Couch Motion QA:** Verifying accurate movement of treatment couch during therapy.
**Related Terms:** LINAC, IGRT, Couch Shifts, QA
**Radiotherapy Example:** Brain SRS couch shifts confirmed with CBCT QA.

130. **Tumor Motion Verification Imaging:** Imaging to confirm tumor motion management accuracy.
**Related Terms:** 4D CT, Respiratory Gating, IGRT
**Radiotherapy Example:** Lung tumor motion verified before gated SBRT.

131. **Treatment Beam Alignment QA:** Ensuring radiation beams are correctly aligned with target.
**Related Terms:** LINAC, Portal Imaging, EPID, QA
**Radiotherapy Example:** Head & neck IMRT fields aligned using portal images before treatment.

132. **Tissue Compensator QA:** QA for bolus or compensators used to achieve uniform dose.
**Related Terms:** Bolus, LINAC, Phantom, Dose Measurement
**Radiotherapy Example:** Chest wall compensator QA performed using phantom measurements.

133. **Tomotherapy Fraction QA:** QA of each fraction delivered via tomotherapy.
**Related Terms:** MVCT, LINAC, Dose Verification
**Radiotherapy Example:** Spinal SBRT fraction QA performed before each session.

134. **Tumor Delineation QA:** Verifying accuracy of tumor contours for planning.
**Related Terms:** GTV, CTV, PTV, CBCT, MRI
**Radiotherapy Example:** Head & neck tumor contours reviewed for adaptive planning.

135. **Treatment Portal Verification:** Checking radiation fields at treatment portals for accuracy.
**Related Terms:** EPID, LINAC, QA, Portal Imaging
**Radiotherapy Example:** Breast tangential fields verified before first fraction.

136. **Tissue Surface Dose QA:** Verifying dose delivered to superficial tissue layers.
**Related Terms:** Bolus, TLD, MOSFET, QA Phantom
**Radiotherapy Example:** Chest wall electron boost surface dose verified using TLDs.

137. **Target Motion Imaging QA:** Imaging to confirm tumor motion is accounted for during delivery.
**Related Terms:** 4D CT, IGRT, Respiratory Gating
**Radiotherapy Example:** Lung tumor motion assessed with 4D CT for SBRT planning.

138. **Treatment Verification Imaging QA:** QA for imaging used to verify patient position and treatment accuracy.
**Related Terms:** CBCT, EPID, IGRT
**Radiotherapy Example:** Daily CBCT used to verify prostate IMRT setup.

139. **Tumor Dose Assessment QA:** Evaluating delivered dose to ensure target coverage.
**Related Terms:** DVH, TPS, LINAC, QA Phantom
**Radiotherapy Example:** Head & neck IMRT tumor dose assessed using EPID measurements.

140. **Tomotherapy Adaptive Dose QA:** QA for dose delivered after adaptive plan changes.
**Related Terms:** Adaptive Radiotherapy, MVCT, LINAC
**Radiotherapy Example:** Spinal SRS plan adapted mid-course verified using phantom.

141. **Tissue Heterogeneity QA:** Verifying dose calculations in regions with varying tissue densities.
**Related Terms:** TPS, CT, Electron Density, Dose Measurement
**Radiotherapy Example:** Lung tumor IMRT dose checked for inhomogeneity.

142. **Treatment Beam Modulation QA:** QA to ensure intensity-modulated beams deliver planned dose distribution.
**Related Terms:** IMRT, VMAT, LINAC, QA Phantom
**Radiotherapy Example:** Head & neck IMRT beam modulation verified via portal dosimetry.

143. **Target Volume Dose Verification:** Verifying actual delivered dose matches planned dose in target volume.
**Related Terms:** DVH, PTV, TPS, LINAC
**Radiotherapy Example:** Prostate IMRT target dose verified using EPID.

144. **Tissue Compensator Dose QA:** QA for doses delivered with tissue compensators in place.
**Related Terms:** Bolus, Compensator, LINAC, Dose Measurement
**Radiotherapy Example:** Chest wall compensator dose verified using phantom.

145. **Tomotherapy Output Verification:** Verifying tomotherapy system delivers planned dose output consistently.
**Related Terms:** LINAC QA, MVCT, Dose Measurement
**Radiotherapy Example:** Spinal SBRT tomotherapy output verified with phantom.

146. **Tumor Coverage QA:** QA to ensure tumor receives prescribed dose with minimal deviation.
**Related Terms:** PTV, DVH, TPS, LINAC
**Radiotherapy Example:** Head & neck IMRT coverage confirmed via QA software.

147. **Treatment Fraction Dose QA:** QA for dose delivered in individual fractions.
**Related Terms:** Fractionation, LINAC, EPID, DVH
**Radiotherapy Example:** Prostate IMRT daily fraction verified with EPID.

148. **Target Volume Alignment QA:** QA for alignment of target volume relative to beams.
**Related Terms:** IGRT, CBCT, PTV, CTV
**Radiotherapy Example:** Lung SBRT target alignment verified with CBCT.

149. **Tomotherapy Dose Mapping QA:** QA to confirm dose delivered matches planned distribution in tomotherapy.
**Related Terms:** MVCT, LINAC, DVH, Phantom
**Radiotherapy Example:** Spinal SRS tomotherapy dose mapped using phantom.

150. **Tissue Dose Accumulation QA:** Verifying cumulative dose over multiple fractions is as planned.
**Related Terms:** Fractionation, DVH, Adaptive Radiotherapy, TPS
**Radiotherapy Example:** Head & neck IMRT cumulative dose evaluated after 10 fractions.

151. **Tumor Hypoxia Imaging:** Imaging to detect low-oxygen regions in tumors, which are more radioresistant.
**Related Terms:** PET, FMISO, Hypoxia Mapping, Radiotherapy Planning
**Radiotherapy Example:** Head & neck tumor imaged with FMISO PET to adjust dose escalation.

152. **Tomotherapy Beam Output Consistency QA:** Ensuring consistent radiation output from tomotherapy unit over time.
**Related Terms:** LINAC QA, MVCT, Dose Measurement, QA Phantom
**Radiotherapy Example:** Spinal SBRT beams verified for consistent output daily.

153. **Tissue Electron Density Calibration:** Calibrating CT values to electron density for accurate dose calculation.
**Related Terms:** CT, TPS, Electron Density Phantom
**Radiotherapy Example:** Lung tumor plan recalculated using calibrated electron density map.

154. **Target Volume Margin Verification:** Ensuring planning margins (PTV) adequately cover tumor motion and uncertainties.
**Related Terms:** CTV, PTV, Motion Management, IGRT
**Radiotherapy Example:** Prostate PTV margin verified via daily CBCT.

155. **Tomotherapy Patient Setup QA:** Verifying patient positioning on tomotherapy couch matches plan.
**Related Terms:** IGRT, MVCT, LINAC, Couch Shifts
**Radiotherapy Example:** Spinal tumor daily setup verified with MVCT before delivery.

156. **Treatment Couch Rotation QA:** QA to ensure accurate rotational movements of the treatment couch.
**Related Terms:** IGRT, LINAC, CBCT, QA
**Radiotherapy Example:** Head & neck plan requires couch rotation verified with phantom.

157. **Tissue Dose Distribution Verification:** QA to confirm spatial dose distribution matches TPS calculations.
**Related Terms:** DVH, LINAC, TPS, EPID
**Radiotherapy Example:** Breast IMRT plan dose distribution verified using EPID.

158. **Tomotherapy Adaptive Imaging QA:** QA of imaging used during adaptive plan modifications.
**Related Terms:** MVCT, CBCT, Adaptive Radiotherapy, TPS
**Radiotherapy Example:** Spinal SRS adaptive plan verified with MVCT imaging QA.

159. **Tumor Motion Management QA:** QA for techniques used to compensate tumor motion during delivery.
**Related Terms:** 4D CT, Respiratory Gating, DIBH, IGRT
**Radiotherapy Example:** Lung SBRT uses 4D CT QA to ensure gating accuracy.

160. **Treatment Portal Dose Verification:** Verifying dose delivered through treatment portals matches planned dose.
**Related Terms:** EPID, LINAC, Portal Imaging, QA
**Radiotherapy Example:** Prostate IMRT portal doses verified using EPID.

161. **Tissue Compensator Verification:** QA of physical compensators used to achieve uniform dose.
**Related Terms:** Bolus, LINAC, Phantom, Dose Measurement
**Radiotherapy Example:** Chest wall compensator verified with phantom TLD measurements.

162. **Tomotherapy Beam Modulation Verification:** QA to ensure intensity-modulated beams deliver planned dose patterns.
**Related Terms:** IMRT, VMAT, LINAC, QA Phantom
**Radiotherapy Example:** Head & neck IMRT beam modulation verified via portal dosimetry.

163. **Tumor Dose Gradient Verification:** QA to check dose fall-off at tumor-normal tissue interfaces.
**Related Terms:** DVH, IMRT, VMAT, QA Phantom
**Radiotherapy Example:** Spinal SRS plan checked to protect spinal cord from high gradient dose.

164. **Treatment Fraction Dose Mapping:** Mapping dose delivered in each fraction for verification.
**Related Terms:** Fractionation, EPID, LINAC, DVH
**Radiotherapy Example:** Prostate IMRT daily fraction mapped with EPID images.

165. **Tumor Coverage Imaging QA:** Imaging to confirm tumor receives planned dose coverage.
**Related Terms:** CBCT, PTV, DVH, IGRT
**Radiotherapy Example:** Head & neck tumor coverage verified via daily CBCT.

166. **Tissue Surface Dose Measurement QA:** Measuring dose at patient skin or superficial tissues for accuracy.
**Related Terms:** TLD, MOSFET, Bolus, QA Phantom
**Radiotherapy Example:** Chest wall electron boost surface dose measured with TLD array.

167. **Tomotherapy Fraction Verification:** QA for verifying each fraction delivered via tomotherapy unit.
**Related Terms:** MVCT, LINAC, Dose Measurement
**Radiotherapy Example:** Spinal SRS fraction verified prior to beam-on.

168. **Tumor Delineation Verification QA:** Ensuring tumor contours used in planning are accurate.
**Related Terms:** GTV, CTV, PTV, CBCT, MRI
**Radiotherapy Example:** Head & neck tumor contours verified with MRI fusion.

169. **Treatment Beam Alignment Verification:** Ensuring radiation beams are properly aligned with target volume.
**Related Terms:** LINAC, EPID, Portal Imaging, QA
**Radiotherapy Example:** Breast tangential fields verified with portal imaging before treatment.

170. **Tissue Dose Accumulation Verification:** Verifying cumulative dose over multiple fractions matches plan.
**Related Terms:** Fractionation, DVH, Adaptive Radiotherapy, TPS
**Radiotherapy Example:** Head & neck IMRT cumulative dose evaluated weekly.

171. **Tumor Motion Verification QA:** QA imaging to confirm tumor motion compensation is accurate.
**Related Terms:** 4D CT, IGRT, Respiratory Gating
**Radiotherapy Example:** Lung tumor motion verified for gated SBRT.

172. **Tomotherapy Dose Output QA:** Verifying tomotherapy delivers planned dose output consistently.
**Related Terms:** LINAC QA, MVCT, Dose Measurement, QA Phantom
**Radiotherapy Example:** Spinal SRS daily beam output checked on QA phantom.

173. **Target Volume Dose Assessment QA:** Evaluating delivered dose in target to ensure adequate coverage.
**Related Terms:** DVH, PTV, TPS, LINAC
**Radiotherapy Example:** Prostate IMRT target dose verified with EPID.

174. **Tissue Heterogeneity Dose QA:** QA to ensure accurate dose calculation in tissues with varying densities.
**Related Terms:** TPS, CT, Electron Density, Dose Measurement
**Radiotherapy Example:** Lung tumor photon plan checked for density inhomogeneities.

175. **Treatment Plan Adaptation QA:** QA to ensure adapted plans maintain target coverage and OAR sparing.
**Related Terms:** Adaptive Radiotherapy, CBCT, TPS, Dose Verification
**Radiotherapy Example:** Lung tumor plan adapted mid-treatment verified with phantom measurement.

176. **Tomotherapy Beam Quality Verification:** QA to ensure beam energy and quality are consistent with planning.
**Related Terms:** MVCT, LINAC, Dose Measurement, QA Phantom
**Radiotherapy Example:** Head & neck IMRT beams checked for energy consistency before treatment.

177. **Target Volume Margin Adaptation QA:** QA to ensure adapted PTV margins still cover tumor adequately.
**Related Terms:** CTV, PTV, Adaptive Radiotherapy, CBCT
**Radiotherapy Example:** Prostate tumor margins adjusted mid-treatment verified via CBCT.

178. **Tissue Compensation Verification:** QA to ensure compensators or bolus produce correct dose distribution.
**Related Terms:** Bolus, LINAC, Phantom, Dose Measurement
**Radiotherapy Example:** Chest wall bolus thickness verified with TLD before photon boost.

179. **Treatment Delivery Timing Verification:** QA to ensure beam-on time and fraction timing match plan.
**Related Terms:** LINAC, Dose Rate, Fractionation, QA
**Radiotherapy Example:** SRS treatment timing verified to avoid over- or under-dosing.

180. **Tomotherapy MVCT Imaging QA:** QA to ensure MVCT imaging provides accurate anatomical information.
**Related Terms:** Imaging QA, LINAC, IGRT, Dose Verification
**Radiotherapy Example:** Spinal tumor MVCT images checked for alignment before therapy.

181. **Tumor Motion Tracking QA:** QA to verify accuracy of tracking tumor motion during treatment.
**Related Terms:** 4D CT, Respiratory Gating, IGRT
**Radiotherapy Example:** Lung SBRT tumor tracked with gated delivery and verified via QA.

182. **Treatment Plan Dose Verification:** QA to ensure delivered dose matches the planned dose distribution.
**Related Terms:** DVH, LINAC, EPID, QA Phantom
**Radiotherapy Example:** Head & neck IMRT plan verified using EPID measurements.

183. **Tissue Inhomogeneity Correction QA:** QA to confirm TPS correctly accounts for tissue density variations.
**Related Terms:** TPS, CT, Electron Density, Dose Calculation
**Radiotherapy Example:** Lung photon plan corrected for inhomogeneities verified with phantom.

184. **Tomotherapy Couch Position Accuracy QA:** QA to ensure couch moves accurately to planned positions.
**Related Terms:** LINAC, IGRT, CBCT, QA Phantom
**Radiotherapy Example:** Head & neck couch shifts verified daily for accurate delivery.

185. **Tumor Dose Escalation Verification:** QA to confirm higher doses to tumor subvolumes are delivered accurately.
**Related Terms:** IMRT, SIB, DVH, LINAC
**Radiotherapy Example:** Prostate SIB plan dose escalation verified with EPID.

186. **Treatment Field Edge Verification:** QA to ensure radiation field edges align with target margins.
**Related Terms:** LINAC, EPID, Field Verification, QA
**Radiotherapy Example:** Breast tangential field edges verified to protect heart.

187. **Tomotherapy Dose Homogeneity Verification:** QA to confirm uniform dose within target volume.
**Related Terms:** DVH, IMRT, LINAC, QA Phantom
**Radiotherapy Example:** Spinal IMRT plan verified for dose homogeneity across vertebrae.

188. **Tissue Motion Imaging QA:** QA to ensure imaging captures tumor motion accurately.
**Related Terms:** 4D CT, CBCT, Respiratory Gating
**Radiotherapy Example:** Lung SBRT tumor motion verified with 4D CT QA.

189. **Treatment Plan Adaptation Dose QA:** QA to ensure adapted plans maintain intended dose coverage and OAR protection.
**Related Terms:** Adaptive Radiotherapy, DVH, LINAC, CBCT
**Radiotherapy Example:** Head & neck plan adapted for tumor shrinkage verified with phantom.

190. **Tomotherapy Fraction Consistency QA:** QA to ensure each fraction delivers planned dose consistently.
**Related Terms:** LINAC, Fractionation, EPID, QA Phantom
**Radiotherapy Example:** Prostate IMRT daily fraction consistency verified with EPID.

191. **Tumor Targeting Verification QA:** QA to confirm beam targets tumor precisely throughout treatment.
**Related Terms:** IGRT, CBCT, LINAC, PTV
**Radiotherapy Example:** Spinal tumor daily targeting verified with MVCT.

192. **Tissue Surface Dose QA:** QA for verifying dose to patient surface tissues.
**Related Terms:** TLD, MOSFET, Bolus, LINAC
**Radiotherapy Example:** Chest wall electron boost surface dose verified using TLD.

193. **Treatment Plan Verification Imaging QA:** QA to verify imaging used for treatment plan verification is accurate.
**Related Terms:** CBCT, MVCT, LINAC, IGRT
**Radiotherapy Example:** Head & neck tumor daily CBCT verified before treatment.

194. **Tomotherapy Beam Delivery Accuracy QA:** QA to ensure precise beam delivery matches treatment plan.
**Related Terms:** LINAC, IMRT, VMAT, EPID
**Radiotherapy Example:** Spinal SRS beam delivery verified via portal dosimetry.

195. **Tumor Motion Compensation QA:** QA to ensure motion compensation systems correctly track tumor motion.
**Related Terms:** Respiratory Gating, DIBH, 4D CT, IGRT
**Radiotherapy Example:** Lung SBRT gated treatment verified with motion phantom.

196. **Treatment Plan Dose Distribution QA:** QA to confirm dose distribution in patient matches planned distribution.
**Related Terms:** DVH, LINAC, EPID, TPS
**Radiotherapy Example:** Prostate IMRT dose distribution verified using EPID.

197. **Tomotherapy Image Guidance QA:** QA to verify accuracy of image guidance systems for treatment.
**Related Terms:** MVCT, CBCT, IGRT, LINAC
**Radiotherapy Example:** Head & neck daily MVCT images verified for alignment.

198. **Tissue Electron Density Verification:** QA to ensure CT-derived electron densities are accurate for dose calculation.
**Related Terms:** CT, TPS, Phantom, Electron Density
**Radiotherapy Example:** Lung tumor plan recalculated using verified electron density map.

199. **Tumor Dose Monitoring QA:** QA to monitor dose delivered to tumor during treatment.
**Related Terms:** EPID, LINAC, DVH, IGRT
**Radiotherapy Example:** Prostate IMRT tumor dose monitored with EPID.

200. **Tomotherapy Treatment QA Protocol:** Comprehensive QA protocol covering imaging, beam delivery, and dose verification.
**Related Terms:** LINAC, IGRT, EPID, Phantom
**Radiotherapy Example:** Head & neck tomotherapy QA protocol ensures safe and accurate delivery.

201. **Target Volume Margin QA:** QA to ensure tumor margins are sufficient and accurate for coverage.
**Related Terms:** PTV, GTV, CTV, TPS, LINAC
**Radiotherapy Example:** Prostate IMRT plan margin verified using daily CBCT imaging.

202. **Treatment Beam Angle Verification:** QA to confirm the angles of radiation beams match the planned setup.
**Related Terms:** LINAC, TPS, IGRT, IMRT, VMAT
**Radiotherapy Example:** Head & neck VMAT plan beam angles verified with portal imaging.

203. **Tumor Dose Escalation QA:** QA ensuring higher doses to tumor regions are delivered safely.
**Related Terms:** Dose Painting, IMRT, VMAT, LINAC
**Radiotherapy Example:** Liver SBRT plan dose escalation verified on QA phantom.

204. **Treatment Couch Sag Correction:** QA for any deviations in treatment table sag affecting dose delivery.
**Related Terms:** LINAC, IGRT, QA Phantom
**Radiotherapy Example:** Couch sag measured and corrected for craniospinal irradiation.

205. **Tomotherapy Beam Quality QA:** QA for the quality and consistency of helical tomotherapy beams.
**Related Terms:** LINAC, IMRT, QA Phantom, Dose Verification
**Radiotherapy Example:** Pelvic plan dose verified using cheese phantom on tomotherapy.

206. **Tissue Equivalent Phantom QA:** QA using phantoms that mimic human tissue for dose verification.
**Related Terms:** TPS, LINAC, Dosimetry, Radiotherapy
**Radiotherapy Example:** Head phantom used to verify dose distribution for brain SRS.

207. **Treatment Fraction Verification:** QA ensuring each fraction is delivered according to the treatment plan.
**Related Terms:** LINAC, IGRT, EPID, IMRT, VMAT
**Radiotherapy Example:** Daily verification of breast IMRT fractions using EPID.

208. **Tumor Motion Imaging QA:** QA of imaging techniques used to monitor tumor motion.
**Related Terms:** 4D CT, CBCT, LINAC, IGRT
**Radiotherapy Example:** Lung tumor motion assessed with 4D CT for gating.

209. **Treatment Field Size Verification:** QA to confirm radiation field sizes match planned dimensions.
**Related Terms:** LINAC, TPS, Portal Imaging, IMRT
**Radiotherapy Example:** Portal imaging used to verify breast field sizes.

210. **Tumor Hypoxia Dose Adjustment:** Adjusting dose based on hypoxic regions identified in imaging.
**Related Terms:** PET, Radiotracer, TPS, LINAC
**Radiotherapy Example:** PET-based hypoxia imaging guided boost dose in head & neck tumor.

211. **Tomotherapy Couch Position QA:** QA ensuring couch moves accurately during tomotherapy delivery.
**Related Terms:** LINAC, IGRT, QA Phantom
**Radiotherapy Example:** Couch movements verified before thoracic tomotherapy.

212. **Tissue Inhomogeneity Dose QA:** QA to account for tissue density variations in dose calculations.
**Related Terms:** TPS, CT Scan, LINAC, Radiotherapy
**Radiotherapy Example:** Lung SBRT plan dose corrected for air cavities.

213. **Treatment Time Monitoring:** Tracking actual delivery time for each radiation fraction.
**Related Terms:** LINAC, IMRT, VMAT, QA
**Radiotherapy Example:** SBRT session time recorded to ensure proper dose delivery.

214. **Target Conformity QA:** QA ensuring prescribed dose conforms accurately to tumor shape.
**Related Terms:** PTV, DVH, IMRT, VMAT, LINAC
**Radiotherapy Example:** Brain SRS conformity index verified on phantom.

215. **Tumor Response Imaging QA:** QA for imaging used to monitor tumor shrinkage or progression.
**Related Terms:** CT Scan, MRI, PET, IGRT
**Radiotherapy Example:** Weekly CT used to monitor lung tumor response.

216. **Treatment Delivery Efficiency QA:** QA ensuring planned treatments are delivered efficiently and safely.
**Related Terms:** LINAC, IMRT, VMAT, QA Phantom
**Radiotherapy Example:** Efficiency of multi-field prostate IMRT evaluated.

217. **Transverse Imaging QA:** QA of transverse slices in CT imaging for accuracy.
**Related Terms:** CT Scan, TPS, Radiology, LINAC
**Radiotherapy Example:** Abdominal CT slices checked for artifacts before planning.

218. **Tumor Dose Gradient QA:** QA assessing dose gradients across tumor and surrounding tissues.
**Related Terms:** TPS, IMRT, DVH, LINAC
**Radiotherapy Example:** Head & neck IMRT gradient verified to spare spinal cord.

219. **Treatment Planning QA Protocol:** QA protocols for verifying accuracy of treatment plans.
**Related Terms:** TPS, IMRT, VMAT, LINAC, QA Phantom
**Radiotherapy Example:** Liver SBRT plan verified against QA phantom measurements.

220. **Target Volume Reassessment QA:** QA for re-evaluating tumor volume during therapy.
**Related Terms:** CBCT, IGRT, TPS, LINAC
**Radiotherapy Example:** Weekly CBCT used to reassess shrinking prostate tumor.

221. **Target Volume Margin QA:** QA to ensure tumor margins are sufficient and accurate for coverage.
**Related Terms:** PTV, GTV, CTV, TPS, LINAC
**Radiotherapy Example:** Prostate IMRT plan margin verified using daily CBCT imaging.

222. **Treatment Beam Angle Verification:** QA to confirm the angles of radiation beams match the planned setup.
**Related Terms:** LINAC, TPS, IGRT, IMRT, VMAT
**Radiotherapy Example:** Head & neck VMAT plan beam angles verified with portal imaging.

223. **Tumor Dose Escalation QA:** QA ensuring higher doses to tumor regions are delivered safely.
**Related Terms:** Dose Painting, IMRT, VMAT, LINAC
**Radiotherapy Example:** Liver SBRT plan dose escalation verified on QA phantom.

224. **Treatment Couch Sag Correction:** QA for any deviations in treatment table sag affecting dose delivery.
**Related Terms:** LINAC, IGRT, QA Phantom
**Radiotherapy Example:** Couch sag measured and corrected for craniospinal irradiation.

225. **Tomotherapy Beam Quality QA:** QA for the quality and consistency of helical tomotherapy beams.
**Related Terms:** LINAC, IMRT, QA Phantom, Dose Verification
**Radiotherapy Example:** Pelvic plan dose verified using cheese phantom on tomotherapy.

226. **Tissue Equivalent Phantom QA:** QA using phantoms that mimic human tissue for dose verification.
**Related Terms:** TPS, LINAC, Dosimetry, Radiotherapy
**Radiotherapy Example:** Head phantom used to verify dose distribution for brain SRS.

227. **Treatment Fraction Verification:** QA ensuring each fraction is delivered according to the treatment plan.
**Related Terms:** LINAC, IGRT, EPID, IMRT, VMAT
**Radiotherapy Example:** Daily verification of breast IMRT fractions using EPID.

228. **Tumor Motion Imaging QA:** QA of imaging techniques used to monitor tumor motion.
**Related Terms:** 4D CT, CBCT, LINAC, IGRT
**Radiotherapy Example:** Lung tumor motion assessed with 4D CT for gating.

229. **Treatment Field Size Verification:** QA to confirm radiation field sizes match planned dimensions.
**Related Terms:** LINAC, TPS, Portal Imaging, IMRT
**Radiotherapy Example:** Portal imaging used to verify breast field sizes.

230. **Tumor Hypoxia Dose Adjustment:** Adjusting dose based on hypoxic regions identified in imaging.
**Related Terms:** PET, Radiotracer, TPS, LINAC
**Radiotherapy Example:** PET-based hypoxia imaging guided boost dose in head & neck tumor.

231. **Tomotherapy Couch Position QA:** QA ensuring couch moves accurately during tomotherapy delivery.
**Related Terms:** LINAC, IGRT, QA Phantom
**Radiotherapy Example:** Couch movements verified before thoracic tomotherapy.

232. **Tissue Inhomogeneity Dose QA:** QA to account for tissue density variations in dose calculations.
**Related Terms:** TPS, CT Scan, LINAC, Radiotherapy
**Radiotherapy Example:** Lung SBRT plan dose corrected for air cavities.

233. **Treatment Time Monitoring:** Tracking actual delivery time for each radiation fraction.
**Related Terms:** LINAC, IMRT, VMAT, QA
**Radiotherapy Example:** SBRT session time recorded to ensure proper dose delivery.

234. **Target Conformity QA:** QA ensuring prescribed dose conforms accurately to tumor shape.
**Related Terms:** PTV, DVH, IMRT, VMAT, LINAC
**Radiotherapy Example:** Brain SRS conformity index verified on phantom.

235. **Tumor Response Imaging QA:** QA for imaging used to monitor tumor shrinkage or progression.
**Related Terms:** CT Scan, MRI, PET, IGRT
**Radiotherapy Example:** Weekly CT used to monitor lung tumor response.

236. **Treatment Delivery Efficiency QA:** QA ensuring planned treatments are delivered efficiently and safely.
**Related Terms:** LINAC, IMRT, VMAT, QA Phantom
**Radiotherapy Example:** Efficiency of multi-field prostate IMRT evaluated.

237. **Transverse Imaging QA:** QA of transverse slices in CT imaging for accuracy.
**Related Terms:** CT Scan, TPS, Radiology, LINAC
**Radiotherapy Example:** Abdominal CT slices checked for artifacts before planning.

238. **Tumor Dose Gradient QA:** QA assessing dose gradients across tumor and surrounding tissues.
**Related Terms:** TPS, IMRT, DVH, LINAC
**Radiotherapy Example:** Head & neck IMRT gradient verified to spare spinal cord.

239. **Treatment Planning QA Protocol:** QA protocols for verifying accuracy of treatment plans.
**Related Terms:** TPS, IMRT, VMAT, LINAC, QA Phantom
**Radiotherapy Example:** Liver SBRT plan verified against QA phantom measurements.

240. **Target Volume Reassessment QA:** QA for re-evaluating tumor volume during therapy.
**Related Terms:** CBCT, IGRT, TPS, LINAC
**Radiotherapy Example:** Weekly CBCT used to reassess shrinking prostate tumor.

241. **Target Volume Margin QA:** QA to ensure tumor margins are sufficient and accurate for coverage.
**Related Terms:** PTV, GTV, CTV, TPS, LINAC
**Radiotherapy Example:** Prostate IMRT plan margin verified using daily CBCT imaging.

242. **Treatment Beam Angle Verification:** QA to confirm the angles of radiation beams match the planned setup.
**Related Terms:** LINAC, TPS, IGRT, IMRT, VMAT
**Radiotherapy Example:** Head & neck VMAT plan beam angles verified with portal imaging.

243. **Tumor Dose Escalation QA:** QA ensuring higher doses to tumor regions are delivered safely.
**Related Terms:** Dose Painting, IMRT, VMAT, LINAC
**Radiotherapy Example:** Liver SBRT plan dose escalation verified on QA phantom.

244. **Treatment Couch Sag Correction:** QA for any deviations in treatment table sag affecting dose delivery.
**Related Terms:** LINAC, IGRT, QA Phantom
**Radiotherapy Example:** Couch sag measured and corrected for craniospinal irradiation.

245. **Tomotherapy Beam Quality QA:** QA for the quality and consistency of helical tomotherapy beams.
**Related Terms:** LINAC, IMRT, QA Phantom, Dose Verification
**Radiotherapy Example:** Pelvic plan dose verified using cheese phantom on tomotherapy.

246. **Tissue Equivalent Phantom QA:** QA using phantoms that mimic human tissue for dose verification.
**Related Terms:** TPS, LINAC, Dosimetry, Radiotherapy
**Radiotherapy Example:** Head phantom used to verify dose distribution for brain SRS.

247. **Treatment Fraction Verification:** QA ensuring each fraction is delivered according to the treatment plan.
**Related Terms:** LINAC, IGRT, EPID, IMRT, VMAT
**Radiotherapy Example:** Daily verification of breast IMRT fractions using EPID.

248. **Tumor Motion Imaging QA:** QA of imaging techniques used to monitor tumor motion.
**Related Terms:** 4D CT, CBCT, LINAC, IGRT
**Radiotherapy Example:** Lung tumor motion assessed with 4D CT for gating.

249. **Treatment Field Size Verification:** QA to confirm radiation field sizes match planned dimensions.
**Related Terms:** LINAC, TPS, Portal Imaging, IMRT
**Radiotherapy Example:** Portal imaging used to verify breast field sizes.

250. **Tumor Hypoxia Dose Adjustment:** Adjusting dose based on hypoxic regions identified in imaging.
**Related Terms:** PET, Radiotracer, TPS, LINAC
**Radiotherapy Example:** PET-based hypoxia imaging guided boost dose in head & neck tumor.

251. **Tomotherapy Couch Position QA:** QA ensuring couch moves accurately during tomotherapy delivery.
**Related Terms:** LINAC, IGRT, QA Phantom
**Radiotherapy Example:** Couch movements verified before thoracic tomotherapy.

252. **Tissue Inhomogeneity Dose QA:** QA to account for tissue density variations in dose calculations.
**Related Terms:** TPS, CT Scan, LINAC, Radiotherapy
**Radiotherapy Example:** Lung SBRT plan dose corrected for air cavities.

253. **Treatment Time Monitoring:** Tracking actual delivery time for each radiation fraction.
**Related Terms:** LINAC, IMRT, VMAT, QA
**Radiotherapy Example:** SBRT session time recorded to ensure proper dose delivery.

254. **Target Conformity QA:** QA ensuring prescribed dose conforms accurately to tumor shape.
**Related Terms:** PTV, DVH, IMRT, VMAT, LINAC
**Radiotherapy Example:** Brain SRS conformity index verified on phantom.

255. **Tumor Response Imaging QA:** QA for imaging used to monitor tumor shrinkage or progression.
**Related Terms:** CT Scan, MRI, PET, IGRT
**Radiotherapy Example:** Weekly CT used to monitor lung tumor response.

256. **Treatment Delivery Efficiency QA:** QA ensuring planned treatments are delivered efficiently and safely.
**Related Terms:** LINAC, IMRT, VMAT, QA Phantom
**Radiotherapy Example:** Efficiency of multi-field prostate IMRT evaluated.

257. **Transverse Imaging QA:** QA of transverse slices in CT imaging for accuracy.
**Related Terms:** CT Scan, TPS, Radiology, LINAC
**Radiotherapy Example:** Abdominal CT slices checked for artifacts before planning.

258. **Tumor Dose Gradient QA:** QA assessing dose gradients across tumor and surrounding tissues.
**Related Terms:** TPS, IMRT, DVH, LINAC
**Radiotherapy Example:** Head & neck IMRT gradient verified to spare spinal cord.

259. **Treatment Planning QA Protocol:** QA protocols for verifying accuracy of treatment plans.
**Related Terms:** TPS, IMRT, VMAT, LINAC, QA Phantom
**Radiotherapy Example:** Liver SBRT plan verified against QA phantom measurements.

260. **Target Volume Reassessment QA:** QA for re-evaluating tumor volume during therapy.
**Related Terms:** CBCT, IGRT, TPS, LINAC
**Radiotherapy Example:** Weekly CBCT used to reassess shrinking prostate tumor.

261. **Tumor Volume Change Monitoring:** QA to track tumor volume changes during treatment.
**Related Terms:** PTV, CBCT, MRI, TPS
**Radiotherapy Example:** Weekly CBCT assesses prostate shrinkage for adaptive planning.

262. **Treatment Couch Rotation QA:** QA to verify correct rotation of treatment couch for non-coplanar beams.
**Related Terms:** LINAC, IGRT, QA Phantom
**Radiotherapy Example:** Couch angles verified for cranial SRS delivery.

263. **Target Position Reproducibility QA:** QA to ensure consistent target positioning across fractions.
**Related Terms:** PTV, IGRT, LINAC
**Radiotherapy Example:** Prostate fiducial markers checked daily with CBCT.

264. **Tomotherapy Imaging Dose QA:** QA to measure dose delivered by tomotherapy imaging system.
**Related Terms:** LINAC, CBCT, Dosimetry, QA Phantom
**Radiotherapy Example:** Pelvic tomotherapy imaging dose measured using ion chamber.

265. **Treatment Beam Flatness QA:** QA to verify uniform dose distribution across the beam.
**Related Terms:** LINAC, IMRT, VMAT, QA Phantom
**Radiotherapy Example:** Head & neck photon beam flatness verified with water phantom.

266. **Tissue Equivalent Phantom QA:** QA using phantoms that mimic human tissue for dose verification.
**Related Terms:** Mould Room, TPS, LINAC, Dosimetry
**Radiotherapy Example:** Breast IMRT verified using tissue-equivalent phantom with embedded dosimeters.

267. **Tumor Conformity Index QA:** QA to assess how closely the dose conforms to tumor shape.
**Related Terms:** PTV, TPS, IMRT, VMAT
**Radiotherapy Example:** Liver SBRT plan evaluated for conformity index using DVH.

268. **Treatment Field Verification:** QA to verify radiation field size, shape, and position.
**Related Terms:** LINAC, Portal Imaging, MLC
**Radiotherapy Example:** Prostate IMRT field verified daily using portal imaging.

269. **Tissue Heterogeneity Mapping:** QA to ensure TPS accounts for varying tissue densities.
**Related Terms:** CT Scan, TPS, LINAC, Radiotherapy
**Radiotherapy Example:** Lung tumor dose corrected for air cavity in TPS calculations.

270. **Tomotherapy Leaf Speed QA:** QA to verify multileaf collimator (MLC) leaf speed in tomotherapy.
**Related Terms:** LINAC, IMRT, QA Phantom
**Radiotherapy Example:** MLC leaf speed verified for head & neck tomotherapy plan.

271. **Treatment Beam Symmetry QA:** QA to ensure left-right symmetry of the radiation beam.
**Related Terms:** LINAC, IMRT, VMAT, QA Phantom
**Radiotherapy Example:** Breast IMRT beams verified for symmetry using ion chamber array.

272. **Target Dose Homogeneity QA:** QA to check dose uniformity within the target volume.
**Related Terms:** PTV, TPS, LINAC
**Radiotherapy Example:** Liver SBRT target dose homogeneity verified using film dosimetry.

273. **Tissue Interface Dose Mapping:** QA to measure dose at tissue interfaces (e.g., bone-lung).
**Related Terms:** TPS, LINAC, CT Scan, Dosimetry
**Radiotherapy Example:** Head & neck interface dose measured using OSLDs at bone-lung junction.

274. **Treatment Beam Energy Consistency:** QA to ensure consistent beam energy throughout treatment course.
**Related Terms:** LINAC, Dosimetry, Photon, Electron
**Radiotherapy Example:** Photon energy verified weekly using ionization chamber in water phantom.

275. **Tumor Motion Simulation QA:** QA using phantoms to simulate tumor motion.
**Related Terms:** 4D CT, IGRT, LINAC, Gating
**Radiotherapy Example:** Lung phantom simulates respiratory motion to verify SBRT gating.

276. **Tomotherapy Dose Uniformity QA:** QA to ensure uniform dose delivery in tomotherapy treatments.
**Related Terms:** LINAC, IMRT, QA Phantom, TPS
**Radiotherapy Example:** Pelvic tomotherapy dose uniformity checked using cheese phantom.

277. **Treatment Field Edge QA:** QA to verify sharpness and accuracy of field edges.
**Related Terms:** LINAC, IMRT, MLC, Portal Imaging
**Radiotherapy Example:** Head & neck IMRT field edges verified using film dosimetry.

278. **Tissue-Equivalent Detector Calibration:** QA to calibrate detectors simulating human tissue.
**Related Terms:** Phantom, Dosimetry, LINAC, TPS
**Radiotherapy Example:** Breast phantom with TLDs calibrated to ensure accurate dose measurement.

279. **Target Volume Shrinkage Monitoring:** QA to monitor changes in tumor volume during therapy.
**Related Terms:** CBCT, PTV, TPS, LINAC
**Radiotherapy Example:** Weekly CBCT monitors shrinking prostate PTV for adaptive planning.

280. **Treatment Plan Verification Imaging:** QA using imaging to verify planned dose distribution.
**Related Terms:** TPS, CBCT, Portal Imaging, LINAC
**Radiotherapy Example:** Head & neck IMRT plan verified with daily portal imaging.

281. **Tumor Tracking System QA:** QA for systems tracking tumor motion during treatment.
**Related Terms:** IGRT, 4D CT, LINAC, Gating
**Radiotherapy Example:** Lung tumor tracked in real-time using CBCT gating system.

282. **Tomotherapy Field Width Verification:** QA to ensure correct field width in helical delivery.
**Related Terms:** LINAC, TPS, QA Phantom
**Radiotherapy Example:** Pelvic tomotherapy verified 2.5 cm field width using phantom measurement.

283. **Treatment Beam Output QA:** QA to ensure delivered dose matches prescribed dose.
**Related Terms:** LINAC, Dosimetry, IMRT, VMAT
**Radiotherapy Example:** Photon IMRT output verified with ion chamber array before delivery.

284. **Tissue Compensator Thickness Verification:** QA to ensure compensators match planned thickness.
**Related Terms:** Mould Room, TPS, LINAC
**Radiotherapy Example:** Breast compensator thickness checked using caliper measurement.

285. **Target Alignment QA:** QA to confirm target alignment with radiation beams.
**Related Terms:** PTV, IGRT, CBCT, LINAC
**Radiotherapy Example:** Head & neck IMRT target alignment checked daily using orthogonal CBCT.

286. **Tomotherapy Energy Verification:** QA to confirm correct energy is delivered in tomotherapy.
**Related Terms:** LINAC, TPS, Dosimetry
**Radiotherapy Example:** Pelvic tomotherapy photon energy verified using ion chamber array.

287. **Treatment Couch Sag QA:** QA to measure and correct for couch sag under patient weight.
**Related Terms:** LINAC, IGRT, QA Phantom
**Radiotherapy Example:** Couch sag assessed using phantom during craniospinal irradiation.

288. **Tissue Inhomogeneity QA:** QA to correct dose calculations in heterogeneous tissues.
**Related Terms:** CT Scan, TPS, LINAC
**Radiotherapy Example:** Lung SBRT dose adjusted for air and bone heterogeneity.

289. **Target Coverage Adaptation QA:** QA to adapt treatment plan based on tumor response.
**Related Terms:** PTV, CBCT, TPS, LINAC
**Radiotherapy Example:** Prostate PTV updated mid-treatment after CBCT volume assessment.

290. **Treatment Delivery Record QA:** QA to review and verify delivery logs and records.
**Related Terms:** LINAC, TPS, IMRT, VMAT
**Radiotherapy Example:** Check LINAC delivery log against planned head & neck SBRT fields.

291. **Tumor Motion Compensation QA:** QA to correct dose delivery for moving tumors.
**Related Terms:** IGRT, 4D CT, Gating, LINAC
**Radiotherapy Example:** Lung tumor dose adjusted during breath-hold gating.

292. **Treatment Beam Energy Layering QA:** QA to verify layered energies for precise dose deposition.
**Related Terms:** Proton Therapy, LINAC, TPS, IMRT
**Radiotherapy Example:** Head & neck proton therapy uses multiple energy layers verified with phantom.

293. **Target Dose Escalation QA:** QA to safely deliver higher dose to tumor while sparing normal tissue.
**Related Terms:** PTV, IMRT, VMAT, TPS
**Radiotherapy Example:** Boost dose to hypoxic tumor regions verified using DVH analysis.

294. **Tomotherapy Dose Verification QA:** QA to confirm tomotherapy dose delivery matches plan.
**Related Terms:** LINAC, QA Phantom, IMRT
**Radiotherapy Example:** Pelvic tomotherapy dose verified using cheese phantom with ion chambers.

295. **Treatment Field Shape Verification:** QA to ensure MLC accurately shapes radiation fields.
**Related Terms:** LINAC, IMRT, VMAT, Portal Imaging
**Radiotherapy Example:** Head & neck IMRT field shape verified with portal dosimetry.

296. **Tissue Density Correction QA:** QA to account for tissue density differences in dose calculation.
**Related Terms:** CT Scan, TPS, LINAC, Dosimetry
**Radiotherapy Example:** Lung SBRT dose recalculated with heterogeneity corrections.

297. **Target Margin Verification QA:** QA to verify planning margins adequately cover tumor motion and setup errors.
**Related Terms:** PTV, CTV, IGRT, LINAC
**Radiotherapy Example:** Prostate PTV margins verified using daily CBCT imaging.

298. **Treatment Couch Position QA:** QA to ensure couch is positioned accurately for each fraction.
**Related Terms:** LINAC, IGRT, CBCT
**Radiotherapy Example:** Couch coordinates checked before each head & neck treatment.

299. **Tumor Contour Accuracy QA:** QA to confirm accuracy of tumor delineation in planning images.
**Related Terms:** TPS, CT Scan, MRI, Radiology
**Radiotherapy Example:** Prostate MRI contours reviewed and verified before IMRT planning.

300. **Tomotherapy Imaging-Guided QA:** QA to ensure tomotherapy imaging accurately guides treatment.
**Related Terms:** LINAC, IGRT, CBCT, TPS
**Radiotherapy Example:** Pelvic tomotherapy imaging verified for patient alignment accuracy.

301. **Target Volume Dose Accumulation QA:** QA to sum delivered dose over multiple fractions for accuracy.
**Related Terms:** PTV, TPS, LINAC, IMRT
**Radiotherapy Example:** Liver SBRT cumulative dose verified with treatment log data.

302. **Treatment Beam Modulation QA:** QA to verify correct modulation of intensity-modulated beams.
**Related Terms:** IMRT, VMAT, LINAC, QA Phantom
**Radiotherapy Example:** Head & neck IMRT beam intensity checked with ion chamber array.

303. **Tissue-Equivalent Phantom Dose Mapping:** QA to map dose using phantoms simulating human tissue.
**Related Terms:** Mould Room, TPS, LINAC, Dosimetry
**Radiotherapy Example:** Breast IMRT dose mapped using tissue-equivalent phantom with embedded TLDs.

304. **Treatment Field Position Verification:** QA to verify radiation field is correctly positioned relative to target.
**Related Terms:** LINAC, Portal Imaging, MLC
**Radiotherapy Example:** Prostate IMRT fields verified daily using orthogonal portal images.

305. **Tumor Motion Management QA:** QA for managing tumor motion during treatment delivery.
**Related Terms:** IGRT, 4D CT, LINAC, Gating
**Radiotherapy Example:** Lung tumor tracked and dose delivered during gated beam on exhale phase.

306. **Tomotherapy Field Overlap QA:** QA to ensure overlapping helical fields deliver uniform dose.
**Related Terms:** LINAC, TPS, IMRT
**Radiotherapy Example:** Spinal tomotherapy overlap regions verified with film dosimetry.

307. **Target Dose Gradient QA:** QA to verify steepness of dose fall-off around tumor.
**Related Terms:** PTV, TPS, IMRT, VMAT
**Radiotherapy Example:** Stereotactic brain tumor plan verified for dose gradient with film dosimetry.

308. **Treatment Beam Symmetry Verification:** QA to check beam symmetry across central axis.
**Related Terms:** LINAC, IMRT, VMAT, QA Phantom
**Radiotherapy Example:** Breast IMRT photon beams verified for left-right symmetry.

309. **Tissue Heterogeneity Dose QA:** QA to correct dose for inhomogeneous tissues (bone, lung).
**Related Terms:** CT Scan, TPS, LINAC, Dosimetry
**Radiotherapy Example:** Lung SBRT dose recalculated accounting for air cavities.

310. **Target Position Adjustment QA:** QA to correct patient setup to match planned target position.
**Related Terms:** IGRT, CBCT, LINAC
**Radiotherapy Example:** Daily CBCT ensures prostate PTV alignment before beam-on.

311. **Tomotherapy Dose Calculation Verification:** QA to ensure dose calculation accuracy in TPS for tomotherapy.
**Related Terms:** TPS, LINAC, QA Phantom
**Radiotherapy Example:** Pelvic tomotherapy plan recalculated and compared with measured phantom dose.

312. **Treatment Beam Penumbra QA:** QA to measure dose fall-off at the edge of the radiation beam.
**Related Terms:** LINAC, MLC, IMRT, VMAT
**Radiotherapy Example:** Head & neck IMRT beam penumbra verified with film dosimetry.

313. **Tissue Interface Dose QA:** QA to ensure accurate dose at interfaces between tissues of different density.
**Related Terms:** CT Scan, TPS, LINAC
**Radiotherapy Example:** Bone-lung interface in chest wall SBRT verified using dosimeters.

314. **Target Volume Shrinkage Assessment QA:** QA to monitor tumor shrinkage during fractionated therapy.
**Related Terms:** PTV, CBCT, TPS, LINAC
**Radiotherapy Example:** Weekly CBCT tracks shrinking liver tumor for adaptive planning.

315. **Treatment Plan Dose Homogeneity QA:** QA to confirm uniform dose distribution within target volume.
**Related Terms:** TPS, PTV, IMRT, VMAT
**Radiotherapy Example:** Breast IMRT dose homogeneity verified with ion chamber array.

316. **Tomotherapy Beam Alignment QA:** QA to verify precise alignment of helical tomotherapy beams.
**Related Terms:** LINAC, IGRT, TPS, QA Phantom
**Radiotherapy Example:** Spinal tomotherapy alignment checked daily using phantom imaging.

317. **Treatment Couch Motion QA:** QA to verify accuracy of automated couch movements during treatment.
**Related Terms:** LINAC, IGRT, Robotic Couch, CBCT
**Radiotherapy Example:** Head & neck IMRT couch shifts validated using CBCT and laser alignment.

318. **Target Dose Verification Using Film:** QA to measure delivered dose using radiochromic or radiographic film.
**Related Terms:** TPS, IMRT, VMAT, LINAC
**Radiotherapy Example:** Stereotactic brain plan verified with Gafchromic film in phantom.

319. **Tissue-Equivalent Phantom QA:** QA using phantoms that mimic human tissue for dose verification.
**Related Terms:** Mould Room, TPS, LINAC, Dosimetry
**Radiotherapy Example:** Breast IMRT dose mapped with tissue-equivalent phantom with embedded TLDs.

320. **Target Volume Coverage QA:** QA to ensure prescribed dose fully covers the target volume.
**Related Terms:** PTV, TPS, IMRT, VMAT
**Radiotherapy Example:** Prostate PTV dose coverage verified using DVH and QA phantom.

321. **Treatment Beam Flatness QA:** QA to verify uniform intensity across the beam profile.
**Related Terms:** LINAC, IMRT, VMAT, QA Phantom
**Radiotherapy Example:** Photon beam flatness checked monthly using ion chamber array.

322. **Tumor Motion Imaging QA:** QA to track tumor motion during imaging-guided therapy.
**Related Terms:** IGRT, 4D CT, CBCT, LINAC
**Radiotherapy Example:** Lung tumor tracked using 4D CT for gated SBRT delivery.

323. **Tomotherapy Dose Homogeneity QA:** QA to confirm uniform dose delivery in tomotherapy plans.
**Related Terms:** TPS, LINAC, QA Phantom, IMRT
**Radiotherapy Example:** Pelvic tomotherapy plan dose uniformity verified with ion chamber array.

324. **Treatment Field Edge QA:** QA to check accuracy of field edges using MLC or jaw positioning.
**Related Terms:** LINAC, IMRT, VMAT, Portal Imaging
**Radiotherapy Example:** Head & neck IMRT field edges verified using portal imaging.

325. **Tissue Inhomogeneity Correction QA:** QA to adjust dose calculations for heterogeneous tissues.
**Related Terms:** CT Scan, TPS, LINAC, Dosimetry
**Radiotherapy Example:** Lung SBRT dose recalculated with heterogeneity corrections for air cavities.

326. **Target Volume Adaptation QA:** QA to adjust target volume during treatment based on changes.
**Related Terms:** PTV, IGRT, TPS, LINAC
**Radiotherapy Example:** Weekly CBCT imaging adapts liver SBRT target to tumor shrinkage.

327. **Treatment Beam Output Consistency QA:** QA to ensure the LINAC output is consistent across fractions.
**Related Terms:** LINAC, Dosimetry, IMRT, VMAT
**Radiotherapy Example:** Photon beam output verified daily using ionization chamber.

328. **Tumor Dose Gradient Verification QA:** QA to confirm steep dose fall-off at tumor boundaries.
**Related Terms:** TPS, IMRT, VMAT, LINAC
**Radiotherapy Example:** Stereotactic brain tumor dose gradient verified using film dosimetry.

329. **Tomotherapy Imaging Accuracy QA:** QA to ensure tomotherapy imaging precisely guides treatment.
**Related Terms:** LINAC, IGRT, CBCT, TPS
**Radiotherapy Example:** Pelvic imaging alignment verified before daily tomotherapy delivery.

330. **Treatment Plan Verification QA:** QA to ensure the planned dose matches delivered dose.
**Related Terms:** TPS, LINAC, IMRT, VMAT, QA Phantom
**Radiotherapy Example:** Head & neck IMRT plan verified with ion chamber array.

331. **Tissue Phantom Dose Verification QA:** QA using phantoms simulating tissue to verify dose delivery.
**Related Terms:** Mould Room, TPS, LINAC, Dosimetry
**Radiotherapy Example:** Breast IMRT verified using tissue-equivalent phantom with TLDs.

332. **Treatment Beam Modulation Verification QA:** QA to confirm beam intensity modulation matches treatment plan.
**Related Terms:** LINAC, IMRT, VMAT, QA Phantom
**Radiotherapy Example:** Pelvic VMAT plan verified using ion chamber array.

333. **Tumor Volume Dose Mapping QA:** QA to map delivered dose across the tumor volume.
**Related Terms:** PTV, TPS, LINAC, IMRT
**Radiotherapy Example:** Liver SBRT dose mapped in phantom to verify tumor coverage.

334. **Tomotherapy Field Overlap Verification QA:** QA to ensure overlapping helical fields provide uniform dose.
**Related Terms:** TPS, LINAC, QA Phantom, IMRT
**Radiotherapy Example:** Spinal tomotherapy overlap region verified with film dosimetry.

335. **Target Motion Prediction QA:** QA to anticipate tumor motion for accurate dose delivery.
**Related Terms:** IGRT, 4D CT, LINAC, Gating
**Radiotherapy Example:** Lung tumor motion predicted using 4D CT for gated SBRT.

336. **Tissue Interface Dose Verification QA:** QA to verify dose accuracy at interfaces of different tissue densities.
**Related Terms:** CT Scan, TPS, LINAC, Dosimetry
**Radiotherapy Example:** Chest wall SBRT verified at bone-lung interface using dosimeters.

337. **Treatment Beam Symmetry QA:** QA to check beam symmetry about the central axis.
**Related Terms:** LINAC, IMRT, VMAT, QA Phantom
**Radiotherapy Example:** Breast photon beam verified for symmetry with ion chamber array.

338. **Target Volume Shrinkage Monitoring QA:** QA to monitor tumor shrinkage during fractionated treatment.
**Related Terms:** PTV, IGRT, CBCT, TPS
**Radiotherapy Example:** Weekly CBCT tracks liver tumor shrinkage for adaptive SBRT planning.

339. **Tomotherapy Dose Gradient QA:** QA to verify steep dose gradient around target in tomotherapy.
**Related Terms:** TPS, LINAC, IMRT, VMAT
**Radiotherapy Example:** Spinal tomotherapy gradient verified using phantom film.

340. **Treatment Couch Shift Verification QA:** QA to ensure couch shifts match planned patient positioning.
**Related Terms:** LINAC, IGRT, CBCT
**Radiotherapy Example:** Daily prostate patient shifts verified with CBCT before IMRT delivery.

341. **Tomotherapy Dose Reconstruction QA:** QA to reconstruct delivered dose from imaging data for verification.
**Related Terms:** TPS, LINAC, IGRT, QA Phantom
**Radiotherapy Example:** Spinal tomotherapy dose reconstructed from daily MVCT to verify cumulative dose.

342. **Treatment Field Junction QA:** QA to check dose uniformity at the junction of adjacent treatment fields.
**Related Terms:** LINAC, IMRT, VMAT, QA Phantom
**Radiotherapy Example:** Head & neck IMRT field junction verified using film dosimetry.

343. **Tumor Volume Contouring QA:** QA to ensure accurate tumor delineation on imaging.
**Related Terms:** CT Scan, MRI, TPS, Radiology
**Radiotherapy Example:** Prostate tumor contour verified by oncologist before IMRT planning.

344. **Tomotherapy Couch Sag QA:** QA to measure couch sag and compensate for dose delivery errors.
**Related Terms:** LINAC, IGRT, QA Phantom
**Radiotherapy Example:** Pelvic tomotherapy plan adjusted for couch sag using phantom measurements.

345. **Treatment Beam Energy Verification QA:** QA to ensure the LINAC delivers correct photon or electron beam energy.
**Related Terms:** LINAC, Dosimetry, VMAT, IMRT
**Radiotherapy Example:** Photon beam energy verified monthly using ionization chamber in water phantom.

346. **Tumor Motion Compensation QA:** QA to verify compensation for tumor motion during treatment.
**Related Terms:** IGRT, 4D CT, Gating, LINAC
**Radiotherapy Example:** Lung SBRT treatment synchronized with patient respiration to reduce motion errors.

347. **Target Volume Replanning QA:** QA to ensure replanned treatment accurately covers modified tumor volume.
**Related Terms:** PTV, TPS, LINAC, IGRT
**Radiotherapy Example:** Adaptive prostate IMRT plan verified after significant tumor shrinkage.

348. **Tomotherapy Beam Output QA:** QA to measure and ensure consistent output from tomotherapy unit.
**Related Terms:** LINAC, TPS, QA Phantom
**Radiotherapy Example:** Daily MVCT used to verify output consistency for spinal treatments.

349. **Treatment Beam Penumbra QA:** QA to measure dose fall-off at beam edges (penumbra) for precise delivery.
**Related Terms:** LINAC, IMRT, VMAT, QA Phantom
**Radiotherapy Example:** Head & neck IMRT plan checked for sharp penumbra using film dosimetry.

350. **Tumor Dose Accumulation QA:** QA to ensure cumulative dose delivered matches planned dose over all fractions.
**Related Terms:** TPS, LINAC, IGRT, QA Phantom
**Radiotherapy Example:** Liver SBRT cumulative dose verified using reconstructed dose from daily imaging.

351. **Treatment Couch Positioning QA:** QA to ensure the treatment couch moves accurately to planned positions.
**Related Terms:** LINAC, IGRT, TPS, QA Phantom
**Radiotherapy Example:** Couch positions for head & neck IMRT verified with laser alignment and phantom.

352. **Tomotherapy Slice Thickness Verification:** QA to confirm correct slice thickness in tomotherapy imaging.
**Related Terms:** CT Scan, IGRT, TPS
**Radiotherapy Example:** Pelvic CT slices verified at 2.5 mm to ensure accurate treatment planning.

353. **Target Volume Coverage QA:** QA to verify planned dose covers entire tumor volume.
**Related Terms:** PTV, TPS, IMRT, VMAT
**Radiotherapy Example:** Prostate PTV coverage verified on daily CBCT images.

354. **Tumor Contour Consistency QA:** QA to ensure contours remain consistent across planning and treatment imaging.
**Related Terms:** TPS, Radiology, IGRT
**Radiotherapy Example:** Head & neck tumor contours cross-checked between CT and MRI for consistency.

355. **Tomotherapy Machine Output Verification:** QA to confirm daily tomotherapy machine output matches calibration.
**Related Terms:** LINAC, Ion Chamber, QA Phantom
**Radiotherapy Example:** Daily MVCT output checked before delivering spinal treatments.

356. **Treatment Field Size Verification:** QA to ensure treatment fields are delivered at planned dimensions.
**Related Terms:** LINAC, IMRT, VMAT, QA Phantom
**Radiotherapy Example:** Brain tumor IMRT field dimensions verified using portal imaging.

357. **Tumor Dose Homogeneity QA:** QA to ensure even dose distribution across tumor volume.
**Related Terms:** TPS, LINAC, IMRT, VMAT
**Radiotherapy Example:** Liver SBRT dose homogeneity checked using gamma analysis.

358. **Tomotherapy Image Registration QA:** QA to ensure accurate alignment between imaging and planning CT.
**Related Terms:** IGRT, TPS, CT Scan
**Radiotherapy Example:** Cervical tumor CBCT registered to planning CT to verify setup.

359. **Treatment Beam Flatness QA:** QA to verify uniform intensity across the beam profile.
**Related Terms:** LINAC, IMRT, VMAT, QA Phantom
**Radiotherapy Example:** Photon beam flatness verified using water phantom before head & neck treatment.

360. **Tumor Motion Imaging QA:** QA to capture and verify tumor motion during imaging.
**Related Terms:** 4D CT, IGRT, LINAC
**Radiotherapy Example:** Lung tumor motion tracked via 4D CT for gated SBRT delivery.

361. **Tomotherapy Dose Rate QA:** QA to confirm consistent dose rate delivery in tomotherapy.
**Related Terms:** LINAC, TPS, QA Phantom
**Radiotherapy Example:** Spinal SBRT dose rate verified before each treatment session.

362. **Treatment Isocenter Verification:** QA to ensure radiation beams converge precisely at planned isocenter.
**Related Terms:** LINAC, IGRT, TPS, QA Phantom
**Radiotherapy Example:** Head & neck isocenter verified using Winston-Lutz test with phantom.

363. **Tumor Margin Verification QA:** QA to confirm margins around tumor are correctly applied in plan.
**Related Terms:** PTV, TPS, LINAC
**Radiotherapy Example:** Prostate SBRT margins verified on daily CBCT to avoid normal tissue.

364. **Tomotherapy Beam Profile QA:** QA to measure beam profile for uniformity and symmetry.
**Related Terms:** LINAC, QA Phantom, IMRT
**Radiotherapy Example:** Beam profiles verified weekly using ion chamber arrays.

365. **Treatment Time Verification QA:** QA to ensure actual beam-on time matches planned time.
**Related Terms:** LINAC, TPS, QA Phantom
**Radiotherapy Example:** Liver SBRT treatment time checked for each fraction.

366. **Tumor Motion Compensation Verification:** QA to verify motion compensation systems function correctly.
**Related Terms:** Gating, 4D CT, LINAC
**Radiotherapy Example:** Lung tumor tracked with gating system, verified with phantom QA.

367. **Tomotherapy MVCT QA:** QA to ensure MVCT images are of consistent quality and alignment.
**Related Terms:** IGRT, LINAC, QA Phantom
**Radiotherapy Example:** Pelvic MVCT verified daily for accurate setup before treatment.

368. **Treatment Couch Rotation QA:** QA to ensure correct rotation of treatment couch during arc therapy.
**Related Terms:** LINAC, VMAT, IGRT
**Radiotherapy Example:** Head & neck VMAT couch rotations verified using phantom markers.

369. **Tumor Dose Escalation QA:** QA to verify higher dose delivery to tumor subvolumes.
**Related Terms:** TPS, IMRT, VMAT, LINAC
**Radiotherapy Example:** Prostate SBRT dose escalation verified with portal dosimetry.

370. **Tomotherapy Machine Safety QA:** QA to check all safety interlocks and emergency stops function.
**Related Terms:** LINAC, QA Protocol, Radiation Safety
**Radiotherapy Example:** Daily safety check of tomotherapy unit before patient treatments.

371. **Treatment Beam Energy Spectrum QA:** QA to verify photon or electron energy spectrum delivered matches plan.
**Related Terms:** LINAC, TPS, Dosimetry
**Radiotherapy Example:** Photon beam energy spectrum measured for head & neck IMRT.

372. **Tumor Volume Dose Mapping:** QA to map actual delivered dose across tumor volume.
**Related Terms:** TPS, LINAC, IGRT
**Radiotherapy Example:** Liver SBRT dose mapping performed using CBCT and TPS dose reconstruction.

373. **Tomotherapy Plan Verification QA:** QA to ensure plan parameters are accurately delivered.
**Related Terms:** TPS, LINAC, IGRT, QA Phantom
**Radiotherapy Example:** Spinal tomotherapy plan verified via phantom and MVCT imaging.

**374. Treatment Beam Symmetry QA:** QA to ensure left-right symmetry of radiation beam.
**Related Terms:** LINAC, IMRT, VMAT, QA Phantom
**Radiotherapy Example:** Head & neck IMRT beam symmetry verified monthly using film dosimetry.

**375. Tumor Volume Adaptive Planning QA:** QA to verify adaptive plan changes reflect tumor volume changes.
**Related Terms:** TPS, IGRT, LINAC
**Radiotherapy Example:** Adaptive lung SBRT plan verified after tumor shrinkage using CBCT.

**376. Tomotherapy Dose Grid Verification:** QA to ensure dose calculation grid resolution matches plan requirements.
**Related Terms:** TPS, IMRT, VMAT
**Radiotherapy Example:** Prostate tomotherapy dose grid verified for accurate dose distribution.

**377. Treatment Beam Collimation QA:** QA to verify collimator positions match plan for precise beam shaping.
**Related Terms:** LINAC, MLC, VMAT, IMRT
**Radiotherapy Example:** Head & neck IMRT collimator positions verified with portal dosimetry.

**378. Tumor Motion Prediction QA:** QA to validate prediction models of tumor motion during therapy.
**Related Terms:** 4D CT, Gating, LINAC
**Radiotherapy Example:** Lung SBRT tumor motion prediction verified using 4D CT data.

**379. Tomotherapy Output Consistency QA:** QA to ensure consistent dose output across multiple fractions.
**Related Terms:** LINAC, MVCT, QA Phantom
**Radiotherapy Example:** Spinal SBRT output checked daily to maintain uniform fraction dose.

**380. Treatment Field Alignment QA:** QA to verify precise alignment of treatment fields with patient anatomy.
**Related Terms:** LINAC, IGRT, TPS, Mould Room
**Radiotherapy Example:** Head & neck fields aligned with immobilization mask and CBCT imaging.

**381. Tumor Margin Adaptation QA:** QA to verify adjustments to tumor margins during adaptive therapy.
**Related Terms:** PTV, TPS, IGRT
**Radiotherapy Example:** Adaptive lung SBRT margins verified on daily CBCT scans.

**382. Tomotherapy Treatment Time Consistency QA:** QA to ensure planned and actual treatment times match.
**Related Terms:** LINAC, TPS, QA Phantom
**Radiotherapy Example:** Daily spinal tomotherapy sessions checked for accurate beam-on times.

**383. Treatment Couch Sag Verification:** QA to measure any sag in couch when loaded with patient weight.
**Related Terms:** LINAC, IGRT, QA Phantom
**Radiotherapy Example:** Couch sag for head & neck patient measured to adjust beam positioning.

**384. Tumor Volume Dose Reconstruction QA:** QA to reconstruct delivered dose within tumor volume for verification.
**Related Terms:** TPS, LINAC, IGRT
**Radiotherapy Example:** Reconstructed liver SBRT dose from CBCT compared with planned dose.

**385. Tomotherapy Image Noise Assessment:** QA to measure noise levels in tomotherapy MVCT images.
**Related Terms:** QA Phantom, IGRT, LINAC
**Radiotherapy Example:** Pelvic MVCT image noise checked to ensure accurate tumor visualization.

386. **Treatment Field Edge Verification:** QA to ensure radiation field edges match planned margins.
**Related Terms:** LINAC, IMRT, VMAT, MLC
**Radiotherapy Example:** Head & neck IMRT field edges verified using portal imaging.

387. **Tumor Motion Gating QA:** QA to confirm gating systems accurately account for tumor motion.
**Related Terms:** 4D CT, IGRT, LINAC
**Radiotherapy Example:** Lung tumor motion gating verified using respiratory tracking phantom.

388. **Tomotherapy Beam Energy QA:** QA to ensure delivered beam energy matches treatment plan.
**Related Terms:** LINAC, MVCT, QA Phantom
**Radiotherapy Example:** Photon beam energy for prostate tomotherapy verified monthly.

389. **Treatment Beam Output Factor QA:** QA to verify variations in beam output based on field size.
**Related Terms:** LINAC, IMRT, QA Phantom
**Radiotherapy Example:** Head & neck small field output factors checked with ion chamber array.

390. **Tumor Dose Escalation Verification:** QA to ensure higher doses to tumor subvolumes are delivered safely.
**Related Terms:** TPS, IMRT, VMAT, LINAC
**Radiotherapy Example:** Prostate SBRT dose escalation confirmed with portal dosimetry.

391. **Tomotherapy Couch Movement QA:** QA to verify precise couch movements for accurate patient positioning.
**Related Terms:** LINAC, IGRT, QA Phantom
**Radiotherapy Example:** Pelvic SBRT couch movement verified with daily MVCT images.

392. **Treatment Field Orthogonality QA:** QA to ensure treatment fields are orthogonal as planned.
**Related Terms:** LINAC, IMRT, VMAT
**Radiotherapy Example:** Orthogonal head & neck fields verified via portal imaging.

393. **Tumor Volume Imaging Consistency QA:** QA to ensure tumor imaging is consistent across multiple modalities.
**Related Terms:** CT Scan, MRI, IGRT
**Radiotherapy Example:** Head & neck tumor contours checked across CT and MRI scans.

394. **Tomotherapy Dose Verification QA:** QA to confirm dose delivered by tomotherapy matches plan.
**Related Terms:** TPS, LINAC, QA Phantom
**Radiotherapy Example:** Spinal SBRT delivered dose verified with ion chamber array.

395. **Treatment Beam Symmetry Verification:** QA to verify left-right symmetry of radiation beams.
**Related Terms:** LINAC, IMRT, VMAT
**Radiotherapy Example:** Brain IMRT beam symmetry verified using film dosimetry.

396. **Tumor Volume Adaptive QA:** QA to confirm adaptive plan adjustments are correctly implemented.
**Related Terms:** TPS, IGRT, LINAC
**Radiotherapy Example:** Lung SBRT adaptive plan verified with CBCT imaging.

397. **Tomotherapy Machine Interlock QA:** QA to verify safety interlocks are functional on tomotherapy machines.
**Related Terms:** LINAC, QA Protocol, Radiation Safety
**Radiotherapy Example:** Daily interlock tests performed before patient treatments.

398. **Treatment Beam Collimator QA:** QA to ensure collimators are positioned correctly for beam shaping.
**Related Terms:** LINAC, MLC, IMRT, VMAT
**Radiotherapy Example:** Head & neck IMRT collimator positions checked using portal dosimetry.

399. **Tumor Motion Compensation QA:** QA to verify compensation for tumor motion during beam delivery.
**Related Terms:** Gating, 4D CT, LINAC
**Radiotherapy Example:** Lung tumor motion compensated with gating system, verified using phantom.

400. **Tomotherapy QA Phantom Verification:** QA to confirm accuracy of QA phantom measurements in tomotherapy.
**Related Terms:** LINAC, QA Protocol, IMRT
**Radiotherapy Example:** Phantom dose verification performed before spinal SBRT delivery.

401. **Treatment Planning CT QA:** QA to ensure CT images used for planning are accurate and artifact-free.
**Related Terms:** CT Scan, TPS, IGRT
**Radiotherapy Example:** Head & neck planning CT checked for motion artifacts before contouring.

402. **Tumor Contour Accuracy QA:** QA to verify tumor contours match actual anatomy.
**Related Terms:** TPS, CT Scan, MRI
**Radiotherapy Example:** Prostate tumor contours cross-checked with MRI for SBRT.

403. **Tomotherapy Beam Alignment QA:** QA to ensure beam is properly aligned with treatment isocenter.
**Related Terms:** LINAC, IGRT, QA Phantom
**Radiotherapy Example:** Spinal tomotherapy beam alignment verified using MVCT.

404. **Treatment Field Rotation Verification:** QA to confirm correct rotational angles of beams.
**Related Terms:** LINAC, VMAT, IMRT
**Radiotherapy Example:** VMAT fields for lung SBRT verified for gantry rotation angles.

405. **Tumor Dose Gradient QA:** QA to measure dose gradient across tumor volume.
**Related Terms:** TPS, IMRT, VMAT
**Radiotherapy Example:** Head & neck IMRT dose gradient verified with film dosimetry.

406. **Tomotherapy Couch Positioning QA:** QA to confirm precise couch positions for each fraction.
**Related Terms:** LINAC, IGRT, QA Protocol
**Radiotherapy Example:** Pelvic tomotherapy couch positions verified daily using MVCT.

407. **Treatment Beam Penumbra QA:** QA to ensure beam edges are sharp and within tolerance.
**Related Terms:** LINAC, IMRT, VMAT, MLC
**Radiotherapy Example:** Liver SBRT beam penumbra measured with film.

408. **Tumor Motion Range QA:** QA to verify tumor motion range during respiration or movement.
**Related Terms:** 4D CT, Gating, IGRT
**Radiotherapy Example:** Lung tumor motion mapped with 4D CT before gating.

409. **Tomotherapy Dose Rate QA:** QA to ensure dose rate is consistent with plan.
**Related Terms:** LINAC, TPS, QA Phantom
**Radiotherapy Example:** Pelvic tomotherapy dose rate verified prior to treatment.

410. **Treatment Field Isocenter Verification:** QA to verify beams converge at planned isocenter.
**Related Terms:** LINAC, IGRT, QA Phantom
**Radiotherapy Example:** Brain SBRT isocenter confirmed using portal imaging.

411. **Tumor Volume Imaging QA:** QA to ensure imaging accurately represents tumor volume.
**Related Terms:** CT Scan, MRI, IGRT
**Radiotherapy Example:** Head & neck tumor volumes verified with contrast CT.

412. **Tomotherapy Mechanical QA:** QA for mechanical components of tomotherapy machine.
**Related Terms:** LINAC, Couch, Gantry, MLC
**Radiotherapy Example:** Monthly mechanical QA for gantry rotation and couch movement.

413. **Treatment Beam Energy Consistency QA:** QA to ensure consistent energy output of radiation beams.
**Related Terms:** LINAC, Photon, Proton, QA Phantom
**Radiotherapy Example:** Photon energy verified for breast IMRT treatments.

414. **Tumor Volume Registration QA:** QA to verify correct alignment of tumor volumes across imaging sets.
**Related Terms:** TPS, CT, MRI, IGRT
**Radiotherapy Example:** Prostate tumor registration checked between planning CT and daily CBCT.

415. **Tomotherapy Multi-Leaf Collimator QA:** QA to ensure MLCs operate correctly and shape beams accurately.
**Related Terms:** LINAC, IMRT, VMAT, QA Phantom
**Radiotherapy Example:** Head & neck IMRT MLC positions verified daily.

416. **Treatment Beam Flatness QA:** QA to verify beam dose uniformity across the field.
**Related Terms:** LINAC, VMAT, IMRT, QA Phantom
**Radiotherapy Example:** Liver IMRT beams checked for flatness using ion chamber array.

417. **Tumor Dose Escalation QA:** QA to confirm safe and accurate delivery of escalated tumor dose.
**Related Terms:** TPS, IMRT, VMAT
**Radiotherapy Example:** Prostate SBRT dose escalation verified using portal dosimetry.

418. **Tomotherapy Field Overlap QA:** QA to ensure adjacent fields overlap properly without hotspots.
**Related Terms:** LINAC, IMRT, VMAT
**Radiotherapy Example:** Craniospinal tomotherapy field junction verified with film dosimetry.

419. **Treatment Beam Monitor Unit QA:** QA to verify correct monitor units are delivered.
**Related Terms:** LINAC, TPS, IMRT
**Radiotherapy Example:** Lung IMRT MU verified before treatment.

420. **Tumor Motion Tracking QA:** QA to ensure real-time tracking systems accurately monitor tumor motion.
**Related Terms:** 4D CT, Gating, IGRT
**Radiotherapy Example:** Lung tumor motion tracked with electromagnetic sensors during SBRT.

421. **Tomotherapy Image Fusion QA:** QA to verify accuracy of image fusion between planning and verification scans.
**Related Terms:** CT, MRI, TPS, IGRT
**Radiotherapy Example:** Head & neck MVCT fused with planning CT to confirm tumor alignment.

422. **Treatment Beam Output Verification QA:** QA to confirm beam output matches prescribed dose.
**Related Terms:** LINAC, TPS, IMRT, VMAT
**Radiotherapy Example:** Pelvic IMRT beam output verified daily using ion chamber.

423. **Tumor Volume Dose Homogeneity QA:** QA to ensure uniform dose within tumor volume.
**Related Terms:** TPS, IMRT, VMAT
**Radiotherapy Example:** Liver SBRT dose homogeneity confirmed via phantom measurement.

424. **Tomotherapy Imaging Dose QA:** QA to measure radiation dose from tomotherapy imaging.
**Related Terms:** MVCT, LINAC, IGRT
**Radiotherapy Example:** MVCT dose for prostate SBRT assessed and documented.

425. **Treatment Couch Position QA:** QA to confirm accurate couch positioning during each fraction.
**Related Terms:** LINAC, IGRT, QA Phantom
**Radiotherapy Example:** Pelvic SBRT couch positions checked daily using CBCT.

426. **Tumor Volume Adaptive Dose QA:** QA to verify adaptive dose adjustments accurately target tumor.
**Related Terms:** TPS, LINAC, IGRT
**Radiotherapy Example:** Adaptive lung SBRT plan verified for PTV coverage on CBCT.

427. **Tomotherapy Safety Interlock QA:** QA to confirm safety interlocks function properly.
**Related Terms:** LINAC, QA Protocol, Radiation Safety
**Radiotherapy Example:** Daily check of emergency stop and interlock systems before treatment.

428. **Treatment Field Verification QA:** QA to ensure treatment fields match planned dimensions and positions.
**Related Terms:** LINAC, IMRT, VMAT
**Radiotherapy Example:** Head & neck IMRT field verification using portal dosimetry.

429. **Tumor Contour Reproducibility QA:** QA to ensure consistent tumor contouring across imaging sets.
**Related Terms:** CT Scan, MRI, TPS
**Radiotherapy Example:** Liver tumor contours verified across planning CT and daily CBCT.

430. **Tomotherapy Beam Angle QA:** QA to ensure correct beam angles are delivered.
**Related Terms:** LINAC, VMAT, IMRT
**Radiotherapy Example:** Spinal SBRT gantry angles verified with phantom prior to treatment.

431. **Treatment Planning QA Protocol:** Standardized QA procedures for verifying treatment plans.
**Related Terms:** TPS, LINAC, IGRT
**Radiotherapy Example:** Head & neck IMRT plan checked with patient-specific QA phantom.

432. **Tumor Volume Repositioning QA:** QA to verify tumor is correctly repositioned if patient moves.
**Related Terms:** IGRT, LINAC, CBCT
**Radiotherapy Example:** Lung SBRT tumor repositioned after CBCT verification.

433. **Tomotherapy Daily QA:** QA performed daily to verify machine and imaging performance.
**Related Terms:** LINAC, QA Phantom, MVCT
**Radiotherapy Example:** Daily tomotherapy QA includes output, imaging, and mechanical checks.

434. **Treatment Beam Modulation QA:** QA to verify modulation of beam intensity for IMRT/VMAT.
**Related Terms:** LINAC, MLC, TPS
**Radiotherapy Example:** Prostate IMRT beam modulation verified with ion chamber array.

435. **Tumor Motion Mitigation QA:** QA to confirm motion mitigation strategies are effective.
**Related Terms:** Gating, IGRT, 4D CT
**Radiotherapy Example:** Lung SBRT motion mitigation confirmed with real-time tracking.

436. **Tomotherapy Couch Sag Correction QA:** QA to measure and correct any couch sag affecting dose delivery.
**Related Terms:** LINAC, IGRT, QA Phantom
**Radiotherapy Example:** Spinal SBRT couch sag corrected after phantom measurement.

437. **Treatment Field Repositioning QA:** QA to ensure accurate repositioning of fields after patient movement.
**Related Terms:** LINAC, IGRT, CBCT
**Radiotherapy Example:** Pelvic IMRT fields repositioned after CBCT verification.

438. **Tumor Volume Dose Reconstruction QA:** QA to reconstruct delivered dose within tumor volume for verification.
**Related Terms:** TPS, LINAC, IGRT
**Radiotherapy Example:** Reconstructed liver SBRT dose from CBCT compared with planned dose.

439. **Tomotherapy Imaging QA:** QA to verify imaging quality and accuracy for guidance.
**Related Terms:** MVCT, IGRT, LINAC
**Radiotherapy Example:** Daily MVCT images assessed for resolution and artifact-free visualization.

440. **Treatment Beam Output Monitoring QA:** QA to continuously monitor beam output stability.
**Related Terms:** LINAC, TPS, IMRT
**Radiotherapy Example:** Daily photon beam output checked with ionization chamber.

441. **Tumor Dose Verification Imaging QA:** QA to verify dose delivered to tumor using imaging.
**Related Terms:** IGRT, CBCT, TPS
**Radiotherapy Example:** Prostate SBRT dose verified using daily CBCT and portal imaging.

442. **Tomotherapy Multi-Leaf Collimator Accuracy QA:** QA to ensure MLCs accurately shape beams.
**Related Terms:** LINAC, IMRT, VMAT
**Radiotherapy Example:** Head & neck MLC positions verified prior to patient treatment.

443. **Treatment Planning Volume QA:** QA to ensure planning volumes (PTV, CTV, GTV) are correctly defined.
**Related Terms:** TPS, CT Scan, MRI
**Radiotherapy Example:** Brain tumor PTV verified with co-registered CT and MRI scans.

444. **Tumor Volume Adaptive Planning QA:** QA for adaptive plan adjustments based on tumor changes.
**Related Terms:** TPS, IGRT, LINAC
**Radiotherapy Example:** Lung SBRT adaptive plan verified daily using CBCT imaging.

445. **Tomotherapy Dose Delivery QA:** QA to verify accurate dose delivery according to plan.
**Related Terms:** LINAC, TPS, QA Phantom
**Radiotherapy Example:** Pelvic SBRT dose delivery checked using ion chamber array.

446. **Treatment Field Intensity QA:** QA to verify field intensity matches the planned dose distribution.
**Related Terms:** IMRT, VMAT, LINAC, TPS
**Radiotherapy Example:** Head & neck IMRT field intensity verified with electronic portal imaging.

447. **Tumor Dose Escalation Imaging QA:** QA to verify imaging supports safe dose escalation.
**Related Terms:** IGRT, CBCT, TPS
**Radiotherapy Example:** Prostate SBRT dose escalation confirmed using daily CBCT.

448. **Tomotherapy Mechanical Stability QA:** QA to ensure mechanical stability of gantry, couch, and MLC.
**Related Terms:** LINAC, QA Protocol, IGRT
**Radiotherapy Example:** Monthly mechanical QA for tomotherapy gantry rotation and couch movement.

449. **Treatment Beam Collimation QA:** QA to confirm collimator positions for accurate field shaping.
**Related Terms:** MLC, LINAC, IMRT, VMAT
**Radiotherapy Example:** Head & neck IMRT collimator positions verified with portal imaging.

450. **Tumor Volume Coverage QA:** QA to ensure full coverage of tumor volume by prescribed dose.
**Related Terms:** TPS, LINAC, IMRT, VMAT
**Radiotherapy Example:** Liver SBRT coverage verified using dose reconstruction on CBCT.

451. **Tomotherapy Beam Delivery Verification QA:** QA to verify that the delivered beam matches the planned parameters.
**Related Terms:** LINAC, TPS, IMRT, VMAT
**Radiotherapy Example:** Head & neck tomotherapy beam delivery verified using phantom measurements.

452. **Treatment Field Overlap Verification QA:** QA to ensure adjacent treatment fields overlap correctly without hotspots.
**Related Terms:** LINAC, IMRT, VMAT
**Radiotherapy Example:** Craniospinal junction verified to prevent overdose at field junctions.

453. **Tumor Motion Compensation QA:** QA to ensure motion compensation techniques accurately track tumor movement.
**Related Terms:** IGRT, Gating, 4D CT
**Radiotherapy Example:** Lung SBRT motion compensation confirmed using real-time tracking system.

454. **Tomotherapy Dose Reconstruction QA:** QA to reconstruct and verify delivered dose in the patient anatomy.
**Related Terms:** TPS, CBCT, LINAC
**Radiotherapy Example:** Liver SBRT dose reconstructed from daily MVCT to compare with planned dose.

455. **Treatment Couch Sag Correction QA:** QA to measure and correct couch sag impacting dose delivery.
**Related Terms:** LINAC, IGRT, QA Phantom
**Radiotherapy Example:** Spinal SBRT couch sag corrected after phantom measurement.

456. **Tumor Volume Repositioning Verification QA:** QA to ensure tumor is correctly repositioned after patient movement.
**Related Terms:** CBCT, IGRT, LINAC
**Radiotherapy Example:** Pelvic IMRT tumor repositioned after CBCT verification before delivery.

457. **Tomotherapy Field Size Verification QA:** QA to verify accuracy of treatment field size and shape.
**Related Terms:** LINAC, MLC, IMRT
**Radiotherapy Example:** Head & neck tomotherapy field size verified with film dosimetry.

458. **Treatment Beam Output Stability QA:** QA to continuously monitor stability of beam output over time.
**Related Terms:** LINAC, IMRT, TPS
**Radiotherapy Example:** Daily photon output checked using ionization chamber array for prostate IMRT.

459. **Tumor Dose Homogeneity Verification QA:** QA to confirm uniform dose distribution within the tumor volume.
**Related Terms:** TPS, IMRT, VMAT
**Radiotherapy Example:** Liver SBRT dose homogeneity verified using patient-specific QA phantom.

460. **Tomotherapy Imaging Dose Verification QA:** QA to assess imaging dose from tomotherapy MVCT or CBCT.
**Related Terms:** MVCT, CBCT, IGRT
**Radiotherapy Example:** Daily imaging dose measured for prostate SBRT to minimize extra exposure.

461. **Treatment Field Repositioning QA:** QA to verify accurate repositioning of fields after patient motion.
**Related Terms:** CBCT, IGRT, LINAC
**Radiotherapy Example:** Pelvic IMRT fields repositioned and verified using CBCT.

462. **Tumor Volume Adaptive Dose Verification QA:** QA to verify adaptive dose adjustments accurately target tumor.
**Related Terms:** TPS, IGRT, LINAC
**Radiotherapy Example:** Lung SBRT adaptive plan verified daily using CBCT.

463. **Tomotherapy Safety Interlock Verification QA:** QA to confirm safety interlocks work properly.
**Related Terms:** LINAC, QA Protocol, Radiation Safety
**Radiotherapy Example:** Daily emergency stop and interlock systems checked before treatment.

464. **Treatment Beam Modulation Verification QA:** QA to verify beam intensity modulation accuracy.
**Related Terms:** MLC, LINAC, IMRT, VMAT
**Radiotherapy Example:** Head & neck IMRT beam modulation verified with ion chamber array.

465. **Tumor Motion Tracking Verification QA:** QA to confirm real-time tracking systems accurately monitor tumor motion.
**Related Terms:** IGRT, 4D CT, Gating
**Radiotherapy Example:** Lung tumor motion tracked with sensors during SBRT delivery.

466. **Tomotherapy Beam Angle Verification QA:** QA to ensure correct delivery of beam angles.
**Related Terms:** LINAC, VMAT, IMRT
**Radiotherapy Example:** Spinal SBRT gantry angles verified with QA phantom.

467. **Treatment Planning QA Checklist:** Standardized QA checklist to verify all aspects of treatment plan.
**Related Terms:** TPS, LINAC, IGRT
**Radiotherapy Example:** Head & neck IMRT plan checked using patient-specific QA phantom checklist.

468. **Tumor Volume Coverage Verification QA:** QA to confirm full coverage of tumor volume by prescribed dose.
**Related Terms:** TPS, LINAC, IMRT, VMAT
**Radiotherapy Example:** Liver SBRT coverage verified using dose reconstruction from CBCT.

469. **Tomotherapy Mechanical Stability Verification QA:** QA to ensure mechanical components (gantry, couch, MLC) are stable.
**Related Terms:** LINAC, QA Protocol, IGRT
**Radiotherapy Example:** Monthly tomotherapy mechanical QA performed for gantry rotation and couch movement.

470. **Treatment Field Collimation Verification QA:** QA to verify collimator positions and field shaping.
**Related Terms:** MLC, LINAC, IMRT, VMAT
**Radiotherapy Example:** Head & neck IMRT collimator positions verified with portal imaging.

471. **Tumor Dose Reconstruction Verification QA:** QA to reconstruct and confirm delivered dose in tumor volume.
**Related Terms:** TPS, CBCT, LINAC
**Radiotherapy Example:** Reconstructed liver SBRT dose compared to planned dose.

472. **Tomotherapy Beam Delivery Accuracy QA:** QA to confirm delivered beams match planned dose and geometry.
**Related Terms:** LINAC, TPS, IMRT
**Radiotherapy Example:** Pelvic SBRT beam delivery verified using phantom dosimetry.

473. **Treatment Couch Position Verification QA:** QA to ensure couch positioning is accurate for each fraction.
**Related Terms:** LINAC, IGRT, QA Phantom
**Radiotherapy Example:** Pelvic IMRT couch positions checked daily using CBCT imaging.

474. **Tumor Volume Adaptive Plan Verification QA:** QA to verify adaptive plan adjustments are delivered accurately.
**Related Terms:** TPS, IGRT, LINAC
**Radiotherapy Example:** Daily lung SBRT adaptive plan verified with CBCT imaging.

475. **Tomotherapy Field Size Accuracy QA:** QA to verify accurate size and shape of treatment fields.
**Related Terms:** LINAC, MLC, IMRT
**Radiotherapy Example:** Head & neck tomotherapy field size verified using film dosimetry.

476. **Treatment Beam Output Verification QA:** QA to confirm beam output matches prescribed dose.
**Related Terms:** LINAC, TPS, IMRT
**Radiotherapy Example:** Prostate IMRT beam output verified daily using ion chamber.

477. **Tumor Dose Homogeneity Verification QA:** QA to confirm uniform dose distribution in tumor.
**Related Terms:** TPS, IMRT, VMAT
**Radiotherapy Example:** Liver SBRT dose homogeneity verified using phantom measurement.

478. **Tomotherapy Imaging Dose Verification QA:** QA to measure dose from imaging procedures in tomotherapy.
**Related Terms:** MVCT, CBCT, IGRT
**Radiotherapy Example:** MVCT imaging dose for prostate SBRT measured and documented.

479. **Treatment Field Repositioning Verification QA:** QA to verify accurate repositioning after patient movement.
**Related Terms:** CBCT, IGRT, LINAC
**Radiotherapy Example:** Pelvic IMRT fields repositioned and verified using CBCT.

480. **Tumor Volume Adaptive Dose Verification QA:** QA to verify adaptive dose adjustments accurately target tumor.
**Related Terms:** TPS, IGRT, LINAC
**Radiotherapy Example:** Lung SBRT adaptive plan verified daily using CBCT.

481. **Tomotherapy Safety Interlock Verification QA:** QA to confirm all safety interlocks function correctly.
**Related Terms:** LINAC, QA Protocol, Radiation Safety
**Radiotherapy Example:** Daily check of emergency stop and interlock systems before treatment.

482. **Treatment Beam Modulation Verification QA:** QA to verify beam intensity modulation accuracy.
**Related Terms:** MLC, LINAC, IMRT, VMAT
**Radiotherapy Example:** Head & neck IMRT beam modulation verified with ion chamber array.

483. **Tumor Motion Tracking Verification QA:** QA to confirm real-time tracking accurately monitors tumor motion.
**Related Terms:** IGRT, 4D CT, Gating
**Radiotherapy Example:** Lung tumor motion tracked with sensors during SBRT delivery.

**484. Tomotherapy Beam Angle Verification QA:** QA to ensure correct beam angles are delivered according to plan.
**Related Terms:** LINAC, VMAT, IMRT
**Radiotherapy Example:** Spinal SBRT gantry angles verified with QA phantom.

**485. Treatment Planning QA Checklist:** Standardized checklist for verifying all aspects of treatment plan.
**Related Terms:** TPS, LINAC, IGRT
**Radiotherapy Example:** Head & neck IMRT plan checked using patient-specific QA phantom checklist.

**486. Tumor Volume Coverage Verification QA:** QA to ensure full coverage of tumor volume by prescribed dose.
**Related Terms:** TPS, LINAC, IMRT, VMAT
**Radiotherapy Example:** Liver SBRT coverage verified using dose reconstruction on CBCT.

**487. Tomotherapy Mechanical Stability Verification QA:** QA to ensure mechanical components are stable and precise.
**Related Terms:** LINAC, QA Protocol, IGRT
**Radiotherapy Example:** Monthly tomotherapy mechanical QA performed for gantry and couch stability.

**488. Treatment Field Collimation Verification QA:** QA to verify accurate field shaping with collimators.
**Related Terms:** MLC, LINAC, IMRT, VMAT
**Radiotherapy Example:** Head & neck IMRT collimator positions verified with portal imaging.

**489. Tumor Dose Reconstruction Verification QA:** QA to reconstruct delivered dose and confirm accuracy.
**Related Terms:** TPS, CBCT, LINAC
**Radiotherapy Example:** Reconstructed liver SBRT dose compared to planned dose.

**490. Tomotherapy Beam Delivery Accuracy QA:** QA to confirm delivered beams match planned dose and geometry.
**Related Terms:** LINAC, TPS, IMRT
**Radiotherapy Example:** Pelvic SBRT beam delivery verified using phantom dosimetry.

**491. Treatment Couch Position Verification QA:** QA to ensure precise couch positioning for each fraction.
**Related Terms:** LINAC, IGRT, QA Phantom
**Radiotherapy Example:** Pelvic IMRT couch positions checked daily using CBCT imaging.

**492. Tumor Volume Adaptive Plan Verification QA:** QA to verify adaptive plan adjustments are accurately delivered.
**Related Terms:** TPS, IGRT, LINAC
**Radiotherapy Example:** Daily lung SBRT adaptive plan verified with CBCT imaging.

**493. Tomotherapy Field Size Accuracy QA:** QA to verify accurate size and shape of treatment fields.
**Related Terms:** LINAC, MLC, IMRT
**Radiotherapy Example:** Head & neck tomotherapy field size verified using film dosimetry.

**494. Treatment Beam Output Verification QA:** QA to confirm beam output matches prescribed dose.
**Related Terms:** LINAC, TPS, IMRT
**Radiotherapy Example:** Prostate IMRT beam output verified daily using ion chamber.

495. **Tumor Dose Homogeneity Verification QA:** QA to confirm uniform dose distribution in tumor.
**Related Terms:** TPS, IMRT, VMAT
**Radiotherapy Example:** Liver SBRT dose homogeneity verified using phantom measurement.

496. **Tomotherapy Imaging Dose Verification QA:** QA to measure dose from imaging procedures in tomotherapy.
**Related Terms:** MVCT, CBCT, IGRT
**Radiotherapy Example:** MVCT imaging dose for prostate SBRT measured and documented.

497. **Treatment Field Repositioning Verification QA:** QA to verify accurate repositioning after patient movement.
**Related Terms:** CBCT, IGRT, LINAC
**Radiotherapy Example:** Pelvic IMRT fields repositioned and verified using CBCT.

498. **Tumor Volume Adaptive Dose Verification QA:** QA to verify adaptive dose adjustments accurately target tumor.
**Related Terms:** TPS, IGRT, LINAC
**Radiotherapy Example:** Lung SBRT adaptive plan verified daily using CBCT.

499. **Tomotherapy Safety Interlock Verification QA:** QA to confirm all safety interlocks function correctly.
**Related Terms:** LINAC, QA Protocol, Radiation Safety
**Radiotherapy Example:** Daily check of emergency stop and interlock systems before treatment.

500. **Treatment Planning Complete QA:** Comprehensive QA encompassing all aspects of treatment planning and verification.
**Related Terms:** TPS, LINAC, IGRT, IMRT, VMAT
**Radiotherapy Example:** Full QA performed for head & neck IMRT plan using phantom, portal imaging, and dose reconstruction.

# U

1. **Ultrasound Imaging in Radiotherapy:** Use of ultrasound to visualize soft tissues for planning or verification.
   **Related Terms:** CT scan, IGRT, Mould Room
   **Radiotherapy Example:** Bladder position monitored using ultrasound before prostate radiotherapy.
2. **Urethral Dose Mapping:** Mapping radiation dose delivered to the urethra to avoid toxicity.
   **Related Terms:** TPS, Dose Volume Histogram (DVH), LINAC
   **Radiotherapy Example:** Prostate IMRT plan evaluated for urethral dose constraints.
3. **Unmodulated Beam Delivery:** Radiation beam delivered without intensity modulation.
   **Related Terms:** LINAC, Photon Beam, Electron Beam
   **Radiotherapy Example:** Conventional radiotherapy for superficial skin lesions using unmodulated photon beams.
4. **Uniformity Index Assessment:** Measure of dose uniformity within the target volume.
   **Related Terms:** TPS, DVH, IMRT, VMAT
   **Radiotherapy Example:** Breast radiotherapy plan checked for uniform dose distribution.
5. **Urinary Bladder Shielding:** Use of shields to protect bladder from unnecessary radiation.
   **Related Terms:** LINAC, Mould Room, Radiotherapy Accessories
   **Radiotherapy Example:** Bladder shield used during pelvic radiotherapy.
6. **Upright Radiotherapy Positioning:** Patient positioned upright for treatment, often for lung or thoracic tumors.
   **Related Terms:** LINAC, IGRT, Immobilization
   **Radiotherapy Example:** Lung tumor treated with upright positioning to reduce diaphragm motion.
7. **User-Defined Beam Modulation:** Operator-customized beam intensity modulation.
   **Related Terms:** LINAC, IMRT, TPS
   **Radiotherapy Example:** Head & neck IMRT plan created with user-defined intensity patterns.
8. **Uterine Dose Assessment:** Evaluating dose received by uterus during pelvic radiotherapy.
   **Related Terms:** TPS, DVH, LINAC
   **Radiotherapy Example:** Gynecological radiotherapy plan evaluated to minimize uterine exposure.
9. **Upper Abdominal Motion Management:** Techniques to reduce tumor motion in upper abdomen during treatment.
   **Related Terms:** IGRT, 4D CT, Gating
   **Radiotherapy Example:** Liver SBRT motion managed with respiratory gating.
10. **Unplanned Dose Verification:** Checking for any unexpected dose deviations during treatment.
    **Related Terms:** TPS, LINAC, IGRT
    **Radiotherapy Example:** Daily portal imaging used to detect unplanned hot spots in head & neck IMRT.
11. **Ultrasound-Guided Setup:** Using ultrasound to guide patient setup before treatment.
    **Related Terms:** IGRT, CT scan, Mould Room
    **Radiotherapy Example:** Bladder position verified with ultrasound before pelvic radiotherapy.

12. **Upright CT Simulation:** Performing CT simulation with patient in upright position.
    **Related Terms:** CT scan, TPS, Radiology
    **Radiotherapy Example:** Thoracic CT simulation done upright to account for lung expansion.
13. **Ureteral Dose Sparing:** Minimizing radiation dose to ureters during pelvic radiotherapy.
    **Related Terms:** TPS, LINAC, DVH
    **Radiotherapy Example:** Pelvic IMRT plan adjusted to reduce ureter dose.
14. **Uniform Beam Profile Verification:** QA to ensure beam has uniform intensity across the field.
    **Related Terms:** LINAC, TPS, Dosimetry
    **Radiotherapy Example:** Photon beam flatness checked before breast radiotherapy.
15. **Upper Thoracic Immobilization:** Immobilizing upper thorax to reduce patient motion during treatment.
    **Related Terms:** Mould Room, IGRT, LINAC
    **Radiotherapy Example:** Head & neck mask with thoracic support used in radiotherapy.
16. **Unintended Organ Dose Measurement:** Measuring dose received by organs outside target volume.
    **Related Terms:** TPS, DVH, LINAC
    **Radiotherapy Example:** Liver dose measured during lung SBRT to assess liver exposure.
17. **User Access Control in TPS:** Restricting TPS access to authorized personnel only.
    **Related Terms:** Radiotherapy Safety, TPS
    **Radiotherapy Example:** Treatment planning edits restricted to physicists and oncologists.
18. **Upper Limb Immobilization:** Immobilizing arms to maintain reproducibility during thoracic radiotherapy.
    **Related Terms:** Mould Room, LINAC, IGRT
    **Radiotherapy Example:** Patient's arms fixed above head during lung radiotherapy.
19. **Urethral Dose Constraint Verification:** Checking that urethral dose is within safe limits.
    **Related Terms:** TPS, DVH, LINAC
    **Radiotherapy Example:** Prostate IMRT plan verified against urethral constraints.
20. **Ultrasonography for Mould Positioning:** Using ultrasound to check position of immobilization molds.
    **Related Terms:** Mould Room, LINAC, IGRT
    **Radiotherapy Example:** Breast radiotherapy mold position verified with ultrasound.
21. **Unidirectional Beam Delivery QA:** QA for single-direction beam delivery to ensure correct dose.
    **Related Terms:** LINAC, TPS, Dosimetry
    **Radiotherapy Example:** Skin lesion treated with electron beam QA verified in one direction.
22. **Upper Abdomen Target Volume Verification:** Ensuring correct dose delivery to upper abdominal tumors.
    **Related Terms:** CT scan, LINAC, IGRT
    **Radiotherapy Example:** Liver SBRT target verified with daily CBCT.
23. **Uterine Motion Assessment:** Evaluating uterine movement during radiotherapy for treatment planning.
    **Related Terms:** IGRT, CT scan, LINAC
    **Radiotherapy Example:** Gynecologic IMRT plan adjusted based on uterine motion assessment.
24. **Unintentional Hotspot Detection:** Detecting areas receiving higher than planned dose.
    **Related Terms:** TPS, LINAC, QA
    **Radiotherapy Example:** Hotspot identified in breast IMRT using film dosimetry.

25. **Upper Body Immobilization QA:** QA to confirm immobilization devices are stable and reproducible.
**Related Terms:** Mould Room, LINAC, IGRT
**Radiotherapy Example:** Head & neck thermoplastic mask checked for stability before treatment.

26. **Ultrasound-Assisted CT Simulation:** Combining ultrasound with CT to improve target localization.
**Related Terms:** CT scan, TPS, IGRT
**Radiotherapy Example:** Bladder tumor localized using ultrasound during CT simulation.

27. **Unmodulated Electron Beam Verification:** QA to verify unmodulated electron beams.
**Related Terms:** LINAC, Dosimetry
**Radiotherapy Example:** Electron beam for chest wall verified with ionization chamber.

28. **Upper Extremity Dose Assessment:** Measuring dose received by arms during thoracic radiotherapy.
**Related Terms:** TPS, LINAC, DVH
**Radiotherapy Example:** Arm dose monitored during breast radiotherapy.

29. **User-Specific QA Protocol:** QA protocol customized for specific patient or treatment site.
**Related Terms:** TPS, LINAC, Dosimetry
**Radiotherapy Example:** Head & neck IMRT patient-specific QA protocol implemented.

30. **Unplanned Beam Interruption QA:** QA for accidental beam stoppages to ensure patient safety.
**Related Terms:** LINAC, QA Protocol, Radiation Safety
**Radiotherapy Example:** Beam interruption during pelvic IMRT verified and logged.

31. **Upper Abdomen Organ Sparing Verification:** Ensuring critical organs in upper abdomen are spared.
**Related Terms:** TPS, DVH, LINAC
**Radiotherapy Example:** Kidney dose monitored during liver SBRT.

32. **Ultrasonic Tissue Interface Assessment:** Assessing tissue interfaces to improve dose calculation.
**Related Terms:** Ultrasound, TPS, Radiology
**Radiotherapy Example:** Bladder-rectum interface evaluated with ultrasound for prostate IMRT.

33. **Upright Immobilization QA:** QA to ensure reproducibility in upright positioning.
**Related Terms:** Mould Room, LINAC, IGRT
**Radiotherapy Example:** Lung SBRT upright positioning verified with imaging.

34. **Unintentional Organ Motion Monitoring:** Tracking unintended motion of organs during therapy.
**Related Terms:** IGRT, 4D CT, LINAC
**Radiotherapy Example:** Liver motion tracked with CBCT during SBRT.

35. **Upper Abdominal Target Volume Dose Verification:** Confirming prescribed dose to target volume.
**Related Terms:** TPS, LINAC, IGRT
**Radiotherapy Example:** Liver SBRT daily dose verified using CBCT and TPS comparison.

36. **Unmodulated Photon Beam QA:** QA to verify uniform photon beam without modulation.
**Related Terms:** LINAC, Dosimetry, TPS
**Radiotherapy Example:** Conventional breast radiotherapy photon beam QA verified using ion chamber.

37. **Upper Thorax Dose Distribution Assessment:** Evaluating dose uniformity in upper thoracic region.
**Related Terms:** TPS, LINAC, DVH
**Radiotherapy Example:** Lung IMRT plan dose distribution checked across upper thorax.

38. **Urinary Bladder Motion Tracking:** Tracking bladder motion to avoid over/under dose.
**Related Terms:** IGRT, CBCT, LINAC
**Radiotherapy Example:** Bladder motion monitored daily for prostate IMRT.

39. **Upper Abdominal Organ Dose Constraint Verification:** Checking critical organ doses are within safe limits.
    **Related Terms:** TPS, DVH, LINAC
    **Radiotherapy Example:** Kidney and liver doses verified during SBRT planning.
40. **Unplanned Dose Logging:** Recording doses received during unexpected events.
    **Related Terms:** TPS, LINAC, Radiation Safety
    **Radiotherapy Example:** Dose from unplanned imaging recorded during pelvic radiotherapy.
41. **Ultrasound-Assisted Target Delineation:** Using ultrasound to improve tumor contouring.
    **Related Terms:** CT scan, TPS, IGRT
    **Radiotherapy Example:** Bladder tumor delineation assisted by ultrasound during CT simulation.
42. **Upright Patient Setup Verification:** Ensuring reproducible upright positioning.
    **Related Terms:** Mould Room, LINAC, IGRT
    **Radiotherapy Example:** Lung SBRT upright setup verified with imaging.
43. **Ureter Dose Constraint Planning:** Planning to keep ureter dose within safe limits.
    **Related Terms:** TPS, DVH, LINAC
    **Radiotherapy Example:** Pelvic IMRT plan adjusted to meet ureter constraints.
44. **Unmodulated Photon Beam Dose Verification:** QA for photon beams delivered without modulation.
    **Related Terms:** LINAC, Dosimetry
    **Radiotherapy Example:** Breast photon beams verified using ion chamber measurements.
45. **Upper Extremity Dose Logging:** Recording dose received by arms during radiotherapy.
    **Related Terms:** TPS, LINAC, DVH
    **Radiotherapy Example:** Arm doses recorded during breast IMRT.
46. **User-Specific Beam Modulation QA:** QA for customized beam modulation for individual patient.
    **Related Terms:** TPS, LINAC, IMRT
    **Radiotherapy Example:** Head & neck IMRT beam intensity pattern verified with QA phantom.
47. **Unintended Organ Dose Logging:** Recording doses received by non-target organs.
    **Related Terms:** TPS, LINAC, DVH
    **Radiotherapy Example:** Kidney dose recorded during liver SBRT for safety documentation.
48. **Upper Abdomen Motion Compensation Verification:** QA to ensure motion compensation techniques work properly.
    **Related Terms:** IGRT, 4D CT, Gating
    **Radiotherapy Example:** Liver tumor motion compensated using respiratory gating verified with CBCT.
49. **Urethral Dose Verification QA:** QA to ensure urethral dose does not exceed constraints.
    **Related Terms:** TPS, DVH, LINAC
    **Radiotherapy Example:** Prostate IMRT plan QA confirms urethral dose is safe.
50. **Upright CT Dose Verification:** QA to verify imaging dose during upright CT simulation.
    **Related Terms:** CT scan, TPS, Radiation Safety
    **Radiotherapy Example:** Thoracic CT dose measured and logged for upright simulation.
51. **Ultrasound-Guided Brachytherapy:** Using ultrasound to guide placement of brachytherapy sources.
    **Related Terms:** Mould Room, LINAC, TPS
    **Radiotherapy Example:** Prostate brachytherapy needle placement guided by transrectal ultrasound.

52. **Upper Abdomen Target Motion Analysis:** Studying motion of tumors in upper abdomen for accurate dose delivery.
**Related Terms:** 4D CT, IGRT, LINAC
**Radiotherapy Example:** Liver SBRT plan adjusted based on motion analysis from 4D CT.

53. **Urethral Sparing Planning:** Planning radiation to minimize dose to urethra.
**Related Terms:** TPS, DVH, IMRT
**Radiotherapy Example:** Prostate IMRT optimized to spare urethra while treating the gland.

54. **Unmodulated Electron Beam QA:** Quality assurance for electron beams without intensity modulation.
**Related Terms:** LINAC, Dosimetry
**Radiotherapy Example:** Electron beam for superficial lesions verified with ionization chamber.

55. **Upper Thorax Dose Verification:** Confirming dose distribution in upper thoracic region.
**Related Terms:** TPS, LINAC, DVH
**Radiotherapy Example:** Lung IMRT plan verified for uniformity in upper thorax.

56. **Unintended Dose Monitoring:** Monitoring dose delivered to organs outside the target.
**Related Terms:** TPS, LINAC, DVH
**Radiotherapy Example:** Kidney dose tracked during liver radiotherapy.

57. **Ultrasonography for Setup QA:** Using ultrasound to verify patient setup before treatment.
**Related Terms:** Mould Room, IGRT, LINAC
**Radiotherapy Example:** Bladder position verified using ultrasound before pelvic radiotherapy.

58. **Upright Immobilization Device Assessment:** QA for upright immobilization devices to ensure reproducibility.
**Related Terms:** Mould Room, LINAC, IGRT
**Radiotherapy Example:** Lung SBRT upright immobilization verified before therapy.

59. **Ureter Dose Logging:** Recording dose received by ureters during treatment.
**Related Terms:** TPS, DVH, LINAC
**Radiotherapy Example:** Pelvic IMRT plan includes ureter dose log for documentation.

60. **Unmodulated Photon Beam Verification:** QA for photon beams delivered without modulation.
**Related Terms:** LINAC, Dosimetry, TPS
**Radiotherapy Example:** Breast radiotherapy photon beam verified with ion chamber.

61. **Upper Body Position Reproducibility:** Ensuring consistent upper body positioning across sessions.
**Related Terms:** Mould Room, LINAC, IGRT
**Radiotherapy Example:** Head & neck mask checked for reproducible positioning each day.

62. **Unintended Organ Motion Logging:** Recording movement of organs that could affect dose delivery.
**Related Terms:** IGRT, 4D CT, LINAC
**Radiotherapy Example:** Liver motion tracked and logged during SBRT sessions.

63. **Upper Abdominal Organ Sparing Planning:** Planning to minimize dose to critical organs in upper abdomen.
**Related Terms:** TPS, DVH, LINAC
**Radiotherapy Example:** Kidney and stomach dose minimized during liver SBRT planning.

64. **Ultrasound-Assisted Mold Alignment:** Using ultrasound to align patient molds for accurate treatment.
**Related Terms:** Mould Room, LINAC, IGRT
**Radiotherapy Example:** Breast immobilization mold positioned using ultrasound verification.

65. **Unplanned Beam Interruption Logging:** Recording details of unexpected beam stoppages.
**Related Terms:** LINAC, Radiation Safety, QA
**Radiotherapy Example:** Pelvic IMRT session interruption logged for safety documentation.

66. **Upper Thorax Motion Compensation:** Techniques to manage motion in upper thorax during treatment.
**Related Terms:** IGRT, 4D CT, Gating
**Radiotherapy Example:** Lung tumor motion mitigated with respiratory gating.

67. **Urethral Dose QA:** QA to confirm urethral dose is within planned constraints.
**Related Terms:** TPS, DVH, LINAC
**Radiotherapy Example:** Prostate IMRT plan QA ensures urethral safety.

68. **Upright Patient Position Verification:** Verifying patient upright positioning for reproducibility.
**Related Terms:** Mould Room, IGRT, LINAC
**Radiotherapy Example:** Thoracic SBRT patient upright setup verified using imaging.

69. **Unmodulated Electron Beam Dose Verification:** QA for electron beams without modulation to ensure correct dose.
**Related Terms:** LINAC, Dosimetry
**Radiotherapy Example:** Chest wall electron beam verified with ion chamber before treatment.

70. **Upper Abdominal Target Dose Verification:** Confirming prescribed dose to upper abdominal tumors.
**Related Terms:** TPS, LINAC, IGRT
**Radiotherapy Example:** Liver SBRT target dose verified using CBCT.

71. **Ultrasonography-Guided Organ Delineation:** Using ultrasound to delineate organ boundaries for treatment planning.
**Related Terms:** CT scan, TPS, Mould Room
**Radiotherapy Example:** Bladder tumor boundaries defined using ultrasound.

72. **Upper Extremity Position Verification:** Ensuring arms are correctly positioned for thoracic radiotherapy.
**Related Terms:** Mould Room, LINAC, IGRT
**Radiotherapy Example:** Patient arms verified above head for breast IMRT.

73. **Unplanned Dose Assessment:** Measuring dose delivered during unplanned events.
**Related Terms:** TPS, LINAC, Radiation Safety
**Radiotherapy Example:** Dose from unplanned imaging tracked during pelvic IMRT.

74. **Upper Abdomen Organ Motion Monitoring:** Tracking motion of critical organs in upper abdomen.
**Related Terms:** IGRT, 4D CT, LINAC
**Radiotherapy Example:** Kidney motion monitored during liver SBRT.

75. **User-Defined Dose Constraints:** Setting custom dose limits for organs and targets in TPS.
**Related Terms:** TPS, DVH, LINAC
**Radiotherapy Example:** Prostate IMRT plan customized for urethra and rectum constraints.

76. **Ultrasound-Guided Immobilization Verification:** Verifying mold and patient position using ultrasound.
**Related Terms:** Mould Room, IGRT, LINAC
**Radiotherapy Example:** Breast mold alignment checked before each session.

77. **Upper Thorax Dose Logging:** Recording delivered dose in upper thorax region.
**Related Terms:** TPS, LINAC, DVH
**Radiotherapy Example:** Lung IMRT plan dose logged for upper thoracic region.

78. **Unintended Hotspot Logging:** Recording locations of unplanned dose hotspots.
**Related Terms:** TPS, Dosimetry, LINAC
**Radiotherapy Example:** Hotspots in breast IMRT logged and evaluated.

79. **Upright CT Dose Monitoring:** Monitoring imaging dose during upright CT simulation.
**Related Terms:** CT scan, Radiation Safety, TPS
**Radiotherapy Example:** Thoracic upright CT scan dose logged for patient safety.

80. **Upper Abdomen Dose Constraint Verification:** Confirming dose to organs in upper abdomen stays within limits.
**Related Terms:** TPS, DVH, LINAC
**Radiotherapy Example:** Kidney and liver doses verified for SBRT plan.

81. **Ultrasound-Assisted Target Verification:** Using ultrasound to confirm tumor position before treatment.
**Related Terms:** IGRT, LINAC, Mould Room
**Radiotherapy Example:** Bladder tumor position verified before each fraction.

82. **Unmodulated Beam QA for LINAC:** QA for LINAC beams delivered without modulation.
**Related Terms:** Dosimetry, TPS, LINAC
**Radiotherapy Example:** Electron beam verified for superficial skin lesion treatment.

83. **Upper Thorax Organ Sparing Planning:** Planning to protect organs in upper thorax from excess dose.
**Related Terms:** TPS, DVH, LINAC
**Radiotherapy Example:** Heart dose minimized during lung IMRT.

84. **Upright Immobilization Verification QA:** QA to confirm upright immobilization device stability.
**Related Terms:** Mould Room, LINAC, IGRT
**Radiotherapy Example:** Lung SBRT upright mask checked for reproducibility.

85. **Unintended Organ Dose QA:** QA to check dose received by non-target organs.
**Related Terms:** TPS, DVH, LINAC
**Radiotherapy Example:** Kidney dose QA performed during liver SBRT planning.

86. **Upper Abdomen Motion Mitigation Verification:** QA to ensure motion mitigation techniques are effective.
**Related Terms:** IGRT, 4D CT, Gating
**Radiotherapy Example:** Respiratory-gated liver SBRT verified for motion mitigation.

87. **Ureter Dose QA:** QA to ensure ureter dose stays within limits.
**Related Terms:** TPS, DVH, LINAC
**Radiotherapy Example:** Pelvic IMRT plan QA confirms ureter safety.

88. **Ultrasound-Guided Fractionation Verification:** Using ultrasound to verify target before each fraction.
**Related Terms:** IGRT, LINAC, Mould Room
**Radiotherapy Example:** Bladder tumor fraction verified daily using ultrasound.

89. **Upper Extremity Dose Monitoring:** Monitoring radiation dose received by arms during treatment.
**Related Terms:** TPS, DVH, LINAC
**Radiotherapy Example:** Arm dose monitored in breast IMRT.

90. **Unmodulated Photon Beam QA Verification:** Verifying unmodulated photon beams for accuracy.
**Related Terms:** LINAC, Dosimetry, TPS
**Radiotherapy Example:** Photon beams checked for flatness in breast treatment.

91. **Upright CT Target Verification:** Using upright CT imaging to confirm tumor location.
**Related Terms:** CT scan, IGRT, TPS
**Radiotherapy Example:** Thoracic tumor verified in upright CT before SBRT.

92. **Upper Thorax Motion Logging:** Recording motion of upper thorax organs during therapy.
**Related Terms:** IGRT, 4D CT, LINAC
**Radiotherapy Example:** Lung motion logged for motion-managed SBRT.

93. **Unplanned Hotspot QA:** QA for unplanned dose hotspots.
**Related Terms:** TPS, Dosimetry, LINAC
**Radiotherapy Example:** Breast IMRT hotspots analyzed using film dosimetry.

94. **Upper Abdomen Target Dose Logging:** Logging dose delivered to upper abdominal targets.
**Related Terms:** TPS, LINAC, DVH
**Radiotherapy Example:** Liver SBRT target dose recorded daily.

95. **Ultrasound-Assisted Organ Sparing Planning:** Planning organ-sparing using ultrasound guidance.
**Related Terms:** TPS, Mould Room, IGRT
**Radiotherapy Example:** Bladder dose minimized during pelvic IMRT using ultrasound guidance.

96. **Upper Thorax Dose Logging QA:** QA to log dose delivered to upper thorax.
**Related Terms:** TPS, LINAC, DVH
**Radiotherapy Example:** Lung IMRT dose QA recorded for upper thorax.

97. **Upright Immobilization Dose Verification:** Verifying delivered dose with upright immobilization.
**Related Terms:** Mould Room, LINAC, TPS
**Radiotherapy Example:** Thoracic SBRT dose verified for upright patient position.

98. **Unmodulated Electron Beam Dose Logging:** Logging dose delivered by unmodulated electron beams.
**Related Terms:** LINAC, Dosimetry
**Radiotherapy Example:** Electron beam dose logged for superficial lesion treatment.

99. **Upper Abdomen Organ Dose QA:** QA to ensure organ dose stays within planned limits.
**Related Terms:** TPS, LINAC, DVH
**Radiotherapy Example:** Kidney and liver dose QA performed for SBRT plan.

100. **Ultrasound-Assisted Beam Alignment:** Using ultrasound to confirm correct beam alignment before treatment.
**Related Terms:** IGRT, LINAC, Mould Room
**Radiotherapy Example:** Bladder tumor beam alignment verified with ultrasound before each fraction.

101. **Upper Pelvis Dose Verification:** Confirming delivered dose in upper pelvic region.
**Related Terms:** TPS, LINAC, DVH
**Radiotherapy Example:** Pelvic IMRT plan verified for upper pelvic dose using CBCT.

102. **Ultrasound-Guided Fiducial Placement:** Using ultrasound to place fiducial markers for IGRT.
**Related Terms:** LINAC, Mould Room, CT scan
**Radiotherapy Example:** Prostate fiducials placed under ultrasound guidance for daily IGRT.

103. **Upper Abdominal Tumor Motion Tracking:** Monitoring motion of upper abdominal tumors during treatment.
**Related Terms:** 4D CT, IGRT, LINAC
**Radiotherapy Example:** Liver SBRT motion tracked with 4D CT and CBCT verification.

104. **Upright Immobilization Dose QA:** QA for dose delivery using upright immobilization devices.
**Related Terms:** Mould Room, LINAC, IGRT
**Radiotherapy Example:** Thoracic SBRT dose verified with upright patient mask in place.

105. **Urethral Dose Logging:** Recording radiation dose delivered to urethra.
**Related Terms:** TPS, DVH, LINAC
**Radiotherapy Example:** Prostate IMRT urethral dose monitored to prevent toxicity.

106. **Unplanned Dose Audit:** Reviewing unintended dose delivered to non-target tissues.
**Related Terms:** LINAC, Radiation Safety, Dosimetry
**Radiotherapy Example:** Pelvic IMRT audit performed after a machine malfunction.

107. **Upper Thorax Organ Sparing Verification:** Confirming organ-sparing techniques are effective in upper thorax.
**Related Terms:** TPS, DVH, LINAC
**Radiotherapy Example:** Heart and lung dose verified for left-sided breast IMRT.

108. **Ultrasound-Assisted Contour Verification:** Using ultrasound to verify organ or tumor contours.
**Related Terms:** CT scan, TPS, Mould Room
**Radiotherapy Example:** Bladder tumor contours verified before planning with ultrasound.

109. **Upper Extremity Dose Logging:** Recording dose received by arms during radiotherapy.
**Related Terms:** TPS, LINAC, DVH
**Radiotherapy Example:** Arm dose logged during breast IMRT to ensure safety.

110. **Unmodulated Photon Beam QA:** QA for photon beams delivered without modulation.
**Related Terms:** LINAC, Dosimetry, TPS
**Radiotherapy Example:** Photon beams verified for flatness and output using ion chamber.

111. **Upright CT Target Verification:** Using upright CT imaging to confirm tumor position.
**Related Terms:** CT scan, IGRT, TPS
**Radiotherapy Example:** Thoracic tumor position verified before SBRT with upright CT.

112. **Upper Abdominal Organ Sparing Planning:** Planning to reduce dose to critical organs in upper abdomen.
**Related Terms:** TPS, DVH, LINAC
**Radiotherapy Example:** Kidney and liver dose minimized for SBRT plan.

113. **Ultrasound-Assisted Beam Verification:** Using ultrasound to confirm beam alignment before therapy.
**Related Terms:** IGRT, LINAC, Mould Room
**Radiotherapy Example:** Bladder tumor beam alignment verified using ultrasound.

114. **Unintended Hotspot QA:** QA to detect unintended high-dose regions.
**Related Terms:** TPS, Dosimetry, LINAC
**Radiotherapy Example:** Breast IMRT hotspots identified and corrected before treatment.

115. **Upper Thorax Motion Logging:** Recording motion of thoracic organs during treatment.
**Related Terms:** IGRT, 4D CT, LINAC
**Radiotherapy Example:** Lung tumor motion logged during respiratory-gated SBRT.

116. **Upright Immobilization Verification:** Verifying upright patient position for treatment reproducibility.
**Related Terms:** Mould Room, LINAC, IGRT
**Radiotherapy Example:** Lung SBRT patient upright mask checked daily for reproducibility.

117. **Upper Abdominal Target Dose Logging:** Recording delivered dose to upper abdominal tumor targets.
**Related Terms:** TPS, LINAC, DVH
**Radiotherapy Example:** Liver SBRT target dose logged daily for accuracy.

118. **Ultrasound-Guided Organ Sparing:** Using ultrasound to minimize dose to critical organs.
**Related Terms:** TPS, Mould Room, IGRT
**Radiotherapy Example:** Bladder dose minimized during pelvic IMRT using ultrasound guidance.

119. **Unmodulated Electron Beam Dose Verification:** QA for electron beams delivered without modulation.
**Related Terms:** LINAC, Dosimetry
**Radiotherapy Example:** Electron beam verified for superficial skin lesion treatment.

120. **Upper Pelvis Organ Dose QA:** QA to ensure upper pelvic organs receive planned dose.
**Related Terms:** TPS, LINAC, DVH
**Radiotherapy Example:** Bladder and rectum dose verified for pelvic IMRT plan.

121. **Ultrasound-Assisted Fractionation Verification:** Verifying target position using ultrasound before each fraction.
**Related Terms:** IGRT, LINAC, Mould Room
**Radiotherapy Example:** Bladder tumor fraction verified daily with ultrasound.

122. **Upper Extremity Position Reproducibility:** Ensuring consistent positioning of arms during treatment.
**Related Terms:** Mould Room, LINAC, IGRT
**Radiotherapy Example:** Arms verified above head for breast IMRT.

123. **Unplanned Dose Assessment:** Measuring unintended dose delivered to non-target tissues.
**Related Terms:** TPS, LINAC, Radiation Safety
**Radiotherapy Example:** Dose from unplanned imaging tracked during pelvic IMRT.

124. **Upper Thorax Dose Logging QA:** QA to log delivered dose in upper thorax region.
**Related Terms:** TPS, LINAC, DVH
**Radiotherapy Example:** Lung IMRT upper thorax dose recorded daily.

125. **Upright CT Dose Monitoring:** Monitoring imaging dose during upright CT simulation.
**Related Terms:** CT scan, Radiation Safety, TPS
**Radiotherapy Example:** Thoracic upright CT scan dose logged for patient safety.

126. **Upper Abdomen Motion Mitigation Verification:** QA to ensure motion mitigation techniques are effective.
**Related Terms:** IGRT, 4D CT, Gating
**Radiotherapy Example:** Respiratory-gated liver SBRT verified for motion mitigation.

127. **Ultrasound-Assisted Immobilization Verification:** Verifying patient molds and position using ultrasound.
**Related Terms:** Mould Room, LINAC, IGRT
**Radiotherapy Example:** Breast mold alignment checked before each fraction.

128. **Unmodulated Photon Beam Dose Logging:** Recording dose delivered by unmodulated photon beams.
**Related Terms:** LINAC, Dosimetry, TPS
**Radiotherapy Example:** Photon beam dose logged for breast IMRT QA.

129. **Upper Abdominal Organ Dose Monitoring:** Monitoring delivered dose to organs in upper abdomen.
**Related Terms:** TPS, LINAC, DVH
**Radiotherapy Example:** Kidney and liver dose monitored during liver SBRT.

130. **Ultrasound-Assisted Target Alignment:** Aligning tumor target using ultrasound before treatment.
**Related Terms:** IGRT, LINAC, Mould Room
**Radiotherapy Example:** Bladder tumor alignment verified daily using ultrasound.

131. **Upper Thorax Motion Compensation:** Techniques to manage motion in upper thorax during therapy.
**Related Terms:** IGRT, 4D CT, Gating
**Radiotherapy Example:** Lung tumor motion compensated using respiratory gating.

132. **Upright Immobilization Dose Logging:** Logging dose delivered using upright immobilization devices.
**Related Terms:** Mould Room, LINAC, TPS
**Radiotherapy Example:** Thoracic SBRT dose logged for upright mask setup.

133. **Unplanned Hotspot Logging:** Recording locations of unintended high-dose regions.
**Related Terms:** TPS, Dosimetry, LINAC
**Radiotherapy Example:** Breast IMRT hotspots logged for correction before treatment.

134. **Upper Abdomen Target Dose QA:** QA to confirm tumor dose in upper abdomen.
**Related Terms:** TPS, LINAC, DVH
**Radiotherapy Example:** Liver SBRT target dose verified for plan accuracy.

135. **Ultrasound-Guided Beam Verification:** Using ultrasound to verify correct beam alignment.
**Related Terms:** IGRT, LINAC, Mould Room
**Radiotherapy Example:** Bladder tumor beam alignment confirmed before treatment.

136. **Unmodulated Electron Beam Dose Logging:** Logging dose delivered by unmodulated electron beams.
**Related Terms:** LINAC, Dosimetry
**Radiotherapy Example:** Electron beam dose logged for skin lesion treatment.

137. **Upper Pelvis Target Dose Monitoring:** Monitoring dose delivered to upper pelvic tumor targets.
**Related Terms:** TPS, LINAC, DVH
**Radiotherapy Example:** Pelvic IMRT upper pelvic target dose tracked.

138. **Ultrasound-Assisted Fraction Verification:** Verifying tumor position using ultrasound before each fraction.
**Related Terms:** IGRT, LINAC, Mould Room
**Radiotherapy Example:** Bladder tumor position verified for each fraction using ultrasound.

139. **Upper Extremity Dose QA:** QA to ensure safe dose to arms during therapy.
**Related Terms:** TPS, LINAC, DVH
**Radiotherapy Example:** Arm dose QA performed during breast IMRT.

140. **Unplanned Dose QA:** QA to assess unintended dose delivered.
**Related Terms:** TPS, LINAC, Radiation Safety
**Radiotherapy Example:** Dose from unplanned imaging or interruptions verified.

141. **Upper Thorax Organ Dose QA:** QA to ensure upper thorax organs receive planned dose.
**Related Terms:** TPS, LINAC, DVH
**Radiotherapy Example:** Heart and lung dose QA performed during breast IMRT.

142. **Upright CT Target QA:** QA for tumor position verification using upright CT.
**Related Terms:** CT scan, IGRT, TPS
**Radiotherapy Example:** Thoracic tumor verified in upright CT for SBRT plan.

143. **Upper Abdomen Dose Constraint QA:** QA to ensure organs in upper abdomen stay within dose limits.
**Related Terms:** TPS, LINAC, DVH
**Radiotherapy Example:** Kidney and liver dose verified for SBRT plan compliance.

144. **Ultrasound-Assisted Organ Motion QA:** QA for organ motion tracking using ultrasound.
**Related Terms:** IGRT, LINAC, Mould Room
**Radiotherapy Example:** Bladder motion tracked before each fraction.

145. **Unmodulated Photon Beam Dose QA:** QA for unmodulated photon beams to ensure correct dose delivery.
**Related Terms:** LINAC, Dosimetry, TPS
**Radiotherapy Example:** Photon beam output verified before breast radiotherapy.

146. **Upper Abdomen Motion Logging QA:** QA to log organ motion in upper abdomen.
**Related Terms:** IGRT, 4D CT, LINAC
**Radiotherapy Example:** Liver motion recorded during SBRT.

147. **Ultrasound-Assisted Immobilization QA:** QA to verify molds and patient position using ultrasound.
**Related Terms:** Mould Room, LINAC, IGRT
**Radiotherapy Example:** Breast mold position checked using ultrasound before each fraction.

148. **Upper Pelvis Organ Sparing QA:** QA to ensure pelvic organs receive safe doses.
**Related Terms:** TPS, LINAC, DVH
**Radiotherapy Example:** Bladder and rectum dose verified during pelvic IMRT QA.

149. **Upright Immobilization QA:** QA for upright patient positioning devices.
**Related Terms:** Mould Room, LINAC, IGRT
**Radiotherapy Example:** Thoracic SBRT upright mask QA verified daily.

150. **Ultrasound-Guided Target Dose Verification:** Verifying dose delivered to target using ultrasound guidance.
**Related Terms:** IGRT, LINAC, Mould Room
**Radiotherapy Example:** Bladder tumor dose verified with ultrasound before treatment.

151. **Uniform Dose Constraint Optimization:** Optimization technique to ensure dose distribution is even across the target volume.
**Related Terms:** DVH, TPS, IMRT planning
**Radiotherapy Example:** TPS optimization ensures uniform dose to prostate PTV while sparing rectum.

152. **Upper Airway Dose Limitation:** Restricting radiation exposure to trachea and nearby upper airway structures.
**Related Terms:** SBRT, OAR sparing, LINAC
**Radiotherapy Example:** Lung SBRT plan adjusted to keep trachea dose within tolerance.

153. **Underdose Detection QA:** QA to detect regions where prescribed dose is not adequately delivered.
**Related Terms:** Portal dosimetry, IMRT QA, DVH
**Radiotherapy Example:** Portal imaging reveals underdosed region in cervical tumor field.

154. **Ureter Dose Assessment:** Evaluating dose delivered to ureter during pelvic or abdominal irradiation.
**Related Terms:** DVH, SBRT, OAR
**Radiotherapy Example:** Kidney SBRT plan reviewed to ensure ureter dose stays below threshold.

155. **Upright Breast Immobilization System:** Mold and support device used for treating breast cancer in upright posture.
**Related Terms:** Mould Room, IGRT, LINAC
**Radiotherapy Example:** Left breast patient immobilized upright to reduce breathing motion for IMRT.

156. **Ultrasound-Based Organ Volume Monitoring:** Tracking organ filling or shrinking using ultrasound during treatment.
**Related Terms:** IGRT, Adaptive RT, Bladder monitoring
**Radiotherapy Example:** Bladder volume checked with ultrasound daily during pelvic RT.

157. **Upper Neck Lymph Node Mapping:** Identification and contouring of upper cervical nodal levels for radiotherapy planning.
**Related Terms:** CT scan, MRI fusion, Contouring
**Radiotherapy Example:** Upper cervical nodal levels II–III contoured for NPC IMRT plan.

158. **Ultralight Thermoplastic Mask:** Lightweight immobilization mask designed for extended comfort.
**Related Terms:** Mould Room, Head & Neck RT, Immobilization
**Radiotherapy Example:** H&N cancer patient fitted with ventilated ultralight mask for 33 fractions.

159. **U159 — Under-table Imaging Mode:** Imaging configuration where detector is positioned under the treatment couch.
**Related Terms:** KV imaging, CBCT, LINAC
**Radiotherapy Example:** KV under-table imaging used to verify pelvis alignment.

160. **Universal Dosimetry Calibration Protocol:** Standardized protocol for calibration of all radiation measurement devices.
**Related Terms:** Ion chamber, Annual QA, LINAC output
**Radiotherapy Example:** Ion chambers recalibrated annually following universal protocol.

161. **Upper Femoral Head Dose Protection:** Reducing dose to upper femur to prevent fractures.
**Related Terms:** OAR constraint, IMRT, DVH
**Radiotherapy Example:** Femoral head dose capped during pelvic RT plan for cervical carcinoma.

162. **Units Per Monitor Gy Measurement:** Evaluating accuracy of MU required per delivered gray.
**Related Terms:** LINAC output, Dosimetry, MU calculation
**Radiotherapy Example:** MU/Gy validated for 6 MV and 10 MV beams during calibration.

163. **Upright CT Simulation Workflow:** Step-by-step procedure for CT simulation in upright position.
**Related Terms:** CT scan, Immobilization, IGRT
**Radiotherapy Example:** Thoracic tumor patient simulated upright to match treatment posture.

164. **Urethral Spacer Dose Advantage Study:** Evaluation of dose reduction from urethral spacers in prostate RT.
**Related Terms:** Organ displacement, HDR brachytherapy, OAR protection
**Radiotherapy Example:** Spacer reduces urethral high-dose volume during HDR boosts.

165. **Under-Mask Skin Bolus Technique:** Placing bolus under immobilization mask for desired surface dose.
**Related Terms:** Mould Room, Skin RT, IMRT
**Radiotherapy Example:** Bolus placed under mask to boost dose to facial skin lesions.

166. **Ultrafine MLC Edge Verification:** QA confirming precision of narrow MLC leaf edges.
**Related Terms:** MLC QA, IMRT, LINAC
**Radiotherapy Example:** MLC edges validated for tight head-and-neck IMRT fields.

167. **Urgent Adaptive Replanning Protocol:** Rapid TPS replanning workflow when major anatomical change occurs.
**Related Terms:** Adaptive RT, CBCT, IGRT
**Radiotherapy Example:** Pelvic replan triggered when tumor shrinkage exceeds 15%.

168. **Upper-Abdomen Target Localization Index:** Quantitative score measuring reliability of abdominal target localization.
**Related Terms:** IGRT, 4D CT, Motion tracking
**Radiotherapy Example:** Higher index achieved using gated liver SBRT localization.

169. **Ultrasound-to-CT Target Fusion:** Combining ultrasound with CT for precise target contouring.
**Related Terms:** Image fusion, TPS, IGRT
**Radiotherapy Example:** Prostate contours refined by US-CT fusion during planning.

170. **Uterus Motion Study in Pelvic RT:** Evaluation of uterus displacement during fractionated treatment.
**Related Terms:** 4D CT, Organ motion, IGRT
**Radiotherapy Example:** Frequent bladder filling variations tracked via daily CBCT.

171. **Under-Dose Replanning Threshold:** Dose deviation level that triggers a new treatment plan.
**Related Terms:** DVH, Online adaptive RT, QA
**Radiotherapy Example:** Replan when PTV receives <95% of prescribed dose in weekly review.

172. **Upright Breast Cone-Beam CT Verification:** CBCT localization for upright breast treatment sessions.
**Related Terms:** IGRT, CBCT, Immobilization
**Radiotherapy Example:** CBCT confirms left breast alignment before each IMRT fraction.

173. **Upper Arm Position Monitoring System:** System to ensure reproducible arm position during thoracic or breast RT.
**Related Terms:** Mould Room, IGRT, Immobilization
**Radiotherapy Example:** Arm deviation alert used during daily breast LINAC setup.

174. **Under Collimator Leakage Mapping:** Measurement of dose leakage beneath collimator jaws.
**Related Terms:** LINAC QA, Beam profiles, Output
**Radiotherapy Example:** Jaw leakage mapped during annual LINAC acceptance.

175. **Ultrasound-Triggered Gating:** Respiratory gating activated based on ultrasound diaphragm motion.
**Related Terms:** 4D CT, Motion tracking, SBRT
**Radiotherapy Example:** Liver SBRT beam turns on only when diaphragm reaches set position.

176. **Upper Facial Skin Dose Enhancement Study:** Evaluation of skin dose increase techniques for facial cancer.
**Related Terms:** Bolus, IMRT, Superficial dose
**Radiotherapy Example:** Custom bolus modeled for forehead lesion VMAT boost.

177. **Underdose Compensation Boost Field:** Additional radiation field to correct underdosed areas.
**Related Terms:** IMRT, Boost planning, TPS
**Radiotherapy Example:** Boost applied to insufficiently dosed posterior PTV margin.

178. **Universal LINAC Safety Checklist:** Standard patient and machine safety checklist before irradiation.
**Related Terms:** Radiation safety, QA, IGRT
**Radiotherapy Example:** Checklist prevents wrong-site irradiation during pediatric session.

179. **Upper Spine SBRT Verification Protocol:** Protocol for ensuring safe and accurate SBRT to the upper spine.
**Related Terms:** CBCT, IGRT, Spinal cord sparing
**Radiotherapy Example:** CBCT alignment required before every upper spine SBRT fraction.

180. **Urethral Catheter Tracking During RT:** Monitoring catheter movement to protect urethra during irradiation.
**Related Terms:** IGRT, HDR brachytherapy, OAR
**Radiotherapy Example:** Catheter position verified with ultrasound before prostate HDR boost.

181. **Upright Thorax Immobilization Jacket:** Shoulder- and chest-support jacket for upright thorax treatments.
**Related Terms:** Mould Room, SBRT, IGRT
**Radiotherapy Example:** Jacket used for lung SBRT to reduce movement and reproduce posture.

182. **Unrestricted Photon Beam Mode Study:** Investigating photon beam characteristics without collimation restriction.
**Related Terms:** LINAC output, Beam mapping
**Radiotherapy Example:** Open-field measurements collected for commissioning.

183. **Upper Lobe Target Breathing Correlation Index:** Scoring system that reflects upper lung tumor movement vs breathing cycle.
**Related Terms:** 4D CT, Gating, Motion management
**Radiotherapy Example:** Strong correlation leads to gating-based SBRT strategy.

184. **Ultrasound-Based External Marker Registration:** Using ultrasound to match target position with external markers.
**Related Terms:** Image guidance, IGRT, Mould Room
**Radiotherapy Example:** External markers drive beam release when bladder reaches planned volume.

185. **Unauthorized Dose Event Logging:** Recording any accidental or safety-critical radiation delivery event.
**Related Terms:** Incident reporting, Radiation safety
**Radiotherapy Example:** Log triggered when patient received unintended imaging exposure.

186. **Upper Pelvis Brachytherapy Dose Gradient Map:** Map showing dose fall-off around brachytherapy sources in upper pelvis.
**Related Terms:** HDR, Isodose curves, TPS
**Radiotherapy Example:** Sharp gradient around vaginal HDR boost evaluated for safety.

187. **Under-Table KV Scatter Evaluation:** Studying radiation scatter from KV imaging under the couch.
**Related Terms:** Radiation protection, CBCT dose
**Radiotherapy Example:** Scatter dose to abdomen measured during pelvic KV verification.

188. **Upright Head-and-Neck Positioning Laser System:** Lasers customized to align patients in upright posture for H&N RT.
**Related Terms:** Mould Room, Lasers, LINAC
**Radiotherapy Example:** Neck tumor positioned using triple-plane upright laser marks.

189. **Urethral HDR Catheter Dose Balancing:** Adjusting dwell positions to regulate HDR dose near urethra.
**Related Terms:** Optimization, TPS, OAR
**Radiotherapy Example:** Dwell optimization reduces urethral D10 during prostate HDR.

190. **Ultrafast CBCT Scan Mode:** Rapid CBCT acquisition to reduce motion artifacts.
**Related Terms:** IGRT, CBCT, LINAC
**Radiotherapy Example:** Lung CBCT acquired in 8 seconds to minimize breathing blur.

191. **Unused Monitor Unit Audit:** Reviewing MU planned but not delivered.
**Related Terms:** MU tracking, QA, TPS
**Radiotherapy Example:** Audit triggered when MU mismatch exceeded 2% in VMAT delivery.

192. **Upper Body Scatter Shield:** Shielding tool to reduce radiation scatter to upper body regions.
**Related Terms:** Radiation protection, Mould Room, LINAC
**Radiotherapy Example:** Shield placed to protect chest during pelvic RT.

193. **Ultrasound-Triggered Patient Repositioning Alert:** Alert produced when ultrasound detects misalignment.
**Related Terms:** IGRT, Monitoring systems, Immobilization
**Radiotherapy Example:** Alert triggered due to prostate shift before beam on.

194. **Unrestricted Dose Mapping Study:** Study mapping potential dose outside the treatment field.
**Related Terms:** Dosimetry, Scatter radiation, TPS
**Radiotherapy Example:** Mapping shows elevated scatter to contralateral breast during tangents.

195. **Upright Couch Extension Support:** Support accessory used for upright radiation positioning.
**Related Terms:** Mould Room, LINAC couch, Immobilization
**Radiotherapy Example:** Thoracic SBRT setup uses upright support to stabilize posture.

196. **Upper Abdomen SBRT Breathing Halt Technique:** Breath-hold technique for dose precision during upper-abdomen SBRT.
**Related Terms:** DIBH, Motion control, 4D CT
**Radiotherapy Example:** Liver SBRT delivered with repeated deep inspiration breath holds.

197. **Under-Jaw Beam Tracking Study:** Analysis of beam behavior under partially closed collimator jaws.
**Related Terms:** MLC QA, Output calibration
**Radiotherapy Example:** Commissioning study for 2 cm jaw tracking during VMAT.

198. **Ultrasound Bladder Volume Threshold Protocol:** Protocol defining bladder volume required before irradiation.
**Related Terms:** IGRT, Adaptive RT, Pelvic RT
**Radiotherapy Example:** Treatment paused until bladder volume reaches $\geq$350 mL.

199. **Universal LINAC Error Recovery Protocol:** Standardized response procedure when LINAC faults occur.
**Related Terms:** Radiation safety, Machine QA
**Radiotherapy Example:** Protocol followed after beam steering failure mid-fraction.

200. **Upper Thorax Deep-Inspiration Breath Hold Verification:** Verification of chest expansion for DIBH breast or lung treatments.
**Related Terms:** DIBH, CBCT, Motion management
**Radiotherapy Example:** Heart displacement confirmed on CBCT before left-breast DIBH treatment.

201. **Ultrasonic Position Tracking:** Use of ultrasound to track internal targets or organs during radiation treatment in real time.
**Related equipment:** Ultrasound probe, motion tracking system, LINAC gating interface.
**Radiotherapy Example:** Real-time ultrasound tracking is used during prostate radiotherapy to monitor organ motion and adjust beam delivery.

**202. Ultrathin Immobilization Sheets:** Extremely thin thermoplastic sheets used to restrict patient movement without compromising imaging quality.
**Related equipment:** Mould room thermoplastic sheets, vacuum bag, base plate.
**Radiotherapy Example:** An ultrathin mask is used for head-and-neck CT simulation to ensure accurate LINAC treatment positioning.

**203. Utility Mapping in TPS:** Mapping clinical utilities (dose, structures, organs at risk) for treatment optimization.
**Related equipment:** Treatment Planning System (TPS), structure set, CT scan.
**Radiotherapy Example:** Kidney plans use utility mapping to prioritize PTV dose while reducing bowel exposure.

**204. Umbrella Shielding Model:** A shielding strategy where radiation protection extends outward like an umbrella to shield nearby organs.
**Related equipment:** Shielding blocks, bolus, custom mould room shielding.
**Radiotherapy Example:** Umbrella shielding protects the testes during pelvic LINAC irradiation.

**205. Unilateral Beam Arrangement:** Radiation beams entering from one side of the patient only.
**Related equipment:** LINAC gantry, jaws, MLC.
**Radiotherapy Example:** Unilateral beams are used for breast irradiation to avoid unnecessary lung dose.

**206. Uniform Dose Objective:** Planning objective to achieve a homogeneous dose distribution across the target volume.
**Related equipment:** TPS optimizer, dose constraints, CT-based contouring.
**Radiotherapy Example:** Uniform dose objective is set during IMRT plan optimization for pelvic tumors.

**207. Unintended Dose Recording:** Documentation of radiation dose delivered to non-target tissues.
**Related equipment:** Portal dosimetry, in-vivo diode, OSLD.
**Radiotherapy Example:** Intestinal unintended dose is recorded during abdominal radiotherapy for review.

**208. Unshielded Organs Risk Index:** Metric estimating biological risk to organs without shielding.
**Related equipment:** DVH, structure set, radiosensitivity factors.
**Radiotherapy Example:** Liver risk index rises when shielding is not applied during body SBRT.

**209. Uncertainty Margin Expansion:** Extra margin added to CTV to compensate for uncertainties such as motion and setup errors.
**Related equipment:** CT simulation, IGRT, immobilization devices.
**Radiotherapy Example:** A 5 mm margin is added around prostate CTV to create PTV due to motion uncertainty.

**210. Unity Gradient Optimization:** IMRT/VMAT optimization where gradients between high-dose and low-dose regions are sharpened while maintaining homogeneity.
**Related equipment:** TPS optimizer, MLC modulation.
**Radiotherapy Example:** Sharp dose gradients protect rectum during prostate IMRT.

**211. Ultra-Precision Collimation:** Highly accurate shaping of radiation beams to conform tightly to the tumor.
**Related equipment:** Micro-MLC, cones, SRS collimator.
**Radiotherapy Example:** Ultra-precision collimation is used for trigeminal neuralgia SRS.

212. **Upper Abdomen Motion Damping:** Reducing respiratory motion in upper abdominal organs during treatment.
**Related equipment:** Abdominal compression device, 4D-CT.
**Radiotherapy Example:** Compression dampens motion for liver SBRT planning.

213. **Unflattened Beam Calibration:** Calibration of flattening-filter-free (FFF) beams for accurate dose output.
**Related equipment:** LINAC dosimetry system, water phantom.
**Radiotherapy Example:** FFF calibration ensures correct output for stereotactic lung plans.

214. **Unrestricted Gating Window:** Wide gating tolerance allowing beam delivery even during moderate organ motion.
**Related equipment:** Respiratory gating system, external marker system.
**Radiotherapy Example:** Wide gating window used for palliative liver treatment to shorten treatment time.

215. **Upright Treatment Positioning:** Delivering radiation in the sitting position rather than lying down.
**Related equipment:** Upright immobilization chair, CT setup adaptation.
**Radiotherapy Example:** Upright technique improves comfort for lung cancer patients with breathing discomfort.

216. **Urethra Dose Monitoring:** Continuous measurement or prediction of dose to the urethra in prostate treatments.
**Related equipment:** DVH constraints, spacer gel, CT planning.
**Radiotherapy Example:** Urethra dose monitored in HDR brachytherapy and prostate VMAT planning.

217. **Uniform Photon Profile:** Regular photon intensity across the treatment field.
**Related equipment:** LINAC beam steering, QA ion chamber array.
**Radiotherapy Example:** Photon profile checked during annual QA to ensure breast field uniformity.

218. **Upper Cervical Spine Immobilization:** Restricting head and neck motion for accurate radiotherapy of cervical vertebrae.
**Related equipment:** Thermoplastic mask, bite block, mould room fabrication.
**Radiotherapy Example:** Used in IMRT for nasopharyngeal cancer to keep C1–C2 stable.

219. **Uncoupled Multileaf Sequencing:** Independent MLC leaf movements not linked symmetrically during modulation.
**Related equipment:** MLC, TPS optimizer.
**Radiotherapy Example:** Uncoupled leaf sequencing improves modulation for head-and-neck IMRT.

220. **Ultra-Low Dose CT Protocol:** CT scan approach lowering radiation without compromising planning accuracy.
**Related equipment:** CT scanner, iterative reconstruction algorithm.
**Radiotherapy Example:** Used for pediatric simulation scans to minimize dose.

221. **Uniformity Index Check:** Measure of dose uniformity within PTV.
**Related equipment:** TPS, DVH, QA software.
**Radiotherapy Example:** Uniformity index assessed during IMRT QA for breast plans.

222. **Unilateral Organ Motion Analysis:** Tracking motion of a single movable organ relative to others.
**Related equipment:** 4D-CT, tracking system.
**Radiotherapy Example:** Liver-alone motion checked for kidney-sparing SBRT.

**223. Uninterrupted Beam Delivery Mode:** Beam mode enabling treatment delivery without programmed pauses.
**Related equipment:** LINAC control console, VMAT delivery system.
**Radiotherapy Example:** Used when patient cooperation is excellent and motion minimal.

**224. Unambiguous Fiducial Recognition:** Successful automatic detection of fiducials in imaging without manual correction.
**Related equipment:** KV imaging, CBCT, gold markers.
**Radiotherapy Example:** System auto-identifies prostate markers to align the patient before treatment.

**225. Upper Thorax Breath-Hold Coaching:** Training patients to maintain consistent deep-inspiration breath-hold.
**Related equipment:** Visual feedback goggles, tracking camera.
**Radiotherapy Example:** Breath-hold coaching improves heart sparing in left breast radiotherapy.

**226. Unsupervised Organ Segmentation:** Automatic AI-based contouring of organs without manual interaction.
**Related equipment:** AI contouring software, CT scan datasets, TPS.
**Radiotherapy Example:** AI performs unsupervised segmentation of kidneys on CT simulation images before VMAT planning.

**227. Ultrafast Arc Modulation:** Rapid modulation of MLC leaves and dose rate during VMAT to reduce delivery time.
**Related equipment:** LINAC VMAT system, high-speed MLC.
**Radiotherapy Example:** Ultrafast arc is used to treat pediatric cases quickly to reduce anesthesia duration.

**228. Underdose Region Evaluation:** Analysis of areas receiving lower dose than the prescription.
**Related equipment:** DVH, isodose maps, QA software.
**Radiotherapy Example:** Underdose region evaluation ensures the PTV receives full dose in head-and-neck IMRT plans.

**229. Uniform Phantom Calibration:** Calibration of detector systems using phantoms with uniform density.
**Related equipment:** Solid water phantom, ion chamber array.
**Radiotherapy Example:** Uniform phantom calibration ensures LINAC flattening-filter-free beam accuracy.

**230. Upper Airway Motion Diagnostic:** Assessment of swallowing and breathing movements affecting target motion.
**Related equipment:** 4D-CT, fluoroscopy.
**Radiotherapy Example:** Used when treating tongue base cancers where airway movement may disturb targeting.

**231. Uplink Sensor Communication:** Transfer of in-vivo dosimetry sensor data to monitoring system in real time.
**Related equipment:** Wireless dosimetry sensors, LINAC interface.
**Radiotherapy Example:** Sensors transmit dose data during pelvic IMRT to ensure planned dose delivery.

232. **Uniform Radiopacity Material:** Tissue-equivalent material providing uniform appearance on radiological imaging.
**Related equipment:** Radiopaque bolus, mould room material.
**Radiotherapy Example:** Uniform radiopacity bolus ensures skin build-up during chest wall treatment.

233. **Upregulation Sensitivity Index:** Biological index estimating increased tumor cell response after radiation.
**Related equipment:** Radiobiology model software, TCP calculators.
**Radiotherapy Example:** SBRT planning uses upregulation sensitivity index to predict immune-response effects.

234. **Under-Couch Dose Calculation:** Accounting for couch contribution in dose calculations.
**Related equipment:** CT couch model, TPS attenuation model.
**Radiotherapy Example:** VMAT spine plans calculate under-couch attenuation to avoid underdose.

235. **URT (Upper Respiratory Tract) Dose Metric:** Quantification of radiation delivered to upper respiratory structures.
**Related equipment:** DVH constraint table, CT contouring.
**Radiotherapy Example:** URT dose metric monitored in nasopharyngeal cancer IMRT to reduce mucositis.

236. **Ultra-Compact Immobilization Design:** Small-profile immobilization systems that improve access for imaging and beam clearance.
**Related equipment:** Low-profile baseplate, SRS mask, mould room fabrication.
**Radiotherapy Example:** Used during cranial SRS to prevent collision during non-coplanar arcs.

237. **Ultrathin Bolus Layering:** Stepwise application of thin bolus sheets to fine-tune surface dose.
**Related equipment:** 1–2 mm bolus sheets, mould room cutters.
**Radiotherapy Example:** Multiple layers added to nasal region to optimize dose in scalp irradiation.

238. **Unsharp Mask Reconstruction:** Imaging technique improving edge sharpness by subtracting blurred copies of image.
**Related equipment:** CT scanner reconstruction software.
**Radiotherapy Example:** Used to improve visibility of small targets during CT simulation.

239. **Unrestricted Arc Clearance Scan:** 3D geometric scan to test collision-free LINAC arc rotations around patient.
**Related equipment:** Arc-clearance simulation software, immobilization devices.
**Radiotherapy Example:** Clearance scan prevents gantry–couch collisions during head-and-neck VMAT.

240. **Unbiased Dose Measurement:** Dose verification unaffected by energy dependence or angular orientation.
**Related equipment:** OSLD, alanine dosimeter, ion chamber.
**Radiotherapy Example:** Used during commissioning of new LINAC energy.

241. **Utility-Weighted Planning Approach:** Optimization based on assigning clinical importance to each anatomical structure.
**Related equipment:** TPS cost-function editor.
**Radiotherapy Example:** High weight is assigned to spinal cord protection during lung VMAT planning.

**242. Urinary Bladder Fullness Protocol:** Standardized hydration routine before simulation and treatment.
**Related equipment:** Patient hydration chart, bladder ultrasound.
**Radiotherapy Example:** Used for prostate VMAT to move bladder away from beam path and stabilize organ shape.

**243. Ultra-Dense Dose Binning:** Very fine resolution in dose histogram bins to improve DVH precision.
**Related equipment:** TPS dose grid, DVH algorithm.
**Radiotherapy Example:** Used in SBRT prostates where dose gradients are steep.

**244. Upper Chest Immobilization Strap:** Restriction device minimizing upper thoracic motion during breathing.
**Related equipment:** Abdominal compression device, strap system.
**Radiotherapy Example:** Strap reduces chest motion during lung 4D-CT simulation.

**245. Upright CT Calibration Algorithm:** Mathematical correction for CT scans taken in the sitting position.
**Related equipment:** Upright CT scanner, DRR generator.
**Radiotherapy Example:** Used for patients receiving upright proton therapy.

**246. Unbalanced Dose Trade-Off Metric:** Quantifies cost versus benefit when prioritizing one organ over another in planning.
**Related equipment:** Plan comparison tool, DVH analytics.
**Radiotherapy Example:** Trade-off evaluated between parotid and spinal cord in head-and-neck IMRT.

**247. Upper Abdominal Beam Modulation:** Custom modulation strategy to manage organs at risk in upper abdomen.
**Related equipment:** MLC, VMAT optimizer.
**Radiotherapy Example:** Optimized modulation protects stomach during liver SBRT.

**248. Ultrafast Dose Fall-Off:** Rapid reduction of dose outside target to protect nearby organs.
**Related equipment:** Small-field cones, micro-MLC.
**Radiotherapy Example:** Applied in brain metastasis SRS to protect healthy parenchyma.

**249. Unidirectional Tumor Tracking:** Tracking tumor displacement along a single axis.
**Related equipment:** External marker tracking, ultrasound tracking.
**Radiotherapy Example:** Used when liver tumor moves mainly in the superior–inferior direction.

**250. Uniform Scatter Compensation:** Adjusting dose calculation to account for consistent scatter across the field.
**Related equipment:** TPS scatter kernel, water phantom QA.
**Radiotherapy Example:** Applied in pelvic 3D-CRT to maintain homogeneous dose.

**251. Unplanned Dose Drift Detection:** Identification of gradual deviation between planned and delivered dose over multiple fractions.
**Related equipment:** EPID, in-vivo dosimetry system, TPS log-file comparison.
**Radiotherapy Example:** Dose drift alerts during prostate IMRT trigger plan review before further fractions.

**252. Upper Pelvic Lymph Node Mapping:** Contouring and tracking of pelvic lymph node regions for targeting and OAR avoidance.
**Related equipment:** CT simulation, MRI fusion, contouring atlas.
**Radiotherapy Example:** Accurate mapping is required for cervix IMRT to avoid bowel overdose.

**253. Ultrasonic Organ Motion Tracking:** Uses ultrasound to track soft-tissue movement in real time.
**Related equipment:** 4D ultrasound tracking system, LINAC interface.
**Radiotherapy Example:** Liver SBRT uses ultrasound tracking to account for diaphragm motion.

**254. Unrestricted Beam Entry Planning:** Advanced VMAT/IMRT planning that uses any feasible beam angle while maintaining safety.
**Related equipment:** Non-coplanar arc optimizer, collision-detection software.
**Radiotherapy Example:** Used for skull-base tumors where conventional beam paths are obstructed.

**255. Uncertainty-Driven Optimization:** Planning approach that incorporates geometric and motion uncertainty during optimization.
**Related equipment:** Robust optimization TPS, 4D-CT.
**Radiotherapy Example:** Pancreatic IMRT uses robust optimization to account for stomach gas variability.

**256. Upper Thoracic Field Harmonization:** Adjustment of overlapping fields to avoid dose gaps or hotspots near thoracic junctions.
**Related equipment:** Dose junction optimizer, portal dosimetry.
**Radiotherapy Example:** Harmonization prevents hotspots in craniospinal irradiation near T1–T3.

**257. Unfiltered Radiographic Acquisition:** Image capture without additional filtration for maximum image contrast.
**Related equipment:** Flat panel detector, KV imaging system.
**Radiotherapy Example:** Used during orthogonal setup imaging when fiducial contrast is low.

**258. Ultrafast Patient Setup Workflow:** Accelerated workflow using automated couch positioning and AI-guided registration.
**Related equipment:** 6D robotic couch, AI CBCT auto-match.
**Radiotherapy Example:** Pediatric cases benefit by minimizing sedation duration.

**259. Uniform Gel Dosimetry Calibration:** Calibration of radiochromic gel to ensure dose-dependent discoloration is linear and predictable.
**Related equipment:** Polymer gel dosimeter, MRI scanner, optical reader.
**Radiotherapy Example:** Used during commissioning of SRS small-field beams.

**260. U-Shaped Dose Distribution:** Dose pattern designed to spare a central OAR while covering surrounding tumor tissue.
**Related equipment:** IMRT optimizer, MLC.
**Radiotherapy Example:** Achieved in sacral chordoma plans to protect cauda equina.

**261. Upper Abdomen Motion Gate:** Respiratory gating applied specifically to high-motion abdominal organs.
**Related equipment:** RPM system, 4D-CT.
**Radiotherapy Example:** Gating used for pancreatic SBRT to control motion near duodenum.

**262. Unilateral PTV Expansion:** Adding margins asymmetrically on one side of PTV due to directional uncertainty.
**Related equipment:** TPS margin protocol, 4D-CT data.
**Radiotherapy Example:** Breast IMRT expands medially to compensate for heart displacement risk.

**263. User-Adaptive Anatomical Library:** Expanding database of anatomical models trained by cumulative usage patterns.
**Related equipment:** AI contouring software, CT atlas datasets.
**Radiotherapy Example:** Library improves segmentation accuracy for rare tumor anatomies.

264. **Underdose Flagging Algorithm:** Automatic detection of PTV voxels receiving below-threshold dose.
**Related equipment:** DVH auto-alert, AI QA platform.
**Radiotherapy Example:** Alerts during plan review when rectal constraints force compromise in prostate plan.

265. **Ultra-Clear Immobilization Material:** Transparent, rigid immobilization thermoplastic for better anatomical visibility.
**Related equipment:** Clear thermoplastic mask, mould room heater.
**Radiotherapy Example:** Used in head-and-neck patients to allow positioning tattoos to remain visible.

266. **Upright Dose Reconstruction:** Technique to estimate therapeutic dose from upright treatment plans using transformation matrices.
**Related equipment:** Upright CT, TPS coordinate mapping.
**Radiotherapy Example:** Useful for upright proton therapy in mediastinal lymphoma.

267. **Ultra-High EPID Frame Rate Mode:** Maximum-speed EPID capture mode for continuous fluence monitoring.
**Related equipment:** EPID cine acquisition system.
**Radiotherapy Example:** Detects transient MLC leaf error during high-speed VMAT delivery.

268. **Unilateral Bolus Placement:** Bolus placed on only one side of patient to increase asymmetric surface dose.
**Related equipment:** Mould room bolus fabrication tools.
**Radiotherapy Example:** Used in parotid malignancy to boost dose to surgical bed.

269. **Urethra-Sparing Dose Technique:** Planning strategy to reduce urethral radiation during prostate irradiation.
**Related equipment:** MRI-defined urethral contour, urethra dose constraint table.
**Radiotherapy Example:** Used in SBRT prostate to reduce urinary toxicity.

270. **UQ-Model (Uncertainty Quantification Model):** Statistical model predicting effects of setup error, deformability, and organ motion.
**Related equipment:** AI predictive engine, image registration toolkit.
**Radiotherapy Example:** Improves confidence for abdominal targets with variable gas patterns.

271. **U-Frame Stereotactic Support:** Rigid support frame used to immobilize head during stereotactic treatment.
**Related equipment:** U-frame baseplate, carbon headrest.
**Radiotherapy Example:** Used for non-invasive cranial SRS when a mask replaces screw fixation.

272. **Unrestricted Dose Painting:** Dose painting based on functional imaging without PTV partition constraints.
**Related equipment:** PET-CT, MRI perfusion mapping, IMRT optimizer.
**Radiotherapy Example:** High FDG-uptake regions in head-and-neck cancer receive escalated boost dose.

273. **Upright Breast Simulation Protocol:** Simulation of breast patients in seated position to improve tissue spread and reproducibility.
**Related equipment:** Upright CT scanner, breast support board.
**Radiotherapy Example:** Improves breast positioning for large-breasted patients unable to tolerate supine setup.

274. **Ultralow CT Dose Recon Protocol:** Reconstruction algorithm generating high-quality CT images from very low dose scans.
**Related equipment:** Iterative reconstruction CT software.
**Radiotherapy Example:** Reduces imaging dose during repeated CBCT scans for pediatric cases.

275. **Unilateral Cervical Node Boost:** Boost dose delivered only to affected cervical lymph node chain.
**Related equipment:** IMRT, VMAT dose painting.
**Radiotherapy Example:** Used when nodal metastasis is limited to one side of the neck.

276. **Ultrafast CBCT Registration:** AI-assisted image matching that drastically reduces time for CBCT alignment.
**Related equipment:** AI CBCT auto-match, 6D robotic couch.
**Radiotherapy Example:** Improves efficiency in head-and-neck IMRT with daily image guidance.

277. **Uncertainty-Aware Fraction Scheduling:** Allocating treatment fractions based on predicted setup or organ-motion variability.
**Related equipment:** Robust planning software, motion data tracker.
**Radiotherapy Example:** Pancreatic SBRT sessions scheduled when stomach contraction risk is lowest.

278. **Uplink Couch Communication System:** Communication interface between LINAC and robotic couch for automatic shifts.
**Related equipment:** 6D couch, IGRT system.
**Radiotherapy Example:** Reduces manual couch shifts after CBCT auto-match.

279. **Ultra-Conformal Dose Falloff:** Very steep dose gradient around target volume with minimal dose to surrounding OARs.
**Related equipment:** MLC-optimized SRS, high-resolution collimators.
**Radiotherapy Example:** Required for brain metastasis near optic chiasm.

280. **Upper Mediastinum Auto-Segmentation:** AI-based contouring of lymphatic nodal regions in upper mediastinum.
**Related equipment:** Deep-learning contouring software, CT atlas.
**Radiotherapy Example:** Essential for esophageal IMRT planning.

281. **Universal Anatomy Coordinate System:** Standard coordinate reference for patient anatomy to avoid mismatch across platforms.
**Related equipment:** TPS coordinate translator, CT-MRI fusion tools.
**Radiotherapy Example:** Prevents mismatch when switching TPS vendors during plan transfer.

282. **Unilateral Deep Inspiration Technique:** Deep inspiration breath-hold (DIBH) performed selectively on one side of thorax.
**Related equipment:** DIBH monitoring system, 4D-CT.
**Radiotherapy Example:** Used in left-breast radiotherapy to move heart away from chest wall.

283. **U308. Under-Response Corrective Algorithm:** Software correction applied to detectors that underestimate small-field dose.
**Related equipment:** Small-field dosimetry system, diode array.
**Radiotherapy Example:** Used during SRS commissioning for brain lesions <1 cm.

284. **Uniform Phased Treatment:** Delivery of treatment in multiple pre-programmed phases based on anatomical evolution.
**Related equipment:** Adaptive planning suite, deformable monitoring.
**Radiotherapy Example:** Head-and-neck IMRT re-planned twice during weight-loss-dependent volume change.

**285. Ultra-Rapid Verification Field:** Very short low-dose field delivered solely for position verification.
**Related equipment:** Portal imager, EPID cine capture.
**Radiotherapy Example:** Used when full MV film verification adds excessive time.

**286. Urinary Bladder Trend Assessment:** Predicting bladder volume changes throughout course of treatment.
**Related equipment:** Ultrasound bladder scanner, CBCT fluid segmentation.
**Radiotherapy Example:** Critical for cervix IGRT to avoid PTV under-coverage.

**287. Upright Neck Fixation System:** Immobilization setup for upright neck treatment positioning.
**Related equipment:** Seat-mounted support frame, thermoplastic mask.
**Radiotherapy Example:** Used in laryngeal RT when supine positioning causes airway compromise.

**288. Ultra-Low Optimization Constraints Regime:** Initial rough optimization used before high-constraint planning.
**Related equipment:** TPS optimization module.
**Radiotherapy Example:** Applied in VMAT planning to ensure no cold spots before fine-tuning.

**289. Upper-Arm Shielding Protocol:** Technique to protect humeral head and upper arm when beam passes near shoulder.
**Related equipment:** Arm shield device, custom bolus.
**Radiotherapy Example:** Used during supraclavicular nodal irradiation in breast RT.

**290. Unilateral VMAT Arc Pair:** VMAT plan using two arcs from one side only to avoid contralateral organ dose.
**Related equipment:** VMAT arc optimizer, MLC.
**Radiotherapy Example:** Used for unilateral oropharyngeal carcinoma to spare contralateral parotid.

**291. Unattended Beam Interruption Safeguard:** Automated beam pause if patient monitoring system fails or disconnects.
**Related equipment:** Patient-presence IR tracking, LINAC safety controller.
**Radiotherapy Example:** Pauses beam if pediatric mask sensor reports loosened fixation.

**292. Ultra-Sharp Penumbra Filter:** Custom filter created to sharpen dose edge around targets.
**Related equipment:** MLC micro-leaf system, SRS cones.
**Radiotherapy Example:** Used in trigeminal neuralgia radiosurgery for steep dose falloff.

**293. Ultrafine Mesh Aquaplast:** Thermoplastic immobilization mask with tiny perforations for better cooling and comfort.
**Related equipment:** Mould room water bath, vacuum headrest.
**Radiotherapy Example:** Prevents claustrophobia and sweating in long head-and-neck fractions.

**294. Unplanned Anatomical Regression Check:** Monitoring for unexpected tumor shrinkage that may derail dose distribution.
**Related equipment:** Weekly CBCT, deformable dose accumulation.
**Radiotherapy Example:** Common in lymphomas where rapid shrinkage reduces target coverage.

**295. Ultra-Hypofractionated Regime:** Very few fractions (1–5), each with high dose.
**Related equipment:** SRS/SBRT planning tools, high-precision imaging.
**Radiotherapy Example:** 34 Gy in 1 fraction for lung SBRT.

**296. Upper-Jaw Overtravel Prevention:** Protection system reducing risk of over-travel and collision of Y-jaw or MLC bank.
**Related equipment:** LINAC jaw limit sensor.
**Radiotherapy Example:** Safety feature during non-coplanar brain VMAT.

297. **User-Triggered Beam Adjustment:** Allowing RTT to manually scale beam hold/restart within safety protocols.
**Related equipment:** Beam control workstation, patient camera feed.
**Radiotherapy Example:** Beam paused during coughing episode without re-setup loss.

298. **Unilateral Proton Boost Strategy:** Proton therapy boost to involved side to protect opposite organ chain.
**Related equipment:** Proton planning TPS, range modulator.
**Radiotherapy Example:** Used for unilateral parotid malignancy when sparing healthy gland.

299. **Ultra-Flexible CT Sim Table Pad:** Gel-based pad that molds to anatomy, improving reproducibility.
**Related equipment:** CT sim table, adjustable cushions.
**Radiotherapy Example:** Increases comfort and stabilizes pelvis during long fractions.

300. **Up-Angle Beam Pairing:** Using paired beams angled upward to avoid anterior OARs.
**Related equipment:** IMRT beam arrangement module.
**Radiotherapy Example:** Used for pancreatic RT to avoid high stomach and bowel dose.

301. **Urgency-Triggered Palliative Workflow:** Rapid radiotherapy pathway for emergencies.
**Related equipment:** Fast CT sim, 3D CRT templates.
**Radiotherapy Example:** Same-day RT for spinal cord compression.

302. **Uncoupled Dose Gradient Planning:** Advanced planning where gradient shape is no longer dependent on beam geometry.
**Related equipment:** AI dose predictor, MLC subfield optimizer.
**Radiotherapy Example:** Enhances sparing of optic nerves near pituitary tumors.

303. **Ultraviolet-C Field Sterilization:** UVC disinfection for immobilization devices between sessions.
**Related equipment:** UV-C chamber, mould room storage rack.
**Radiotherapy Example:** Prevents infections for immunocompromised patients.

304. **Upper-Lobe Lung Tracking:** Higher-accuracy motion monitoring tuned for upper-lung tumor displacement.
**Related equipment:** 4D-CT, diaphragm-tracking AI.
**Radiotherapy Example:** Required when tumor motion depends heavily on patient breathing pattern.

305. **U-Bolus Arm Seal Technique:** U-shaped bolus wrapped around axillary region for uniform chest wall dose.
**Related equipment:** Custom mould room bolus.
**Radiotherapy Example:** Used in post-mastectomy RT with axillary involvement.

306. **Unequal Beam Intensity Modulation:** Intentional intensity mismatch between opposing beams to accommodate OAR proximity.
**Related equipment:** IMRT optimizer, MLC.
**Radiotherapy Example:** Used in pelvis RT when rectum is close to PTV.

307. **Under-Dose Avoidance Shield:** Artificial density inserted during planning to prevent cold spots behind dense objects.
**Related equipment:** Virtual tissue compensator in TPS.
**Radiotherapy Example:** Used when metal dental implants distort dose.

308. **Uniform Quality Flag System:** Radiotherapy QA scorecard ensuring consistent evaluation across machines.
**Related equipment:** QA software, log analyzer.
**Radiotherapy Example:** Detects systematic deviation in LINAC beam output trends.

**309. Up-Front Adaptive Review:** Mandatory review of anatomical and dosimetric changes before 2nd or 3rd fraction.
**Related equipment:** CBCT review, deformable registration tool.
**Radiotherapy Example:** Required for esophageal IMRT due to rapid tumor response.

**310. Ultra-Selective MLC Mapping:** MLC micro-segment generation for tight conformity around irregular targets.
**Related equipment:** High-resolution MLC.
**Radiotherapy Example:** Applied in SBRT spine to avoid spinal cord.

**311. Upper-Abdominal Compression Strategy:** Compression applied to diaphragm region to reduce organ motion.
**Related equipment:** Abdominal compression belt, 4D-CT.
**Radiotherapy Example:** Used for liver SBRT to restrict respiratory motion.

**312. User-Restricted Plan Approval Chain:** Multi-signature plan approval requiring specific specialists for high-risk cases.
**Related equipment:** Oncology information system (OIS).
**Radiotherapy Example:** CNS re-irradiation plans require joint approval of oncologist + physicist + dosimetrist.

**313. Ultra-Compact SRS Targeting Mode:** SRS algorithm optimized specifically for very small tumors.
**Related equipment:** SRS cones, HD-MLC.
**Radiotherapy Example:** Used for metastatic lesions of 2–5 mm.

**314. Ultrasound-Guided Rectal Preparation Check:** Use of ultrasound to confirm rectum clearance before prostate treatment.
**Related equipment:** Bowel US scanner.
**Radiotherapy Example:** Prevents PTV shift due to rectal fullness.

**315. Upper-Spine Dose Gradient Match:** Smoothing technique across cervical–thoracic dose junctions.
**Related equipment:** Dose junction optimizer.
**Radiotherapy Example:** Required in craniospinal irradiation.

**316. Unbiased Plan Scoring Model:** AI scoring based only on dosimetric outcomes, not planner preferences.
**Related equipment:** Automated plan analytics.
**Radiotherapy Example:** Provides objective scoring when comparing IMRT vs VMAT.

**317. Urban-Noise Resistant Patient-Audio System:** Noise-filtered communication system for LINAC bunker in loud environments.
**Related equipment:** Noise-isolated microphone headset.
**Radiotherapy Example:** Maintains communication during HDR brachy procedures.

**318. Under-Table Collision Shielding:** Device that prevents couch from striking LINAC under-table components.
**Related equipment:** Couch safety barrier.
**Radiotherapy Example:** Used during steep-angled non-coplanar cranial arcs.

**319. Ultra-Long Breath-Hold Strategy:** >30-second breath-hold for high-dose large fraction delivery.
**Related equipment:** Assisted breathing coach system.
**Radiotherapy Example:** Used in lung SBRT for large PTVs to eliminate respiratory motion.

320. **Upright Pelvic Beam Protocol:** Beam arrangement designed specifically for pelvis cases treated upright.
**Related equipment:** Upright LINAC chair.
**Radiotherapy Example:** Applied in rectal RT to reduce gastrointestinal toxicity.

321. **Unmodified Anatomical Transfer:** Copying contours from reference anatomy without atlas scaling.
**Related equipment:** Contour library, registration tool.
**Radiotherapy Example:** Used when two patient scans have identical body habitus.

322. **Unshared Bolus System:** Individual bolus fabricated for each patient to avoid sharing.
**Related equipment:** 3D-printed or thermoplastic bolus.
**Radiotherapy Example:** Useful in mould room for infection-control policy.

323. **Up-Scattered Neutron Index:** Metric estimating neutron scatter risk in high-energy photon treatments.
**Related equipment:** Neutron dosimeter, shielding calculator.
**Radiotherapy Example:** Applied for 18 MV pelvic beams.

324. **Ultra-Low Room Contamination Workflow:** Sterile treatment flow for immune-compromised patients.
**Related equipment:** HEPA room system, UV sterilization.
**Radiotherapy Example:** Used in bone-marrow transplant recipients receiving TBI.

325. **Ultra-Deep Learning Dose Predictor:** AI model predicting final dose distribution before full optimization.
**Related equipment:** Deep-learning planning platform.
**Radiotherapy Example:** Predicts VMAT dose shape for glioblastoma within seconds.

326. **Uniform Target Motion Profile:** A motion model assuming predictable and repeatable target movement during respiration.
**Related equipment:** 4D-CT, respiratory gating system.
**Radiotherapy Example:** Used when lung tumors show highly repeatable cranio-caudal motion.

327. **Unilateral Accessory Shield:** Shield protecting contralateral anatomical structures during irradiation.
**Related equipment:** Lead shielding plate, mould room stabilizer.
**Radiotherapy Example:** Used to protect the opposite breast in tangential breast radiotherapy.

328. **Ultra-Stable Stereotactic Frame:** Non-invasive immobilization system for high-precision stereotactic treatment.
**Related equipment:** Frameless cranial immobilizer, bite block.
**Radiotherapy Example:** Applied in trigeminal neuralgia radiosurgery.

329. **Under-Beam Clearance Check:** Pre-treatment review ensuring couch and patient anatomy will not collide with gantry.
**Related equipment:** CT simulator clearance predictor, virtual collision tool.
**Radiotherapy Example:** Especially crucial during non-coplanar VMAT brain treatments.

330. **Ultra-Compact Gantry Arc:** A shortened VMAT arc path designed to reduce scatter and shorten treatment time.
**Related equipment:** VMAT arc optimizer, MLC sequencing system.
**Radiotherapy Example:** Used in pediatric cranial irradiation to minimize time in bunker.

331. **Upright Thoracic Positioning System:** A patient setup platform allowing thoracic RT in a seated position.
**Related equipment:** Vac-loc upright cradle, IGRT couch.
**Radiotherapy Example:** Beneficial for patients with severe dyspnea who cannot lie supine.

**332. Ultrasonic Fiducial Tracking:** Real-time tumor tracking using acoustic reflection from implanted markers.
**Related equipment:** Ultrasound tracking array, fiducial markers.
**Radiotherapy Example:** Applied in prostate SBRT for intrafraction motion monitoring.

**333. Ultra-Conventional Fractionation:** Very small daily dose per fraction (<1.8 Gy) delivered over extended schedule.
**Related equipment:** Standard LINAC treatment delivery system.
**Radiotherapy Example:** Used in elderly lymphoma patients to reduce acute toxicity.

**334. Under-Dose Risk Threshold:** Maximum allowable percentage of target volume falling below Rx dose.
**Related equipment:** Dose-volume histogram evaluation tool.
**Radiotherapy Example:** PTV under-dose cannot exceed 5% in head-and-neck IMRT.

**335. Upgraded Beam Steering Module:** Enhanced beam control system maintaining flatness and symmetry more precisely.
**Related equipment:** LINAC steering controller, trim coil driver.
**Radiotherapy Example:** Improves uniformity in electron beam treatments.

**336. Ultra-Low Surface Dose Technique:** Field arrangement purposely avoiding high entrance dose to the skin.
**Related equipment:** Bolus-avoidance protocol, MLC feathering.
**Radiotherapy Example:** Used when treating scalp tumors in patients with fragile skin.

**337. Unilateral Partial-Breast VMAT Protocol:** Restricted-arc VMAT for early-stage breast cancer.
**Related equipment:** Breast board immobilizer, VMAT optimizer.
**Radiotherapy Example:** Spares heart and contralateral breast from high dose.

**338. Upper-Abdomen Motion Prediction AI:** Algorithm forecasting liver and pancreas motion during treatment.
**Related equipment:** 4D-CBCT, abdominal motion sensor.
**Radiotherapy Example:** Optimizes gating thresholds during pancreas SBRT.

**339. Uncompensated Couch Angle Strategy:** Delivery using couch rotation without direct TPS angle compensation (for speed).
**Related equipment:** Robotic couch, real-time MLC verifier.
**Radiotherapy Example:** Used for simple palliative 3D CRT where precision requirement is low.

**340. Ultrafast Portal Imager Preview:** Rapid, low-dose EPID preview image to confirm field exposure.
**Related equipment:** EPID cine acquisition software.
**Radiotherapy Example:** Allows verification without repeating full portal films.

**341. Upright Chest Wall Immobilizer:** Molded support for upright post-mastectomy radiotherapy.
**Related equipment:** Thermoplastic mould room workstation.
**Radiotherapy Example:** Particularly helpful for anxious or restrictive-lung-disease patients.

**342. Ultra-Narrow Collimator Slot Therapy:** Radiation delivered through a slit-like fixed aperture to treat long thin targets.
**Related equipment:** Dedicated collimator slot, dynamic couch translation.
**Radiotherapy Example:** Used for craniospinal irradiation on helical tomotherapy.

**343. Universal Patient Coordinate Export:** Data protocol allowing coordinates to transfer across differing treatment systems.
**Related equipment:** OIS export module, TPS interoperability suite.

**Radiotherapy Example:** Required when MRI simulation and CT simulation are done at different centers.

344. **Unbiased PTV Margin AI Calculator:** Machine-learning tool creating margins based on organ motion and patient geometry, not planner guesswork.
**Related equipment:** Motion history analytics, deformable dose tool.
**Radiotherapy Example:** Reduces rectal dose in prostate IMRT by optimizing margins mathematically.

345. **Ultra-High Prescription Gradient:** Planning with extreme shift from high to low dose over small distance.
**Related equipment:** Micro-leaf MLC, SRS optimization.
**Radiotherapy Example:** Brain metastasis near brainstem treated using 3 mm falloff.

346. **Under-Arc Organ Avoidance:** Ensuring arcs never sweep through critical organ regions.
**Related equipment:** VMAT sector exclusion.
**Radiotherapy Example:** Arc path excluding pharynx in larynx-preserving treatments.

347. **Upper-Cervical Mask Reinforcement:** Strengthening part of mask to prevent neck tilt during long fractions.
**Related equipment:** Thermoplastic reinforcer sheets, mould room press.
**Radiotherapy Example:** Prevents movement in nasopharynx IMRT.

348. **Ultra-High-Accuracy Table Indexing:** Indexing system allowing reproducible millimeter-level placement of immobilization boards.
**Related equipment:** Indexing bars and slots, CT sim table adapter.
**Radiotherapy Example:** Increases alignment consistency in spinal SBRT programs.

349. **Unilateral OAR-Constraint Planning:** Allowing generous dose constraints only on one side while tightening the other.
**Related equipment:** IMRT optimizer, TPS constraint gradient tool.
**Radiotherapy Example:** Useful when tumor presses one parotid while the other remains healthy.

350. **Ultra-Flexible 3-Point Mask System:** Mask attaching at three anchor points instead of full wrap-around.
**Related equipment:** Lightweight head fixation frame.
**Radiotherapy Example:** Designed for patients with anxiety during head-and-neck RT.

351. **Upright Pelvis CBCT Workflow:** IGRT protocol designed for seated pelvis treatments.
**Related equipment:** Upright CBCT arm or rotating patient platform.
**Radiotherapy Example:** Used for prostate patients unable to lie flat.

352. **Unmodifiable Dose-Constraint Warning:** Safety rule preventing changes to OAR constraints beyond recommended tolerance.
**Related equipment:** TPS locked-constraint mode.
**Radiotherapy Example:** Stops accidental relaxation of spinal cord dose limit.

353. **Upgraded Beam Output Stabilizer:** Component maintaining dose reproducibility despite temperature or RF variations.
**Related equipment:** LINAC monitor chamber feedback loop.
**Radiotherapy Example:** Keeps ±1% daily dose consistency for all photon energies.

354. **Ultra-Short Fraction Delivery Mode:** Fast-delivery algorithm shortening beam-on time while preserving modulation.
**Related equipment:** HFA-VMAT mode, dual-layer MLC.
**Radiotherapy Example:** Cuts delivery time in lung SBRT from 12 to 6 minutes.

355. **Uniform Midline Dose Check:** Ensuring midline depth receives correct dose in 3D conformal planning.
**Related equipment:** Water-equivalent phantom with midline detector.
**Radiotherapy Example:** Used for whole brain irradiation.

356. **Under-Breast Tissue Air-Gap Fill:** Eliminating air pocket under breast that may cause underdose.
**Related equipment:** Customized bolus, pad support.
**Radiotherapy Example:** Prevents cold regions in obese breast patients.

357. **U-Shaped Couch Support Cradle:** Cradle that supports pelvis and lumbar region without shifting patient position.
**Related equipment:** Vacuum body mold.
**Radiotherapy Example:** Helps maintain posture in long pelvic IMRT sessions.

358. **Unmanned Daily QA Station:** Automated QA system requiring no manual technician input.
**Related equipment:** Autonomous dosimetry phantom, cloud QA software.
**Radiotherapy Example:** Performs LINAC output and symmetry checks at 6 AM automatically.

359. **Ultra-Fine Bolus Surface Scan:** High-resolution 3D scan to fabricate perfectly conformal bolus.
**Related equipment:** 3D optical scanner, 3D printer.
**Radiotherapy Example:** Used for nasal and auricular skin cancers.

360. **Upright Abdominal Compression Seat:** Sitting-based device compressing abdomen to reduce tumor motion.
**Related equipment:** Breath-monitor system + compression module.
**Radiotherapy Example:** Liver SBRT with 12-second breath-hold cycles.

361. **Ultra-Wide Field CBCT Protocol:** CBCT scan capturing thorax + abdomen simultaneously.
**Related equipment:** Wide-panel CBCT imager.
**Radiotherapy Example:** Used for TBI setup to view whole trunk.

362. **Unilateral Dose Hotspot Allowance:** Accepting higher dose in a limited zone to protect a sensitive bilateral organ.
**Related equipment:** Hotspot management tool in TPS.
**Radiotherapy Example:** Permitted hotspot in parotid region to protect brainstem.

363. **Up-Scaled Fraction Resolution:** Increasing fraction count to minimize biological toxicity.
**Related equipment:** Standard LINAC.
**Radiotherapy Example:** 30 fractions instead of 15 for elderly head-and-neck patient.

364. **Unfiltered MRI-Sim Protocol:** MRI simulation without noise-reduction filters to preserve spatial edges.
**Related equipment:** MRI-Sim + RT immobilization mask.
**Radiotherapy Example:** Important when identifying optic chiasm and optic nerve border.

365. **Ultra-High Dose Prediction Kernel:** Calculation engine optimized for large-dose per fraction accuracy.
**Related equipment:** SBRT TPS solver.
**Radiotherapy Example:** Required for >15 Gy fractions in spine SBRT.

366. **Upper-Neck Adaptive CBCT Algorithm:** Special adaptive workflow focusing on varying neck soft tissues.
**Related equipment:** Adaptive RTP platform.
**Radiotherapy Example:** Tracks tumor shrinkage and lymph node reduction over fractions.

**367. Under-Correction Safety Filter:** Blocking setup shifts that exceed safe movement threshold.
**Related equipment:** 6D couch lockout system.
**Radiotherapy Example:** Prevents patient asymmetry during pelvic couch rotation.

**368. Ultra-Precise Electron Cut-Out Mapping:** Digitized shape matching for electron treatment apertures.
**Related equipment:** Electron cut-out scanner + milling unit.
**Radiotherapy Example:** Used for scalp and parotid skin cancers.

**369. Upright Tumor Biopsy-to-RT Workflow:** Direct scheduling pipeline reducing time from biopsy to first treatment.
**Related equipment:** Radiology + RT OIS interoperability.
**Radiotherapy Example:** Reduces disease progression risk for rapidly growing tumors.

**370. Universal QA Priority Tagging:** Labeling system categorizing QA issues by urgency and effect on patient safety.
**Related equipment:** QA ticket management software.
**Radiotherapy Example:** Beam symmetry deviation classified as "high priority".

**371. Unrestricted Arc Gantry-Avoidance Set:** Gantry path programmed to avoid only specified forbidden zones.
**Related equipment:** VMAT sector optimizer.
**Radiotherapy Example:** Arc avoids tracheostomy tube region during neck RT.

**372. Ultra-Low Spatial Uncertainty Mask:** Mask constructed to limit head translation to under 1 mm.
**Related equipment:** Carbon-fiber reinforced RT mask.
**Radiotherapy Example:** Required for single-fraction brain SRS.

**373. Updated Stereotactic Dose Library:** Collection of SRS dose templates clinically validated for various targets.
**Related equipment:** TPS plan library tool.
**Radiotherapy Example:** New pineal region SRS dose model added from clinical trial.

**374. Under-Dose Visual Heatmap:** Color-coded map highlighting PTV cold spots.
**Related equipment:** TPS heatmap visualization.
**Radiotherapy Example:** Helps planners fix dose drop near surgical cavity wall.

**375. Ultra-Rapid Linac Beam Recovery:** Restarting beam delivery quickly after automatic safety interruption.
**Related equipment:** Smart beam-restart controller.
**Radiotherapy Example:** Minimizes treatment time when interruptions occur due to coughing or patient motion.

**376. Ultrafast Beam Imaging:** Real-time capture of radiation beam shape and field during delivery.
**Related equipment:** EPID, LINAC imaging panel.
**Radiotherapy Example:** Used to verify VMAT kidney plan MLC motion frame-by-frame during treatment.

**377. Upper Thoracic Spine Collimation:** Specialized beam shaping for spine treatment to avoid lung and ribs.
**Related equipment:** MLC, dynamic wedges.
**Radiotherapy Example:** Applied while irradiating T5–T8 spine metastasis to reduce lung dose.

378. **Unrestricted Radiology Transfer Protocol:** Imaging import method supporting all DICOM sources without conversion.
**Related equipment:** PACS, DICOM import module.
**Radiotherapy Example:** Allows CT/MRI from outside hospitals to load directly into TPS for planning.

379. **Ultralow Motion Tracking Mode:** Algorithm detecting extremely small internal shifts during treatment.
**Related equipment:** Surface tracking systems, respiratory motion monitoring.
**Radiotherapy Example:** Used in SBRT pancreas to stop the beam when abdominal motion exceeds limit.

380. **Uplift Skin Dose Control:** Dose enhancement technique for superficial areas to maintain coverage.
**Related equipment:** Bolus, beam angle modifiers.
**Radiotherapy Example:** Used in chest wall RT to ensure adequate dose to surgical scar.

381. **Uniform Bone Density Override:** Assigning fixed HU values to bone for more accurate dose calculation.
**Related equipment:** TPS HU override tool.
**Radiotherapy Example:** Required for hip prosthesis cases to prevent dose error.

382. **Uracil Radiosensitization Model:** Biological model predicting radiosensitizing effect of fluorouracil derivatives.
**Related equipment:** Radiobiology modeling module.
**Radiotherapy Example:** Used when building concurrent chemoradiation regimen for GI tumors.

383. **Uncut Immobilization Neck Support:** Neck rest used without trimming to improve long-term stability.
**Related equipment:** Thermoplastic masks, headrests.
**Radiotherapy Example:** Supports patients with tremors during head-and-neck RT.

384. **U409. Ultrasafe Electrical Isolation Module:** Prevents electrical feedback damage during high-power beam delivery.
**Related equipment:** LINAC electrical board.
**Radiotherapy Example:** Activated during high-MU FFF SBRT treatments.

385. **Upgraded Dose Kernel Library:** Updated dataset used for high-accuracy TPS dose calculation.
**Related equipment:** TPS planning system library.
**Radiotherapy Example:** Installed after LINAC acceptance for improved dose computation.

386. **Urinary Spacer Technique:** Insertion of hydrogel to push bladder/rectum away from prostate.
**Related equipment:** Hydrogel injector, ultrasound guidance.
**Radiotherapy Example:** Used in prostate VMAT to reduce rectal toxicity.

387. **Uterus Adaptive Workflow:** Daily plan adaptation to account for uterus mobility.
**Related equipment:** CBCT, MRI fusion, adaptive TPS.
**Radiotherapy Example:** Applied in cervical cancer RT when uterus shifts significantly.

388. **Unilateral Neck Immobilization Template:** Mask shaping template for one-side neck support.
**Related equipment:** Thermoplastic mask, mould room tools.
**Radiotherapy Example:** Used in parotid gland RT to avoid unnecessary immobilization of the opposite side.

389. **Ultrafine Skin Wire Marking:** Very thin wire used to mark surgical scars or lesions on CT scan.
**Related equipment:** Skin wire marker / lead wire.
**Radiotherapy Example:** Used in chest wall CT simulation to mark scar for boost field.

**390. U-Shaped Brain SRS Arc Path:** Arc path avoiding lenses and optic pathways while covering brain target.
**Related equipment:** VMAT SRS planning optimizer.
**Radiotherapy Example:** Used for pituitary adenoma to minimize optic nerve damage.

**391. Unstable Patient Position Alert:** Motion warning system when patient shifts beyond tolerance.
**Related equipment:** Surface guidance camera, LINAC interlock.
**Radiotherapy Example:** Halts beam delivery when patient moves during head-and-neck RT.

**392. Ultra-Compliant Vacuum Mattress:** Vacuum cushion forming anatomic support to limit movement.
**Related equipment:** Vac-loc cushions, immobilization pumps.
**Radiotherapy Example:** Common in liver SBRT with abdominal compression.

**393. Uncut Aperture Collimator Mode:** Manual MLC aperture mode without auto-optimization.
**Related equipment:** MLC panel control.
**Radiotherapy Example:** Used in emergency palliative spine radiotherapy when time is limited.

**394. Upper Airway Target Boost:** High dose boost to airway portion with recurrence risk.
**Related equipment:** Boost plan, VMAT arcs.
**Radiotherapy Example:** Used in laryngeal cancer treatment to improve local control.

**395. Under-Couch Dose Compensation Module:** Dose correction algorithm for attenuation caused by treatment couch.
**Related equipment:** TPS couch model, couch attenuation data.
**Radiotherapy Example:** Used for pelvic VMAT when beams pass through couch.

**396. Unilateral Pelvic Field Technique:** Radiation technique treating only one side of the pelvis while sparing the opposite side.
**Related equipment:** MLC shaping, asymmetric jaws, wedge compensators.
**Radiotherapy Example:** Used for unilateral pelvic lymph node RT in prostate cancer recurrence.

**397. Unsharp Mask Edge Detection:** Image enhancement method improving edge visibility on CT/MRI for contour precision.
**Related equipment:** TPS image preprocessing tool, radiology workstations.
**Radiotherapy Example:** Used to clearly visualize pancreas-tumor interface during planning.

**398. Upper Abdomen Compression Plate:** Compression device reducing diaphragmatic motion to limit organ movement.
**Related equipment:** Abdominal compression belt, overlay board.
**Radiotherapy Example:** Applied in liver SBRT to reduce breathing-induced tumor displacement.

**399. Ultrahigh Dose Verification Cycle:** QA loop for extremely high dose-per-fraction treatments.
**Related equipment:** EPID, phantom with ion chambers.
**Radiotherapy Example:** Required before delivering 24 Gy single-fraction SBRT.

**400. Urethral Dose Restriction Protocol:** Planning method to limit radiation dose to the urethra during prostate RT.
**Related equipment:** Catheter markers, urethra contouring tools.
**Radiotherapy Example:** Used in HDR brachytherapy plans to reduce risk of urinary toxicity.

**401. Unified CT-MRI Registration Workflow:** Combined registration pipeline to fuse CT and MRI seamlessly for delineation.
**Related equipment:** Image fusion module in TPS.
**Radiotherapy Example:** Used for brain tumor plans for MRI-based contouring and CT-based dose calculation.

402. **Urgent Radiotherapy Pathway:** Fast-track workflow for emergencies requiring immediate treatment.
**Related equipment:** Rapid planning algorithm, palliative RT templates.
**Radiotherapy Example:** Applied for spinal cord compression needing same-day RT.

403. **Upper Airway Shielding Protocol:** Shielding practice to spare upper airway tissues during head-and-neck RT.
**Related equipment:** Bolus, lead shield, customized cutouts.
**Radiotherapy Example:** Used in oropharyngeal RT to protect soft palate in specific cases.

404. **Ultrawide Field Dose Tracking:** Real-time dose calculation for treatment fields wider than standard LINAC width.
**Related equipment:** Extended EPID, wide-field film detector.
**Radiotherapy Example:** Used in craniospinal irradiation requiring large overlapping fields.

405. **Unilateral Breast Immobilization Pod:** Stabilized breast support designed for single-side breast irradiation.
**Related equipment:** Breast board, arm support, tilt system.
**Radiotherapy Example:** Used in left-sided breast RT while maintaining reproducible posture.

406. **Underwire Artifact Correction:** Algorithm for removing CT artifacts caused by bra underwire or metal implants.
**Related equipment:** Metal artifact reduction (MAR) software.
**Radiotherapy Example:** Applied before planning when patients forget to remove bras for CT simulation.

407. **Upward Field Junction Optimization:** Optimization technique for upper field junction in multi-isocenter irradiation.
**Related equipment:** Feathering algorithm, independent jaw control.
**Radiotherapy Example:** Used in craniospinal RT to avoid hotspot at cervical–thoracic junction.

408. **Ultrasound-Guided Organ Position Mapping:** Real-time tracking of organ location using ultrasound during treatment.
**Related equipment:** US probe, surface tracking workstation.
**Radiotherapy Example:** Used in prostate RT to verify bladder filling before each fraction.

409. **Uniform Lung Heterogeneity Model:** Dose correction model accounting for lung tissue density variations.
**Related equipment:** Monte-Carlo dose calculation module.
**Radiotherapy Example:** Applied in lung VMAT to improve predicted vs. delivered dose agreement.

410. **Ultrafast Adaptive Override:** Instant HU override mode during adaptive radiotherapy when organ filling changes.
**Related equipment:** Adaptive TPS, CBCT deformable registration.
**Radiotherapy Example:** Used when bladder volume increases significantly between fractions.

411. **Utility Power Backup Interlock:** Safety feature preventing beam delivery during unstable electrical supply.
**Related equipment:** LINAC UPS, beam hold circuit.
**Radiotherapy Example:** Interrupts treatment automatically during voltage dip to protect patient safety.

412. **Unilateral Boost Field IMRT:** Technique applying additional dose only to a selected side of symmetric region.
**Related equipment:** IMRT optimizer, cone-down boost geometry.
**Radiotherapy Example:** Used to boost only one cervical lymph node chain.

**413. Ultracontour Target Refinement:** Extra-fine contour correction using edge recognition and atlas overlays.
**Related equipment:** AI segmentation module.
**Radiotherapy Example:** Helps refine optic chiasm contours during glioma RT planning.

**414. Upright Radiotherapy Simulation:** CT simulation conducted in sitting/upright posture using special scanner.
**Related equipment:** Upright CT chair, immobilization frame.
**Radiotherapy Example:** Used when patients cannot lie flat due to respiratory distress.

**415. Ultra-Shield Neutron Filter:** Accessory minimizing secondary neutron dose from high-energy photon beams.
**Related equipment:** Neutron absorbing plates (borated plastic).
**Radiotherapy Example:** Installed during 18 MV treatment for pelvic RT to reduce neutron scatter.

**416. Unilateral Orbital Dose Constraint:** Limiting dose to unaffected eye during orbital radiation for tumors.
**Related equipment:** VMAT optimizer, bolus shield.
**Radiotherapy Example:** Used in lacrimal gland RT to keep contralateral optic nerve sparing.

**417. U-Arm Isocentric Control:** Robotic arm system maintaining isocenter precision while rotating imaging plane.
**Related equipment:** Orthopedic U-arm radiography frame.
**Radiotherapy Example:** Assists orthogonal X-ray imaging for pelvis IGRT.

**418. Urgent CT Simulation Slot:** Reserved scheduling block for emergency radiotherapy patients.
**Related equipment:** CT simulator priority scheduler.
**Radiotherapy Example:** Used for patients requiring same-day planning because of airway compromise.

**419. Ultra-Close Target-OAR Gradient:** Treatment plan requiring steep dose gradient near critical organ.
**Related equipment:** SRS optimizer, micro-MLC.
**Radiotherapy Example:** Applied for trigeminal neuralgia RT to protect brainstem.

**420. Uniform Phased IMRT Ring:** Ring-shaped control structure distributing intermediate dose around PTV.
**Related equipment:** Structure set with ring ROI.
**Radiotherapy Example:** Used in prostate IMRT to reduce hot spots.

**421. Ultraspeed Patient Turnaround Mode:** Rapid workflow for high-volume treatment centers.
**Related equipment:** Automatic couch indexing, auto-setup imaging.
**Radiotherapy Example:** Practiced in busy head-and-neck clinics to shorten daily schedule.

**422. Upright Immobilization Head Mask:** Thermoplastic mask designed for vertical seated position.
**Related equipment:** Upright treatment chair.
**Radiotherapy Example:** Used for patients with respiratory dysfunction unable to lie flat.

**423. Unthreaded Catheter Fixation:** Catheter securing technique for HDR brachytherapy without tissue threading.
**Related equipment:** Catheter fixation buttons, adhesive disc.
**Radiotherapy Example:** Used in breast IORT catheter placements.

424. **Ultra-Fine Detector Spacing Array:** QA array with high detector density for precise fluence measurement.
**Related equipment:** SRS MapCHECK, high-resolution ion chamber array.
**Radiotherapy Example:** Used for stereotactic brain QA before 4 mm small-target VMAT delivery.

425. **Upgraded LINAC Beam Model Validation:** Validation of new beam model after service/upgrade to ensure dosimetric accuracy.
**Related equipment:** Water phantom, ion chambers, TPS model update.
**Radiotherapy Example:** Performed after replacement of LINAC flattening filter or MLC calibration.

426. **Ultra-Precision MLC Leaf Gap Calibration:** Highly sensitive verification of MLC leaf gap to prevent dose errors in small targets.
**Related equipment:** High-resolution EPID, SRS MapCHECK.
**Radiotherapy Example:** Essential before delivering single-isocenter multiple brain metastasis SRS.

427. **Unilateral Lung Shielding Technique:** Shielding one lung to reduce pulmonary toxicity during chest irradiation.
**Related equipment:** Custom blocks, MLC shielding.
**Radiotherapy Example:** Used when treating mediastinal lymphoma while sparing one lung.

428. **Ultrafast CT Motion Freezing:** CT mode capturing images in <0.25 seconds to eliminate breathing motion.
**Related equipment:** Ultrafast 4D CT scanner.
**Radiotherapy Example:** Improves pancreatic SBRT planning by eliminating motion artifacts.

429. **Uniform Neck Bolus Application:** Even application of bolus material across curvature of neck to enhance surface dose.
**Related equipment:** Gel bolus, sculpted bolus mask.
**Radiotherapy Example:** Used in head-and-neck RT to increase dose to skin-involved nodes.

430. **Underdose Recovery Strategy:** Workflow for compensating missed dose in previous fractions while protecting OARs.
**Related equipment:** Adaptive TPS, dose accumulation software.
**Radiotherapy Example:** Used when a patient misses a SBRT fraction and requires safe replanning.

431. **Upright Thoracic Simulation System:** CT scanning installation that enables patients to be simulated sitting upright.
**Related equipment:** Vertical CT couch, vacuum back support.
**Radiotherapy Example:** Used for lung cancer patients with severe dyspnea unable to lie down.

432. **Ultralow MRI Dose Marker Protocol:** MRI-visible markers inserted without radiation exposure for localization.
**Related equipment:** Plastic fiducial MRI marker, non-metallic implants.
**Radiotherapy Example:** Used for prostate MR-guided radiotherapy instead of gold fiducials.

433. **Unventilated Lung Mapping:** Mapping areas of lung not participating in ventilation to prevent dose concentration.
**Related equipment:** VQ scan fusion, PET/CT, MRI ventilation mapping.
**Radiotherapy Example:** Applied in lung RT to spare ventilated regions and prevent pneumonitis.

434. **Universal Beam Energy Cross-Check:** Standardized benchmarking of beam energies across multiple LINACs.
**Related equipment:** Reference ion chamber, water phantom.
**Radiotherapy Example:** Required when multiple LINACs are used interchangeably for same patient.

435. **Upper Spine Field Split Optimization:** Optimization of field split line for craniospinal irradiation to avoid hot/cold spots.
**Related equipment:** Automated feathering algorithm, junction optimizer.
**Radiotherapy Example:** Used during pediatric CNS RT to adjust cervical junction each week.

436. **Ultrafine Optic Nerve Contouring Protocol:** Maximizing contour resolution around optic nerve to prevent radiation-induced neuropathy.
**Related equipment:** High-resolution MRI fusion.
**Radiotherapy Example:** Used for base-of-skull and orbital tumor planning.

437. **Urethrogram-Guided Prostate Localization:** Bladder-filled urethrogram technique to visualize urethra during simulation.
**Related equipment:** Contrast catheter, fluoroscopy-CT hybrid imaging.
**Radiotherapy Example:** Helps reduce urethral toxicity during HDR brachytherapy.

438. **Uncertainty-Weighted Dose Mapping:** Assigns dose weighting based on motion and deformation uncertainties.
**Related equipment:** 4D dose accumulation tools.
**Radiotherapy Example:** Used in liver VMAT where breathing introduces variable motion.

439. **Upright Immobilization Thermoplastic Casting:** Custom immobilization mask fabricated in sitting posture for repeatable setup.
**Related equipment:** Thermoplastic sheet, overhead frame.
**Radiotherapy Example:** Used when airway obstruction prevents supine head-and-neck setup.

440. **Unprescribed Residual Dose Registry:** Documentation system for unintended low-dose radiation to outside-target structures.
**Related equipment:** Dose-volume histogram reporting tools.
**Radiotherapy Example:** Required by quality committees for pediatric body irradiation.

441. **Upstream Beam Monitor QA:** QA validating pre-target beam sensor measuring photon fluence before exiting head.
**Related equipment:** Monitor chamber, redundant ion chamber.
**Radiotherapy Example:** Checks LINAC monitor chamber accuracy before patient beam delivery.

442. **Ultrawide Couch-Kick Collision Check:** Ensures couch kicks used in non-coplanar plans do not collide with gantry or patient.
**Related equipment:** Virtual collision simulation in TPS.
**Radiotherapy Example:** Used in trigeminal neuralgia radiosurgery to avoid crashing at 322°.

443. **Upper Airway Dose Preservation Rule:** Planning rule ensuring safe tolerance doses for larynx, pharynx, and epiglottis.
**Related equipment:** OAR dose priority templates.
**Radiotherapy Example:** Prevents xerostomia and dysphagia in oropharyngeal cancer RT.

444. **Undistorted Pelvic MRI Transfer:** MRI acquisition without geometric distortion for direct CT fusion.
**Related equipment:** Pelvic MRI distortion correction software.
**Radiotherapy Example:** Required for brachytherapy planning in cervical cancer.

445. **Ultraclear CT Metal Artifact Reduction Mode:** CT scanning mode designed to eliminate streaking caused by implants.
**Related equipment:** MAR algorithm, iterative reconstruction.
**Radiotherapy Example:** Helps contour spinal canal in patients with metal rods.

446. **Universal Immobilization Index:** Measuring index on immobilization boards to replicate exact patient position daily.
**Related equipment:** Mask indexing holes, couch latch system.
**Radiotherapy Example:** Ensures breast board position is identical each fraction.

447. **Under-Dose Hotspot Alert:** TPS warning when under-dose appears within high-dose target volume.
**Related equipment:** Dose violation reporting tool.
**Radiotherapy Example:** Automatically signals planner to correct cold spot in VMAT prostate RT.

448. **Upright Deep Inspiration Breath-Hold Platform:** DIBH system for upright radiation posture with real-time lung volume tracking.
**Related equipment:** Surface guidance camera system.
**Radiotherapy Example:** Lowers heart dose in left-breast cancer when patient cannot lie down.

449. **Ultra-High DRR Reconstruction:** High-resolution reconstruction of digitally reconstructed radiographs for IGRT.
**Related equipment:** TPS DRR module, MV/KV imaging.
**Radiotherapy Example:** Helps match ribs and spine precisely before lung RT.

450. **U-Shaped Mandible Shield:** Shield contoured to protect mandible during oral cavity RT.
**Related equipment:** Custom mould room fabricated shield.
**Radiotherapy Example:** Prevents osteoradionecrosis risk during tongue cancer RT.

451. **Unilateral Kidney Dose Stop Protocol:** Special restriction to limit dose to one kidney during abdominal irradiation.
**Related equipment:** Dose-limiting structure with high priority.
**Radiotherapy Example:** Used for para-aortic nodal RT sparing the right kidney.

452. **Urgency-Adjusted Radiotherapy Scheduling:** Scheduling algorithm based on clinical urgency priority.
**Related equipment:** Oncology treatment queue digital scheduler.
**Radiotherapy Example:** Metastatic spinal compression treated before routine pelvic RT.

453. **Uniform Adaptive Plan Switching:** Switching between pre-computed plans depending on bladder/filling conditions.
**Related equipment:** Plan library adaptive radiotherapy system.
**Radiotherapy Example:** Used in bladder cancer to deliver plan based on daily bladder volume.

454. **Upper Extremity Immobilization Module:** Shoulder/arm positioning system for thoracic and breast RT.
**Related equipment:** Arm shuttle, T-bar immobilizer.
**Radiotherapy Example:** Used in lung SBRT to clear arms from beam path.

455. **Ultrasensitive TLD Patch Monitoring:** Very sensitive skin-placed TLD for patient in-vivo dosimetry.
**Related equipment:** Lithium fluoride TLD badge.
**Radiotherapy Example:** Measures exit dose during pediatric AP/PA abdominal fields.

456. **Upgraded MLC Speed Verification:** QA ensuring upgraded MLC leaves move at correct speed during dynamic delivery.
**Related equipment:** Log file analysis, high-speed camera.
**Radiotherapy Example:** Ensures lung SABR VMAT does not lose modulation quality.

457. **Upper Abdomen Motion Surrogate:** External surrogate indicating internal organ motion trend.
**Related equipment:** Respiratory belt, marker block.
**Radiotherapy Example:** Used during liver SBRT gating to pause beam at stable breathing phase.

**458. Ultrathin Surface Bolus Film:** Very thin bolus sheet increasing superficial dose without contour distortion.
**Related equipment:** 1–2 mm hydrogel bolus film.
**Radiotherapy Example:** Used for scalp irradiation without altering isocenter.

**459. Underwater LINAC Leak Check:** Leak inspection for electron applicators using water pool test.
**Related equipment:** Water tank, diode detector.
**Radiotherapy Example:** Detects electron applicator leakage before clinical use.

**460. Ultralow Scatter Beam Profile:** Beam profile clinically optimized to reduce lateral scatter dose.
**Related equipment:** Flattening-filter-free mode.
**Radiotherapy Example:** Improves dose fall-off in lung and liver SBRT.

**461. Universal Patient Safety Timeout:** Mandatory pause to verify patient identity and treatment plan before irradiation.
**Related equipment:** Digital verification checklist.
**Radiotherapy Example:** Prevents wrong-site RT events across all treatment rooms.

**462. Upright CT Isocenter Marking:** Marking system ensuring reproducible isocenter location in upright scans.
**Related equipment:** Vertical laser projection system.
**Radiotherapy Example:** Used for upright palliative thorax RT.

**463. Ultrasound-Only Prostate IGRT:** Image-guided prostate RT using ultrasound instead of X-ray for localization.
**Related equipment:** Clarity™ or similar US IGRT platform.
**Radiotherapy Example:** Avoids X-ray dose in routine prostate tracking.

**464. Uterine Motion Gating:** Beam gating based on uterine motion pattern during gynecologic RT.
**Related equipment:** US or MRI motion tracking.
**Radiotherapy Example:** Used in uterine sarcoma RT to account for respiratory and bladder motion.

**465. Ultra-Dense 3D Printing Shell:** High-density printed shielding shell to reduce unplanned dose.
**Related equipment:** 3D mould room printer.
**Radiotherapy Example:** Printed for protecting ears during parotid RT.

**466. Under-Beam Couch Attenuation Modeling:** TPS algorithm that includes dose effects of couch during beam delivery.
**Related equipment:** Couch model import module.
**Radiotherapy Example:** Improves accuracy of posterior fields in lung VMAT.

**467. Universal Couch Index Lock:** A universal locking index to eliminate patient setup variation.
**Related equipment:** Indexed immobilization board.
**Radiotherapy Example:** Ensures exact pelvis setup throughout IMRT course.

**468. Upper Trachea Sparing Technique:** Beam shaping to avoid high doses to upper trachea during neck RT.
**Related equipment:** VMAT control points, high priority OAR.
**Radiotherapy Example:** Prevents long-term airway fibrosis in laryngeal cancer RT.

**469. Upright Orthogonal X-Ray Workflow:** Imaging workflow to acquire orthogonal kV images while patient is sitting.
**Related equipment:** U-arm imaging paired with upright CT.
**Radiotherapy Example:** Used for upright lung stereotactic treatments.

**470. Unscheduled Fraction Deviation Protocol:** Safety workflow triggered when treatment fraction deviates from prescription.
**Related equipment:** MOSAIQ / ARIA quality alert system.
**Radiotherapy Example:** Flags if a fraction is accidentally given twice or skipped.

**471. Ultra-Rapid Physics Chart Review:** Fast-tracked physics review for emergency treatment starts.
**Related equipment:** Automated QA checklist system.
**Radiotherapy Example:** Required when initiating overnight RT for bleeding tumors.

**472. Upper Abdomen Organ Deformation Model:** Predicts daily stomach, liver, and bowel shape changes for adaptive RT.
**Related equipment:** Deformable image registration (DIR).
**Radiotherapy Example:** Used for pancreas RT replanning triggered by organ shifts.

**473. Uncertainty-Balanced Beam Modulation:** Beam modulation accounting for daily motion variation to reduce risk of misses.
**Related equipment:** Probabilistic TPS optimizer.
**Radiotherapy Example:** Reduces PTV margin in lung SBRT without compromising coverage.

**474. Universal Post-Treatment Survey System:** Standardized patient-reported outcome tracking after radiotherapy.
**Related equipment:** Digital toxicity monitoring platform.
**Radiotherapy Example:** Documents late toxicity patterns in breast and prostate RT.

**475. Unconditionally Safe Shutdown Mode:** Emergency LINAC shutdown ensuring beam termination even during software failure.
**Related equipment:** Hardwired emergency stop switch, beam fail-safe circuit.
**Radiotherapy Example:** Activates instantly when couch collision is detected mid-treatment.

**476. Uncertainty propagation (noun):** Process of tracking how individual uncertainties affect final dose calculations.
**Related Terms:** Error analysis, Robust planning.
**Example in Radiotherapy:** Used to evaluate cumulative setup and range errors.

**477. Under-response correction (noun):** Adjustment applied when detectors report lower than true dose.
**Related Terms:** Detector calibration, Dosimetric correction.
**Example in Radiotherapy:** Applied during small-field dosimetry.

**478. Uniform dose coverage (noun):** Even distribution of prescribed dose throughout the target.
**Related Terms:** Homogeneity index, PTV coverage.
**Example in Radiotherapy:** Required for conventional fractionation plans.

**479. Ultrasound-based localization (noun):** Use of ultrasound to identify internal anatomy before treatment.
**Related Terms:** IGRT, Soft-tissue guidance.
**Example in Radiotherapy:** Prostate position verified prior to beam delivery.

**480. Uplink data transfer (noun):** Transmission of treatment or monitoring data to control systems.
**Related Terms:** System interface, Real-time monitoring.
**Example in Radiotherapy:** Couch position data sent to LINAC controller.

**481. Upper airway sparing (noun):** Technique to reduce dose to trachea and laryngeal structures.
**Related Terms:** OAR protection, Dose constraints.
**Example in Radiotherapy:** Applied in head-and-neck IMRT.

482. **Upper abdominal motion control (noun):** Methods used to limit respiratory motion in abdominal targets.
**Related Terms:** Gating, Compression.
**Example in Radiotherapy:** Used during liver SBRT.

483. **Ultrafine dose grid (noun):** High-resolution spatial grid for dose calculation.
**Related Terms:** Dose resolution, TPS accuracy.
**Example in Radiotherapy:** Used for stereotactic planning.

484. **Unilateral target coverage (noun):** Dose coverage applied to one side of an anatomical structure.
**Related Terms:** Asymmetric planning, Beam arrangement.
**Example in Radiotherapy:** Used for unilateral tonsillar cancer.

485. **Urethra-sparing optimization (noun):** Planning strategy to minimize dose to the urethra.
**Related Terms:** OAR constraints, IMRT optimization.
**Example in Radiotherapy:** Common in prostate SBRT.

486. **Ultrashort delivery time (noun):** Very brief beam-on time for a treatment fraction.
**Related Terms:** High dose rate, Efficiency.
**Example in Radiotherapy:** Achieved using VMAT or FFF beams.

487. **Upper thoracic stabilization (noun):**
Immobilization technique limiting motion of upper chest.
**Related Terms:** Immobilization device, Reproducibility.
**Example in Radiotherapy:** Used in lung and breast treatments.

488. **Unintended exposure assessment (noun):** Evaluation of dose delivered outside the intended volume.
**Related Terms:** Incident analysis, QA review.
**Example in Radiotherapy:** Performed after imaging or setup deviations.

489. **Ultrasound signal alignment (noun):** Matching ultrasound reference images to planning anatomy.
**Related Terms:** Image registration, IGRT.
**Example in Radiotherapy:** Used in prostate localization systems.

490. **Upper extremity positioning (noun):** Placement of arms to avoid beam interference.
**Related Terms:** Patient setup, Immobilization.
**Example in Radiotherapy:** Arms raised during thoracic treatments.

491. **Uniform beam output (noun):** Consistent radiation intensity across the treatment field.
**Related Terms:** Flatness, Beam symmetry.
**Example in Radiotherapy:** Verified during machine QA.

492. **Under-dosage risk (noun):** Likelihood of delivering less than prescribed dose.
**Related Terms:** Cold spot, Target miss.
**Example in Radiotherapy:** Considered when margins are reduced.

493. **Ultrasound-assisted verification (noun):** Confirmation of anatomy using ultrasound before treatment.
**Related Terms:** Image guidance, Setup verification.
**Example in Radiotherapy:** Bladder filling checked before pelvic RT.

494. **Upper-body motion monitoring (noun):** Tracking patient movement in thoracic and neck regions.
**Related Terms:** Motion management, Surface imaging.
**Example in Radiotherapy:** Used during stereotactic treatments.

495. **Unbiased dose comparison (noun):** Dose evaluation free from systematic measurement bias.
**Related Terms:** Independent verification, QA.
**Example in Radiotherapy:** Comparing TPS dose with phantom measurements.

496. **Utility-based plan ranking (noun):** Plan comparison method based on clinical priorities.
**Related Terms:** Decision metrics, Optimization.
**Example in Radiotherapy:** Used to select best IMRT plan.

497. **Ultralow imaging dose (noun):** Minimal radiation dose used for verification imaging.
**Related Terms:** Imaging optimization, Patient safety.
**Example in Radiotherapy:** Applied in pediatric IGRT.

498. **Upper abdomen organ protection (noun):** Strategies to limit dose to stomach, liver, or kidneys.
**Related Terms:** OAR sparing, Planning constraints.
**Example in Radiotherapy:** Critical in pancreatic SBRT.

499. **Unplanned interruption handling (noun):** Procedure for managing unexpected beam stops.
**Related Terms:** Safety protocol, Treatment continuity.
**Example in Radiotherapy:** Fraction resumed after interruption review.

500. **Ultrasound-guided motion tracking (noun):** Real-time monitoring of internal organ movement using ultrasound.
**Related Terms:** Motion tracking, Adaptive RT.
**Example in Radiotherapy:** Used for prostate motion monitoring.

# V

1. **VMAT (Volumetric Modulated Arc Therapy):** Rotational radiotherapy technique that delivers modulated dose while the gantry rotates continuously around the patient.
   **Related equipment:** LINAC, MLC, EPID, TPS.
   **Radiotherapy Example:** Used for prostate cancer to reduce bladder and rectum dose compared to 3D-CRT.
2. **Vacuum Immobilization Bag:** A mouldable bag that becomes rigid after air is removed to create a custom patient support.
   **Related equipment:** Vacuum pump, mould room immobilization tools.
   **Radiotherapy Example:** Used to immobilize whole body during pediatric craniospinal irradiation.
3. **Verification Film:** Radiographic film used to verify field shape, position, and MLC accuracy during QA.
   **Related equipment:** Film cassette, densitometer.
   **Radiotherapy Example:** Used to validate electron cutout patterns before first treatment.
4. **Verification Simulation:** A repeat CT scan or imaging session used to confirm correct setup before treatment begins.
   **Related equipment:** CT simulator, lasers, immobilization devices.
   **Radiotherapy Example:** Required for adaptive replanning in head-and-neck patients after weight loss.
5. **Virtual Simulation:** Planning technique using CT images to simulate treatment geometrically without physical fluoroscopy.
   **Related equipment:** CT simulator, TPS.
   **Radiotherapy Example:** Used to mark isocenter and field borders digitally for breast RT.
6. **Voxel:** 3D volumetric pixel representing a small cube of imaging data in CT or MRI.
   **Related equipment:** CT/MRI scanner, TPS.
   **Radiotherapy Example:** Dose is calculated per voxel for DVH generation.
7. **Virtual Isocenter:** Secondary reference point used to position patients when true isocenter is not within the body.
   **Related equipment:** LINAC lasers, coordinate shift tool.
   **Radiotherapy Example:** Used when treating total skin electron therapy.
8. **Vertebral Body Sparing:** Technique used to reduce dose to vertebrae to prevent growth impairment in children.
   **Related equipment:** VMAT / IMRT optimization, immobilization board.
   **Radiotherapy Example:** Applied in pediatric abdominal RT.
9. **Varian LINAC:** Brand of medical linear accelerator widely used in radiotherapy delivery.
   **Related equipment:** MLC, kV/MV imaging, CBCT.
   **Radiotherapy Example:** Performs IMRT, VMAT, SRS, and SBRT for multiple cancer types.
10. **Vertical Couch Shift:** Vertical movement of treatment couch used for patient alignment prior to beam-on.
    **Related equipment:** 6D robotic couch.
    **Radiotherapy Example:** Corrects supine setup error during spinal SBRT.

11. **Ventilation Image Fusion:** Fusion of ventilation scan with CT/dose plan to spare functional lung regions.
    **Related equipment:** 4D-CT, SPECT, PET, MRI ventilation.
    **Radiotherapy Example:** Used in NSCLC RT to prevent radiation pneumonitis.
12. **Verification Checklist:** Patient-specific safety confirmation review performed before first treatment.
    **Related equipment:** ARIA / MOSAIQ workflow software.
    **Radiotherapy Example:** Ensures imaging plan matches dose plan configuration.
13. **Van Herk Margin Formula:** Formula used to calculate CTV-PTV margin based on systematic and random setup errors.
    **Related equipment:** IGRT log data, couch shift statistics.
    **Radiotherapy Example:** Margin determination for prostate planning.
14. **Volumetric Segmentation:** 3D contouring of organs and targets on CT/MRI datasets.
    **Related equipment:** TPS contouring tools, auto-segmentation AI.
    **Radiotherapy Example:** Used to define GTV and OARs in brain tumor planning.
15. **Visual Field Matching:** Visual comparison of field junctions during multi-field planning.
    **Related equipment:** Beam's-eye-view tool in TPS.
    **Radiotherapy Example:** Important in craniospinal irradiation to prevent hot/cold spots.
16. **Vascular Dose Limiting:** Planning rule to minimize radiation dose to major blood vessels.
    **Related equipment:** CTA fusion, OAR auto-priority.
    **Radiotherapy Example:** Used in pancreas and liver SBRT to prevent vessel stenosis.
17. **Voluntary Breath-Hold:** Patient voluntarily holds breath to move selected organs away from target.
    **Related equipment:** SGRT system, DIBH camera gating.
    **Radiotherapy Example:** Used in left-breast radiotherapy to reduce heart dose.
18. **Vertebral Body Matching:** Matching of bony landmarks instead of tumors for IGRT alignment.
    **Related equipment:** CBCT / kV-kV imaging.
    **Radiotherapy Example:** Used when treating spinal metastasis where soft tissue visibility is limited.
19. **Variable Dose Rate Arc:** Modulated arc delivery with changing dose rate per gantry angle for better dose shaping.
    **Related equipment:** LINAC dynamic dose control.
    **Radiotherapy Example:** Used in VMAT for pelvic and brain plans.
20. **V20 Lung Parameter:** Percentage of lung receiving ≥20 Gy; key predictor of pneumonitis risk.
    **Related equipment:** DVH analysis.
    **Radiotherapy Example:** Limited to ≤30% in lung cancer RT.
21. **Vaginal Cylinder:** Applicator used to deliver HDR brachytherapy to the vaginal cuff.
    **Related equipment:** Ir-192 HDR afterloader, CT-based applicator scan.
    **Radiotherapy Example:** Used after hysterectomy for endometrial cancer.
22. **Vertebral Localization Box:** Radiopaque marker tool helping to identify vertebra numbering on CT.
    **Related equipment:** CT simulator, localization strip.
    **Radiotherapy Example:** Ensures correct level during spinal radiotherapy.
23. **Visual Toxicity Scale:** Patient-reported scale to document treatment-related visual impairment.
    **Related equipment:** EMR toxicity form.
    **Radiotherapy Example:** Used during optic pathway glioma irradiation.
24. **Virtual Bolus:** Planning bolus artificially added in TPS to shape dose without real bolus placement.
    **Related equipment:** TPS virtual bolus tool.
    **Radiotherapy Example:** Used in chest wall RT to create smooth surface dose fall-off.

25. **Volumetric Marker Seeds:** Fiducial markers implanted to improve tumor localization during image guidance.
**Related equipment:** Gold markers, ultrasound, CBCT.
**Radiotherapy Example:** Implanted in prostate to track motion during treatment.

26. **Voluntary Motion Suppression:** Reduction of body movement using conscious patient control during radiotherapy.
**Related equipment:** SGRT cameras, breath-hold monitors, immobilization boards.
**Radiotherapy Example:** Patient asked to stay still without sedation during whole-brain radiation to avoid setup error.

27. **Ventral Dose Avoidance:** Dose optimization strategy to reduce dose to anterior organs while treating posterior tumors.
**Related equipment:** IMRT/VMAT optimizer, OAR shaping constraints.
**Radiotherapy Example:** Used in rectal cancer radiotherapy to protect the bladder and small bowel.

28. **Volumetric Reconstruction:** Creation of 3D internal anatomy model from multiple CT slices for planning.
**Related equipment:** CT simulation software, TPS fusion tools.
**Radiotherapy Example:** Enables accurate 3D tumor delineation for liver SBRT.

29. **Varian Portal Vision:** Electronic portal imaging device mounted on Varian LINACs to verify treatment fields.
**Related equipment:** EPID, LINAC imaging arm.
**Radiotherapy Example:** Used for daily field verification in pelvic IMRT.

30. **Virtual Reality Patient Education:** Use of VR to help patients understand radiotherapy workflow and reduce anxiety.
**Related equipment:** VR headset, treatment room 3D simulation software.
**Radiotherapy Example:** Pediatric patients shown VR demonstration of LINAC before first treatment.

31. **Voxel-Based Dose Accumulation:** Summation of dose delivered across fractions accounting for anatomical changes.
**Related equipment:** Deformable registration software, 4D CT.
**Radiotherapy Example:** Used in adaptive radiotherapy to evaluate delivered vs planned dose to parotid glands.

32. **Vacuum Cushion Calibration:** Verification that vacuum bags maintain rigidity and shape across treatment course.
**Related equipment:** Vacuum mould room devices, seal integrity tester.
**Radiotherapy Example:** Ensures reproducible posture in pediatric craniospinal irradiation.

33. **Volumetric Density Correction:** TPS correction of dose calculation according to tissue density variations.
**Related equipment:** CT calibration phantom, Monte Carlo algorithm.
**Radiotherapy Example:** Improves lung SBRT accuracy by adjusting for air-lung density differences.

34. **Vertebral Beam Junction QA:** QA ensuring seamless overlap of beams covering long spine segments.
**Related equipment:** Film phantom, 2D array dosimeter.
**Radiotherapy Example:** Used in craniospinal irradiation to prevent hot/cold spots at junctions.

35. **Video-Based Patient Monitoring:** Real-time visual monitoring of patient during treatment for safety and motion control.
    **Related equipment:** Closed-circuit camera, intercom.
    **Radiotherapy Example:** Therapist watches patient during total-body irradiation to ensure compliance with hand/arm positions.
36. **Ventilation-Weighted Dose Planning:** Incorporating lung ventilation maps into dose optimization to spare functional regions.
    **Related equipment:** 4D CT, PET-ventilation, SPECT-ventilation.
    **Radiotherapy Example:** Used in NSCLC radiotherapy to minimize pneumonitis risk.
37. **Virtual Isodose Display:** Graphic TPS display of isodose lines across anatomical slices for plan review.
    **Related equipment:** TPS plan viewer, DVH tools.
    **Radiotherapy Example:** Used to review heart dose distribution during left-breast therapy.
38. **Volume Expansion Margin:** Extra margin added to target volume to account for geometric uncertainty.
    **Related equipment:** IGRT statistics, TPS margin tool.
    **Radiotherapy Example:** CTV to PTV margin set according to prostate motion data.
39. **Virtual Laser System:** Software simulation used to align reference lines when physical lasers are unavailable.
    **Related equipment:** CT simulator software.
    **Radiotherapy Example:** Used during offline CT contouring when patient was positioned without lasers.
40. **Volumetric Hotspot Control:** Technique to reduce high-dose zones within PTV using optimization constraints.
    **Related equipment:** IMRT optimizer, dose-shaping tool.
    **Radiotherapy Example:** Prevents hotspots in head-and-neck plans around salivary glands.
41. **Vertebral Body Contouring Protocol:** Standard guideline for drawing vertebra contours for planning and IGRT matching.
    **Related equipment:** TPS manual contouring tools, auto-segmentation models.
    **Radiotherapy Example:** Used for spinal metastasis SBRT fusion-matching.
42. **Volumetric Position Correction:** Patient shift adjustment based on 3D anatomy comparison rather than single-point alignment.
    **Related equipment:** CBCT fusion system, 6D robotic couch.
    **Radiotherapy Example:** Applied in pancreas SBRT where soft tissue matching is required.
43. **Vacuum Table Positioning:** Securing and labeling vacuum immobilization systems to ensure reproducible couch alignment.
    **Related equipment:** Mould room immobilization table, body markers.
    **Radiotherapy Example:** Ensures same pelvis rotation for all fractions of cervical cancer radiotherapy.
44. **Visual Target Verification:** Therapist-performed visual cross-checking of digital field and patient setup before beam-on.
    **Related equipment:** On-board imaging, ARIA/MOSAIQ verification list.
    **Radiotherapy Example:** Used prior to every brain SRS treatment to prevent mismatch.
45. **Vascular Dose Reconstruction:** Dose estimation specifically to blood vessels to predict radiation-induced stenosis risk.
    **Related equipment:** CTA MRI fusion, TPS contouring.
    **Radiotherapy Example:** Applied in pancreatic and liver SBRT near major arteries.

46. **Volume-Preserving Optimization:** Algorithm designed to protect functional anatomy while maintaining target coverage.
    **Related equipment:** Biological optimization engine, organ viability maps.
    **Radiotherapy Example:** Used to protect hippocampus during whole-brain radiotherapy.

47. **Varian PerfectPitch Couch:** Six-degrees-of-freedom robotic treatment couch used for precise positioning.
    **Related equipment:** LINAC IGRT system, couch motion controller.
    **Radiotherapy Example:** Used to correct rotational errors during spine SBRT.

48. **Video-Assisted Mould Fabrication:** Use of video reference recording to ensure reproducible immobilization creation.
    **Related equipment:** Mould room cameras, thermoplastic masks, vacuum cushions.
    **Radiotherapy Example:** Ensures repeated mask fabrication consistency in pediatrics.

49. **Volumetric Biological Dose Model:** Dose prediction model including tissue repair and sensitivity variations across volume.
    **Related equipment:** Biologically-based TPS calculator.
    **Radiotherapy Example:** Helps select doses for re-irradiation of recurrent head-and-neck cancer.

50. **Verification Dose Recording:** Documentation of delivered dose compared with planned dose across treatment course.
    **Related equipment:** R&V system, EPID dosimetry, MOSAIQ, ARIA.
    **Radiotherapy Example:** Required for adaptive planning decision-making in lung cancer IMRT.

51. **Voxel-Level Dose Painting:** Selectively delivering non-uniform dose intensities within the tumor based on biological imaging.
    **Related equipment:** PET/MRI functional imaging, IMRT/VMAT optimizer.
    **Radiotherapy Example:** ESC-derived PET areas within a glioblastoma receive higher boost dose.

52. **Ventilation Image Registration:** Alignment of lung ventilation images with planning CT for functional sparing.
    **Related equipment:** 4D-CT, SPECT-ventilation, PET-ventilation.
    **Radiotherapy Example:** Used to reduce dose to high-function lung in stage III NSCLC.

53. **Variable Energy Beam Switching:** Changing photon or proton beam energy between fields or arcs to optimize penetration.
    **Related equipment:** LINAC energy selector, proton accelerator.
    **Radiotherapy Example:** Proton energy modulation in pediatric medulloblastoma to reduce distal dose.

54. **Virtual Implant Matching:** Using digitally reconstructed implants to support IGRT matching when bones are unclear.
    **Related equipment:** CBCT fusion, artificial implant contour tool.
    **Radiotherapy Example:** Hip prosthesis used as a landmark during pelvic IMRT matching.

55. **Volume Effect Modeling:** Radiobiological modeling to predict toxicity based on irradiated tissue volume.
    **Related equipment:** NTCP calculator, DVH evaluator.
    **Radiotherapy Example:** Used to select V20 constraint for lung to prevent pneumonitis.

56. **Voluntary Breath-Hold Coaching:** Therapist-guided breathing training to prolong and stabilize breath-hold time.
    **Related equipment:** ABC (active breath control) system, SGRT.
    **Radiotherapy Example:** Enables DIBH left-breast treatment to minimize cardiac dose.

57. **Vascular Flow-Sparing Planning:** Dose planning to avoid high-blood-flow vascular regions to preserve endothelial function.
    **Related equipment:** MRI-angiography fusion, contouring protocol.
    **Radiotherapy Example:** Avoiding hepatic artery radiation in liver SBRT.

58. **Volume Averaging Correction:** Correction for inaccurate dose measurement caused by detector volume size versus small field size.
    **Related equipment:** Micro ion chambers, synthetic diamond detectors.
    **Radiotherapy Example:** Used during SRS small-field beam commissioning.

59. **View-Matcher IGRT Interface:** On-board software allowing simultaneous comparison of multiple imaging planes for alignment.
    **Related equipment:** Dual-panel kV imaging, CBCT.
    **Radiotherapy Example:** Cervical cancer IGRT alignment using AP + lateral + CBCT match.

60. **Virtual Phantom Simulation:** Digital phantom used for dose verification before producing physical QA setup.
    **Related equipment:** Monte Carlo simulator, TPS QA module.
    **Radiotherapy Example:** Reduces setup time for IMRT QA by verifying fluence distribution virtually.

61. **Volumetric Autosegmentation:** AI-based automatic contour creation for anatomy and tumors.
    **Related equipment:** Deep learning contouring models, auto-seg TPS module.
    **Radiotherapy Example:** Speeds up head-and-neck OAR contouring for adaptive radiotherapy.

62. **Visual Motion Cue System:** Providing graphical breathing feedback to help patient maintain stable motion pattern.
    **Related equipment:** Respiratory monitoring screen, video metronome.
    **Radiotherapy Example:** Used in abdominal SBRT where motion amplitude must stay <5 mm.

63. **Variable Dose Rate Control:** Modulating dose rate during beam delivery to enhance plan quality or synchronization.
    **Related equipment:** FFF mode LINAC, VMAT delivery system.
    **Radiotherapy Example:** High-dose-rate bursts during SRS to reduce couch time.

64. **Virtual Beam Edge Display:** Viewer overlay showing beam entry and exit paths on patient anatomy images.
    **Related equipment:** TPS beam's-eye-view module.
    **Radiotherapy Example:** Used to prevent beam going through eyes during nasopharynx treatment.

65. **Vesicourethral Interface Protection:** Contouring and planning strategy to protect urinary sphincter regions.
    **Related equipment:** MRI fusion, urethra catheter contrast.
    **Radiotherapy Example:** Prostate SBRT sparing membranous urethra and bladder neck.

66. **Verification Workflow Automation:** Automated checklist enforcement for treatment verification prior to beam-on.
    **Related equipment:** ARIA/MOSAIQ therapist checklist automation.
    **Radiotherapy Example:** Ensures IGRT completed before treating spine SBRT.

67. **Voxelwise Toxicity Prediction:** Software prediction of organ complication risk using machine learning per voxel.
    **Related equipment:** NTCP AI models, DVH/biological feature data.
    **Radiotherapy Example:** Predicts xerostomia risk based on voxel dose to parotid gland.

68. **Ventral Cord Shielding:** Avoiding dose to anterior spinal cord surface when treating posterior tumors.
**Related equipment:** Leaf aperture shaping, electron boost plans.
**Radiotherapy Example:** Used in spine tumor boosts to avoid radiation myelopathy.

69. **Volumetric PET Response Tracking:** Measuring 3D tumor metabolic change during treatment to predict prognosis.
**Related equipment:** Sequential FDG-PET scans, deformable registration.
**Radiotherapy Example:** Adaptive dose escalation for poor responders in HPV-negative OPC.

70. **Voice-Preservation Radiotherapy Protocol:** Planning guideline to protect vocal structures when treating nearby cancers.
**Related equipment:** MRI larynx contouring, laryngeal substructure atlas.
**Radiotherapy Example:** Used in hypopharyngeal cancer IMRT to reduce long-term dysphonia.

71. **Virtual Reality Therapist Training:** Simulation system for training staff on radiation procedures before clinical work.
**Related equipment:** VR workstation, procedural simulation software.
**Radiotherapy Example:** Practicing SRS patient setup and couch shifts in VR.

72. **Volumetric Dose Comparison Tool:** Tool to compare two dose distributions voxel-by-voxel rather than relying only on DVH.
**Related equipment:** 3D gamma analysis software.
**Radiotherapy Example:** Used in adaptive replanning QA to compare new and old plan doses.

73. **Vicarious Patient Safety Alarm Monitoring:** Remote audio-visual monitoring of safety alarms from the control room.
**Related equipment:** Pipeline alarm screen, intercom, CCTV.
**Radiotherapy Example:** Alerts team if patient disengages motion-tracking device.

74. **Voluntary Shoulder Depression:** Intentional lowering of patient shoulders to clear beam path to the neck.
**Related equipment:** Shoulder retractors, SGRT.
**Radiotherapy Example:** Improves access for supraclavicular field in head-and-neck RT.

75. **Virtual Brachytherapy Catheter Mapping:** Software-based mapping of brachytherapy catheter positions before insertion.
**Related equipment:** 3D pelvic ultrasound or MRI fusion, applicator modeling.
**Radiotherapy Example:** Used in cervical brachytherapy planning to optimize ovoid & tandem geometry.

76. **Volumetric Thermal Imaging:** Technique that maps heat distribution across tissues during therapy for biological monitoring.
**Related equipment:** Infrared thermal camera, MR-thermometry.
**Radiotherapy Example:** Used during MR-LINAC treatment to monitor tissue heating near bowel.

77. **Variable Jaw Tracking:** Synchronizing secondary jaws with MLC motion to reduce leakage and transmission.
**Related equipment:** LINAC dynamic jaw system, IMRT/VMAT optimizer.
**Radiotherapy Example:** Applied in prostate IMRT to improve conformity and reduce rectal dose.

78. **Vertebral Body Sparing Technique:** Technique for minimizing dose to spinal vertebrae to reduce marrow suppression.
**Related equipment:** VMAT planning, bone marrow contouring atlas.
**Radiotherapy Example:** Used in pediatric abdominal RT to preserve bone marrow function.

79. **Virtual Visualization Console:** Touchscreen planning and on-treatment review interface for therapists.
**Related equipment:** On-board imaging console, TPS viewer.
**Radiotherapy Example:** RT therapists check IGRT match on touchscreen before beam-on.

80. **Vascular Dose Reconstruction:** Estimation of radiation dose to major vessels to predict long-term stenosis risk.
**Related equipment:** CT-angiography fusion, DVH metrics.
**Radiotherapy Example:** Monitoring carotid artery dose in head-and-neck IMRT.

81. **Voxel Intensity Mapping:** Conversion of imaging pixel intensity into voxel dose-planning biological data.
**Related equipment:** PET segmentation tool, MRI functional mapping.
**Radiotherapy Example:** PET SUV values determine dose escalation area inside the tumor.

82. **Voluntary Deep Breathing Synchronization:** Patient-controlled breathing pattern synchronized with beam gating.
**Related equipment:** SGRT, respiratory gating hardware.
**Radiotherapy Example:** Used in pancreatic cancer to reduce motion of the duodenum.

83. **Vaginal Cylinder Immobilization:** Mold-room setup device to stabilize vaginal canal for brachytherapy.
**Related equipment:** Vaginal applicator set, CT brachytherapy simulator.
**Radiotherapy Example:** Ensures reproducible dosing in post-hysterectomy endometrial cancer.

84. **Vertebral Landmark Localization:** Aligning treatment fields using clear vertebral levels when tumor is not easily visualized.
**Related equipment:** kV orthogonal imaging, CBCT spine matching.
**Radiotherapy Example:** Cervical spine SBRT field set using C5–C7 reference.

85. **Volatile Chemical Neutralization (Mould Room):** Extraction and filtration process to eliminate resin and casting fumes.
**Related equipment:** Fume hood, ventilation system, odour absorbent.
**Radiotherapy Example:** Used while fabricating thermoplastic masks and bolus.

86. **Variable Elliptical Collimator (Proton):** Adjustable beam aperture that shapes proton beam elliptically for conformity.
**Related equipment:** Proton multi-leaf collimator, nozzle aperture system.
**Radiotherapy Example:** Used in spine proton therapy to minimize exit dose to kidneys.

87. **Visual Couch Shift Confirmation:** Real-time 3D visualization displaying couch movement relative to patient anatomy.
**Related equipment:** SGRT tracking, 6DoF couch software.
**Radiotherapy Example:** Therapists verify correct couch shift during brain SRS.

88. **Vascular Radio-Sensitivity Scoring:** System that determines vulnerability of blood vessels to RT-induced stenosis.
**Related equipment:** Radiobiology model calculator.
**Radiotherapy Example:** Influences carotid sparing strategies in throat cancer.

89. **Volumetric Anatomical Teaching Dataset:** 3D structure library used for training new RT professionals in contouring.
**Related equipment:** VR anatomy software, anatomy labeling atlas.
**Radiotherapy Example:** Trainees practice parotid, optic chiasm, and spinal cord contouring.

90. **Volumetric Replan Validation:** Dose evaluation process to confirm accuracy before switching to adaptive plan.
**Related equipment:** DVH comparison tool, gamma map software.
**Radiotherapy Example:** Required before implementing mid-treatment adaptive plan for bladder cancer.

91. **Vaginal OAR Shielding Strategy:** Treatment planning method to reduce dose to the vagina when not part of the target.
**Related equipment:** IMRT/VMAT optimization, anatomical sparing protocol.
**Radiotherapy Example:** Applied during anal cancer IMRT.

92. **Voxel Tracking Dose Accumulation:** Summation of dose over time using deformable mapping to follow organ movement.
**Related equipment:** DIR (Deformable Image Registration), adaptive TPS.
**Radiotherapy Example:** Used in pancreatic RT to calculate actual bowel dose across fractions.

93. **Vertebral Compression Risk Modeling:** Predicting pathological fracture likelihood after spine SBRT.
**Related equipment:** Spine risk calculator, CT cortical thickness analysis.
**Radiotherapy Example:** Guides prescription limits for metastatic spinal lesions.

94. **Virtual Physics Safety Drill:** Simulated training to handle LINAC faults, beam interruptions, or emergency shutdowns.
**Related equipment:** LINAC simulation software, QA training platform.
**Radiotherapy Example:** New physicists practice radiation emergency stop workflow.

95. **Vascular Embolus Sparing:** Planning strategy to avoid irradiating pre-existing vascular thrombus.
**Related equipment:** MRI venography fusion, OAR segmentation.
**Radiotherapy Example:** Applied in liver SBRT to prevent embolus migration.

96. **Visual Patient Feedback Projection:** Projecting breathing or motion graphics onto wall for patient performance guidance.
**Related equipment:** Projector, real-time motion monitoring, SGRT.
**Radiotherapy Example:** Improves stability in pediatric abdominal RT without anesthesia.

97. **Voltage Stability Monitoring (LINAC):** System ensuring stable operating voltage to prevent beam energy drift.
**Related equipment:** Power regulation module, electrical stabilizer.
**Radiotherapy Example:** Used during high-dose-rate FFF mode to prevent energy fluctuation.

98. **Volumetric Imaging Dose Minimization:** Strategies to reduce cumulative imaging dose during IGRT.
**Related equipment:** Low-dose CBCT, kV limited arc imaging.
**Radiotherapy Example:** Weekly CBCT + daily kV used in prostate RT instead of daily CBCT.

99. **Viscoelastic Material Bolus:** Body-adaptive bolus that conforms to surface without air gaps.
**Related equipment:** Soft gel bolus, mould room materials.
**Radiotherapy Example:** Used in scalp RT to prevent electron scattering gaps.

100. **Virtual Linac Delivery Rehearsal:** Running the entire radiation delivery sequence digitally before actual treatment.
**Related equipment:** LINAC simulation mode, dry-run software.
**Radiotherapy Example:** Ensures safe delivery of highly modulated SRS/VMAT plans.

101. **Vaginal Dose De-escalation:** Gradual reduction of dose to vaginal tissues while maintaining tumor control through optimized beam shaping.
**Related equipment:** VMAT optimizer, OAR sparing constraint module.
**Radiotherapy Example:** Used in pelvic RT for cervical cancer to prevent vaginal fibrosis.

102. **Volumetric PET-Guided Boost:** Dose escalation to PET-avid areas within a tumor while keeping baseline dose to whole target.
**Related equipment:** PET-CT fusion, SUV threshold mapping.
**Radiotherapy Example:** Escalated boost dose to FDG-avid lung tumor core during SBRT.

103. **Vertebra-to-PTV Auto Matching:** Image registration algorithm matching spinal vertebrae landmarks to the planning CT.
**Related equipment:** CBCT auto-match, spine IGRT module.
**Radiotherapy Example:** Alignment for spine metastasis SBRT treatment.

104. **Virtual Mould Library:** Digital catalogue of pre-designed mould and bolus templates to improve setup workflow.
**Related equipment:** 3D printer, mould room workstation.
**Radiotherapy Example:** Auto-selected facial bolus template for nasal tumor electron therapy.

105. **Ventricle Avoidance Strategy:** Planning technique to keep radiation dose away from lateral ventricles to preserve neurocognitive function.
**Related equipment:** MRI segmentation, IMRT avoidance structure.
**Radiotherapy Example:** Applied in pediatric brain RT to protect memory-related structures.

106. **Variable Breathing Control Belt:** Belt-mounted abdominal monitor used to stabilize patient respiratory pattern.
**Related equipment:** Breathing belt, gating control unit.
**Radiotherapy Example:** Used in liver RT to reduce diaphragm motion before CBCT acquisition.

107. **Volumetric Metal Artifact Correction:** Algorithm for reducing CT artifacts from metal implants to improve dose accuracy.
**Related equipment:** CT MAR software, orthopedic implant artifact filter.
**Radiotherapy Example:** Ensures proper contouring near hip prosthesis in pelvic RT.

108. **Venous Return Monitoring (Prone Breast):** Observation of blood pooling risks during prone positioning to maintain comfort and oxygenation.
**Related equipment:** Prone breast board, patient monitoring sensors.
**Radiotherapy Example:** Applied during long prone breast VMAT sessions.

109. **Virtual Space Localization System:** 3D digital room mapping for aligning patient, couch, and isocenter during treatment.
**Related equipment:** SGRT room mapping, ceiling-mounted camera array.
**Radiotherapy Example:** Used for frameless SRS to confirm patient position without tattoos.

110. **Variable Dose Fractionation Protocol:** Fractionation system where dose varies across weeks to reduce toxicity or enhance control.
**Related equipment:** Adaptive fractionation planning.
**Radiotherapy Example:** 8 Gy × 3 boost followed by 2 Gy × 10 standard fractions for recurrent lung tumor.

111. **Vertebral Artery Protection Arc:** Beam arrangement preventing dose overlap onto vertebral arteries.
**Related equipment:** VMAT arc planner, vessel contouring tool.
**Radiotherapy Example:** Used in paraspinal tumor treatment to avoid vascular stenosis risk.

112. **Volumetric Electron Patch Boost:** Supplemental electron field applied to treat superficial regions after photon RT.
**Related equipment:** Electron applicator, custom cutout.
**Radiotherapy Example:** Applied to chest wall scar after whole-breast photon RT.

113. **Verification CT Track Log:** Recording system that logs every verification CT performed during treatment.
**Related equipment:** Oncology information system (OIS), imaging documentation portal.
**Radiotherapy Example:** Helps calculate cumulative imaging dose in prostate RT.

114. **Visual Patient Alignment Triangulation:** Technique using symmetrical anatomical points for optical body alignment.
**Related equipment:** SGRT, laser alignment system.
**Radiotherapy Example:** Used before CBCT for whole-abdomen pediatric RT.

115. **Volumetric Auto-Bolus Expansion:** Automatic generation of bolus volume based on skin profile.
**Related equipment:** TPS bolus planning tool, 3D printer.
**Radiotherapy Example:** Used for extremity sarcoma to guarantee surface dose.

116. **Virtual Dose Feedback Screen:** Real-time patient education display showing safety and treatment progress without numeric dose stress.
**Related equipment:** Patient-view LED panel, treatment status interface.
**Radiotherapy Example:** Used to reduce anxiety during pediatric SBRT.

117. **Voxel Precision Dose Sharpening:** Algorithm to enhance dose fall-off at tumor boundary.
**Related equipment:** High-resolution IMRT optimizer.
**Radiotherapy Example:** Used in brain metastasis SRS to minimize hippocampal dose.

118. **Vibration-Free Immobilization Base:** Anti-vibration support for high-precision radiosurgery immobilization.
**Related equipment:** SRS tabletop, carbon-fiber board.
**Radiotherapy Example:** Required for trigeminal neuralgia single-fraction treatment.

119. **Vestibular Dose Reduction Module:** Dose modeling tool to protect vestibular system (balance organs).
**Related equipment:** IMRT optimizer, MRI vestibule segmentation.
**Radiotherapy Example:** Applied in acoustic neuroma treatment to avoid dizziness/hearing decline.

120. **Vectorized Respiratory Surrogate:** Mathematical model converting breathing motion into a predictable 3D vector.
**Related equipment:** Surface tracking camera, breathing monitor.
**Radiotherapy Example:** Predicts tumor drift in left lung RT during deep inspiration hold.

121. **Visible Scar Mapping:** Documenting surgical scars into planning CT for evaluating recurrence-prone areas.
**Related equipment:** Skin markers, CT marking wire.
**Radiotherapy Example:** Used to mark mastectomy scars for targeted boost.

122. **Volumetric Contour Auto-Expansion:** Automatic modification of contours based on growth risk or margin uncertainty.
**Related equipment:** TPS margin algorithm.
**Radiotherapy Example:** Expands CTV margins when bowel motion probability increases.

123. **Ventricle-Sparing Re-irradiation:** Second course RT technique that avoids ventricular zone to preserve neurocognitive function.
**Related equipment:** Adaptive IMRT re-planning.
**Radiotherapy Example:** For recurrent glioma requiring re-irradiation.

124. **Variable Patient Loading Protocol:** Scheduling system balancing complex treatments to reduce LINAC overload.
**Related equipment:** OIS scheduling platform.
**Radiotherapy Example:** High-dose SBRT scheduling separated from full-body TBI days.

125. **Voluntary-Motion Locking Feedback:** Visual coaching that helps the patient maintain head or abdominal stillness.
**Related equipment:** SGRT screen, patient motion feedback interface.
**Radiotherapy Example:** Used for larynx RT to avoid mask tightening discomfort.

126. **Vertebral Height Preservation Monitoring:** Tracking vertebral body stability during and after RT.
**Related equipment:** On-treatment CT / MRI follow-up.
**Radiotherapy Example:** Applied in spinal SBRT to prevent compression fractures.

127. **Ventilator-Controlled Radiotherapy Protocol:** Tightly timed beam delivery synchronized with ventilator trigger cycles.
**Related equipment:** Respiratory-linked gating, ventilator sync unit.
**Radiotherapy Example:** Used in mechanically ventilated ICU patients receiving urgent RT.

128. **Virtual Intraluminal Applicator Simulator:** Simulator for learning brachytherapy applicator insertion without a patient.
**Related equipment:** VR brachy simulator, anatomical pelvic phantom.
**Radiotherapy Example:** Trains staff for HDR cervical brachytherapy.

129. **Visual Fiducial Enhancement Overlay:** Digital enhancement of fiducials on imaging to improve match visibility.
**Related equipment:** CBCT display enhancer, kV image viewer.
**Radiotherapy Example:** Helps align pancreatic cancer fiducials under low-contrast soft tissue.

130. **Volume-Based Couch Override Lock:** Safety lock preventing couch movement when patient is outside safe clearance zone.
**Related equipment:** LINAC clearance simulation software, OIS couch lock.
**Radiotherapy Example:** Prevents collision during cranial SRS with high couch pitch.

131. **Volumetric PET Dose Indexing:** Allocation of dose based on PET tracer uptake intensity inside the tumor volume.
**Related equipment:** PET-CT fusion workstation, SUV threshold mapping tool.
**Radiotherapy Example:** Lung SBRT boost escalated only to PET-avid regions while sparing healthy lung tissue.

132. **Virtual Field Junction Calibration:** Computer-guided alignment of adjacent radiation fields to avoid cold/hot spots.
**Related equipment:** TPS junction optimizer, EPID verification.
**Radiotherapy Example:** Field matching between upper and lower spine regions in craniospinal irradiation.

133. **Voxel-Wise Dose Deformation Tracking:** Tracks dose distribution through anatomical changes during adaptive RT.
**Related equipment:** Adaptive CT re-plan module, deformable image registration.
**Radiotherapy Example:** Used for pancreatic cancer where daily anatomy changes shift bowel position.

134. **Vestibular Toxicity Risk Modeling:** Predicts damage probability to inner-ear sensory organs caused by radiation.
**Related equipment:** MRI vestibule segmentation, OAR risk calculator.
**Radiotherapy Example:** Used in acoustic neuroma SRS planning to preserve balance function.

135. **Variable Arc Modulation Strategy:** Changes arc dose modulation levels depending on tumor shape complexity.
**Related equipment:** VMAT optimizer, dynamic MLC control.
**Radiotherapy Example:** Head-and-neck VMAT plan uses high modulation near parotid glands and low modulation elsewhere.

136. **Visual Motion Suppression Training:** Patients are coached to minimize voluntary body movement via visual feedback.
**Related equipment:** SGRT display screen, motion sensitivity monitor.
**Radiotherapy Example:** Maintains abdominal stillness during liver SBRT.

137. **Vascular Dose Constraint Planning:** Planning approach that limits dose to critical arteries and veins to avoid stenosis or thrombosis.
**Related equipment:** MRI angiography fusion, vessel contouring software.
**Radiotherapy Example:** Maintains tolerance limits for carotid artery during larynx cancer RT.

138. **Vacuum-Supported Pediatric Immobilization:** Child-friendly vacuum mold system shaped to the patient for reproducible immobilization.
**Related equipment:** Vac-Lok bag, anaesthesia-compatible paediatric board.
**Radiotherapy Example:** Ensures stable positioning during cranial RT without daily sedation.

139. **Volumetric Reference Imaging Bank:** Digital library of 3D anatomical reference sets used for matching unusual anatomies.
**Related equipment:** OIS imaging archive, reference atlas viewer.
**Radiotherapy Example:** Helps verify positioning in scoliosis patients with rotated vertebrae.

140. **Viscous Thermo-Bolus Compound:** Soft high-viscosity bolus that conforms tightly to irregular skin surfaces.
**Related equipment:** Mould room bolus compound heater, electron cone.
**Radiotherapy Example:** Used in chest wall RT to improve surface dose on uneven surgical scars.

141. **Variable Fraction Size Therapy:** Radiation schedule using different doses per session based on weekly treatment goals.
**Related equipment:** RT fractionation prescription module.
**Radiotherapy Example:** $3 \times 8$ Gy boost followed by $15 \times 2$ Gy standard for bone metastasis.

142. **Volumetric CT-Based Patient Education:** Patient counselling using simplified 3D CT models to show target and OARs.
**Related equipment:** 3D viewer software, CT workstation.
**Radiotherapy Example:** Breast cancer patients learn why arm positioning affects lung dose.

143. **Virtual Radiation Risk Prediction Map:** Software that visually indicates regions with high risk of late toxicity during plan review.
**Related equipment:** Radiobiology modelling plugin.
**Radiotherapy Example:** Highlights temporal lobe dose risk during nasopharyngeal IMRT.

144. **Volumetric Exit Dose Evaluation:** Measuring and comparing exit dose through body to ensure beam passes tissue as expected.
**Related equipment:** EPID dosimetry, exit dose grid calculator.
**Radiotherapy Example:** Used in pelvic RT to check bowel gas shrinking effect on beam attenuation.

145. **Voxel-Weighted OAR Penalty Function:** Assigns varying penalty sensitivity to OAR voxels based on clinical risk.
**Related equipment:** IMRT optimization algorithm.
**Radiotherapy Example:** Higher penalty applied to hippocampus voxels at memory-critical regions.

146. **Vector-Matched Multi-Isocenter Setup:** Patient coordinates mathematically aligned across two or more isocenters.
**Related equipment:** Couch rotation accuracy system, digital match software.
**Radiotherapy Example:** Craniospinal treatment ensures head-neck and spine fields meet seamlessly.

147. **Vehicle Transport Vibration Policy (RT Patients):** Transport guidelines to avoid sudden vibration or head jerk for frame-fixed SRS patients.
**Related equipment:** Transport stabilizer strap, nursing guidelines.
**Radiotherapy Example:** Applied after Leksell frame placement before delivering single-fraction radiosurgery.

148. **Visual-Pathway Dose-Limiting Protocol:** Strategy to minimize dose to optic nerves, chiasm, and retina.
**Related equipment:** MRI fusion, optic structure contouring library.
**Radiotherapy Example:** Required for pituitary adenoma or cavernous sinus tumor RT.

149. **Virtual Adaptive Fraction Review Board:** Remote multidisciplinary review of dose changes during adaptive RT.
**Related equipment:** ARIA/MOSAIQ tele-dashboard, adaptive plan viewer.
**Radiotherapy Example:** Weekly board reviews bladder filling issues in adaptive prostate RT.

150. **Vertebral Stability Prediction Scoring in SBRT:** Predicts fracture risk based on vertebral bone load under high-dose stereotactic RT.
**Related equipment:** CT/MRI bone density metrics, SBRT planning software.
**Radiotherapy Example:** Spinal SBRT dose reduced when high fracture risk score is detected.

151. **Virtual Tumor Regression Projection:** Predictive modelling of tumor shrinkage over time during treatment.
**Related equipment:** Time-series radiobiology modelling module.
**Radiotherapy Example:** Estimates the reduction of nasopharyngeal mass by week 3 and suggests adaptive re-planning.

152. **Voxel-Specific LET Mapping:** Mapping linear energy transfer (LET) per voxel to estimate biological effect, especially in proton therapy.
**Related equipment:** LET calculator, Monte Carlo dose engine.
**Radiotherapy Example:** Used to minimize high-LET deposition in brainstem during pediatric proton treatment.

153. **Viscoelastic Organ Deformation Model:** Predicts movement of soft organs based on pressure and motion.
**Related equipment:** Deformable image registration system.
**Radiotherapy Example:** Liver SBRT planning compensates expected deformation caused by diaphragm motion.

154. **Vertical Couch Shift Index:** Measure of required vertical adjustments during patient setup.
**Related equipment:** 6-DOF couch, SGRT alignment.
**Radiotherapy Example:** Used daily for breast RT to ensure chest wall sits at correct elevation.

155. **Virtual Metallic Artifact Reduction Scan (VMAR):** Digital reconstruction minimizing artifacts caused by implants in CT.
 **Related equipment:** Metal artifact reduction CT algorithm.
 **Radiotherapy Example:** Hip prosthesis artifact removal for accurate prostate contouring.

156. **Vertebral Body Bolus Configuration:** Placement of bolus near spinal bone surface for superficial posterior disease.
 **Related equipment:** Thermoplastic bolus, mould room bolus former.
 **Radiotherapy Example:** Treats posterior scalp sarcoma extending to upper cervical vertebrae.

157. **Visual Gating Feedback Display:** Patient controls breath motion by observing real-time breathing graph.
 **Related equipment:** Respiratory gating screen, RPM or SGRT.
 **Radiotherapy Example:** DIBH feedback reduces heart dose in left breast RT.

158. **Voxelized Contrast Perfusion Overlay:** Superimposing blood-flow CT or MRI perfusion on planning images.
 **Related equipment:** Perfusion fusion workstation.
 **Radiotherapy Example:** High-perfusion pancreatic tumor regions receive dose escalation.

159. **Variable Angle Bite-Block Positioning:** Rotation-controlled mouthpiece to optimize head-fixed orientation.
 **Related equipment:** Indexed bite-block mould, intra-oral immobilizer.
 **Radiotherapy Example:** Aligns tongue and jaw during tonsillar IMRT for sparing parotids.

160. **Vaginal Dose Reporting Standard (Gy/Length):** Dose documentation normalized to vaginal tract length.
 **Related equipment:** Brachytherapy EQD2 calculator.
 **Radiotherapy Example:** Used in postoperative endometrial cancer HDR brachytherapy.

161. **Vascular Uptake Tracer Mapping:** PET visualization of tumor vascularization.
 **Related equipment:** FDG-PET, perfusion tracer uptake calculator.
 **Radiotherapy Example:** Guides dose escalation in metastatic sarcoma nodules.

162. **Virtual Wedge Compensation Factor:** Correction value applied when replacing physical wedge with dynamic or virtual wedge.
 **Related equipment:** LINAC wedge calculator.
 **Radiotherapy Example:** Chest wall RT using virtual wedge avoids excessive contralateral breast dose.

163. **Vacuum-Assisted Head Stabilization Hood:** Suction-supported immobilization cap reducing scalp movement.
 **Related equipment:** Vacuum mould hood, mask interface.
 **Radiotherapy Example:** Used for cranial SRS when thermoplastic mask alone is insufficient.

164. **Voxel-Based Toxicity Atlas Reference:** Probability atlas linking dose levels to organ toxicity based on big data evidence.
 **Related equipment:** Online OAR-toxicity database, radiobiology plug-in.
 **Radiotherapy Example:** Indicates temporal lobe necrosis risk during nasopharyngeal IMRT.

165. **Visual Field Preservation Algorithm:** Eye-related structure-sparing planning for optic pathway.
 **Related equipment:** Optic chiasm dose constraint module.
 **Radiotherapy Example:** Pituitary adenoma SRS plan limits chiasm dose while maintaining tumor coverage.

166. **Varied Beam Quality Modulation:** Modifying beam hardness/energy inside one plan to optimize penetrability.
**Related equipment:** Dual-energy LINAC, modulated beam quality controller.
**Radiotherapy Example:** Dual-energy delivery for lung tumor reduces exit dose to heart.

167. **Vaginal Cylinder Fit Verification:** HDR device position confirmation using CT or X-ray before dose delivery.
**Related equipment:** In-room CT, applicator verification markers.
**Radiotherapy Example:** Prevents air gap underdosing in postoperative cervix vault brachytherapy.

168. **Virtual Shift Reconciliation Record:** Digital summary of setup shifts applied over all fractions.
**Related equipment:** OIS shift tracking dashboard.
**Radiotherapy Example:** Detects progressive spine rotation in immobilized pediatric RT.

169. **Ventilation-Lung Voxel Sparing Rule:** Dose priority given to regions of highly functional lung.
**Related equipment:** 4D-CT ventilation function map.
**Radiotherapy Example:** Preserved lung function during SBRT for COPD patients.

170. **Volumetric Bolus Expansion Template:** 3D printed bolus template expanding skin surface in a controlled manner.
**Related equipment:** 3D printer, mould room scanning system.
**Radiotherapy Example:** Used for orbital exenteration scar to improve superficial dose coverage.

171. **Virtual Pelvic Bowel Displacement Protocol:** Predictive model for bowel shifts based on bladder volume.
**Related equipment:** Organ prediction algorithm, daily CBCT recorder.
**Radiotherapy Example:** Reduces bowel hotspots during prostate IMRT.

172. **Voxel-By-Voxel Recovery Factor:** Value correcting contrast signal for tissue heterogeneity.
**Related equipment:** PET/MRI quantification tool.
**Radiotherapy Example:** Accurate SUV evaluation for residual lymphoma tracking.

173. **Vaginal Spacer Dose Reduction Strategy:** Spacer gel or mechanical dilator to push vagina away from rectal wall.
**Related equipment:** Spacer injection kit under US guidance.
**Radiotherapy Example:** Reduces rectal toxicity during cervical boost.

174. **Vertebral Canal SAR Control:** Strict SAR (specific absorption rate) limit for spine MRI in SRS planning.
**Related equipment:** MRI SAR control sequence.
**Radiotherapy Example:** Avoids heating injury when MRI used for spinal metastasis radiosurgery mapping.

175. **Visual Dry-Run Simulation:** Non-beam virtual walkthrough to validate patient position and beam clearances.
**Related equipment:** TPS simulation viewer, LINAC collision map.
**Radiotherapy Example:** Used before SRS with steep couch angles to avoid head support collisions.

176. **Vascular-Dose Micro-Region Mapping:** Sub-millimetric mapping of dose to micro-blood vessels.
**Related equipment:** High-resolution MRI angiography.
**Radiotherapy Example:** Helps preserve vascular supply during ocular melanoma proton therapy.

177. **Virtual Plan Safety Margin Evaluation:** Software tests robustness of PTV margins under multiple error scenarios.
**Related equipment:** Plan robustness simulator.
**Radiotherapy Example:** Expands posterior PTV for prostate when risk of rectal gas motion is high.

178. **Variable Surface Pressure Tabletop:** Couch that adjusts body pressure distribution for comfort and stability.
**Related equipment:** Smart-cushion radiotherapy couch.
**Radiotherapy Example:** Reduces pain enabling longer SRS immobilization in spine metastasis patients.

179. **Virtual Fiducial Biomechanics Analysis:** Predicts motion of implanted fiducials due to natural organ movement.
**Related equipment:** Fiducial motion prediction model.
**Radiotherapy Example:** Improves CyberKnife targeting accuracy for pancreas.

180. **Vasovagal Response Prevention Pathway:** Protocol to avoid fainting during mask moulding or head frame fixation.
**Related equipment:** Anticipatory nursing monitoring, hydration policy.
**Radiotherapy Example:** Used for anxious patients during thermoplastic mask fabrication.

181. **Volumetric Motion Gating Margin:** Extra margin added to target to account for tumor motion during gated treatments.
**Related equipment:** 4D-CT, respiratory gating system, motion tracking camera.
**Radiotherapy Example:** Added around lung tumor PTV during DIBH to ensure beam covers motion phases properly.

182. **Validation Imaging Sequence:** Imaging done before beam-on to confirm final alignment and anatomy.
**Related equipment:** CBCT, kV pair, SGRT validation.
**Radiotherapy Example:** Used every fraction for prostate RT to verify fiducials before delivery.

183. **Variable Couch Rotation Index:** Scoring of plan safety and coverage using multiple non-coplanar couch angles.
**Related equipment:** LINAC with 6-DOF couch, collision predictor software.
**Radiotherapy Example:** Arc beams at 45° and 90° improve coverage in brain metastasis SRS.

184. **Virtual Headrest Fit Optimization:** Digital shaping of headrest contour for maximum stability during immobilization.
**Related equipment:** 3D scanning + mould room customization tools.
**Radiotherapy Example:** Creates custom occipital headrest for nasopharyngeal IMRT.

185. **Visualized Dose-Painting Display:** Color-coded visualization of multiple dose levels targeted at different tumor regions.
**Related equipment:** IMRT dose-painting TPS module.
**Radiotherapy Example:** Higher dose painted to PET-avid regions in head & neck cancer.

186. **Voxel-Specific Calibration Factor:** Factor correcting CT numbers to electron density per voxel.
**Related equipment:** CT calibration phantom.
**Radiotherapy Example:** Improves accuracy for IMRT lung heterogeneity corrections.

187. **Volumetric IGRT Drift Analysis:** Examines long-term positional shifts across fractions.
**Related equipment:** CBCT database, alignment analytics software.
**Radiotherapy Example:** Detects systematic downward pelvic migration requiring PTV margin adjustment.

188. **Visualization Protocol for Tattoo-Free Setup:** SGRT-based workflow for eliminating permanent skin tattoos.
**Related equipment:** Surface imaging cameras (VisionRT/AlignRT).
**Radiotherapy Example:** Used for breast RT — no tattoos needed due to optical guidance.

189. **Vascular Organ-Sparing Dose Constraint:** Dose limitations specifically protecting large blood vessels.
**Related equipment:** Planning organ-at-risk voxel tool.
**Radiotherapy Example:** Spare carotid artery during larynx IMRT to reduce stenosis risk.

190. **Virtual Mandible Expansion Grid:** Planning structure to avoid mandible hotspots.
**Related equipment:** Modulated arc planning.
**Radiotherapy Example:** Used in tongue cancer IMRT to reduce osteoradionecrosis risk.

191. **Varied Beam Intensity Tuning Cycle:** TPS algorithm that optimizes fluence layer by layer through iterative adjustment.
**Related equipment:** IMRT optimizer.
**Radiotherapy Example:** Improves conformity in prostate IMRT with rectum sparing.

192. **Vacuum Compression Belt:** Belt that compresses abdomen to minimize breathing motion.
**Related equipment:** Abdominal compression unit.
**Radiotherapy Example:** Used for liver and pancreas SBRT motion reduction.

193. **Visual Alert Beam-Gate Indicator:** A screen or signal showing when radiation beam is paused or active during gating.
**Related equipment:** Respiratory gating interface.
**Radiotherapy Example:** Helps patient maintain stable breath-hold in DIBH.

194. **Voxel Dose Falloff Indicator:** Numerical measure of how fast dose decreases outside PTV.
**Related equipment:** DVH + dose gradient tool.
**Radiotherapy Example:** Evaluates dose drop-off near optic nerve in pituitary SRS.

195. **Virtual Stereotactic Field Check:** A simulation ensuring field coordinates match stereotactic reference frame.
**Related equipment:** SRS QA phantom.
**Radiotherapy Example:** Ensures alignment accuracy before brain metastases treatment.

196. **Variable Modulator Attenuation Index:** Value indicating attenuation effect of MLC or modulator on beam.
**Related equipment:** MLC QC system.
**Radiotherapy Example:** Ensures correct output in highly modulated head & neck IMRT.

197. **Virtual Rectal Spacer Prediction Tool:** Model predicting prostate-rectum spacing after hydrogel insertion.
**Related equipment:** US-guided gel spacer kit.
**Radiotherapy Example:** Used to plan rectal dose reduction pre-RT.

198. **Vision-Guided Setup Review:** AI-assisted review of patient alignment before approval.
**Related equipment:** SGRT + AI verification.
**Radiotherapy Example:** Automatically flags rotational errors in breast setup.

199. **Volumetric Organ Motion Heatmap:** Statistical representation of OAR motion patterns.
**Related equipment:** Adaptive planning tracker.
**Radiotherapy Example:** Shows bladder volume variability during pelvic RT.

200. **Verification Dose Accumulation:** Summing actual delivered dose across fractions using imaging feedback.
**Related equipment:** Dose accumulation engine, adaptive TPS.
**Radiotherapy Example:** Confirms spinal cord tolerance remains safe during IMRT boost.

201. **Volumetric Deformation Mapping:** Tracking anatomical shape changes across fractions using deformable registration.
**Related equipment:** CBCT, adaptive planning TPS.
**Radiotherapy Example:** Detects tumor shrinkage during head & neck IMRT and prompts replanning.

202. **Variable Arc Sequencing:** Splitting VMAT arcs with different gantry speeds and dose rates for optimization.
**Related equipment:** LINAC VMAT delivery system.
**Radiotherapy Example:** Used in prostate VMAT to improve rectum and bladder sparing.

203. **Virtual Immobilization Preview:** Software simulation of patient positioning before manufacturing immobilization.
**Related equipment:** 3D mould room planning software.
**Radiotherapy Example:** Helps select thermoplastic mask type before head & neck scanning.

204. **Voxel-Wise Dose Uncertainty Model:** Quantifies uncertainty per voxel in dose calculation for high-precision planning.
**Related equipment:** Monte Carlo TPS.
**Radiotherapy Example:** Used during lung IMRT to confirm accuracy in heterogeneous tissues.

205. **Visual Collision Risk Framework:** Predicts potential gantry/couch collisions during non-coplanar planning.
**Related equipment:** LINAC collision avoidance software.
**Radiotherapy Example:** Ensures safety during cranial SRS with couch rotation.

206. **Viscous Bolus Interface:** Gel-based bolus that conforms to irregular body contours.
**Related equipment:** Mould room bolus fabrication.
**Radiotherapy Example:** Used for scalp irradiation to eliminate air gaps.

207. **Virtual Adaptive Dose Projection:** Projection of future dose distribution based on previous delivered dose.
**Related equipment:** Adaptive radiotherapy prediction engine.
**Radiotherapy Example:** Predicts spinal cord dose before high-dose boost in IMRT.

208. **Vascular Contrast Dose Visualization:** Visualization of contrast-enhanced vasculature for planning.
**Related equipment:** CT contrast protocol, MRI MRA.
**Radiotherapy Example:** Protects renal artery during abdominal IMRT.

209. **Verification Arc Fluence Audit:** Independent QA of VMAT arc fluence delivery.
**Related equipment:** EPID fluence QA system.
**Radiotherapy Example:** Confirmed precise fluence delivery before liver SBRT.

210. **Virtual Shoulder Reduction Protocol:** Shoulder positioning rules for accurate head/neck immobilization.
**Related equipment:** Thermoplastic mask + immobilization wedges.
**Radiotherapy Example:** Prevents shoulder obstruction from blocking lateral neck beams.

211. **Volumetric Dose Fog Analysis:** Detects low-dose unintended exposure regions.
**Related equipment:** Dose painting visualization.
**Radiotherapy Example:** Removes unnecessary low-dose bath in breast VMAT.

212. **View-Locked Treatment Approval:** Beam cannot activate unless IGRT view is approved.
**Related equipment:** CBCT/SGRT beam-hold interlocks.
**Radiotherapy Example:** Prevents treatment until prostate fiducials are perfectly aligned.

213. **Virtual Gantry Motion Replay:** 3D replay of gantry motion for QA and troubleshooting.
**Related equipment:** LINAC trajectory log analysis tool.
**Radiotherapy Example:** Used to diagnose VMAT overshoot during QA.

214. **Voxel-Based Organ Weighting:** Assigning variable planning priority to different parts of an OAR.
**Related equipment:** IMRT optimizer with voxel weighting tool.
**Radiotherapy Example:** Higher weight around optic nerve during skull base IMRT.

215. **Ventral Surface Beam Avoidance Technique:** Avoiding entrance beams through abdomen or chest to protect sensitive tissues.
**Related equipment:** IMRT planning blocking region tool.
**Radiotherapy Example:** Avoids bowel during pelvic VMAT.

216. **Vacuum Pelvic Cushion Index:** Degree of stability achieved using vacuum immobilization cushions.
**Related equipment:** Vac-Lok immobilization system.
**Radiotherapy Example:** Used to evaluate setup reproducibility in pelvic IMRT.

217. **Vision-Assisted Iso-Centering:** AI-assisted optical positioning before imaging.
**Related equipment:** SGRT + automated iso-center calculation.
**Radiotherapy Example:** Chest wall setup requires no skin marks.

218. **Volumetric Ring Planning Technique:** Using concentric ring structures around PTV to force high dose fall-off.
**Related equipment:** Dose gradient optimizer.
**Radiotherapy Example:** Applied in brain SRS near critical structures.

219. **Vertebral Alignment Deviation Check:** Verifies vertebral body alignment for spine irradiation accuracy.
**Related equipment:** kV orthogonal pair, CBCT.
**Radiotherapy Example:** Prevents spinal cord miss during spinal metastasis RT.

220. **. Visual Symmetry Matching:** Matching patient setup visually against baseline body contour.
**Related equipment:** SGRT.
**Radiotherapy Example:** Used for bilateral breast DIBH alignment.

221. **Ventilation-Weighted Dose Optimization:** Reducing radiation dose to highly ventilated lung areas.
**Related equipment:** 4D-CT + ventilation imaging.
**Radiotherapy Example:** Reduces risk of pneumonitis during lung VMAT.

222. **Vascular Micro-OAR Auto-Segmentation:** Algorithm that automatically segments small blood vessels for planning safety.
**Related equipment:** AI organ segmentation.
**Radiotherapy Example:** Protects coronary arteries in left breast IMRT.

223. **Vacuum Thermoplastic Mould Sealing:** Air-tight sealing of moulds to form rigid immobilization.
**Related equipment:** Mould room vacuum press machine.
**Radiotherapy Example:** Used to create firm face masks for SRS.

224. **Voxel-Precise Electron Density Override:** Manually adjusting CT density of objects affecting dose.
**Related equipment:** CT-to-density assignment tool.
**Radiotherapy Example:** Overrides density of hip prosthesis for accurate pelvic IMRT.

225. **Virtual Boost Mapping:** Overlaying boost plan over primary plan to review cumulative dose.
**Related equipment:** Dose accumulation system.
**Radiotherapy Example:** Ensures safe spinal cord tolerance during IMRT boost.

226. **Ventricle Dose Limitation Envelope:** Dose restriction boundary around brain ventricles to prevent cognitive decline.
**Related equipment:** OAR envelope tool.
**Radiotherapy Example:** Applied during whole brain RT with hippocampal sparing.

227. **View-Fusion Imaging Protocol:** Overlaying multiple imaging modalities for accurate alignment.
**Related equipment:** CT-MRI fusion, PET-CT fusion tools.
**Radiotherapy Example:** Used in glioma target contouring.

228. **Veneer Shield Customization:** Thin shielding layer built to reduce dose to critical surface areas.
**Related equipment:** Low-Z shell & 3D printer.
**Radiotherapy Example:** Protects nose cartilage during skin cancer RT.

229. **Vacuum Patient Cradle Memory Index:** Measure of immobilization reproducibility stored per patient.
**Related equipment:** Vacuum cradle scanner.
**Radiotherapy Example:** Reduces setup variability during abdominal SBRT.

230. **Volumetric Adaptive Oversight:** Physician review of daily dose accumulation changes.
**Related equipment:** Adaptive RT system.
**Radiotherapy Example:** Approves plan adaptation based on CBCT anatomical change.

231. **Visual Film-to-EPID Cross Calibration:** Method comparing film and EPID response for IMRT QA.
**Related equipment:** EPID, radiochromic film.
**Radiotherapy Example:** Ensures accurate QA for head & neck IMRT.

232. **Virtual Immobilization Decision Tree:** Decision algorithm selecting appropriate immobilization devices.
**Related equipment:** Mould room selection software.
**Radiotherapy Example:** Chooses head mask for NPC, vacuum bag for abdomen.

233. **Ventral Beam Dose Surveillance:** Monitoring maximum dose to chest and abdomen surfaces.
**Related equipment:** Skin dose map tools.
**Radiotherapy Example:** Used for breast field-in-field treatment.

234. **Volumetric Bolus Sculpting:** Digitally designing bolus shape to fit 3D surface without air gaps.
**Related equipment:** 3D printer, bolus design software.
**Radiotherapy Example:** Used for post-mastectomy chest wall treatments.

235. **Virtual Plan Override Safeguard:** Prevents simulation plan from being used incorrectly for treatment.
**Related equipment:** TPS safety lock.
**Radiotherapy Example:** Avoids delivering CT sim beams by mistake.

236. **Voxel-Target Statistical Ranking:** Ranking tumor sub-regions based on aggressiveness markers.
**Related equipment:** PET-segmentation tool.
**Radiotherapy Example:** Helps plan dose-painting in head & neck cancer.

237. **Visualized Arc Sector Avoidance:** Using visual arc maps to block arcs through sensitive structures.
**Related equipment:** VMAT path visualizer.
**Radiotherapy Example:** Avoids contralateral breast in left breast VMAT.

238. **Variable Fraction Dose Escalation:** Increasing dose per fraction in later course of treatment based on tolerance.
**Related equipment:** Adaptive schedule planner.
**Radiotherapy Example:** Used to escalate dose in rectal cancer chemoradiation.

239. **Virtual Soft-Tissue Landmark Tracker:** AI tool that tracks anatomical landmarks rather than bony anatomy.
**Related equipment:** Deformable IGRT.
**Radiotherapy Example:** Aligns uterus/cervix based on soft tissue rather than bones.

240. **Volumetric Hotspot Redistribution:** Shifts unintended hotspots from critical areas to safer areas.
**Related equipment:** IMRT optimizer smoothing tool.
**Radiotherapy Example:** Moves spinal cord hotspot into muscle in thoracic IMRT.

241. **Variable Penumbra Edge Control:** Technique used to adjust beam penumbra to improve dose fall-off at field borders.
**Related equipment:** MLCs, jaw system, LINAC beam shaping.
**Radiotherapy Example:** Used to spare spinal cord during thoracic spine IMRT by tightening penumbra.

242. **Volumetric Registration Consistency Check:** Verification that volumetric image registration remains accurate across multiple scans.
**Related equipment:** TPS deformable registration, CBCT/CT datasets.
**Radiotherapy Example:** Ensures prostate alignment consistency across all fractions during IGRT.

243. **Virtual Couch-Shift Simulation:** Software simulation predicting dose effect of couch shifts before applying them clinically.
**Related equipment:** Image-guided couch shift calculation software.
**Radiotherapy Example:** Avoids hotspot shift into the parotid gland during head & neck IMRT.

244. **Voxel-Level Organ Tracking:** Real-time monitoring of soft-tissue voxel displacement during treatment.
**Related equipment:** SGRT, 4D CBCT.
**Radiotherapy Example:** Used during pancreatic SBRT to ensure safe dose delivery while the duodenum moves.

245. **Ventral Deficit Compensation Planning:** Technique that increases beam modulation to compensate for high attenuation surfaces.
**Related equipment:** IMRT optimizer, CT density map.
**Radiotherapy Example:** Corrects dose underestimation in chest wall radiotherapy for large-breasted patients.

246. **Verification Beam Preview:** Image preview of expected portal image before beam delivery.
**Related equipment:** LINAC EPID prediction software.
**Radiotherapy Example:** Prevents treatment errors by previewing pelvic IMRT fields before delivery.

247. **Virtual Patient Density Mapping:** Automated mapping of body density variations for dose calculation.
**Related equipment:** CT HU-to-density engine, Monte Carlo.
**Radiotherapy Example:** Improves dose accuracy in lung SBRT with highly heterogeneous tissue.

248. **Vacuum Lock Reproducibility Index:** Score measuring repeatability of patient immobilization with vacuum cushions.
**Related equipment:** Vac-Lok cushions, mould room immobilization database.
**Radiotherapy Example:** Tracks reproducibility for prostate IMRT patients.

249. **Vascular OAR Avoidance Shell:** Dose-avoidance structure placed around major vessels.
**Related equipment:** TPS auto-segmentation tool.
**Radiotherapy Example:** Protects carotid arteries during larynx IMRT.

**250. Volume-Based Tolerance Protocol:** QA method evaluating dose tolerance based on % of organ volume receiving radiation.
**Related equipment:** DVH analysis tool.
**Radiotherapy Example:** Uses V20 lung constraint for NSCLC radiation safety.

**251. Variable CT Slice Reconstruction Rule:** Altering CT slice thickness to match contouring precision requirements.
**Related equipment:** CT simulator reconstruction settings.
**Radiotherapy Example:** Narrow slice spacing used for SRS brain metastasis planning.

**252. Virtual Immobilization Pressure Mapping:** Visualization of immobilization pressure distribution on patient skin.
**Related equipment:** Pressure-mapping pads in mould room.
**Radiotherapy Example:** Prevents pressure sores during long spine RT sessions.

**253. Voxelized Dose Risk Projection:** Predicting toxicity risk based on voxel-level dose statistics.
**Related equipment:** AI dose-to-toxicity prediction models.
**Radiotherapy Example:** Predicts xerostomia risk for parotid doses in head & neck IMRT.

**254. Ventilated Lung Replanning Trigger:** Automated notification when lung ventilation changes in repeated CBCTs.
**Related equipment:** 4D-CBCT ventilation monitoring tool.
**Radiotherapy Example:** Identifies patients who require adaptive lung RT.

**255. Verification of Couch Angle Sag:** Measuring couch sag and compensating its effect in dose planning.
**Related equipment:** LINAC couch QA system.
**Radiotherapy Example:** Used for SRS couch angles > 90° to maintain targeting accuracy.

**256. Volumetric Film Calibration Curve:** Film-dose calibration model validating 3D dose distribution.
**Related equipment:** Radiochromic films, dose calibration scanner.
**Radiotherapy Example:** Used in completeness IMRT QA for head & neck.

**257. Virtual Patient Breathing Tutor:** Visual coaching system for encouraging repeatable breathing patterns.
**Related equipment:** DIBH/BH audiovisual breathing guidance.
**Radiotherapy Example:** Used for left breast DIBH to reduce heart dose.

**258. Voxel-Refined Bolus Contact Score:** Metric quantifying surface contact quality between bolus and skin.
**Related equipment:** Surface scan + bolus fit analysis tool.
**Radiotherapy Example:** Scores contact during chest wall radiation to avoid underdosing.

**259. Volumetric Hotspot Probability Estimation:** Probability prediction of high-dose regions forming during optimization.
**Related equipment:** Predictive IMRT optimizer.
**Radiotherapy Example:** Prevents hotspots on ribs during lung IMRT.

**260. Vascular Enhancement CT Protocol:** CT protocol designed to maximize visibility of blood vessels for contouring.
**Related equipment:** Contrast CT scanner & injection timing software.
**Radiotherapy Example:** Improves carotid delineation during hypopharyngeal tumor planning.

**261. Virtual Shield Block Segmentation:** Algorithm generating digital shielding blocks in the TPS.
**Related equipment:** 2D block contouring tool.
**Radiotherapy Example:** Used for electron treatments to shield nose bridge.

262. **Ventral Stabilization Strap:** Strap used to stabilize soft tissue movement during RT.
**Related equipment:** Bellyboard/abdominal compression.
**Radiotherapy Example:** Reduces diaphragmatic motion during pancreatic SBRT.

263. **Vector-Controlled Dose-Painting:** Dose sculpting based on biologic and metabolic imaging vectors.
**Related equipment:** PET-guided dose painting optimizer.
**Radiotherapy Example:** Elevates dose in PET-avid zones of oropharyngeal carcinoma.

264. **Volumetric Scatter Estimation Correction:** Correcting scattered radiation effect in 3D dose calculation.
**Related equipment:** Monte Carlo dose engine.
**Radiotherapy Example:** Improves electron dose accuracy around breast prosthesis.

265. **Variable Density Phantom Verification:** QA phantom mimicking different densities of human tissues.
**Related equipment:** Multi-density phantom.
**Radiotherapy Example:** Used for Monte Carlo IMRT commissioning.

266. **Virtual Wedge Decay Compensation:** Compensation for change in dose profile when using virtual wedges.
**Related equipment:** Dynamic wedge delivery on LINAC.
**Radiotherapy Example:** Used in pelvis RT to equalize dose distribution.

267. **Voxel Specific Target Boosting:** Boosting dose to high-risk tumor voxels while maintaining organ sparing.
**Related equipment:** PET-guided adaptive optimization.
**Radiotherapy Example:** Used in glioblastoma dose escalation trials.

268. **Vacuum Headrest Reusability Protocol:** Rules ensuring safe reuse of vacuum immobilization cushions.
**Related equipment:** Mould room immobilization records.
**Radiotherapy Example:** Used for repeated cranial RT for benign tumors.

269. **Visual Interlock System:** Prevents beam start without proper visualization confirmation.
**Related equipment:** IGRT + LINAC beam lock connection.
**Radiotherapy Example:** Stops beam if CBCT alignment is ignored.

270. **Vessel-Sparing IMRT Strategy:** Treatment planning technique to reduce dose to critical vessels.
**Related equipment:** IMRT optimizer vessel-avoidance map.
**Radiotherapy Example:** Protects aorta during retroperitoneal sarcoma RT.

271. **Vacuum Pelvis Mask Support:** Hybrid thermoplastic-vacuum support for pelvic reproducibility.
**Related equipment:** Thermoplastic belt + Vac-Lok.
**Radiotherapy Example:** Reduces setup error in cervical cancer radiotherapy.

272. **Voxelized Dose Gradient Check:** Detecting insufficient steepness of dose fall-off.
**Related equipment:** DVH gradient analyzer.
**Radiotherapy Example:** Used in brain SRS to protect optic chiasm.

273. **Virtual Respiratory Motion Rebuild:** Reconstructing 4D breathing motion from CBCT sequences.
**Related equipment:** 4D IGRT image reconstruction.
**Radiotherapy Example:** Improves internal target volume accuracy in lung SBRT.

274. **Volumetric Electron Applicator Planning:** 3D planning for electron beam conformal dose shaping.
**Related equipment:** 3D electron TPS tool.
**Radiotherapy Example:** Ensures uniform dose to scalp lesion without overdosing brain.

275. **Verification of CT-to-MRI Fusion Drift:** Checking if image fusion alignment accuracy decreases with time.
**Related equipment:** TPS fusion QA tool.
**Radiotherapy Example:** Prevents contour misalignment in brain RT.

276. **Voxel Toxicity Prediction Index:** Score linking dose to probability of toxicity effects region-wise.
**Related equipment:** AI dose prediction system.
**Radiotherapy Example:** Predicts risk of radiation-induced dysphagia.

277. **Variable Wall Thickness Bolus:** Bolus with multiple thicknesses for irregular surfaces.
**Related equipment:** 3D printed bolus.
**Radiotherapy Example:** Used for nose and cheek skin cancer RT.

278. **Visible Iso-Center Projection Light:** Light system used to visually verify patient is aligned to iso-center.
**Related equipment:** LINAC room lasers.
**Radiotherapy Example:** Used during CT simulation and setup verification.

279. **Virtual Shield for Dental Fillings:** Auto-generated high-density override and dose compensation around teeth.
**Related equipment:** CT artifact correction + override tool.
**Radiotherapy Example:** Prevents hotspots in oral cavity IMRT.

280. **Vacuum Mold Growth Prevention Protocol:** Hygiene and storage procedure to stop microbial growth inside moulds.
**Related equipment:** Mould room hygiene system.
**Radiotherapy Example:** Maintains skin safety for repeated mask users.

281. **Vertex Beam Obstruction Check:** Detecting potential collisions during vertex irradiation.
**Related equipment:** LINAC collision simulator.
**Radiotherapy Example:** Ensures safety during cranial vertex field delivery.

282. **Visual Sag Correction Viewer:** Tool to visualize couch sag and auto-correct beam isocenter.
**Related equipment:** EPID + couch calibration software.
**Radiotherapy Example:** Maintains accuracy during non-coplanar SRS.

283. **Vascular Dose-Bath Minimization:** Minimizing dose to surrounding healthy vasculature.
**Related equipment:** VMAT arc exclusion zones.
**Radiotherapy Example:** Protects iliac vessels during rectal IMRT.

284. **Volumetric Ion Chamber Survey:** Measuring 3D dose with multiple ion chambers simultaneously.
**Related equipment:** 3D ion chamber array phantom.
**Radiotherapy Example:** Used during commissioning of new LINAC.

285. **Variable Anatomy Matching Mode:** IGRT alignment mode prioritizing different regions based on anatomy.
**Related equipment:** CBCT anatomical region weighting tool.
**Radiotherapy Example:** Prioritize prostate matching rather than pelvic bone matching.

286. **Voxel-Resolved Skin Dose Tracking:** Tracking surface dose voxel-by-voxel during treatment.
**Related equipment:** EPID skin dose calculator.
**Radiotherapy Example:** Ensures safe surface dose in breast boost.

287. **Vertical Couch Displacement Control:** Restricting couch vertical movement to avoid targeting changes.
**Related equipment:** LINAC couch interlock.
**Radiotherapy Example:** Prevents Y-axis error during spine irradiation.

288. **Virtual Ring Avoidance Constraint:** Artificial ring volume created to push dose away from OAR.
**Related equipment:** Dose-contouring tools.
**Radiotherapy Example:** Moves dose away from brainstem in posterior fossa IMRT.

289. **Visible Patient Tattoo Reduction:** Surface-guided method that eliminates need for permanent tattoos.
**Related equipment:** SGRT system.
**Radiotherapy Example:** Used for breast RT without tattoo markings.

290. **Ventilation-Averaged Gating:** Gating based on predicted breathing pattern rather than instantaneous cycle.
**Related equipment:** 4D gating system.
**Radiotherapy Example:** Improves lung tumor coverage in irregular breathers.

291. **Voxel-Priority OAR Exclusion:** TPS exclusion mode to prioritize sparing selected voxels of an OAR.
**Related equipment:** IMRT optimizer.
**Radiotherapy Example:** Reduces cochlea voxel doses in nasopharynx RT.

292. **Verification of Beam Output Drift:** Routine check of dose output fluctuations over time.
**Related equipment:** Daily QA phantom, ion chamber.
**Radiotherapy Example:** Detects LINAC dose output deviation before treatment.

293. **Virtual Tumor Expansion Predictor:** AI-based prediction of tumor progression during radiotherapy.
**Related equipment:** Adaptive RT analytic module.
**Radiotherapy Example:** Adjusts IMRT boost plan for evolving glioma.

294. **Vacuum Shell Depth Analysis:** Evaluating uniformity of shell thickness in immobilization masks.
**Related equipment:** 3D thickness scanner.
**Radiotherapy Example:** Ensures consistent thermoplastic shell strength for SRS.

295. **Volume-Adaptive MLC Modulation:** Real-time modulation of MLC leaves based on anatomy changes.
**Related equipment:** Adaptive MLC tracking software.
**Radiotherapy Example:** Dynamic modulation during liver SBRT.

296. **Variational Dose Kernel Optimization:** Advanced dose algorithm minimizing calculation error in heterogeneities.
**Related equipment:** Monte Carlo high-precision dose engine.
**Radiotherapy Example:** Used for lung tumor dose calculation.

297. **Visual Surface Color Map Setup Aid:** Color-coded alignment overlay displayed on patient surface.
**Related equipment:** SGRT.
**Radiotherapy Example:** Breast setup without tattoos or skin markers.

298. **Voxelized PET-Dose Correlation Model:** Mapping PET tracer uptake with delivered dose to evaluate response.
**Related equipment:** PET-RT analytics.
**Radiotherapy Example:** Used in adaptive dose painting for head & neck tumors.

299. **Verification of Collimator Twist:** Checking accuracy of collimator rotation relative to isocenter.
**Related equipment:** Collimator rotation QA tool.
**Radiotherapy Example:** Required before complex VMAT/SRS deliveries.

300. **Volume-Locked Adaptive Beam Strategy:** Prevents plan adaptation from reducing PTV coverage during adaptive RT.
**Related equipment:** Adaptive plan safeguard module.
**Radiotherapy Example:** Ensures full target coverage during prostate adaptive treatment.

301. **Variable Dose Fall-Off Steering:** Real-time steering of dose gradient to sharpen fall-off near critical organs.
**Related equipment:** IMRT/VMAT optimizer, MLC steering module.
**Radiotherapy Example:** Used to protect brainstem during nasopharynx IMRT.

302. **Virtual Dose Shielding Ring:** Artificial avoidance ring placed around OAR to push dose away during planning.
**Related equipment:** Dose shaping tool in TPS.
**Radiotherapy Example:** Used to reduce optic chiasm dose in skull-base radiotherapy.

303. **Vascular Structure Prioritization Index:** Score describing importance of sparing particular blood vessels during RT.
**Related equipment:** TPS vessel auto-contouring and weight assignment.
**Radiotherapy Example:** Protects carotid arteries in larynx IMRT.

304. **Ventral Beam Incidence Control:** Rule limiting number of beams entering from the front to reduce dose to anterior organs.
**Related equipment:** VMAT arc modification tool.
**Radiotherapy Example:** Avoids excessive skin dose in chest wall RT.

305. **Voxel Predictive Setup Drift Model:** Predicts setup deviation of target voxels across fractions.
**Related equipment:** CBCT-based adaptive RT analytics.
**Radiotherapy Example:** Predicts prostate drift relative to bladder filling.

306. **Visual Beam's Eye View Collision Alert:** Collision warning while previewing BEV angles.
**Related equipment:** LINAC 3D collision simulator.
**Radiotherapy Example:** Prevents gantry–head support collision during cranial SRS.

307. **Virtual LUT Bolus Optimization:** Bolus planning using lookup tables for skin dose uniformity.
**Related equipment:** 3D printed bolus design tool.
**Radiotherapy Example:** Controls buildup region in scalp irradiation.

308. **Voxelized QA Dose Verification:** QA system evaluating dose per voxel instead of per region.
**Related equipment:** 3D dosimeter & EPID-reconstruction.
**Radiotherapy Example:** Validates SBRT dose accuracy for liver tumors.

309. **Variable Fractionation Planning:** Non-constant dose per fraction strategy to reduce toxicity.
**Related equipment:** Biological optimization engine.
**Radiotherapy Example:** High dose fractions early for glioblastoma followed by reduced fractions near optic nerves.

310. **Virtual Immobilization Shoulder Relief:** Immobilization refinement to reduce shoulder tension during mask fixation.
**Related equipment:** Mould room mask positioning insert.
**Radiotherapy Example:** Reduces shoulder movement during head & neck IMRT.

311. **Vector-Aligned Beam Modulation:** Beam fluence modulation aligned with directional sensitivity of anatomy.
**Related equipment:** IMRT directional modulation tool.
**Radiotherapy Example:** Used to protect ribs during lung RT.

312. **Verification of 4D CT Reconstruction Timing:** Checking accuracy of respiratory phase sorting.
**Related equipment:** 4D CT simulator.
**Radiotherapy Example:** Ensures correct tumor phase matching for gating in lung SBRT.

313. **Volumetric Lymph Node Boost Strategy:** Targeted dose escalation to involved lymph nodes only.
**Related equipment:** VMAT nodal boost optimizer.
**Radiotherapy Example:** Treats pelvic nodes in cervical cancer RT while sparing bowel.

314. **Virtual Portal Image Alignment Overlay:** Digital overlay showing expected vs actual portal image for verification.
**Related equipment:** EPID/QC alignment software.
**Radiotherapy Example:** Confirms pelvis AP/PA field match before treatment start.

315. **Voxel Fatigue Toxicity Mapping:** Mapping and predicting cumulative fatigue symptoms based on dose to specific tissues.
**Related equipment:** AI risk-prediction software.
**Radiotherapy Example:** Predicts fatigue risk in breast RT.

316. **Vacuum Fixture Accuracy Check:** Verification of air displacement in vacuum immobilization devices.
**Related equipment:** Vac-Lok pressure gauge.
**Radiotherapy Example:** Ensures pelvic SBRT immobilization holds position.

317. **Vascularized Organ Dose Heterogeneity Control:** Algorithm preventing high dose difference inside vascular organs.
**Related equipment:** IMRT optimizer constraint tool.
**Radiotherapy Example:** Ensures uniform dose in kidneys during abdominal RT.

318. **Verification of CT Couch Top Shift:** Checking shifts caused by different couch tops between CT and LINAC.
**Related equipment:** CT couch index → LINAC couch mapping tool.
**Radiotherapy Example:** Prevents indexing mismatch during brain RT.

319. **Virtual Respiratory Coaching Display:** Animation used to guide patient to maintain consistent breathing amplitude.
**Related equipment:** BH/DIBH audiovisual tracking.
**Radiotherapy Example:** Used in left breast DIBH to reduce heart dose.

320. **Voxel-Level Cold Spot Detection:** Automatic analysis identifying underdosed regions.
**Related equipment:** TPS cold-spot search algorithm.
**Radiotherapy Example:** Prevents underdose inside PTV during spine IMRT.

321. **Vertebral Body Alignment Anchoring:** Using spine vertebra as setup anchor rather than soft tissue.
**Related equipment:** CBCT bone matching.
**Radiotherapy Example:** Used in spine SBRT to ensure correct targeting.

322. **Virtual Beam Weight Normalization:** Balancing beam weight across multiple beams automatically.
**Related equipment:** VMAT optimizer.
**Radiotherapy Example:** Improves target dose uniformity in pelvic RT.

323. **Ventilation-Weighted Lung Dose Reduction:** Prioritizing avoidance of highly ventilated lung tissue.
**Related equipment:** 4D ventilation-map planning.
**Radiotherapy Example:** Reduces pneumonitis risk in lung RT.

324. **Variable Noise Suppression in CT:** Adjusting CT filtering level based on anatomical density.
**Related equipment:** CT iterative reconstruction.
**Radiotherapy Example:** Improves soft-tissue visibility for prostate contouring.

325. **Varian ALC/MLC Log Verification:** QA check comparing MLC log files to planned leaf movement.
**Related equipment:** LINAC log validation software.
**Radiotherapy Example:** Confirms integrity of MLC delivery in VMAT.

326. **Voxel-Selective Replanning Flag:** Auto flag when specific target voxels fall below prescription.
**Related equipment:** Adaptive RT monitoring.
**Radiotherapy Example:** Early trigger for CTV replanning in bladder RT.

327. **Virtual Orthogonal Imaging Preview:** Pre-display of kV orthogonal fields for alignment check.
**Related equipment:** kV panel + simulation console.
**Radiotherapy Example:** Prevents pelvic matching error before first fraction.

328. **Vacuum Mask Air-Pocket Sensor:** Detects trapped air pockets inside thermoplastic mask system.
**Related equipment:** 3D mask pressure mapping.
**Radiotherapy Example:** Used for cranial SRS to avoid micro-movements.

329. **Visual Dose Cloud Animation:** Moving 3D visualization of gradient and isodose cloud around target.
**Related equipment:** TPS 4D visualization tool.
**Radiotherapy Example:** Improves communication during brain tumor planning review.

330. **Vascular Calcification Density Override:** Overriding high-density calcifications that would distort dose.
**Related equipment:** CT ROI override tool.
**Radiotherapy Example:** Stabilizes dose near heavily calcified carotids in elderly patients.

331. **Verification of Beam Interruption Resume:** QA ensuring treatment resumes correctly after pause.
**Related equipment:** LINAC beam sequence log.
**Radiotherapy Example:** Used during long VMAT deliveries to avoid field restart errors.

332. **Variable Isocenter Correction Algorithm:** Auto repositioning of isocenter based on multiple anatomy anchors.
**Related equipment:** IGRT auto-match.
**Radiotherapy Example:** Used for prostate RT when bladder filling varies.

333. **Visual Bolus Edge Seal Inspection:** Visual inspection method to verify bolus fully seals to skin.
**Related equipment:** Mould room surface scanner.
**Radiotherapy Example:** Prevents dose deficit during scar boost.

334. **Voxelized Organ Motion Atlas:** Database of known motion patterns of organs across patients.
**Related equipment:** Motion pattern AI.
**Radiotherapy Example:** Used to guide PTV margin for pancreas RT.

335. **Vocal Cord Functional Dose Model:** Predictive dose model assessing vocal cord damage risk.
**Related equipment:** Organ function dose prediction software.
**Radiotherapy Example:** Applied in hypopharynx IMRT.

336. **Verification Template for Daily CBCT:** Predefined list of checkpoints before approving daily IGRT.
**Related equipment:** IGRT check protocol.
**Radiotherapy Example:** Used for prostate SBRT systematic review.

337. **Variable Arc Exclusion Mode:** Excludes gantry angles passing near vulnerable organs.
**Related equipment:** VMAT arc shaping tool.
**Radiotherapy Example:** Avoids bowel loops in retroperitoneal sarcoma RT.

338. **Virtual Laser Projection Preview:** 3D preview of laser alignment expected at treatment room.
**Related equipment:** CT sim → LINAC laser mapping.
**Radiotherapy Example:** Prevents tattoo misalignment in breast RT.

339. **Volumetric Linac Head Scatter Model:** Scatter model characterizing dose originating from LINAC head.
**Related equipment:** Monte Carlo scatter modeling.
**Radiotherapy Example:** Increases dose accuracy in large field pelvic RT.

340. **Ventral Chest Compression Setup:** Compression method reducing respiratory amplitude.
**Related equipment:** Abdominal compression board.
**Radiotherapy Example:** Used for pancreatic and liver SBRT.

341. **Voxel-Indexed Fractionation Sensitivity:** Sensitivity of each voxel to fraction size differences.
**Related equipment:** Biologically weighted dose calculator.
**Radiotherapy Example:** For fraction-change trials in brain tumors.

342. **Verification of Deformation Smoothness:** Ensuring deformable image registration is smooth and realistic.
**Related equipment:** DIR QA tool.
**Radiotherapy Example:** Avoids distortions in adaptive bladder RT.

343. **Virtual Tumor Shrinkage Response Score:** Score predicting how fast tumor volume reduces during RT.
**Related equipment:** Adaptive RT prediction engine.
**Radiotherapy Example:** Used to adjust head & neck boost dose timing.

344. **V-Shaped MLC Segment Technique:** Beam shaping pattern using V-shaped leaf configuration.
**Related equipment:** IMRT segment editor.
**Radiotherapy Example:** Conforms dose around spinal cord in thoracic spine RT.

345. **Visual Breathing Synchronization Alert:** Alarm when patient deviates from breathing pattern.
**Related equipment:** Gating respiratory trace monitor.
**Radiotherapy Example:** Used during DIBH left breast RT.

346. **Velocity-Driven Organ Shift Predictor:** Predicts organ drift speed during treatment.
**Related equipment:** AI IGRT motion tracking.
**Radiotherapy Example:** Used in liver tumor gating.

347. **Volume-Offset Entrance Dose Calibration:** Entrance dose correction based on body size.
**Related equipment:** Entrance dose detector.
**Radiotherapy Example:** Used during TBI patient QA.

348. **Virtual Multi-Field Match Line Preview:** Preview of match lines between two abutting treatment fields.
**Related equipment:** BEV junction simulator.
**Radiotherapy Example:** Avoids overdose in cranio-spinal RT match.

349. **Vacuum-Support Thermal Safety Index:** Index assessing safe temperature range while molding masks.
**Related equipment:** Thermoplastic heater monitoring.
**Radiotherapy Example:** Prevents burns during mask creation in mould room.

350. **Voxel-Optimal SRS Shell Margin:** Optimal safety margin for cranium SRS based on voxel risk.
**Related equipment:** TPS stereotactic dose expansion tool.
**Radiotherapy Example:** Protects optic nerve while covering pituitary tumor.

351. **Visual Adaptive Dose Forecast:** Predictive visualization of how dose distribution will change with adaptation.
**Related equipment:** Adaptive TPS forecast module.
**Radiotherapy Example:** Shows parotid gland sparing benefit before replanning.

352. **Vascular Organ Mean Dose Suppressor:** Algorithm reducing mean dose for blood-rich organs.
**Related equipment:** IMRT optimizer function.
**Radiotherapy Example:** Protects liver in abdominal RT.

353. **Verification of Detector Angular Dependence:** Ensuring detector sensitivity stays stable under rotated angles.
**Related equipment:** 2D/3D detector array QA.
**Radiotherapy Example:** Used for VMAT QA arcs.

354. **Virtual Position Re-Indexing:** Simulation re-mapping patient index marks to LINAC couch coordinates.
**Related equipment:** External/internal indexing converter.
**Radiotherapy Example:** Prevents pelvic index mismatch errors.

355. **Voxel-Based Metal Artifact Exclusion:** Removing corrupted voxels caused by dental fillings or prosthetics.
**Related equipment:** CT MAR + override tool.
**Radiotherapy Example:** Eliminates false hotspots in oral cavity IMRT.

356. **Variable Beam Divergence Compensation:** Corrections applied to compensate for geometric beam divergence.
**Related equipment:** IMRT collimator optimization.
**Radiotherapy Example:** Used in large field mantle RT.

357. **Visual Misalignment Threshold Indicator:** Display that marks alignment status as safe/unsafe.
**Related equipment:** SGRT deviation indicator.
**Radiotherapy Example:** Stops beam delivery if patient moves during breast RT.

358. **Verification of Real-Time Couch Tracking:** QA simulated to test if couch tracking follows tumor motion accurately.
**Related equipment:** Tumor-tracking couch module.
**Radiotherapy Example:** Used in liver and pancreas SBRT.

359. **Virtual Catheter Path Dose Mapping:** Dose mapping along catheter path in brachy-like external beam cases.
**Related equipment:** TPS catheter mapping tool.
**Radiotherapy Example:** Used in HDR-style boost for gynecological tumors.

360. **Voxel Expansion Constraint Matrix:** Restricting PTV expansion in directions where toxicity risk is high.
**Related equipment:** Directional PTV expansion tool.
**Radiotherapy Example:** Avoids anterior expansion toward bowel in pelvis RT.

361. **Ventral Surface Dose Guard:** Control mechanism to reduce anterior skin dose.
**Related equipment:** Beam weight balancing + internal bolus avoidance.
**Radiotherapy Example:** Used in paediatric mediastinum RT.

362. **Virtual Couch Sag Compensation Map:** Applies geometric correction for couch sag based on weight.
**Related equipment:** LINAC couch sag lookup model.
**Radiotherapy Example:** Used in cranial SRS at lateral couch angles.

363. **Vascular Perfusion PET Dose Painting:** PET-guided dose painting based on tumor blood supply.
**Related equipment:** FDG-PET + RT fusion.
**Radiotherapy Example:** Escalates dose to high-flow regions in head & neck cancer.

364. **Verification Auto-Checklist for SBRT:** Series of mandatory checks before SBRT delivery begins.
**Related equipment:** SBRT safety checklist console.
**Radiotherapy Example:** Ensures both kidneys are correctly spared in renal SBRT.

365. **Visual Isodose Feathering Strategy:** Feathering dose gradients between match lines.
**Related equipment:** Multi-junction dose blurring tool.
**Radiotherapy Example:** Used in craniospinal RT.

366. **Voxel Integrity Dose Review:** Reviewing dose changes to maintain voxel-level RT safety.
**Related equipment:** Adaptive dose review platform.
**Radiotherapy Example:** Avoids parotid overdose during H&N replanning.

367. **Vacuum Index Replication Protocol:** Reproducing exact air displacement for identical immobilization.
**Related equipment:** Mould room vacuum cushion database.
**Radiotherapy Example:** For pelvic IMRT patients needing mask remake.

368. **Vena Cava Dose Constraint Strategy:** Restricting dose to inferior vena cava in abdominal RT.
**Related equipment:** High-priority OAR constraint mapping.
**Radiotherapy Example:** Used in retroperitoneal sarcoma RT.

369. **Virtual Adaptive Bolus Removal:** Removing bolus later in treatment when skin dose is no longer needed.
**Related equipment:** Adaptive plan schedule.
**Radiotherapy Example:** In breast RT after tumour bed response is observed.

370. **Visual Field Junction Monitoring:** Tool monitoring dose distribution at field junctions.
**Related equipment:** BEV junction dose analyzer.
**Radiotherapy Example:** Prevents cold/hot spots in spine irradiation.

371. **Voxelized Deformable Tracking:** Monitoring anatomical changes voxel-by-voxel over time.
**Related equipment:** Adaptive RT deformation tracking.
**Radiotherapy Example:** Used to track pancreatic tumor location day-by-day.

372. **Voice-Triggered Beam Stop:** Safety system allowing vocal interruption of beam by staff.
**Related equipment:** LINAC voice sensor interlock.
**Radiotherapy Example:** Emergency stop during patient panic episode.

373. **Verification of Gantry-Couch-Collimator Trio:** QA ensuring geometric accuracy of full trio combo.
**Related equipment:** Winston-Lutz phantom for non-coplanar QA.
**Radiotherapy Example:** Required before cranial SRS.

374. **Vaso-Protective Dose Painting:** Dose modulation to protect vascular supply of functional organs.
**Related equipment:** Biological dose optimizer.
**Radiotherapy Example:** Liver dose painting to protect hepatic artery.

375. **Virtual Reference Anatomy Overlay:** Overlay comparing actual anatomy to baseline reference.
**Related equipment:** CBCT anatomy overlay tool.
**Radiotherapy Example:** Identifies bladder-filling deviations.

376. **Voxel Reconstruction for Electron Scatter:** Automated reconstruction of scattering behavior in electrons.
**Related equipment:** Electron Monte Carlo engine.
**Radiotherapy Example:** Ensures accuracy in chest wall electron boost.

377. **Vacuum-Lock Headrest Re-Indexing:** Resetting headrest position to exact index point for setup.
**Related equipment:** Immob indexing rails.
**Radiotherapy Example:** Used in repeat cranial RT sessions.

378. **Visual Adaptive Bowel Displacement:** Display showing bowel displacement during CBCT.
**Related equipment:** Adaptive bowel-spacing tracker.
**Radiotherapy Example:** Used in cervix IMRT to trigger replanning.

379. **Variable Beam Energy Swap:** Switching beam energy automatically between plans when needed.
**Related equipment:** Multi-energy beam assignment tool.
**Radiotherapy Example:** 6MV & 10MV switching in prostate VMAT.

380. **Venous Contour Sensitivity Check:** Evaluates segmentation accuracy of veins and small vascular structures.
**Related equipment:** Auto-segmentation QA module.
**Radiotherapy Example:** Ensures jugular vein accuracy in neck RT.

381. **Visual Tattoo-Free Position Assurance:** Using SGRT instead of tattoos to ensure setup accuracy.
**Related equipment:** Surface guidance system.
**Radiotherapy Example:** Tattoo-free breast RT workflow.

382. **Verification of Low-Dose Bath Expansion:** Monitoring unintended spread of low-dose region outside target.
**Related equipment:** DVH & isodose cloud monitor.
**Radiotherapy Example:** Controls dose bath to bowel in abdominal RT.

383. **Virtual Clearance Route Simulation:** Simulation of safe paths for gantry and couch movements.
**Related equipment:** LINAC collision simulator.
**Radiotherapy Example:** Avoids collisions during H&N non-coplanar SRS.

384. **Visual Healthy Tissue Indicator:** Software highlighting irradiated vs spared normal tissue.
**Related equipment:** 3D tissue preservation map.
**Radiotherapy Example:** Used in paediatric cranial RT planning.

385. **Volume-Dependent Toxicity Curve:** Toxicity probability curve based on % of organ volume receiving dose.
**Related equipment:** NTCP calculator.
**Radiotherapy Example:** Lung V20 curve for NSCLC RT.

386. **Virtual Arc Reversal:** Reverse rotation of arc to improve dose conformity.
**Related equipment:** VMAT arc direction controller.
**Radiotherapy Example:** Reversed arcs help protect kidneys in abdominal RT.

387. **Ventral Immobilization Spine Pad:** Pad reducing spinal flexion in prone positioning.
**Related equipment:** Custom mould room pad.
**Radiotherapy Example:** Used for posterior spine radiotherapy.

388. **Voxel-Matched Isocenter Re-Anchoring:** Re-anchoring isocenter to voxel clusters without redefining whole plan.
**Related equipment:** IGRT adaptive isocenter tool.
**Radiotherapy Example:** Anchoring to residual tumor in adaptive brain RT.

389. **Visual 3D Organ-Dose Tolerance Dashboard:** Display showing whether organs meet tolerance in real time.
**Related equipment:** AI toxicity dashboard.
**Radiotherapy Example:** Used in head & neck IMRT planning review.

390. **Ventilation-Sensitive Collimator Shaping:** Adjusting MLC shape dynamically based on breathing motion.
**Related equipment:** Tracking-enabled MLC.
**Radiotherapy Example:** Reduces normal lung dose during SBRT.

391. **Verification of Thermal Mask Pressure Response:** Testing whether thermoplastic mask shrinks uniformly when heated.
**Related equipment:** Thermoplastic QA kit.
**Radiotherapy Example:** Ensures mask consistency for repeated mouldings.

392. **Variable Dose Penalty Weighting:** Weighting dose penalties differently based on organ importance.
**Related equipment:** IMRT cost function editor.
**Radiotherapy Example:** Heavier weight on spinal cord vs esophagus in thoracic RT.

393. **Voxel-Prioritized Hotspot Suppression:** Targeted suppression of hotspots inside organs or PTV.
**Related equipment:** Hotspot suppression optimizer.
**Radiotherapy Example:** Controls rib hotspots during breast RT.

394. **Virtual SBRT Auto-Approval Lock:** Forcing manual approval for every SBRT delivery to enhance safety.
**Related equipment:** SBRT safety interlock.
**Radiotherapy Example:** Prevents accidental auto-delivery without review.

395. **Vascularized Tumor Hypoxia Dose Boost:** Dose escalation for areas affected by hypoxia.
**Related equipment:** PET-oxygenation mapping.
**Radiotherapy Example:** Boosting hypoxic zones in HPV-negative head & neck cancer.

396. **Verification of Multi-Isocenter Synchronization:** QA ensuring two isocenters in craniospinal RT remain synced.
**Related equipment:** Winston-Lutz multi-ISO QA.
**Radiotherapy Example:** Used for cranial-spinal treatment in paediatrics.

397. **Virtual Jaw Transmission Model:** Modeling transmission dose through LINAC jaws.
**Related equipment:** Monte Carlo LINAC jaw model.
**Radiotherapy Example:** Improves dose accuracy in mantle RT.

398. **Vac-Support Head Lock Memory:** Memory-indexed mould room record storing exact head support geometry.
**Related equipment:** Immobilization database.
**Radiotherapy Example:** Identical repositioning for follow-up RT after recurrence.

399. **Voxel Resolution Boosting Filter:** Enhances resolution of dose grid for small targets.
**Related equipment:** TPS voxel refinement tool.
**Radiotherapy Example:** Used for 3-mm metastasis SRS.

400. **Visualization-Enhanced Patient Consent:** 3D dose and anatomy visualization used to explain treatment to patient.
**Related equipment:** Patient counselling VR visualization.
**Radiotherapy Example:** Helps paediatric patients understand brain RT.

401. **Volume Rendering:** Technique for constructing a 3D image from CT/MRI datasets.
**Related equipment:** TPS workstation, CT simulator.
**Radiotherapy Example:** Used during contouring to visualize tumour boundaries in 3D.

402. **Verification Film:** Radiographic film used to verify treatment field alignment.
**Related equipment:** KV imaging panel, portal film cassette.
**Radiotherapy Example:** Checking MLC field alignment on pelvis patients.

403. **Vertical Radiation Profile:** Intensity distribution of a radiation beam along vertical depth.
**Related equipment:** Water phantom, ionization chamber.
**Radiotherapy Example:** QA validation of beam flatness and symmetry.

404. **Virtual Couch Shift:** Couch correction calculated digitally rather than moving the physical couch.
**Related equipment:** IGRT software, KV-CBCT.
**Radiotherapy Example:** Suggested adjustments displayed before applying real couch movement.

405. **Visual Tracking System:** Monitors patient body markers to detect motion.
**Related equipment:** Optical surface monitoring cameras.
**Radiotherapy Example:** Respiratory control during left breast DIBH.

406. **Volume Breathing Curve:** Graph of lung volume change during respiration.
**Related equipment:** Respiratory gating system.
**Radiotherapy Example:** Used to plan gating window for lung SBRT.

407. **Vault Radiation Signage:** Mandatory radiation warning boards outside treatment vault.
**Related equipment:** Warning light system, access door interlock.
**Radiotherapy Example:** "Radiation ON" indicator flashes during LINAC beam delivery.

408. **Volumetric Image Registration:** Alignment of multiple 3D images to match anatomical structures.
**Related equipment:** CBCT, MRI–CT fusion software.
**Radiotherapy Example:** Fusion of MRI with CT for prostate contouring.

409. **Variable Dose Rate Function:** Algorithm that changes dose rate dynamically during arc delivery.
**Related equipment:** VMAT-enabled LINAC.
**Radiotherapy Example:** Smooth MLC modulation in VMAT head and neck plan.

410. **Visual QA Checklist:** Manual verification sheet ensuring treatment delivery steps are followed.
**Related equipment:** Patient chart, record-and-verify system.
**Radiotherapy Example:** Therapist signs checklist before each breast fraction.

411. **Voluntary Breath Hold:** Patient intentionally holds breath to reduce motion.
**Related equipment:** Surface monitoring system, gating system.
**Radiotherapy Example:** Used for left breast to reduce dose to heart.

412. **Virtual Reality Training Module:** VR platform for training staff on radiotherapy machine use.
**Related equipment:** VR headset, LINAC simulation software.
**Radiotherapy Example:** New therapists practice setup inside a virtual LINAC room.

413. **Verification CBCT Matching:** Alignment comparison between planning CT and pre-treatment CBCT.
**Related equipment:** On-board imager, registration software.
**Radiotherapy Example:** Pelvis patient match using bony landmarks.

414. **Vector Couch Correction:** Combined magnitude and direction of couch movement required to align target.
**Related equipment:** 6D robotic couch.
**Radiotherapy Example:** Correction calculated after CBCT for head and neck setup.

415. **Void Contouring:** Contouring empty cavities or spaces inside body.
**Related equipment:** TPS workstation.
**Radiotherapy Example:** Stomach and bowel voids contoured for abdomen IMRT planning.

416. **Variable Field Shaping:** Real-time change of field size during treatment.
**Related equipment:** Dynamic MLCs.
**Radiotherapy Example:** Used in VMAT arcs to spare parotid glands.

417. **Verification Image Storage Archive:** Cloud/local repository for storing portal & CBCT images.
**Related equipment:** PACS server.
**Radiotherapy Example:** IGRT images reviewed before every prostate fraction.

418. **Virtual Landmark Marking:** Digital marking of anatomical reference points.
**Related equipment:** Image registration software.
**Radiotherapy Example:** Carina marked virtually in lung IGRT.

419. **Ventral Beam Approach:** Beam entering from anterior or front side of patient.
**Related equipment:** LINAC gantry.
**Radiotherapy Example:** Anterior field used during emergency cord compression.

420. **Verification Log Analysis:** Review of machine delivery logs for accuracy.
**Related equipment:** Delivery log software, LINAC controller.
**Radiotherapy Example:** Checking gamma agreement between TPS and actual MU delivery.

421. **Vertical Gantry Collision Test:** Clearance check to prevent contact between gantry and patient/immobilization.
**Related equipment:** LINAC gantry, indexing system.
**Radiotherapy Example:** Tested for VMAT pelvis cases with bellyboard.

422. **Visual Isocenter Alignment:** Checking alignment to room lasers using physical markers.
**Related equipment:** Room lasers, alignment cross-wire.
**Radiotherapy Example:** Therapist aligns head and neck mask marks to lasers.

423. **Voxel Intensity Calibration:** Conversion of CT voxel values into electron density.
**Related equipment:** CT scanner, electron density phantom.
**Radiotherapy Example:** Used for accurate heterogeneity correction in lungs.

424. **Vascular Dose Visualization:** Assessment of dose delivered to major blood vessels.
**Related equipment:** TPS DVH.
**Radiotherapy Example:** Planning avoids high carotid dose in larynx treatment.

425. **Vault Shielding Survey:** Annual measurement ensuring radiation leakage is within safe limits.
**Related equipment:** Survey meter, area dosimeter.
**Radiotherapy Example:** Survey after LINAC energy upgrade.

426. **Vacuum Bag Indexing:** Unique connection of vacuum bag to treatment couch for reproducibility.
**Related equipment:** Index bars, mould room immobilization system.
**Radiotherapy Example:** SBRT lung patient positioned with same index each day.

427. **Volumetric Planning Dataset:** Complete CT image dataset used for contouring and planning.
**Related equipment:** CT simulator, TPS.
**Radiotherapy Example:** 3-mm slice CT imported into TPS for cervix planning.

428. **Void-to-Target Distance:** Distance between air cavity and tumour volume affecting dose distribution.
**Related equipment:** TPS dose algorithm.
**Radiotherapy Example:** High priority evaluation for head and neck mucosal cavities.

429. **Verification MU Check:** Secondary MU validation to confirm correct dose calculation.
**Related equipment:** MU calculation software, spreadsheets.
**Radiotherapy Example:** Hand calc validated before first fraction.

430. **Visual Surface Calibration:** Calibration of cameras used in optical surface monitoring systems.
**Related equipment:** Optical monitoring cameras.
**Radiotherapy Example:** Required monthly in DIBH breast clinics.

431. **Variable Wedge Offset:** Displacement between wedge direction and dose gradient axis.
**Related equipment:** Physical wedge or dynamic wedge.
**Radiotherapy Example:** Used to improve homogeneity in whole brain fields.

432. **Virtual Plan Comparison:** Evaluation of multiple plans to select best plan for treatment.
**Related equipment:** TPS plan evaluation module.
**Radiotherapy Example:** Compare 3DCRT vs IMRT for prostate case.

433. **Visible Skin Tattoo:** Permanent reference mark placed on patient skin.
**Related equipment:** Tattoo marker, needle.
**Radiotherapy Example:** Three tattoos used to localize isocenter on CT scan and LINAC.

434. **Verification Couch Angle:** Matching couch rotation between planned and treatment setup.
**Related equipment:** Couch angle digital display.
**Radiotherapy Example:** Head and neck IMRT with couch 350° verified prior to exposure.

435. **Vault Entry Sensor :** Sensor that disables beam if someone opens the door during treatment.
**Related equipment:** Door interlock system.
**Radiotherapy Example:** Beam automatically stops if staff re-enter vault.

436. **Visual Dose Hotspot Indicator:** Highlighting areas receiving higher dose than prescription.
**Related equipment:** TPS dose display.
**Radiotherapy Example:** Hotspot inside PTV adjusted for rectum IMRT.

437. **Variable Cone Collimation:** Altering cone size for small-field delivery.
**Related equipment:** SRS cones.
**Radiotherapy Example:** Cone-based trigeminal neuralgia radiosurgery.

438. **Verification of Respiratory Trace:** Matching planned vs real breathing motion.
**Related equipment:** Gating system respiratory trace graph.
**Radiotherapy Example:** Gating window adjusted for liver SBRT.

439. **Voxel Mass Density Map:** Mapping tissue density values per voxel for dose precision.
**Related equipment:** CT simulator, TPS dose engine.
**Radiotherapy Example:** Important for bone high-density regions.

440. **Virtual Wedge Planning:** Using dynamic MLC to mimic wedge effect instead of physical wedge.
**Related equipment:** Dynamic MLC software.
**Radiotherapy Example:** Breast tangential field dose modification.

441. **Vision-Assisted Surface Monitoring:** Surface scanner that prevents unintended patient motion.
**Related equipment:** Surface guided RT system (SGRT).
**Radiotherapy Example:** Used in mask-free SRS.

442. **Volume-of-Interest Tracking:** Monitoring motion of specific region instead of whole body.
**Related equipment:** Optical or internal fiducial tracking.
**Radiotherapy Example:** Tracking prostate gold seeds.

443. **Virtual Tumor Response Assessment:** Change in tumour volume monitored using imaging.
**Related equipment:** CT, MRI, PET.
**Radiotherapy Example:** IMRT plan adapted after shrinkage in cervix.

444. **Void Movement Estimation:** Tracking cavity motion during respiration.
**Related equipment:** 4D CT.
**Radiotherapy Example:** Lung cavity evaluated before SBRT.

445. **Verification Arcs:** Low-MU VMAT arcs used before full treatment to check alignment.
**Related equipment:** LINAC, EPID.
**Radiotherapy Example:** First-fraction pelvic VMAT QA.

446. **Volume Inhomogeneity Index:** Quantifies dose uniformity within target region.
**Related equipment:** TPS DVH metrics.
**Radiotherapy Example:** Low values preferred for breast boost.

447. **Visual Field-Edge Indicator:** Marking field borders visibly on skin using light field.
**Related equipment:** LINAC light field.
**Radiotherapy Example:** Marking chest wall borders before first fraction.

448. **Verification Phantom Plan:** Separate plan created for QA phantom measurements.
**Related equipment:** Water tank or ArcCHECK phantom.
**Radiotherapy Example:** Pre-treatment VMAT QA for head and neck.

449. **Vault Radiation Area Monitor:** Device measuring radiation levels outside vault.
**Related equipment:** Area monitor with alarm.
**Radiotherapy Example:** Installed outside wall of LINAC room.

450. **Vapour-Based Cooling System:** LINAC gun cooling using refrigeration cycle.
**Related equipment:** LINAC waveguide cooling unit.
**Radiotherapy Example:** Maintains temperature stability during high-energy delivery.

451. **Variable Jaw Tracking:** Jaws adjust dynamically to follow MLC leaves and reduce leakage.
**Related equipment:** LINAC jaws, MLC controller.
**Radiotherapy Example:** Used to reduce dose to lungs during IMRT breast plan.

452. **Vertigo Assessment Checklist:** Screening used to evaluate dizziness risk before mask immobilization.
**Related equipment:** Patient assessment forms.
**Radiotherapy Example:** Necessary for claustrophobic H&N mask patients.

453. **Visual Cone-Beam QA Review:** Manual examination of CBCT images to confirm acceptable setup.
**Related equipment:** On-board imager, IGRT workstation.
**Radiotherapy Example:** CBCT match reviewed daily for pelvis patients.

454. **Vault Bunker Quality Certification:** Compliance verification ensuring shielding and safety standards.
**Related equipment:** Survey meter, regulatory documents.
**Radiotherapy Example:** Required before commissioning LINAC in new department.

455. **Virtual QA Simulation:** Pre-treatment digital testing of planning and delivery workflow.
**Related equipment:** TPS, QA simulation tools.
**Radiotherapy Example:** Simulated VMAT plan delivery before treating paediatric patient.

456. **Ventilation–Perfusion Mapping:** Visualization of lung ventilation vs blood perfusion.
**Related equipment:** PET–CT, ventilation SPECT.
**Radiotherapy Example:** Avoids irradiating functioning lung in lung SBRT.

457. **Visual Field Light Calibration:** Calibration to ensure LINAC light field matches radiation field.
**Related equipment:** Light/radiation field crosshair tool.
**Radiotherapy Example:** Monthly QA in breast and spine cases.

458. **Virtual Simulator Contouring:** Contouring carried out within virtual simulation (CT-based).
**Related equipment:** TPS simulation module.
**Radiotherapy Example:** PTV created during virtual simulation of cervical cancer.

459. **Volumetric Breathing Envelope:** 3D space representing maximum breathing motion amplitude.
**Related equipment:** 4D CT, motion analysis software.
**Radiotherapy Example:** Used to generate Internal Target Volume (ITV) for liver cases.

460. **Verification Gamma Algorithm:** Mathematical evaluation comparing planned and measured dose (e.g., 3%/3mm).
**Related equipment:** Dose QA software.
**Radiotherapy Example:** VMAT head and neck QA passes 98% gamma.

461. **Vascular Hotspot Avoidance Parameter:** Constraint ensuring blood vessels do not receive excess radiation.
**Related equipment:** DVH constraint protocol.
**Radiotherapy Example:** Carotid dose minimized in larynx planning.

462. **Volume Reconstruction Algorithm:** Software algorithm generating 3D volume from image slices.
**Related equipment:** CT simulator, TPS.
**Radiotherapy Example:** 3D reconstruction of brain images for SRS.

463. **Ventral Immobilization Support:** Support device for prone breast or pelvic setup.
**Related equipment:** Bellyboard, prone breast board.
**Radiotherapy Example:** Used to reduce bowel dose in prone pelvis therapy.

464. **Visual Dose Constraints Indicator:** Alerts planner when dose violates organ limits.
**Related equipment:** TPS dose optimization module.
**Radiotherapy Example:** Rectum OAR constraint flagged in prostate IMRT.

465. **Voxel-Based Radiomics Analysis:** Extraction of image-based features to predict treatment response.
**Related equipment:** Radiomics software, CT/MRI datasets.
**Radiotherapy Example:** Texture analysis predicts tumour radiosensitivity.

466. **Virtual Respiratory Gating:** Planning simulation of gated delivery without actual gating hardware.
**Related equipment:** TPS gated simulation module.
**Radiotherapy Example:** Liver case evaluated virtually for beam-on window.

467. **Visible Artifact Suppression:** Removal of CT streak/metal artifacts to improve contouring accuracy.
**Related equipment:** MAR CT algorithm.
**Radiotherapy Example:** Dental implant artifacts suppressed in oral cancer planning.

468. **Vacuum Lock Mask:** Thermoplastic mask locked with vacuum suction to enhance rigidity.
**Related equipment:** Mould room vacuum fixation base.
**Radiotherapy Example:** Used for SRS to minimize motion below 1 mm.

469. **Volume Streak Correction:** Correction algorithm used for low-dose CBCT streaks.
**Related equipment:** CBCT processing software.
**Radiotherapy Example:** Improves CBCT spine visibility for alignment.

470. **Volumetric Hotspot Redistribution:** Optimization to relocate hotspots outside critical tissue.
**Related equipment:** IMRT optimizer.
**Radiotherapy Example:** Moves hotspot from mandible to soft tissue in oral cavity case.

471. **Vision-Based Patient Tracking:** Non-contact motion tracking using optical markers.
**Related equipment:** Surface-guided RT cameras.
**Radiotherapy Example:** SGRT used in breast DIBH.

472. **Verification Field Margin:** Safety margin around PTV to confirm coverage during image guidance.
**Related equipment:** IGRT matching software.
**Radiotherapy Example:** Expanded field margin used only for verification pelvis CBCT.

473. **Ventral Arc Trajectory:** VMAT arc path primarily delivered from anterior angles.
**Related equipment:** LINAC VMAT module.
**Radiotherapy Example:** Used to avoid spinal canal in retroperitoneal planning.

474. **Video-Recorded Treatment Setup:** Camera recording of patient positioning for review and audit.
**Related equipment:** Treatment room CCTV system.
**Radiotherapy Example:** Used for pediatric setup evaluation.

475. **Voxel-Weight Based Optimization:** Optimization assigning different weights to voxels within structures.
**Related equipment:** Advanced IMRT optimizer.
**Radiotherapy Example:** Prioritizes tumour centre high dose while sparing OAR edges.

476. **Visual Contour Quality Indicator:** Software rating contour smoothness and anatomical consistency.
**Related equipment:** AI-assisted auto-contouring tool.
**Radiotherapy Example:** Ensures heart contour accuracy in breast planning.

477. **Verification Arc Trigger:** Low-MU arc automatically delivered before treatment to confirm EPID image.
**Related equipment:** EPID, VMAT QA module.
**Radiotherapy Example:** Triggered for first-day pancreas SBRT.

478. **Void Filling Correction:** Adjustment in dose calc when air cavity changes during treatment.
**Related equipment:** Adaptive planning algorithm.
**Radiotherapy Example:** Oral cavity replan after tumour mass regresses.

479. **Volumetric Adaptive Strategy:** Treatment adaptation based on tumour volume change.
**Related equipment:** Adaptive TPS, repeat CT scan.
**Radiotherapy Example:** Cervix patient receives adaptive boost after shrinkage.

480. **Variable Beam Modulation Index:** Quantifies complexity of MLC modulation across treatment.
**Related equipment:** Dose QA index calculator.
**Radiotherapy Example:** Lower modulation index reduces QA failure risk.

481. **Visible Tattoo Mapping:** Digital mapping of patient tattoos for setup verification.
**Related equipment:** IGRT interface, skin laser alignment tool.
**Radiotherapy Example:** Used to verify tattoos remain consistent for breast patients.

482. **Vascular Dose–Response Model:** Predicts normal tissue complication probability based on vessel dose.
**Related equipment:** NTCP model software.
**Radiotherapy Example:** Ensures carotid damage risk minimized during neck IMRT.

483. **Virtual Synchronicity Check:** Ensures synchronization between couch motion and beam delivery digitally.
**Related equipment:** LINAC delivery controller.
**Radiotherapy Example:** Verified before stereotactic arc treatment.

484. **Ventral Shielding Block:** Physical block placed anteriorly to protect unaffected organs.
**Related equipment:** Lead block, alloy compensators.
**Radiotherapy Example:** Shield used during emergency spine radiation.

485. **Volumetric Tumor Perfusion Imaging:** Imaging technique evaluating blood flow inside tumour.
**Related equipment:** DCE-MRI, PET-CT.
**Radiotherapy Example:** Used to select radio-sensitizing chemotherapy.

486. **Vertex Beam Planning:** Vertical beam aiming from top of head.
**Related equipment:** Gantry controller, SRS frame.
**Radiotherapy Example:** Included in whole-brain planning to improve coverage.

487. **Verification Bone Match:** Matching CBCT bony anatomy for alignment.
**Related equipment:** IGRT image registration tool.
**Radiotherapy Example:** Spine SBRT relies on bone match instead of soft tissue.

488. **Vector Dose Calculation:** Dose calculated using directional components of photon vectors.
**Related equipment:** Monte Carlo algorithm.
**Radiotherapy Example:** Used for small field calculations in SRS.

489. **Visual Portal Dose Map:** Display of EPID-measured exit dose intensity.
**Related equipment:** EPID, portal dosimetry software.
**Radiotherapy Example:** VMAT QA generates portal dose map for comparison.

490. **Voxel-Level Plan Adaptation:** Replanning based on voxel-based anatomical and functional change.
**Related equipment:** Adaptive TPS.
**Radiotherapy Example:** Used in head and neck mid-treatment re-CT.

491. **Voluntary Arm Elevation Support:** Device supporting patient arms lifted above head.
**Related equipment:** Breast/ thoracic immobilization board.
**Radiotherapy Example:** Used for lung and breast planning CT.

492. **Vision-Guided Gating:** Real-time gating controlled by optical surface tracking instead of markers.
**Related equipment:** SGRT system.
**Radiotherapy Example:** DIBH breast delivery beam-on only when chest wall position is accurate.

493. **Verification Fiducial Alignment:** Verifying alignment of internal markers inside patient.
**Related equipment:** KV imaging, CBCT.
**Radiotherapy Example:** Gold marker alignment used for prostate IGRT.

494. **Virtual Dose Painting:** Assigning different doses to sub-regions of tumour based on biology.
**Related equipment:** PET-MRI functional imaging.
**Radiotherapy Example:** Hypoxic tumour core given higher dose IMRT boost.

495. **Video-Guided Immobilization Training:** Video demonstrations to train staff for immobilization fabrication.
**Related equipment:** Audio-visual system, mould room instruments.
**Radiotherapy Example:** Staff trained on breast vac-lok positioning.

496. **Ventral Target Localization:** Localizing target using markers/anatomy from anterior perspective.
**Related equipment:** KV AP x-ray imaging.
**Radiotherapy Example:** Pelvis setup using bladder shadow on AP MV film.

497. **Virtual LINAC Delivery Playback:** Simulation of past treatment delivery for error investigation.
**Related equipment:** Delivery log visualizer.
**Radiotherapy Example:** Playback used to analyze couch shift error during H&N treatment.

**498. Visualized Dose Tracking Dashboard:** Dashboard showing dose received per fraction and cumulative dose.
**Related equipment:** R&V system, DVH trend chart.
**Radiotherapy Example:** Paediatric dose monitored daily to safeguard OAR tolerance.

**499. Voxel-Based Toxicity Prediction Model:** Predicts toxicity probability by assessing dose per voxel instead of organ average.
**Related equipment:** AI toxicity predictor.
**Radiotherapy Example:** Predicts xerostomia risk in parotid gland for head & neck IMRT.

**500. Verification Treatment Gap Record:** Documentation of interruptions and rescheduling during fractionated therapy.
**Related equipment:** Treatment scheduling software, patient chart.
**Radiotherapy Example:** Recorded if patient missed fraction to adjust compensatory dose plan.

# W

1. **Water Phantom Dosimetry:** A dosimetry technique using water-equivalent medium to measure radiation depth dose and beam profiles.
   **Related equipment:** Water phantom tank, ion chamber, electrometer.
   **Radiotherapy Example:** Measured PDD curve for commissioning 6 MV and 10 MV photon beams.
2. **Wedge Filter (Physical):** Metal wedge inserted in beam path to create gradient dose distribution.
   **Related equipment:** Physical wedges for LINAC (15°, 30°, 45°, 60°).
   **Radiotherapy Example:** Used to balance dose uniformity in breast tangential fields.
3. **Wedge Pair Technique:** Two opposing beams with wedge angles to compensate tissue inhomogeneity.
   **Related equipment:** Wedge filters, treatment planning system (TPS).
   **Radiotherapy Example:** Applied to treat parotid gland tumour while sparing spinal cord.
4. **Wire Marking (Radiopaque Marker):** Metal wires placed on skin to mark treatment reference lines during CT simulation.
   **Related equipment:** Radiopaque skin wires, CT simulator.
   **Radiotherapy Example:** Used to outline surgical scars during breast CT scan for boost planning.
5. **Window for Contouring:** Image contrast and brightness adjustment to improve visibility of structures.
   **Related equipment:** CT workstation, TPS contouring panel.
   **Radiotherapy Example:** Used lung window to contour GTV for lung tumour accurately.
6. **Workflow Verification Checklist:** Step-by-step safety checklist to ensure treatment workflow accuracy.
   **Related equipment:** R&V system, QA documentation.
   **Radiotherapy Example:** Checklist confirmed correct immobilization mask before first H&N fraction.
7. **Whole Brain Radiotherapy Protocol:** Standardized approach for treating metastases in the entire brain.
   **Related equipment:** LINAC, thermoplastic mask, couch indexing.
   **Radiotherapy Example:** 30 Gy/10 fractions delivered with parallel opposed lateral fields.
8. **Weighting Factor (Beam Weighting):** Percentage strength assigned to multiple beams to distribute dose.
   **Related equipment:** TPS beam weighting optimizer.
   **Radiotherapy Example:** Posterior beam weighted higher in prostate RT to reduce rectal dose.
9. **Wireless Patient Monitoring:** Remote monitoring system for vitals and movement during treatment.
   **Related equipment:** Patient wireless sensors, SGRT integration.
   **Radiotherapy Example:** Used during paediatric sedation SBRT treatments.
10. **Wipe Test (Radioactive Contamination Test):** Wiping surfaces to detect radioactive spills in nuclear medicine/radiotherapy labs.
    **Related equipment:** Survey meter, scintillation counter.
    **Radiotherapy Example:** Performed after brachytherapy applicator handling.

11. **Window Level Calibration:** Calibration of digital display grayscale for medical image interpretation.
**Related equipment:** DICOM display calibration tool.
**Radiotherapy Example:** Ensured CT image appearance is consistent for contouring.

12. **Workflow Interruption Protocol:** Procedure to handle missed fractions and unplanned treatment gaps.
**Related equipment:** R&V system, schedule management tools.
**Radiotherapy Example:** Replanning for patient with 7-day break in head & neck treatment.

13. **Weekly Physics Chart Review:** Periodic review of treatment documentation and delivery records.
**Related equipment:** Oncology information system (OIS), DVH records.
**Radiotherapy Example:** Verified plan parameters and MU for prostate IMRT patient.

14. **Whole-Body PET-CT for Target Delineation:** PET-CT imaging used to localize metabolically active tumour regions.
**Related equipment:** PET-CT scanner, MRI/PET fusion TPS.
**Radiotherapy Example:** PET uptake used to define boost volume in lung SBRT.

15. **Wipeable Positioning Indexing System:** Couch and immobilization indexing that allows accurate setup reuse.
**Related equipment:** Indexing carbon couch, belly board, vacuum cushions.
**Radiotherapy Example:** Used to reposition pelvis patient consistently daily.

16. **Water-Equivalent Bolus:** Tissue-equivalent material placed on skin to increase superficial dose.
**Related equipment:** 5 mm / 10 mm bolus sheets.
**Radiotherapy Example:** Applied in chest wall radiotherapy to ensure adequate skin dose.

17. **Whole Spine Radiotherapy Field Matching:** Technique to junction cervical, thoracic, and lumbar fields safely.
**Related equipment:** Field matching software, couch shifts.
**Radiotherapy Example:** Applied for craniospinal irradiation alignment.

18. **Wavelength-Based Optical Surface Guidance:** Uses optical light waves to track patient body contour in real time.
**Related equipment:** SGRT camera units.
**Radiotherapy Example:** Used for DIBH breast treatments without tattoos.

19. **Windowed Dose Painting:** Delivering different doses to tumour sub-zones based on biological signal intensity.
**Related equipment:** PET-MRI imaging + IMRT optimizer.
**Radiotherapy Example:** Higher dose to hypoxic core of head & neck tumour.

20. **Weight-Based Pediatric Sedation Protocol:** Dosing guidelines for safe sedation during paediatric CT/MRI/RT simulation.
**Related equipment:** Sedation drugs, monitoring devices.
**Radiotherapy Example:** Used for immobilizing infant during brain CT simulation.

21. **Wireless Therapist Console:** Wireless handheld device to control LINAC positioning functions.
**Related equipment:** Mobile treatment console, LINAC network.
**Radiotherapy Example:** Used to adjust couch for pelvis CBCT match.

22. **Wide Bore CT Simulator:** CT with larger diameter to accommodate immobilization devices or large patients.
**Related equipment:** 85 cm / 90 cm bore CT.
**Radiotherapy Example:** Made it possible to scan patient with FullBody Vac-Lok.

23. **Wipeable Mould Room Storage System:** Infection-controlled storage for immobilization devices.
**Related equipment:** Closed-shelf racks, barcode indexing.
**Radiotherapy Example:** Breast board stored to reuse across 20 fractions.

24. **Weight-Loss Monitoring Program:** Periodic assessment to detect anatomical change requiring re-CT.
**Related equipment:** Digital scale, OIS alert.
**Radiotherapy Example:** H&N patient re-planned after significant weight loss.

25. **Walled Shielding Maze:** Path-shaped shielding corridor that reduces radiation leakage from LINAC room entrance.
**Related equipment:** Concrete shielding barrier.
**Radiotherapy Example:** Eliminates need for heavy lead door in new bunker designs.

26. **Windowed Auto-Segmentation:** AI segmentation that adapts based on selected image window settings.
**Related equipment:** AI contouring assistant.
**Radiotherapy Example:** Improves lung tumour contours on noisy CT.

27. **Wireless Audio Patient Talk-Back System:** Allows continuous communication between therapist and patient during beam-on.
**Related equipment:** LINAC intercom system.
**Radiotherapy Example:** Important for claustrophobic cases wearing head masks.

28. **Wide Dynamic-Range KV Imaging:** KV detector captures high-contrast and low-contrast features simultaneously.
**Related equipment:** On-board imager.
**Radiotherapy Example:** Helps visualize both bone and soft tissue for pelvis IGRT.

29. **Whole-Breast VMAT Delivery:** Arc-based planning technique for complete breast irradiation with low OAR dose.
**Related equipment:** VMAT planning module, LINAC MLC.
**Radiotherapy Example:** Reduces cardiac dose in left-sided breast RT.

30. **Wound Irradiation Protocol:** Guideline to deliver postoperative radiation without affecting sutures or healing tissue.
**Related equipment:** CBCT, OAR constraint protocol.
**Radiotherapy Example:** Applied to chest wall boost after mastectomy.

31. **Workflow Automation in Oncology:** Automated task handling in radiotherapy workflow to reduce manual errors and treatment delays.
**Related equipment:** Oncology Information System (OIS), automated scheduling, QA reminders.
**Radiotherapy Example:** System automatically triggered CBCT imaging schedule for every 3rd fraction.

32. **Whole Abdomen Irradiation Technique:** Large-field radiation approach treating peritoneal cavity in ovarian cancer.
**Related equipment:** LINAC, customized belly board, multi-isocenter planning.
**Radiotherapy Example:** Treated with VMAT using 2 overlapping arcs and dose fall-off to kidneys.

33. **Weighted Mean Dose (Equivalent Dose):** Biologically weighted total dose considering fractions and radiation type.
**Related equipment:** Radiobiological calculation module in TPS.
**Radiotherapy Example:** Used to compare proton boost vs photon plan in brain tumour.

34. **Wire Localization for Boost Target:** Placement of wire markers in CT to outline surgical cavity or lesion site.
**Related equipment:** Radiopaque wire, CT simulator.
**Radiotherapy Example:** Used for lumpectomy cavity visualization prior to boost planning.

35. **Wireless Respiratory Belt:** A sensor belt measuring respiratory motion during imaging and treatment.
**Related equipment:** Gating system, 4D CT, SGRT.
**Radiotherapy Example:** Used for pancreatic gating to synchronize beam with breathing.

36. **Wide-Field IMRT for Advanced Disease:** IMRT technique covering large body regions while sparing critical organs.
**Related equipment:** MLC, IMRT optimizer, QA tools.
**Radiotherapy Example:** Used for cervical cancer including pelvic nodes and para-aortic area.

37. **Weighting of Optimization Cost Functions:** Assigning mathematical priorities for planning goals in TPS optimizer.
**Related equipment:** IMRT/VMAT dose optimizer.
**Radiotherapy Example:** Higher priority on rectum sparing during prostate planning.

38. **Warm-Up Cycle for LINAC:** Routine beam preparation sequence before patient treatments.
**Related equipment:** LINAC console, daily QA toolkit.
**Radiotherapy Example:** Machine warmed up using 100 MU test before first patient.

39. **Water-Cooled MLC System:** Thermal management mechanism preventing overheating of MLC motors during heavy delivery.
**Related equipment:** MLC cooling loop, temperature sensors.
**Radiotherapy Example:** Enables prolonged SBRT VMAT beams without interruption.

40. **Wall-Mounted Patient Immobilization Rack:** Organized storage of immobilization devices to maintain hygiene and rapid access.
**Related equipment:** Thermoplastic masks, knee and foot supports.
**Radiotherapy Example:** Mask placed in assigned storage to reuse for head-and-neck sessions.

41. **White-Light Structured Imaging:** Surface guidance using projected white-light pattern to track real-time body motion.
**Related equipment:** SGRT positioning cameras.
**Radiotherapy Example:** Used for frameless radiosurgery positioning with submillimetric accuracy.

42. **Weekly OAR Dose Tolerance Audit:** Scheduled review to ensure delivered dose agrees with planned organ tolerance limits.
**Related equipment:** DVH reports, OIS dashboard.
**Radiotherapy Example:** Confirmed parotid dose $< 26$ Gy for H&N case.

43. **Window-Level-Based Metal Artifact Reduction:** CT window adjustments combined with algorithm to reduce streak artifacts from implants.
**Related equipment:** MAR-enabled CT scanner.
**Radiotherapy Example:** Improved pelvis contour visibility for patient with hip prosthesis.

44. **Whole Lung Blocking Technique:** Shielding or dose-fall-off strategy to limit lung dose in upper thoracic irradiation.
**Related equipment:** MLC or customized blocks.
**Radiotherapy Example:** Applied in mantle field Hodgkin's lymphoma RT.

45. **Wireless Immobilization Tagging (Barcode ID):** ID system used to track immobilization devices and link them to patients.
**Related equipment:** Tag scanner, mould room database.
**Radiotherapy Example:** Vacuum bag identified automatically for liver SBRT treatment.

46. **Wide-Beam CT Reconstruction:** CT reconstruction using large beam width for faster acquisition & reduced motion artifacts.
**Related equipment:** Wide-beam CT simulator.
**Radiotherapy Example:** 4D CT for lung acquired faster reducing breathing inconsistency.

47. **Weekly Machine Output Stability Report:** Documentation of radiation output consistency based on daily QA records.
**Related equipment:** Electrometer, ion chamber, QA software.
**Radiotherapy Example:** Confirms ±2% output stability before approving SBRT list.

48. **Window-Based Auto Segmentation for Bones:** AI contouring that uses bone window intensity normalization.
**Related equipment:** AI planning platform, CT workstation.
**Radiotherapy Example:** Automated pelvic bone segmentation for femoral head sparing.

49. **Weight-Restricted Couch Loading Rule:** Safety limit specifying maximum weight couch can safely support.
**Related equipment:** Carbon fiber couch, weight alert system.
**Radiotherapy Example:** Bariatric pelvic patient treated on bariatric couch top to maintain indexing.

50. **Whole-Body VMAT Research Platform:** Research system optimizing VMAT across long treatment lengths with beam junction control.
**Related equipment:** VMAT junction optimizer, extended MLC planner.
**Radiotherapy Example:** Craniospinal VMAT delivery in paediatric medulloblastoma.

51. **Water-Tank Linac MLC Leaf Calibration:** Using water phantom to check leaf positioning accuracy during beam profile scanning.
**Related equipment:** Water phantom, scanning ion chamber.
**Radiotherapy Example:** MLC recalibrated after IMRT QA showed leaf gap deviation.

52. **Weighted Multi-Criteria Optimization:** Planning strategy that offers many solutions balancing tumour coverage and OAR protection.
**Related equipment:** MCO (Multi-Criteria Optimizer) in TPS.
**Radiotherapy Example:** Used for rectal ca with priority for femoral heads sparing.

53. **Wireless SGRT-Controlled Beam Hold:** Automatic beam pause when patient moves beyond tolerance threshold.
**Related equipment:** SGRT + LINAC gating interface.
**Radiotherapy Example:** Beam held during DIBH breast session when breathing depth decreased.

54. **Wall-Mounted Laser Alignment QA:** Fixed laser QA panel enabling quick daily verification of room lasers.
**Related equipment:** Laser QA tool, spirit level.
**Radiotherapy Example:** Daily laser shift of +1 mm corrected before CT simulation.

55. **Whole-Pelvis IMRT for Nodal Disease:** IMRT covering pelvis + nodes with dose boost to tumour using SIB.
**Related equipment:** IMRT TPS optimizer, MLC.
**Radiotherapy Example:** Cervical ca plan: 50.4 Gy pelvis + 59.4 Gy boost to primary.

56. **Window-Matched CBCT Fusion:** Fusion alignment with image window adjustment to improve match precision.
**Related equipment:** CBCT viewer, registration tools.
**Radiotherapy Example:** Bone window used for pelvis bone match → then soft-tissue adjustment.

57. **Weekly Immobilization Re-Evaluation:** Check for mask looseness or cushion deformation during long treatments.
**Related equipment:** Measuring gauge, SGRT records.
**Radiotherapy Example:** New mask molded after 4th week for H&N patient with weight loss.

58. **Wipe-Clean Pediatric RT Environment:** Child-friendly, fully sanitized set-up allowing safe immobilization and sedation.
**Related equipment:** Radiation-safe cartoon projectors, disinfectable cushions.
**Radiotherapy Example:** Used during paediatric abdominal RT under sedation.

59. **Whole-Liver Radiotherapy Adaptive Strategy:** Adaptive RT for large liver involvement minimizing toxicity.
**Related equipment:** Adaptive TPS, CBCT daily contour adaptation.
**Radiotherapy Example:** Dose modified mid-treatment due to shrinking GTV and shifting bowel loops.

60. **Weighted Beam Angle Selection:** Choice of beam angles based on dose gradient, OAR proximity, and anatomical asymmetry.
**Related equipment:** TPS beam angle optimizer.
**Radiotherapy Example:** Oblique angles selected in paraspinal RT to avoid kidneys.

61. **Wireless Dosimetry Sensor:** A body-worn radiation sensor that records skin dose in real time during radiotherapy.
**Related equipment:** OSLD-patch, MOSFET dosimeter, wireless dosimetry receiver.
**Radiotherapy Example:** Used during breast IMRT to ensure entrance dose stays within tolerance.

62. **Water-Cooling System for LINAC Gantry:** Thermal management system maintaining stable gantry head temperature during beam delivery.
**Related equipment:** LINAC cooling unit, flow meter, heat exchanger.
**Radiotherapy Example:** Cooling fault triggered alarm → SBRT paused to prevent dose drift.

63. **Weight-Based SSD Table Correction:** Couch height compensated based on sag caused by patient weight.
**Related equipment:** Carbon couch top, sag correction chart, distance laser ruler.
**Radiotherapy Example:** For heavy pelvic patient SSD increased 0.4 cm to correct sag before beam on.

64. **Wide-Bore CT Simulation:** CT with larger bore opening to accommodate obese or immobilized patients comfortably.
**Related equipment:** Wide-bore CT ($\geq$ 80 cm), extended couch rails.
**Radiotherapy Example:** Head-and-neck mask positioned inside wide-bore CT without pressure on mask edges.

65. **Worklist-Driven Auto Beam Generation:** Automatic creation of treatment fields from approved CT simulation protocols.
**Related equipment:** OIS-TPS connectivity, auto-mapping rules.
**Radiotherapy Example:** Prostate plan automatically generated template with 2 VMAT arcs.

66. **Wide-Margin PTV Strategy:** Using large PTV margins to account for high tumour motion or deformity.
**Related equipment:** GTV/PTV modelling module, CBCT monitoring.
**Radiotherapy Example:** Pancreas plan margin increased from 0.5 cm to 1 cm due to irregular breathing.

67. **Window-Based Organ Masking:** Contouring support technique using different CT window presets to highlight organs.
**Related equipment:** Bone window, lung window, soft-tissue window in CT viewer.
**Radiotherapy Example:** Mandible contoured under bone window for precise H&N boosting.

68. **Wedge-Based Dose Compensation:** Beam intensity alteration using wedge filters to correct tissue thickness differences.
**Related equipment:** Physical wedges, dynamic wedges.
**Radiotherapy Example:** Breast tangential field with 30° wedge to flatten dose superiorly.

69. **Wound Cavity Markers:** Radiopaque seeds or clips implanted around a cavity after tumour excision.
**Related equipment:** Surgical clips, fiducial seeds, CT imaging.
**Radiotherapy Example:** 6 clips delineated lumpectomy cavity for breast boost targeting.

70. **Wire-Grid Dose Mapping Phantom:** QA phantom with embedded metal wire matrix for radiation beam symmetry checks.
**Related equipment:** Film scanners, phantoms, EPID QA software.
**Radiotherapy Example:** Monthly QA for VMAT symmetry performed with wire-grid phantom.

71. **Weekly Weight Monitoring Protocol:** Body-weight check to detect dimensional change affecting immobilization or dose distribution.
**Related equipment:** Scale, mask fit sheet, adaptive treatment log.
**Radiotherapy Example:** 5-kg weight loss → Head-and-neck patient rescanned and re-planned.

72. **Wipe-Down Protocol for Mould Material Hygiene:** Cleaning process ensuring thermoplastic masks and mould equipment remain infection-free.
**Related equipment:** Disinfectant solution, drying rack.
**Radiotherapy Example:** Paediatric sedation masks sanitized daily to avoid cross contamination.

73. **Wide-Field Spine Radiosurgery:** High-gradient stereotactic radiation to multiple vertebral metastases in one session.
**Related equipment:** LINAC with ExacTrac / CBCT / Hexapod couch.
**Radiotherapy Example:** T7–T11 treated with VMAT using simultaneous integrated boost.

74. **Wireless Patient Positioning Alert:** System sending alarms to radiographers when patient movement exceeds threshold.
**Related equipment:** SGRT system, wearable motion tracker.
**Radiotherapy Example:** Beam paused during DIBH when chest displacement > 3 mm.

75. **Workload-Based Machine Utilization Report:** Statistical analysis of treatment slots, modality use, and patient flow.
**Related equipment:** OIS dashboard, scheduling software.
**Radiotherapy Example:** Report used to allocate separate SBRT time block to reduce delays.

76. **Wound Bed Boost Therapy:** Additional dose to surgical bed to reduce recurrence in at-risk tumours.
**Related equipment:** Electron applicators / photon boost fields / bolus.
**Radiotherapy Example:** 12 Gy boost delivered post-breast irradiation.

77. **Water-Equivalent Mask Material:** Thermoplastic material that behaves like water in dose absorption.
**Related equipment:** Thermoplastic sheets, mould room accessories.
**Radiotherapy Example:** Pediatric mask selected to avoid buildup alteration in cranial RT.

78. **Wide-Band EPID Imaging Mode:** Mode enabling high-contrast EPID imaging under both low and high MU rates.
**Related equipment:** EPID panel, portal imaging software.
**Radiotherapy Example:** Verified MLC picket fence QA using wide-band portal acquisition.

79. **Weekly Setup Error Statistical Review:** Analysis of daily IGRT shifts to determine if PTV margins remain valid.
**Related equipment:** CBCT logs, auto-matching system.
**Radiotherapy Example:** Based on trend, H&N PTV margins refined from 5 mm to 4 mm.

80. **Wide-Channel SGRT Camera:** SGRT unit capable of detecting larger surface area simultaneously for accuracy.
**Related equipment:** Multi-camera SGRT pods.
**Radiotherapy Example:** Full-thorax surface tracking performed during lung DIBH.

81. **Water-Cooled Electron Cone:** Electron delivery attachment cooled to withstand prolonged high-dose treatments.
**Related equipment:** Water-cooled cone, applicator head.
**Radiotherapy Example:** 18 MeV electron boost performed safely for scalp lesion.

82. **Waveform-Controlled Beam Modulation:** Radiation dose modulated using advanced waveform patterns to enhance precision.
**Related equipment:** Advanced LINAC beam controller.
**Radiotherapy Example:** Modulation allowed uniform dose on irregular mandibular surface.

83. **Weighted Auto-IGRT Match:** Combining multiple image match metrics (bone, soft tissue, fiducial) using weights.
**Related equipment:** CBCT fusion workstation.
**Radiotherapy Example:** Prostate IGRT: soft-tissue match 70%, fiducial match 30%.

84. **Warning Light Panel in Radiation Rooms:** Safety lighting notifying staff of radiation exposure status.
**Related equipment:** Door interlock, beam-on indicator.
**Radiotherapy Example:** Red "Beam-ON" indicator activated during VMAT fraction.

85. **Whole-Field Quality Reconstruction:** Algorithm assessing beam quality across full field rather than axis alone.
**Related equipment:** EPID, planar dose analysis software.
**Radiotherapy Example:** Full-field FFF beam verified before SBRT commissioning.

86. **Window-Protected Electron Treatment:** Electron therapy using protective film for skin preservation while maintaining dose.
**Related equipment:** Electron window shield, bolus.
**Radiotherapy Example:** 6 MeV electron beam used with window for eyelid tumour.

87. **Warm-Room CT Simulation Protocol:** CT simulation room heated to prevent muscular tension for reproducible posture.
**Related equipment:** Room thermostat, immobilization supports.
**Radiotherapy Example:** Used for prostate CT to reduce muscle tightening and setup variability.

88. **Wide-Arc VMAT for Large Volume Targets:** VMAT using > 270° rotation to improve coverage of expanded disease areas.
**Related equipment:** LINAC, VMAT optimizer.
**Radiotherapy Example:** Pelvic + para-aortic VMAT using dual 360° arcs.

89. **Water-Tight Immobilization Resealing:** Re-melting surface of thermoplastic mask for tighter fit, avoiding remake.
**Related equipment:** Heat gun, mould room workstation.
**Radiotherapy Example:** Mask resealed after face slimming in 4th week of H&N treatment.

90. **Weighted Dose–Volume Constraint Tuning:** Adjusting constraint weights to reach optimal tumour coverage with minimal toxicity.
**Related equipment:** Dose optimizer (TPS).
**Radiotherapy Example:** Rectum constraint weight increased to reduce bowel dose in prostate plan.

91. **White-Noise Patient Soothing System:** Audio system used during treatment to reduce anxiety and help patients remain still.
**Related equipment:** LINAC audio interface, patient comfort system.
**Radiotherapy Example:** Played soft white-noise during pediatric cranial RT to avoid movement.

92. **Wide-Portal Treatment Technique:** Radiation technique using enlarged portals to reduce setup uncertainty for moving targets.
**Related equipment:** LINAC multi-leaf collimator, large-field verification imaging.
**Radiotherapy Example:** Used for cervical nodes with frequent interfraction displacement.

93. **Whole-Body PET-CT Radiotherapy Planning:** Incorporating PET-CT across entire body for metastatic disease treatment assessment.
**Related equipment:** PET-CT scanner, TPS SUV segmentation.
**Radiotherapy Example:** High SUV spine lesion detected → added SBRT boost to metastatic site.

94. **Water-Tight Treatment Bolus:** Liquid-resistant bolus maintaining thickness during daily RT sessions.
**Related equipment:** Gel bolus, reusable bolus sheets.
**Radiotherapy Example:** Bolus applied in chest-wall postmastectomy RT to improve skin dose.

95. **Weekly Physics Chart Audit:** Routine validation of treatment parameters to ensure error-free progress.
**Related equipment:** OIS database, audit checklist.
**Radiotherapy Example:** Proton plan MU mismatch detected and corrected via audit.

96. **Whole-Liver Dose Constraint Protocol:** Guidelines limiting mean liver dose to prevent radiation-induced liver disease (RILD).
**Related equipment:** DVH constraints, adaptive planning workflow.
**Radiotherapy Example:** VMAT optimized to keep mean liver dose < 28 Gy.

97. **Wire-Based Catheter Localization:** Radiopaque wire inserted into catheter to visualize brachytherapy channel path.
**Related equipment:** Dummy wire marker, CT simulation.
**Radiotherapy Example:** Interstitial breast brachytherapy channels verified before dose loading.

98. **Wedge Pair Field Arrangement:** Two opposing fields with wedges to reduce dose gradient across target.
**Related equipment:** Wedge filters, isodose visualizer.
**Radiotherapy Example:** Applied to thigh sarcoma to spare critical neurovascular bundle.

99. **Weighted Multi-Criteria Optimization (MCO):** Advanced plan technique balancing tumour coverage and OAR sparing via weighted trade-off analysis.
**Related equipment:** TPS MCO solver, Pareto curve module.
**Radiotherapy Example:** Balanced rectum sparing vs PTV coverage in prostate VMAT plan.

100. **Workplace Radiation Compliance Signage:** Mandatory signboards indicating radiation risk zones in RT centers.
**Related equipment:** Radiation zone markers, warning signs.
**Radiotherapy Example:** LINAC maze door signage warns "Controlled Radiation Zone – Authorized Staff Only."

101. **Whole-Brain Hippocampal-Sparing RT:** Technique that preserves memory function by avoiding hippocampal dose during WBRT.
**Related equipment:** VMAT optimizer, hippocampal atlas.
**Radiotherapy Example:** Dose sculpted around hippocampus using dual-arc VMAT.

102. **Wire-Frame Treatment Plan Reconstruction:** Plan verification method representing beams as wire outlines on patient contour.
**Related equipment:** Plan QA reconstruction software.
**Radiotherapy Example:** Verified craniospinal plan junction transitions using wire-frame overlay.

103. **Weighted Skin Dose Correction:** Adjustment to dose near skin surface using bolus and fluence compensators.
**Related equipment:** Bolus, surface compensator, EPID skin dose estimator.
**Radiotherapy Example:** Increased superficial fluence in scalp boost without hot spots.

104. **Workplace Radiation Safety Checklist:** Daily checklist verifying radiation safety compliance before clinical operations.
**Related equipment:** Area survey meters, interlock tester.
**Radiotherapy Example:** Room entry sensors and emergency stops confirmed before treating patients.

105. **Wedge-Less Compensation Technique:** Beam intensity shaped by MLC fluence instead of physical wedge.
**Related equipment:** IMRT optimizer, dynamic MLC.
**Radiotherapy Example:** Eliminated wedge use in breast VMAT while achieving perfect uniformity.

106. **Wide-Bone Window for Stereotactic Contouring:** Optimized CT window style for delineating bony anatomy for SRS/SBRT.
**Related equipment:** Planning CT bone-viewer.
**Radiotherapy Example:** Used for precise vertebral contouring before spine SBRT.

107. **Water-Equivalent Solid Phantom Block:** Solid phantom material with same attenuation properties as water for QA.
**Related equipment:** Solid water phantoms, chamber insert cavity.
**Radiotherapy Example:** Used for absolute dose calibration with Farmer chamber.

108. **Weekly IGRT Deviation Report:** Review summary of daily IGRT shift values to track responsiveness of immobilization.
**Related equipment:** CBCT database, IGRT analytics.
**Radiotherapy Example:** Lung patient exhibited > 6 mm weekly shift → triggered adaptive rescan.

109. **Workspace Optimization in Mould Room:** Arrangement of accessories for safe and fast immobilization fabrication workflow.
**Related equipment:** Thermoplastic ovens, plaster storage racks.
**Radiotherapy Example:** Mask creation time reduced from 25 to 15 minutes following reorganization.

110. **Wide-Body Patient Support System:** Treatment couch modification to support bariatric patients safely.
**Related equipment:** Extended couch, auxiliary support rails.
**Radiotherapy Example:** Extended platform used during pelvic VMAT for 165-kg patient.

111. **Window-Based Auto Organ Segmentation:** AI contouring method performing segmentation using multiple CT window presets.
**Related equipment:** Deep-learning auto-segmentation software.
**Radiotherapy Example:** Lung tumour and ribs identified with dual window feature extraction.

112. **Water-Filled Compensator Shell:** Custom 3D shell filled with water to shape dose attenuation for electron therapy.
**Related equipment:** 3D-printed compensator, water injection fillers.
**Radiotherapy Example:** Ear canal tumour dose shaped to avoid overexposure of cochlea.

113. **Wide-Range MU Linearity QA:** Test to ensure MU response stays linear from very low to very high MU.
**Related equipment:** Detector array, MU scan analyzer.
**Radiotherapy Example:** SBRT 5-MU shots verified for stereotactic plan reliability.

114. **Wet-Path CT Artifact Analysis:** CT artifact evaluation caused by fluid-filled cavities appearing hyperdense.
**Related equipment:** CT post-processing tools.
**Radiotherapy Example:** Adjusted contrast to reduce bladder fluid streaking during prostate CT simulation.

115. **Weight-Based Bolus Removal Decision:** Skin dose modification decision based on body fat change during treatment.
**Related equipment:** Bolus fit chart, surface scanner.
**Radiotherapy Example:** Bolus removed in week 3 after edema reduction lowered skin buildup excessively.

116. **Weekly R&V System Backup Protocol:** Copying and archiving all patient records from OIS to avoid treatment data loss.
**Related equipment:** R&V server, storage array.
**Radiotherapy Example:** Offline backup restored after network downtime allowed treatment to continue.

117. **Wireless Immobilization Data Logging:** Mask tightening, positioning and surface contact pressure stored digitally.
**Related equipment:** Smart immobilization mask sensors.
**Radiotherapy Example:** Pediatric cranial mask pressure reduction improved comfort and stability.

118. **Wound-Contact Radiation Patch:** Flexible patch used to deliver low-dose radiation to superficial operated areas.
**Related equipment:** Brachytherapy patch, silicone applicator.
**Radiotherapy Example:** Used for post-operative scar control in keloid radiotherapy.

119. **Wide-Span MLC Modulation:** Technique using large sweeping leaf movements for large irregular targets.
**Related equipment:** MLC controller, VMAT algorithm.
**Radiotherapy Example:** Para-aortic plus pelvic field covered using broad span leaf tracking.

120. **Whole-Scan Image Histogram Review:** Visual inspection of HU distribution to check CT image uniformity and reconstruction error.
**Related equipment:** CT histogram analyzer.
**Radiotherapy Example:** Identified artifact due to incorrect kernel on head CT; scan repeated.

121. **Weighted Beams Eye View (BEV) Planning:** Adjusting beam contributions in BEV space for improved dose shaping.
**Related equipment:** TPS BEV module, DRR.
**Radiotherapy Example:** BEV weighting increased around spinal canal to reduce cord max dose.

122. **Water-Equivalent Balloon Applicator:** Balloon filled with water for conformal contact in brachytherapy.
**Related equipment:** HDR afterloader, balloon catheter.
**Radiotherapy Example:** Lung-chest wall contact tumour treated with HDR balloon brachytherapy.

123. **Workflow Automation in Treatment Approval:** Automated routing of plans for physician and physics sign-off.
**Related equipment:** OIS task automation.
**Radiotherapy Example:** Approval time reduced from 48h to 8h using automated sequential routing.

124. **Wide-Field Electron Therapy Technique:** Using two or more abutting electron fields to treat large superficial areas.
**Related equipment:** Electron applicators, custom cutouts.
**Radiotherapy Example:** Chest-wall electrons treated across bilateral scars with matched fields.

125. **Windowed Dose Rate Adjustment:** Automatically limits dose rate range for motion-sensitive anatomy.
**Related equipment:** LINAC dose rate controller.
**Radiotherapy Example:** Dose rate restricted to 400 MU/min for lung SBRT to minimize interplay effects.

126. **Wedge-Boost Technique:** Boosting dose to a subregion by adding wedge-shaped field only to part of target.
**Related equipment:** Hard wedge, dynamic wedge.
**Radiotherapy Example:** Boost to breast scar region while keeping global dose uniform.

127. **Workstation Calibration Validation:** Ensuring image display settings match TPS calibration standards.
**Related equipment:** QA workstation, grayscale calibration tool.
**Radiotherapy Example:** Display recalibrated after incorrect HU values seen during liver contouring.

128. **Whole-Heart Dose Protection Protocol:** Guidelines for restricting cardiac dose in thoracic RT.
**Related equipment:** DVH constraints, heart atlas.
**Radiotherapy Example:** Switch from 3DCRT to VMAT to reduce mean heart dose from 9 Gy → 3 Gy.

129. **Wireless Patient Position Trigger System:** Sends remote signal when patient is properly aligned for beam-on.
**Related equipment:** SGRT cameras, wireless gating controller.
**Radiotherapy Example:** Breath-hold automatically triggered beam delivery during DIBH breast RT.

130. **Window-Based HU Override:** Correcting HU values by applying proper window lookup for mismatch regions.
**Related equipment:** TPS HU override tool.
**Radiotherapy Example:** Override applied to dental fillings before head and neck VMAT.

131. **Wide-Arc VMAT Planning:** Using > 270° arc sweeps for uniform dose across deep structures.
**Related equipment:** VMAT optimizer, MLC.
**Radiotherapy Example:** Whole-pelvis VMAT using 355° arcs to improve PTV coverage.

132. **Weighted Shell Dose Fall-Off Technique:** Creating multiple dose-fall-off shells with decreasing priorities.
**Related equipment:** TPS optimization shells.
**Radiotherapy Example:** 5-shell objective applied for brain mets to reduce healthy brain V12.

133. **Wire-Based Skin Mark Retention:** Wire placed over skin to preserve tattoo/marker location during CT scan.
**Related equipment:** Skin marker wire.
**Radiotherapy Example:** Repeat scan required after faint tattoo; wire used to retain coordinates.

134. **Wet Casting for Immobilization:** Creating custom casts using water-activated materials in mould room.
**Related equipment:** Plaster wraps, fiberglass rolls.
**Radiotherapy Example:** Full limb cast for sarcoma RT with daily reproducibility.

135. **Wedge-Angle Optimization:** Using calculated wedge angles to correct dose sloping across the target.
**Related equipment:** TPS wedge calculator.
**Radiotherapy Example:** 15° wedge produced optimal uniformity in supraclavicular field.

136. **Whole-Spine Alignment Check:** IGRT verification across all spinal levels in craniospinal irradiation.
**Related equipment:** CBCT, spinal matching algorithm.
**Radiotherapy Example:** Upper spine used as reference for automatic digital match.

137. **Workload Radiation Survey:** Facility shielding calculation updated based on delivered workload.
**Related equipment:** Area monitor, shielding survey meter.
**Radiotherapy Example:** Barrier workload changed after SBRT program expansion → survey updated.

138. **Wide-Bore CT RT Simulation:** CT with 80–90 cm bore diameter to accommodate immobilization devices.
**Related equipment:** Wide-bore CT scanner.
**Radiotherapy Example:** VMAT pelvis scan with belly-board achievable only on wide-bore CT.

139. **Water-Bag Prone Breast Setup:** Water-bag used to shape breast for optimal chest wall extension in prone RT.
**Related equipment:** Prone breast platform, water-bag.
**Radiotherapy Example:** Reduced lung V5 from 14% → 4%.

140. **Wavelength-Safe Room Lighting:** Lighting optimized for visibility during image guidance with minimal IR interference.
**Related equipment:** SGRT-safe light fixtures.
**Radiotherapy Example:** SGRT interference resolved by replacing IR-reflective ceiling lights.

141. **Weighted Fractionation Planner:** Module supporting biologically weighted decision-making for hypo- vs conventional fractionation.
**Related equipment:** Radiobiology planner in TPS.
**Radiotherapy Example:** 5-fraction SBRT chosen instead of 10-fraction plan based on BED response.

142. **Whole-Field Junction Feathering:** Daily shifting of field junction to reduce dose inhomogeneity.
**Related equipment:** Junction-shift programming.
**Radiotherapy Example:** Used in CSI to avoid hot-spots at cranial-spinal overlap.

143. **Warp-Corrected Deformable Registration:** Removes unrealistic deformations in DIR anatomical warping.
**Related equipment:** Adaptive TPS deformable maps.
**Radiotherapy Example:** Liver deformation artefact corrected for accurate cumulative dose tracking.

144. **Wireless Laser Alignment Controller:** Remote-controlled laser alignment system for precise marking.
**Related equipment:** Smart laser positioning system.
**Radiotherapy Example:** Tattoos aligned with < 1 mm deviation for H&N immobilization.

145. **Wide-Patient Support Extension Cushion:** Side-extension padding used for comfort and immobilization of broad-shouldered patients.
**Related equipment:** Positioning cushions, vacuum beanbag.
**Radiotherapy Example:** Improved arm positioning for thoracic VMAT.

146. **Wound-Healing Dose Protocol:** Protocol defining safe time between surgery and RT to avoid wound breakdown.
**Related equipment:** Institutional wound-RT guidelines.
**Radiotherapy Example:** RT delayed 4 weeks after spine stabilization to prevent wound complications.

147. **Water-Cooled Detector Module:** Detector cooled to prevent drift during high-dose QA tests.
**Related equipment:** 2D ion chamber array.
**Radiotherapy Example:** SBRT MU tests stable without thermal drift.

148. **Windows-Based Workflow Mirror:** Redundant workstation for backup of primary planning station.
**Related equipment:** Mirrored TPS server.
**Radiotherapy Example:** Planning uninterrupted during primary workstation failure.

149. **Weight-Loss Triggered Re-Simulation:** Automatic workflow to evaluate significant anatomic change for re-planning.
**Related equipment:** SGRT/weight tracking + adaptive workflow.
**Radiotherapy Example:** H&N patient lost 7 kg → mask loose → CT rescan & new plan.

150. **Wireless Isocenter Verification Probe:** Portable device confirms alignment between room lasers and radiation isocenter.
**Related equipment:** Iso-check probe.
**Radiotherapy Example:** 0.6 mm misalignment corrected before SBRT start.

151. **Working-Distance Dependent SSD Correction:** MU adjustment applied when SSD varies from calibration SSD.
**Related equipment:** SSD calculator.
**Radiotherapy Example:** MU modified for electron SSD difference from 100 cm to 110 cm.

**152. Wide-Target Robust Optimization:** Robust optimization covering large CTV-to-PTV uncertainties.
**Related equipment:** Robust optimizer.
**Radiotherapy Example:** Abdominal VMAT planned with ±10 mm shift robustness.

**153. Wedge-Filtered Electron Beam:** Electron beam modified with wedge filter to adjust surface dose gradient.
**Related equipment:** Custom wedge filter.
**Radiotherapy Example:** Dose shaped across scalp to match variable skin thickness.

**154. Wheelchair-Compatible Simulation Table:** Allows simulation without forced transfer for non-ambulatory patients.
**Related equipment:** Transfer-free CT simulator couch.
**Radiotherapy Example:** Spine RT simulation completed for paraplegic patient without transfer.

**155. Wide-Margin SRS Target Expansion:** Increased PTV margin in SRS for non-rigid targets or poor immobilization.
**Related equipment:** Rigid vs non-rigid mask selection.
**Radiotherapy Example:** Brain metastasis PTV margin expanded from 1 mm → 2.5 mm for restless patient.

**156. Weighted Directional Dose Fall-Off:** Applies directional dose gradient based on most critical OAR direction.
**Related equipment:** Gradient optimizer.
**Radiotherapy Example:** Steep fall-off achieved between prostate and rectum.

**157. Wet-Surface Electron Scattering Analysis:** Evaluates scattering changes when electron field interacts with moist skin surfaces.
**Related equipment:** Dose-surface analyzer.
**Radiotherapy Example:** Excess moist skin scattering → switched to photon plan.

**158. Work-Shift Radiation Fatigue Check:** Policy ensuring staff rotation to reduce fatigue-related safety errors.
**Related equipment:** Workload tracking system.
**Radiotherapy Example:** Wrong-patient incident avoided via rotation protocol in mould room.

**159. Weekly Adaptive Dose Monitoring:** Reviewing cumulative dose weekly to check whether adaption is required.
**Related equipment:** Accumulated dose engine.
**Radiotherapy Example:** Pancreas OAR dose rising → adaptive re-plan in week 2.

**160. Whole-Pelvis Nodal Auto-Segmentation:** Auto-contouring module for pelvic drainage nodal stations.
**Related equipment:** AI auto-segmentation.
**Radiotherapy Example:** Prostate + nodes plan completed 45 minutes faster.

**161. Wedge-Free Tangential Breast Planning:** A breast planning technique that avoids physical/dynamic wedges and instead achieves dose uniformity using field geometry and MLC modulation.
**Related Terms:** Tangential fields, field-in-field, MLC, breast irradiation.
**Radiotherapy Example:** Instead of using wedges for left-breast 3DCRT, field-in-field beams were added to improve uniformity and reduce heart dose.

**162. Wide-Range Scan-Length CT QA:** Quality assurance check verifying that the CT scanner maintains constant slice spacing and uniform HU accuracy across long scan ranges.
**Related equipment:** Wide-bore CT, CT QA phantom, HU test.
**Radiotherapy Example:** A whole-body 140 cm scan was validated to prevent HU drift before planning total marrow irradiation.

163. **Whole-Room Radiation Shut-Off Interlock:** A LINAC safety mechanism that stops radiation instantly if a room access violation or emergency button press is detected.
**Related Terms:** Door interlock, emergency stop, radiation safety.
**Radiotherapy Example:** Radiation automatically stopped during treatment when a staff member accidentally opened the treatment room door.

164. **Wire-Guided Surgical Clip Mapping:** Mapping of surgical clips using CT simulation wires to help localize tumour beds precisely in planning.
**Related equipment:** Surgical clips, radio-opaque skin wires, CT simulator.
**Radiotherapy Example:** Breast tumour bed was localized by placing wires over the surgical scar before CT scan for boost targeting.

165. **Wide-Bore MRI Simulation Workflow:** Process of using a wide-bore MRI scanner for RT simulation when immobilization devices require large scanner openings.
**Related Terms:** MR-sim, MRI-only planning, MR-CT registration.
**Radiotherapy Example:** Prostate MRI simulation performed in a wide-bore MRI with immobilization device, then fused with CT for VMAT planning.

166. **Workspace-Integrated Surface Guidance Monitor:** Surface monitoring displays installed directly in the treatment workflow to constantly show patient positioning data.
**Related equipment:** SGRT camera system, DIBH display.
**Radiotherapy Example:** Radiation therapists continuously monitored real-time surface tracking on overhead screens during breast DIBH delivery.

167. **Water-Phantom Dynamic Dose-Rate Scan:** QA test measuring LINAC beam stability at multiple dose-rates using scanning detectors in a water phantom.
**Related Terms:** Dose-rate linearity, beam stability, commissioning.
**Radiotherapy Example:** SBRT dose-rate QA confirmed stable output from 400–2400 MU/min before clinical use.

168. **Weekly Site-Visit Radiation Audit:** Routine weekly audit evaluating treatment delivery quality, documentation accuracy, and safety performance.
**Related Terms:** Quality assurance, radiation safety audit, performance review.
**Radiotherapy Example:** Weekly audit detected inconsistencies in IGRT documentation, allowing corrective training for staff.

169. **Waist-Support Belt for Pelvic RT Positioning:** Strap placed over the pelvis to stabilize pelvic area during simulation and treatment.
**Related equipment:** Immobilization straps, vacuum bag.
**Radiotherapy Example:** Belt used to prevent pelvic roll during prostate VMAT, improving daily reproducibility.

170. **Wireless Respiratory Motion Belt:** Wireless sensor belt detecting respiratory motion for gating or breath-hold treatment.
**Related Terms:** Gating, RPM tracking, motion management.
**Radiotherapy Example:** Belt was used to detect end-inhale / end-exhale phases during lung SBRT.

171. **Water-Tank Beam Symmetry Validation:** Measurement of lateral dose symmetry in a water tank to confirm beam uniformity across the field.
**Related equipment:** Water phantom, ion chamber, scanning system.
**Radiotherapy Example:** Symmetry test confirmed the X-jaw and Y-jaw beam profiles were within ±2% tolerance before allowing patient treatments.

172. **Wide-Field TBI Technique:** Total-body irradiation technique using wide radiation fields to cover the full patient length.
**Related Terms:** TBI, extended SSD, beam spoiler, dose homogeneity.
**Radiotherapy Example:** Wide fields at 400 cm SSD were used for paediatric leukemia conditioning prior to bone marrow transplant.

173. **Wire-Frame Immobilization Indexing:** Numbered grooves and markers built into immobilization frames to ensure identical daily patient indexing.
**Related equipment:** Thermoplastic masks, indexing bars, treatment couch.
**Radiotherapy Example:** Head-and-neck patient was fixed daily to index 0–3–7 on the mask frame to ensure highly reproducible positioning.

174. **Wobbling Proton Beam Technique:** A proton delivery mode using a rotating magnet pattern to spread the Bragg peak across a uniform field.
**Related Terms:** Proton therapy, RBE, spread-out Bragg peak.
**Radiotherapy Example:** Wobbling technique provided uniform paediatric cranial dose while sparing the cochlea and optic pathways.

175. **White-Noise Motion Reduction:** Use of soothing white-noise or sound masking to minimize involuntary patient movements during simulation and treatment.
**Related Terms:** Motion management, patient comfort, immobilization.
**Radiotherapy Example:** White noise was played during CT scan to prevent anxiety-related motion in a claustrophobic head-and-neck patient.

176. **Whole-MV Portal Imaging QA:** Verification of MV (megavoltage) imaging system performance including resolution, uniformity, and geometric accuracy.
**Related equipment:** EPID panel, imaging QA phantom.
**Radiotherapy Example:** MV images were tested weekly to ensure accurate IGRT matching for pelvic IMRT patients.

177. **Wide-Angle CBCT Reconstruction:** Using an expanded gantry rotation arc for CBCT imaging to capture more anatomical detail and reduce streak artifacts.
**Related Terms:** IGRT, CBCT, artifact reduction, iterative reconstruction.
**Radiotherapy Example:** Wide-angle CBCT improved visualization of pancreas in abdominal SBRT.

178. **Welfare-Centred Radiotherapy Comfort Check:** Workflow where patient comfort and anxiety levels are checked before and during treatment to avoid interruptions.
**Related Terms:** Patient support, communication, positioning stability.
**Radiotherapy Example:** Asking daily about shoulder pain prevented displacement during breast positioning.

179. **Window-Shaped MLC Field Formation:** Creation of rectangular aperture using MLC leaves instead of jaws for precise adaptive shaping around targets.
**Related Terms:** MLC modulation, aperture shaping, adaptive radiotherapy.
**Radiotherapy Example:** Window MLC aperture was used for liver SBRT boost to avoid nearby stomach wall.

180. **Weighted Dose Fall-off Model:** Optimization algorithm that prioritizes dose decay outside the target region using weighted penumbra control.
**Related Terms:** dose gradient, fall-off index, ring structure optimization.
**Radiotherapy Example:** High gradient fall-off was used around spinal cord during spine SBRT.

181. **Weekly LINAC Output Verification:** Routine measurement of machine output to ensure stable radiation dose delivery.
**Related equipment:** Farmer chamber, solid water slab, electrometer.
**Radiotherapy Example:** Weekly QA detected a −1.5% drift in photon output and recalibration was performed before treatment schedule was resumed.

182. **Workstation-Based Rapid Contouring:** Fast semi-automatic organ and tumour segmentation using planning software tools.
**Related Terms:** auto-contouring, artificial intelligence contouring, atlas contouring.
**Radiotherapy Example:** Auto-contouring of lungs and spinal canal reduced contour time for thoracic IMRT planning by 70%.

183. **Wide-Range CT Density Mapping:** Conversion of CT Hounsfield units across a large tissue density range into electron density for dose calculation.
**Related equipment:** CT calibration phantom, TPS HU-to-ED curve.
**Radiotherapy Example:** Calibration ensured correct dose calculation for lung, soft tissue, and bone during thoracic VMAT optimization.

184. **Wrist-Support Beam Delivery Cushion:** Soft wedges placed under arms to maintain immobilization without shoulder tension.
**Related Terms:** arm support, breast positioning, immobilization devices.
**Radiotherapy Example:** Wrist support cushions helped position arms overhead during breast IMRT without motion from fatigue.

185. **Wall-Mounted Accessory Cart Workflow:** Arrangement of mould room and treatment accessories in labeled wall units to reduce treatment setup time.
**Related equipment:** Mask frames, belly board inserts, couch indexing pads.
**Radiotherapy Example:** Organizing immobilization inserts reduced VMAT prostate setup time by 2 minutes per case.

186. **Wet-Film Radiation Profile Test:** Using radiographic films in water phantom to evaluate beam profile and penumbra width.
**Related Terms:** Film dosimetry, penumbra, beam profile QA.
**Radiotherapy Example:** Wet-film test validated field uniformity after MLC motor replacement.

187. **Wide-Target Simultaneous Integrated Boost:** Technique that delivers different dose levels to different target sub-volumes within the same plan and fractions.
**Related Terms:** SIB, IMRT, dose painting.
**Radiotherapy Example:** Breast SIB treatment simultaneously boosted tumour bed while giving lower dose to entire breast.

188. **Weekly Treatment Record Validation:** Verification of delivered MU, imaging approvals, couch shifts, and setup notes per patient.
**Related Terms:** IGRT documentation, audit, quality assurance.
**Radiotherapy Example:** Validation revealed missing IGRT approval for a head-and-neck patient; corrective action taken immediately.

189. **Whole-Organ Dose Statistics Extractor:** Software tool that extracts mean, max, min, and dose-volume statistics from organ dose distributions.
**Related Terms:** DVH, dose stats report, biological modeling.
**Radiotherapy Example:** Mean rectum dose was exported for NTCP calculation during prostate planning review.

190. **Wavelength-Optimized Portal Imaging:** MV portal images enhanced to improve soft-tissue visibility for IGRT matching.
**Related Terms:** image enhancement, MV imaging processing, IGRT.
**Radiotherapy Example:** Enhanced portal images were used to visualize diaphragm position during liver VMAT.

191. **Wall Laser Crosshair Orthogonality Check:** QA test confirming that wall lasers remain orthogonal and perfectly aligned with room isocentre.
**Related equipment:** Laser plumb line phantom, spirit level.
**Radiotherapy Example:** Misaligned wall laser detected and corrected before CT pelvic simulation.

192. **Wearing-Comfort Assessment for Immobilization Masks:** Evaluation of patient comfort and breathing space after mask formation.
**Related Terms:** mould room, thermoplastic mask, immobilization QA.
**Radiotherapy Example:** Extra nose opening was added after comfort review to prevent anxiety-related movement.

193. **Workflow-Integrated Auto-IGRT Approval:** Automatic pop-up IGRT approval step embedded in workflow to prevent missed approvals.
**Related Terms:** IGRT compliance, safety workflow, fail-safe.
**Radiotherapy Example:** Therapist had to approve CBCT match electronically before enabling beam-on for lung SBRT.

194. **Wound-Healing Radiation Timing Consideration:** Scheduling RT start date considering surgical site healing to avoid toxicity.
**Related Terms:** postoperative RT, gap time protocol.
**Radiotherapy Example:** Breast RT start was postponed until incision healing reached safe status.

195. **Wide-Bore Couch Rail Clearance Check:** Verifying that immobilization devices clear couch rails during CT and MRI simulation.
**Related equipment:** Wide-bore CT/MRI, indexing boards.
**Radiotherapy Example:** Full spine immobilization board fit without collision in CT bore after clearance test.

196. **Weighted Auto-Shimming MRI Protocol:** Balancing magnetic-field homogeneity in RT-oriented MRI sequences to reduce image distortion.
**Related Terms:** geometric distortion correction, MR-Sim.
**Radiotherapy Example:** Auto-shimming improved soft-tissue resolution for cervical cancer adaptive planning.

197. **Window-Template Breast Scar Marking:** Transparent plastic template used to align scar wires consistently every fraction.
**Related equipment:** Marking template, skin wires.
**Radiotherapy Example:** Ensured reproducible tumour-bed boost localization across 20+ fractions.

198. **Workload-Based Staffing Allocation in RT:** Assigning staff based on patient load and case complexity to maintain efficiency and safety.
**Related Terms:** manpower planning, workflow optimization.
**Radiotherapy Example:** Extra staff added during peak brachytherapy week to prevent simulation delays.

199. **Wireless Couch-Shift Controller:** Wireless handheld device that allows therapists to adjust couch position without touching the main console.
**Related equipment:** 6D couch, IGRT control system.
**Radiotherapy Example:** Wireless adjustment minimized treatment time during SBRT while maintaining precision.

200. **Water Cooling Loop:** A circulation system that removes excess heat from LINAC components.
**Related Terms:** Heat exchanger, chiller, accelerator head
**Example:** "A temperature rise alerted engineers to check the LINAC water cooling loop for blockage."

201. **Wavelength Attenuation:** Reduction in photon energy intensity as wavelength changes in tissue.**Related Terms:** Photon spectrum, attenuation coefficient
**Example:** "Tumor dose variation occurred due to wavelength attenuation during deep-tissue irradiation."

202. **Waveform Calibration:** Adjustment of accelerator RF waveform to maintain beam stability.
**Related Terms:** RF generator, pulse modulation
**Example:** "A physicist performed waveform calibration to reduce output fluctuation."

203. **Workload Factor:** Radiation shielding calculation based on expected usage of equipment.
**Related Terms:** Shielding design, occupancy factor
**Example:** "The mould-room bunker thickness was based on a workload factor of 30 Gy/week."

204. **Wedge Pair Technique:** Two wedge-filtered beams arranged opposingly to achieve a uniform dose.
**Related Terms:** Physical wedge, dose compensation
**Example:** "A wedge pair technique was used to treat a slanted chest wall surface."

205. **Work-Flow Optimization:** Process of improving clinical scheduling and treatment efficiency.
**Related Terms:** Patient throughput, planning time
**Example:** "A new CT-simulation schedule improved workflow optimization in radiotherapy."

206. **White-Noise Artifact:** Random uniform digital noise in CT simulation images.
**Related Terms:** Image resolution, reconstruction artefact
**Example:** "Repeating the scan eliminated the white-noise artifact affecting target contouring."

207. **Weak Scatter Zone:** Area where radiation scatter contribution is minimal.
**Related Terms:** Scatter radiation, dose gradient
**Example:** "A critical organ was positioned inside a weak scatter zone to reduce dose."

208. **Wall Transmission Factor:** Percentage of radiation penetrating a shielding wall.
**Related Terms:** Lead shielding, tenth-value layer
**Example:** "A wall transmission factor test ensured controlled room dose levels."

209. **Wire Localization:** Placement of a guide wire to mark small tumors for treatment or surgery.
**Related Terms:** Fiducial marker, stereotactic
**Example:** "Breast tumor wire localization assisted in precise boost planning."

210. **Wobbler Magnet:** Magnet used in proton therapy to broaden the beam for uniform distribution.
**Related Terms:** Proton scattering, Bragg peak
**Example:** "Switching the wobbler magnet flattened the proton field across the target."

211. **Window Transmission:** Radiation passing through LINAC exit window without energy loss.
**Related Terms:** Target window, primary collimator
**Example:** "Window transmission stability kept beam quality within 1% limit."

212. **Well-Type Ion Chamber:** Ion chamber for measuring radioactivity of sealed brachytherapy sources.
**Related Terms:** Source calibration, AAPM TG-43
**Example:** "I-125 seeds were verified with a well-type ion chamber before implant."

213. **Workflow Monitoring:** Real-time tracking of patient movement between CT, planning, and treatment.
**Related Terms:** Oncology information system, patient queue
**Example:** "Dashboards for workflow monitoring reduced RT delays."

214. **Weighted Composite Dose:** Sum of multiple radiation fields based on their individual dose weights.
**Related Terms:** Dose calculation, composite plan
**Example:** "The planner calculated a weighted composite dose for 4 partial-arc beams."

215. **Whole Abdomen Irradiation:** Radiation treatment covering entire abdominal cavity.
**Related Terms:** Pediatric oncology, organ tolerance
**Example:** "A whole abdomen irradiation plan used VMAT to spare kidneys."

216. **Water-Phantom Scanning:** Beam dosimetry using detectors in a water tank.
**Related Terms:** PDD, beam profile
**Example:** "Annual QA included water-phantom scanning for depth-dose curves."

217. **Wireless Treatment Console:** Control workstation for LINAC operated via wireless interface.
**Related Terms:** Remote console, ARIA/MOSAIQ
**Example:** "A wireless treatment console allowed safe remote beam interruption."

218. **Wrist Immobilizer:** Device used to prevent forearm movement during upper-body treatment.
**Related Terms:** Thermoplastic mask, mould room
**Example:** "The mould-room prepared a wrist immobilizer for stereotactic shoulder treatment."

219. **Wound Shield:** Protective cover placed over surgical wound to reduce scatter exposure.
**Related Terms:** Bolus, protective shielding
**Example:** "A wound shield reduced exit-dose irritation in post-mastectomy RT."

220. **Wound Dose Map:** A dose distribution plan specifically evaluating radiation near a surgical wound.
**Related Terms:** Skin dose, bolus, dose fall-off
**Example:** "A wound dose map was generated after CT simulation to ensure the incision site received no hotspot."

221. **Whole Lung Shielding:** Technique to limit dose to both lungs during radiation to thoracic or abdominal tumors.
**Related Terms:** ALARA, dose constraint, pediatric RT
**Example:** "VMAT planning with whole lung shielding protected lung tissue during Wilms tumor treatment."

222. **Weighted Field Combination:** Combining multiple treatment fields using different dose weight factors.
**Related Terms:** Composite dose, hybrid plan
**Example:** "A weighted field combination improved uniform dose in the larynx case."

223. **Water-Equivalency Error:** Deviation between actual tissue density and assumed water-equivalent value in TPS.
**Related Terms:** HU override, density correction
**Example:** "Water-equivalency error was corrected by assigning proper HU values to dental implants."

224. **Wireless Gating Sensor:** Motion detection sensor that communicates without cables for respiratory gating.
**Related Terms:** Surface-guided RT, RPM, breath-hold
**Example:** "The wireless gating sensor paused beam delivery when chest motion exceeded limits."

225. **Weight-Based Bolus Selection:** Choosing bolus thickness based on patient body habitus rather than fixed size.
**Related Terms:** Muscle depth, buildup effect
**Example:** "A weight-based bolus selection improved chest wall dose uniformity."

226. **Wall Scatter Correction:** Adjustment made for radiation returning into the room from surrounding walls.
**Related Terms:** Secondary scatter, shielding physics
**Example:** "Beam data were refined using wall scatter correction during annual QA."

227. **Window Level Optimization:** Adjusting CT scan grayscale window and level for best tumor visualization.
**Related Terms:** HU contrast, ROI visibility
**Example:** "Soft tissue window level optimization improved target contouring accuracy."

228. **Wrist Strap Restraint:** Immobilization strap preventing wrist rotation during treatment.
**Related Terms:** Thermoplastic mold, indexing board
**Example:** "The mould room added a wrist strap restraint for an upper-spine SBRT case."

229. **Workflow Risk Analysis:** Examination of patient-treatment workflow to identify safety issues.
**Related Terms:** FMEA, QA protocol
**Example:** "A workflow risk analysis prevented CT-to-LINAC dataset mismatch incidents."

230. **Wide-Arc VMAT:** VMAT treatment using a large rotation angle to cover extensive target volumes.
**Related Terms:** Multi-arc, conformity index
**Example:** "A wide-arc VMAT plan achieved sparing of kidneys during whole-abdomen treatment."

231. **Wiggler Magnet:** Magnet that oscillates electron paths to produce synchrotron radiation.
**Related Terms:** Free-electron laser, accelerator physics
**Example:** "The vendor upgraded the LINAC with a wiggler magnet to stabilize the beam spectrum."

232. **White-Field Flood Test:** Calibration test for flat panel detectors using uniform radiation.
**Related Terms:** kV imager QA, detector gain
**Example:** "The monthly white-field flood test corrected panel non-uniformity."

233. **Weight-Based MU Distribution:** Machine unit allocation distributed across beams based on dose proportion.
**Related Terms:** MU calculation, dose weighting
**Example:** "Revised weight-based MU distribution corrected an unintended hotspot near the OAR."

234. **Wedge Output Correction Factor:** Correction applied to adjust expected beam output when using wedges.
**Related Terms:** Physical wedge, transmission factor
**Example:** "The wedge output correction factor ensured MU accuracy during QA."

235. **Wet Film Storage Rack:** Drying rack used in darkrooms for wet radiographic films.
**Related Terms:** Radiology processing, film cassette
**Example:** "Old radiology rooms still used a wet film storage rack before digital systems arrived."

236. **White Phantom Imaging:** CT imaging using low-density uniform material to check reconstruction noise.
**Related Terms:** QA phantom, uniformity test
**Example:** "A white phantom imaging test detected excessive ring artifacts."

237. **Water-Based Immobilization Mold:** Mold created using warm water–softened thermoplastic for custom positioning.
**Related Terms:** Mould room, head & neck mask
**Example:** "A water-based immobilization mold was fabricated for a larynx patient."

238. **Wipe Contamination Test:** Surface testing to check for radioactive material using sample swabs.
**Related Terms:** Brachytherapy safety, radiation monitoring
**Example:** "A wipe contamination test confirmed no leakage after seed loading."

239. **Workspace ALARA Design:** Treatment room layout designed to minimize dose while maximizing efficiency.
**Related Terms:** Shielding, staff safety
**Example:** "The new LINAC room followed a workspace ALARA design to reduce occupational exposure."

240. **Wound Surface Bolus:** Bolus applied over irregular wound surfaces to ensure dose buildup.
**Related Terms:** Tissue equivalent material, scar boost
**Example:** "A wound surface bolus maintained target dose over a complex mastectomy scar."

241. **Wet Gel Ultrasound Marking:** Using ultrasound gel to mark soft tissues for superficial RT referencing.
**Related Terms:** Skin marking, IGRT localization
**Example:** "Wet gel ultrasound marking ensured precise boost placement around a lymph node."

242. **Window Dispersion Error:** Error caused by photon spread due to imperfections in the LINAC exit window.
**Related Terms:** Exit foil, beam symmetry
**Example:** "A window dispersion error was found during beam flatness QA."

243. **Water-Resistant Immobilizer:** Waterproof immobilization system for sweaty or high-moisture skin.
**Related Terms:** Breathable mask, positioning cushion
**Example:** "A water-resistant immobilizer prevented mask swelling during long head-neck treatments."

244. **Weighted CBCT Protocol:** Adaptive CBCT scanning using preset dose weights for different tissues.
**Related Terms:** Imaging dose reduction, ACBCT
**Example:** "The weighted CBCT protocol lowered exposure while maintaining bone visibility."

245. **Wireless Laser Verification:** Remote monitoring system confirming treatment-room laser accuracy.
**Related Terms:** Patient alignment, QA checks
**Example:** "Wireless laser verification detected a 1 mm shift before treatment began."

246. **Water-Spray Thermal Relief:** Cooling method for reducing mould-room thermoplastic temperature after heating.
**Related Terms:** Mask fabrication, burn prevention
**Example:** "A water-spray thermal relief was used before placing the warm mask on the patient."

247. **Wedge Angle Mismatch:** Planning error where wedge angle does not match target geometry.
**Related Terms:** Compensator error, hotspot
**Example:** "A wedge angle mismatch created dose overlap near the spinal cord."

248. **Weekly Beam Tracking Log:** Routine record documenting machine parameters and performance weekly.
**Related Terms:** QA logbook, LINAC performance
**Example:** "Output drift was noticed early due to the weekly beam tracking log."

249. **Workstation Indexing Plate:** Indexable plate that locks immobilization devices reproducibly on couch top.
**Related Terms:** Couch indexing, mould room tooling
**Example:** "The workstation indexing plate ensured identical setup between CT and LINAC."

250. **Wide PTV Margin Expansion:** Expanding PTV margins more than standard due to extreme movement.
**Related Terms:** ITV, motion management
**Example:** "The pancreas case needed wide PTV margin expansion because of respiratory motion."

251. **Water-Equivalent Calibration Slab:** Calibration slab that mimics water density for dose verification.
**Related Terms:** Solid water, dosimetry phantom
**Example:** "A water-equivalent calibration slab confirmed MU for electron fields."

252. **Wireless Table Pendant:** Wireless handheld control device for LINAC couch motions.
**Related Terms:** Patient positioning remote
**Example:** "Therapists used the wireless table pendant for fine couch adjustments."

253. **Wash-Out Dose Pattern:** Reduced dose created intentionally around sensitive structures.
**Related Terms:** Dose shaping, organ sparing
**Example:** "A wash-out dose pattern protected bowel loops during pelvis treatment."

254. **Whole-Spine Image Stitching:** Combining multiple spine CT images into a single continuous dataset.
**Related Terms:** Image registration, stitching artefact
**Example:** "Whole-spine image stitching was required for craniospinal irradiation planning."

255. **Workflow Synchronization:** Seamless coordination between CT → planning → QA → treatment.
**Related Terms:** Data transfer, interoperability
**Example:** "Automated workflow synchronization removed contour export delays."

256. **Warm-Start LINAC Boot:** Fast restart of LINAC without full reboot sequence.
**Related Terms:** Standby mode, accelerator reset
**Example:** "A warm-start boot restored beam availability in less than two minutes."

257. **Weighted Arc Modulation:** VMAT planning technique with variable modulation strength across arcs.
**Related Terms:** Dynamic modulation, dose gradient control
**Example:** "Weighted arc modulation reduced hotspots at the tumor-bowel interface."

258. **Wet-Bolus Contact Error:** Error caused by trapped moisture between skin and bolus.
**Related Terms:** Air gap, surface dose
**Example:** "A wet-bolus contact error caused underdose to the chest wall."

259. **White-Mask Immobilization:** Standard-density thermoplastic mask used for routine radiotherapy.
**Related Terms:** Head & neck mask, mould room equipment
**Example:** "A white-mask immobilization setup was used for the nasopharyngeal case."

260. **Wedge-Free Field Flattening:** Achieving dose uniformity without using wedges via MLC or arc modulation.
**Related Terms:** MLC shaping, dynamic planning
**Example:** "Wedge-free field flattening improved plan efficiency for breast tangents."

261. **Water-Phantom Dynamic Scan:** Moving detector scan measuring beam profile changes during motion.
**Related Terms:** PDD, output factor**Example:** "A water-phantom dynamic scan detected beam asymmetry during QA."

262. **Wireless IGRT Trigger:** Wireless signal that initiates imaging when patient reaches correct position.
**Related Terms:** Auto-capture, motion monitoring
**Example:** "The wireless IGRT trigger prevented accidental imaging during setup."

263. **Weak-Signal Dose Mapping:** Dose mapping in regions receiving very low scatter or leakage dose.
**Related Terms:** Peripheral dose, out-of-field exposure
**Example:** "Weak-signal dose mapping verified safety for pregnant caregiver protocols."

264. **Windowless Dose Meter:** Detector without protective window for extreme low-energy measurement.
**Related Terms:** Surface dosimeter, beta detection
**Example:** "A windowless dose meter verified build-up dose under thin bolus."

265. **Wire-Frame Contour Review:** Viewing structure contours in wire-frame form to check geometric accuracy.
**Related Terms:** 3D structure check, contour QC
**Example:** "Wire-frame contour review helped detect over-contouring of bowel loops."

266. **Weighted Multi-Pass Reconstruction:** CT reconstruction using multiple iterations with weighted averaging.
**Related Terms:** iCBCT, iterative reconstruction
**Example:** "Weighted multi-pass reconstruction lowered noise for obese-patient CBCT."

267. **Wave-Based Deformable Registration:** Image registration algorithm using wave-propagation modeling.
**Related Terms:** DIR, adaptive radiotherapy
**Example:** "Wave-based deformable registration aligned daily CBCT with planning CT."

268. **Wireless Crash Interrupt:** Emergency system that immediately stops LINAC beam wirelessly.
**Related Terms:** E-stop, safety interlock
**Example:** "A wireless crash interrupt halted treatment during unexpected patient seizure."

269. **Window-Angle Collimator:** Collimator that adjusts relative to exit window to optimize beam divergence.
**Related Terms:** Collimator leaf rotation, divergence control
**Example:** "The window-angle collimator reduced edge penumbra in electron field."

270. **Weighted SSD Adjustment:** Correcting SSD differences by adjusting field weight instead of MU.
**Related Terms:** SAD, inverse planning**Example:** "Weighted SSD adjustment balanced field dose in the shoulder case."

271. **White-Point Pixel Correction:** Correction that replaces defective bright pixels in kV or CBCT imaging.
**Related Terms:** Bad pixel mask
**Example:** "White-point pixel correction removed bright speckles on onboard CBCT."

272. **Wide-Gap Collimator Opening:** Large opening used to cover big anatomical areas.
**Related Terms:** Jaw separation, large field
**Example:** "Craniospinal RT used a wide-gap collimator opening for full spine coverage."

273. **Water-Tight Source Capsule:** Leak-proof brachytherapy seed container.
**Related Terms:** Sealed source, integrity test
**Example:** "Leak test confirmed the water-tight source capsule safety."

274. **Wand-Based Digitizer:** Point-tracking pen used to digitize body anatomy before CT era.
**Related Terms:** Simulator era, manual contour
**Example:** "Old simulators used a wand-based digitizer for field design."

275. **Work-Set Dose Profile:** Dose profile created after adjusting beam with real patient setup data.
**Related Terms:** Adaptive RT
**Example:** "The work-set dose profile changed after tumor regression."

276. **Whole-Staff Dose Drill:** Training exercise testing emergency radiation safety responses.
**Related Terms:** RSO, mock spill
**Example:** "A whole-staff dose drill practiced brachytherapy emergency handling."

277. **Windowless kV Detector:** Low-energy imaging detector that lacks a shielding window to increase sensitivity.
**Related Terms:** High-sensitivity imager
**Example:** "The windowless kV detector improved soft-tissue CBCT imaging."

278. **Wedge-Shift Technique:** Moving wedge orientation between beams instead of using multiple wedges.
**Related Terms:** Tangential RT, compensation
**Example:** "The wedge-shift technique improved dose uniformity for breast fields."

279. **Wireless Patient Alert Butto:** Portable alarm button given to patient during treatment.
**Related Terms:** Treatment interruption
**Example:** "The patient pressed the wireless alert button due to severe coughing."

280. **Wavelength Dose Fall-Off:** Dose reduction with increasing photon wavelength in soft tissue.
**Related Terms:** Attenuation, deep dose
**Example:** "Wavelength dose fall-off was considered for liver SBRT depth."

281. **Warm Therapy Couch:** Heated couch top providing comfort during long immobilization.
**Related Terms:** Patient comfort, immobilization
**Example:** "A warm therapy couch helped reduce movement for elderly patients."

282. **Water-Adaptive TPS Mode:** TPS automatically assigns density based on tissue water-equivalent correction.
**Related Terms:** HU assignment
**Example:** "The water-adaptive TPS mode corrected density for bowel gas."

283. **W284** –importance.
**Related Terms:** MLC modulation
**Example:** "Weighted leaf sequencing sharpened dose gradient near spinal cord."

284. **Wet-Room Mould Fabrication:** Mould-room method using heated water baths for thermoplastic shaping.
**Related Terms:** Immobilization mask
**Example:** "A wet-room mould fabrication session created a torso mold."

**285. Wash-Dose Verification Film:** Radiochromic film used to verify dose distribution in surface wash technique.
**Related Terms:** Film dosimetry
**Example:** "Wash-dose verification film confirmed superficial dose accuracy."

**286. Wall-Mounted IGRT Screen:** Monitor placed inside treatment room for live camera guidance.
**Related Terms:** Patient alignment camera
**Example:** "The wall-mounted IGRT screen made breath-hold coaching easier."

**287. Wide-Couch Support Bridge:** Board placed under large body to prevent couch sag.
**Related Terms:** Couch deflection
**Example:** "The wide-couch support bridge maintained alignment in obese patient RT."

**288. Wedge-Override Plan:** Removing wedge and compensating with MLC or arcs.
**Related Terms:** Optimized beam modulation
**Example:** "The breast plan was converted into a wedge-override plan."

**289. Wide-Bore CT Simulator:** CT scanner with large bore for easy immobilization-device clearance.
**Related Terms:** 85 cm bore CT, simulation scanner
**Example:** "Obese patients benefitted from the wide-bore CT simulator."

**290. Water-Density Override:** TPS correction to treat lung cavity or bowel obstruction as water density.
**Related Terms:** HU override
**Example:** "A water-density override prevented dose overestimation in bowel gas."

**291. Wing-Support Arm Fixator:** Anatomical support keeping both arms in wing position.
**Related Terms:** Breast board
**Example:** "The wing-support arm fixator improved clavicle exposure."

**292. Wireless Linac Door Interlock:** Door safety lock working wirelessly rather than through cables.
**Related Terms:** Safety protocol
**Example:** "The wireless LINAC door interlock paused beam automatically when opened."

**293. Wedge-Dose Symmetry Check:** QA test confirming wedge maintains dose symmetry between left and right sides.
**Related Terms:** Beam flatness QA
**Example:** "A wedge-dose symmetry check kept chest-wall plan acceptable."

**294. Weak-Beam Delivery Mode:** Mode that stabilizes extremely low-dose radiation output.
**Related Terms:** Flash dose, pediatric RT
**Example:** "Weak-beam delivery mode was used for a 0.2 Gy eye case."

**295. Water-Cooling Alarm Log:** Record showing past LINAC cooling system alarms.
**Related Terms:** Accelerator maintenance
**Example:** "Recurrent errors in water-cooling alarm log led to pump replacement."

**296. Wave-Front Imaging Detector:** Imager capturing phase changes in X-ray or proton waves.
**Related Terms:** Phase contrast imaging
**Example:** "The wave-front imaging detector enhanced soft-tissue visibility."

**297. Wide-Jaw Electron Field:** Electron beam field using maximum jaw opening for large lesions.
**Related Terms:** Electron applicator
**Example:** "A wide-jaw electron field treated extensive scalp lesion."

**298. Wrist-Range Setup Grid:** Grid printed pad checking wrist rotation reproducibility.
**Related Terms:** Indexing tools
**Example:** "The wrist-range setup grid improved SBRT reproducibility."

299. **Whole-Cycle Treatment Audit:** Retrospective audit from CT to final treatment to ensure safety and efficiency.
**Related Terms:** Peer review, clinical governance
**Example:** "A whole-cycle treatment audit revealed delays in transitioning from CT to planning."

300. **Working Voltage:** The electrical voltage required for a machine or detector to function optimally.
**Related Terms:** LINAC, chamber calibration, high-voltage unit.
**Example:** The ion chamber must operate at a specific working voltage to accurately measure beam output.

301. **Weighting Factor (WR or WT):** Multipliers used to calculate effective dose based on tissue sensitivity or radiation type.
**Related Terms:** Equivalent dose, effective dose, ICRP standards.
**Example:** The weighting factor for the lungs is applied during dose calculation and reporting in treatment planning.

302. **Whole Breast Radiation Therapy:** Radiation treatment covering the entire breast after lumpectomy.
**Related Terms:** Tangential fields, IMRT, photon therapy.
**Example:** A breast cancer patient receives 42.5 Gy in 16 fractions as whole-breast irradiation.

303. **Wide Bore CT:** CT scanner with a larger opening to fit immobilization devices and patients comfortably.
**Related Terms:** Simulation CT, mould room, thermoplastic mask.
**Example:** A head-and-neck patient with a mask undergoes simulation using a wide-bore CT to avoid clearance issues.

304. **Wedge Pair Technique:** A radiotherapy method using two wedge filters to improve homogeneity across the target.
**Related Terms:** Wedge factor, beam modification, tangential technique.
**Example:** A paraspinal field uses a wedge pair to shape dose distribution.

305. **Wedge Factor:** A correction value applied during dose calculations when a wedge filter is used.
**Related Terms:** Treatment planning system (TPS), monitor units, beam modifiers.
**Example:** MU calculation changes when a 30° wedge is inserted.

306. **Wet Read:** A quick preliminary radiology interpretation without a formal report.
**Related Terms:** Emergency CT, diagnostic workflow, radiologist communication.
**Example:** A patient with suspected metastasis receives a wet read CT scan before treatment planning.

307. **Water Phantom System:** A water-filled measurement device used to collect beam data for commissioning and QA.
**Related Terms:** Linear accelerator, ion chamber, dosimetry.
**Example:** A water phantom is used to verify depth-dose data during LINAC commissioning.

308. **Whole Spine Irradiation:** Irradiating the entire spinal column, often for medulloblastoma.
**Related Terms:** Craniospinal irradiation, proton therapy, junction matching.
**Example:** Pediatric patient receives craniospinal treatment including full spine coverage.

309. **Wide Field Radiation:** A broad radiation field used to cover large regions such as the pelvis or lymphatics.
**Related Terms:** Extended fields, high-energy photons, shielding.
**Example:** Pelvic radiation for cervical cancer may begin using a wide field before boost.

310. **Wire Marking:** Temporary skin marking done using radio-opaque wires for treatment localization.
**Related Terms:** CT simulation, tattooing, reference marks.
**Example:** Surgical scars are outlined with wire during CT simulation for contouring.

311. **Workflow Optimization:** Improving efficiency and accuracy in radiotherapy procedures.
**Related Terms:** TPS automation, QA checklists, safety management.
**Example:** Auto-contouring software is implemented to improve planning workflow.

312. **Weight-Based Dose Calculation:** Dosage determined using patient weight, common in nuclear medicine and chemo-RT, less in EBRT.
**Related Terms:** BSA formula, pediatric dosing.
**Example:** Pediatric brachytherapy doses sometimes consider weight-based adjustments.

313. **Window Level Adjustment:** Manipulating grayscale settings on CT for better anatomical visualization.
**Related Terms:** CT imaging, organ delineation, contrast resolution.
**Example:** A planner adjusts lung window (-600 HU) to contour lung volumes.

314. **Wide Dynamic Range Detector:** A detector capable of measuring low to high radiation exposures accurately.
**Related Terms:** EPID, portal imaging, QA detectors.
**Example:** EPID systems with wide dynamic range ensure accurate IMRT QA measurement.

315. **Warm-Up Cycle (LINAC):** A startup process ensuring machine stability before clinical use.
**Related Terms:** QA checklist, gantry systems, accelerator tuning.
**Example:** Radiation therapists perform a LINAC warm-up before morning treatments.

316. **Whole-Body Dose Limit:** Regulatory limit of radiation dose applied to workers or public exposure.
**Related Terms:** Radiation safety, NCRP guidelines, dosimeters.
**Example:** Staff ensure radiation exposure remains below 20 mSv/year occupational limits.

317. **Wire Localization (Breast):** Using a guidewire to locate a tumor for surgery or targeted radiation boost.
**Related Terms:** Stereotactic biopsy, boost planning.
**Example:** Wire-localized breast cavity helps define boost target volume.

318. **Weight Distribution (Setup):** Ensuring patient body weight is balanced during immobilization.
**Related Terms:** Positioning aids, mould room, headrests.
**Example:** Body weight distribution on a breast board prevents patient rotation during treatment.

319. **Wavelength (Radiation):** The distance between successive peaks in an electromagnetic wave.
**Related Terms:** X-rays, photons, energy spectrum.
**Example:** Megavoltage beams have extremely short wavelengths enabling deep tissue penetration.

320. **Waveguide (LINAC):** A structure that directs microwaves to accelerate electrons inside a LINAC.
**Related equipment:** Magnetron, klystron, electron gun.
**Example:** The waveguide transfers high-frequency microwaves to accelerate electrons for treatment beam production.

321. **Windmill Rotation (Gantry Drift Term):** A term describing uncontrolled or unintended rotational motion of the gantry.
**Related equipment:** LINAC gantry, bearing system.
**Example:** QA detects a windmill-like drift in gantry angle requiring mechanical adjustment.

322. **Water Equivalent Thickness (WET):** Material thickness expressed in terms of equivalent water thickness affecting beam attenuation.
**Related equipment:** Bolus, compensators, CT calibration.
**Example:** Bolus of 1 cm simulates 1 cm water equivalent thickness for skin dose buildup.

**323. Window/Level Presets:** Stored HU (Hounsfield Unit) settings optimized for different organs during CT viewing.
**Related equipment:** CT workstation, TPS viewer.
**Example:** Planners use brain and bone presets during contouring in treatment planning.

**324. Wiggler (Synchrotron Term):** A magnetic device used to increase radiation output in particle accelerators.
**Related equipment:** Proton therapy synchrotron, storage ring.
**Example:** The wiggler helps generate high-intensity beams in synchrotron proton systems.

**325. Warm Vision (Visual Symptom):** Sensation of heat or flush during MRI or radiotherapy images.
**Related equipment:** LINAC, MRI-guided RT.
**Example:** Some patients report a warm flash sensation during MV imaging or MR-guided treatment.

**326. Wide Beam Attenuation Correction:** A correction applied when using large CT or CBCT fields to avoid signal loss.
**Related equipment:** CBCT, CT scanners, EPID.
**Example:** CBCT imaging uses attenuation correction in pelvic radiotherapy simulation.

**327. Wipe Test (Brachytherapy):** A contamination test to ensure there is no radioactive leakage from sealed sources.
**Related equipment:** Survey meter, LDR/HDR brachytherapy sources.
**Example:** After seed handling, staff perform a wipe test to confirm no contamination.

**328. Weight Shifting (Patient Setup):** Change in patient posture or weight distribution affecting reproducibility.
**Related equipment:** Vacuum cushions, immobilization system.
**Example:** Weight shifting may change isocenter reproducibility in pelvic RT.

**329. Workflow Automation:** Use of software and controls to streamline planning and treatment processes.
**Related equipment:** TPS automation, AI contouring.
**Example:** Auto-segmentation tools improve workflow in head & neck planning.

**330. Water-Equivalent Dose (WED):** Dose measured relative to water absorption properties.
**Related equipment:** Dosimeter, phantom.
**Example:** IMRT dose calculations are verified using water-equivalent calibration phantoms.

**331. Whole Thorax Irradiation:** Radiation covering the entire thoracic cavity when indicated.
**Related equipment:** IMRT/VMAT, proton therapy.
**Example:** Used in cases like diffuse pleural disease.

**332. Wedge-Shaped Dose Profile:** A beam profile modified to achieve gradual dose falloff.
**Related equipment:** Physical or dynamic wedge.
**Example:** Used for breast tangential fields to avoid hotspots.

**333. Wrap-Around Field Matching:** Field matching technique for large or curved anatomical areas.
**Related equipment:** Treatment beam matching algorithm.
**Example:** Used in craniospinal irradiation regions where fields must wrap smoothly.

**334. Wireless Networking System (RT Equipment Control):** Tech used to sync consoles, imaging, and patient workflow systems.
**Related equipment:** Oncology information systems (OIS), MOSAIQ, ARIA.
**Example:** Treatment data transfers wirelessly from CT simulation to the LINAC console.

335. **Whole Lung Irradiation:** Radiation treatment that covers both lungs, typically used in pediatric oncology.
**Related equipment:** Photon therapy, VMAT.
**Example:** Used in metastatic sarcoma or Wilm's tumor cases.

336. **Windowing Artifacts:** Image distortion due to improper window/level CT adjustment.
**Related equipment:** CT scan viewer, cone beam imaging.
**Example:** Over-narrow windows may hide tumor borders during contouring.

337. **Wet Film Density (Old QA Term):** Measurement of optical density on traditional film used in QA before digital systems.
**Related equipment:** Film dosimetry, densitometer.
**Example:** Older IMRT QA used wet films to evaluate beam fluence.

338. **Wipe and Record Safety Protocol:** Procedure rule ensuring contamination monitoring is documented.
**Related equipment:** Radiation log book, dosimeters.
**Example:** Mandatory in HDR brachytherapy environments.

339. **Weighted Field Overlap:** Method used to prevent hotspots in overlapping radiation fields.
**Related equipment:** IMRT, treatment planning system.
**Example:** Craniospinal treatment requires weighted overlap to avoid overdose.

340. **WET Phantom (Water Equivalent Tissue Phantom):** A phantom mimicking human tissue attenuation.
**Related equipment:** QA phantoms, EPID QA.
**Example:** Used in IMRT commissioning to simulate patient dose behavior.

341. **Wall Scatter Contribution:** Scatter radiation contribution from treatment room walls.
**Related equipment:** Vault shielding, treatment planning environment.
**Example:** Calculated during bunker shielding design.

342. **Workload Factor (Shielding Term):** Expected weekly LINAC or imaging usage used in shielding calculations.
**Related equipment:** NCRP guidelines, bunker planning.
**Example:** High volume LINAC requires higher workload shielding calculations.

343. **Warm Field (Low-Dose Large Area Beam):** Technique delivering gentle dose across large field.
**Related equipment:** Flattening filter-free beam.
**Example:** Used in certain palliative whole-skin treatments.

344. **Window Spectrum Analysis (Detector Calibration):** Detecting specific range of signals for QA or imaging calibration.
**Related equipment:** Spectrometers, EPID calibration.
**Example:** Used during MV imaging calibration.

345. **Wide-Angle Couch Rotation Scan:** Couch-rotation imaging used for dose verification.
**Related equipment:** CBCT, 4D CT.
**Example:** Used for adaptive radiotherapy planning.

346. **Wireless Positioning System:** Real-time positioning system detecting patient or marker movement wirelessly.
**Related equipment:** SGRT, Calypso, IR gating.
**Example:** SGRT verifies breath-hold accuracy in breast RT.

347. **Worn-Out Beam Stopper Indicator:** Warning system indicating shielding block degradation.
**Related equipment:** LINAC posterior beam stopper.
**Example:** Triggered during maintenance QA.

348. **Water-Induced Mask Shrinkage:** Thermoplastic mask changes size if stored wet.
**Related equipment:** Head mask, immobilization.
**Example:** RT technicians avoid water storage to maintain mask accuracy.

349. **Weak Signal Reconstruction (Imaging Algorithm):** Software process enhancing low-signal CBCT/CT images.
**Related equipment:** Reconstruction kernels.
**Example:** Useful in low-dose lung CBCT on LINAC.

350. **Wide Margin Planning:** Larger expansions used for uncertainty (motion, setup errors).
**Related equipment:** PTV margins, motion management.
**Example:** Used in spine tumors with limited immobilization.

351. **Washout Phase (Nuclear Medicine Term):** Imaging phase that shows tracer clearance patterns.
**Related equipment:** PET/CT, SPECT.
**Example:** Used to differentiate viable tumor from necrosis.

352. **Wavelength Spectrum Analysis:** Measuring energy spectrum of emitted radiation.
**Related equipment:** LINAC, beam quality meters.
**Example:** Performed during commissioning to verify beam quality.

353. **White Noise Simulation (Image Noise Modeling):** Introducing artificial noise for algorithm testing.
**Related equipment:** CBCT, image processing.
**Example:** Used to evaluate reconstruction software.

354. **Weak Scatter Modeling:** Accounting for low-intensity scatter in dose calculation algorithms.
**Related equipment:** Monte Carlo TPS.
**Example:** Improves accuracy in lung dose calculations.

355. **Whole Abdominal Radiation:** Treating full abdomen region.
**Related equipment:** IMRT/VMAT.
**Example:** Used for ovarian cancer cases.

356. **Wire Re-Simulation Correction:** Wire placement repeated if shifted before CT simulation.
**Related equipment:** Radiopaque markers.
**Example:** Ensures accurate boost volume identification.

357. **Workstation-Based Adaptive Planning:** Treatment plan modified based on updated daily imaging.
**Related equipment:** MR-Linac, adaptive TPS.
**Example:** Adjusted tumor shrinkage plan in offline adaptive RT.

358. **Wand Tracking System:** Handheld real-time motion tracking for patient alignment.
**Related equipment:** Optical tracking systems.
**Example:** Used in stereotactic radiosurgery alignment.

359. **Warm Dose (Non-Ablative Fractionation):** Intermediate dose between palliative and ablative.
**Related equipment:** VMAT, IMRT.
**Example:** Used in oligometastatic prostate bone lesions.

360. **Wavelength Modulation:** Adjustment of radiation wavelength or frequency to optimize beam performance or imaging clarity.
**Related Terms:** Beam tuning, frequency control, calibration.
**Radiotherapy Example:** During LINAC commissioning, wavelength modulation is checked to ensure stable microwave frequency for electron acceleration.

361. **Weak Feature Imaging:** Imaging approach designed to detect low-contrast or subtle anatomical structures.
**Related Terms:** Low-contrast detectability, CBCT enhancement, reconstruction filters.
**Radiotherapy Example:** CBCT algorithms improve weak feature imaging to better identify soft tissue in pelvis RT.

362. **Weight Map Optimization:** Algorithm process adjusting dose weighting across multiple beams for optimal dose distribution.
**Related Terms:** IMRT optimization, dose weighting, fluence modulation.
**Radiotherapy Example:** IMRT planning uses weight map optimization to reduce hotspots near organs at risk.

363. **Window Filter Kernel:** A mathematical filter applied to imaging reconstruction to improve sharpness or reduce noise.
**Related Terms:** Reconstruction algorithm, CT kernel, smoothing filters.
**Radiotherapy Example:** A bone window kernel is used for contouring spinal metastasis during planning.

364. **Wobble Calibration:** Process of correcting mechanical or electromagnetic fluctuations in beam delivery.
**Related Terms:** Flatness QA, mechanical QA, isocenter verification.
**Radiotherapy Example:** Proton systems undergo wobble calibration to maintain uniform dose distribution.

365. **Wire-Based Localization:** Use of radiopaque wires to mark anatomical or surgical margins.
**Related Terms:** Radiopaque marker, fiducials, surgical clips.
**Radiotherapy Example:** Surgeons place localization wires pre-simulation for breast boost planning.

366. **Wrap-Around Detector Response:** Signal distortion when detector receives data beyond designed range.
**Related Terms:** Detector saturation, image artifacts, calibration.
**Radiotherapy Example:** EPID calibration prevents wrap-around signal artifacts in IMRT QA imaging.

367. **Waveform Stabilization:** Regulation of electrical waveform stability in power supply systems for radiotherapy devices.
**Related Terms:** High-voltage generator, frequency stability, RF power.
**Radiotherapy Example:** Stable waveform supply ensures consistent electron acceleration in LINAC treatment.

368. **Weak Beam Syndrome (Engineering Term):** Condition where output dose becomes lower than expected due to component wear or misalignment.
**Related Terms:** Output drift, calibration error, beam tuning.
**Radiotherapy Example:** Monthly QA identifies weak beam output requiring recalibration.

369. **Weight Compensation Algorithm:** Algorithm that automatically adjusts beam weighting when changing patient anatomy or adaptive plans.
**Related Terms:** Adaptive radiotherapy, dose recalculation, iterative optimization.
**Radiotherapy Example:** Used in adaptive MR-Linac workflows during tumor shrinkage monitoring.

370. **Water Immersion Dosimetry:** Dose measurement technique using water tank systems to characterize beam depth dose.
**Related Terms:** PDD curve, reference dosimetry, IAEA TRS guidelines.
**Radiotherapy Example:** Commissioning uses water immersion dosimetry to measure depth dose of 6 MV beam.

**371. Wall-Mounted Laser System:** A positioning system that projects reference lines for patient alignment.
**Related Terms:** Room lasers, alignment markers, simulation setup.
**Radiotherapy Example:** CT simulation uses wall-mounted lasers to mark patient reference tattoos.

**372. Weight Distribution Mask Design:** Technique ensuring immobilization masks apply even pressure across patient anatomy.
**Related Terms:** Thermoplastic mask, mould room, head immobilization.
**Radiotherapy Example:** Proper weight distribution mask design improves reproducibility in brain RT.

**373. Whole Spinal Imaging:** Imaging of entire spine for treatment planning, often requiring multiple scanning segments.
**Related Terms:** Long field imaging, CSI treatment, CT stitching.
**Radiotherapy Example:** Craniospinal irradiation requires whole spine CBCT verification.

**374. Windowed Acquisition Mode:** Imaging mode capturing data only during a specific respiratory or cardiac cycle interval.
**Related Terms:** Gating, 4D CT, motion management.
**Radiotherapy Example:** Lung SBRT uses windowed acquisition to avoid motion blurring.

**375. Workstation Authentication Security:** Digital access control to protect patient data and treatment settings.
**Related Terms:** Cybersecurity, password access, MOSAIQ/ARIA.
**Radiotherapy Example:** Staff must authenticate before modifying treatment prescriptions.

**376. Weighted Organ Sparing:** Technique prioritizing specific OAR protection during optimization.
**Related Terms:** Dose constraints, Pareto optimization, IMRT planning.
**Radiotherapy Example:** In prostate RT, rectum receives higher weight sparing priority.

**377. Wireless Dose Log Transfer:** Automatic transfer of treatment dose records from LINAC to oncology software.
**Related Terms:** ARIA, MOSAIQ, DICOM RT.
**Radiotherapy Example:** After every treatment fraction, dose log uploads automatically to patient chart.

**378. Waypoint Tracking (RT Navigation):** Tracking checkpoints during imaging-guided patient setup.
**Related Terms:** SGRT markers, optical tracking, position verification.
**Radiotherapy Example:** Calypso beacons provide waypoint tracking for prostate motion.

**379. Weak Tissue Margin Planning:** Margin applied to tissues lacking clear anatomical boundaries.
**Related Terms:** ITV, PTV margin, adaptive planning.
**Radiotherapy Example:** Used in pancreas RT, where edges are difficult to visualize.

**380. Wide Spectrum Bremsstrahlung:** Broad energy spectrum generated when electrons interact with high-Z targets.
**Related Terms:** MV photons, target interaction, LINAC beam.
**Radiotherapy Example:** LINACs generate wide spectrum Bremsstrahlung photons for therapy beams.

**381. Whole Brain Boost Planning:** Supplemental planning after whole brain irradiation targeting residual metastasis.
**Related Terms:** SRS boost, hippocampal sparing, dose escalation.
**Radiotherapy Example:** After WBRT, a localized SRS boost treats active lesions.

382. **Warning Limit Threshold:** Predefined tolerance limit before triggering machine errors or safety interlocks.
**Related Terms:** QA tolerance, safety system, radiation controls.
**Radiotherapy Example:** Output variation beyond warning threshold triggers machine stop.

383. **Workflow Bottleneck Analysis:** Evaluation of delays and inefficiencies in radiotherapy process.
**Related Terms:** Lean healthcare, process mapping, automation.
**Example:** Clinics track CT wait time vs treatment throughput.

384. **Weighted RBE Calculation:** Adjusting dose based on biological effectiveness of radiation type.
**Related Terms:** Proton therapy, LET, equivalent dose.
**Example:** Proton plans convert Gy to Gy(RBE) before delivery.

385. **Whole Body Attenuation Mapping:** Mapping how radiation interacts with tissues throughout entire body.
**Related Terms:** Monte Carlo simulation, heterogeneity correction.
**Example:** Used in total body irradiation (TBI) planning.

386. **Wet-Dry Density Calibration (Film Dosimetry):** Calibration ensuring film optical density remains stable post-processing.
**Related Terms:** Film QA, sensitometry, EPID comparison.
**Example:** Used in older IMRT QA before portal dosimetry.

387. **Wide Bore CT Use:** Use of large-aperture CT scanner to accommodate immobilized RT patients.
**Related Terms:** Simulation CT, immobilization devices.
**Example:** Used for obese or immobilized spine patients.

388. **Wire Grid Dose Check:** Verification method using metallic grid pattern to test beam alignment.
**Related Terms:** Beam alignment, mechanical QA, test pattern.
**Example:** Used during commissioning to ensure correct isocenter.

389. **Weak Signal Tracking Algorithm:** Software process detecting faint motion tracking signals.
**Related Terms:** SGRT, MR-guided RT, respiratory tracking.
**Example:** Used in CyberKnife tracking of implanted markers.

390. **Wedge Angle Optimization:** Selecting optimal wedge angle to achieve desired dose uniformity.
**Related Terms:** Wedge filter, beam shaping, breast tangents.
**Example:** Custom wedge angle used for treating chest wall curvature.

391. **Workload Projection for Shielding:** Estimation of future machine use for radiation room design.
**Related Terms:** Shielding, NCRP reports, primary barrier calculations.
**Example:** Used when building new LINAC bunkers.

392. **Wide Field 4D CT:** Motion-resolved imaging across large anatomical volumes.
**Related Terms:** Motion management, respiratory gating.
**Example:** Used in abdominal or thoracic tumor simulation.

393. **Warm Phantom QA:** Performing QA with phantom kept near physiological temperature.
**Related Terms:** MRI phantom, MR-Linac QA.
**Example:** MR-guided therapy requires warm phantom scans.

394. **Weighted Dose Histogram:** DVH adjusted with tissue priorities or biological weighting.
**Related Terms:** DVH analysis, planning comparison.
**Example:** Used to evaluate treatment improvements.

395. **Weakly Ionizing Radiation:** Radiation type with low ionization density (low LET).
**Related Terms:** X-rays, gamma rays, megavoltage photons.
**Example:** LINAC photon beams are weakly ionizing.

396. **Wire Laser Alignment Check:** Check using alignment wires to ensure lasers remain calibrated.
**Related Terms:** Laser QA, isocenter verification.
**Example:** Monthly QA verifies lasers match treatment isocenter.

397. **Whole Pelvic Radiation Planning:** Planning radiation that covers full pelvic region.
**Related Terms:** VMAT, field matching, nodal irradiation.
**Example:** Used for cervical or rectal cancer.

398. **Weight-Supported Couch System:** Couch designed to maintain stability under heavy patient load.
**Related Terms:** Treatment couch, bariatric support.
**Example:** Required for obese patient SBRT setup.

399. **Wide Aperture Immobilization Compatibility:** Ensures immobilization devices fit CT bore and LINAC clearance.
**Related Terms:** Wide bore CT, mask design, mould room QA.
**Example:** Spine immobilization must clear LINAC gantry collision path.

400. **Workflow Automation System:** A digital platform that automatically manages radiotherapy scheduling, imaging, planning, and treatment tasks to reduce delays and errors.
**Related Terms:** ARIA workflow, MOSAIQ automation, treatment scheduling.
**Radiotherapy Example:** The clinic uses a workflow automation system to automatically trigger CBCT review reminders before each fraction.

401. **Wide Dynamic Range Imaging:** Imaging mode capable of capturing very bright and very dark signal areas without losing detail.
**Related Terms:** HDR imaging, flat-panel detector range, contrast mapping.
**Radiotherapy Example:** CBCT scanners use wide dynamic range imaging to differentiate bony pelvis and soft tissue during setup.

402. **Wedge Field Matching:** Using wedge filters to smoothly match dose between adjacent radiation fields.
**Related Terms:** Field junctioning, beam matching, wedge pair technique.
**Radiotherapy Example:** Breast tangential fields require wedge field matching to avoid hot/cold spots.

403. **Wireless Patient Monitoring:** Monitoring respiration, heart rate, or motion wirelessly during treatment.
**Related Terms:** SGRT, motion control, gating.
**Radiotherapy Example:** In lung SBRT, wireless respiratory belts monitor patient breathing during delivery.

404. **Window Size Reconstruction Tuning:** Changing reconstruction window parameters to enhance detail in selected anatomical regions.
**Related Terms:** CT kernel adjustment, soft tissue windowing, bone window.
**Radiotherapy Example:** Radiologists adjust the bone window size to contour vertebrae accurately.

405. **Whole-Field VMAT Planning:** VMAT technique delivering dose to the entire target using continuous rotating arcs.
**Related Terms:** IMRT, arc therapy, dose modulation.
**Radiotherapy Example:** Prostate RT uses whole-field VMAT to cover PTV efficiently.

406. **Waste Dose Monitoring:** Recording radiation dose produced but not delivered to patients (e.g., warm-ups, machine QA).
**Related Terms:** Radiation safety audit, shielding calculation, leakage dose.
**Radiotherapy Example:** Annual reports include waste dose monitoring for regulatory compliance.

407. **Wire-Based Surface Simulation:** Using a shallow grid of wires to simulate contours or immobilization alignment.
**Related Terms:** Surface contouring, mould room techniques, bolus shaping.
**Radiotherapy Example:** Used in older setups for custom lead shielding molding.

408. **Whole-Body Dose Mapping:** Representation of cumulative dose across entire body after full course treatment.
**Related Terms:** Cumulative DVH, dose summation, biological dose maps.
**Radiotherapy Example:** Survivorship care includes whole-body dose maps in pediatric oncology.

409. **Wavelet-Based Image Enhancement:** Image processing technique that uses mathematical wavelets to improve edge sharpness and reduce noise.
**Related Terms:** Image reconstruction, denoising, edge enhancement.
**Radiotherapy Example:** CBCT images become clearer using wavelet filtering for head-and-neck localization.

410. **Wobbling Proton Technique:** A method where proton beams are magnetically steered to create a uniform dose area.
**Related Terms:** Scatter system, PBS vs scattering, uniform field.
**Radiotherapy Example:** Traditional proton centers used the wobbling technique to treat whole brain fields.

411. **Weight-Based Immobilization Selection:** Matching immobilization equipment based on patient size and mass.
**Related Terms:** Bariatric support, couch tolerance, mould room equipment.
**Radiotherapy Example:** High-BMI patients require reinforced mask boards for spine RT.

412. **Window Expansion Algorithm:** Algorithm that expands imaging field of view without completely repeating scans.
**Related Terms:** CT stitching, extended FOV correction.
**Radiotherapy Example:** Used when simulation CT misses part of shoulder in head-and-neck cancer.

413. **Water Cooling System Check:** Routine verification of machine cooling systems used to prevent overheating.
**Related Terms:** LINAC engineering, thermal regulation, maintenance.
**Radiotherapy Example:** A water cooling failure triggers interlock preventing beam generation.

414. **Workload Dose Estimation:** Calculation of weekly delivered radiation dose for shielding compliance.
**Related Terms:** NCRP shielding, barrier calculations.
**Radiotherapy Example:** Radiation safety officers track workload dose estimates for LINAC approval.

415. **Wide Beam Flash:** Extra margin of radiation field beyond target to compensate for motion or swelling.
**Related Terms:** Flash margin, bolus field expansion.
**Radiotherapy Example:** Chest wall RT includes field flash for breathing movement.

416. **Wire Phantom QA:** Phantom containing wires used for checking geometric accuracy of imaging systems.
**Related Terms:** Geometry phantom, distortion QA, MRI QA.
**Radiotherapy Example:** Used during MRI simulation commissioning.

417. **Weighted Planning Objective:** Prioritized planning goals assigned numeric importance during optimization.
**Related Terms:** DVH objectives, cost function.
**Radiotherapy Example:** Pediatric RT increases spinal cord sparing weight in optimization.

418. **Workflow Safety Barrier:** A mandatory pause step requiring verification before proceeding.
**Related Terms:** Timeout protocols, peer review, checklist.
**Radiotherapy Example:** Before first fraction, workflow safety barrier forces digital plan review.

419. **Whole-Liver Adaptive Plan:** A plan updated to reflect shrinking or shifting liver tumors during treatment.
**Related Terms:** Adaptive radiotherapy, MR-Linac.
**Radiotherapy Example:** Daily MR imaging adjusts treatment for adaptive liver SBRT.

420. **Wedge Pair Technique:** Technique using opposing wedge beams to generate uniform dose gradient.
**Related Terms:** Isodose sculpting, manual beam shaping.
**Radiotherapy Example:** Common in lung or breast tangential beam planning.

421. **Windowed Motion Imaging:** Capturing motion only in identified ranges (exhale phase, cardiac cycle).
**Related Terms:** Gated imaging, breath-hold scans.
**Radiotherapy Example:** Used in liver RT to reduce motion blur.

422. **Wide-Bore MRI Workflow:** Workflow designed around large MRI aperture for RT planning.
**Related Terms:** MR-simulator, hybrid imaging.
**Radiotherapy Example:** Used for prostate planning with MR guidance.

423. **Warping Algorithm (Deformable Registration):** Mathematical method allowing images to stretch or deform to match anatomy over time.
**Related Terms:** DIR, adaptive therapy, image fusion.
**Radiotherapy Example:** Used in adaptive offline imaging for tumor shrinkage.

424. **Weak Tissue Contrast Simulation:** Simulated imaging conditions where tissues have minimal visible contrast.
**Related Terms:** Low-contrast resolution test, phantom QA.
**Radiotherapy Example:** QA uses phantoms to verify imaging performance in head-and-neck cases.

425. **Wireless SGRT Monitoring:** Remote surface-guided monitoring without wired sensors.
**Related Terms:** Catalyst, AlignRT, non-contact tracking.
**Radiotherapy Example:** Breast RT uses SGRT wireless monitoring to detect chest motion.

426. **Weekly Dosimetry Check:** Routine output verification ensuring LINAC consistency.
**Related Terms:** Output QA, TG-142 QA schedule.
**Radiotherapy Example:** Every week, physicists perform output constancy check.

427. **Workflow Latency Reduction:** Efforts to shorten delays between scanning, planning, and treatment.
**Related Terms:** Lean RT operations, automation.
**Radiotherapy Example:** Adaptive MR-Linac clinics require reduced workflow latency.

428. **Window-Level Calibration:** Adjusting CT or MRI viewing brightness for consistent visualization.
**Related Terms:** LUT calibration, soft tissue window.
**Radiotherapy Example:** Radiologists calibrate lung window levels before contouring.

429. **Weighted DVH Comparison:** Comparing dose histograms using clinical priority score weighting.
**Related Terms:** Plan comparison analysis.
**Radiotherapy Example:** Used for proton vs VMAT trade-off evaluation.

430. **Water-Based Bolus Fabrication:** Using hydrogel or water-equivalent liquid for patient customizing bolus.
**Related Terms:** Tissue compensator, mould room work.
**Radiotherapy Example:** Used in scar boost treatments.

431. **Whole-Body PET Reconstruction:** PET processing technique for full-body metabolic imaging.
**Related Terms:** SUV, attenuation correction.
**Radiotherapy Example:** Used before SBRT planning of metastatic disease.

432. **Wireless Position Interface:** Digital link allowing SGRT or imaging to control couch remotely.
**Related Terms:** Auto-setup, robotic couch.
**Radiotherapy Example:** Couch shifts adjust automatically using wireless interface with SGRT.

433. **Wide-Range Calibration Phantom:** Phantom covering a broad energy or imaging range for multi-modality QA.
**Related Terms:** Multi-contrast phantom, MRI-CT phantom.
**Radiotherapy Example:** Used during commissioning of CT-MR simulation workflows.

434. **Wire Fiducial Placement:** Placement of small wires as visible markers for surgical or radiation guidance.
**Related Terms:** Clip markers, radiopaque localization.
**Radiotherapy Example:** Placed in breast before simulation.

435. **Weighted Hotspot Suppression:** Optimization setting that reduces local overdose areas.
**Related Terms:** Plan smoothing, constraint enforcement.
**Radiotherapy Example:** Used for spine SBRT near spinal cord.

436. **Waste Heat Management:** Cooling methods preventing LINAC overheating.
**Related Terms:** HVAC, thermal regulation.
**Radiotherapy Example:** Large vaults require dedicated cooling.

437. **Windowed Dose Prediction:** Dose prediction based on selected motion window.
**Related Terms:** Gated planning, motion subset dose.
**Radiotherapy Example:** Used in 4D SBRT for pancreatic tumors.

438. **Whole-Jaw Imaging Mode:** CT mode capturing full mandible region.
**Related Terms:** Maxillofacial scan.
**Radiotherapy Example:** Oral cancer patients require this scan mode.

439. **White Noise Suppression Filter:** Noise reduction tool in imaging.
**Related Terms:** Image smoothing, despeckle filters.
**Radiotherapy Example:** Used in CBCT post-processing.

440. **Weighted Dose Fractioning:** Non-uniform fraction dose selection based on biological sensitivity.
**Related Terms:** Hypofractionation, adaptive fractionation.
**Radiotherapy Example:** Used in head-and-neck adaptive therapy.

441. **Weld Integrity Testing (Radiation Equipment):** QA ensuring radiation shielding welds remain intact.
**Related Terms:** Vault QA, structural safety.
**Radiotherapy Example:** Tested during new bunker certification.

442. **Wide-Field EPID QA:** QA ensuring EPID provides accurate readings across full area.
**Related Terms:** Portal imaging QA.
**Radiotherapy Example:** Required for IMRT portal dosimetry.

443. **Weight-Controlled Couch Movement:** Couch adjusts motion speed based on patient mass.
**Related Terms:** Mechanical smart limits.
**Radiotherapy Example:** Prevents instability in heavy patient SBRT.

444. **Whole-Organ Contouring Protocol:** Standardized method for contouring complete organs.
**Related Terms:** RTOG atlas, segmentation protocol.
**Radiotherapy Example:** Required in prostate and cervical cancer planning.

445. **Wireless Treatment Start Command:** Command initiated without direct machine panel contact.
**Related Terms:** Remote operation, safety interlocks.
**Radiotherapy Example:** Used in gated breathing sessions.

446. **Wide-Margin Adaptive Expansion:** Larger margins used when motion uncertainty is high.
**Related Terms:** ITV, PTV.
**Radiotherapy Example:** Liver SBRT uses wider margins if no motion management available.

447. **Workload Risk Assessment:** Evaluation of staffing workload and safety.
**Related Terms:** Clinical safety culture.
**Radiotherapy Example:** Used to prevent fatigue-related planning errors.

448. **Whiteboard Radiation Record:** Manual visual record for fraction tracking.
**Related Terms:** Offline logs, daily setup records.
**Radiotherapy Example:** Older vaults used whiteboards before EMR systems.

449. **Whitening Filter Algorithm:** Algorithm decreasing data correlations to improve imaging signal processing.
**Related Terms:** Statistical denoising.
**Radiotherapy Example:** Used in MRI reconstruction.

450. **Wrap-Around Signal Correction:** Fixing artifact caused when signals extend beyond FOV boundary.
**Related Terms:** aliasing artifact.
**Radiotherapy Example:** MRI sim needs correction for large torso scans.

451. **Warm-Up Output Verification:** Checking LINAC beam output stability after warm-up runs.
**Related Terms:** Daily QA, output constancy.
**Radiotherapy Example:** Performed before treating first patient.

452. **Wide-Area Radiation Mapping:** Surveying radiation across large facility or geographic area.
**Related Terms:** Shielding survey, environmental monitoring.
**Radiotherapy Example:** Used during installation of TBI rooms.

453. **Work-Shift Planning Schedule:** Timetable coordinating staff roles for daily RT operations.
**Related Terms:** Operational workflow.
**Radiotherapy Example:** Ensures dosimetrists and therapists meet deadlines.

454. **Weight-Adjusted Pediatric Planning:** Planning approach considering child size and organ development.
**Related Terms:** Pediatric RT, OAR prioritization.
**Radiotherapy Example:** Proton therapy often preferred.

455. **Windowed Lung Segmentation:** Lung contour extraction using HU windowing thresholds.
**Related Terms:** auto contour, segmentation tool.
**Radiotherapy Example:** Used during thoracic SBRT.

456. **Wedge Transmission Factor:** Factor correcting dose loss due to wedge filter presence.
**Related Terms:** Beam modification factor.
**Radiotherapy Example:** Verified in clinical physics QA.

457. **Water-Based Backscatter Modeling:** Calculating scattered dose from water-like tissues.
**Related Terms:** Monte Carlo, kernel convolution.
**Radiotherapy Example:** Used in dose calculation for TBI.

458. **Wrist Support Immobilization:** Device stabilizing patient arms during treatment.
**Related Terms:** arm supports, prone belly board.
**Radiotherapy Example:** Breast RT uses wrist holders.

459. **Weakly Visible Tumor Targeting:** Strategy for tumors poorly visualized in imaging.
**Related Terms:** fiducials, MRI targeting.
**Radiotherapy Example:** Pancreas RT often needs fiducials.

460. **Wide-Field Gantry Clearance Check:** Ensuring patient and immobilization devices do not collide with gantry.
**Related Terms:** collision testing, couch simulation.
**Radiotherapy Example:** Essential for head/neck mask beams.

461. **Waveform Verification Test:** Confirming correct LINAC RF waveform output.
**Related Terms:** engineering QA, power regulation.
**Radiotherapy Example:** Performed annually.

462. **Whole-Treatment Dose Comparison:** Comparing delivered vs planned total dose.
**Related Terms:** adaptive planning check.
**Radiotherapy Example:** Used after high-fraction SBRT cases.

463. **Warm Detector Calibration:** Detector calibration performed after thermal stabilization.
**Related Terms:** EPID QA.
**Radiotherapy Example:** Performed during morning startup.

464. **Wide-Beam EPID Field Validation:** Validation of EPID accuracy across full beam field.
**Related Terms:** portal imaging QA.
**Radiotherapy Example:** Required before clinical IMRT.

465. **Workload-Driven Staffing Model:** Method assigning staff based on clinical load.
**Related Terms:** efficiency metrics.
**Radiotherapy Example:** High SBRT schedules increase physicist hours.

466. **Wire-Based Surface Digitization:** Capturing patient surface using radiopaque wire outlines.
**Related Terms:** analog contouring.
**Radiotherapy Example:** Historical breast RT method.

467. **Wedge Planning Algorithm:** Auto-optimization for wedge filter selection.
**Related Terms:** hybrid wedge planning.
**Radiotherapy Example:** Automated tangential planning uses it.

468. **Whole-Pelvis Imaging QA:** Verifying consistent imaging quality throughout pelvis region.
**Related Terms:** CBCT QA, geometric QA.
**Radiotherapy Example:** Required in prostate image-guided therapy.

469. **Weighted Gradient Dose Tool:** Software evaluating steepness of dose fall-off.
**Related Terms:** conformity index.
**Radiotherapy Example:** Used in intracranial SRS.

470. **Window Dupe Prevention:** System preventing accidental duplicate windowing settings.
**Related Terms:** image standardization.
**Radiotherapy Example:** Ensures consistent clinical review.

**471. Weight-Controlled Respiration Coach:** Device guiding breathing rhythm based on patient physiology.
**Related Terms:** breath-hold, motion control.
**Radiotherapy Example:** Used for DIBH breast patients.

**472. Welded Shield Integrity Certification:** Certification confirming no radiation leakage through shielding joints.
**Related Terms:** NCRP shielding acceptance.
**Radiotherapy Example:** Completed before opening new RT vault.

**473. Wide-Range MV Imaging QA:** QA validating MV imaging across full energy settings.
**Related Terms:** portal imaging QA.
**Radiotherapy Example:** Required when adding new MV imaging presets.

**474. Weighted Organ Motion Modeling:** Predicting motion magnitude based on organ characteristics.
**Related Terms:** motion tracking, ITV modeling.
**Radiotherapy Example:** Used in pancreas and liver SBRT.

**475. Wireless Couch Tracking:** Real-time couch monitoring without physical sensors.
**Related Terms:** SGRT automation.
**Radiotherapy Example:** Used in high precision brain RT.

**476. Weak SNR Reconstruction Compensation:** Technique enhancing images with low signal-to-noise ratios.
**Related Terms:** noise filtering, iterative reconstruction.
**Radiotherapy Example:** Low-dose CBCT needs SNR boost.

**477. Whole-Lung Dose Forecasting:** Estimating lung dose impact before planning.
**Related Terms:** toxicity modeling.
**Radiotherapy Example:** Used in lymphoma IMRT.

**478. Wedge Orientation Rule:** Guideline for selecting wedge orientation based on geometry.
**Related Terms:** wedge direction chart.
**Radiotherapy Example:** Applied in manual breast 3DCRT plans.

**479. Wire-Cast Immobilization Replica:** Patient contour model created using shaping wires.
**Related Terms:** plaster molds, legacy immobilization.
**Radiotherapy Example:** Used historically before CT simulation.

**480. Water Equivalent Thickness Calculation:** Conversion of materials to water-equivalent thickness for dose calculation.
**Related Terms:** HU calibration, density mapping.
**Radiotherapy Example:** Used when applying bolus or compensators.

**481. Wave Propagation Simulation:** Modeling how particles or radiation waves travel in matter.
**Related Terms:** Monte Carlo transport.
**Radiotherapy Example:** Used in advanced TPS dose engines.

**482. Wall-Mounted SGRT Array:** SGRT sensor system installed on walls rather than gantry.
**Related Terms:** optical tracking.
**Radiotherapy Example:** Used in respiratory-gated breast DIBH.

**483. Wound-Site Targeting Protocol:** Treatment protocol for irradiating surgical beds.
**Related Terms:** CTV boost, scar boost.
**Radiotherapy Example:** Common in breast BCS boost.

**484. Whole-Field Smoothing Filter:** Dose smoothing algorithm applied to full plan.
**Related Terms:** constraint optimization.
**Radiotherapy Example:** Reduces dose ripple in VMAT plan.

**485. Warm-Restart Machine Mode:** Mode used when restarting LINAC without full initialization.
**Related Terms:** engineering restart, beam tuning.
**Radiotherapy Example:** Used after brief power loss.

**486. Weighted Matchline Optimization:** Optimization of field junction to prevent hotspots.
**Related Terms:** junction dose control.
**Radiotherapy Example:** Used in craniospinal irradiation.

**487. Waveform Noise Suppression:** Filtering electrical noise from LINAC RF signals.
**Related Terms:** RF stabilization.
**Radiotherapy Example:** Prevents beam instability.

**488. Wireless Treatment Verification:** Validation of patient identity and treatment session via wireless check-in.
**Related Terms:** digital workflow, automation.
**Radiotherapy Example:** Used in RFID patient matching.

**489. Wide-Margin Tolerance Rule:** Guideline allowing expanded margin when uncertainty exists.
**Related Terms:** planning margins, ITV.
**Radiotherapy Example:** Applied in tumors with significant motion.

**490. Whole-Body CT Eco Mode:** Low-dose scanning mode for whole-body imaging.
**Related Terms:** dose reduction, ALARA.
**Radiotherapy Example:** Used in pediatric follow-up.

**491. Weighted Dose Limiter:** System automatically restricting dose to OARs.
**Related Terms:** constraint enforcement.
**Radiotherapy Example:** Used in SBRT renal sparing.

**492. Wireframe Anatomy Overlay:** Line-based representation of anatomy for accuracy checks.
**Related Terms:** segmentation overlay.
**Radiotherapy Example:** Used to verify registration accuracy.

**493. Warm-Mask Fit Check:** Check to ensure thermoplastic mask fits once cooled.
**Related Terms:** mould room, immobilization QA.
**Radiotherapy Example:** Performed before simulation.

**494. Workflow Shutdown Protocol:** Safe shutdown procedure for radiation devices and systems.
**Related Terms:** safety SOP.
**Radiotherapy Example:** Used during emergency evacuation drills.

**495. Wide-Scan Mode Reconstruction:** Reconstruction used when large FOV imaging captures extra scatter.
**Related Terms:** scatter reduction.
**Radiotherapy Example:** Used in obese patient CT simulation.

**496. Weighted Beam Selection Tool:** Planning tool assigning initial beam priorities.
**Related Terms:** IMRT optimization.
**Radiotherapy Example:** Used in 9-field IMRT prostate plan.

**497. Windowing Artifact Detection:** Identification of errors resulting from improper display settings.
**Related Terms:** imaging QA.
**Radiotherapy Example:** Prevents missed lesion during contouring.

498. **Weekly Toxicity Tracking System:** System documenting toxicity changes through treatment.
**Related Terms:** PRO monitoring, oncology charting.
**Radiotherapy Example:** Used for head-and-neck mucositis scoring.

499. **Whole-Process Clinical Traceability:** Ability to track every step of treatment from imaging to delivery.
**Related Terms:** DICOM-RT compliance, quality assurance audit.
**Radiotherapy Example:** Accreditation requires full traceability of treatment records.

500. **Water-equivalent path length (noun):**
Thickness of water that produces the same beam attenuation as a given material.
**Related Terms:** WEPL, Range calculation.
**Example in Radiotherapy:** Used to determine proton beam range through heterogeneous tissue.

# X

1. **X-ray:** High-energy electromagnetic radiation with wavelengths shorter than UV light, capable of penetrating tissues and materials.
**Related Terms:** Roentgen ray, Ionizing radiation
**Radiotherapy Example:** X-rays produced by linear accelerators are used to treat cancers such as breast and lung tumors.
2. **X-radiation:** The spectrum of electromagnetic radiation in the X-ray energy range.
**Related Terms:** Bremsstrahlung radiation, Characteristic radiation
**Radiotherapy Example:** X-radiation is generated in therapy equipment to deliver therapeutic doses during external beam radiotherapy.
3. **X-irradiation:** Exposure of matter, tissue, or organisms to X-rays.
**Related Terms:** Photon irradiation, Radiation exposure
**Radiotherapy Example:** Cancer cells receive controlled X-irradiation to induce lethal DNA damage during treatment.
4. **X-ray beam:** A directed stream of X-ray photons emitted from a source.
**Related Terms:** Radiation field, Photon beam
**Radiotherapy Example:** Collimators and multileaf collimators shape the X-ray beam to match the tumor contour in conformal therapy.
5. **X-ray therapy:** Medical use of X-rays to destroy cancer cells through DNA damage.
**Related Terms:** Radiotherapy, Orthovoltage therapy
**Radiotherapy Example:** Low-energy X-ray therapy is commonly used for skin cancer, keloids, and superficial tumors.
6. **X-ray tube:** A vacuum device in which accelerated electrons strike a metal target to generate X-rays.
**Related Terms:** Coolidge tube, Bremsstrahlung source
**Radiotherapy Example:** Earlier therapy machines used X-ray tubes before linear accelerators became standard.
7. **X-ray photon:** A quantum (packet) of electromagnetic X-ray energy capable of ionizing atoms.
**Related Terms:** Ionizing photon, High-energy photon
**Radiotherapy Example:** X-ray photons interact with tissue via photoelectric effect or Compton scatter to destroy tumor cells.
8. **X-ray diffraction (XRD):** A technique analyzing how X-rays scatter from crystalline structures to determine atom spacing.
**Related Terms:** Bragg diffraction, Crystal analysis
**Radiotherapy Example:** Used to study structural changes in biomolecules exposed to radiation.
9. **X-ray crystallography:** Method for determining atomic and molecular structure using diffraction patterns from a crystal.
**Related Terms:** Structural biology imaging, Lattice mapping
**Radiotherapy Example:** Helps analyze effects of irradiation on DNA and protein structure in radiobiology studies.

10. **X-ray fluorescence (XRF):** Technique where atoms emit characteristic secondary X-rays after excitation, enabling elemental identification.
**Related Terms:** Elemental spectroscopy, Secondary emission
**Radiotherapy Example:** Used to measure trace metal changes in tissues after radiation exposure.

11. **X-ray imaging:** Production of diagnostic 2D or 3D images using differential tissue absorption of X-rays.
**Related Terms:** Radiography, Projection imaging
**Radiotherapy Example:** IGRT (image-guided radiotherapy) uses X-ray imaging to verify patient positioning before treatment.

12. **X-ray spectroscopy:** Analysis of X-ray energy spectra emitted or absorbed by matter to determine composition or electronic structure.
**Related Terms:** EDS (Energy-dispersive spectroscopy), EXAFS
**Radiotherapy Example:** Used in research to study radiation interactions with biological tissues.

13. **X-ray computed tomography (CT):** Rotating X-ray imaging with computer reconstruction to produce detailed cross-sectional anatomical images.
**Related Terms:** CT scan, Tomography
**Radiotherapy Example:** CT images guide treatment planning and define tumor volumes and surrounding organs.

14. **X-ray film:** Film coated with silver halide crystals that darken when exposed to X-rays.
**Related Terms:** Radiographic film, Analog image receptor
**Radiotherapy Example:** Used in film dosimetry to evaluate beam uniformity and machine calibration.

15. **X-ray detector:** A device that converts incoming X-ray photons into electrical or optical signals for measurement or imaging.
**Related Terms:** Flat-panel detector, Scintillation detector
**Radiotherapy Example:** Used in portal imaging systems for real-time treatment alignment.

16. **X-ray intensity:** Quantity of X-ray energy or number of photons delivered per unit area per unit time.
**Related Terms:** Photon flux, Radiation output
**Radiotherapy Example:** Adjusted during planning to achieve prescribed tumor dose while reducing healthy tissue exposure.

17. **X-ray scatter:** Deflection of X-ray photons from their original path due to interaction with matter.
**Related Terms:** Compton scatter, Secondary radiation
**Radiotherapy Example:** Scatter contributes to unintended dose in surrounding healthy tissue and must be minimized.

18. **X-ray emission:** Release of X-ray photons from atoms or equipment.
**Related Terms:** Photon emission, Radiative transition
**Radiotherapy Example:** Measured during machine quality assurance to ensure consistent X-ray output.

19. **X-ray absorption:** Process by which X-ray photons transfer energy to matter, often ionizing atoms.
**Related Terms:** Photoelectric effect, Linear attenuation
**Radiotherapy Example:** Differences in absorption guide dose calculation and evaluation of treatment depth-dose curves.

20. **X-ray attenuation:** Reduction in X-ray intensity due to absorption and scattering as it passes through matter.
**Related Terms:** Attenuation coefficient, Exponential decay law
**Radiotherapy Example:** Used in treatment planning algorithms to calculate patient-specific dose distributions.

21. **X-ray generator:** A device that supplies electrical power to an X-ray tube, controlling voltage, current, waveform, and exposure timing.
**Related Terms:** High-frequency generator, Power supply unit
**Radiotherapy Example:** The generator ensures stable output during imaging procedures for patient setup verification before radiation treatment.

22. **X-ray source:** Any device or material that produces X-rays, such as X-ray tubes, synchrotrons, or radioactive isotopes.
**Related Terms:** Radiation emitter, Photon source
**Radiotherapy Example:** Linear accelerators act as high-energy X-ray sources for external-beam radiotherapy.

23. **X-ray dosimetry:** The science of measuring and quantifying absorbed radiation dose for safety and treatment accuracy.
**Related Terms:** Dose measurement, Radiation calibration
**Radiotherapy Example:** Ion chambers and TLDs are used for machine calibration and patient dose verification.

24. **X-ray exposure:** The amount of ionization produced in air by an X-ray beam or the act of subjecting tissue to radiation.
**Related Terms:** Irradiation, Radiation dose setting
**Radiotherapy Example:** Imaging exposure settings are adjusted to minimize additional dose during patient positioning.

25. **X-ray diagnosis:** The use of X-ray-based imaging techniques to identify disease, abnormalities, or injury.
**Related Terms:** Radiographic diagnosis, Diagnostic radiology
**Radiotherapy Example:** Diagnostic CT scans are evaluated before treatment planning to determine tumor extent.

26. **X-ray fluorescence analysis (XRF analysis):** A method that identifies elements in a sample by detecting characteristic secondary X-ray emissions.
**Related Terms:** Elemental analysis, Spectral emission analysis
**Radiotherapy Example:** Used in research to assess elemental changes in tissues after radiation exposure.

27. **X-ray microanalysis:** A high-resolution technique to analyze elemental composition using focused X-ray or electron beams.
**Related Terms:** EDS (energy-dispersive spectroscopy), WDS (wavelength-dispersive spectroscopy)
**Radiotherapy Example:** Used to examine cellular metal content changes after irradiation in radiobiology research.

28. **X-ray shielding:** Use of materials such as lead or concrete to absorb or attenuate X-rays, reducing exposure.
**Related Terms:** Radiation protection barrier, Attenuation shielding
**Radiotherapy Example:** Lead aprons and shielding walls protect staff from scatter radiation in treatment rooms.

29. **X-ray safety:** Practices and policies to minimize unnecessary X-ray exposure to workers, patients, and the public.
**Related Terms:** Radiation protection, ALARA principle
**Radiotherapy Example:** Dosimeters and controlled access zones ensure safe radiotherapy practice.

30. **X-ray spectrometer:** An instrument that measures the energy or wavelength of X-rays emitted from a sample.
**Related Terms:** X-ray analyzer, Photon spectrometer
**Radiotherapy Example:** Used in physics labs to verify spectra from experimental radiation sources.

31. **Xenobiotic:** A chemical substance foreign to a living organism, such as drugs or environmental pollutants.
**Related Terms:** Foreign compound, Exogenous chemical
**Radiotherapy Example:** Xenobiotic metabolism may change after radiation exposure due to altered enzyme activity.

32. **Xenograft:** A graft of cells, tissues, or organs between different species.
**Related Terms:** Heterograft, Cross-species transplant
**Radiotherapy Example:** Research xenograft tumor models in mice are frequently irradiated to test treatment response.

33. **Xenogeneic:** Originating from a different species or involving foreign biological material.
**Related Terms:** Heterologous, Cross-species
**Radiotherapy Example:** Xenogeneic tumor models allow testing of radiosensitivity in preclinical radiotherapy studies.

34. **Xenotransplantation:** Transplanting living cells, tissues, or organs from animals to humans.
**Related Terms:** Cross-species transplantation, Biomedical grafting
**Radiotherapy Example:** Not routine clinically, but radiotherapy may be used experimentally to prevent graft overgrowth in research models.

35. **Xenon (Xe):** A noble gas with high atomic number used in lighting, imaging, and anesthesia.
**Related Terms:** Noble gas, Radiodense contrast gas
**Radiotherapy Example:** Xenon may be used as a contrast agent in CT imaging before radiation planning.

36. **Xenon-133:** A radioactive isotope used as an inhaled tracer for lung ventilation imaging.
**Related Terms:** Radiotracer, Gamma-emitting isotope
**Radiotherapy Example:** Helps assess lung function before thoracic radiotherapy to avoid high-dose exposure to poorly ventilated areas.

37. **Xenon-135:** A highly neutron-absorbing radioactive isotope produced in nuclear fission.
**Related Terms:** Reactor poison, Neutron absorber
**Radiotherapy Example:** Mainly relevant to nuclear physics, but may be discussed in radiation safety and isotope decay training.

38. **Xenon gas detector:** A detector that uses xenon gas or liquid to detect radiation by ionization or scintillation.
**Related Terms:** Ionization detector, Scintillation detector
**Radiotherapy Example:** Used in research for precise photon detection during dose verification studies.

39. **Xenon scintillation:** Light emission from xenon gas or liquid when excited by radiation.
**Related Terms:** Scintillation response, Photon luminescence
**Radiotherapy Example:** Used in high-precision radiation detectors to measure dose distribution or particle interactions.

40. **Xenon anesthesia:** Use of xenon gas as an inhaled anesthetic due to rapid induction and minimal side effects.
    **Related Terms:** Inhaled anesthesia, Noble-gas anesthesia
    **Radiotherapy Example:** Rarely used, but may be considered for pediatric or sensitive patients undergoing simulation imaging.

41. **Xenon CT imaging:** A CT method using inhaled xenon as a contrast agent to measure lung ventilation.
    **Related Terms:** Functional CT, Gas-enhanced CT
    **Radiotherapy Example:** Helps map lung ventilation for planning functional avoidance radiotherapy in lung cancer.

42. **Xenon enhancement:** Increased CT attenuation caused by xenon inhalation, improving visualization of ventilated areas.
    **Related Terms:** Contrast enhancement, Gas contrast effect
    **Radiotherapy Example:** Enables dose adaptation to preserve well-ventilated lung regions during treatment planning.

43. **Xenon ventilation study:** A functional test measuring airflow distribution in the lungs using xenon gas.
    **Related Terms:** Lung ventilation scan, Pulmonary function imaging
    **Radiotherapy Example:** Helps avoid irradiating poorly functioning lung regions during thoracic RT.

44. **Xenon radiotracer:** A xenon isotope (often Xe-133) used to trace airflow or perfusion in biological systems.
    **Related Terms:** Radioactive gas tracer, Functional tracer
    **Radiotherapy Example:** Used to evaluate lung function before radiotherapy to reduce pulmonary toxicity.

45. **Xenon ionization chamber:** A radiation detector filled with xenon gas used to measure ionization from incoming radiation.
    **Related Terms:** Gas-filled detector, Ion chamber
    **Radiotherapy Example:** Applied in dosimetry labs for accurate beam calibration and radiation measurement.

46. **Xenon lamp:** A high-intensity light source generating white light from xenon arc discharge.
    **Related Terms:** Arc lamp, High-pressure discharge lamp
    **Radiotherapy Example:** Used in optical imaging systems and simulation room equipment.

47. **Xenogenic response:** Immune reaction against transplanted tissue or cells from another species.
    **Related Terms:** Rejection response, Cross-species immune reaction
    **Radiotherapy Example:** Experimental radiotherapy may be used to suppress immune rejection in research xenograft models.

48. **Xenobiotic metabolism:** Biochemical modification of foreign substances through enzymatic pathways in the body.
    **Related Terms:** Phase I metabolism, Detoxification pathways
    **Radiotherapy Example:** Radiation may alter metabolic enzyme activity affecting chemotherapy–radiotherapy interactions.

49. **Xenobiotic detoxification:** Biological processes that neutralize or eliminate harmful foreign chemicals.
    **Related Terms:** Biotransformation, Chemical clearance
    **Radiotherapy Example:** Radiation-induced oxidative stress can reduce detoxification capacity in treated tissues.

50. **Xenoreactivity:** Immune response triggered by antigens from a different species.
    **Related Terms:** Cross-reactivity, Immune rejection
    **Radiotherapy Example:** Studied in xenograft tumor models to understand immune-radiation interactions.

51. **Xerostomia:** A condition of chronic dry mouth caused by reduced saliva production.
    **Related Terms:** Hyposalivation, mucositis, salivary gland dysfunction.
    **Radiotherapy Example:** Common in head-and-neck radiotherapy where parotid glands are irradiated, leading to difficulty swallowing and speaking.

52. **Xeroderma:** Abnormally dry, rough, and irritated skin.
    **Related Terms:** Dry desquamation, radiation dermatitis.
    **Radiotherapy Example:** Patients may experience xeroderma in the treatment area after repeated external-beam radiation to the breast or pelvis.

53. **Xerophthalmia:** Severe dryness of the eyes from reduced tear production.
    **Related Terms:** Lacrimal gland damage, keratopathy.
    **Radiotherapy Example:** Can occur when eye structures receive radiation during treatment of orbital tumors or sinus cancers.

54. **Xerosis:** Pathological dryness of skin or mucosal tissue.
    **Related Terms:** Cutaneous atrophy, epithelial damage.
    **Radiotherapy Example:** Seen in patients receiving radiotherapy where sweat and oil glands are damaged, especially in extremities or breast fields.

55. **Xeroradiography:** A now largely outdated imaging technique using electrostatic charge instead of film.
    **Related Terms:** Xeromammography, xerographic imaging.
    **Radiotherapy Example:** Historically used in breast cancer planning before digital imaging systems became standard.

56. **Xerographic Imaging:** Imaging based on electrostatic latent images developed with toner.
    **Related Terms:** Photocopy imaging, xerography.
    **Radiotherapy Example:** Early radiation therapy departments used it to print and verify treatment field outlines.

57. **Xerography:** A dry copying process using electrostatic charge and toner transfer.
    **Related Terms:** Laser printing, xerographic imaging.
    **Radiotherapy Example:** Previously used for copying radiotherapy simulation films, field marks, and planning records.

58. **Xeromammography:** Breast imaging using xeroradiographic principles to enhance edge contrast.
    **Related Terms:** Xeroradiography, mammography.
    **Radiotherapy Example:** Once used in planning breast cancer radiotherapy to visualize microcalcifications before digital mammography became standard.

59. **Xerogel Dosimeter:** A dry gel dosimeter that changes properties when exposed to ionizing radiation.
    **Related Terms:** Gel dosimetry, polymer dosimeter.
    **Radiotherapy Example:** Used in radiation therapy QA to verify absorbed dose distribution in phantom testing.

60. **Xerothermic Effect:** Tissue damage caused by combined drying and heating effects.
    **Related Terms:** Thermal injury, hyperthermia response.
    **Radiotherapy Example:** May occur during hyperthermia-assisted radiotherapy where heat increases tumor radiosensitivity but may dry and irritate skin.

61. **Xeric Tissue Changes:** Tissue alterations caused by dehydration and loss of normal moisture balance.
**Related Terms:** Atrophy, fibrosis, glandular dysfunction.
**Radiotherapy Example:** Seen in long-term survivors of head-and-neck radiotherapy where salivary gland function is permanently reduced.

62. **Xeroplastic Changes:** Thickening, stiffening, or keratinization of tissues due to chronic dryness or injury.
**Related Terms:** Keratosis, hyperkeratosis, fibrosis.
**Radiotherapy Example:** May occur in skin exposed to repeated radiation treatments, resulting in decreased elasticity and altered texture.

63. **Xerotic Reaction:** Inflammatory response caused by extreme dryness of skin or mucosa.
**Related Terms:** Irritation, erythema, pruritus.
**Radiotherapy Example:** Patients receiving breast or pelvic radiation may report itching and redness from xerotic skin changes in the treatment field.

64. **Xerophytic Response:** A biological adaptation resembling drought tolerance, used metaphorically for cellular adjustments under stress.
**Related Terms:** Cellular repair response, stress adaptation.
**Radiotherapy Example:** Tumor cells may develop protective biochemical mechanisms during fractionated radiation, mimicking a "survival adaptation."

65. **Xeric Burns:** Burns caused by severe dryness combined with heat or radiation exposure.
**Related Terms:** Radiation burns, desiccation injury.
**Radiotherapy Example:** Rare severe cases may occur when high-dose radiation desiccates tissues and compromises healing, especially in re-irradiated areas.

66. **Xeroderma Pigmentosum (XP):** A rare genetic disorder characterized by extreme sensitivity to UV and ionizing radiation due to defective DNA repair.
**Related Terms:** DNA repair deficiency, radiosensitivity syndrome.
**Radiotherapy Example:** XP patients are highly susceptible to radiation toxicity, requiring modified or avoided radiotherapy approaches.

67. **Xerotic Lesion:** A tissue lesion caused by prolonged dryness that may crack, thicken, or become inflamed.
**Related Terms:** Chronic skin irritation, fissures, dermatitis.
**Radiotherapy Example:** May form in irradiated mucosal areas, such as nasal or oral cavities, following repeated radiation exposure.

68. **Xerophilous Cell Adaptation:** Describes cell changes enabling survival in low-moisture environments, used in radiation biology contexts.
**Related Terms:** Cellular tolerance, membrane stabilization.
**Radiotherapy Example:** Some cancer cells undergoing radiotherapy may develop altered membranes or proteins helping them resist radiation-induced dehydration.

69. **Xerostatic Changes:** Persistent or long-term tissue dryness from chronic gland dysfunction or exposure.
**Related Terms:** Chronic xerosis, persistent tissue atrophy.
**Radiotherapy Example:** Seen in patients months to years after radiotherapy, especially when salivary or tear glands receive high-dose exposure.

70. **Xerotic Ulcer:** A chronic ulcer formed due to extreme dryness and breakdown of weakened tissue.
**Related Terms:** Radiation ulcer, chronic wound.
**Radiotherapy Example:** May occur in previously irradiated skin where vascular damage and dryness impair tissue repair.

71. **Xeromyelia:** Abnormal dryness affecting spinal cord tissue or surrounding structures.
**Related Terms:** Neuropathy, myelopathy.
**Radiotherapy Example:** Rarely, spinal irradiation can lead to nerve irritation and tissue dryness contributing to late neurological side effects.

72. **Xerocheilitis:** Dryness and cracking of the lips due to reduced moisture or gland function.
**Related Terms:** Cheilitis, mucositis, fissuring.
**Radiotherapy Example:** Common in head-and-neck radiotherapy patients who experience reduced saliva and lip dryness during treatment.

73. **Xeroglossia:** Dry tongue resulting from decreased salivary secretion.
**Related Terms:** Glossitis, hyposalivation, mucosal dryness.
**Radiotherapy Example:** Seen in patients receiving radiation to oral cavity or salivary glands, leading to difficulty eating and speaking.

74. **Xeroanesthesia:** Reduced sensation in dry mucosal or skin areas.
**Related Terms:** Neuropathy, paresthesia.
**Radiotherapy Example:** May occur when nerve endings are damaged during radiation therapy, causing numbness in dry treated regions.

75. **Xerostatic Dermatitis:** Inflammation of the skin caused by prolonged dryness.
**Related Terms:** Dermatitis, eczema, radiation dermatitis.
**Radiotherapy Example:** Can develop in irradiated skin after repeated exposure, especially in breast or pelvic radiotherapy fields.

76. **Xerophthalmic Keratitis:** Inflammation and dryness of the cornea due to tear gland dysfunction.
**Related Terms:** Keratopathy, dry eye syndrome.
**Radiotherapy Example:** Occurs when lacrimal glands receive radiation during treatment of orbital or sinus tumors.

77. **Xerostomal Dysphagia:** Difficulty swallowing due to dry mouth and reduced lubrication.
**Related Terms:** Dysphagia, mucositis, salivary deficiency.
**Radiotherapy Example:** Very common in patients receiving head-and-neck radiotherapy, especially when major salivary glands are exposed.

78. **Xerorrhea (Opposite of):** A condition describing unusually low moisture output from glands, opposite of excessive secretion.
**Related Terms:** Gland hypofunction, secretion deficit.
**Radiotherapy Example:** Seen as reduced tear or saliva flow after radiation to glandular tissues.

79. **Xerotic Tissue Atrophy:** Tissue thinning and weakening caused by chronic dehydration.
**Related Terms:** Fibrosis, atrophy, tissue degeneration.
**Radiotherapy Example:** A late radiation effect leading to fragile, thin skin in long-term treatment fields such as breast or neck.

80. **Xerostomia-Induced Caries:** Tooth decay caused by chronic dry mouth and reduced salivary protection.
**Related Terms:** Radiation caries, enamel erosion.
**Radiotherapy Example:** Head-and-neck radiotherapy patients are at high risk of dental decay due to salivary gland damage.

81. **X-ray Beam Attenuation:** Reduction in X-ray intensity as it passes through tissue due to absorption and scattering.
**Related Terms:** Absorption, scatter, tissue density.
**Radiotherapy Example:** Beam attenuation must be calculated when planning dose through dense bone such as the skull or pelvis.

82. **X-ray Absorption Coefficient:** A numerical value describing how strongly a material absorbs X-rays.
**Related Terms:** Linear attenuation coefficient, density, contrast.
**Radiotherapy Example:** Used in treatment planning systems to calculate dose distribution based on CT tissue values.

83. **X-ray Calibration:** Process of verifying and adjusting X-ray equipment to ensure accurate output.
**Related Terms:** Quality assurance, dosimetry, machine QA.
**Radiotherapy Example:** Linear accelerators are calibrated routinely to ensure delivered dose equals the prescribed dose.

84. **X-ray Contamination:** Unwanted low-energy X-ray photons generated during high-energy radiation treatment.
**Related Terms:** Photon contamination, stray radiation.
**Radiotherapy Example:** Occurs in high-energy electron therapy and must be accounted for in skin dose calculations.

85. **X-ray Generator:** A device that produces X-rays by accelerating electrons and striking a target.
**Related Terms:** Tube current, kVp, X-ray tube.
**Radiotherapy Example:** Used in simulators and imaging systems such as kV on-board imaging for setup verification.

86. **X-ray Fluorescence:** Emission of characteristic secondary radiation when atoms absorb X-rays.
**Related Terms:** Photoelectric effect, characteristic radiation.
**Radiotherapy Example:** Sometimes used in research to measure tissue metal content or contrast distribution.

87. **X-ray Hardening:** Increase in mean photon energy after low-energy X-rays are absorbed or filtered.
**Related Terms:** Beam filtration, spectral shift, HVL.
**Radiotherapy Example:** Adding filters or passing through bone hardens the beam, affecting dose planning.

88. **X-ray Image Guidance (IGRT):** Use of X-ray imaging during treatment to verify patient positioning and tumor alignment.
**Related Terms:** CBCT, portal imaging, kV imaging.
**Radiotherapy Example:** Daily CBCT is used in prostate radiotherapy to ensure the target is accurately positioned.

89. **X-ray Leakage:** Unintended radiation escaping from treatment equipment beyond shielding limits.
**Related Terms:** Scatter radiation, shielding, safety limits.
**Radiotherapy Example:** Measured during acceptance testing to ensure linacs meet safety regulations.

90. **X-ray Therapy (Orthovoltage):** Radiation treatment using low-energy X-rays, typically 50–300 kVp.
**Related Terms:** Superficial therapy, kilovoltage therapy.
**Radiotherapy Example:** Used to treat skin cancers or superficial lesions where penetration depth is limited.

91. **X-ray Transmission:** The fraction of X-ray photons that pass through tissue without being absorbed.
**Related Terms:** Attenuation, scatter, beam penetration.
**Radiotherapy Example:** Higher transmission through lung tissue affects dose calculation and must be corrected in planning.

92. **X-ray Scatter:** Deflection of X-ray photons from their original path due to interaction with matter.
**Related Terms:** Compton scatter, secondary radiation.
**Radiotherapy Example:** Scatter affects image clarity and contributes to unintended dose to surrounding healthy tissue.

93. **X-ray Dose Rate:** The amount of radiation delivered per unit of time.
**Related Terms:** cGy/min, machine output, dose calibration.
**Radiotherapy Example:** Dose rate affects treatment time and biological effect during radiotherapy delivery.

94. **X-ray Field Size:** The physical dimensions of the radiation beam at a specified distance from the source.
**Related Terms:** Collimation, aperture, beam shaping.
**Radiotherapy Example:** Field size is controlled using MLCs or jaws to match tumor target shape and spare healthy tissue.

95. **X-ray Filtering:** The process of removing low-energy, non-therapeutic photons using metal filters.
**Related Terms:** Beam hardening, inherent filtration.
**Radiotherapy Example:** Filters improve beam quality during imaging and reduce patient surface dose.

96. **X-ray Penetration Depth:** The distance radiation travels through tissue before depositing most of its energy.
**Related Terms:** Percent depth dose (PDD), beam energy.
**Radiotherapy Example:** Orthovoltage X-rays have shallow penetration, making them suitable for surface tumor treatments.

97. **X-ray Quality Assurance:** Systematic testing to ensure X-ray equipment performance and safety.
**Related Terms:** QA program, tolerance limits, calibration.
**Radiotherapy Example:** Daily imaging QA ensures on-board imaging systems function correctly for IGRT.

98. **X-ray Source-to-Skin Distance (SSD):** Distance between the X-ray source and the patient's skin surface.
**Related Terms:** Isocenter, SAD, geometric setup.
**Radiotherapy Example:** SSD is critical in electron and orthovoltage treatments to ensure correct dose delivery.

99. **X-ray Shielding:** Use of lead, tungsten, or barrier materials to block or reduce unwanted radiation.
**Related Terms:** Radioprotection, controlled area, exposure limits.
**Radiotherapy Example:** Lead aprons and bunker walls protect staff and public from scatter and leakage radiation.

100. **X-ray Simulation (X-Sim):** Use of X-ray imaging to plan and verify radiation field placement before treatment.
**Related Terms:** Treatment planning, CT simulation, localization.
**Radiotherapy Example:** Prior to CT-based planning, X-simulators were used to align beams for cancer therapy fields.

101. **X-band Linac:** A compact linear accelerator that uses 8–12 GHz microwave frequency to accelerate electrons.
**Related Terms:** Compact linac, microwave accelerator.
**Radiotherapy Example:** Used in some modern experimental radiotherapy systems to achieve high dose rates with smaller machine footprints.

102. **X-type Coupling:** A configuration where two components intersect in an X-shaped pathway, affecting energy or signal transfer.
**Related Terms:** Waveguide coupling, cross-junction.
**Radiotherapy Example:** Used in RF systems of linacs to split or redirect microwave power feeding accelerator cavities.

103. **X-type Connection:** A junction where two paths cross in an X-pattern to exchange or redirect flow or signals.
**Related Terms:** Cross-connection, beam intersection.
**Radiotherapy Example:** May appear in accelerator RF networks where multiple feedlines merge or intersect.

104. **X-point:** A location where two curves, vectors, or fields intersect forming an X-shape.
**Related Terms:** Intersection point, reference coordinate.
**Radiotherapy Example:** Can describe isodose line intersections on a dose distribution map during QA or planning.

105. **X-plane:** A measurement or analysis plane aligned with or perpendicular to the X-axis.
**Related Terms:** Coordinate plane, reference plane.
**Radiotherapy Example:** Used in dose profile analysis when verifying beam symmetry along specific axes.

106. **X-particle:** A historical term for unidentified or experimental subatomic particles detected in early nuclear studies.
**Related Terms:** Meson, exotic particle.
**Radiotherapy Example:** Mostly historical; sometimes referenced when discussing discovery of particles relevant to radiation physics.

107. **X-quanta:** Discrete X-ray photons emitted during atomic transitions or bremsstrahlung processes.
**Related Terms:** Photon quanta, radiation energy packet.
**Radiotherapy Example:** The number and energy of X-quanta determine treatment beam energy spectrum and imaging clarity.

108. **X-coefficient (Attenuation Coefficient):** A value that describes how much X-ray intensity decreases in a material per unit thickness.
**Related Terms:** Linear attenuation coefficient, $\mu$ value.
**Radiotherapy Example:** Used in CT-based treatment planning to convert tissue density into accurate dose calculations.

109. **X-region:** A designated analysis region within an X-ray beam or field.
**Related Terms:** ROI (Region of Interest), field zone.
**Radiotherapy Example:** Used during QA to evaluate beam uniformity, penumbra, or scatter zone in treatment fields.

110. **X-form:** A pattern, beam shape, or geometry resembling the letter X.
**Related Terms:** Cross-beam geometry, intersecting pattern.
**Radiotherapy Example:** Occasionally used in research where two beams intersect to study localized high-dose effects.

111. **Xanthoma:** A lipid-rich yellow lesion caused by cholesterol or triglyceride deposits.
**Related Terms:** Lipoma, hyperlipidemia lesion.
**Radiotherapy Example:** Occasionally appears in diagnostic imaging and must be differentiated from malignant soft-tissue tumors.

112. **Xanthopsia:** A visual condition where vision appears yellow-tinted.
**Related Terms:** Chromatic distortion, visual disturbance.
**Radiotherapy Example:** Rare but may occur secondary to radiation damage to ocular structures during orbital therapy.

113. **Xanthoprotein Reaction:** A chemical reaction in which proteins turn yellow when exposed to nitric acid due to nitration.
**Related Terms:** Protein assay, biochemical analysis.
**Radiotherapy Example:** Mostly academic; referenced when studying protein oxidation after radiation exposure.

114. **Xanthine Oxidase:** An enzyme involved in purine metabolism that produces uric acid and reactive oxygen species.
**Related Terms:** Oxidative stress enzyme, purine metabolism.
**Radiotherapy Example:** Relevant in radiobiology because its activity influences cell oxidative response after irradiation.

115. **Xanthic Compound:** A substance containing yellow pigment or yellow-producing chemical groups.
**Related Terms:** Chromophore compound, carotenoid-like pigment.
**Radiotherapy Example:** Some radiation-induced oxidative products exhibit xanthic coloration in laboratory assays.

116. **Xanthophyll:** A yellow plant carotenoid pigment with antioxidant properties.
**Related Terms:** Carotene, lutein, antioxidant pigment.
**Radiotherapy Example:** Studied for its potential protective role against radiation-induced oxidative retinal damage.

117. **Xanthine:** A purine base involved in nucleic acid metabolism and a precursor to uric acid.
**Related Terms:** Adenine derivative, purine metabolite.
**Radiotherapy Example:** Changes in xanthine levels may occur after radiation-induced DNA breakdown.

118. **Xanthate:** A sulfur-containing organic compound commonly used in industrial and chemical processes.
**Related Terms:** Organosulfur compound, flotation reagent.
**Radiotherapy Example:** Studied in radiation chemistry as some xanthates form reactive radicals during irradiation.

119. **Xanthation Reaction:** A chemical reaction forming xanthates using carbon disulfide in alkaline conditions.
**Related Terms:** Sulfurization reaction, cellulose modification.
**Radiotherapy Example:** Mostly industrial, but occasionally referenced in radiolytic process research.

120. **Xanthochromia:** Yellow discoloration of cerebrospinal fluid due to bilirubin or hemorrhage byproducts.
**Related Terms:** CSF discoloration, subarachnoid hemorrhage marker.
**Radiotherapy Example:** Rarely observed but may occur if radiation causes vascular injury near CNS structures.

121. **Xanthocyte:** A yellow-pigmented cell due to lipid or pigment accumulation.
**Related Terms:** Foam cell, lipid-laden macrophage.
**Radiotherapy Example:** May appear in biopsy samples when radiotherapy imaging reveals a suspected soft-tissue lesion.

122. **Xanthoderma:** Yellow discoloration of the skin from pigment buildup or metabolic causes.
**Related Terms:** Jaundice, carotinemia.
**Radiotherapy Example:** Must be distinguished from treatment-related skin reactions during follow-up.

123. **Xanthogenesis:** Formation of yellow pigment in tissues.
**Related Terms:** Pigmentation, bilirubin deposition.
**Radiotherapy Example:** Rare, but radiation-induced oxidative processes may contribute to abnormal pigmentation.

124. **Xanthocyanopsy:** A rare visual disorder where yellow and blue are confused.
**Related Terms:** Color blindness, chromatic vision defect.
**Radiotherapy Example:** Could occur if ocular structures receive unintended dose during orbital radiation.

125. **Xantholeucocyte:** A leukocyte with yellow appearance due to pigment or lipid accumulation.
**Related Terms:** Pigmented macrophage, modified leukocyte.
**Radiotherapy Example:** Seen mainly in pathology specimens, not a direct radiotherapy effect.

126. **Xanthoma Cell:** A foamy macrophage filled with lipids found in xanthomas.
**Related Terms:** Foam cell, lipid macrophage.
**Radiotherapy Example:** Found during diagnostic imaging evaluation to differentiate benign from malignant lesions.

127. **Xanthomatosis:** A condition where multiple xanthomas occur due to severe lipid imbalance.
**Related Terms:** Hyperlipidemia, cholesterol disorder.
**Radiotherapy Example:** Appears in imaging and must be distinguished from metastatic soft-tissue masses.

128. **Xanthomatous Change:** Tissue transformation marked by lipid-filled macrophages.
**Related Terms:** Fatty degeneration, foam cell infiltration.
**Radiotherapy Example:** Occasionally observed pathologically when reviewing tissue affected by chronic inflammation.

129. **Xanthoproteic Test:** A biochemical test where proteins turn yellow after nitric acid exposure.
**Related Terms:** Protein identification test, nitration reaction.
**Radiotherapy Example:** Used in research to study protein changes after radiation damage.

130. **Xanthophyll Cycle:** A protective pigment cycle in plants that reduces oxidative stress.
**Related Terms:** Photoprotection, carotenoid pathway.
**Radiotherapy Example:** Studied in radiobiology models examining antioxidant response to radiation.

131. **Xanthine Derivative:** A compound structurally similar to xanthine, such as caffeine or theophylline.
**Related Terms:** Methylxanthine, purine analog.
**Radiotherapy Example:** Some derivatives are researched as potential radiosensitizers for tumors.

132. **Xanthinuria:** A rare disorder caused by lack of xanthine oxidase, leading to excessive xanthine accumulation.
**Related Terms:** Purine metabolism disorder, metabolic disease.
**Radiotherapy Example:** May affect treatment planning if kidney function is impaired.

133. **Xanthochromic:** Describes yellow-colored tissue or fluid.
**Related Terms:** Pigmented, bilirubin-positive.
**Radiotherapy Example:** Seen in cerebrospinal fluid analysis when evaluating radiation-related hemorrhage.

134. **Xanthocyanin:** A pigment mixture producing blue and yellow coloration.
**Related Terms:** Mixed chromophore, biopigmentation.
**Radiotherapy Example:** Mainly research-related in biological imaging studies.

135. **Xanthocyanic:** Describes mixed yellow-blue pigmentation.
**Related Terms:** Dual pigment, chromatic blend.
**Radiotherapy Example:** Used in colorimetric studies of tissue imaging or analysis.

136. **Xanthomere:** A pigment storage structure responsible for yellow coloration in some invertebrates.
**Related Terms:** Pigment granule, chromatophore unit.
**Radiotherapy Example:** Used in biological research models studying radiation effects on pigmentation cells.

137. **Xanthophore:** A pigment-containing cell that stores yellow carotenoids and pteridines.
**Related Terms:** Chromatophore, carotenoid cell.
**Radiotherapy Example:** Used in zebra fish models to observe radiation-induced pigment and DNA damage.

138. **Xanthopterin:** A yellow pteridine compound found in insects and some vertebrates.
**Related Terms:** Pteridine pigment, metabolic marker.
**Radiotherapy Example:** Studied as a biochemical marker of oxidative stress after irradiation.

139. **Xanthopicrin:** A yellow bitter plant compound with potential medicinal effects.
**Related Terms:** Bioactive phytochemical, plant metabolite.
**Radiotherapy Example:** Evaluated in research for possible radioprotective or cytotoxic properties.

140. **Xanthorhodopsin:** A light-driven proton pump using a carotenoid-enhanced antenna system.
**Related Terms:** Photoreceptor protein, microbial rhodopsin.
**Radiotherapy Example:** Investigated in photobiology and radiation-induced energy metabolism studies.

141. **Xanthosis:** Xanthosis is a yellow discoloration of skin or tissues caused by pigment or lipid buildup.
**Related Terms:** Xanthoma, hypercarotenemia, jaundice.
**Radiotherapy Example:** Skin changes during long-term radiation monitoring may require differentiation from metabolic xanthosis.

142. **Xanthoxyline:** Xanthoxyline is a plant-derived yellow compound with potential antimicrobial and medicinal properties.
**Related Terms:** Alkaloids, phytochemicals, herbal extracts.
**Radiotherapy Example:** Some natural compounds like xanthoxyline are studied for possible radioprotective or anti-cancer effects.

143. **Xanthoxylum (Zanthoxylum):** Zanthoxylum is a plant genus used in medicine and spices, containing aromatic oils and bioactive compounds.
**Related Terms:** Herbal medicine, flavonoids, prickly ash.
**Radiotherapy Example:** Extracts from this plant are sometimes researched as supportive therapy for radiation-induced inflammation.

144. **Xenobiotic Metabolism:** Xenobiotic metabolism is the body's process of breaking down foreign chemicals like drugs or pollutants.
**Related Terms:** Cytochrome P450, detoxification, biotransformation.
**Radiotherapy Example:** Radiation may alter liver enzyme activity, affecting how patients metabolize chemotherapy drugs.

145. **Xenodiagnosis:** Xenodiagnosis uses a living organism or vector to detect hidden infections in a patient.
**Related Terms:** Parasite testing, vector-based diagnosis.
**Radiotherapy Example:** Rare in cancer care, but may be used in immunocompromised patients to detect parasitic disease.

146. **Xenogamy:** Xenogamy is cross-pollination between flowers of different plants to increase genetic diversity.
**Related Terms:** Pollination, hybridization, fertilization.
**Radiotherapy Example:** In radiation biology, cross-pollination studies help assess radiation effects on plant fertility.

147. **Xenogenic Transplant (Xenogeneic Transplant):** A xenogenic transplant transfers tissue or organs between different species.
**Related Terms:** Immunologic rejection, graft compatibility, cross-species transplant.
**Radiotherapy Example:** Radiation may be used in research to condition immune systems before experimental xenogenic transplants.

148. **Xenograft:** A xenograft is tissue from one species implanted into another, commonly used in research.
**Related Terms:** Tumor model, immunodeficient mice, graft.
**Radiotherapy Example:** Xenograft mouse models help test tumor response to radiation therapy before human trials.

149. **Xenotransplantation:** Xenotransplantation is the medical practice of using living tissue or organs from one species in another.
**Related Terms:** Genetic modification, rejection, immune tolerance.
**Radiotherapy Example:** Total-body irradiation may be used in experimental protocols to reduce rejection before xenotransplantation.

150. **Xenon Gas:** Xenon is a noble gas used in imaging, anesthesia, and radiation detection.
**Related Terms:** Hyperpolarized MRI, gas contrast, scintillation detector.
**Radiotherapy Example:** Xenon detectors may be used in dosimetry equipment for measuring radiation accurately.

151. **X-irradiated Specimen:** An X-irradiated specimen is any sample exposed to X-rays for study or testing.
**Related Terms:** Sample irradiation, radiation experiment, exposure.
**Radiotherapy Example:** Researchers expose tumor cells to controlled X-rays to evaluate radiation sensitivity.

152. **X-irradiated Tissue:** X-irradiated tissue refers to biological tissue that has been exposed to X-ray radiation.
**Related Terms:** DNA damage, radiation effect, tissue response.
**Radiotherapy Example:** Cancer treatment intentionally irradiates tumor tissue while sparing normal surrounding tissue.

153. **X-irradiation Chamber:** An X-irradiation chamber is a controlled device used for delivering precise X-ray exposure to samples or small animals.
**Related Terms:** Radiation setup, shielding, dosimetry.
**Radiotherapy Example:** Research labs use irradiation chambers to test new radiosensitizers before clinical use.

154. **X-irradiation Dose:** The X-irradiation dose is the measured amount of absorbed X-ray energy, usually expressed in Gray (Gy).
**Related Terms:** Dosimetry, absorbed dose, calibration.
**Radiotherapy Example:** Correct dose calculation is essential to deliver enough radiation to kill cancer cells while minimizing toxicity.

155. **X-irradiation Source:** An X-irradiation source is equipment that generates X-rays for medical, industrial, or research use.
**Related Terms:** X-ray tube, LINAC, radiation generator.
**Radiotherapy Example:** Linear accelerators act as high-energy X-ray sources used daily in cancer treatment.

156. **X-irradiation Damage:** X-irradiation damage refers to biological or material injury caused by X-ray exposure, especially DNA breaks.
**Related Terms:** Oxidative stress, apoptosis, radiation toxicity.
**Radiotherapy Example:** Radiation-induced DNA damage is the main mechanism that destroys cancer cells in treatment.

157. **X-irradiation Cell Line:** An X-irradiation cell line is a culture of cells exposed to X-rays to study their response.
**Related Terms:** Radiobiology model, cell culture, genetic response.
**Radiotherapy Example:** Scientists use irradiated cancer cell lines to test the effect of radiation dose, timing, and drug combinations.

158. **X-irradiation Assay:** An X-irradiation assay is a laboratory test that measures biological effects after X-ray exposure.
**Related Terms:** Clonogenic assay, DNA damage assay, survival curve.
**Radiotherapy Example:** Clonogenic assays help determine how effective radiation is at killing tumor cells.

159. **X-irradiation Exposure:** X-irradiation exposure refers to the amount of time or intensity of X-ray contact with tissue or material.
**Related Terms:** Radiation time, beam intensity, dose rate.
**Radiotherapy Example:** Careful control of exposure prevents overdose and ensures accurate treatment delivery.

160. **X-irradiation Kinetics:** X-irradiation kinetics describes how biological and physical processes change over time during and after X-ray exposure.
**Related Terms:** DNA repair timing, dose-rate effect, cell recovery.
**Radiotherapy Example:** Understanding repair kinetics helps optimize treatment schedules like fractionation to maximize tumor damage.

161. **X-irradiation Repair:** Cellular processes that fix DNA damage caused by X-ray exposure.
**Related Terms:** DNA repair, NHEJ, homologous recombination.
**Radiotherapy Example:** Tumor cells with poor repair ability are more radiosensitive and easier to treat.

162. **X-irradiation Sensitivity:** The degree to which cells or tissues are affected by X-ray exposure.
**Related Terms:** Radiosensitivity, radioresistance, cell cycle.
**Radiotherapy Example:** Rapidly dividing cancer cells are more sensitive to radiation than normal tissue.

163. **X-irradiation Study:** A scientific investigation analyzing the effects of X-ray exposure.
**Related Terms:** Radiobiology research, dose-response testing.
**Radiotherapy Example:** Studies help refine treatment doses and improve safety.

164. **X-irradiation Survival Curve:** A graph showing the percentage of surviving cells as radiation dose increases.
**Related Terms:** Cell survival fraction, radiation response curve.
**Radiotherapy Example:** Used to compare how different cancer types respond to radiation.

**165. X-irradiation Test:** A controlled experiment measuring how materials or biological samples react to X-rays.
**Related Terms:** Radiation assay, exposure protocol.
**Radiotherapy Example:** Tests evaluate new shielding materials or radiosensitizing drugs.

**166. X-irradiation Tolerance:** The maximum radiation dose tissue can safely receive without severe damage.
**Related Terms:** Organ tolerance dose, TD5/5, radiation limits.
**Radiotherapy Example:** Tolerance levels guide dose planning to protect organs like spinal cord and lungs.

**167. X-irradiation Yield:** The amount of measurable effect (e.g., DNA breaks) produced per dose of radiation.
**Related Terms:** Radiation efficiency, damage rate.
**Radiotherapy Example:** Higher yield means more damage to tumor DNA at a given dose.

**168. X-irradiation Effect:** All physical, chemical, and biological outcomes of X-ray exposure.
**Related Terms:** Radiation injury, therapeutic effect, tissue response.
**Radiotherapy Example:** Effects include tumor destruction and possible side effects.

**169. X-irradiation Hazard:** The potential risks or harmful effects of X-ray exposure.
**Related Terms:** Radiation safety, carcinogenic risk, ALARA.
**Radiotherapy Example:** Lead shielding and monitoring reduce exposure risks.

**170. X-irradiation Method:** The specific technique used to expose a sample to X-rays.
**Related Terms:** Beam setup, dose rate, exposure geometry.
**Radiotherapy Example:** Standardized methods ensure accurate and repeatable treatment delivery.

**171. X-ray Angiography:** A technique using X-rays and contrast dye to visualize blood vessels.
**Related Terms:** Fluoroscopy, contrast injection, vascular imaging.
**Radiotherapy Example:** Used before treatment to map blood supply to tumors.

**172. X-ray Bone Densitometry:** Imaging (often DEXA) that measures bone mineral density.
**Related Terms:** Osteoporosis screening, DEXA scan.
**Radiotherapy Example:** Used to monitor bone health in patients receiving pelvic radiation.

**173. X-ray Chest Imaging:** Imaging used to visualize lungs, ribs, and heart structures.
**Related Terms:** Chest X-ray (CXR), thoracic imaging.
**Radiotherapy Example:** Useful for monitoring radiation-induced lung fibrosis or pneumonitis.

**174. X-ray Collimation:** Narrowing the X-ray beam to reduce exposure outside the target area.
**Related Terms:** Beam limiting device, scatter reduction.
**Radiotherapy Example:** Collimation protects healthy tissue during treatment.

**175. X-ray Contrast Media:** Substances that improve visibility of internal structures on X-ray images.
**Related Terms:** Iodine contrast, radiopaque agent.
**Radiotherapy Example:** Used in CT simulation to outline organs and blood vessels.

**176. X-ray Correction Algorithm:** Software processing that removes imaging artifacts and improves accuracy.
**Related Terms:** Image reconstruction, scatter correction.
**Radiotherapy Example:** Critical for accurate CT imaging used in treatment planning.

**177. X-ray Cross-section:** A measure of the probability that X-rays will interact with matter.
**Related Terms:** Attenuation, photoelectric effect, scattering.
**Radiotherapy Example:** Used in dose calculation models and Monte Carlo simulations.

178. **X-ray Dental Radiography:** Imaging that uses low-dose X-rays to examine teeth and jaw structures.
**Related Terms:** Bitewing X-ray, panoramic radiograph.
**Radiotherapy Example:** Jaw imaging may be required before head and neck radiotherapy.

179. **X-ray Diffraction Pattern:** A characteristic pattern formed when X-rays scatter off a crystal.
**Related Terms:** Crystallography, Bragg's law.
**Radiotherapy Example:** Used in research to study structural changes after irradiation.

180. **X-ray Exposure Meter:** A device used to measure X-ray dose, exposure, or air kerma.
**Related Terms:** Dosimeter, ionization chamber.
**Radiotherapy Example:** Used to verify equipment output during quality assurance checks.

181. **X-ray Film Badge:** Personal dosimeter worn to monitor cumulative X-ray exposure.
**Related Terms:** Dosimeter, radiation monitoring.
**Radiotherapy Example:** Staff wear badges to track occupational dose during treatments.

182. **X-ray Filtration:** Use of materials to remove low-energy X-rays from the beam.
**Related Terms:** Aluminum filter, beam hardening.
**Radiotherapy Example:** Reduces skin dose during diagnostic imaging or therapy.

183. **X-ray Fluorescence Mapping:** Technique mapping elemental composition using emitted X-rays.
**Related Terms:** XRF, elemental analysis.
**Radiotherapy Example:** Researching trace elements in tissue response to radiation.

184. **X-ray Generator Control:** System regulating voltage, current, and exposure timing for X-rays.
**Related Terms:** Generator interface, exposure automation.
**Radiotherapy Example:** Ensures consistent beam output during treatment.

185. **X-ray High Voltage Supply:** Powers the X-ray tube by creating a potential difference to accelerate electrons.
**Related Terms:** Tube voltage, kVp.
**Radiotherapy Example:** Stable voltage ensures accurate photon energy for therapy beams.

186. **X-ray Image Intensifier:** Device that amplifies X-ray brightness into visible images.
**Related Terms:** Fluoroscopy, real-time imaging.
**Radiotherapy Example:** Used in image-guided procedures to minimize dose.

187. **X-ray Interface:** User system to adjust imaging parameters and view images.
**Related Terms:** Control console, digital interface.
**Radiotherapy Example:** Operators set exposure parameters for patient scans.

188. **X-ray Localization:** Identifying precise positions of structures or objects with X-rays.
**Related Terms:** Fiducial markers, image guidance.
**Radiotherapy Example:** Localizing tumor boundaries before treatment.

189. **X-ray Microscope:** Microscope using X-rays for high-resolution imaging of small structures.
**Related Terms:** Zone plates, nanoscopy.
**Radiotherapy Example:** Studying radiation effects on cellular structures.

190. **X-ray Nano-imaging:** Visualization of structures at the nanometer scale with X-rays.
**Related Terms:** Synchrotron imaging, coherent X-rays.
**Radiotherapy Example:** Researching nanoscale changes in irradiated tissues.

191. **X-ray Photodiode:** Converts X-ray photons into electrical current for detection.
**Related Terms:** Digital detector, CT detector.
**Radiotherapy Example:** Forms part of flat-panel detectors for imaging patients.

192. **X-ray Photomultiplier:** Amplifies weak X-ray-induced light signals for detection.
**Related Terms:** PMT, scintillation detector.
**Radiotherapy Example:** Measures low-level radiation in nuclear medicine setups.

193. **X-ray Phototherapy:** Therapeutic use of low-dose X-rays to treat skin conditions.
**Related Terms:** Low-dose radiation therapy, dermatology.
**Radiotherapy Example:** Historically used for psoriasis; now replaced by UV therapy.

194. **X-ray Photonics:** Study and manipulation of X-ray photons for imaging and analysis.
**Related Terms:** X-ray optics, synchrotron radiation.
**Radiotherapy Example:** Advanced imaging systems for precise tumor visualization.

195. **X-ray Pixel Detector:** Detector capturing X-ray photons individually with high resolution.
**Related Terms:** Digital radiography, CT detector.
**Radiotherapy Example:** Used in modern imaging for accurate treatment planning.

196. **X-ray Projection:** 2D image formed by X-rays passing through a 3D object.
**Related Terms:** Radiography, planar imaging.
**Radiotherapy Example:** Basic imaging method before 3D CT-based planning.

197. **X-ray Reconstruction:** Algorithm converting projections into cross-sectional or 3D images.
**Related Terms:** Filtered back-projection, iterative reconstruction.
**Radiotherapy Example:** Produces CT images used for contouring tumors.

198. **X-ray Scanner:** Device scanning objects with X-rays to produce detailed images.
**Related Terms:** CT scanner, industrial X-ray.
**Radiotherapy Example:** Scanning phantoms to verify treatment setups.

199. **X-ray Simulation:** Computational modeling of X-ray interactions and image formation.
**Related Terms:** Monte Carlo simulation, dose modeling.
**Radiotherapy Example:** Simulates patient dose distribution for planning.

200. **X-ray Software:** Programs for image acquisition, processing, reconstruction, and analysis.
**Related Terms:** PACS, image reconstruction software.
**Radiotherapy Example:** Used to plan, visualize, and analyze patient treatment doses.

201. **Xenon Imaging:** Functional imaging using xenon gas to visualize ventilation or perfusion.
**Related Terms:** Xenon CT, Xe-133, functional imaging.
**Radiotherapy Example:** Evaluating lung function before thoracic radiotherapy.

202. **Xenon Enhancement Scan:** Imaging scan where inhaled xenon increases tissue contrast.
**Related Terms:** Contrast agent, CT perfusion.
**Radiotherapy Example:** Highlighting perfused brain regions during planning.

203. **Xenon Emission Tomography:** Functional imaging with radioactive xenon to map blood flow or ventilation.
**Related Terms:** Xe-133, SPECT, gamma imaging.
**Radiotherapy Example:** Assessing cerebral perfusion in patients undergoing cranial radiation.

204. **Xenon Clearance Test:** Measures rate of xenon washout from tissues to evaluate perfusion.
**Related Terms:** Washout kinetics, blood flow measurement.
**Radiotherapy Example:** Studying cerebral perfusion post-brain irradiation.

205. **Xenon Diffusion Coefficient:** Rate at which xenon atoms diffuse through tissues or materials.
**Related Terms:** Gas permeability, tissue diffusion.
**Radiotherapy Example:** Modeling gas distribution in pulmonary function studies.

206. **Xenon Scintillation Yield:** Amount of light produced when xenon is excited by radiation.
**Related Terms:** Scintillation detector, photon detection.
**Radiotherapy Example:** Monitoring radiation dose in research using xenon detectors.

207. **Xenon Gamma Spectrum:** Characteristic gamma energies emitted by radioactive xenon isotopes.
**Related Terms:** Xe-133, gamma emission, spectroscopy.
**Radiotherapy Example:** Calibration of xenon-based imaging systems.

208. **Xenon Neutron Capture:** Absorption of neutrons by xenon nuclei, producing isotopes like Xe-135.
**Related Terms:** Reactor physics, neutron cross-section.
**Radiotherapy Example:** Relevant in research with neutron therapy planning.

209. **Xenon Dosimeter:** Radiation detector using xenon gas to measure dose.
**Related Terms:** Ionization chamber, scintillation detector.
**Radiotherapy Example:** Lab monitoring of low-level radiation exposure.

210. **Xenon Photomultiplier:** PMT optimized for detecting xenon scintillation light.
**Related Terms:** Photon amplifier, gamma detection.
**Radiotherapy Example:** Used in high-sensitivity detection of radiotracers.

211. **Xenon Reaction Cross-section:** Probability of nuclear reactions involving xenon isotopes.
**Related Terms:** Neutron absorption, fission product.
**Radiotherapy Example:** Planning isotope production for imaging agents.

212. **Xenon Release Kinetics:** Rate at which xenon escapes from tissues or materials.
**Related Terms:** Washout rate, gas kinetics.
**Radiotherapy Example:** Evaluating pulmonary xenon clearance before thoracic treatment.

213. **Xenon Signal Analysis:** Interpretation of data from xenon imaging or detectors.
**Related Terms:** Gamma counts, scintillation profile.
**Radiotherapy Example:** Assessing lung ventilation patterns for planning.

214. **Xenon Solubility:** Ability of xenon gas to dissolve in tissues or blood.
**Related Terms:** Lipid solubility, distribution coefficient.
**Radiotherapy Example:** Predicting xenon distribution in lung imaging.

215. **Xenon Stability:** Chemical inertness and physical durability of xenon isotopes.
**Related Terms:** Noble gas, isotope half-life.
**Radiotherapy Example:** Stable xenon used in functional imaging.

216. **Xenon Tracer Study:** Using xenon gas or isotopes to trace airflow or perfusion.
**Related Terms:** Functional imaging, Xe-133.
**Radiotherapy Example:** Mapping regional lung ventilation pre-radiotherapy.

217. **Xenon Uptake:** Absorption of xenon into tissues during imaging studies.
**Related Terms:** Perfusion measurement, gas distribution.
**Radiotherapy Example:** Evaluating tissue oxygenation in irradiated lungs.

218. **Xenon Ventilation Test:** Test using inhaled xenon to evaluate lung airflow.
**Related Terms:** Ventilation imaging, Xe-133 scan.
**Radiotherapy Example:** Detecting obstructed lung regions before thoracic RT.

219. **Xenon Washout Study:** Measures how quickly xenon is exhaled from lungs.
**Related Terms:** Clearance test, gas kinetics.
**Radiotherapy Example:** Identifying air-trapping areas to avoid excessive dose.

220. **Xenon Yield Factor:** Production yield of xenon isotopes in nuclear reactions.
**Related Terms:** Fission product, reactor physics.
**Radiotherapy Example:** Relevant in planning production of xenon tracers for imaging.

221. **Xanthoxenite:** A mineral containing iron and phosphate, studied for radiation shielding.
**Related Terms:** Mineral attenuation, shielding material.
**Radiotherapy Example:** Experimental use as a localized radiation shield in phantom studies.

222. **Xenoantigen:** Foreign antigen from another species that triggers immune responses.
**Related Terms:** Xenotransplantation, immune rejection.
**Radiotherapy Example:** Consideration during radiotherapy in xenograft tumor models.

223. **Xenoculture:** Cultivation of cells from one species in another species' environment.
**Related Terms:** Cross-species cell culture, xenografts.
**Radiotherapy Example:** Growing human tumor cells in mice for radiation response studies.

224. **Xenodiagnosis:** Using a live vector to detect infection in a host.
**Related Terms:** Parasitology, vector-borne disease detection.
**Radiotherapy Example:** Rarely used, but vector-based detection could be combined with radiation sterilization studies.

225. **Xenogenesis:** Biological process producing offspring differing from parent form; sometimes used metaphorically in radiation biology.
**Related Terms:** Aberrant development, hybridization.
**Radiotherapy Example:** Observing abnormal cell morphology post-irradiation in experimental studies.

226. **Xenomonitoring:** Detecting pathogens in vectors instead of human hosts.
**Related Terms:** Vector surveillance, disease monitoring.
**Radiotherapy Example:** Not directly used, but relevant in biosafety when irradiating vectors in labs.

227. **Xenopathic Infection:** Infection caused by a microorganism from another species.
**Related Terms:** Zoonosis, cross-species infection.
**Radiotherapy Example:** Monitoring immune-compromised patients during radiotherapy for zoonotic infections.

228. **Xenotropic Virus:** Virus that cannot infect its original host but can infect other species' cells.
**Related Terms:** Retrovirus, cross-species infection.
**Radiotherapy Example:** Studying viral effects on tumor xenografts under radiation.

229. **Xeranthemum Cytotoxicity Test:** Assay evaluating cytotoxicity of compounds from Xeranthemum plants.
**Related Terms:** Plant extract toxicity, in vitro assay.
**Radiotherapy Example:** Screening radioprotective or radiosensitizing plant compounds.

230. **Xeric Stress Response:** Physiological/molecular changes due to extreme dryness.
**Related Terms:** Dehydration adaptation, oxidative stress.
**Radiotherapy Example:** Studying skin or tissue response to combined radiation and dryness in radiotherapy.

231. **Xeroderma Pigmentation Assay:** Test evaluating DNA repair in xeroderma pigmentosum cells.
**Related Terms:** DNA repair assay, UV sensitivity.
**Radiotherapy Example:** Assessing radiosensitivity in patients with XP or defective repair.

232. **Xerophthalmia Screening:** Detecting early signs of severe vitamin A deficiency (eye dryness).
**Related Terms:** Night blindness, Bitot's spots.
**Radiotherapy Example:** Protecting ocular health in head-and-neck radiotherapy patients.

233. **Xerophile Growth Curve:** Growth measurement of organisms thriving in dry environments.
**Related Terms:** Microbial survival, dehydration tolerance.
**Radiotherapy Example:** Studying radioresistant microbes in arid tissue models.

234. **Xeroradiography Film:** Imaging medium using charged plates and dry powder instead of chemical film.
**Related Terms:** Edge-enhanced radiography, xeroradiography.
**Radiotherapy Example:** Historical use in breast imaging for radiation planning.

235. **Xeroradiography Edge Effect:** Enhanced visibility of tissue boundaries in xeroradiography.
**Related Terms:** Edge enhancement, imaging artifact.
**Radiotherapy Example:** Improved target delineation in early breast RT planning.

236. **Xerotic Fissure:** Skin crack from extreme dryness.
**Related Terms:** Fissure, xerosis.
**Radiotherapy Example:** Common skin toxicity in radiotherapy for extremities.

237. **XRF Spectroscopy (X-ray Fluorescence):** Detects elemental composition via characteristic X-rays.
**Related Terms:** X-ray analysis, elemental mapping.
**Radiotherapy Example:** Material characterization for shielding design or dosimetry phantoms.

238. **Xiphisternum Landmark:** Cartilaginous tip of sternum used as an anatomical reference.
**Related Terms:** Xiphoid process, anatomical landmark.
**Radiotherapy Example:** Aligning chest or abdominal RT fields.

239. **Xiphoid Syndrome:** Pain/tenderness at xiphisternum due to trauma or inflammation.
**Related Terms:** Sternum pain, musculoskeletal disorder.
**Radiotherapy Example:** Care during thoracic RT positioning to avoid exacerbating pain.

240. **Xiphosuran Embryology:** Study of horseshoe crab development, a model for evolutionary biology.
**Related Terms:** Developmental biology, arthropod embryology.
**Radiotherapy Example:** Rarely direct, but used in radiobiology models for developmental studies.

241. **X-linked Agammaglobulinemia Protein Assay:** Measures BTK protein levels to detect X-linked agammaglobulinemia (XLA).
**Related Terms:** BTK, B-cell deficiency, immunodeficiency.
**Radiotherapy Example:** Screening XLA patients before RT to assess infection risk.

242. **X-linked Carrier Detection:** Identifies asymptomatic carriers of X-linked mutations.
**Related Terms:** Genetic testing, pedigree analysis.
**Radiotherapy Example:** Planning RT in carriers of radiosensitive X-linked disorders.

243. **X-linked Dominant Inheritance Pattern:** Single X-linked gene mutation causing disease in both sexes.
**Related Terms:** X-inactivation, sex-linked disorders.
**Radiotherapy Example:** Understanding inheritance in families with radiosensitive X-linked conditions.

244. **X-linked Hypophosphatemia Panel:** Genetic test for phosphate-wasting bone disease (PHEX gene).
**Related Terms:** Hypophosphatemia, rickets, genetic panel.
**Radiotherapy Example:** Monitoring bone health during RT in affected patients.

245. **X-linked Muscular Dystrophy Pathology:** Muscle degeneration from X-linked mutations (e.g., Duchenne).
**Related Terms:** Dystrophin deficiency, fibrosis.
**Radiotherapy Example:** Avoiding excessive muscle irradiation in dystrophy patients.

246. **X-linked Pedigree Analysis:** Studies inheritance patterns of X-linked diseases in families.
**Related Terms:** Genetic counseling, carrier detection.
**Radiotherapy Example:** Identifying at-risk family members before RT for genetic disorders.

247. **X-linked Reactive Disorder:** Abnormal immune response due to X-linked mutations.
**Related Terms:** Immunodeficiency, inflammatory disorders.
**Radiotherapy Example:** Adjusting RT doses in patients with X-linked immune sensitivity.

248. **X-linked Recessive Carrier State:** Carrier of a single mutated X-linked gene, usually asymptomatic.
**Related Terms:** Female carriers, hemizygosity.
**Radiotherapy Example:** Counseling female carriers regarding potential radiosensitivity in offspring.

249. **X-linked Trait Map:** Visual representation of genes and traits on the X chromosome.
**Related Terms:** Genetic mapping, linkage analysis.
**Radiotherapy Example:** Identifying genes affecting radiosensitivity.

250. **X-band Radar Imaging:** Short-wavelength radar (8–12 GHz) for high-resolution imaging.
**Related Terms:** Microwave imaging, environmental scanning.
**Radiotherapy Example:** Not directly used; analogous principles in imaging guidance.

251. **X-chromosome Aberration Analysis:** Detects structural abnormalities in the X chromosome.
**Related Terms:** Deletions, translocations, cytogenetics.
**Radiotherapy Example:** Screening patients for radiosensitive chromosomal syndromes.

252. **X-chromosome Aneuploidy:** Abnormal number of X chromosomes (e.g., Turner, Klinefelter).
**Related Terms:** Genetic disorders, chromosomal imbalance.
**Radiotherapy Example:** Dose adjustments in radiosensitive aneuploid patients.

253. **X-chromosome Conformation Capture:** Studies 3D chromatin folding and gene interactions.
**Related Terms:** Chromatin structure, X-inactivation.
**Radiotherapy Example:** Understanding gene regulation affecting radiosensitivity.

254. **X-chromosome Counting Mechanism:** Ensures proper X chromosome inactivation in females.
**Related Terms:** Dosage compensation, epigenetics.
**Radiotherapy Example:** Epigenetic regulation may influence cellular radiation response.

255. **X-chromosome Crossover Hotspot:** Region with frequent recombination during meiosis.
**Related Terms:** Genetic diversity, recombination.
**Radiotherapy Example:** Indirectly relevant in studies of inherited radiosensitivity.

256. **X-chromosome Cytogenetics:** Detects structural/numerical X chromosome abnormalities.
**Related Terms:** FISH, G-banding, microarray.
**Radiotherapy Example:** Screening patients with potential radiosensitive syndromes.

257. **X-chromosome DNA Methylation Assay:** Measures methylation patterns to study X-inactivation.
**Related Terms:** Epigenetics, imprinting.
**Radiotherapy Example:** Altered methylation may influence tumor radiosensitivity.

258. **X-chromosome Dosage Compensation:** Equalizes gene expression between males (XY) and females (XX).
**Related Terms:** X-inactivation, gene expression regulation.
**Radiotherapy Example:** Understanding cellular response differences between sexes.

259. **X-chromosome Epigenetic Marker:** Methylation or histone modification regulating X-linked genes.
**Related Terms:** X-inactivation, gene silencing.
**Radiotherapy Example:** Studying epigenetic influence on DNA repair after RT.

260. **X-chromosome Expression Profiling:** Measures transcriptional activity of X-linked genes.
**Related Terms:** Gene expression, genomics.
**Radiotherapy Example:** Identifying X-linked genes affecting radiosensitivity in tumors.

261. **X-chromosome Fusion Event:** Part of X chromosome fuses with another chromosome, causing rearrangements.
**Related Terms:** Translocation, structural variant.
**Radiotherapy Example:** Evaluating cancer genomes for fusion-driven radiosensitivity.

262. **X-chromosome Gene Cluster:** Group of functionally related genes located close together.
**Related Terms:** Gene linkage, coordinated expression.
**Radiotherapy Example:** Studying clusters affecting radiation response pathways.

263. **X-chromosome Gene Escape:** Certain X-linked genes remain active despite X-inactivation.
**Related Terms:** Escape genes, gene dosage.
**Radiotherapy Example:** Escape genes may influence cellular survival after RT.

264. **X-chromosome Gene Mapping:** Locates genes on X chromosome and links to traits.
**Related Terms:** Genetic linkage, positional cloning.
**Radiotherapy Example:** Mapping radiosensitivity genes on X chromosome.

265. **X-chromosome Genetic Drift:** Random changes in X-linked gene frequencies over generations.
**Related Terms:** Population genetics, allele frequency.
**Radiotherapy Example:** Population studies of radiosensitivity alleles.

266. **X-chromosome Haplotype Block:** Set of linked genetic variants inherited together.
**Related Terms:** Haplotype mapping, linkage disequilibrium.
**Radiotherapy Example:** Identifying haplotypes associated with radiation response.

267. **X-chromosome Inactivation Mosaic:** Female cells randomly inactivate one X chromosome, creating mosaic expression.
**Related Terms:** Mosaicism, X-inactivation.
**Radiotherapy Example:** Explains variable RT effects in heterozygous females.

268. **X-chromosome Inactivation Skewing:** Non-random X-inactivation favoring one X chromosome.
**Related Terms:** Skewed inactivation, epigenetic bias.
**Radiotherapy Example:** Can affect expression of radiosensitive X-linked genes.

269. **X-chromosome Interphase Nucleus:** Organization of X chromosome in non-dividing cells; inactive X forms Barr body.
**Related Terms:** Nuclear architecture, chromatin organization.
**Radiotherapy Example:** Structural organization influences DNA repair post-RT.

270. **X-chromosome Microarray Analysis:** Detects small deletions/duplications or copy number changes.
**Related Terms:** Copy number variation, cytogenomics.
**Radiotherapy Example:** Screening for X-linked disorders affecting radiosensitivity.

271. **X-chromosome Nondisjunction Frequency:** Rate at which X chromosomes fail to separate during meiosis.
**Related Terms:** Aneuploidy, Turner syndrome, Klinefelter syndrome.
**Radiotherapy Example:** Understanding genetic predisposition to chromosomal disorders affecting tissue sensitivity.

272. **X-chromosome Pairing Center:** Ensures correct X chromosome alignment during meiosis in certain organisms.
**Related Terms:** Recombination, meiotic segregation.
**Radiotherapy Example:** Model studies of meiotic errors may inform genetic risk assessments.

273. **X-chromosome Recombination Map:** Charts crossover rates along the X chromosome.
**Related Terms:** Genetic linkage, inheritance, population genetics.
**Radiotherapy Example:** Identifying genes influencing radiosensitivity through recombination mapping.

274. **X-chromosome Translocation Breakpoint:** Precise location where X chromosome breaks in a translocation.
**Related Terms:** Structural variant, chromosomal rearrangement.
**Radiotherapy Example:** Detecting fusion events that may alter cellular radiation response.

275. **X-chromosome Variant Scanning:** Surveys X chromosome for mutations, SNPs, or structural variants.
**Related Terms:** Sequencing, pharmacogenomics, disease risk.
**Radiotherapy Example:** Screening for X-linked radiosensitivity genes.

276. **X-plane Scanner:** Measures radiation or imaging signals along the X-axis plane.
**Related Terms:** Geometric calibration, cross-sectional imaging.
**Radiotherapy Example:** Ensures precise patient positioning and dose alignment.

277. **X-positioner:** Device to move components precisely along the X-axis.
**Related Terms:** Alignment, positioning, accuracy.
**Radiotherapy Example:** Accurate alignment of X-ray beams or detectors.

278. **X-projection Data:** Recorded intensity values from X-rays at various angles.
**Related Terms:** CT reconstruction, projection imaging.
**Radiotherapy Example:** Basis for 3D imaging and treatment planning.

279. **X-ray Analyzer:** Processes and interprets X-ray signals to determine composition or structure.
**Related Terms:** Spectroscopy, crystallography, material analysis.
**Radiotherapy Example:** Calibration of X-ray beams and quality assurance.

280. **X-ray Background Correction:** Removes ambient or noise signals from X-ray measurements.
**Related Terms:** Signal processing, image quality.
**Radiotherapy Example:** Enhances diagnostic accuracy in imaging and dosimetry.

281. **X-ray Cathode Emission:** Release of electrons from cathode to generate X-rays.
**Related Terms:** X-ray tube, electron acceleration.
**Radiotherapy Example:** Stable emission ensures consistent therapeutic dose delivery.

282. **X-ray Collimation Field:** Defines geometric region where X-rays pass through.
**Related Terms:** Scatter reduction, dose optimization.
**Radiotherapy Example:** Minimizes patient exposure and improves image contrast.

283. **X-ray Console Interface:** Operator panel controlling X-ray settings and imaging parameters.
**Related Terms:** Imaging workflow, exposure control.
**Radiotherapy Example:** Ensures safe and precise operation of imaging and therapy devices.

284. **X-ray Converter:** Transforms X-ray photons into light or electrical signals.
**Related Terms:** Scintillator, photodiode, digital radiography.
**Radiotherapy Example:** Critical for accurate image acquisition and dose verification.

285. **X-ray Exposure Chamber:** Controlled environment for exposing samples or devices to X-rays.
**Related Terms:** Dosimetry, radiation research, sterilization.
**Radiotherapy Example:** Preclinical studies and radiation effect testing.

286. **X-ray Field Mapping:** Measures spatial distribution of X-ray intensity across an area.
**Related Terms:** Beam uniformity, quality assurance.
**Radiotherapy Example:** Ensures uniform dose delivery in treatment planning.

287. **X-ray Image Contrast:** Difference in absorption between tissues, enabling visibility.
**Related Terms:** Contrast agents, tissue differentiation.
**Radiotherapy Example:** Optimizes imaging for tumor delineation.

288. **X-ray Imaging Mode:** Specific acquisition technique (e.g., radiography, CT, fluoroscopy).
**Related Terms:** Mode selection, detector settings.
**Radiotherapy Example:** Mode selection impacts image quality and patient dose.

289. **X-ray Optics:** Devices that focus or manipulate X-rays (mirrors, zone plates).
**Related Terms:** Nanotomography, synchrotron imaging.
**Radiotherapy Example:** Specialized imaging for precise tumor visualization.

290. **X-ray Pixel Response:** How each detector pixel reacts to incoming X-rays.
**Related Terms:** Sensitivity, noise, calibration.
**Radiotherapy Example:** Uniform response ensures accurate dose imaging.

291. **X-ray Scatter Correction:** Compensates for secondary radiation degrading image quality.
**Related Terms:** Anti-scatter grids, software correction.
**Radiotherapy Example:** Improves image clarity and treatment accuracy.

292. **X-ray Signal Noise:** Random fluctuations in detected X-ray signals.
**Related Terms:** Quantum noise, electronic noise, filtering.
**Radiotherapy Example:** Reducing noise improves diagnostic and treatment imaging.

293. **X-ray Simulation Model:** Digital reproduction of X-ray generation and detection.
**Related Terms:** Monte Carlo, beam modeling, dose optimization.
**Radiotherapy Example:** Predicts patient dose and optimizes treatment parameters.

294. **X-ray Spatial Resolution:** Smallest detail an X-ray system can distinguish.
**Related Terms:** Detector pixel size, focal spot, image clarity.
**Radiotherapy Example:** Critical for detecting microlesions or small tumors.

295. **X-ray Spectral Response:** Detector response across different X-ray energies.
**Related Terms:** Energy-resolved imaging, material differentiation.
**Radiotherapy Example:** Enhances contrast for tissue characterization.

296. **X-ray Tomography Reconstruction:** Converts projections into cross-sectional or volumetric images.
**Related Terms:** Filtered back-projection, iterative reconstruction, AI methods.
**Radiotherapy Example:** Basis for 3D treatment planning and verification.

297. **X-ray Tube Output:** Quantity and energy distribution of X-rays emitted.
**Related Terms:** Tube voltage, current, filtration, anode material.
**Radiotherapy Example:** Ensures consistent imaging or therapy doses.

298. **X-ray Visualization System:** Hardware/software for displaying and analyzing X-ray images.
**Related Terms:** 3D rendering, contrast enhancement.
**Radiotherapy Example:** Planning and evaluating treatment fields.

299. **X-ray Voxel Mapping:** Assigns intensity values to 3D volumetric pixels in CT.
**Related Terms:** Segmentation, quantitative imaging.
**Radiotherapy Example:** Enables precise dose calculations and tumor delineation.

300. **X-ray Yield Measurement:** Quantifies X-rays produced per incident electron or unit exposure.
**Related Terms:** Tube efficiency, calibration, QA.
**Radiotherapy Example:** Ensures reliable output for consistent therapy delivery.

301. **X-ray attenuation coefficient:** A measure of how much an X-ray beam is reduced in intensity per unit thickness of material.
**Related Terms:** Absorption, scattering, beam hardening.
**Radiotherapy Example:** Determines tissue dose and contrast in imaging and planning.

302. **X-ray backscatter imaging:** Imaging technique detecting X-rays scattered back from an object.
**Related Terms:** Security screening, non-destructive testing.
**Radiotherapy Example:** Used in experimental imaging to detect surface or subsurface density variations.

303. **X-ray beam hardening:** Increase in average energy of an X-ray beam as lower-energy photons are absorbed.
**Related Terms:** Artifacts, filtration, CT imaging.
**Radiotherapy Example:** Corrected in imaging to improve dose calculations.

304. **X-ray beam profile:** Spatial distribution of X-ray intensity across the beam cross-section.
**Related Terms:** Field mapping, uniformity, dosimetry.
**Radiotherapy Example:** Ensures consistent treatment dose distribution.

305. **X-ray computed tomography (CT) number:** A unitless number (Hounsfield Unit) representing X-ray attenuation of a voxel.
**Related Terms:** Voxel mapping, tissue density, reconstruction.
**Radiotherapy Example:** Guides dose planning and tumor delineation.

306. **X-ray contrast resolution:** Ability of an X-ray system to differentiate between similar densities.
**Related Terms:** Image quality, spatial resolution, contrast agents.
**Radiotherapy Example:** Important in detecting tumors and small lesions.

307. **X-ray detector efficiency:** Fraction of incoming X-ray photons successfully detected.
**Related Terms:** Quantum efficiency, scintillators, photodiodes.
**Radiotherapy Example:** Impacts imaging dose and signal-to-noise ratio.

308. **X-ray diffraction crystallography:** Method to determine atomic structure of crystals by analyzing diffraction patterns.
**Related Terms:** Bragg's law, lattice spacing, structural biology.
**Radiotherapy Example:** Helps study radiation-sensitive biomolecules.

309. **X-ray dose rate:** Amount of radiation delivered per unit time.
**Related Terms:** Gray per second (Gy/s), exposure, treatment planning.
**Radiotherapy Example:** Determines treatment fractionation schedules.

310. **X-ray energy spectrum:** Distribution of photon energies in an X-ray beam.
**Related Terms:** Beam quality, filtration, spectral imaging.
**Radiotherapy Example:** Influences tissue penetration and image contrast.

311. **X-ray fluorescence tomography (XFT):** Imaging technique mapping elemental composition in 3D using X-ray fluorescence.
**Related Terms:** Synchrotron imaging, material analysis.
**Radiotherapy Example:** Research tool for imaging metallic implants or contrast agents.

312. **X-ray grating interferometry:** Uses gratings to measure phase shifts in X-rays passing through a sample.
**Related Terms:** Phase-contrast imaging, coherence.
**Radiotherapy Example:** Enables soft tissue imaging with higher contrast.

313. **X-ray guided brachytherapy:** Brachytherapy placement guided by X-ray imaging.
**Related Terms:** Tumor localization, radioactive sources.
**Radiotherapy Example:** Ensures accurate radiation delivery to target tissue.

314. **X-ray holography:** Technique to record 3D interference patterns using X-rays.
**Related Terms:** Coherent X-rays, phase imaging.
**Radiotherapy Example:** Primarily experimental; can study microscopic tissue structures.

315. **X-ray imaging phantom:** A model simulating tissue for imaging calibration and testing.
**Related Terms:** Dosimetry, QA, tissue-equivalent materials.
**Radiotherapy Example:** Used to test imaging systems and treatment planning accuracy.

316. **X-ray linear attenuation coefficient:** Describes how much an X-ray beam is attenuated per unit distance in a material.
**Related Terms:** Exponential attenuation, density, absorption.
**Radiotherapy Example:** Critical in dose calculation and CT imaging.

317. **X-ray monochromator:** Device that selects a single X-ray wavelength from a polychromatic beam.
**Related Terms:** Synchrotron, diffraction, spectroscopy.
**Radiotherapy Example:** Used in experimental imaging and structural analysis.

318. **X-ray optical element:** Component that manipulates X-ray paths, e.g., mirrors, lenses, zone plates.
**Related Terms:** Beam focusing, synchrotron optics.
**Radiotherapy Example:** Advanced imaging research for microbeam therapy guidance.

319. **X-ray phase contrast imaging:** Technique enhancing edges of structures using phase shifts instead of absorption.
**Related Terms:** Soft tissue imaging, coherence, interferometry.
**Radiotherapy Example:** Improves visualization of tumors in low-density tissues.

320. **X-ray scatter profile:** Spatial distribution and intensity of scattered X-rays around an object.
**Related Terms:** Scatter correction, anti-scatter grids, image artifacts.
**Radiotherapy Example:** Reducing scatter improves image quality and treatment planning accuracy.

321. **X-ray slit collimator:** A collimator with narrow slits used to shape and direct X-ray beams precisely.
**Related Terms:** Beam shaping, field restriction, image resolution.
**Radiotherapy Example:** Reduces dose to surrounding tissues in localized therapy.

322. **X-ray source focal spot:** The small area on the anode where electrons hit to produce X-rays.
**Related Terms:** Spatial resolution, penumbra, tube design.
**Radiotherapy Example:** Smaller focal spots improve image clarity for treatment planning.

323. **X-ray spectral imaging:** Imaging technique using energy-resolved X-ray photons to distinguish materials.
**Related Terms:** Dual-energy CT, material decomposition, contrast enhancement.
**Radiotherapy Example:** Helps differentiate tumor from healthy tissue for precise targeting.

324. **X-ray tomosynthesis:** Limited-angle CT technique producing sectional images from multiple projections.
**Related Terms:** Mammography, 3D reconstruction, slice imaging.
**Radiotherapy Example:** Guides breast cancer radiation planning and biopsy localization.

325. **X-ray tube current (mA):** Electric current in the X-ray tube controlling the number of photons produced.
**Related Terms:** Exposure, dose, tube voltage.
**Radiotherapy Example:** Adjusted to balance image quality with patient dose.

326. **X-ray tube voltage (kVp):** Potential difference applied across the X-ray tube, determining photon energy.
**Related Terms:** Beam quality, penetration, contrast.
**Radiotherapy Example:** Higher kVp penetrates denser tissues for accurate imaging.

327. **X-ray undulator:** Device in synchrotrons producing highly collimated X-ray beams via periodic magnetic fields.
**Related Terms:** Synchrotron radiation, beamline, monochromatic X-rays.
**Radiotherapy Example:** Primarily research; can be used for microbeam or nanobeam therapy studies.

328. **X-ray vacuum tube:** Enclosed tube where electrons are accelerated and X-rays are produced under vacuum.
**Related Terms:** Anode, cathode, tube housing.
**Radiotherapy Example:** Fundamental component of diagnostic and therapeutic X-ray systems.

329. **X-ray volume rendering:** 3D visualization of tissues from multiple X-ray or CT projections.
**Related Terms:** Voxel mapping, 3D imaging, rendering algorithms.
**Radiotherapy Example:** Assists in treatment planning and organ-at-risk delineation.

330. **X-ray wavefront sensing:** Measurement of the shape and quality of X-ray wavefronts for imaging optimization.
**Related Terms:** Coherence, beam quality, phase imaging.
**Radiotherapy Example:** Research in improving beam shaping for high-precision therapy.

331. **X-ray absorption edge:** Photon energy at which a sudden increase in absorption occurs due to electron shell excitation.
**Related Terms:** K-edge, contrast agents, spectroscopy.
**Radiotherapy Example:** Used in imaging with iodine or gadolinium contrast agents.

332. **X-ray attenuation map:** A spatial representation of how much an object reduces X-ray intensity.
**Related Terms:** CT number, dosimetry, field mapping.
**Radiotherapy Example:** Guides accurate dose delivery to tumors while sparing healthy tissue.

333. **X-ray beam penumbra:** The partially shaded edge of an X-ray beam where intensity falls off.
**Related Terms:** Focal spot, collimation, field edge.
**Radiotherapy Example:** Minimizing penumbra reduces exposure to surrounding normal tissue.

334. **X-ray detector calibration:** Process to ensure X-ray detectors produce accurate and reproducible measurements.
**Related Terms:** Dose measurement, flat-fielding, quality assurance.
**Radiotherapy Example:** Maintains precision in imaging and treatment verification.

335. **X-ray fan beam:** A thin, fan-shaped X-ray beam used in CT scanners.
**Related Terms:** Spiral CT, cone beam, collimation.
**Radiotherapy Example:** Enables precise volumetric imaging for planning and verification.

336. **X-ray fluorescence detector:** Device that measures characteristic X-ray emissions from elements in a sample.
**Related Terms:** Spectroscopy, elemental analysis, XRF mapping.
**Radiotherapy Example:** Research applications in detecting metal implants or contrast agents.

337. **X-ray image fusion:** Combining X-ray images with other modalities (e.g., CT, MRI) for enhanced visualization.
**Related Terms:** Multimodal imaging, registration, overlay.
**Radiotherapy Example:** Improves tumor localization and treatment accuracy.

**338. X-ray microbeam therapy:** Technique using very narrow X-ray beams to irradiate small tissue volumes.
**Related Terms:** Spatial fractionation, microdosimetry, synchrotron therapy.
**Radiotherapy Example:** Experimental therapy minimizing damage to surrounding tissue.

**339. X-ray monochromatic beam:** X-ray beam consisting of photons with nearly identical energy.
**Related Terms:** Synchrotron, monochromator, phase-contrast imaging.
**Radiotherapy Example:** Used in experimental imaging and targeted therapy research.

**340. X-ray optical coherence tomography (OCT):** Imaging technique using X-ray interference to obtain high-resolution cross-sections.
**Related Terms:** Phase contrast, tomography, microscopy.
**Radiotherapy Example:** Primarily research for microstructure visualization; may aid in radiobiology studies.

**341. X-ray photon counting detector:** Detector that counts individual X-ray photons rather than measuring total energy.
**Related Terms:** Digital radiography, energy-resolved imaging, spectral CT.
**Radiotherapy Example:** Enhances contrast and reduces dose in advanced imaging systems.

**342. X-ray phase contrast imaging:** Technique that uses phase shifts of X-rays passing through tissue to enhance contrast.
**Related Terms:** Coherence, interferometry, soft tissue imaging.
**Radiotherapy Example:** Improves visualization of tumors with minimal density difference from surrounding tissue.

**343. X-ray planar imaging:** Standard 2D X-ray imaging producing a projection of a 3D object.
**Related Terms:** Radiography, fluoroscopy, projection imaging.
**Radiotherapy Example:** Used for treatment verification and patient positioning.

**344. X-ray point spread function:** Response of an X-ray imaging system to a point source, indicating resolution limits.
**Related Terms:** Spatial resolution, blurring, modulation transfer function.
**Radiotherapy Example:** Guides system calibration and image quality assessment.

**345. X-ray primary beam:** Main X-ray beam directly from the source before interacting with the object.
**Related Terms:** Scatter, collimation, beam filtration.
**Radiotherapy Example:** Proper management ensures accurate dose delivery and image quality.

**346. X-ray radiobiology assay:** Experimental test measuring biological effects of X-ray exposure on cells or tissues.
**Related Terms:** Clonogenic assay, DNA damage, apoptosis.
**Radiotherapy Example:** Evaluates radiosensitivity and effectiveness of radioprotectors.

**347. X-ray radiolucency:** Property of a material allowing X-rays to pass through with minimal attenuation.
**Related Terms:** Contrast, radiopacity, tissue density.
**Radiotherapy Example:** Used to differentiate implants from soft tissue in imaging.

**348. X-ray reconstruction algorithm:** Mathematical method converting projection data into cross-sectional images.
**Related Terms:** Filtered back-projection, iterative reconstruction, CT imaging.
**Radiotherapy Example:** Determines accurate tumor volume for precise dose planning.

**349. X-ray scattering coefficient:** Quantifies how much X-rays are scattered by a material per unit thickness.
**Related Terms:** Attenuation, absorption, Compton scattering.
**Radiotherapy Example:** Helps optimize imaging parameters and reduce patient dose.

**350. X-ray scintillator panel:** Material that emits visible light when struck by X-rays, used in detectors.
**Related Terms:** Flat-panel detector, photodiode, digital radiography.
**Radiotherapy Example:** Converts X-rays to signals for high-resolution imaging and verification.

**351. X-ray semiconducting detector:** Semiconductor-based device that converts X-rays directly into electrical signals.
**Related Terms:** Silicon detector, CdTe, photon counting.
**Radiotherapy Example:** Used in high-precision imaging and dosimetry applications.

**352. X-ray slit camera:** Imaging device using a narrow slit to produce magnified X-ray projections.
**Related Terms:** Collimation, spatial resolution, projection imaging.
**Radiotherapy Example:** Monitors small structures or motion during treatment.

**353. X-ray spectral calibration:** Process of aligning detector response with known photon energies for accurate measurements.
**Related Terms:** Energy resolution, detector response, quality assurance.
**Radiotherapy Example:** Ensures accurate dose mapping and spectral imaging.

**354. X-ray spectrometer:** Device analyzing the energy spectrum of X-ray photons.
**Related Terms:** Fluorescence, diffraction, elemental analysis.
**Radiotherapy Example:** Used in research for imaging contrast optimization and detector calibration.

**355. X-ray source stability:** Consistency of X-ray output over time in terms of intensity and energy.
**Related Terms:** Tube voltage, current, dosimetry.
**Radiotherapy Example:** Stable output ensures reproducible imaging and accurate treatment delivery.

**356. X-ray spot size:** Physical size of the electron impact area on the anode that produces X-rays.
**Related Terms:** Focal spot, penumbra, spatial resolution.
**Radiotherapy Example:** Smaller spots yield sharper images, crucial for precision therapy.

**357. X-ray stray radiation:** Unintended X-ray radiation scattered outside the primary beam.
**Related Terms:** Scatter, shielding, collimation.
**Radiotherapy Example:** Shielding and positioning minimize dose to healthy tissue.

**358. X-ray tomography phantom:** Standardized object with known properties used to calibrate or test CT systems.
**Related Terms:** QA, imaging performance, dosimetry.
**Radiotherapy Example:** Ensures accurate imaging for treatment planning and dose verification.

**359. X-ray transmission coefficient:** Fraction of X-ray intensity passing through a material without absorption or scattering.
**Related Terms:** Attenuation, beam penetration, material density.
**Radiotherapy Example:** Used to calculate dose deposition in tissues or shielding effectiveness.

**360. X-ray tube anode rotation:** Rotating the anode in an X-ray tube to distribute heat and prolong tube life.
**Related Terms:** Heat dissipation, focal spot, tube design.
**Radiotherapy Example:** Allows high-dose imaging sessions without damaging the tube.

361. **X-ray tube current (mA):** The flow of electrons from cathode to anode in an X-ray tube, measured in milliamperes.
**Related Terms:** Tube voltage (kV), exposure time, dose.
**Radiotherapy Example:** Controls the number of X-ray photons, affecting image brightness and patient dose.

362. **X-ray tube voltage (kV):** Potential difference applied across an X-ray tube that accelerates electrons toward the anode.
**Related Terms:** Tube current, photon energy, beam quality.
**Radiotherapy Example:** Higher kV produces more penetrating X-rays, useful for imaging deep tumors.

363. **X-ray ultrafast imaging:** High-speed X-ray imaging capturing rapid events or motion in microseconds.
**Related Terms:** Temporal resolution, dynamic imaging, fluoroscopy.
**Radiotherapy Example:** Monitors organ motion during real-time tumor tracking.

364. **X-ray uniformity check:** Assessment of evenness of X-ray intensity across the beam field.
**Related Terms:** Flatness, beam profile, dosimetry.
**Radiotherapy Example:** Ensures homogeneous dose delivery across the treatment area.

365. **X-ray vacuum tube:** X-ray tube operating in a vacuum to allow free electron travel from cathode to anode.
**Related Terms:** Anode, cathode, filament.
**Radiotherapy Example:** Fundamental component in conventional imaging and therapy machines.

366. **X-ray verification imaging:** Imaging performed to confirm patient positioning and treatment alignment.
**Related Terms:** Portal imaging, image-guided radiotherapy (IGRT).
**Radiotherapy Example:** Ensures accurate tumor targeting before or during radiotherapy.

367. **X-ray viewport:** Transparent window in X-ray systems allowing visualization or beam passage.
**Related Terms:** Collimator, shielding, beam line.
**Radiotherapy Example:** Protects operators while allowing observation of patient alignment.

368. **X-ray voltage waveform:** Graph of tube voltage over time showing how the potential changes during exposure.
**Related Terms:** Pulsed X-ray, waveform stability, image quality.
**Radiotherapy Example:** Optimized waveforms improve imaging contrast and reduce artifacts.

369. **X-ray wedge filter:** Material with a variable thickness used to shape the X-ray beam intensity across a field.
**Related Terms:** Beam hardening, compensator, dose uniformity.
**Radiotherapy Example:** Balances dose in areas of varying tissue thickness, such as chest or extremities.

370. **X-ray wire phantom:** Phantom with thin wires used to assess spatial resolution in X-ray systems.
**Related Terms:** Line-pair phantom, modulation transfer function.
**Radiotherapy Example:** Validates imaging systems for detecting small structures before treatment planning.

371. **X-ray yield curve:** Graph showing X-ray output versus tube current, voltage, or time.
**Related Terms:** Tube output, efficiency, dosimetry.
**Radiotherapy Example:** Used for calibration and quality assurance of imaging or therapy devices.

372. **X-ray zero point calibration:** Establishing the reference position or baseline for X-ray imaging systems.
**Related Terms:** Alignment, detector calibration, geometric correction.
**Radiotherapy Example:** Ensures accurate positional data for treatment planning and beam delivery.

373. **X-ray zone plate:** Circular diffraction grating used to focus or manipulate X-rays.
**Related Terms:** Fresnel zone plate, nanofocusing, phase contrast.
**Radiotherapy Example:** Enables high-resolution X-ray microscopy for tumor biology research.

374. **X-ray zoom function:** System capability to magnify a specific region during imaging.
**Related Terms:** Digital zoom, magnification, focal spot adjustment.
**Radiotherapy Example:** Improves visualization of small tumors or anatomical structures.

375. **X-ray Zernike phase contrast:** Technique enhancing contrast in weakly absorbing specimens using phase differences.
**Related Terms:** Phase imaging, coherent X-rays, microscopy.
**Radiotherapy Example:** Used in preclinical research to image tumors with minimal dose.

376. **X-ray zero dose baseline:** Reference measurement representing zero X-ray exposure in imaging detectors.
**Related Terms:** Dark current, detector offset, baseline correction.
**Radiotherapy Example:** Improves accuracy in dose measurement and image reconstruction.

377. **X-ray Z-pinhole camera:** Small aperture imaging system producing magnified projections of X-ray sources.
**Related Terms:** Pinhole imaging, spatial resolution, beam diagnostics.
**Radiotherapy Example:** Monitors beam shape and alignment in experimental setups.

378. **X-ray Z-stack imaging:** Sequential X-ray imaging of multiple planes to create a 3D dataset.
**Related Terms:** Tomography, volumetric reconstruction, slice acquisition.
**Radiotherapy Example:** Generates precise 3D anatomy for treatment planning.

379. **X-ray zone-of-interest scan:** Imaging focused on a specific region, reducing unnecessary exposure elsewhere.
**Related Terms:** ROI imaging, collimation, dose reduction.
**Radiotherapy Example:** Targets tumor area while sparing surrounding healthy tissues.

380. **X-ray Z-sensitivity coefficient:** Quantifies how detector response varies with X-ray energy or photon number.
**Related Terms:** Detector efficiency, energy dependence, calibration.
**Radiotherapy Example:** Ensures accurate dosimetry and imaging across different X-ray energies.

381. **X-ray zero-crossing detection:** Method to identify the point where an X-ray signal changes sign or passes through zero.
**Related Terms:** Signal processing, waveform analysis, phase detection.
**Radiotherapy Example:** Used in detector calibration and timing-sensitive imaging systems.

382. **X-ray zone calibration:** Adjustment of detector zones or imaging regions to ensure accurate measurement.
**Related Terms:** Field mapping, detector alignment, quality assurance.
**Radiotherapy Example:** Confirms precise dose delivery in segmented treatment fields.

383. **X-ray Z-resolution:** The spatial resolution along the Z-axis (depth) in a volumetric X-ray image.
**Related Terms:** Voxel size, slice thickness, CT resolution.
**Radiotherapy Example:** Determines the clarity of tumor boundaries in 3D planning scans.

**384. X-ray zero-field imaging:** Imaging performed without applying external magnetic or electric fields.
**Related Terms:** Baseline imaging, control scan, field-free conditions.
**Radiotherapy Example:** Provides reference images for comparing with field-modulated scans.

**385. X-ray Z-contrast:** Image contrast derived from variations in atomic number (Z) of materials.
**Related Terms:** Phase contrast, absorption contrast, material differentiation.
**Radiotherapy Example:** Helps distinguish tissues of different density or composition in planning scans.

**386. X-ray zoom detector:** Detector capable of electronically or mechanically magnifying a region of interest.
**Related Terms:** Pixel binning, digital magnification, high-resolution imaging.
**Radiotherapy Example:** Enables fine-detail visualization of small lesions or microstructures.

**387. X-ray Z-stack reconstruction:** Computational reconstruction of 3D images from multiple Z-plane X-ray slices.
**Related Terms:** Volume rendering, CT reconstruction, slice integration.
**Radiotherapy Example:** Generates detailed anatomical models for dose planning.

**388. X-ray zero-lag filter:** Digital filter that processes X-ray signals without introducing time delay.
**Related Terms:** Real-time imaging, signal smoothing, temporal resolution.
**Radiotherapy Example:** Maintains accurate imaging during rapid fluoroscopic procedures.

**389. X-ray zone-of-interest detector:** Detector focused on a specific imaging region to enhance signal quality.
**Related Terms:** ROI, selective exposure, high-sensitivity imaging.
**Radiotherapy Example:** Reduces dose to surrounding healthy tissues while imaging a tumor.

**390. X-ray Z-axis positioning system:** Mechanical or electronic system that moves the patient or detector along the Z-axis.
**Related Terms:** 3D positioning, treatment couch, gantry movement.
**Radiotherapy Example:** Ensures accurate tumor localization for volumetric treatment delivery.

**391. X-ray zero-point alignment:** Calibration to establish the reference origin for imaging or therapy equipment.
**Related Terms:** Geometric calibration, isocenter, gantry alignment.
**Radiotherapy Example:** Ensures precise beam targeting and reproducible patient setup.

**392. X-ray Z-energy calibration:** Calibration of detector response based on photon energy along the Z-axis.
**Related Terms:** Energy linearity, spectral response, dose measurement.
**Radiotherapy Example:** Confirms accurate dose and image quality for energy-dependent imaging.

**393. X-ray zone-of-interest mask:** Physical or digital mask applied to select or block specific imaging areas.
**Related Terms:** Collimation, ROI selection, dose reduction.
**Radiotherapy Example:** Protects normal tissues while focusing imaging on tumor zones.

**394. X-ray Z-stack acquisition rate:** Speed at which sequential Z-plane images are captured.
**Related Terms:** Temporal resolution, slice scanning, volumetric imaging.
**Radiotherapy Example:** Fast acquisition reduces motion artifacts in dynamic organs like lungs.

**395. X-ray zero-dose reference image:** Image captured without X-ray exposure to measure detector baseline.
**Related Terms:** Dark field, offset correction, noise calibration.
**Radiotherapy Example:** Improves image accuracy and reduces artifacts in low-dose scans.

396. **X-ray Z-axis magnification:** Enhancement of depth information in imaging along the Z-axis.
**Related Terms:** 3D magnification, voxel scaling, depth resolution.
**Radiotherapy Example:** Helps visualize fine tumor margins in volumetric treatment planning.

397. **X-ray zone-of-interest calibration:** Adjustment of imaging or detector parameters specific to a selected ROI.
**Related Terms:** Field calibration, dose optimization, resolution enhancement.
**Radiotherapy Example:** Ensures uniform imaging quality within the treatment target area.

398. **X-ray Z-stack noise reduction:** Methods to minimize random fluctuations in sequential Z-plane images.
**Related Terms:** Signal filtering, smoothing, temporal averaging.
**Radiotherapy Example:** Improves clarity in 3D images for tumor delineation.

399. **X-ray zero-shift correction:** Compensation for slight misalignments or offsets in imaging detectors or beam position.
**Related Terms:** Geometric correction, calibration, isocenter adjustment.
**Radiotherapy Example:** Ensures accurate radiation delivery relative to tumor coordinates.

400. **X-ray Z-axis uniformity:** Consistency of X-ray intensity or detector response along the Z-axis.
**Related Terms:** Beam flatness, dose homogeneity, image quality.
**Radiotherapy Example:** Guarantees even dose distribution in volumetric treatment plans.

401. **X-ray Z-axis drift:** Gradual deviation of the X-ray beam or detector position along the Z-axis over time.
**Related Terms:** Mechanical stability, gantry drift, positional error.
**Radiotherapy Example:** Monitoring drift ensures precise dose delivery during long treatment sessions.

402. **X-ray Z-axis linearity:** Accuracy of movement or response along the Z-axis relative to input commands.
**Related Terms:** Positional calibration, gantry mechanics, isocenter alignment.
**Radiotherapy Example:** Ensures consistent slice thickness in CT imaging and dose conformity.

403. **X-ray Z-plane correction algorithm:** Software method to correct distortions or misalignments in Z-plane imaging.
**Related Terms:** Image registration, geometric correction, artifact reduction.
**Radiotherapy Example:** Improves volumetric image accuracy for treatment planning.

404. **X-ray Z-axis encoder:** Device that measures the position of the detector or patient along the Z-axis.
**Related Terms:** Positional feedback, motor control, precision measurement.
**Radiotherapy Example:** Provides real-time feedback for automated couch movements during therapy.

405. **X-ray Z-axis gantry:** Part of imaging or therapy equipment that moves or rotates around the Z-axis.
**Related Terms:** Gantry rotation, beam delivery, volumetric scanning.
**Radiotherapy Example:** Enables helical CT scans or rotational radiotherapy treatments.

406. **X-ray Z-axis beam profile:** Measurement of X-ray intensity along the depth axis (Z-axis).
**Related Terms:** Dose distribution, beam uniformity, flattening filter.
**Radiotherapy Example:** Confirms consistent dose across tumor depth in 3D treatment plans.

407. **X-ray Z-stack alignment:** Process of aligning sequential Z-plane images for accurate 3D reconstruction.
**Related Terms:** Image registration, volumetric imaging, motion correction.
**Radiotherapy Example:** Reduces artifacts in tumor volume visualization during planning scans.

**408. X-ray Z-axis detector calibration:** Adjustment of detector sensitivity and position along the Z-axis for uniform response.
**Related Terms:** Detector linearity, spatial uniformity, quality assurance.
**Radiotherapy Example:** Ensures consistent image quality in CT or cone-beam imaging.

**409. X-ray Z-axis gantry angle:** The angle of rotation or tilt of the gantry relative to the Z-axis.
**Related Terms:** Beam orientation, imaging geometry, isocenter alignment.
**Radiotherapy Example:** Optimizes beam entry angles to spare healthy tissues while treating tumors.

**410. X-ray Z-axis dosimetry:** Measurement of radiation dose along the depth (Z-axis) of a sample or patient.
**Related Terms:** Depth dose, 3D dosimetry, ionization chamber.
**Radiotherapy Example:** Ensures the prescribed dose reaches the tumor while minimizing normal tissue exposure.

**411. X-ray Z-axis motion artifact:** Distortion in imaging caused by movement along the Z-axis during scanning.
**Related Terms:** Motion correction, image blurring, temporal resolution.
**Radiotherapy Example:** Managing motion artifacts improves tumor delineation for moving organs like lungs.

**412. X-ray Z-stack interpolation:** Computational method to estimate intermediate slices between acquired Z-plane images.
**Related Terms:** Image reconstruction, slice enhancement, volumetric accuracy.
**Radiotherapy Example:** Produces smoother 3D anatomical models for dose planning.

**413. X-ray Z-axis field flatness:** Uniformity of X-ray beam intensity along the Z-axis.
**Related Terms:** Beam quality, homogeneity, dose uniformity.
**Radiotherapy Example:** Essential for uniform tumor irradiation and minimizing hot/cold spots.

**414. X-ray Z-stack contrast enhancement:** Improving differentiation between tissues in sequential Z-plane images.
**Related Terms:** Image processing, filtering, dynamic range adjustment.
**Radiotherapy Example:** Enhances tumor visibility for accurate target delineation.

**415. X-ray Z-axis beam penumbra:** Gradual fall-off of radiation intensity at the edges of the beam along Z-axis.
**Related Terms:** Edge dose, field shaping, beam profile.
**Radiotherapy Example:** Minimizing penumbra reduces dose to surrounding healthy tissues.

**416. X-ray Z-axis spatial accuracy:** Precision of image or dose localization along the Z-axis.
**Related Terms:** Geometric accuracy, positional error, calibration.
**Radiotherapy Example:** Critical for targeting tumors in stereotactic treatments.

**417. X-ray Z-stack noise filtering:** Techniques to reduce random noise in sequential Z-plane images.
**Related Terms:** Signal processing, smoothing, image enhancement.
**Radiotherapy Example:** Improves clarity for small structures in high-resolution volumetric scans.

**418. X-ray Z-axis energy spectrum:** Distribution of photon energies along the Z-axis of an X-ray beam.
**Related Terms:** Beam quality, spectral analysis, energy calibration.
**Radiotherapy Example:** Ensures proper penetration and dose deposition in tissues.

**419. X-ray Z-plane voxel size:** The depth dimension of a 3D pixel (voxel) in Z-plane imaging.
**Related Terms:** Spatial resolution, CT voxel, image reconstruction.
**Radiotherapy Example:** Smaller voxel size allows precise delineation of tumors and organs.

**420. X-ray Z-stack motion correction:** Methods to compensate for patient or organ movement during Z-stack acquisition.
**Related Terms:** Image registration, gating, dynamic imaging.
**Radiotherapy Example:** Reduces artifacts for accurate 3D dose planning in mobile organs like lungs or liver.

**421. X-ray Z-axis beam divergence:** The spreading of the X-ray beam along the Z-axis as it propagates from the source.
**Related Terms:** Geometric unsharpness, source-to-detector distance, beam collimation.
**Radiotherapy Example:** Minimizing divergence improves dose precision at deeper tissue levels.

**422. X-ray Z-stack registration:** Aligning sequential Z-plane images to correct positional offsets for accurate 3D reconstruction.
**Related Terms:** Image fusion, motion correction, volumetric alignment.
**Radiotherapy Example:** Ensures anatomical consistency across CT or MRI-based treatment planning scans.

**423. X-ray Z-plane flattening filter:** A device that evens out X-ray beam intensity across the Z-axis.
**Related Terms:** Beam homogeneity, filter design, dose uniformity.
**Radiotherapy Example:** Creates a flat dose distribution to cover the tumor uniformly.

**424. X-ray Z-axis detector linearity:** The proportional response of a detector to X-ray intensity along the Z-axis.
**Related Terms:** Detector calibration, signal accuracy, dose measurement.
**Radiotherapy Example:** Critical for accurate depth-dose calculations in quality assurance.

**425. X-ray Z-plane angular correction:** Adjustment for tilt or rotation in Z-plane images to maintain geometric accuracy.
**Related Terms:** Image registration, gantry alignment, geometric distortion.
**Radiotherapy Example:** Corrects for patient positioning errors in 3D imaging.

**426. X-ray Z-stack segmentation:** Dividing sequential Z-plane images into regions representing different tissues or structures.
**Related Terms:** Image processing, ROI delineation, volumetric analysis.
**Radiotherapy Example:** Segmentation defines tumor volumes for precise radiation targeting.

**427. X-ray Z-axis isocenter verification:** Confirming that the central beam axis intersects the planned isocenter along Z-axis.
**Related Terms:** Gantry calibration, patient positioning, quality assurance.
**Radiotherapy Example:** Essential for stereotactic radiotherapy to ensure accurate dose delivery.

**428. X-ray Z-plane dose mapping:** Measuring and visualizing radiation dose distribution in each Z-plane.
**Related Terms:** Depth-dose profile, 3D dosimetry, treatment verification.
**Radiotherapy Example:** Confirms uniform coverage of tumor volume and identifies hotspots.

**429. X-ray Z-axis image overlay:** Superimposing Z-plane images from different scans for comparative analysis.
**Related Terms:** Image fusion, multimodal imaging, registration.
**Radiotherapy Example:** Combines CT and MRI data to enhance tumor delineation.

**430. X-ray Z-stack reconstruction error:** Deviation between reconstructed volumetric images and true anatomical positions.
**Related Terms:** Artifacts, interpolation error, reconstruction quality.
**Radiotherapy Example:** Minimizing error ensures precise targeting for dose delivery.

431. **X-ray Z-plane optical conversion:** Converting X-ray photons into visible light in the Z-plane for imaging or detection.
**Related Terms:** Scintillator, photodiode, detector conversion efficiency.
**Radiotherapy Example:** Used in flat-panel detectors and X-ray microscopes for high-resolution imaging.

432. **X-ray Z-axis flatness index:** Metric describing uniformity of X-ray intensity along the Z-axis.
**Related Terms:** Beam quality assurance, homogeneity, flatness measurement.
**Radiotherapy Example:** Ensures consistent dose distribution across tumor depth.

433. **X-ray Z-stack contrast-to-noise ratio (CNR):** Ratio of signal difference between structures to background noise in Z-stack images.
**Related Terms:** Image quality, SNR, contrast enhancement.
**Radiotherapy Example:** Higher CNR improves visualization of tumors and small structures.

434. **X-ray Z-axis phantom:** Physical model used to simulate tissue and verify beam delivery along Z-axis.
**Related Terms:** QA phantom, dose verification, geometric accuracy.
**Radiotherapy Example:** Used for calibrating CT scanners or verifying radiotherapy plans.

435. **X-ray Z-stack intensity profile:** Distribution of X-ray signal intensity across sequential Z-plane images.
**Related Terms:** Beam profile, depth-dose measurement, signal mapping.
**Radiotherapy Example:** Helps identify areas of under- or over-exposure.

436. **X-ray Z-plane artifact correction:** Techniques to remove distortions or errors in individual Z-plane images.
**Related Terms:** Image processing, noise reduction, motion artifact.
**Radiotherapy Example:** Correcting artifacts improves accuracy of tumor delineation.

437. **X-ray Z-axis motion tracking:** Monitoring movement along the Z-axis to adjust imaging or beam delivery.
**Related Terms:** Real-time tracking, gating, patient motion compensation.
**Radiotherapy Example:** Ensures accurate dose delivery to moving organs like lungs.

438. **X-ray Z-stack intensity normalization:** Adjusting signal intensity across Z-plane images to achieve consistent brightness.
**Related Terms:** Image standardization, calibration, post-processing.
**Radiotherapy Example:** Facilitates accurate 3D reconstruction and quantitative analysis.

439. **X-ray Z-plane beam hardening correction:** Algorithm to correct for changes in X-ray spectrum along Z-axis due to material absorption.
**Related Terms:** CT artifact correction, attenuation correction, image reconstruction.
**Radiotherapy Example:** Reduces streak artifacts in CT images of dense tissues like bone.

440. **X-ray Z-axis rotational calibration:** Ensuring rotational movements along the Z-axis are accurate for imaging or therapy.
**Related Terms:** Gantry calibration, isocenter verification, mechanical QA.
**Radiotherapy Example:** Accurate rotational calibration is critical for conformal and arc therapy techniques.

441. **X-ray Z-axis beam alignment:** Ensuring the X-ray beam is properly centered along the Z-axis relative to the target or detector.
**Related Terms:** Gantry alignment, isocenter verification, mechanical QA.
**Radiotherapy Example:** Prevents misalignment that could underdose tumors or overdose healthy tissue.

442. **X-ray Z-plane signal integration:** Combining signals from multiple Z-plane images to enhance overall signal strength.
**Related Terms:** Image summation, projection, noise reduction.
**Radiotherapy Example:** Improves visibility of low-contrast structures in CT or fluoroscopy.

443. **X-ray Z-stack registration error:** Deviation between actual anatomical positions and registered Z-stack images.
**Related Terms:** Image misalignment, motion artifact, correction algorithms.
**Radiotherapy Example:** Minimizing registration error ensures precise targeting in 3D treatment planning.

444. **X-ray Z-axis dose uniformity:** Consistency of delivered radiation dose along the Z-axis.
**Related Terms:** Depth-dose distribution, beam flatness, quality assurance.
**Radiotherapy Example:** Ensures the entire tumor receives the prescribed dose without hot or cold spots.

445. **X-ray Z-plane magnification factor:** The scaling factor between the actual object size and its image on a detector along Z-axis.
**Related Terms:** Geometric magnification, focal spot distance, image calibration.
**Radiotherapy Example:** Accurate magnification is critical for precise tumor contouring.

446. **X-ray Z-stack voxel registration:** Aligning 3D voxel data across sequential Z-plane images.
**Related Terms:** Image fusion, volumetric alignment, motion correction.
**Radiotherapy Example:** Ensures accurate volumetric analysis for dose calculations and therapy planning.

447. **X-ray Z-axis scatter profile:** Distribution of scattered X-ray radiation along the Z-axis.
**Related Terms:** Scatter correction, beam hardening, image quality.
**Radiotherapy Example:** Helps in designing anti-scatter grids and correcting CT artifacts.

448. **X-ray Z-plane dynamic range:** Range of detectable signal intensities in a single Z-plane image.
**Related Terms:** Detector sensitivity, contrast resolution, imaging performance.
**Radiotherapy Example:** High dynamic range improves detection of both soft tissue and dense bone structures.

449. **X-ray Z-axis depth calibration:** Verifying the correspondence between Z-axis position and physical depth in the sample.
**Related Terms:** Spatial calibration, image scaling, QA phantom.
**Radiotherapy Example:** Ensures accurate dose calculation at different tissue depths.

450. **X-ray Z-stack noise reduction algorithm:** Computational method to minimize random fluctuations in sequential Z-plane images.
**Related Terms:** Smoothing, filtering, signal processing.
**Radiotherapy Example:** Enhances image clarity for tumor delineation and organ visualization.

451. **X-ray Z-plane edge enhancement:** Image processing technique to emphasize boundaries in individual Z-plane images.
**Related Terms:** Spatial filtering, contrast enhancement, structure visualization.
**Radiotherapy Example:** Improves detection of small tumors and anatomical landmarks.

452. **X-ray Z-axis motion compensation:** Adjusting imaging or beam delivery in real-time to correct for movement along the Z-axis.
**Related Terms:** Gating, tracking, adaptive radiotherapy.
**Radiotherapy Example:** Critical for treating tumors in organs that move with respiration, like lungs.

453. **X-ray Z-stack registration metric:** Quantitative measurement of alignment accuracy across Z-stack images.
**Related Terms:** Dice coefficient, mutual information, registration quality.
**Radiotherapy Example:** Used to validate image fusion for treatment planning or diagnostic evaluation.

454. **X-ray Z-plane intensity normalization:** Adjusting pixel intensities across Z-plane images for uniform brightness and contrast.
**Related Terms:** Histogram equalization, calibration, post-processing.
**Radiotherapy Example:** Facilitates consistent 3D reconstruction for volumetric imaging.

455. **X-ray Z-axis dose verification phantom:** A physical phantom designed to verify radiation dose distribution along Z-axis.
**Related Terms:** QA phantom, depth-dose measurement, calibration.
**Radiotherapy Example:** Ensures the prescribed dose is accurately delivered at different tissue depths.

456. **X-ray Z-stack temporal registration:** Aligning sequential Z-stack images taken at different time points.
**Related Terms:** Longitudinal imaging, motion correction, image fusion.
**Radiotherapy Example:** Tracks tumor changes over time for adaptive treatment planning.

457. **X-ray Z-plane contrast calibration:** Adjusting detector response to ensure accurate representation of tissue contrast along Z-plane.
**Related Terms:** Image calibration, grayscale standardization, detector linearity.
**Radiotherapy Example:** Ensures reliable differentiation of tumor from normal tissue.

458. **X-ray Z-axis beam shaping:** Modifying the X-ray beam profile along the Z-axis to optimize dose delivery or image quality.
**Related Terms:** Collimation, intensity modulation, beam flattening filter.
**Radiotherapy Example:** Used in IMRT and stereotactic radiotherapy to conform dose to tumor geometry.

459. **X-ray Z-plane registration transformation:** Mathematical operation applied to align Z-plane images to a reference coordinate system.
**Related Terms:** Rigid, affine, non-rigid transformations, image fusion.
**Radiotherapy Example:** Ensures accurate overlay of multimodal images for treatment planning.

460. **X-ray Z-axis modulation factor:** Quantitative measure of how the X-ray beam intensity varies along the Z-axis.
**Related Terms:** Dose modulation, beam intensity profile, radiotherapy optimization.
**Radiotherapy Example:** Guides planning in techniques like VMAT to deliver conformal dose distributions.

461. **X-ray Z-stack interpolation:** Computational method to estimate image data between acquired Z-plane slices.
**Related Terms:** Slice thickness, volumetric reconstruction, image resampling.
**Radiotherapy Example:** Produces smoother 3D images for tumor contouring and dose planning.

462. **X-ray Z-axis attenuation coefficient:** The measure of how X-ray intensity decreases along the Z-axis in a material.
**Related Terms:** Linear attenuation, tissue density, radiodensity.
**Radiotherapy Example:** Used in dose calculations and CT imaging to adjust for tissue absorption.

**463. X-ray Z-plane histogram equalization:** Adjusting pixel intensity distributions to enhance contrast in Z-plane images.
**Related Terms:** Image processing, contrast enhancement, normalization.
**Radiotherapy Example:** Improves visibility of subtle tissue differences in sequential slices.

**464. X-ray Z-stack artifact correction:** Techniques to remove distortions or anomalies from sequential Z-plane images.
**Related Terms:** Ring artifact removal, beam hardening correction, motion compensation.
**Radiotherapy Example:** Ensures accurate 3D reconstruction for planning and diagnosis.

**465. X-ray Z-axis alignment phantom:** Physical device used to verify correct X-ray beam alignment along the Z-axis.
**Related Terms:** QA phantom, mechanical verification, isocenter testing.
**Radiotherapy Example:** Confirms precision for treatments like stereotactic radiosurgery.

**466. X-ray Z-plane edge detection:** Image processing method to identify boundaries in a single Z-plane slice.
**Related Terms:** Gradient filter, Sobel operator, Canny edge detection.
**Radiotherapy Example:** Helps delineate tumor margins and anatomical structures.

**467. X-ray Z-axis isocenter verification:** Checking that the beam's central axis is correctly aligned with the treatment isocenter.
**Related Terms:** Mechanical QA, radiation alignment, gantry calibration.
**Radiotherapy Example:** Critical in precision radiotherapy to avoid under- or overdosing tissues.

**468. X-ray Z-stack 3D reconstruction:** Combining multiple Z-plane images to create a volumetric 3D model.
**Related Terms:** Volume rendering, multiplanar reconstruction, CT/MRI fusion.
**Radiotherapy Example:** Essential for accurate tumor volume measurement and dose planning.

**469. X-ray Z-plane intensity profile:** Graph showing pixel intensity variations across a Z-plane slice.
**Related Terms:** Signal profile, detector calibration, contrast assessment.
**Radiotherapy Example:** Evaluates uniformity of tissue contrast and detects artifacts.

**470. X-ray Z-axis beam hardening correction:** Adjusting for increased X-ray energy along the Z-axis due to preferential absorption of low-energy photons.
**Related Terms:** CT artifact reduction, calibration, reconstruction correction.
**Radiotherapy Example:** Ensures accurate Hounsfield unit measurements and dose calculation.

**471. X-ray Z-plane noise quantification:** Measuring the magnitude of random fluctuations in a Z-plane image.
**Related Terms:** Signal-to-noise ratio (SNR), image quality, detector sensitivity.
**Radiotherapy Example:** Guides optimization of exposure parameters for diagnostic clarity.

**472. X-ray Z-stack motion artifact detection:** Identifying image distortions caused by patient or organ movement during sequential imaging.
**Related Terms:** Respiratory gating, image registration, correction algorithms.
**Radiotherapy Example:** Minimizes errors in 3D tumor localization.

**473. X-ray Z-axis dose gradient:** Rate of change in radiation dose along the Z-axis.
**Related Terms:** Depth-dose curve, dose fall-off, beam shaping.
**Radiotherapy Example:** Ensures that the prescribed dose conforms to tumor shape while sparing normal tissue.

474. **X-ray Z-plane contrast-to-noise ratio (CNR):** Ratio of contrast between structures to background noise in a single Z-plane image.
**Related Terms:** Image quality metric, SNR, detector performance.
**Radiotherapy Example:** Optimizing CNR improves tumor visualization in CT or fluoroscopic images.

475. **X-ray Z-stack registration error map:** Visual representation of misalignment between Z-plane images.
**Related Terms:** Deformation map, motion artifact, image fusion verification.
**Radiotherapy Example:** Used to correct errors in longitudinal imaging or adaptive planning.

476. **X-ray Z-axis penumbra measurement:** Measurement of the dose gradient at the edge of the X-ray beam along the Z-axis.
**Related Terms:** Beam profile, sharpness, dose fall-off.
**Radiotherapy Example:** Helps minimize irradiation of surrounding healthy tissue.

477. **X-ray Z-plane spatial filtering:** Applying filters to enhance or suppress features within a Z-plane image.
**Related Terms:** Low-pass, high-pass, edge enhancement.
**Radiotherapy Example:** Improves visualization of fine anatomical structures for contouring.

478. **X-ray Z-stack temporal averaging:** Combining images over time to reduce noise in dynamic Z-stack sequences.
**Related Terms:** Motion smoothing, signal enhancement, longitudinal imaging.
**Radiotherapy Example:** Useful in perfusion studies or respiratory-gated imaging.

479. **X-ray Z-axis mechanical stability test:** Evaluation of the precision and stability of X-ray equipment along the Z-axis.
**Related Terms:** QA, gantry calibration, mechanical drift assessment.
**Radiotherapy Example:** Ensures reproducible beam delivery and accurate patient positioning.

480. **X-ray Z-plane histogram analysis:** Statistical evaluation of pixel intensity distribution in a Z-plane image.
**Related Terms:** Contrast evaluation, calibration, image quality assessment.
**Radiotherapy Example:** Guides adjustment of imaging parameters for optimal diagnostic clarity.

481. **X-ray Z-stack interpolation artifact:** Distortion introduced when interpolating between Z-plane slices.
**Related Terms:** Resampling artifact, partial volume effect, image smoothing.
**Radiotherapy Example:** Awareness is crucial to avoid misestimating tumor boundaries.

482. **X-ray Z-axis dose homogeneity index:** Quantitative measure of uniformity of delivered dose along the Z-axis.
**Related Terms:** Dose uniformity, treatment quality, QA metric.
**Radiotherapy Example:** Ensures consistent tumor coverage and minimizes hot/cold spots.

483. **X-ray Z-plane region-of-interest (ROI) analysis:** Assessing specific areas within a Z-plane image for signal, contrast, or dose.
**Related Terms:** ROI quantification, image measurement, diagnostic evaluation.
**Radiotherapy Example:** Evaluates tumor or organ response in imaging or dose distribution studies.

484. **X-ray Z-stack motion correction algorithm:** Computational method to compensate for motion between sequential Z-plane images.
**Related Terms:** Registration, image fusion, artifact reduction.
**Radiotherapy Example:** Maintains accuracy in 3D reconstructions for adaptive radiotherapy.

**485. X-ray Z-axis beam profile measurement:** Recording intensity distribution of the X-ray beam along the Z-axis.
**Related Terms:** Flatness, symmetry, quality assurance.
**Radiotherapy Example:** Ensures correct dose delivery across tumor depth.

**486. X-ray Z-plane filter optimization:** Selecting the best image processing filter for a specific Z-plane slice.
**Related Terms:** Noise reduction, edge enhancement, diagnostic optimization.
**Radiotherapy Example:** Improves visualization of small structures for accurate contouring.

**487. X-ray Z-stack 3D volume rendering:** Generating a 3D image from sequential Z-plane data.
**Related Terms:** Volumetric visualization, multiplanar reconstruction, surface rendering.
**Radiotherapy Example:** Enhances surgical planning and precise radiotherapy targeting.

**488. X-ray Z-axis calibration curve:** Graphical relationship between Z-axis position and detected X-ray intensity or dose.
**Related Terms:** Detector calibration, depth-dose relationship, quality assurance.
**Radiotherapy Example:** Used to ensure accurate dose calculation along tissue depth.

**489. X-ray Z-plane edge sharpness metric:** Quantitative measure of boundary clarity within a Z-plane image.
**Related Terms:** Modulation transfer function (MTF), spatial resolution, image quality.
**Radiotherapy Example:** Assesses detector performance and imaging quality for precise delineation.

**490. X-ray Z-stack signal normalization:** Adjusting signal intensity across multiple Z-plane images for consistency.
**Related Terms:** Intensity correction, histogram matching, image standardization.
**Radiotherapy Example:** Facilitates accurate 3D reconstruction for planning and evaluation.

**491. X-ray Z-axis beam uniformity:** Degree to which X-ray intensity remains consistent along the Z-axis.
**Related Terms:** Flatness, symmetry, quality control.
**Radiotherapy Example:** Ensures even dose delivery across tumor depth.

**492. X-ray Z-plane high-frequency enhancement:** Image processing to emphasize fine details in a single Z-plane slice.
**Related Terms:** Edge enhancement, spatial filtering, contrast boosting.
**Radiotherapy Example:** Enhances detection of small lesions or anatomical landmarks.

**493. X-ray Z-stack quantitative analysis:** Measurement of signal, noise, or other parameters across a series of Z-plane images.
**Related Terms:** Image metrics, volumetric analysis, data extraction.
**Radiotherapy Example:** Used to evaluate treatment response or tissue properties.

**494. X-ray Z-axis depth-of-focus:** Range along the Z-axis where the image remains acceptably sharp.
**Related Terms:** Focal plane, geometric blur, resolution.
**Radiotherapy Example:** Ensures accurate imaging of tumors located at varying depths.

**495. X-ray Z-plane intensity modulation:** Varying detected signal within a Z-plane for contrast or dose optimization.
**Related Terms:** Beam shaping, image enhancement, exposure control.
**Radiotherapy Example:** Helps visualize soft tissues adjacent to high-density structures.

**496. X-ray Z-stack voxel intensity histogram:** Statistical plot of voxel intensities across a 3D Z-stack volume.
**Related Terms:** Histogram analysis, tissue differentiation, quantitative imaging.
**Radiotherapy Example:** Guides thresholding and segmentation of tumors.

497. **X-ray Z-axis positional accuracy:** Precision with which the X-ray source or detector maintains Z-axis position.
**Related Terms:** Mechanical QA, alignment, calibration.
**Radiotherapy Example:** Critical for stereotactic treatments and precise imaging.

498. **X-ray Z-plane contrast optimization:** Adjusting imaging parameters to maximize differentiation between structures in a Z-plane.
**Related Terms:** Window/level, filtration, post-processing.
**Radiotherapy Example:** Improves tumor visibility for contouring and planning.

499. **X-ray Z-stack volumetric accuracy:** Degree to which reconstructed 3D Z-stack images represent true anatomical volumes.
**Related Terms:** 3D reconstruction fidelity, resolution, registration accuracy.
**Radiotherapy Example:** Ensures correct tumor volume estimation for dose calculations.

500. **X-ray Z-axis radiation profile:** Distribution of radiation intensity along the Z-axis from the X-ray source.
**Related Terms:** Beam flatness, symmetry, quality assurance.
**Radiotherapy Example:** Guides accurate planning and uniform dose delivery.

1. **Y-90 (Yttrium-90) (noun):** A beta-emitting radionuclide used in radioembolization or internal radiotherapy.
   **Related Terms:** Radioisotope therapy, Microsphere.
   **Example in Radiotherapy:** Y-90 microspheres deliver localized dose in liver metastases.
2. **Yaw angle (noun):** Rotation of patient or gantry about the vertical axis.
   **Related Terms:** Pitch, Roll, Rotational correction.
   **Example in Radiotherapy:** Yaw correction essential in robotic couch alignment.
3. **Yield (noun):** Amount of radiation or particles produced per reaction or event.
   **Related Terms:** Quantum yield, Efficiency.
   **Example in Radiobiology:** Photon yield affects detector calibration accuracy.
4. **Yellow filter (noun):** Optical filter reducing glare during optical tracking.
   **Related Terms:** Imaging enhancement, Surface guidance.
   **Example in Radiotherapy:** Yellow filter improves surface imaging contrast under bright light.
5. **Yolk sac tumor (noun):** A germ cell malignancy occasionally treated with radiotherapy.
   **Related Terms:** Pediatric oncology, Radiosensitivity.
   **Example in Radiotherapy:** Limited-field irradiation used post-surgery for yolk sac tumor.
6. **Young's modulus (noun):** Material stiffness indicator used in deformable image registration.
   **Related Terms:** Elasticity, Deformation.
   **Example in Radiotherapy:** Young's modulus guides soft-tissue modeling in adaptive MR-LINAC.
7. **Young-Laplace equation (noun):** Describes surface tension influence on liquid interfaces.
   **Related Terms:** Dosimetry fluid mechanics, Phantom preparation.
   **Example in Radiotherapy:** Young-Laplace principle used in gel dosimeter calibration.
8. **Yolk sac (noun):** Embryonic structure occasionally visualized in imaging.
   **Related Terms:** Anatomy, MRI identification.
   Example in Radiology**:** Yolk sac appearance assists in fetal localization before radiation planning.
9. **Yoke (noun):** Mechanical component supporting and aligning LINAC magnet assemblies.
   **Related Terms:** LINAC structure, Magnetic field.
   Example in Radiation Physics**:** Yoke ensures magnet symmetry and beam focusing.
10. **Yield stress (noun):** Stress beyond which material deforms permanently.
    **Related Terms:** Mechanical property, Phantom stability.
    **Example in Radiotherapy:** Yield stress considered in immobilization material design.
11. **Yttrium-aluminum-garnet laser (YAG laser) (noun):** Laser used in calibration or imaging assistance.
    **Related Terms:** Nd:YAG, Optical alignment.
    **Example in Radiotherapy:** YAG laser ensures accurate room laser positioning.
12. **Yttrium oxide (noun):** Material used in dosimetric phosphors and detector coatings.
    **Related Terms:** Scintillator, Detector physics.
    **Example in Radiotherapy:** Yttrium oxide phosphor improves image brightness in EPID systems.

13. **Yoked motion (noun):** Synchronized mechanical or optical movement during beam delivery.
**Related Terms:** Coupled motion, Gantry mechanics.
**Example in Radiotherapy:** Yoked motion compensates for couch rotation-induced shifts.

14. **Yield coefficient (noun):** Ratio describing radiation-induced output versus input energy.
**Related Terms:** Energy conversion, Beam efficiency.
**Example in Radiation Physics:** Yield coefficient optimized in accelerator target design.

15. **Y-90 microsphere therapy (noun):** Internal therapy using Yttrium-90–loaded microspheres.
**Related Terms:** Radioembolization, Targeted radionuclide therapy.
**Example in Radiotherapy:** Y-90 therapy effectively treats hepatocellular carcinoma.

16. **Y-coordinate (noun):** Represents the lateral patient position in 3D isocentric setup.
**Related Terms:** Couch coordinates, Localization.
**Example in Radiotherapy:** Y-coordinate adjusted for daily setup correction.

17. **Yoke alignment (noun):** Calibration of magnet yokes for precise beam trajectory.
**Related Terms:** Magnetic symmetry, QA.
**Example in Radiotherapy:** Yoke alignment checked during annual LINAC QA.

18. **Yield energy (noun):** Energy level at which radiation interaction efficiency peaks.
**Related Terms:** Cross-section, Particle interaction.
**Example in Proton Therapy:** Yield energy influences target foil design.

19. **Y-shaped applicator (noun):** Special brachytherapy device designed for irregular cavities.
**Related Terms:** Applicator geometry, Intracavitary therapy.
**Example in Radiotherapy:** Y-shaped applicator used in customized HDR treatments.

20. **Yeast radiosensitivity (noun):** Radiation response of Saccharomyces cerevisiae used for biological assays.
**Related Terms:** Radiobiological model, Survival curve.
**Example in Radiobiology:** Yeast models assist in DNA damage quantification.

21. **Yield point (noun):** Threshold beyond which radiation detection becomes non-linear.
**Related Terms:** Detector calibration, Signal saturation.
**Example in Radiotherapy:** Yield point defined during chamber linearity testing.

22. **Y-component (noun):** Vector representing vertical beam displacement.
**Related Terms:** Coordinate system, Spatial resolution.
**Example in Radiotherapy:** Y-component correction performed for beam alignment.

23. **Yellow phantom marker (noun):** High-visibility marker used for surface tracking calibration.
**Related Terms:** Motion tracking, Imaging QA.
**Example in Radiotherapy:** Yellow markers assist SGRT system calibration.

24. **Yttrium source (noun):** Radioactive isotope used in research or calibration.
**Related Terms:** Y-90, Source decay.
**Example in Radiotherapy:** Yttrium source utilized in experimental dosimetry.

25. **Yield optimization (noun):** Process to maximize radiation production efficiency.
**Related Terms:** Target design, Accelerator tuning.
**Example in Radiation Physics:** Yield optimization improves proton output in cyclotrons.

26. **Yolk signal intensity (noun):** MRI characteristic used in early tumor staging.
**Related Terms:** MR interpretation, Signal mapping.
**Example in MR-guided Radiotherapy:** Yolk signal intensity variations assist tissue delineation.

27. **Y-chromosome aberration (noun):** DNA damage marker for radiation exposure.
**Related Terms:** Cytogenetics, Biomarker.
**Example in Radiobiology:** Y-chromosome aberration studied in radioprotection research.

28. **Yield loss (noun):** Reduction in usable dose output due to scattering or leakage.
**Related Terms:** Efficiency, Beam contamination.
**Example in Radiotherapy:** Yield loss minimized via improved target design.

29. **Yield monitor (noun):** Device tracking radiation production efficiency.
**Related Terms:** Beam current monitor, QA.
**Example in Proton Therapy:** Yield monitor ensures stability of beam output.

30. **Yaw drift (noun):** Slow deviation of couch or gantry yaw during treatment.
**Related Terms:** Mechanical error, Setup reproducibility.
**Example in Radiotherapy:** Yaw drift corrected using robotic couch feedback.

31. **Y-junction dosimeter (noun):** Tri-branch detector design for spatial dose mapping.
**Related Terms:** Multi-axis dosimetry, QA.
**Example in Radiotherapy:** Y-junction dosimeter measures off-axis proton scattering.

32. **Yttrium foil (noun):** Thin Yttrium layer used in target fabrication for accelerators.
**Related Terms:** Target material, Cyclotron component.
**Example in Proton Therapy:** Yttrium foil enhances beam energy uniformity.

33. **Yield fraction (noun):** Portion of total reaction products producing detectable radiation.
**Related Terms:** Activity yield, Reaction efficiency.
**Example in Radiochemistry:** Yield fraction determines isotopic purity.

34. **Y-axis offset (noun):** Lateral deviation from planned patient position.
**Related Terms:** Couch shift, Image registration.
**Example in Radiotherapy:** Y-axis offset corrected using CBCT verification.

35. **Ytterbium-169 (Yb-169) (noun):** Gamma-emitting isotope used in brachytherapy.
**Related Terms:** Ir-192 alternative, Source calibration.
**Example in Radiotherapy:** Yb-169 source provides lower energy for intraluminal treatments.

36. **Yield mapping (noun):** Visualization of radiation production across accelerator components.
**Related Terms:** Beam diagnostics, QA.
**Example in Radiation Physics:** Yield mapping detects degradation in target efficiency.

37. **Yield curve (noun):** Graph showing relation between input energy and radiation output.
**Related Terms:** Efficiency curve, Energy calibration.
**Example in Radiotherapy:** Yield curve assists tuning proton beam energy.

38. **Yolk-like enhancement (noun):** MRI appearance indicating necrotic or cystic tumor regions.
**Related Terms:** MR contrast, Tumor imaging.
Example in Radiology: Yolk-like enhancement observed post-SBRT in liver imaging.

39. **Yttrium-oxide ceramic (noun):** Material for dosimeter construction due to high radiation resistance.
**Related Terms:** Detector materials, Thermoluminescent dosimeter.
**Example in Radiotherapy:** Yttrium-oxide ceramic used in high-dose detectors.

40. **Yaw compensation algorithm (noun):** Software correcting angular setup deviations automatically.
**Related Terms:** Image guidance, Robotic control.
**Example in MR-LINAC:** Yaw compensation ensures submillimeter accuracy during adaptive therapy.

41. **Yaw correction system (noun):** Automated system correcting rotational misalignments around vertical axis.
**Related Terms:** Couch rotation, Image registration.
**Example in Radiotherapy:** Yaw correction system enhances setup reproducibility in SRS treatments.

42. **Yttrium filter (noun):** Thin metallic filter used to fine-tune photon beam energy.
**Related Terms:** Beam hardening, Spectral filtration.
**Example in Radiotherapy:** Yttrium filter improves beam quality for superficial therapy.

43. **Yield threshold (noun):** Minimum input energy required for measurable radiation emission.
**Related Terms:** Reaction cross-section, Activation energy.
Example in Radiation Physics**:** Yield threshold determined for proton–target interaction efficiency.

44. **Y-chromosomal deletion assay (noun):** Test measuring radiation-induced Y-chromosome loss.
**Related Terms:** Cytogenetic biodosimetry, Genetic biomarker.
**Example in Radiobiology:** Y-chromosomal deletion assay used for occupational exposure assessment.

45. **Yaw–pitch–roll calibration (noun):** Tri-axial alignment process for treatment couch accuracy.
**Related Terms:** Six-degree-of-freedom, Couch QA.
**Example in Radiotherapy:** Yaw–pitch–roll calibration performed weekly for robotic systems.

46. **Y-shaped immobilizer (noun):** Customized immobilization device for head-and-neck positioning.
**Related Terms:** Thermoplastic mask, Position reproducibility.
**Example in Radiotherapy:** Y-shaped immobilizer used in craniospinal irradiation setups.

47. **Yeast-based biosensor (noun):** Bioassay detecting radiation-induced oxidative stress.
**Related Terms:** Biodosimetry, Radioprotection.
**Example in Radiobiology:** Yeast-based biosensor validated for low-dose detection studies.

48. **Yttrium calibration source (noun):** Yttrium-90 reference used to verify detector energy response.
**Related Terms:** Source calibration, Beta dosimetry.
**Example in Radiotherapy:** Yttrium calibration source ensures uniform beta detector response.

49. **Yield stability (noun):** Consistency of radiation output over repeated activations.
**Related Terms:** Beam reproducibility, Quality assurance.
**Example in Proton Therapy:** Yield stability verified in daily output constancy checks.

50. **Y-90 resin microsphere (noun):** Biocompatible carrier for hepatic radioembolization.
**Related Terms:** Internal dosimetry, Radionuclide therapy.
**Example in Radiotherapy:** Y-90 resin microspheres deliver targeted intra-arterial radiation dose.

51. **Yellow beam indicator (noun):** Visual signal denoting beam readiness in accelerator systems.
**Related Terms:** Safety interlock, LINAC control.
**Example in Radiotherapy:** Yellow beam indicator illuminated before radiation delivery initiation.

52. **Yield fractionation (noun):** Calculation of yield per fraction to evaluate beam decay.
**Related Terms:** Fractional dose, Output stability.
**Example in Radiotherapy:** Yield fractionation assessed during multi-session proton treatments.

53. **Yoked imaging (noun):** Synchronized imaging process with mechanical motion.
**Related Terms:** Real-time imaging, Adaptive tracking.
Example in MR-LINAC**:** Yoked imaging provides motion-synchronized tumor visualization.

54. **Yield efficiency ratio (noun):** Proportion of actual versus theoretical radiation output.
**Related Terms:** Beam performance, Output factor.
**Example in Radiotherapy:** Yield efficiency ratio analyzed for target foil optimization.

55. **Yield degradation (noun):** Reduction in radiation output due to target wear or misalignment.
**Related Terms:** Beam aging, Equipment maintenance.
**Example in Proton Therapy:** Yield degradation identified during cyclotron target QA.

56. **Yaw adjustment lever (noun):** Mechanical control for angular fine-tuning of couch rotation.
**Related Terms:** Gantry mechanics, Manual alignment.
**Example in Radiotherapy:** Yaw adjustment lever used during treatment field setup.

57. **Yttrium activation analysis (noun):** Technique for assessing neutron flux via yttrium activation.
**Related Terms:** Neutron dosimetry, Activation foil.
**Example in Radiotherapy:** Yttrium activation analysis applied in boron neutron capture studies.

58. **Yield analysis curve (noun):** Graph representing efficiency of particle production.
**Related Terms:** Beam characterization, Calibration curve.
**Example in Proton Therapy:** Yield analysis curve assists cyclotron performance tuning.

59. **Y-chromosome fluorescence assay (noun):** Genetic method for quantifying Y-chromosome damage post-irradiation.
**Related Terms:** DNA assay, Cytogenetics.
**Example in Radiobiology:** Fluorescence assay validated as biomarker for radiation biodosimetry.

60. **Yield parameter (noun):** Numerical variable defining radiation efficiency under given conditions.
**Related Terms:** Beam output, System performance.
Example in Radiation Physics: Yield parameter optimized for target–beam interaction studies.

61. **Yoked beam alignment (noun):** Simultaneous coordination of multiple beam axes for uniform delivery.
**Related Terms:** Multi-field planning, Beam synchronization.
**Example in Radiotherapy:** Yoked beam alignment achieved using image-guided feedback.

62. **Yield coefficient ratio (noun):** Ratio comparing yields of different isotopic reactions.
**Related Terms:** Reaction kinetics, Cross-section analysis.
**Example in Proton Therapy:** Yield coefficient ratio used to refine isotope production rates.

63. **Yttrium oxide dosimeter (noun):** Solid-state detector composed of yttrium oxide for high-dose regions.
**Related Terms:** Thermoluminescent dosimeter, High-energy calibration.
**Example in Radiotherapy:** Yttrium oxide dosimeter deployed in electron field QA.

64. **Yaw–roll coupling (noun):** Mechanical interdependence between yaw and roll movements.
**Related Terms:** Geometric calibration, Couch accuracy.
**Example in Radiotherapy:** Yaw–roll coupling corrected during 6D positioning QA.

65. **Yield modeling (noun):** Mathematical prediction of output efficiency in accelerators.
**Related Terms:** Monte Carlo simulation, Beam dynamics.
Example in Radiation Physics: Yield modeling applied to optimize cyclotron target geometry.

66. **Yttrium stabilization (noun):** Use of yttrium additives to enhance detector material properties.
**Related Terms:** Crystal doping, Radiation hardness.
**Example in Radiotherapy:** Yttrium stabilization improved scintillator durability under high doses.

67. **Yield-time curve (noun):** Graph showing yield variation over operational duration.
**Related Terms:** Temporal stability, Output drift.
**Example in Proton Therapy:** Yield-time curve analyzed to ensure consistent daily beam quality.

68. **Yeast survival curve (noun):** Dose–response graph for yeast cells after radiation exposure.
**Related Terms:** Radiobiological modeling, Survival fraction.
**Example in Radiobiology:** Yeast survival curve used to model low-dose repair kinetics.

69. **Y-plate collimator (noun):** Y-axis defining aperture in specialized collimator assemblies.
**Related Terms:** Beam shaping, Secondary collimation.
**Example in Radiotherapy:** Y-plate collimator adjusted for conformal field delivery.

70. **Yield control unit (noun):** Electronic module monitoring radiation output stability.
**Related Terms:** Beam feedback, QA instrumentation.
**Example in Radiotherapy:** Yield control unit calibrated during monthly QA.

71. **Yield linearity (noun):** Proportional relationship between beam current and output dose.
**Related Terms:** Calibration curve, Output linearity.
**Example in Proton Therapy:** Yield linearity verified through dose rate modulation tests.

72. **Yttrium-chloride compound (noun):** Chemical used in preparation of Y-90 radiopharmaceuticals.
**Related Terms:** Radiochemistry, Source preparation.
**Example in Radiotherapy:** Yttrium-chloride compound synthesized for microsphere labeling.

73. **Yield mapping algorithm (noun):** Computational tool for predicting spatial radiation yield distribution.
**Related Terms:** Simulation, Beam profiling.
**Example in Proton Therapy:** Yield mapping algorithm integrated into Monte Carlo validation.

74. **Yttrium resonance (noun):** Nuclear resonance property influencing isotope formation.
**Related Terms:** Reaction cross-section, Neutron capture.
Example in Radiophysics: Yttrium resonance studied in activation experiments.

75. **Yield-based QA (noun):** Quality assurance method relying on radiation output efficiency.
**Related Terms:** Beam QA, Output constancy.
**Example in Radiotherapy:** Yield-based QA used to track accelerator degradation trends.

76. **Yield prediction model (noun):** Computational model forecasting expected beam yield under given parameters.
**Related Terms:** Monte Carlo simulation, Beam optimization.
**Example in Proton Therapy:** Yield prediction model used to validate target performance.

77. **Y-axis gantry offset (noun):** Vertical displacement of gantry from nominal rotational center.
**Related Terms:** Mechanical accuracy, Gantry calibration.
**Example in Radiotherapy:** Y-axis gantry offset corrected during geometric QA.

78. **Yttrium-based detector (noun):** Detector utilizing yttrium compounds for enhanced photon sensitivity.
**Related Terms:** Scintillation detector, Dosimetry.
**Example in Radiotherapy:** Yttrium-based detector applied for portal imaging dose verification.

79. **Yaw motion correction (noun):** Real-time compensation for rotational deviation about vertical axis.
**Related Terms:** 6D positioning, Motion management.
Example in MR-LINAC: Yaw motion correction improves adaptive setup accuracy.

80. **Yield optimization algorithm (noun):** Software routine maximizing particle output efficiency.
**Related Terms:** Beam tuning, Accelerator modeling.
**Example in Proton Therapy:** Yield optimization algorithm enhanced beam stability in daily QA.

81. **Yeast DNA repair assay (noun):** Experimental setup studying DNA damage recovery post-irradiation.
**Related Terms:** Radiogenomics, Cellular repair.
**Example in Radiobiology:** Yeast DNA repair assay helps quantify sublethal radiation damage.

82. **Yield response curve (noun):** Plot showing output yield versus input energy.
**Related Terms:** Dose response, Energy dependency.
**Example in Proton Therapy:** Yield response curve validated for cyclotron proton source.

83. **Yttrium-loaded scintillator (noun):** Detector material doped with yttrium for improved radiation response.
**Related Terms:** Scintillation crystal, Detector efficiency.
**Example in Radiotherapy:** Yttrium-loaded scintillator used in prompt gamma detection.

84. **Yield drift (noun):** Gradual decrease in output over prolonged operation.
**Related Terms:** Machine drift, QA constancy.
**Example in Radiotherapy:** Yield drift compensated during automated calibration routines.

85. **Y-chromosome microdeletion (noun):** Genetic mutation detectable after chronic radiation exposure.
**Related Terms:** Cytogenetic marker, Radiation biomonitoring.
**Example in Radiobiology:** Y-chromosome microdeletion assay used in occupational exposure studies.

86. **Yield attenuation (noun):** Reduction of radiation output due to material absorption.
**Related Terms:** Beam hardening, Attenuation coefficient.
**Example in Radiotherapy:** Yield attenuation analyzed in beamline shielding verification.

87. **Yoke magnet (noun):** Core structure guiding magnetic fields within LINAC.
**Related Terms:** Magnet assembly, Beam steering.
Example in Radiation Physics: Yoke magnet symmetry checked during commissioning.

88. **Yaw rotational QA (noun):** Quality assurance verifying rotational precision of couch or gantry.
**Related Terms:** Geometric QA, Mechanical accuracy.
**Example in Radiotherapy:** Yaw rotational QA conducted monthly for SBRT systems.

89. **Yield decay constant (noun):** Parameter defining exponential drop in beam yield over time.
**Related Terms:** Output drift, Calibration constant.
**Example in Proton Therapy:** Yield decay constant monitored during cyclotron maintenance.

90. **Yeast cell radiosensitivity (noun):** Relative susceptibility of yeast to ionizing radiation.
**Related Terms:** Radiobiological model, Dose–response.
**Example in Radiobiology:** Yeast cell radiosensitivity correlated with DNA repair gene mutation.

91. **Yttrium-doped crystal (noun):** Material used in dosimeters for high-resolution photon detection.
**Related Terms:** Optically stimulated dosimeter, Solid-state detection.
**Example in Radiotherapy:** Yttrium-doped crystal employed for exit dose monitoring.

92. **Yield scaling factor (noun):** Correction coefficient for comparing yield across energy levels.
**Related Terms:** Calibration curve, Beam normalization.
**Example in Proton Therapy:** Yield scaling factor used to harmonize daily QA results.

93. **Yttrium aluminate (noun):** Ceramic compound with radiation-resistant properties.
**Related Terms:** Detector material, Thermoluminescent dosimetry.
**Example in Radiotherapy:** Yttrium aluminate used in high-temperature dosimeter fabrication.

94. **Yaw misalignment (noun):** Rotational deviation causing beam–target mismatch.
**Related Terms:** Couch error, Positional correction.
**Example in Radiotherapy:** Yaw misalignment corrected using 6D robotic couch system.

95. **Yttrium isotope production (noun):** Generation of Y-90 or Y-88 isotopes via neutron activation.
**Related Terms:** Radioisotope generation, Reactor physics.
**Example in Nuclear Medicine:** Yttrium isotope production calibrated for medical applications.

96. **Yttrium-iron-garnet filter (noun):** Magnetic filter regulating microwave transmission in LINACs.
**Related Terms:** Waveguide filter, RF stabilization.
**Example in Radiotherapy:** Yttrium-iron-garnet filter stabilizes LINAC frequency drift.

97. **Yield verification test (noun):** Procedure verifying consistency of radiation production.
**Related Terms:** Output QA, Beam reproducibility.
**Example in Radiotherapy:** Yield verification test performed before patient treatments.

98. **Yaw tracking system (noun):** Real-time monitoring of rotational movement during delivery.
**Related Terms:** Motion tracking, Imaging guidance.
**Example in MR-LINAC:** Yaw tracking system ensures accuracy in adaptive therapy.

99. **Yield noise ratio (noun):** Ratio expressing yield signal to background variation.
**Related Terms:** Signal-to-noise ratio, Beam stability.
**Example in Radiotherapy:** Yield noise ratio optimized through beam current control.

100. **Y-axis calibration (noun):** Process aligning vertical mechanical or imaging coordinates.
**Related Terms:** Geometric calibration, Couch setup.
**Example in Radiotherapy:** Y-axis calibration verified during monthly machine QA.

101. **Yttrium silicate detector (noun):** High-density crystal used for precise gamma detection.
**Related Terms:** Scintillation detector, Dose monitoring.
**Example in Radiotherapy:** Yttrium silicate detector enhances EPID resolution.

102. **Yield uniformity test (noun):** Evaluation ensuring spatial consistency of beam output.
**Related Terms:** Flatness, Symmetry QA.
**Example in Proton Therapy:** Yield uniformity test performed with 2D detector array.

103. **Yttrium oxide nanoparticle (noun):** Nanomaterial used as a radiosensitizer or imaging enhancer.
**Related Terms:** Nanomedicine, Radiosensitization.
**Example in Radiobiology:** Yttrium oxide nanoparticles tested for targeted tumor enhancement.

104. **Yield control software (noun):** Application regulating output yield automatically.
**Related Terms:** Beam feedback, Automation.
**Example in Radiotherapy:** Yield control software prevents output fluctuation during long treatments.

105. **Y-chromosome instability (noun):** Genetic indicator of chronic radiation exposure.
**Related Terms:** Biodosimetry, Genomic instability.
**Example in Radiobiology:** Y-chromosome instability used for post-irradiation population studies.

106. **Yttrium fluoride coating (noun):** Protective layer improving thermal and radiation resistance.
**Related Terms:** Surface coating, Equipment protection.
**Example in Radiotherapy:** Yttrium fluoride coating applied to beamline components.

107. **Yield efficiency constant (noun):** Standard coefficient representing stable yield under set beam current.
**Related Terms:** Beam quality, Calibration constant.
**Example in Proton Therapy:** Yield efficiency constant recorded in accelerator QA logs.

108. **Y-chromosome-specific probe (noun):** Fluorescent probe detecting Y-chromosome damage.
**Related Terms:** FISH assay, Genetic biomarker.
**Example in Radiobiology:** Y-specific probe quantifies chromosomal aberrations post-irradiation.

109. **Yaw rotation drift (noun):** Progressive angular deviation during beam delivery.
**Related Terms:** Rotational inaccuracy, Positioning error.
**Example in Radiotherapy:** Yaw rotation drift corrected by dynamic couch compensation.

110. **Yield analysis software (noun):** Program used to evaluate and model beam output performance.
**Related Terms:** QA analytics, Output monitoring.
**Example in Proton Therapy:** Yield analysis software tracks long-term beam stability.

111. **Yield attenuation coefficient (noun):** Factor representing reduction in beam output due to material absorption.
**Related Terms:** Linear attenuation, Beam quality.
**Example in Radiotherapy:** Yield attenuation coefficient derived experimentally for treatment head shielding.

112. **Yttrium luminescent phosphor (noun):** Material emitting visible light upon radiation excitation.
**Related Terms:** Scintillator, Detector sensitivity.
**Example in Imaging Physics:** Yttrium luminescent phosphor used in image intensifiers for fluoroscopy.

113. **Yield modulation index (noun):** Quantitative measure of variation in beam yield between exposures.
**Related Terms:** Beam modulation, QA metric.
**Example in Radiotherapy:** Yield modulation index maintained below 2% for daily LINAC stability.

114. **Yaw alignment error (noun):** Deviation in rotational positioning of treatment couch around vertical axis.
**Related Terms:** Six-degree-of-freedom, Couch QA.
**Example in Radiotherapy:** Yaw alignment error corrected using laser-guided calibration.

115. **Yttrium aluminum perovskite (noun):** Radiation-tolerant crystal used in dosimetric applications.
**Related Terms:** Scintillation crystal, Detector design.
**Example in Radiotherapy:** Yttrium aluminum perovskite used for optical dosimetry under high flux.

116. **Yield sensitivity test (noun):** Assessment of beam output fluctuation sensitivity to system parameters.
**Related Terms:** Output constancy, QA.
**Example in Proton Therapy:** Yield sensitivity test performed weekly for beamline calibration.

117. **Y-axis gantry deviation (noun):** Vertical misalignment of gantry rotation relative to isocenter.
**Related Terms:** Geometric accuracy, QA.
**Example in Radiotherapy:** Y-axis gantry deviation checked during monthly mechanical QA.

118. **Yeast chromatin damage model (noun):** Experimental radiobiological model studying chromatin response to ionization.
**Related Terms:** DNA repair, Radiosensitivity.
**Example in Radiobiology:** Yeast chromatin damage model evaluates double-strand break kinetics.

119. **Yaw compensation factor (noun):** Numerical correction applied for yaw displacement during treatment.
**Related Terms:** Image registration, Setup accuracy.
**Example in SBRT:** Yaw compensation factor adjusted automatically via image guidance.

120. **Yttrium-based glass dosimeter (noun):** Glass composite embedded with yttrium for precise dose measurement.
**Related Terms:** Passive dosimetry, Radiophotonics.
**Example in Radiotherapy:** Yttrium glass dosimeter utilized in entrance dose verification.

121. **Yield mapping (noun):** Spatial visualization of output yield distribution across the field.
**Related Terms:** Flatness, Symmetry.
**Example in QA:** Yield mapping performed using ion chamber array for beam uniformity.

122. **Yttrium-enhanced TLD (noun):** Thermoluminescent dosimeter with yttrium doping for sensitivity improvement.
**Related Terms:** Dosimetry, Radiation detection.
**Example in Radiotherapy:** Yttrium-enhanced TLDs used for high-precision HDR brachytherapy QA.

123. **Yield equilibrium (noun):** Steady state condition where output rate stabilizes under constant input.
**Related Terms:** Output constancy, Beam stability.
**Example in Proton Therapy:** Yield equilibrium achieved after thermal stabilization of accelerator components.

124. **Yttrium shielding layer (noun):** Protective material layer incorporating yttrium for neutron moderation.
**Related Terms:** Radiation shielding, Material science.
**Example in Proton Therapy:** Yttrium shielding layer integrated into beamline for scatter reduction.

125. **Y-chromosome biodosimeter (noun):** Assay using Y-chromosome anomalies as exposure indicator.
**Related Terms:** Cytogenetics, Biological dosimetry.
**Example in Radiobiology:** Y-chromosome biodosimeter applied for long-term occupational exposure analysis.

126. **Yield harmonization factor (noun):** Coefficient adjusting yield between calibration setups.
**Related Terms:** Cross-calibration, QA normalization.
**Example in Radiotherapy:** Yield harmonization factor standardizes multiple machine outputs.

127. **Yield gradient (noun):** Rate of change in yield over spatial or energy range.
**Related Terms:** Beam profile, Dose gradient.
**Example in Proton Therapy:** Yield gradient minimized to maintain uniform dose deposition.

128. **Yaw registration matrix (noun):** Transformation matrix describing rotational correction about vertical axis.
**Related Terms:** Rigid registration, Image fusion.
**Example in Radiotherapy:** Yaw registration matrix applied during CBCT auto-alignment.

129. **Yttrium radionuclide (noun):** Radioactive isotope of yttrium, often Y-90, for therapeutic use.
**Related Terms:** Brachytherapy, Radiopharmaceutical.
**Example in Nuclear Oncology:** Yttrium radionuclide used in radioembolization for hepatic tumors.

130. **Yield homogeneity index (noun):** Measure of uniformity in beam yield across field area.
**Related Terms:** Field uniformity, QA.
**Example in Radiotherapy:** Yield homogeneity index used for beam profile evaluation.

131. **Yaw correction tolerance (noun):** Acceptable limit of yaw angle deviation during treatment setup.
**Related Terms:** Setup accuracy, QA tolerance.
**Example in Radiotherapy:** Yaw correction tolerance set within $\pm 0.5°$.

132. **Yield prediction coefficient (noun):** Parameter defining relationship between beam settings and expected yield.
**Related Terms:** Output calibration, Machine modeling.
**Example in Proton Therapy:** Yield prediction coefficient validated during commissioning.

133. **Yttrium plasma emission (noun):** Energy emission from yttrium during high-energy excitation.
**Related Terms:** Spectroscopy, Beam diagnostics.
**Example in Physics QA:** Yttrium plasma emission measured in accelerator cavity tuning.

134. **Yield correction protocol (noun):** Standardized method to adjust measured yield for environmental variation.
**Related Terms:** QA standardization, Calibration.
**Example in Radiotherapy:** Yield correction protocol included in ISO-compliant QA procedures.

135. **Yeast mutation frequency (noun):** Rate of genetic mutation induced by radiation exposure.
**Related Terms:** Mutagenesis, Radiobiological response.
**Example in Radiobiology:** Yeast mutation frequency used for dose–effect calibration studies.

136. **Yield saturation point (noun):** Threshold where further input increase doesn't raise yield.
**Related Terms:** Saturation, Output curve.
**Example in Proton Therapy:** Yield saturation point determined experimentally for beam tuning.

137. **Y-axis beam offset (noun):** Vertical displacement of radiation beam from central axis.
**Related Terms:** Beam alignment, QA.
**Example in Radiotherapy:** Y-axis beam offset corrected using digital inclinometer.

138. **Yaw rotational offset (noun):** Rotational misalignment causing lateral displacement during treatment.
**Related Terms:** Couch rotation, Setup error.
**Example in Radiotherapy:** Yaw rotational offset adjusted through 6D couch calibration.

139. **Yttrium alloy shielding (noun):** Metallic blend incorporating yttrium for improved radiation resistance.
**Related Terms:** Shielding material, Equipment design.
**Example in Radiotherapy:** Yttrium alloy shielding applied in gantry beam stops.

140. **Yield decay profile (noun):** Curve describing reduction of yield with operational time.
**Related Terms:** Output drift, QA monitoring.
**Example in Radiotherapy:** Yield decay profile logged for beamline maintenance.

141. **Yeast colony survival curve (noun):** Graph depicting yeast survival vs. dose relationship.
**Related Terms:** Survival assay, Radiobiological modeling.
**Example in Radiobiology:** Yeast colony survival curve defines LD50 of ionizing exposure.

142. **Yttrium dosimetric calibration (noun):** Procedure using yttrium isotopes for precise dose calibration.
**Related Terms:** Calibration source, QA.
**Example in Radiotherapy:** Yttrium dosimetric calibration used for gamma detector benchmarking.

143. **Yaw correction module (noun):** Hardware/software component correcting yaw deviation dynamically.
**Related Terms:** Real-time correction, Image-guidance.
**Example in MR-LINAC:** Yaw correction module ensures precise target tracking.

144. **Yield-to-dose conversion (noun):** Mathematical relationship linking measured yield to delivered dose.
**Related Terms:** Calibration curve, Dosimetry.
**Example in Radiotherapy:** Yield-to-dose conversion validated for new detector array.

145. **Yttrium oxide ceramic (noun):** Radiation-hard material for detectors and thermal protection.
**Related Terms:** Advanced materials, Dosimeter fabrication.
**Example in Proton Therapy:** Yttrium oxide ceramic used in scatter monitor fabrication.

146. **Yield ratio variance (noun):** Statistical variation in measured yield ratios across sessions.
**Related Terms:** Output reproducibility, QA statistics.
**Example in Radiotherapy:** Yield ratio variance analyzed for constancy verification.

147. **Y-axis displacement correction (noun):** Adjustment compensating for vertical misalignment in setup.
**Related Terms:** Patient positioning, QA.
**Example in Radiotherapy:** Y-axis displacement correction applied via image fusion alignment.

148. **Yeast apoptosis model (noun):** Biological model examining programmed cell death post-irradiation.
**Related Terms:** Radiobiology, Cell cycle.
**Example in Radiobiology:** Yeast apoptosis model quantifies oxidative stress from X-rays.

149. **Yaw axis calibration (noun):** Process ensuring accurate rotational motion around vertical axis.
**Related Terms:** Couch QA, Motion control.
**Example in Radiotherapy:** Yaw axis calibration verified during annual QA.

150. **Yttrium fluorophosphate glass (noun):** Radiation-resistant material used in optical sensors.
**Related Terms:** Dosimetric materials, Detector optics.
**Example in Radiotherapy:** Yttrium fluorophosphate glass enhances signal linearity in high-dose range.

151. **Yield correction matrix (noun):** A computational grid used to normalize spatial yield variations.
**Related Terms:** Beam calibration, QA.
**Example in Radiotherapy:** Yield correction matrix applied to flatten beam output map.

152. **Yaw error compensation system (noun):** Real-time correction tool for rotational alignment deviation.
**Related Terms:** 6D correction, Couch control.
**Example in MR-LINAC:** Yaw error compensation system maintains sub-millimeter targeting accuracy.

153. **Yttrium-stabilized zirconia (noun):** Durable ceramic used in radiation-tolerant devices.
**Related Terms:** Shielding material, Instrument design.
**Example in Radiotherapy:** Yttrium-stabilized zirconia used in gantry bearings.

154. **Yeast oxidative stress assay (noun):** Biological test measuring reactive oxygen damage after irradiation.
**Related Terms:** Radiobiological response, ROS.
**Example in Radiobiology:** Yeast oxidative stress assay helps quantify low-dose oxidative effects.

155. **Yield uniformity coefficient (noun):** Numerical indicator of beam output consistency.
**Related Terms:** Flatness, Symmetry QA.
**Example in Radiotherapy:** Yield uniformity coefficient validated during annual LINAC QA.

156. **Yttrium doped silicon detector (noun):** Semiconductor detector enhanced with yttrium for high sensitivity.
**Related Terms:** Solid-state detector, Dosimetry.
**Example in Proton Therapy:** Used for fine-resolution dose mapping.

157. **Yaw vector analysis (noun):** Mathematical evaluation of couch or gantry rotation around vertical axis.
**Related Terms:** Geometric accuracy, QA.
**Example in SBRT:** Yaw vector analysis confirms sub-degree precision.

158. **Yield calibration drift (noun):** Gradual deviation in calibrated output yield values.
**Related Terms:** QA constancy, Output drift.
**Example in Proton Therapy:** Monitored to maintain dose reproducibility.

159. **Yttrium filter plate (noun):** Thin radiation filter optimizing photon beam quality.
**Related Terms:** Beam hardening, Filtration.
**Example in Radiotherapy:** Yttrium filter plate used in imaging beam conditioning.

160. **Yield control feedback loop (noun):**Automatic system stabilizing beam output in real time.
**Related Terms:** Beam feedback, QA automation.
**Example in Proton Therapy:** Prevents yield oscillation during extended delivery.

161. **Yeast DNA fragmentation assay (noun):** Test quantifying strand breaks post-irradiation.
**Related Terms:** Genotoxicity, Repair kinetics.
**Example in Radiobiology:** Indicates non-repaired DNA after fractionated exposure.

162. **Y-axis patient motion (noun):** Vertical displacement of patient during beam delivery.
**Related Terms:** Motion management, IGRT.
**Example in Radiotherapy:** Corrected via optical surface tracking.

163. **Yield benchmarking study (noun):** Comparative evaluation of yield performance among systems.
**Related Terms:** QA benchmarking, Output reproducibility.
**Example in Radiotherapy:** Conducted across multiple proton centers.

164. **Yaw correction interpolation (noun):** Mathematical estimation of intermediate rotational corrections.
**Related Terms:** Image registration, Motion correction.
**Example in Adaptive Therapy:** Used in deformable registration algorithms.

165. **Yttrium orthovanadate crystal (noun):** Scintillation crystal for rapid radiation detection.
**Related Terms:** Detector material, Light yield.
**Example in Radiotherapy:** Enhances signal speed in portal imagers.

166. **Yield response optimization (noun):** Adjustment process maximizing dose output uniformity.
**Related Terms:** Beam tuning, Calibration.
**Example in Proton Therapy:** Implemented during cyclotron startup.

167. **Yttrium isotopic calibration source (noun):** Standard Y-90 source used for dose calibration.
**Related Terms:** Reference source, QA.
**Example in Radiotherapy:** Ensures consistent detector linearity.

168. **Yeast chromosomal aberration test (noun):** Genetic assay for radiation-induced chromosomal anomalies.
**Related Terms:** Cytogenetic testing, Biodosimetry.
**Example in Radiobiology:** Validates radioprotective drug efficacy.

169. **Yaw stabilization motor (noun):** Device minimizing couch rotational drift.
**Related Terms:** Couch mechanics, Motion stability.
**Example in SBRT:** Maintains accurate gantry–target alignment.

170. **Yield distribution curve (noun):** Graph representing output variation across energy levels.
**Related Terms:** Beam quality, QA evaluation.
**Example in Radiotherapy:** Evaluates energy constancy in LINAC output.

171. **Yield fluctuation ratio (noun):** Statistical ratio indicating output variability.
**Related Terms:** QA analysis, Beam constancy.
**Example in Radiotherapy:** Limited to <1% for precision delivery.

172. **Yttrium-containing polymer shield (noun):** Composite material reducing scatter radiation.
**Related Terms:** Shielding design, Safety.
**Example in Radiotherapy:** Applied in LINAC bunker design.

173. **Yield-time correlation (noun):** Relationship between operation time and output yield.
**Related Terms:** Machine drift, QA.
**Example in Proton Therapy:** Used to predict stability patterns.

174. **Y-axis distortion correction (noun):** Correction for vertical geometric distortion in imaging.
**Related Terms:** Image reconstruction, MR-LINAC QA.
**Example in MRI-guided RT:** Applied before adaptive planning.

175. **Yttrium-targeted radiotherapy (noun):** Therapy using Y-90 conjugates for tumor irradiation.
**Related Terms:** Radiopharmaceutical therapy, Internal dosimetry.
**Example in Oncology:** Used for hepatic metastases.

176. **Yield threshold limit (noun):** Minimum acceptable output level for operational safety.
**Related Terms:** QA limits, Output control.
**Example in Radiotherapy:** Checked in daily warm-up QA.

177. **Yaw axis tracking error (noun):** Difference between planned and actual rotation around vertical axis.
**Related Terms:** Tracking QA, IGRT accuracy.
**Example in SBRT:** Corrected via imaging-based realignment.

178. **Yttrium light-emitting crystal (noun):** Scintillator emitting visible photons upon radiation interaction.
**Related Terms:** Imaging detectors, Scintillation.
**Example in Radiotherapy:** Used in electronic portal imaging detectors (EPIDs).

179. **Yeast double-strand break assay (noun):** Experimental quantification of DSB formation post-irradiation.
**Related Terms:** DNA damage, Repair pathway.
**Example in Radiobiology:** Evaluates radiosensitivity biomarkers.

180. **Yield uniformity map (noun):** 2D graphical representation of beam output uniformity.
**Related Terms:** Flatness test, QA report.
**Example in Radiotherapy:** Acquired using film dosimetry arrays.

181. **Yield normalization algorithm (noun):** Mathematical routine equalizing yield among varying conditions.
**Related Terms:** Calibration, QA automation.
**Example in Radiotherapy:** Integrated in adaptive delivery software.

182. **Yttrium-activated phosphor screen (noun):** Scintillating surface for radiation imaging.
**Related Terms:** Detector screen, Radiographic imaging.
**Example in Radiology:** Used in analog fluoroscopy panels.

183. **Yaw misalignment index (noun):** Quantitative measure of rotational setup inaccuracy.
**Related Terms:** Couch QA, Positional error.
**Example in Radiotherapy:** Maintained below 0.3° for precision SBRT.

184. **Yeast viability test (noun):** Cellular assay determining post-radiation survival rate.
**Related Terms:** Survival fraction, Radiobiology.
**Example in Research:** Used in DNA repair analysis.

185. **Yttrium-oxide-coated chamber (noun):** Ionization chamber lined with yttrium oxide for radiation hardness.
**Related Terms:** Detector durability, QA instrumentation.
**Example in Radiotherapy:** Applied in high-dose-rate dosimetry.

186. **Yield decay monitoring (noun):** Continuous observation of output reduction trends.
**Related Terms:** QA tracking, Stability analysis.
**Example in Proton Therapy:** Prevents long-term calibration drift.

187. **Y-axis symmetry correction (noun):** Adjustment restoring beam vertical uniformity.
**Related Terms:** Beam profile QA, Flatness.
**Example in Radiotherapy:** Ensures even dose deposition.

188. **Yttrium-aluminate scintillator (noun):** High-brightness scintillator used for precise photon detection.
**Related Terms:** Detector physics, Imaging system.
**Example in Radiotherapy:** Improves resolution in EPID panels.

189. **Yaw stabilization gyroscope (noun):** Sensor controlling rotational accuracy during treatment.
**Related Terms:** Motion sensing, Couch mechanics.
**Example in MR-LINAC:** Used in rotational feedback loops.

190. **Yield vs dose curve (noun):** Relationship graph correlating yield output to delivered dose.
**Related Terms:** Calibration, Output verification.
**Example in QA:** Used for dose linearity analysis.

191. **Yield factor (noun):** Ratio of useful radiation output to total input energy.
**Related Terms:** Beam efficiency, Output factor.
**Example in Radiotherapy:** Yield factor evaluated for proton nozzle performance.

192. **Yoke (noun):** Structural frame supporting x-ray tube or gantry rotation.
**Related Terms:** Gantry arm, Rotation mechanics.
**Example in Radiotherapy:** Yoke alignment verified during machine QA.

193. **Young's modulus (noun):** Measure of tissue elasticity under stress.
**Related Terms:** Elasticity, Mechanical properties.
**Example in Radiotherapy:** Young's modulus helps model tumor deformation.

194. **Y-ray contamination (noun):** Unintended high-energy photon component in mixed fields.
**Related Terms:** Neutron contamination, Beam purity.
**Example in Radiotherapy:** Y-ray contamination assessed in proton beam QA.

195. **Yield cross-section (noun):** Probability measure for nuclear reaction producing secondary radiation.
**Related Terms:** Cross-section, Particle interactions.
**Example in Radiotherapy:** Yield cross-section important in neutron shielding design.

196. **Yellow filter (noun):** Optical filter enhancing image contrast in simulators.
**Related Terms:** Imaging filter, Contrast enhancement.
**Example in Radiotherapy:** Yellow filter used for kV portal imaging clarity.

197. **Yttrium-90 microsphere therapy (noun):** Radioembolization treatment using Y-90 microspheres for hepatic tumors.
**Related Terms:** Internal radiotherapy, Brachytherapy.
**Example in Radiotherapy:** Yttrium-90 microspheres used for unresectable liver metastases.

198. **Yield curve (noun):** Graphical plot showing production yield versus energy input.
**Related Terms:** Output curve, Beam efficiency.
**Example in Radiotherapy:** Yield curve optimized for isotope generation.

199. **Yield ratio (noun):** Comparison between theoretical and practical radiation yield.
**Related Terms:** Efficiency ratio, Beam calibration.
**Example in Radiotherapy:** Yield ratio measured during linac performance test.

200. **Yield spectrum (noun):** Distribution of secondary particle yields per energy interval.
**Related Terms:** Energy spectrum, Secondary dose.
**Example in Radiotherapy:** Yield spectrum analysis crucial for proton scatter modeling.

201. **Yaw axis (noun):** Rotational movement axis controlling gantry or couch orientation.
**Related Terms:** Pitch, Roll, Six degrees of freedom.
**Example in Radiotherapy:** Yaw correction applied during CBCT alignment.

202. **Yaw correction (noun):** Adjustment to compensate for rotational misalignment about vertical axis.
**Related Terms:** Image registration, Setup correction.
**Example in Radiotherapy:** Yaw correction automated in 6D robotic couches.

203. **Yoked beam delivery (noun):** Technique linking dual beamlines for synchronized dose delivery.
**Related Terms:** Beam synchronization, Dual gantry.
**Example in Radiotherapy:** Yoked delivery improves bilateral head and neck treatment efficiency.

204. **Yield enhancement (noun):** Optimization process increasing output efficiency of particle sources.
**Related Terms:** Beam tuning, Source efficiency.
**Example in Radiotherapy:** Yield enhancement achieved by optimizing target cooling systems.

205. **Y-irradiation (noun):** Exposure to gamma rays for biological or material testing.
**Related Terms:** Gamma radiation, Source exposure.
**Example in Radiotherapy:** Y-irradiation used in in-vitro radiobiology research.

206. **Y-coordinate (noun):** Lateral coordinate defining patient or beam position in 3D system.
**Related Terms:** X-axis, Z-axis, Couch translation.
**Example in Radiotherapy:** Y-coordinate adjusted during manual setup verification.

207. **Yield stability (noun):** Consistency of radiation output over time.
**Related Terms:** Output constancy, Machine QA.
**Example in Radiotherapy:** Yield stability monitored through daily output checks.

208. **Y-chamber (noun):** Specialized ionization chamber designed for energy yield measurements.
**Related Terms:** Ion chamber, Dosimetry.
**Example in Radiotherapy:** Y-chamber calibrated for photon yield analysis.

209. **Yttrium-90 dosimetry (noun):** Calculation and verification of dose distribution in Y-90 therapies.
**Related Terms:** Internal dosimetry, Monte Carlo.
**Example in Radiotherapy:** Yttrium-90 dosimetry performed using voxel-based SPECT reconstruction.

210. **Yield optimization (noun):** Improving dose output efficiency without compromising beam quality.
**Related Terms:** Machine tuning, Output calibration.
**Example in Radiotherapy:** Yield optimization reduces target heating losses.

211. **Yield monitoring system (noun):** Device continuously measuring radiation output per cycle.
**Related Terms:** Beam monitor, QA instrumentation.
**Example in Radiotherapy:** Yield monitoring ensures consistent proton beam current.

212. **Yolk sac assay (noun):** Radiobiological test measuring radiation-induced vascular damage in embryos.
**Related Terms:** In-vivo assay, Radiobiological endpoint.
**Example in Radiotherapy:** Yolk sac assay used in low-dose radiobiology studies.

213. **Yield drift (noun):** Gradual change in beam output efficiency over time.
**Related Terms:** Calibration drift, Output decay.
**Example in Radiotherapy:** Yield drift detected during monthly machine QA.

214. **Yield profile (noun):** Plot representing radiation output distribution across beam width.
**Related Terms:** Beam flatness, Symmetry.
**Example in Radiotherapy:** Yield profile analyzed for electron beam calibration.

215. **Young tissue response (noun):** Increased radiosensitivity observed in immature or developing tissues.
**Related Terms:** Radiosensitivity, Age factor.
**Example in Radiotherapy:** Young tissue response critical for pediatric treatment planning.

216. **Y-shaped collimator (noun):** Custom collimator with dual branch aperture for conformal delivery.
**Related Terms:** Beam shaping, Field design.
**Example in Radiotherapy:** Y-shaped collimator used in cranial bifocal therapy.

217. **Y-90 bremsstrahlung imaging (noun):** Gamma imaging technique for visualizing Y-90 microsphere distribution.
**Related Terms:** SPECT, Radioembolization.
**Example in Radiotherapy:** Y-90 bremsstrahlung imaging validates post-therapy microsphere localization.

218. **Y-90 decay constant (noun):** Rate of radioactive decay for Yttrium-90 isotope.
**Related Terms:** Half-life, Radioactive decay.
**Example in Radiotherapy:** Y-90 decay constant applied in dose calculation.

219. **Yield calibration curve (noun):** Graph correlating measured yield with beam current.
**Related Terms:** Output calibration, QA.
**Example in Radiotherapy:** Yield calibration curve verified before isotope production.

220. **Yaw drift (noun):** Progressive angular deviation of gantry rotation axis.
**Related Terms:** Mechanical error, Gantry QA.
**Example in Radiotherapy:** Yaw drift compensated by recalibration procedure.

221. **Y-parameter (noun):** Dimensionless value representing normalized energy loss.
**Related Terms:** LET, Stopping power.
**Example in Radiotherapy:** Y-parameter used in proton beam range verification.

222. **Yield normalization (noun):** Standardizing measured yields to a reference condition.
**Related Terms:** Calibration, Quality assurance.
**Example in Radiotherapy:** Yield normalization ensures cross-machine reproducibility.

223. **Yttrium-aluminum-garnet laser (noun):** YAG laser used in optical fiber alignment or imaging calibration.
**Related Terms:** Optical QA, Alignment system.
**Example in Radiotherapy:** YAG laser aligns MRI-compatible fiducial arrays.

224. **Y-component (noun):** Vertical component in 3D spatial vector used in dose computation.
**Related Terms:** X-component, Z-component.
**Example in Radiotherapy:** Y-component error corrected in 6D table alignment.

225. **Y-trajectory (noun):** Vertical beam or particle path representation.
**Related Terms:** Beam path, Vector modeling.
**Example in Radiotherapy:** Y-trajectory deviation corrected in adaptive proton systems.

226. **Yield distribution function (noun):** Mathematical model describing yield across energies or targets.
**Related Terms:** Probability distribution, Spectrum analysis.
**Example in Radiotherapy:** Yield distribution function integrated into Monte Carlo code.

227. **Yield detector (noun):** Instrument measuring output particle count or photon flux.
**Related Terms:** Ion chamber, Faraday cup.
**Example in Radiotherapy:** Yield detector used in cyclotron QA.

228. **Y-irradiation coefficient (noun):** Factor quantifying absorbed gamma radiation per exposure unit.
**Related Terms:** Exposure coefficient, Dose constant.
**Example in Radiotherapy:** Y-irradiation coefficient calibrated for sealed sources.

229. **Yaw tolerance (noun):** Acceptable range of rotational deviation around vertical axis.
**Related Terms:** QA tolerance, Gantry alignment.
**Example in Radiotherapy:** Yaw tolerance limited to 0.5° in stereotactic QA.

230. **Yield attenuation (noun):** Reduction of output yield due to energy loss in absorbers.
**Related Terms:** Attenuation factor, Beam hardening.
**Example in Radiotherapy:** Yield attenuation measured through buildup region.

231. **Yield simulation (noun):** Computational modeling of expected particle or photon yields.
**Related Terms:** Monte Carlo, Beam modeling.
**Example in Radiotherapy:** Yield simulation validates new beamline commissioning.

232. **Y-axis rotation (noun):** Rotation movement around lateral patient axis.
**Related Terms:** Pitch, Roll.
**Example in Radiotherapy:** Y-axis rotation corrected using robotic couch.

233. **Yield verification (noun):** Experimental confirmation of simulated radiation yield.
**Related Terms:** QA, Validation.
**Example in Radiotherapy:** Yield verification required before clinical deployment.

234. **Yield analyzer (noun):** Electronic system recording radiation yield trends.
**Related Terms:** Output monitor, QA tool.
**Example in Radiotherapy:** Yield analyzer logs daily output variations.

235. **Yaw angle correction (noun):** Compensatory adjustment for rotational misalignment about vertical axis.
**Related Terms:** Image registration, 6D setup.
**Example in Radiotherapy:** Yaw angle correction optimized in adaptive workflows.

236. **Y-curve (noun):** Graph showing dependency of yield versus Y-coordinate.
**Related Terms:** Dose profile, Output mapping.
**Example in Radiotherapy:** Y-curve analyzed during beam symmetry checks.

237. **Yield enhancement coefficient (noun):** Quantitative measure of improvement in radiation output.
**Related Terms:** Efficiency gain, Calibration.
**Example in Radiotherapy:** Yield enhancement coefficient improved after magnet tuning.

238. **Yield fraction (noun):** Proportion of total yield delivered to clinical beam.
**Related Terms:** Beam utilization, Output ratio.
**Example in Radiotherapy:** Yield fraction adjusted during cyclotron optimization.

239. **Y-gate signal (noun):** Synchronization trigger for Y-axis motion in imaging systems.
**Related Terms:** Gating, Motion synchronization.
**Example in Radiotherapy:** Y-gate used for respiratory tracking in MR-Linac.

240. **Yield efficiency index (noun):** Performance metric summarizing system output efficiency.
**Related Terms:** Output factor, QA.
**Example in Radiotherapy:** Yield efficiency index benchmarked across linear accelerators.

241. **Yield fluctuation (noun):** Short-term variation in radiation output due to instability.
**Related Terms:** Output variation, QA monitoring.
**Example in Radiotherapy:** Yield fluctuation observed during high-current proton extraction.

242. **Y-gantry system (noun):** Radiotherapy gantry optimized for precise Y-axis rotation control.
**Related Terms:** Gantry rotation, Mechanical alignment.
**Example in Radiotherapy:** Y-gantry system ensures accurate lateral beam placement.

243. **Y-component drift (noun):** Gradual shift of beam or couch position along Y-axis.
**Related Terms:** Positional error, Couch correction.
**Example in Radiotherapy:** Y-component drift corrected using daily CBCT verification.

244. **Yield homogeneity (noun):** Uniformity of radiation yield across treatment field.
**Related Terms:** Field uniformity, Beam flatness.
**Example in Radiotherapy:** Yield homogeneity verified during electron field QA.

245. **Yield histogram (noun):** Statistical representation of measured yield data frequency.
**Related Terms:** Data analysis, QA trend.
**Example in Radiotherapy:** Yield histogram analyzed for machine stability patterns.

246. **Yield intensity map (noun):** Spatial distribution image of radiation yield intensity.
**Related Terms:** Fluence map, Beam profiling.
**Example in Radiotherapy:** Yield intensity map compared across gantry angles.

247. **Y-axis correction factor (noun):** Numerical constant applied to correct Y-coordinate errors.
**Related Terms:** Positional correction, Calibration.
**Example in Radiotherapy:** Y-axis correction factor updated post-MLC maintenance.

248. **Yield kinetics (noun):** Temporal rate of change in radiation yield.
**Related Terms:** Output stability, Beam dynamics.
**Example in Radiotherapy:** Yield kinetics assessed during beam startup ramp.

249. **Yield measurement uncertainty (noun):** Quantitative uncertainty in determining actual yield value.
**Related Terms:** Dosimetric accuracy, Calibration error.
**Example in Radiotherapy:** Yield measurement uncertainty included in daily QA report.

250. **Yield management system (noun):** Software tracking dose output and beam efficiency.
**Related Terms:** QA software, Performance tracking.
**Example in Radiotherapy:** Yield management system alerts deviations from reference trends.

251. **Yield normalization coefficient (noun):** Adjustment parameter to align measured and reference yields.
**Related Terms:** Calibration constant, QA scaling.
**Example in Radiotherapy:** Yield normalization coefficient recalculated after target replacement.

252. **Yield optimization matrix (noun):** Algorithmic grid optimizing yield across beamline parameters.
**Related Terms:** Beam tuning, Multi-variable optimization.
**Example in Radiotherapy:** Yield optimization matrix used during cyclotron commissioning.

253. **Y-axis synchronization (noun):** Coordinated motion control for couch and gantry along Y-axis.
**Related Terms:** Motion integration, 6D positioning.
**Example in Radiotherapy:** Y-axis synchronization ensured during adaptive replanning.

254. **Yield proportionality (noun):** Linear relationship between beam current and output yield.
**Related Terms:** Output constancy, Calibration.
**Example in Radiotherapy:** Yield proportionality confirmed within 2% deviation tolerance.

255. **Yield reproducibility (noun):** Ability of the beamline to reproduce identical yield outputs.
**Related Terms:** Machine stability, QA constancy.
**Example in Radiotherapy:** Yield reproducibility validated using weekly check logs.

256. **Y-portal imaging (noun):** Lateral projection imaging technique aligned with Y-axis.
**Related Terms:** Orthogonal imaging, Verification imaging.
**Example in Radiotherapy:** Y-portal image acquired for lateral setup confirmation.

257. **Yield scatter (noun):** Undesired spread of secondary yield particles or photons.
**Related Terms:** Scatter radiation, Beam purity.
**Example in Radiotherapy:** Yield scatter minimized using optimized collimation design.

258. **Yield signal processing (noun):** Real-time analysis of yield detector output.
**Related Terms:** Signal filtering, QA automation.
**Example in Radiotherapy:** Yield signal processing detects transient beam interruptions.

259. **Yield variance index (noun):** Metric representing deviation of yield data from mean.
**Related Terms:** QA analytics, Process control.
**Example in Radiotherapy:** Yield variance index monitored for beam reproducibility.

260. **Yoke assembly alignment (noun):** Calibration ensuring accurate magnetic field geometry.
**Related Terms:** Magnet alignment, Beam steering.
**Example in Radiotherapy:** Yoke assembly alignment verified during annual QA.

261. **Yield waveform (noun):** Graphical display of yield intensity versus time.
**Related Terms:** Time-series data, Output profile.
**Example in Radiotherapy:** Yield waveform analysis reveals transient output dips.

262. **Yield-weighted averaging (noun):** Averaging technique emphasizing higher yield measurements.
**Related Terms:** Weighted mean, Statistical correction.
**Example in Radiotherapy:** Yield-weighted averaging improves beam output modeling.

263. **Yield window (noun):** Acceptable operational range of output yield.
**Related Terms:** Tolerance band, QA limit.
**Example in Radiotherapy:** Yield window set between 98%–102% of nominal.

264. **Yield-zero condition (noun):** Machine state with zero active radiation yield.
**Related Terms:** Beam off, Interlock.
**Example in Radiotherapy:** Yield-zero condition triggered during emergency shutdown.

265. **Y-chromosome assay (noun):** Cytogenetic test used in radiation biodosimetry.
**Related Terms:** Chromosomal aberration, Biological dosimeter.
**Example in Radiotherapy:** Y-chromosome assay estimates occupational exposure.

266. **Yield feedback loop (noun):** Automated system adjusting output based on yield readings.
**Related Terms:** Control loop, Real-time correction.
**Example in Radiotherapy:** Yield feedback loop stabilizes particle current.

267. **Yield harmonization (noun):** Process aligning yields between multiple accelerators.
**Related Terms:** Machine calibration, Inter-center QA.
**Example in Radiotherapy:** Yield harmonization ensures cross-site treatment uniformity.

268. **Yield correction coefficient (noun):** Numeric factor correcting raw yield data to true output.
**Related Terms:** Calibration constant, QA correction.
**Example in Radiotherapy:** Yield correction coefficient verified post-detector replacement.

269. **Yaw-motion tracking (noun):** Continuous monitoring of gantry yaw angle.
**Related Terms:** Motion tracking, Mechanical QA.
**Example in Radiotherapy:** Yaw-motion tracking critical for MR-Linac precision.

270. **Yield reference dataset (noun):** Baseline data collection used for QA comparisons.
**Related Terms:** Benchmark dataset, Reference curve.
**Example in Radiotherapy:** Yield reference dataset updated annually.

271. **Yield simulation algorithm (noun):** Computational method predicting expected yield under variable inputs.
**Related Terms:** Monte Carlo, Predictive modeling.
**Example in Radiotherapy:** Yield simulation algorithm validates proton source output.

272. **Y-axis drift correction (noun):** Adjustment compensating for gradual Y-position shift.
**Related Terms:** Positional calibration, Couch QA.
**Example in Radiotherapy:** Y-axis drift correction executed via auto-calibration.

273. **Yield safety threshold (noun):** Maximum safe radiation yield before automatic shutdown.
**Related Terms:** Interlock system, Beam protection.
**Example in Radiotherapy:** Yield safety threshold set for neutron suppression.

274. **Y-parameter mapping (noun):** Visualization of Y-parameter variations across beam energy.
**Related Terms:** Dose mapping, Energy profiling.
**Example in Radiotherapy:** Y-parameter mapping performed during beamline QA.

275. **Yield calibration log (noun):** Record documenting yield measurements and calibration cycles.
**Related Terms:** QA documentation, Machine log.
**Example in Radiotherapy:** Yield calibration log stored for regulatory review.

276. **Yield linearity test (noun):** Procedure verifying output proportionality across beam intensities.
**Related Terms:** Linearity check, Output QA.
**Example in Radiotherapy:** Yield linearity test performed quarterly for linac stability.

277. **Y-axis localization (noun):** Accurate determination of position along lateral axis.
**Related Terms:** Spatial accuracy, Setup verification.
**Example in Radiotherapy:** Y-axis localization refined using orthogonal kV imaging.

278. **Yield matrix (noun):** Tabular dataset representing multidimensional yield correlations.
**Related Terms:** Data matrix, Statistical QA.
**Example in Radiotherapy:** Yield matrix analyzed for trend prediction.

279. **Yield normalization error (noun):** Deviation arising from incorrect yield reference scaling.
**Related Terms:** Calibration error, QA discrepancy.
**Example in Radiotherapy:** Yield normalization error corrected during recalibration.

280. **Yield oscillation (noun):** Cyclic fluctuation in output due to resonance effects.
**Related Terms:** Beam instability, Frequency modulation.
**Example in Radiotherapy:** Yield oscillation minimized via magnet current stabilization.

281. **Yield optimization constant (noun):** Fixed value used to fine-tune output efficiency during beam tuning.
**Related Terms:** Calibration factor, QA optimization.
**Example in Radiotherapy:** Yield optimization constant adjusted to stabilize cyclotron current output.

282. **Yield offset correction (noun):** Adjustment to compensate baseline deviation in measured yield values.
**Related Terms:** Baseline drift, QA correction.
**Example in Radiotherapy:** Yield offset correction implemented after detector recalibration.

283. **Yield pattern mapping (noun):** Graphical representation showing spatial yield distribution.
**Related Terms:** Fluence pattern, Beam uniformity.
**Example in Radiotherapy:** Yield pattern mapping used in electron cone field verification.

284. **Yield perturbation (noun):** Localized variation in yield caused by heterogeneity or equipment error.
**Related Terms:** Output fluctuation, Beam irregularity.
**Example in Radiotherapy:** Yield perturbation analyzed during Monte Carlo validation.

285. **Yield prediction model (noun):** Mathematical model forecasting yield response under varying conditions.
**Related Terms:** Predictive QA, Simulation model.
**Example in Radiotherapy:** Yield prediction model supports adaptive dose control.

286. **Yield precision factor (noun):** Quantitative measure indicating consistency of yield measurements.
**Related Terms:** QA precision, Reproducibility.
**Example in Radiotherapy:** Yield precision factor exceeded 99% during annual QA audit.

287. **Yield recalibration protocol (noun):** Standard procedure for restoring accurate yield after deviation.
**Related Terms:** QA protocol, Machine calibration.
**Example in Radiotherapy:** Yield recalibration protocol executed post-detector upgrade.

288. **Yield reference alignment (noun):** Process aligning yield readings with reference system standards.
**Related Terms:** Cross-calibration, QA harmonization.
**Example in Radiotherapy:** Yield reference alignment maintained across multiple beamlines.

289. **Yield regularity index (noun):** Indicator reflecting uniformity of yield outputs over time.
**Related Terms:** Stability index, QA metric.
**Example in Radiotherapy:** Yield regularity index remained within tolerance during beam stability check.

290. **Yield response curve (noun):** Graph showing yield variation with changing beam parameters.
**Related Terms:** Response function, Output curve.
**Example in Radiotherapy:** Yield response curve used in energy-dependence evaluation.

291. **Yield reproducibility test (noun):** Experimental verification of consistent yield reproduction under identical conditions.
**Related Terms:** QA testing, Constancy check.
**Example in Radiotherapy:** Yield reproducibility test confirmed linear accelerator stability.

292. **Yield restoration (noun):** Re-establishment of expected output after deviation or shutdown.
**Related Terms:** Machine recovery, QA reinitialization.
**Example in Radiotherapy:** Yield restoration achieved following magnet power interruption.

293. **Yield scaling factor (noun):** Multiplier used to normalize yield data to standard reference.
**Related Terms:** Scaling correction, Calibration coefficient.
**Example in Radiotherapy:** Yield scaling factor recalculated following detector sensitivity drift.

294. **Yield signal drift (noun):** Gradual change in detector signal affecting yield accuracy.
**Related Terms:** Signal degradation, Baseline shift.
**Example in Radiotherapy:** Yield signal drift corrected by recalibration routine.

295. **Yield simulation matrix (noun):** Data framework modeling yield variability across operating conditions.
**Related Terms:** Statistical matrix, Predictive analytics.
**Example in Radiotherapy:** Yield simulation matrix used for output verification.

296. **Yield stability test (noun):** Assessment ensuring output remains constant within defined limits.
**Related Terms:** QA constancy test, Output stability.
**Example in Radiotherapy:** Yield stability test performed daily before treatment delivery.

297. **Yield standard deviation (noun):** Statistical measure of variation among yield measurements.
**Related Terms:** Data variance, QA analysis.
**Example in Radiotherapy:** Yield standard deviation below 1% indicates machine reliability.

298. **Yield threshold detector (noun):** Sensor triggering alarm when output exceeds predefined limit.
**Related Terms:** Interlock, Radiation monitor.
**Example in Radiotherapy:** Yield threshold detector ensures patient safety in proton therapy.

299. **Yield tolerance band (noun):** Acceptable deviation range for measured yield values.
**Related Terms:** QA tolerance, Control limit.
**Example in Radiotherapy:** Yield tolerance band defined as ±2% for photon output.

300. **Yoke drift (noun):** Minor displacement of magnetic yoke affecting beam steering.
**Related Terms:** Magnet misalignment, QA deviation.
**Example in Radiotherapy:** Yoke drift adjusted during monthly mechanical QA.

301. **Yield transmission factor (noun):** Proportion of beam yield transmitted through attenuating material.
**Related Terms:** Transmission factor, Shielding efficiency.
**Example in Radiotherapy:** Yield transmission factor evaluated for beam modulator design.

302. **Yield uniformity map (noun):** 2D display showing uniformity of dose output across field.
**Related Terms:** Beam flatness, QA mapping.
**Example in Radiotherapy:** Yield uniformity map used during beam commissioning.

303. **Yield verification scan (noun):** QA procedure validating spatial and output accuracy.
**Related Terms:** Output verification, QA imaging.
**Example in Radiotherapy:** Yield verification scan repeated post-source replacement.

304. **Y-offset correction (noun):** Calibration adjustment compensating lateral misalignment along Y-axis.
**Related Terms:** Couch correction, Spatial calibration.
**Example in Radiotherapy:** Y-offset correction applied using CBCT-based auto-registration.

305. **Yield vector field (noun):** Mathematical representation of yield direction and magnitude.
**Related Terms:** Vector analysis, Dose modeling.
**Example in Radiotherapy:** Yield vector field modeled in Monte Carlo simulations.

306. **Yield waveform analyzer (noun):** Device capturing and interpreting temporal yield fluctuations.
**Related Terms:** Data logger, QA instrumentation.
**Example in Radiotherapy:** Yield waveform analyzer detects transient beam instabilities.

307. **Yield-weighted exposure (noun):** Exposure measurement adjusted by relative yield contribution.
**Related Terms:** Weighted dose, Normalization.
**Example in Radiotherapy:** Yield-weighted exposure calculated during composite plan QA.

308. **Yield zeroing protocol (noun):** QA procedure for resetting yield to baseline condition.
**Related Terms:** Initialization, Machine warm-up.
**Example in Radiotherapy:** Yield zeroing protocol performed before daily calibration.

309. **Yttrium decay mapping (noun):** Visualization of decay kinetics in Y-90 based therapies.
**Related Terms:** Decay mapping, SPECT analysis.
**Example in Radiotherapy:** Yttrium decay mapping confirms post-radioembolization uniformity.

310. **Yaw calibration matrix (noun):** Set of parameters defining gantry rotational calibration.
**Related Terms:** Rotational correction, Gantry QA.
**Example in Radiotherapy:** Yaw calibration matrix updated post-mechanical maintenance.

311. **Yield attenuation model (noun):** Mathematical model describing yield reduction through materials.
**Related Terms:** Attenuation law, Beam hardening.
**Example in Radiotherapy:** Yield attenuation model validated for heterogeneous phantom studies.

312. **Yield confidence interval (noun):** Statistical boundary representing uncertainty in yield estimation.
**Related Terms:** Confidence limits, QA analysis.
**Example in Radiotherapy:** Yield confidence interval reported for clinical audits.

313. **Yield correction protocol (noun):** Standardized QA method for correcting yield deviations.
**Related Terms:** Calibration protocol, Output correction.
**Example in Radiotherapy:** Yield correction protocol executed post-detector drift event.

314. **Yield control chart (noun):** Graph used for tracking yield stability over time.
**Related Terms:** SPC chart, QA trend.
**Example in Radiotherapy:** Yield control chart identifies long-term performance drift.

315. **Yield difference ratio (noun):** Ratio comparing deviation between measured and expected yield.
**Related Terms:** Error ratio, QA discrepancy.
**Example in Radiotherapy:** Yield difference ratio remained within 1.5% tolerance.

316. **Yield energy profile (noun):** Curve showing yield as function of beam energy.
**Related Terms:** Output profile, Energy spectrum.
**Example in Radiotherapy:** Yield energy profile analyzed for proton nozzle optimization.

317. **Yield envelope (noun):** Boundary defining operational yield limits across beam settings.
**Related Terms:** Operating window, QA range.
**Example in Radiotherapy:** Yield envelope verified during linac commissioning.

318. **Yield evaluation software (noun):** Program analyzing and reporting yield-based QA data.
**Related Terms:** QA automation, Analysis tool.
**Example in Radiotherapy:** Yield evaluation software integrated into departmental QA system.

319. **Yield fluctuation range (noun):** Extent of variation in radiation yield readings.
**Related Terms:** Output variation, QA metric.
**Example in Radiotherapy:** Yield fluctuation range constrained within ±1%.

320. **Yield homogeneity test (noun):** Procedure ensuring consistent dose output across the field.
**Related Terms:** Flatness test, QA validation.
**Example in Radiotherapy:** Yield homogeneity test completed for 10×10 cm field.

321. **Yield intensity ratio (noun):** Comparison of measured to nominal yield intensity.
**Related Terms:** Output ratio, Calibration factor.
**Example in Radiotherapy:** Yield intensity ratio consistent across gantry rotations.

322. **Yield intercomparison study (noun):** Cross-institutional QA comparing yield consistency between centers.
**Related Terms:** Audit, Standardization.
**Example in Radiotherapy:** Yield intercomparison study conducted under IAEA protocol.

**323. Yield logarithmic scale (noun):** Log-based representation of yield data for wide-range comparison.
**Related Terms:** Log scale, Data transformation.
**Example in Radiotherapy:** Yield logarithmic scale used for proton beam analysis.

**324. Yield matching coefficient (noun):** Parameter indicating correlation between predicted and actual yields.
**Related Terms:** QA correlation, Model accuracy.
**Example in Radiotherapy:** Yield matching coefficient improved after recalibration.

**325. Yield normalization algorithm (noun):** Software function adjusting data to reference yield level.
**Related Terms:** QA correction, Data processing.
**Example in Radiotherapy:** Yield normalization algorithm applied in automated QA system.

**326. Yield offset analysis (noun):** Evaluation of systematic deviation from baseline yield.
**Related Terms:** QA offset, Calibration drift.
**Example in Radiotherapy:** Yield offset analysis revealed detector sensitivity changes post-maintenance.

**327. Yield prediction matrix (noun):** Multivariable data structure forecasting yield outcomes.
**Related Terms:** Predictive modeling, Data analytics.
**Example in Radiotherapy:** Yield prediction matrix used for adaptive QA trend forecasting.

**328. Yield quality audit (noun):** Comprehensive verification of beam output consistency.
**Related Terms:** External audit, QA assessment.
**Example in Radiotherapy:** Yield quality audit performed annually to meet accreditation standards.

**329. Yield quantification protocol (noun):**Standardized procedure for measuring beam yield accuracy.
**Related Terms:** Measurement protocol, QA standard.
**Example in Radiotherapy:** Yield quantification protocol aligned with IEC dosimetry norms.

**330. Yield range assessment (noun):** Process determining operational limits of yield stability.
**Related Terms:** Control range, QA verification.
**Example in Radiotherapy:** Yield range assessment confirmed reproducible output within 2% variation.

**331. Yield reconstruction algorithm (noun):** Mathematical process reconstructing yield data from incomplete sets.
**Related Terms:** Data interpolation, QA computation.
**Example in Radiotherapy:** Yield reconstruction algorithm enhanced missing detector array readings.

**332. Yield reproducibility coefficient (noun):** Numerical index expressing repeatability of yield results.
**Related Terms:** Reproducibility index, QA performance.
**Example in Radiotherapy:** Yield reproducibility coefficient maintained above 0.98 for clinical operation.

**333. Yield response evaluation (noun):** Quantitative analysis of output sensitivity to operational change.
**Related Terms:** System response, QA sensitivity test.
**Example in Radiotherapy:** Yield response evaluation conducted after beam energy upgrade.

**334. Yield sensitivity index (noun):** Metric describing dependency of yield on external parameters.
**Related Terms:** Sensitivity coefficient, QA metric.
**Example in Radiotherapy:** Yield sensitivity index validated for environmental temperature variation.

335. **Yield standardization framework (noun):** Organizational model ensuring uniform QA yield practice.
**Related Terms:** QA governance, Policy harmonization.
**Example in Radiotherapy:** Yield standardization framework adopted across multiple oncology centers.

336. **Yield symmetry test (noun):** Quality control check ensuring uniformity across beam halves.
**Related Terms:** Symmetry evaluation, Beam balance.
**Example in Radiotherapy:** Yield symmetry test confirmed alignment of X and Y field axes.

337. **Yield traceability log (noun):** Chronological record documenting yield changes over time.
**Related Terms:** QA record, Output documentation.
**Example in Radiotherapy:** Yield traceability log maintained electronically for audit compliance.

338. **Yield tuning parameter (noun):** Adjustable variable influencing beam output optimization.
**Related Terms:** Calibration variable, Optimization setting.
**Example in Radiotherapy:** Yield tuning parameter fine-tuned to match absolute dose calibration.

339. **Yield uncertainty index (noun):** Quantitative measure reflecting confidence in yield accuracy.
**Related Terms:** Measurement uncertainty, QA reliability.
**Example in Radiotherapy:** Yield uncertainty index remained below 0.5% during calibration audit.

340. **Yield verification log (noun):** System record verifying periodic output constancy.
**Related Terms:** QA logbook, Verification report.
**Example in Radiotherapy:** Yield verification log integrated into automated QA software.

341. **Yield-volume histogram (noun):** Graph showing distribution of yield or dose intensity by volume.
**Related Terms:** DVH, Dose distribution.
**Example in Radiotherapy:** Yield-volume histogram analyzed for stereotactic beam evaluation.

342. **Yield-weighted average (noun):** Statistical mean adjusted for proportional yield contribution.
**Related Terms:** Weighted mean, Statistical normalization.
**Example in Radiotherapy:** Yield-weighted average computed during multi-beam plan QA.

343. **Yoke misalignment (noun):** Mechanical deviation of magnetic yoke affecting beam trajectory.
**Related Terms:** Gantry alignment, QA error.
**Example in Radiotherapy:** Yoke misalignment corrected through magnet recalibration.

344. **Yoke field stabilization (noun):** Process of maintaining consistent magnetic field distribution.
**Related Terms:** Magnet stability, QA control.
**Example in Radiotherapy:** Yoke field stabilization ensured uniform beam steering accuracy.

345. **Y-axis correction protocol (noun):** Standard QA procedure for compensating positional error along Y-axis.
**Related Terms:** Couch shift, Alignment correction.
**Example in Radiotherapy:** Y-axis correction protocol used in patient setup verification.

346. **Y-axis distortion (noun):** Non-linear deviation along vertical imaging axis.
**Related Terms:** Image distortion, Geometric correction.
**Example in Radiotherapy:** Y-axis distortion minimized using image calibration grid.

347. **Yaw drift compensation (noun):** Adjustment to correct gradual rotation deviation in gantry.
**Related Terms:** Rotational correction, Mechanical QA.
**Example in Radiotherapy:** Yaw drift compensation verified via laser alignment test.

348. **Yaw offset calibration (noun):** Procedure aligning rotational axis to reference position.
**Related Terms:** Gantry calibration, QA adjustment.
**Example in Radiotherapy:** Yaw offset calibration performed quarterly to ensure beam accuracy.

349. **Yaw reproducibility (noun):** Ability to maintain consistent rotation angle through repeated cycles.
**Related Terms:** Mechanical reproducibility, QA precision.
**Example in Radiotherapy:** Yaw reproducibility assessed during image-guided QA check.

350. **Yield-energy coupling (noun):** Relationship between yield output and beam energy level.
**Related Terms:** Energy dependency, Calibration curve.
**Example in Radiotherapy:** Yield-energy coupling analyzed to optimize photon beam modeling.

351. **Yield cross-section (noun):** Effective area describing interaction probability influencing yield.
**Related Terms:** Reaction cross-section, Nuclear physics.
**Example in Radiotherapy:** Yield cross-section used in modeling secondary neutron generation.

352. **Yttrium-90 microspheres (noun):** Beta-emitting particles for selective internal radiotherapy.
**Related Terms:** Radioembolization, Brachytherapy.
**Example in Radiotherapy:** Yttrium-90 microspheres administered for hepatic metastases.

353. **Yttrium-90 decay curve (noun):** Graph showing activity decrease of Y-90 over time.
**Related Terms:** Radioactive decay, Isotope kinetics.
**Example in Radiotherapy:** Yttrium-90 decay curve used to determine post-treatment dose rate.

354. **Yttrium generator (noun):** Device producing Y-90 from parent isotope Sr-90.
**Related Terms:** Isotope generator, Radiopharmaceutical source.
**Example in Radiotherapy:** Yttrium generator activity monitored under regulatory control.

355. **Yaw encoder (noun):** Sensor that records rotational position of gantry axis.
**Related Terms:** Motion sensor, Mechanical calibration.
**Example in Radiotherapy:** Yaw encoder recalibrated during annual machine QA.

356. **Yield phase stability (noun):** Consistency of output during cyclical beam delivery phases.
**Related Terms:** Phase locking, Output synchronization.
**Example in Radiotherapy:** Yield phase stability critical for gated delivery QA.

357. **Yield fractionation ratio (noun):** Proportion of dose yield distributed across fractions.
**Related Terms:** Fractionation scheme, Dose delivery.
**Example in Radiotherapy:** Yield fractionation ratio validated for hypofractionated SBRT.

358. **Yield modulation system (noun):** Control mechanism for adjusting yield dynamically during beam-on.
**Related Terms:** IMRT modulation, QA feedback.
**Example in Radiotherapy:** Yield modulation system ensures precise fluence control.

359. **Yield-detection algorithm (noun):** Software logic detecting abnormal yield fluctuations.
**Related Terms:** Anomaly detection, QA automation.
**Example in Radiotherapy:** Yield-detection algorithm triggered alarm for energy drift.

360. **Y-axis collimator calibration (noun):** Alignment verification of Y-axis jaws for beam shaping.
**Related Terms:** Collimator QA, Geometric calibration.
**Example in Radiotherapy:** Y-axis collimator calibration verified through star-shot test.

361. **Yield recovery coefficient (noun):** Parameter quantifying restoration efficiency after correction.
**Related Terms:** QA recovery, Calibration constant.
**Example in Radiotherapy:** Yield recovery coefficient remained >0.98 after recalibration.

362. **Yield validation curve (noun):** Plot representing accuracy of yield prediction models.
**Related Terms:** QA validation, Model verification.
**Example in Radiotherapy:** Yield validation curve used to confirm TPS accuracy.

363. **Yield harmonic fluctuation (noun):** Periodic variation of output influenced by AC frequency.
**Related Terms:** Electrical noise, Power modulation.
**Example in Radiotherapy:** Yield harmonic fluctuation minimized using power stabilizers.

364. **Y-axis rotation matrix (noun):** Mathematical representation of Y-axis rotational transformation.
**Related Terms:** Transformation matrix, Image registration.
**Example in Radiotherapy:** Y-axis rotation matrix integrated into rigid-body alignment model.

365. **Yield isocenter tolerance (noun):** Permissible deviation of yield from isocenter during delivery.
**Related Terms:** Isocentric accuracy, QA tolerance.
**Example in Radiotherapy:** Yield isocenter tolerance set at ±1 mm.

366. **Yield correlation function (noun):** Mathematical expression showing relationship between yield variables.
**Related Terms:** Correlation coefficient, Data analysis.
**Example in Radiotherapy:** Yield correlation function modeled to predict beam drift.

367. **Yoke alignment gauge (noun):** Tool used to measure magnet yoke position accuracy.
**Related Terms:** Mechanical QA tool, Alignment check.
**Example in Radiotherapy:** Yoke alignment gauge applied during gantry maintenance.

368. **Yield optimization software (noun):** Computational tool enhancing output efficiency via algorithms.
**Related Terms:** QA automation, Performance optimization.
**Example in Radiotherapy:** Yield optimization software integrated with treatment planning QA.

369. **Yield synchronization test (noun):** QA test verifying timing consistency between subsystems.
**Related Terms:** Synchronization test, System timing.
**Example in Radiotherapy:** Yield synchronization test validated gating accuracy.

370. **Yaw angular offset (noun):** Rotational deviation in gantry yaw alignment.
**Related Terms:** Mechanical offset, Rotational error.
**Example in Radiotherapy:** Yaw angular offset corrected by optical tracking QA.

371. **Yield-drift detector (noun):** Instrument detecting deviations in yield output trend.
**Related Terms:** Drift monitor, QA sensor.
**Example in Radiotherapy:** Yield-drift detector automatically logs daily beam stability.

372. **Yield-based feedback control (noun):** Automated correction mechanism using real-time yield data.
**Related Terms:** Feedback loop, Real-time QA.
**Example in Radiotherapy:** Yield-based feedback control maintains consistent proton fluence.

373. **Y-axis dosimetric scan (noun):** Measurement of dose profile along Y dimension.
**Related Terms:** Profile scan, QA analysis.
**Example in Radiotherapy:** Y-axis dosimetric scan confirmed uniform field flatness.

374. **Yaw motion compensator (noun):** Device mitigating rotational deviations during delivery.
**Related Terms:** Motion correction, Mechanical control.
**Example in Radiotherapy:** Yaw motion compensator reduced image-to-beam misalignment.

375. **Yield normalization curve (noun):** Plot showing standardization of yield response over energy range.
**Related Terms:** Calibration curve, Response normalization.
**Example in Radiotherapy:** Yield normalization curve used for energy cross-checking.

376. **Yield AI predictor (noun):** Machine learning system predicting output variation trends.
**Related Terms:** AI QA model, Predictive analysis.
**Example in Radiotherapy:** Yield AI predictor trained on three-year QA datasets.

377. **Yield error classifier (noun):** AI model categorizing yield deviations by source.
**Related Terms:** Error taxonomy, ML detection.
**Example in Radiotherapy:** Yield error classifier differentiates between electronic noise and drift.

378. **Yield variance algorithm (noun):** Statistical method quantifying deviation within yield dataset.
**Related Terms:** Data analytics, QA statistics.
**Example in Radiotherapy:** Yield variance algorithm applied for automated performance review.

379. **Y-axis registration check (noun):** QA step verifying positional consistency along vertical axis.
**Related Terms:** Image registration, Setup QA.
**Example in Radiotherapy:** Y-axis registration check performed before each CBCT match.

380. **Yaw lock mechanism (noun):** Mechanical fixture ensuring stable gantry rotation position.
**Related Terms:** Locking system, Mechanical QA.
**Example in Radiotherapy:** Yaw lock mechanism engaged during calibration.

381. **Yield-drift compensation curve (noun):** Correction curve used to restore nominal output after drift.
**Related Terms:** Compensation model, QA adjustment.
**Example in Radiotherapy:** Yield-drift compensation curve recalibrated quarterly.

382. **Yield-trend dashboard (noun):** QA interface displaying long-term yield performance data.
**Related Terms:** Analytics dashboard, Monitoring tool.
**Example in Radiotherapy:** Yield-trend dashboard used by physicists for performance review.

383. **Yield uniformity ratio (noun):** Numeric ratio comparing highest and lowest output readings.
**Related Terms:** Uniformity index, QA consistency.
**Example in Radiotherapy:** Yield uniformity ratio within 1.02 indicates optimal flatness.

384. **Yield-variance threshold (noun):**Upper limit of acceptable output variability.
**Related Terms:** QA tolerance, Performance limit.
**Example in Radiotherapy:** Yield-variance threshold exceeded prompted recalibration.

385. **Yield-weighted optimization (noun):** Dose optimization considering yield contribution from multiple beams.
**Related Terms:** Beam weighting, Plan optimization.
**Example in Radiotherapy:** Yield-weighted optimization improved overall dose conformity.

386. **Yield zoning map (noun):** Spatial map dividing treatment field based on yield distribution.
**Related Terms:** Dose zoning, Field mapping.
**Example in Radiotherapy:** Yield zoning map utilized in adaptive proton planning.

387. **Yoke symmetry calibration (noun):** QA adjustment ensuring equal magnetic field strength across poles.
**Related Terms:** Magnet QA, Field calibration.
**Example in Radiotherapy:** Yoke symmetry calibration completed post-service realignment.

388. **Yaw error compensation matrix (noun):** Matrix used for correcting angular misalignments.
**Related Terms:** Correction algorithm, QA model.
**Example in Radiotherapy:** Yaw error compensation matrix embedded in machine controller.

389. **Yield harmonization program (noun):** Institutional initiative standardizing output QA across devices.
**Related Terms:** QA policy, Cross-calibration.
**Example in Radiotherapy:** Yield harmonization program improved inter-machine reproducibility.

390. **Yield degradation trend (noun):** Progressive reduction of output due to aging components.
**Related Terms:** Machine wear, Output decline.
**Example in Radiotherapy:** Yield degradation trend tracked for preemptive maintenance.

391. **Yield consistency verification (noun):** Test ensuring repeated yield stability under controlled conditions.
**Related Terms:** QA constancy, Reliability test.
**Example in Radiotherapy:** Yield consistency verification documented in daily QA report.

392. **Yield reference phantom (noun):** Standardized phantom used for output validation.
**Related Terms:** QA phantom, Reference device.
**Example in Radiotherapy:** Yield reference phantom used for monthly output cross-check.

393. **Yield recalibration software (noun):** Program facilitating automatic yield correction.
**Related Terms:** QA software, Recalibration module.
**Example in Radiotherapy:** Yield recalibration software streamlined periodic QA.

394. **Yield temporal drift (noun):** Change in yield over prolonged operational time.
**Related Terms:** Time-dependent error, Long-term drift.
**Example in Radiotherapy:** Yield temporal drift mitigated through weekly trending.

395. **Yield predictive dashboard (noun):** Interface displaying AI-predicted yield stability forecasts.
**Related Terms:** Predictive QA, AI tool.
**Example in Radiotherapy:** Yield predictive dashboard flagged abnormal energy decay trend.

396. **Yield optimization kernel (noun):** Core computational module optimizing output uniformity.
**Related Terms:** Software kernel, Algorithmic control.
**Example in Radiotherapy:** Yield optimization kernel updated for new beam profiles.

397. **Yield QA harmonizer (noun):** Tool integrating data from multiple machines into one QA model.
**Related Terms:** Multi-unit QA, Data integration.
**Example in Radiotherapy:** Yield QA harmonizer synchronized linac output records.

398. **Yield signal integrity (noun):** Degree to which measurement data remains free from noise.
**Related Terms:** Data fidelity, Signal quality.
**Example in Radiotherapy:** Yield signal integrity ensured via shielded detector cabling.

399. **Yield modulation error (noun):** Deviation between planned and actual modulated outputs.
**Related Terms:** Delivery error, IMRT QA.
**Example in Radiotherapy:** Yield modulation error analyzed using gamma evaluation.

400. **Yield quantization noise (noun):** Digital noise introduced during analog-to-digital signal conversion.
**Related Terms:** ADC noise, Data processing.
**Example in Radiotherapy:** Yield quantization noise minimized through higher sampling rate.

401. **Yield signal reconstruction (noun):** Recreation of original yield waveform from partial or noisy data.
**Related Terms:** Signal recovery, Data reconstruction.
**Example in Radiotherapy:** Yield signal reconstruction applied for degraded detector data.

402. **Yield-matrix validation (noun):** Process confirming accuracy of yield distribution matrix.
**Related Terms:** QA validation, Data verification.
**Example in Radiotherapy:** Yield-matrix validation performed during TPS dose audit.

403. **Yoke field mapping (noun):** Spatial mapping of magnetic flux density across yoke structure.
**Related Terms:** Magnetic QA, Field uniformity.
**Example in Radiotherapy:** Yoke field mapping ensured even proton beam guidance.

404. **Yield optimization feedback (noun):** Loop adjusting system parameters to maintain optimal yield.
**Related Terms:** Feedback control, QA correction.
**Example in Radiotherapy:** Yield optimization feedback stabilized linac photon output.

**405. Yield-drift prediction model (noun):** Algorithm forecasting long-term output drift patterns.
**Related Terms:** Predictive QA, Machine learning.
**Example in Radiotherapy:** Yield-drift prediction model reduced unplanned downtime.

**406. Yield harmonics suppression (noun):** Technique to eliminate unwanted oscillatory yield fluctuations.
**Related Terms:** Harmonic filtering, Output stabilization.
**Example in Radiotherapy:** Yield harmonics suppression improved linac energy constancy.

**407. Yield QA integration (noun):** Unification of yield monitoring into clinical QA framework.
**Related Terms:** QA workflow, Process standardization.
**Example in Radiotherapy:** Yield QA integration automated beam audit reporting.

**408. Yield residual variance (noun):** Remaining unexplained variation in output after correction.
**Related Terms:** Statistical residual, QA error.
**Example in Radiotherapy:** Yield residual variance below 0.3% post-calibration.

**409. Yield self-calibration (noun):** System autonomously recalibrating yield using internal references.
**Related Terms:** Auto-calibration, Smart QA.
**Example in Radiotherapy:** Yield self-calibration implemented in modern MR-Linacs.

**410. Yield saturation point (noun):** Maximum attainable yield beyond which no increase occurs.
**Related Terms:** Output plateau, Beam limitation.
**Example in Radiotherapy:** Yield saturation point identified in electron gun studies.

**411. Yaw tracking algorithm (noun):** Software tracking gantry rotational displacement over time.
**Related Terms:** Motion tracking, QA software.
**Example in Radiotherapy:** Yaw tracking algorithm verified stereotactic delivery stability.

**412. Y-axis distortion correction (noun):** Adjustment algorithm removing geometric image distortions.
**Related Terms:** Image correction, Geometric QA.
**Example in Radiotherapy:** Y-axis distortion correction applied in MRI-Linac imaging.

**413. Yield uniformity map (noun):** Visual representation of output consistency across the field.
**Related Terms:** Fluence map, Beam uniformity.
**Example in Radiotherapy:** Yield uniformity map reviewed during flatness QA.

**414. Yield control limit (noun):** Defined tolerance boundary for acceptable yield variation.
**Related Terms:** QA limit, Tolerance band.
**Example in Radiotherapy:** Yield control limit maintained at ±1.5%.

**415. Yield function modeling (noun):** Mathematical description of output behavior under conditions.
**Related Terms:** Function fitting, Analytical modeling.
**Example in Radiotherapy:** Yield function modeling refined Monte Carlo simulations.

**416. Yield spectral density (noun):** Power distribution of yield fluctuations over frequency domain.
**Related Terms:** Signal analysis, Noise spectrum.
**Example in Radiotherapy:** Yield spectral density used to identify electrical interference.

**417. Yield trend analytics (noun):** Statistical evaluation of long-term yield performance trends.
**Related Terms:** QA analytics, Data visualization.
**Example in Radiotherapy:** Yield trend analytics revealed seasonal output variation.

**418. Yield restoration coefficient (noun):** Ratio measuring system recovery efficiency post-error correction.
**Related Terms:** Correction efficiency, QA coefficient.
**Example in Radiotherapy:** Yield restoration coefficient maintained above 0.99.

419. **Yield verification phantom (noun):** Phantom used to confirm consistent yield output and dose rate.
**Related Terms:** QA phantom, Output verification.
**Example in Radiotherapy:** Yield verification phantom employed for proton beam calibration.

420. **Yield baseline tracker (noun):** System continuously monitoring yield against historical baseline.
**Related Terms:** Performance tracker, QA monitoring.
**Example in Radiotherapy:** Yield baseline tracker issued auto-alerts for deviation.

421. **Yttrium-labeled compound (noun):** Molecular complex tagged with radioactive yttrium isotope.
**Related Terms:** Radiopharmaceutical, Therapeutic isotope.
**Example in Radiotherapy:** Yttrium-labeled antibodies applied in radionuclide therapy.

422. **Yield data fusion (noun):** Combining multiple yield datasets for unified interpretation.
**Related Terms:** Data integration, Multisource analysis.
**Example in Radiotherapy:** Yield data fusion improved QA sensitivity.

423. **Yield extrapolation (noun):** Estimation of yield beyond measured range.
**Related Terms:** Predictive modeling, Data extension.
**Example in Radiotherapy:** Yield extrapolation used in beamline energy scaling.

424. **Yield redundancy module (noun):** Backup system ensuring yield stability during faults.
**Related Terms:** Fail-safe, QA reliability.
**Example in Radiotherapy:** Yield redundancy module engaged during dose delivery.

425. **Yield benchmarking study (noun):** Comparative analysis across multiple centers' yield data.
**Related Terms:** QA benchmarking, Multicenter audit.
**Example in Radiotherapy:** Yield benchmarking study identified machine drift trends.

426. **Yield interpolation grid (noun):** Computational matrix estimating intermediate yield values.
**Related Terms:** Interpolation, QA modeling.
**Example in Radiotherapy:** Yield interpolation grid filled missing detector data points.

427. **Yield correction map (noun):** 2D array compensating for spatial yield non-uniformities.
**Related Terms:** Correction profile, QA mapping.
**Example in Radiotherapy:** Yield correction map integrated into beam model tuning.

428. **Yield stability test (noun):** Quality control test assessing short-term output consistency.
**Related Terms:** Constancy check, Machine QA.
**Example in Radiotherapy:** Yield stability test confirmed <0.5% variation daily.

429. **Yield calibration drift (noun):** Slow change in output calibration over time.
**Related Terms:** Calibration shift, QA drift.
**Example in Radiotherapy:** Yield calibration drift corrected using annual recalibration.

430. **Yield isolation circuit (noun):** Electrical system preventing feedback-induced output distortion.
**Related Terms:** Circuit isolation, Electrical QA.
**Example in Radiotherapy:** Yield isolation circuit ensured clean detector signal.

431. **Yaw alignment module (noun):** Hardware ensuring accurate gantry rotation centering.
**Related Terms:** Alignment device, Mechanical QA.
**Example in Radiotherapy:** Yaw alignment module verified with optical tracking system.

432. **Yield harmonization algorithm (noun):** Mathematical model aligning yield data across systems.
**Related Terms:** Standardization, Data normalization.
**Example in Radiotherapy:** Yield harmonization algorithm integrated into cloud QA.

433. **Yield-response curve (noun):** Graph of yield variation versus control variable.
**Related Terms:** Calibration curve, System response.
**Example in Radiotherapy:** Yield-response curve established for new energy mode.

434. **Y-axis resolution (noun):** Spatial precision of imaging or measurement along Y-direction.
**Related Terms:** Spatial resolution, Image quality.
**Example in Radiotherapy:** Y-axis resolution improved with finer reconstruction voxel size.

435. **Yield detector calibration (noun):** Process ensuring detector accuracy for yield measurement.
**Related Terms:** Detector QA, Output calibration.
**Example in Radiotherapy:** Yield detector calibration conducted monthly with reference chamber.

436. **Yield-dose correlation (noun):** Relationship between measured yield and absorbed dose.
**Related Terms:** Calibration correlation, Dosimetry link.
**Example in Radiotherapy:** Yield-dose correlation validated for MR-Linac photon beams.

437. **Yield correction audit (noun):** Independent review verifying applied yield corrections.
**Related Terms:** External QA, Audit process.
**Example in Radiotherapy:** Yield correction audit approved during accreditation.

438. **Yield-geometry alignment (noun):** Synchronization of spatial beam geometry with yield field.
**Related Terms:** Isocenter alignment, Beam QA.
**Example in Radiotherapy:** Yield-geometry alignment verified by portal dosimetry.

439. **Yield signal drift (noun):** Gradual shift in signal baseline during operation.
**Related Terms:** Drift error, Electronic instability.
**Example in Radiotherapy:** Yield signal drift corrected via recalibration filter.

440. **Yield thermal compensation (noun):** Adjustment accounting for temperature-dependent output changes.
**Related Terms:** Thermal drift, Environmental QA.
**Example in Radiotherapy:** Yield thermal compensation applied for cyclotron cooling cycles.

441. **Yield variance correction (noun):** Statistical adjustment reducing variability in yield data.
**Related Terms:** Variance stabilization, QA correction.
**Example in Radiotherapy:** Yield variance correction enhanced beam constancy analysis.

442. **Yield feedback analysis (noun):** Study of response behavior in feedback-controlled yield systems.
**Related Terms:** Control dynamics, QA feedback.
**Example in Radiotherapy:** Yield feedback analysis optimized closed-loop dose delivery.

443. **Yaw calibration profile (noun):** Data chart mapping rotational calibration precision.
**Related Terms:** Calibration log, Rotational QA.
**Example in Radiotherapy:** Yaw calibration profile stored in machine QA database.

444. **Yield adjustment tolerance (noun):** Allowable deviation range during recalibration procedures.
**Related Terms:** QA tolerance, Adjustment limit.
**Example in Radiotherapy:** Yield adjustment tolerance set at ±1%.

445. **Yield optimization controller (noun):** Automated control module maximizing beam stability.
**Related Terms:** Feedback controller, System optimization.
**Example in Radiotherapy:** Yield optimization controller improved adaptive proton delivery.

446. **Y-axis scanner (noun):** Device scanning radiation profile along Y-coordinate.
**Related Terms:** Profile scanner, Beam QA.
**Example in Radiotherapy:** Y-axis scanner recorded off-axis dose uniformity.

447. **Yield normalization audit (noun):** Process verifying proper normalization between detectors or machines.
**Related Terms:** Inter-comparison, QA validation.
**Example in Radiotherapy:** Yield normalization audit standardized multi-center QA.

448. **Yield stability coefficient (noun):** Numeric index defining beam stability over time.
**Related Terms:** Stability index, QA parameter.
**Example in Radiotherapy:** Yield stability coefficient consistently >0.99.

449. **Yield signal comparator (noun):** Circuit comparing live yield to reference level.
**Related Terms:** Comparator circuit, QA hardware.
**Example in Radiotherapy:** Yield signal comparator triggered alert at 2% deviation.

450. **Yttrium dosimetry standard (noun):** Reference protocol for Y-90 dose measurement.
**Related Terms:** Isotope dosimetry, Calibration protocol.
**Example in Radiotherapy:** Yttrium dosimetry standard aligned with IAEA TRS guidelines.

451. **Yield-drift compensator (noun):** Device counteracting long-term yield deviation.
**Related Terms:** Drift controller, Stability correction.
**Example in Radiotherapy:** Yield-drift compensator minimized proton source decay effects.

452. **Yield validation software (noun):** Program assessing QA compliance of yield data.
**Related Terms:** QA software, Data validation.
**Example in Radiotherapy:** Yield validation software automated audit report generation.

453. **Yield correction algorithm (noun):** Computational model adjusting raw yield readings.
**Related Terms:** QA correction, Signal processing.
**Example in Radiotherapy:** Yield correction algorithm implemented in TPS calibration.

454. **Yield consistency index (noun):** Metric defining reproducibility of yield outputs.
**Related Terms:** QA index, Reproducibility test.
**Example in Radiotherapy:** Yield consistency index >0.97 indicates excellent stability.

455. **Yield recovery log (noun):** Documentation of yield restoration after faults.
**Related Terms:** Maintenance record, QA history.
**Example in Radiotherapy:** Yield recovery log archived post-service intervention.

456. **Yield equalization process (noun):** Procedure balancing outputs across multiple beams.
**Related Terms:** Output balancing, QA harmonization.
**Example in Radiotherapy:** Yield equalization process standardized arc segment fluences.

457. **Yield attenuation factor (noun):** Ratio quantifying yield loss through attenuating medium.
**Related Terms:** Transmission factor, Dosimetric correction.
**Example in Radiotherapy:** Yield attenuation factor measured for compensator QA.

458. **Yield accuracy audit (noun):** Comprehensive assessment validating measurement precision.
**Related Terms:** QA audit, Calibration review.
**Example in Radiotherapy:** Yield accuracy audit performed biannually for compliance.

459. **Yield isolation transformer (noun):** Electrical transformer preventing interference between circuits.
**Related Terms:** Isolation device, Electrical QA.
**Example in Radiotherapy:** Yield isolation transformer ensured detector circuit protection.

460. **Yield proportional detector (noun):** Sensor whose output linearly correlates with incident dose rate.
**Related Terms:** Ion chamber, Linear detector.
**Example in Radiotherapy:** Yield proportional detector used for output calibration.

461. **Yttrium-labeled resin (noun):** Microsphere medium used for selective internal radiation therapy.
**Related Terms:** SIRT, Brachytherapy agent.
**Example in Radiotherapy:** Yttrium-labeled resin applied in hepatocellular carcinoma cases.

462. **Yield modulation controller (noun):** Hardware modulating dose rate in real time.
**Related Terms:** Dose rate control, QA electronics.
**Example in Radiotherapy:** Yield modulation controller ensured uniform pulsed delivery.

463. **Yield-variance mapping (noun):** Graphical visualization of output fluctuation zones.
**Related Terms:** QA mapping, Trend visualization.
**Example in Radiotherapy:** Yield-variance mapping identified low-stability gantry positions.

464. **Yield detector noise ratio (noun):** Signal-to-noise metric in detector output.
**Related Terms:** SNR, QA signal quality.
**Example in Radiotherapy:** Yield detector noise ratio exceeded 40 dB post-calibration.

465. **Yield deviation alert (noun):** Automated warning for exceeding yield tolerance.
**Related Terms:** QA alarm, System alert.
**Example in Radiotherapy:** Yield deviation alert triggered at ±2% output shift.

466. **Yield variance plot (noun):** Graph showing variation of yield with time or condition.
**Related Terms:** QA trend chart, Performance graph.
**Example in Radiotherapy:** Yield variance plot reviewed during monthly QA.

467. **Yield phase modulation (noun):** Output control method altering phase for smoother delivery.
**Related Terms:** Phase adjustment, Beam modulation.
**Example in Radiotherapy:** Yield phase modulation enhanced gated therapy precision.

468. **Yield calibration coefficient (noun):** Constant linking measured signal to true yield.
**Related Terms:** Calibration factor, QA constant.
**Example in Radiotherapy:** Yield calibration coefficient verified annually.

469. **Yield balance report (noun):** Summary report comparing reference and measured outputs.
**Related Terms:** QA report, Audit summary.
**Example in Radiotherapy:** Yield balance report filed after beam tuning.

470. **Yaw feedback control (noun):** System maintaining stable rotational positioning.
**Related Terms:** Servo control, Motion QA.
**Example in Radiotherapy:** Yaw feedback control improved robotic couch precision.

471. **Yield modulation matrix (noun):** Data grid controlling fluence variation.
**Related Terms:** IMRT matrix, Fluence control.
**Example in Radiotherapy:** Yield modulation matrix optimized for VMAT delivery.

472. **Yield QA verification tool (noun):** Software ensuring compliance with QA yield thresholds.
**Related Terms:** QA verification, Automated auditing.
**Example in Radiotherapy:** Yield QA verification tool integrated with cloud database.

473. **Yield monitoring dashboard (noun):** Digital interface visualizing real-time yield data.
**Related Terms:** QA dashboard, Performance monitoring.
**Example in Radiotherapy:** Yield monitoring dashboard flagged abnormal drift trend.

474. **Yield precision index (noun):** Metric quantifying repeatability and exactness of yield.
**Related Terms:** Accuracy index, QA precision.
**Example in Radiotherapy:** Yield precision index remained above 0.99.

475. **Yield range compensator (noun):** Device adjusting for range-dependent output variation.
**Related Terms:** Range shifter, Proton QA.
**Example in Radiotherapy:** Yield range compensator fine-tuned for distal edge control.

476. **Yield QA summary (noun):** Compiled report of QA yield results and trends.
**Related Terms:** QA documentation, Summary report.
**Example in Radiotherapy:** Yield QA summary appended to monthly physicist review.

477. **Yaw stabilization protocol (noun):** Standard procedure ensuring rotational constancy.
**Related Terms:** Mechanical QA, Setup reproducibility.
**Example in Radiotherapy:** Yaw stabilization protocol executed before high-precision treatments.

478. **Yield reconstruction map (noun):** 2D visualization reconstructed from detector array signals.
**Related Terms:** Beam map, QA reconstruction.
**Example in Radiotherapy:** Yield reconstruction map verified uniform electron beam spread.

479. **Yield-variance control loop (noun):** Automated system maintaining yield within tolerance band.
**Related Terms:** Feedback loop, Stability control.
**Example in Radiotherapy:** Yield-variance control loop ensured adaptive correction.

480. **Yield field compensator (noun):** Physical device equalizing non-uniform beam output.
**Related Terms:** Compensator, Beam flattening.
**Example in Radiotherapy:** Yield field compensator customized for irregular tumor shapes.

481. **Yield detector calibration file (noun):** Data record storing detector-specific correction factors.
**Related Terms:** QA file, Calibration data.
**Example in Radiotherapy:** Yield detector calibration file updated post-service.

482. **Yield uniformity coefficient (noun):** Ratio expressing degree of output evenness.
**Related Terms:** Flatness metric, QA indicator.
**Example in Radiotherapy:** Yield uniformity coefficient ≥0.98 considered optimal.

483. **Yield monitoring probe (noun):** Portable device measuring localized output.
**Related Terms:** QA probe, Detector device.
**Example in Radiotherapy:** Yield monitoring probe checked dose symmetry.

484. **Yield detector drift test (noun):** Routine checking long-term detector stability.
**Related Terms:** Stability test, QA calibration.
**Example in Radiotherapy:** Yield detector drift test confirmed negligible deviation.

485. **Yield normalization factor (noun):** Scaling constant aligning data to reference.
**Related Terms:** Normalization, QA factor.
**Example in Radiotherapy:** Yield normalization factor applied for inter-machine comparison.

486. **Yield verification algorithm (noun):** Software verifying compliance of measured yield data.
**Related Terms:** QA verification, Algorithmic check.
**Example in Radiotherapy:** Yield verification algorithm automated QA record review.

487. **Yield pattern recognition (noun):** AI-based system identifying irregular yield behaviors.
**Related Terms:** Pattern detection, Predictive QA.
**Example in Radiotherapy:** Yield pattern recognition detected early magnetron fault.

488. **Yield constancy chart (noun):** Graph tracking daily output stability.
**Related Terms:** Constancy log, QA chart.
**Example in Radiotherapy:** Yield constancy chart posted near console.

489. **Yield calibration audit (noun):** External review verifying calibration accuracy.
**Related Terms:** Accreditation audit, QA review.
**Example in Radiotherapy:** Yield calibration audit cleared by national authority.

490. **Yield verification dose test (noun):** Physical test confirming calculated vs measured dose.
**Related Terms:** Dose QA, Output verification.
**Example in Radiotherapy:** Yield verification dose test matched within 1%.

491. **Yield optimization matrix (noun):** Computational grid adjusting fluence for uniformity.
**Related Terms:** Optimization, Beam modeling.
**Example in Radiotherapy:** Yield optimization matrix fine-tuned arc delivery.

492. **Yield QA integration module (noun):** Software integrating QA data across departments.
**Related Terms:** QA integration, Centralized database.
**Example in Radiotherapy:** Yield QA integration module unified linac QA records.

493. **Yield synchronization error (noun):** Mismatch in timing between yield and delivery command.
**Related Terms:** Sync error, Control latency.
**Example in Radiotherapy:** Yield synchronization error corrected via firmware update.

494. **Yield statistical control chart (noun):** SPC tool for ongoing yield monitoring.
**Related Terms:** Statistical process control, QA monitoring.
**Example in Radiotherapy:** Yield control chart showed process capability index of 1.3.

495. **Yield correlation coefficient (noun):** Statistical measure of linear relationship between variables.
**Related Terms:** Pearson coefficient, Data analysis.
**Example in Radiotherapy:** Yield correlation coefficient between detectors was 0.999.

496. **Yield verification chamber (noun):** Ion chamber used to confirm absolute output.
**Related Terms:** Reference chamber, QA device.
**Example in Radiotherapy:** Yield verification chamber recalibrated annually.

497. **Yield monitoring log (noun):** Record documenting daily output checks.
**Related Terms:** QA logbook, Performance record.
**Example in Radiotherapy:** Yield monitoring log reviewed monthly by physicist.

498. **Yield normalization matrix (noun):** Grid applying normalization factors across detector array.
**Related Terms:** Correction matrix, QA modeling.
**Example in Radiotherapy:** Yield normalization matrix corrected detector sensitivity bias.

499. **Yield QA compliance report (noun):** Document summarizing QA conformity to standards.
**Related Terms:** QA documentation, Compliance audit.
**Example in Radiotherapy:** Yield QA compliance report submitted to accrediting board.

500. **Yield variance summary (noun):** Final statistical report summarizing yield fluctuation data.
**Related Terms:** Variance report, QA summary.
**Example in Radiotherapy:** Yield variance summary confirmed stable proton source output.

# Z

1. **Z-Axis Calibration (noun):** Process ensuring longitudinal movement accuracy of imaging or treatment systems.
   **Related Terms:** Couch translation, Isocenter verification.
   **Example in Radiotherapy:** Z-axis calibration was verified during the MR-Linac QA procedure.
2. **Z-Axis Deviation (noun):** Error along the longitudinal axis during image-guided setup.
   **Related Terms:** Setup error, Image registration.
   **Example in Radiotherapy:** Z-axis deviation beyond 2 mm prompted re-imaging before treatment delivery.
3. **Z-Axis Resolution (noun):** Determines image clarity along the longitudinal plane.
   **Related Terms:** Slice thickness, Spatial resolution.
   **Example in Radiotherapy:** High Z-axis resolution improved CBCT target visualization.
4. **Z-Axis Shift Correction (noun):** Adjustment to compensate for longitudinal displacement.
   **Related Terms:** Couch offset, Translational correction.
   **Example in Radiotherapy:** The therapist applied Z-axis shift correction to match the liver SBRT target.
5. **Z-Direction Dose Fall-Off (noun):** Rate of dose decrease along the longitudinal axis.
   **Related Terms:** Penumbra, Dose gradient.
   **Example in Radiotherapy:** Proton distal Z-direction fall-off was sharper than that of photon beams.
6. **Z-Motion Artifact (noun):** Image distortion from patient or couch motion along Z-axis.
   **Related Terms:** Motion blurring, Artifact reduction.
   **Example in Radiotherapy:** Z-motion artifacts were minimized by breath-hold imaging.
7. **Z-Plane Registration (noun):** Alignment of image slices in the longitudinal plane.
   **Related Terms:** Image fusion, Alignment accuracy.
   **Example in Radiotherapy:** Z-plane registration enhanced target matching precision.
8. **Z-Distance Verification (noun):** Procedure confirming geometric accuracy in the longitudinal direction.
   **Related Terms:** QA geometry, Couch calibration.
   **Example in Radiotherapy:** Z-distance verification ensured correct proton beam range delivery.
9. **Z-Score Normalization (noun):** Statistical technique standardizing datasets for radiobiological analysis.
   **Related Terms:** Data normalization, Statistical modeling.
   **Example in Radiotherapy:** Tumor control probability data were processed using Z-score normalization.
10. **Zonal Dose Analysis (noun):** Evaluation of dose distribution across anatomical zones.
    **Related Terms:** Isodose mapping, Region-based QA.
    **Example in Radiotherapy:** Zonal dose analysis confirmed uniform delivery in the cranial field.
11. **Zonal Heterogeneity (noun):** Variation in tissue density or composition within a region.
    **Related Terms:** Tissue inhomogeneity, Dose perturbation.
    **Example in Radiotherapy:** Zonal heterogeneity impacted proton range accuracy.

12. **Zero-Dose Region (noun):** Anatomical area intentionally excluded from radiation exposure.
**Related Terms:** Shielding zone, Dose avoidance.
**Example in Radiotherapy:** The pacemaker pocket was maintained as a zero-dose region.
13. **Zero-Degree Gantry (noun):** Reference beam angle used for calibration.
**Related Terms:** Mechanical isocenter, QA baseline.
**Example in Radiotherapy:** Zero-degree gantry position was used for mechanical QA testing.
14. **Zero-Flux Boundary (noun):** Surface where no particles cross during simulation.
**Related Terms:** Boundary condition, Monte Carlo modeling.
**Example in Radiotherapy:** Monte Carlo code used a zero-flux boundary for dose calculation.
15. **Zero-Point Drift (noun):** Gradual baseline shift in detector readings.
**Related Terms:** Detector calibration, Signal stability.
**Example in Radiotherapy:** Zero-point drift correction was applied before chamber measurement.
16. **Zero-Offset Correction (noun):** Adjustment eliminating baseline signal bias in detectors.
**Related Terms:** Output calibration, Baseline alignment.
**Example in Radiotherapy:** The chamber's zero-offset correction was verified daily.
17. **Zenith Angle (noun):** Angle between vertical reference and beam axis.
**Related Terms:** Non-coplanar geometry, Gantry rotation.
**Example in Radiotherapy:** The therapist used a 25° zenith angle to avoid lung overlap.
18. **Zeeman Effect (noun):** Magnetic field–induced spectral line splitting.
**Related Terms:** MR signal shift, Magnetic resonance physics.
**Example in Radiotherapy:** The Zeeman effect influenced MR-Linac frequency calibration.
19. **Zeff (Effective Atomic Number) (noun):** Weighted average atomic number representing photon interaction likelihood.
**Related Terms:** Attenuation coefficient, Tissue equivalence.
**Example in Radiotherapy:** Zeff was used to calibrate tissue-equivalent bolus materials.
20. **Zeta Potential (noun):** Electrokinetic potential influencing nanoparticle stability.
**Related Terms:** Radiopharmaceutical delivery, Surface charge.
**Example in Radiotherapy:** Zeta potential modified the biodistribution of gold nanoparticles.
21. **Zinc Oxide Nanoparticle (noun):** Nanoparticle with radiosensitizing and antioxidant properties.
**Related Terms:** Nanodosimetry, Radiomodifiers.
**Example in Radiotherapy:** Zinc oxide nanoparticles enhanced DNA damage in hypoxic tumors.
22. **Zonal Energy Deposition (noun):** Localized pattern of energy transfer within tissue regions.
**Related Terms:** Microdosimetry, LET mapping.
**Example in Radiotherapy:** Zonal energy deposition profiles informed biological dose modeling.
23. **Zone of Uncertainty (noun):** Region with ambiguous margin due to organ motion.
**Related Terms:** PTV expansion, Motion margin.
**Example in Radiotherapy:** The diaphragm created a zone of uncertainty in liver SBRT.
24. **Zone-Based Planning (noun):** Method dividing target into subregions for tailored dosing.
**Related Terms:** Dose painting, Adaptive radiotherapy.
**Example in Radiotherapy:** Zone-based planning was applied for heterogeneous tumor volumes.
25. **Zernike Polynomial Reconstruction (noun):** Mathematical function describing optical aberrations in imaging.
**Related Terms:** Image correction, Beam shaping.
**Example in Radiotherapy:** Zernike polynomial analysis refined CBCT reconstruction accuracy.

26. **Zero-Leakage Shielding (noun):** Design criterion preventing radiation escape beyond safe limits.
**Related Terms:** Vault design, Shielding efficiency.
**Example in Radiotherapy:** Zero-leakage shielding was validated through neutron survey tests.

27. **Zonal Motion Management (noun):** Strategy to account for organ motion within specific regions.
**Related Terms:** Gating, Tracking, 4D imaging.
**Example in Radiotherapy:** Zonal motion management improved dose conformity in lung SBRT.

28. **Zonal Temperature Correction (noun):** Compensation for temperature variation affecting detector sensitivity.
**Related Terms:** Environmental correction, Chamber calibration.
**Example in Radiotherapy:** The chamber applied zonal temperature correction before proton QA.

29. **Zonal Radiobiological Weighting (noun):** Application of different RBE values across tissue zones.
**Related Terms:** RBE modeling, Biological optimization.
**Example in Radiotherapy:** Zonal radiobiological weighting enhanced proton therapy planning accuracy.

30. **Zero-Dose Verification (noun):** Confirmation that shielded structures receive negligible dose.
**Related Terms:** QA check, Secondary scatter analysis.
**Example in Radiotherapy:** Zero-dose verification confirmed pacemaker protection.

31. **Zonal Adaptive Margin (noun):** Region-specific margin adjusted for differential motion.
**Related Terms:** Adaptive planning, Motion robustness.
**Example in Radiotherapy:** The zonal adaptive margin reduced rectal dose in prostate treatment.

32. **Zonal Proton Fluence Map (noun):** Spatial fluence distribution of protons within zones.
**Related Terms:** Fluence modulation, Beam scanning.
**Example in Radiotherapy:** Zonal proton fluence map validated scanning precision.

33. **Zygomatic Avoidance Arc (noun):** Trajectory minimizing dose to zygomatic bone.
**Related Terms:** Non-coplanar beam, OAR sparing.
**Example in Radiotherapy:** Zygomatic avoidance arc was applied in brain VMAT.

34. **Z-Weighted Dose Map (noun):** Dose visualization emphasizing longitudinal dose variations.
**Related Terms:** Dose visualization, 3D mapping.
**Example in Radiotherapy:** Z-weighted dose maps aided adaptive SBRT verification.

35. **Zonal Verification QA (noun):** Quality assurance evaluating performance across system zones.
**Related Terms:** Segmental QA, Machine QA.
**Example in Radiotherapy:** Zonal verification QA detected couch drift in the Z-plane.

36. **Z-Dose Symmetry (noun):** Assessment of uniformity along the longitudinal beam axis.
**Related Terms:** Beam symmetry, QA metrics.
**Example in Radiotherapy:** Z-dose symmetry was checked during daily output calibration.

37. **Zonal Beam Hardening (noun):** Selective increase in beam energy due to tissue thickness.
**Related Terms:** Beam filtration, Attenuation.
**Example in Radiotherapy:** Zonal beam hardening caused minor CT number distortion.

38. **Z-Coordinate Registration (noun):** Alignment of treatment and imaging coordinate systems in the longitudinal axis.
**Related Terms:** Image fusion, Spatial accuracy.
**Example in Radiotherapy:** Z-coordinate registration ensured MR-Linac precision alignment.

39. **Z-Displacement Error (noun):** Mismatch between planned and delivered couch position along Z-axis.
    **Related Terms:** Setup deviation, Translational error.
    **Example in Radiotherapy:** Z-displacement error beyond 1 mm triggered repositioning.
40. **Z-Field Aperture (noun):** Field opening dimension in the longitudinal direction.
    **Related Terms:** Collimator jaw, Beam shaping.
    **Example in Radiotherapy:** Z-field aperture was optimized for spinal IMRT.
41. **Zonal Attenuation Map (noun):** Representation of attenuation coefficients across different longitudinal zones.
    **Related Terms:** CT number map, Electron density correction.
    **Example in Radiotherapy:** Zonal attenuation map improved adaptive planning accuracy.
42. **Zero-Beam Reference (noun):** Standard calibration setup for beam output verification.
    **Related Terms:** Reference dosimetry, QA baseline.
    **Example in Radiotherapy:** Zero-beam reference was recorded during commissioning.
43. **Zonal Dose Deviation (noun):** Variation between planned and measured dose across defined zones.
    **Related Terms:** Gamma analysis, QA audit.
    **Example in Radiotherapy:** Zonal dose deviation within 2% indicated good plan accuracy.
44. **Zonal Density Mapping (noun):** Tissue density evaluation along the Z-axis for planning accuracy.
    **Related Terms:** Hounsfield calibration, CT-to-density conversion.
    **Example in Radiotherapy:** Zonal density mapping refined lung heterogeneity correction.
45. **Zonal Motion Envelope (noun):** Defined boundary of organ movement in longitudinal dimension.
    **Related Terms:** 4D imaging, Motion management.
    **Example in Radiotherapy:** Zonal motion envelope used for gating window .
46. **Zonal Dose Constraint (noun):** Maximum permissible dose within a specific anatomical zone.
    **Related Terms:** Dose limit, OAR constraint.
    **Example in Radiotherapy:** Zonal dose constraint applied to avoid spinal overexposure.
47. **Zonal Dose Homogeneity (noun):** Degree of dose uniformity within a specific region.
    **Related Terms:** Homogeneity index, Dose distribution.
    **Example in Radiotherapy:** Zonal dose homogeneity improved through reoptimization.
48. **Zonal Tissue Correction (noun):** Adjustment of dose calculation for tissue inhomogeneity.
    **Related Terms:** Heterogeneity correction, Density scaling.
    **Example in Radiotherapy:** Zonal tissue correction was applied for lung SBRT planning.
49. **Zonal Proton Stopping Power (noun):** Effective energy loss parameter per tissue region.
    **Related Terms:** Range uncertainty, Proton dosimetry.
    **Example in Radiotherapy:** Zonal proton stopping power reduced distal range errors.
50. **Zonal LET Distribution (noun):** Spatial variation of Linear Energy Transfer across treatment zones.
    **Related Terms:** LET mapping, RBE modeling.
    **Example in Radiotherapy:** Zonal LET distribution used in biologically weighted planning.
51. **Z-Plane Dose Gradient (noun):** Rate of dose change along the longitudinal axis.
    **Related Terms:** Dose fall-off, Sharpness index.
    **Example in Radiotherapy:** Proton Z-plane dose gradient was validated through Monte Carlo simulation.
52. **Z-Resolution Phantom (noun):** Calibration device assessing longitudinal imaging resolution.
    **Related Terms:** QA phantom, Image quality.
    **Example in Radiotherapy:** Z-resolution phantom tested CBCT slice reconstruction.

53. **Zonal Distortion Correction (noun):** Image correction to compensate for non-linear spatial distortion.
**Related Terms:** MR-Linac QA, Geometric fidelity.
**Example in Radiotherapy:** MR images underwent zonal distortion correction for accuracy.

54. **Zonal Motion Artifact (noun):** Image blur from regional organ motion along Z-axis.
**Related Terms:** Respiratory artifact, 4DCT.
**Example in Radiotherapy:** Zonal motion artifacts were minimized using gating.

55. **Zero-Gradient Field (noun):** Region in MRI with uniform magnetic strength.
**Related Terms:** MR imaging, Field uniformity.
**Example in Radiotherapy:** MR-Linac design maintains zero-gradient field around isocenter.

56. **Zonal Beam Intensity Map (noun):** Profile of beam fluence across longitudinal zones.
**Related Terms:** Intensity modulation, Beam shaping.
**Example in Radiotherapy:** Zonal intensity map adjusted to improve target coverage.

57. **Zonal Scatter Correction (noun):** Algorithm correcting for photon or proton scatter in specific regions.
**Related Terms:** Image correction, Monte Carlo.
**Example in Radiotherapy:** Zonal scatter correction improved PET-based dose verification.

58. **Zonal QA Benchmark (noun):** Standardized reference for multi-zone system performance testing.
**Related Terms:** QA protocol, Performance validation.
**Example in Radiotherapy:** Zonal QA benchmark compared MR-Linac data to vendor baseline.

59. **Zero-Drift Ion Chamber (noun):** Detector with negligible long-term signal drift.
**Related Terms:** Chamber stability, Calibration.
**Example in Radiotherapy:** Zero-drift ion chamber used for high-precision QA.

60. **Zonal Dose Optimization (noun):** Selective improvement of dose within anatomical subregions.
**Related Terms:** Adaptive planning, Dose painting.
**Example in Radiotherapy:** Zonal optimization refined liver target conformity.

61. **Zonal Output Constancy (noun):** Uniformity of machine output in different beam zones.
**Related Terms:** Output calibration, Beam QA.
**Example in Radiotherapy:** Zonal output constancy test performed weekly.

62. **Zero-Noise Image Mode (noun):** Imaging configuration minimizing electronic and quantum noise.
**Related Terms:** Image SNR, Quality enhancement.
**Example in Radiotherapy:** Zero-noise mode improved MR-guided image clarity.

63. **Zonal RBE Calibration (noun):** Adjustment of biological dose weighting across proton zones.
**Related Terms:** RBE modeling, Proton biology.
**Example in Radiotherapy:** Zonal RBE calibration validated using Monte Carlo-based data.

64. **Zonal Tissue Compensation (noun):** Technique for balancing dose through irregular density.
**Related Terms:** Bolus compensation, Density correction.
**Example in Radiotherapy:** Zonal compensation used for breast tangential setup.

65. **Zonal Verification Image (noun):** Radiographic image capturing specific longitudinal section for QA.
**Related Terms:** Portal imaging, IGRT verification.
**Example in Radiotherapy:** Zonal verification image confirmed lung lesion matching.

66. **Z-Direction Penumbra (noun):** Partial shadow region along longitudinal beam fall-off.
**Related Terms:** Dose gradient, Beam edge.
**Example in Radiotherapy:** Proton Z-direction penumbra analyzed using film dosimetry.

67. **Zonal Adaptive Replanning (noun):** Partial plan modification addressing regional changes.
**Related Terms:** ART, Dose adaptation.
**Example in Radiotherapy:** Zonal adaptive replanning adjusted tumor regression volume.

68. **Zonal Image Fusion (noun):** Localized image registration for improved anatomical alignment.
**Related Terms:** Multimodality fusion, Target accuracy.
**Example in Radiotherapy:** Zonal fusion between MRI and CT guided contour adaptation.

69. **Zonal Dose Constraint Report (noun):** QA document summarizing dose limit adherence by region.
**Related Terms:** Plan evaluation, QA audit.
**Example in Radiotherapy:** Zonal constraint report submitted during chart round review.

70. **Zonal Monte Carlo Simulation (noun):** Localized computational modeling of dose deposition.
**Related Terms:** Monte Carlo, Particle transport.
**Example in Radiotherapy:** Zonal Monte Carlo used for pediatric proton planning.

71. **Zonal Plan Verification (noun):** Evaluation of plan accuracy for specific anatomical sections.
**Related Terms:** QA check, Dose validation.
**Example in Radiotherapy:** Zonal plan verification confirmed liver SBRT delivery accuracy.

72. **Zonal Plan Adaptation (noun):** Partial plan modification for anatomy-specific changes.
**Related Terms:** Adaptive radiotherapy, Plan update.
**Example in Radiotherapy:** Zonal plan adaptation was performed after tumor shrinkage.

73. **Zonal Tissue Sampling (noun):** Extraction of tissue data by anatomical region for analysis.
**Related Terms:** Radiobiological sampling, Biopsy mapping.
**Example in Radiotherapy:** Zonal tissue sampling supported voxel-based RBE modeling.

74. **Zonal Uniformity Index (noun):** Metric describing dose evenness within a zone.
**Related Terms:** Homogeneity index, QA metric.
**Example in Radiotherapy:** Zonal uniformity index met tolerance for spinal IMRT fields.

75. **Zonal Weighted DVH (noun):** Dose-volume histogram normalized per anatomical zone.
**Related Terms:** DVH analysis, Dose statistics.
**Example in Radiotherapy:** Zonal weighted DVH improved target comparison across patients.

76. **Zero-Field Output Check (noun):** Test to confirm zero radiation when the beam is disabled.
**Related Terms:** Safety interlock, Output QA.
**Example in Radiotherapy:** Zero-field output check ensured beam shut-off integrity.

77. **Zonal Field Matching (noun):** Technique aligning adjacent radiation fields in the longitudinal axis.
**Related Terms:** Junction dose, Field matching.
**Example in Radiotherapy:** Zonal field matching optimized craniospinal irradiation.

78. **Zonal Neutron Leakage (noun):** Neutron scatter within specific longitudinal areas of a vault.
**Related Terms:** Radiation protection, Shielding analysis.
**Example in Radiotherapy:** Zonal neutron leakage was measured during proton QA.

79. **Zero-Sum Dose Distribution (noun):** Balanced dose trade-off ensuring OAR protection without target compromise.
**Related Terms:** Plan optimization, Dose balancing.
**Example in Radiotherapy:** Zero-sum distribution achieved between spinal cord and PTV.

80. **Zonal Dose Painting (noun):** Assigning different dose levels within target subregions.
**Related Terms:** Dose escalation, Functional imaging.
**Example in Radiotherapy:** Zonal dose painting targeted hypoxic tumor cores.

81. **Zonal Scatter Profile (noun):** Representation of scattered radiation intensity per zone.
**Related Terms:** Scatter correction, QA imaging.
**Example in Radiotherapy:** Zonal scatter profile verified shielding adequacy.

82. **Zonal Energy Spectrum (noun):** Range of beam energies across anatomical regions.
**Related Terms:** Beam modulation, Spectral analysis.
**Example in Radiotherapy:** Zonal energy spectrum optimized for tissue heterogeneity.

83. **Zonal Air Gap Correction (noun):** Adjustment accounting for varying air gaps along Z-axis.
**Related Terms:** Bolus correction, Setup QA.
**Example in Radiotherapy:** Zonal air gap correction refined skin dose prediction.

84. **Zonal Alignment Deviation (noun):** Error in field positioning along defined longitudinal sections.
**Related Terms:** Setup deviation, Image guidance.
**Example in Radiotherapy:** Zonal alignment deviation was corrected using CBCT.

85. **Zonal Attenuation Curve (noun):** Graph representing attenuation variation by region.
**Related Terms:** Linear attenuation, Beam hardening.
**Example in Radiotherapy:** Zonal attenuation curves guided proton range calibration.

86. **Zonal Biophysical Model (noun):** Model defining regional variations in biological response.
**Related Terms:** Radiobiological modeling, RBE.
**Example in Radiotherapy:** Zonal biophysical models improved LET-weighted dose predictions.

87. **Zonal Dose Calibration Phantom (noun):** Phantom designed for region-specific dose calibration tests.
**Related Terms:** QA phantom, Dosimetry calibration.
**Example in Radiotherapy:** Zonal phantom verified IMRT output consistency.

88. **Zonal Dose Gradient Index (noun):** Quantitative measure of dose fall-off steepness by zone.
**Related Terms:** Gradient index, Plan evaluation.
**Example in Radiotherapy:** Zonal gradient index used in SRS plan review.

89. **Zonal Dose Overlap (noun):** Intersection of high-dose volumes between adjacent zones.
**Related Terms:** Field junction, Overlap management.
**Example in Radiotherapy:** Zonal dose overlap minimized via feathering technique.

90. **Zonal Dose Symmetry Check (noun):** Test evaluating left-right and longitudinal dose uniformity.
**Related Terms:** Symmetry QA, Flatness test.
**Example in Radiotherapy:** Zonal symmetry check performed during beam commissioning.

91. **Zonal Magnetic Interference (noun):** Magnetic field disturbances in MR-Linac by region.
**Related Terms:** Field mapping, MR QA.
**Example in Radiotherapy:** Zonal interference measured with magnetic probes.

92. **Zonal MRI Geometric Distortion (noun):** Spatial error in MR imaging across longitudinal slices.
**Related Terms:** MR QA, Geometric correction.
**Example in Radiotherapy:** Zonal distortion map generated before contouring.

93. **Zonal Output Factor (noun):** Machine output variation at specific longitudinal zones.
**Related Terms:** Output calibration, QA analysis.
**Example in Radiotherapy:** Zonal output factor compared to baseline monthly.

94. **Zonal Proton Fluence Deviation (noun):** Difference in expected and measured proton fluence.
**Related Terms:** Beam QA, Dose monitoring.
**Example in Radiotherapy:** Zonal fluence deviation analyzed via log-file QA.

95. **Zonal Range Uncertainty (noun):** Variation in proton penetration depth across zones.
**Related Terms:** Range verification, Uncertainty modeling.
**Example in Radiotherapy:** Zonal range uncertainty minimized using in-room imaging.

96. **Zonal RBE Map (noun):** Distribution of relative biological effectiveness values per region.
**Related Terms:** RBE modeling, Proton biology.
**Example in Radiotherapy:** Zonal RBE map used for biologically weighted optimization.

97. **Zonal Scatter Dose (noun):** Secondary radiation dose accumulated in adjacent zones.
**Related Terms:** Scatter component, Dose leakage.
**Example in Radiotherapy:** Zonal scatter dose calculated for pediatric head cases.

98. **Zonal Structural Mask (noun):** Binary overlay defining regions of interest for plan analysis.
**Related Terms:** Segmentation, Contour validation.
**Example in Radiotherapy:** Zonal structural mask applied during AI contouring review.

99. **Zonal Verification Log (noun):** QA record tracking daily performance of specific machine zones.
**Related Terms:** QA documentation, Audit trail.
**Example in Radiotherapy:** Zonal verification log archived for NABH compliance.

100. **Zonal Weighting Function (noun):** Mathematical weighting applied to emphasize specific anatomical regions in optimization.
**Related Terms:** Dose weighting, Objective function.
**Example in Radiotherapy:** Zonal weighting function enhanced target coverage.

101. **Zonal Proton Energy Modulation (noun):** Variation of proton energy in defined depth regions for uniform dose distribution.
**Related Terms:** Range modulation, SOBP.
**Example in Radiotherapy:** Zonal proton energy modulation achieved a spread-out Bragg peak.

102. **Zonal MR Gradient Compensation (noun):** Correction for magnetic gradient distortions across spatial zones.
**Related Terms:** MR correction, Distortion mapping.
**Example in Radiotherapy:** Zonal MR gradient compensation refined image registration accuracy.

103. **Zonal QA Benchmarking Protocol (noun):** Standard procedure comparing QA data across treatment zones.
**Related Terms:** QA validation, Benchmark dataset.
**Example in Radiotherapy:** Zonal QA benchmarking ensured inter-machine uniformity.

104. **Zero-Point Dosimeter Drift (noun):** Deviation in dosimeter baseline when no radiation is present.
**Related Terms:** Dosimeter calibration, QA check.
**Example in Radiotherapy:** Zero-point dosimeter drift corrected before beam output measurement.

105. **Zonal PET Activity Mapping (noun):** Mapping of metabolic activity within anatomical zones using PET.
**Related Terms:** Functional imaging, Dose painting.
**Example in Radiotherapy:** Zonal PET mapping guided adaptive plan updates.

106. **Zonal Dose Audit Sheet (noun):** Document summarizing zone-wise dose audit results.
**Related Terms:** QA documentation, Dose verification.
**Example in Radiotherapy:** Zonal dose audit sheet reviewed before accreditation visit.

107. **Zonal Motion Quantification (noun):** Measurement of anatomical motion magnitude in specific zones.
**Related Terms:** Motion tracking, 4D QA.
**Example in Radiotherapy:** Zonal motion quantification identified diaphragm excursion.

108. **Zonal Field Overlap Index (noun):** Quantifies field intersection between neighboring zones.
**Related Terms:** Junction QA, Field matching.
**Example in Radiotherapy:** Zonal overlap index optimized spinal field matching.

109. **Zero-Scatter Field Verification (noun):** Check ensuring scatter-free delivery in test fields.
**Related Terms:** Beam QA, Phantom check.
**Example in Radiotherapy:** Zero-scatter field verification validated electron cone performance.

110. **Zonal Biophysical Calibration Model (noun):** Calibration algorithm adjusting dose by local biological response.
**Related Terms:** RBE model, Biophysical correction.
**Example in Radiotherapy:** Zonal calibration model refined proton plan accuracy.

111. **Zonal Dose Adaptation Algorithm (noun):** Algorithm modifying dose based on anatomical zone variations.
**Related Terms:** Adaptive planning, AI optimization.
**Example in Radiotherapy:** Zonal adaptation algorithm reduced liver dose heterogeneity.

112. **Zonal QA Tolerance Table (noun):** Reference of acceptable QA deviation limits per zone.
**Related Terms:** QA policy, Verification protocol.
**Example in Radiotherapy:** Zonal tolerance table approved during internal audit.

113. **Zonal Plan Conformity Index (noun):** Numerical measure of plan conformity within each anatomical zone.
**Related Terms:** Conformity index, Plan quality.
**Example in Radiotherapy:** Zonal conformity index exceeded departmental standards.

114. **Zonal MRI Co-Registration Report (noun):** Document detailing MR-CT fusion accuracy by zones.
**Related Terms:** Image fusion, Registration QA.
**Example in Radiotherapy:** Zonal co-registration report reviewed before contour approval.

115. **Zonal Dose Symmetry Phantom (noun):** Phantom designed for verifying dose uniformity across zones.
**Related Terms:** QA phantom, Symmetry check.
**Example in Radiotherapy:** Zonal symmetry phantom validated daily QA outputs.

116. **Zonal Field Drift Log (noun):** Record of gradual machine output drift by field zone.
**Related Terms:** Output tracking, QA log.
**Example in Radiotherapy:** Zonal field drift log analyzed during maintenance.

117. **Zero-Tolerance Error Policy (noun):** Strict QA protocol forbidding any dose deviation beyond limits.
**Related Terms:** QA policy, Compliance.
**Example in Radiotherapy:** Zero-tolerance policy applied to SBRT verification.

118. **Zonal Dose Accumulation Map (noun):** Cumulative dose distribution chart across zones.
**Related Terms:** Dose summation, QA verification.
**Example in Radiotherapy:** Zonal accumulation map reviewed for composite plan.

119. **Zonal Adaptive Workflow (noun):** Structured procedure for performing regional adaptive planning.
**Related Terms:** Online adaptation, Workflow design.
**Example in Radiotherapy:** Zonal adaptive workflow reduced replan time.

120. **Zonal MR Artifact Correction (noun):** Process of eliminating MR image distortions per region.
**Related Terms:** Image QA, Geometric correction.
**Example in Radiotherapy:** Zonal artifact correction improved contour precision.

121. **Zonal Radiobiological Dose Model (noun):** Predictive model linking dose and biological response per zone.
**Related Terms:** LQ model, Radiobiology.
**Example in Radiotherapy:** Zonal dose model refined hypoxic tissue dose weighting.

122. **Zonal Proton LET Map (noun):** Visualization of LET variations across treatment zones.
**Related Terms:** LET distribution, Proton therapy.
**Example in Radiotherapy:** Zonal LET map assisted in RBE-weighted plan review.

123. **Zonal QA Traceability Record (noun):** Archive ensuring all QA data can be traced by zone.
**Related Terms:** QA documentation, Audit trail.
**Example in Radiotherapy:** Zonal traceability record maintained for ISO certification.

124. **Zonal Dose Correction Factor (noun):** Adjustment multiplier for measured dose per anatomical zone.
**Related Terms:** Dose calibration, Correction coefficient.
**Example in Radiotherapy:** Zonal correction factors updated monthly.

125. **Zonal Dose Deconvolution (noun):** Mathematical process to separate overlapping dose contributions.
**Related Terms:** Dose analysis, Image reconstruction.
**Example in Radiotherapy:** Zonal deconvolution clarified overlapping IMRT beams.

126. **Zonal Energy Calibration Table (noun):** Reference sheet defining energy calibration constants per zone.
**Related Terms:** Beam calibration, QA setup.
**Example in Radiotherapy:** Zonal energy calibration table updated quarterly.

127. **Zonal QA Response Curve (noun):** Graph showing QA parameter response across zones.
**Related Terms:** QA sensitivity, System performance.
**Example in Radiotherapy:** Zonal response curve verified beam stability.

128. **Zero-Dose Control Region (noun):** Area intentionally shielded from radiation exposure.
**Related Terms:** Dose sparing, Shielding.
**Example in Radiotherapy:** Zero-dose control region ensured lens protection.

129. **Zonal Verification Index (noun):** Metric expressing percentage of verified plan points per zone.
**Related Terms:** Gamma index, QA analysis.
**Example in Radiotherapy:** Zonal verification index met 98% passing rate.

130. **Zonal Output Stability Chart (noun):** Graph displaying daily output constancy by zone.
**Related Terms:** Machine QA, Output constancy.
**Example in Radiotherapy:** Zonal stability chart used for linearity evaluation.

131. **Zonal Dose Rate Map (noun):** A spatial visualization showing instantaneous dose rates across defined anatomical zones.
**Related Terms:** Dose mapping, 4D QA.
**Example in Radiotherapy:** The zonal dose rate map identified hotspots near the chest wall.

132. **Zonal Ionization Profile (noun):** Distribution of ionization intensity in each treatment zone.
**Related Terms:** Ion chamber profiling, Dose distribution.
**Example in Radiotherapy:** The zonal ionization profile ensured homogeneity during QA checks.

133. **Zonal Beam Flatness Report (noun):** Document showing uniformity of radiation beam intensity by region.
**Related Terms:** Beam uniformity, QA documentation.
**Example in Radiotherapy:** The zonal beam flatness report confirmed tolerance within ±2%.

134. **Zonal Dose Linearization Chart (noun):** Graph correlating measured dose and prescribed dose per zone.
**Related Terms:** Dose calibration, QA chart.
**Example in Radiotherapy:** The linearization chart verified accurate IMRT delivery.

135. **Zonal QA Acceptance Record (noun):** Official log of verified QA tests for individual machine zones.
**Related Terms:** QA checklist, Accreditation file.
**Example in Radiotherapy:** Zonal QA acceptance record signed after annual calibration.

136. **Zonal Output Variation Index (noun):** Metric quantifying daily output fluctuation across treatment zones.
**Related Terms:** Machine stability, Beam QA.
**Example in Radiotherapy:** The variation index remained below 1% for three months.

137. **Zonal Monte Carlo Kernel (noun):** Simulation dataset modeling photon or proton transport per anatomical zone.
**Related Terms:** Dose engine, Particle transport.
**Example in Radiotherapy:** Zonal Monte Carlo kernel validated in liver SBRT planning.

138. **Zonal Isocenter Verification Sheet (noun):** Document confirming isocenter alignment for zone-specific setups.
**Related Terms:** Mechanical QA, Position verification.
**Example in Radiotherapy:** The verification sheet confirmed submillimeter accuracy.

139. **Zonal Dose Homogeneity Factor (noun):** Ratio expressing uniformity of absorbed dose in a zone.
**Related Terms:** Homogeneity index, Plan evaluation.
**Example in Radiotherapy:** Homogeneity factor improved with adaptive reoptimization.

140. **Zonal Plan Consistency Matrix (noun):** Comparative grid ensuring consistency among multiple plan revisions.
**Related Terms:** Plan audit, Adaptive QA.
**Example in Radiotherapy:** The consistency matrix validated adaptive replan quality.

141. **Zonal Dose Reconstruction Log (noun):** Chronological record of reconstructed dose distributions.
**Related Terms:** Dose recalculation, Verification log.
**Example in Radiotherapy:** Reconstruction logs aided in patient-specific QA reviews.

142. **Zonal Proton Depth Profile (noun):** Graph plotting proton energy deposition by depth per zone.
**Related Terms:** Bragg curve, Proton range.
**Example in Radiotherapy:** Depth profile revealed distal edge misalignment.

143. **Zonal Imaging QA Control Sheet (noun):** Checklist validating imaging system performance zone-wise.
**Related Terms:** Imaging QA, CBCT verification.
**Example in Radiotherapy:** Imaging QA control sheet reviewed before SBRT setup.

144. **Zonal Dose Uniformity Chart (noun):** Tabulated values indicating uniform dose coverage per region.
**Related Terms:** Dose map, QA data.
**Example in Radiotherapy:** Uniformity chart ensured consistent breast field coverage.

145. **Zonal Adaptive Optimization Loop (noun):** Automated iterative process adjusting plans by zone response.
**Related Terms:** Adaptive radiotherapy, AI optimization.
**Example in Radiotherapy:** Adaptive optimization loop recalculated daily liver dose.

146. **Zonal Beam Steering Correction (noun):** Fine-tuning of beam direction in zone-specific QA.
**Related Terms:** Beam alignment, QA calibration.
**Example in Radiotherapy:** Beam steering correction completed after gantry QA.

147. **Zonal QA Protocol Validation Sheet (noun):** Official record certifying compliance with QA procedures.
**Related Terms:** Validation report, QA policy.
**Example in Radiotherapy:** Validation sheet filed post-annual QA audit.

148. **Zonal Field Output Report (noun):** Summary of beam output data categorized by zones.
**Related Terms:** Output constancy, QA trend.
**Example in Radiotherapy:** Zonal field report showed linear output behavior.

149. **Zonal Imaging Reconstruction Grid (noun):** Digital grid aiding zone-based image reformation.
**Related Terms:** Reconstruction matrix, Image QA.
**Example in Radiotherapy:** Reconstruction grid enhanced MR-CT fusion precision.

150. **Zonal Dose Verification Record (noun):** Patient-specific QA record documenting verified zone doses.
**Related Terms:** Verification file, QA archive.
**Example in Radiotherapy:** Record submitted during IROC audit.

151. **Zonal Range Uncertainty Chart (noun):** Graph representing proton range deviations per tissue zone.
**Related Terms:** Range uncertainty, Proton QA.
**Example in Radiotherapy:** Chart guided adaptive plan re-evaluation.

152. **Zonal Detector Response Factor (noun):** Calibration constant correlating detector signal to dose regionally.
**Related Terms:** Detector calibration, QA response.
**Example in Radiotherapy:** Response factor confirmed linear sensitivity in MR-Linac field.

153. **Zonal Dose Volume Histogram (noun):** Graph plotting dose versus volume for each anatomical zone.
**Related Terms:** DVH, Plan evaluation.
**Example in Radiotherapy:** Zonal DVH guided PTV margin assessment.

154. **Zonal Output Linearity Test (noun):** Quality test confirming dose output proportionality.
**Related Terms:** Linearity QA, Machine performance.
**Example in Radiotherapy:** Test results submitted to physics QA report.

155. **Zonal RBE Weighting Table (noun):** Data sheet mapping RBE values across zones.
**Related Terms:** Radiobiological correction, Proton planning.
**Example in Radiotherapy:** Table applied to brain tumor RBE calculations.

156. **Zonal LET Distribution Map (noun):** Spatial map showing LET gradients within each zone.
**Related Terms:** LET analysis, Proton therapy.
**Example in Radiotherapy:** Distribution map used for RBE adjustment.

157. **Zonal MR-Linac Field Uniformity Report (noun):** Document detailing magnetic field uniformity per imaging zone.
**Related Terms:** MR QA, Field mapping.
**Example in Radiotherapy:** Report reviewed during MR safety audit.

158. **Zonal Dose Calibration Certificate (noun):** Certification confirming valid dose calibration by region.
**Related Terms:** Calibration validation, QA document.
**Example in Radiotherapy:** Certificate archived under national QA guidelines.

159. **Zonal Data Integrity Audit (noun):** Audit ensuring data consistency across all machine zones.
**Related Terms:** QA traceability, Data validation.
**Example in Radiotherapy:** Audit confirmed no missing dosimetric records.

160. **Zonal Electron Density Map (noun):** 3D map of relative electron density per region.
**Related Terms:** CT calibration, Density correction.
**Example in Radiotherapy:** Density map used for Monte Carlo simulation input.

161. **Zonal Uncertainty Matrix (noun):** Tabular representation of geometric and dosimetric uncertainties by zone.
**Related Terms:** Error propagation, QA modeling.
**Example in Radiotherapy:** The uncertainty matrix aided margin calculation for adaptive prostate RT.

162. **Zonal Dose Drift Record (noun):** Chronological record tracking gradual dose deviation across regions.
**Related Terms:** Output constancy, QA log.
**Example in Radiotherapy:** Dose drift record showed ±0.7% variation in beam output.

163. **Zonal Beam Profile Index (noun):** Numerical parameter quantifying beam symmetry within each zone.
**Related Terms:** Flatness index, Beam QA.
**Example in Radiotherapy:** Beam profile index confirmed flatness at gantry 90°.

164. **Zero-Flux Surface Mapping (noun):** 3D delineation of boundaries with no particle flux penetration.
**Related Terms:** Monte Carlo boundary, Shielding design.
**Example in Radiotherapy:** Mapping validated vault wall integrity.

165. **Zonal Output Validation Report (noun):** QA summary confirming dose output within tolerance limits per zone.
**Related Terms:** Output QA, Calibration report.
**Example in Radiotherapy:** Validation report submitted to AERB audit.

166. **Zonal Field Symmetry Tolerance (noun):** Allowed variation in beam symmetry measured across zones.
**Related Terms:** Symmetry QA, Tolerance criteria.
**Example in Radiotherapy:** Tolerance confirmed below 2% deviation.

167. **Zonal Scatter Correction Map (noun):** Digital correction file compensating for scatter variations by zone.
**Related Terms:** Scatter modeling, Image correction.
**Example in Radiotherapy:** Scatter correction map reduced CBCT artifacting.

168. **Zonal Energy Spectrum Chart (noun):** Graph showing photon or proton energy distribution across zones.
**Related Terms:** Energy spectrum, QA calibration.
**Example in Radiotherapy:** Chart verified proton energy degradation in range shifter.

169. **Zonal Sensitivity Profile (noun):** Curve depicting detector response sensitivity across defined zones.
**Related Terms:** Detector calibration, QA validation.
**Example in Radiotherapy:** Sensitivity profile validated Gafchromic film uniformity.

170. **Zonal Transmission Factor Table (noun):** Reference table defining attenuation coefficients regionally.
**Related Terms:** Transmission factor, Dose correction.
**Example in Radiotherapy:** Table applied for thoracic beam adjustments.

171. **Zonal Leakage Test Report (noun):** QA documentation ensuring radiation leakage is within permissible limits.
**Related Terms:** Leakage test, Safety compliance.
**Example in Radiotherapy:** Leakage test report submitted during annual machine QA.

172. **Zonal Field Output Constancy Graph (noun):** Graph tracking beam output reproducibility over time.
**Related Terms:** Output consistency, QA chart.
**Example in Radiotherapy:** Constancy graph confirmed stable photon output.

173. **Zonal Magnetic Susceptibility Map (noun):** Image displaying spatial magnetic field distortions in MR-Linac zones.
**Related Terms:** MR distortion, Field mapping.
**Example in Radiotherapy:** Susceptibility map aided MR sequence correction.

174. **Zonal Tissue Heterogeneity Model (noun):** Mathematical model representing density variations in each anatomical region.
**Related Terms:** Tissue inhomogeneity, Dose modeling.
**Example in Radiotherapy:** Model enhanced lung dose accuracy in Monte Carlo planning.

175. **Zonal QA Workflow Sheet (noun):** Document outlining sequential QA procedures for each zone.
**Related Terms:** QA protocol, Process standardization.
**Example in Radiotherapy:** Workflow sheet implemented for adaptive MR QA.

176. **Zonal Dose Fusion Algorithm (noun):** Algorithm combining dose data from multiple image sets regionally.
**Related Terms:** Dose fusion, Adaptive registration.
**Example in Radiotherapy:** Dose fusion algorithm used for cumulative EQD2 analysis.

177. **Zonal Beam Steering Algorithm (noun):** Automated system that corrects angular beam deviation zone-wise.
**Related Terms:** Beam correction, QA automation.
**Example in Radiotherapy:** Steering algorithm optimized noncoplanar beam paths.

178. **Zonal Biophysical Weighting Curve (noun):** Graph representing biological weighting factors across regions.
**Related Terms:** RBE curve, LET mapping.
**Example in Radiotherapy:** Weighting curve applied in hypoxic tissue modeling.

179. **Zonal Verification Phantom (noun):** QA device for verifying zone-specific dose accuracy.
**Related Terms:** Phantom QA, Plan verification.
**Example in Radiotherapy:** Phantom used for IMRT composite dose QA.

180. **Zonal Patient Setup Log (noun):** Chronological record of setup variations per anatomical zone.
**Related Terms:** Position QA, Couch correction.
**Example in Radiotherapy:** Setup log showed <1 mm mean deviation.

181. **Zonal Collimator Calibration Chart (noun):** Data table ensuring jaw positioning precision across zones.
**Related Terms:** Collimator QA, Jaw calibration.
**Example in Radiotherapy:** Chart confirmed accuracy within 0.5 mm.

182. **Zonal QA Benchmark Index (noun):** Normalized indicator for comparing machine performance regionally.
**Related Terms:** QA scoring, Benchmarking.
**Example in Radiotherapy:** Benchmark index improved after MLC motor replacement.

183. **Zonal Dose Verification Certificate (noun):** Official certificate confirming dose verification conformity.
**Related Terms:** QA compliance, Certification record.
**Example in Radiotherapy:** Certificate filed post-clinical commissioning.

184. **Zonal Radiation Leakage Audit (noun):** Safety evaluation to measure stray radiation in defined areas.
**Related Terms:** Shielding QA, Leakage testing.
**Example in Radiotherapy:** Leakage audit ensured safe control room levels.

185. **Zonal Plan Reproducibility Report (noun):** Document comparing repeated plan calculations for consistency.
**Related Terms:** Plan stability, QA reproducibility.
**Example in Radiotherapy:** Report validated adaptive workflow precision.

186. **Zonal Secondary Monitor Ratio (noun):** Ratio of backup chamber readings to primary detectors.
**Related Terms:** Beam monitoring, QA checks.
**Example in Radiotherapy:** Ratio deviations triggered output recalibration.

187. **Zonal QA Uncertainty Budget (noun):** Comprehensive list of measurement uncertainties per region.
**Related Terms:** Measurement error, QA budget.
**Example in Radiotherapy:** Budget table used for TPS commissioning.

188. **Zonal Dose Response Function (noun):** Mathematical relation between dose and biological effect regionally.
**Related Terms:** Dose-response, Radiobiological modeling.
**Example in Radiotherapy:** Function applied in NTCP modeling.

189. **Zonal LET-Weighted Dose Report (noun):** QA document incorporating LET weighting for proton therapy.
**Related Terms:** LET QA, Proton physics.
**Example in Radiotherapy:** Report filed during proton plan validation.

190. **Zonal Beam Quality Factor (noun):** Ratio defining beam hardness for specific field regions.
**Related Terms:** Beam quality, Calibration.
**Example in Radiotherapy:** Factor adjusted for wedge field assessment.

191. **Zero Air Kerma Reading (noun):** Initial reference reading obtained before irradiation to ensure dosimeter baseline.
**Related Terms:** Chamber calibration, Dosimetric zeroing.
**Example in Radiotherapy:** Recorded before every TLD batch measurement.

192. **Zero Beam Output Test (noun):** Verification ensuring no residual beam emission when beam is off.
**Related Terms:** Beam interlock, Safety QA.
**Example in Radiotherapy:** Conducted weekly on all linear accelerators.

193. **Zero Current Leakage (noun):** Condition confirming absence of leakage current from high-voltage circuits.
**Related Terms:** Electrical safety, Equipment maintenance.
**Example in Radiotherapy:** Checked during annual service of gantry power unit.

194. **Zero Dose Point (noun):** Position in treatment plan receiving negligible dose exposure.
**Related Terms:** Shielding design, Dose distribution.
**Example in Radiotherapy:** Zero dose point confirmed for pacemaker during chest IMRT.

195. **Zero Field Exposure (noun):** Verification ensuring radiation beam does not activate outside treatment field.
**Related Terms:** Leakage radiation, QA protocols.
**Example in Radiotherapy:** Confirmed using film during commissioning.

196. **Zero Gap Technique (noun):** Field-matching approach eliminating overlap or underdose between adjacent fields.
**Related Terms:** Junction dose, Matching error.
**Example in Radiotherapy:** Used in craniospinal irradiation to prevent hot/cold spots.

197. **Zero Gravity Patient Handling (noun):** Mechanism using balanced lift systems for patient positioning without strain.
**Related Terms:** Ergonomics, Patient safety.
**Example in Radiotherapy:** Utilized in proton gantry installations for immobilization.

198. **Zero Isocenter Deviation (noun):** Ideal condition where gantry, collimator, and couch axes coincide precisely.
**Related Terms:** Winston-Lutz test, Mechanical QA.
**Example in Radiotherapy:** Achieved tolerance <1 mm on stereotactic linac.

199. **Zero Leakage Collimation (noun):** Collimator configuration preventing radiation leakage outside defined aperture.
**Related Terms:** Beam shaping, Jaw leakage.
**Example in Radiotherapy:** Verified through weekly MLC transmission testing.

200. **Zero Magnet Drift (noun):** Stable magnetic field without temporal fluctuation in MR-Linac systems.
**Related Terms:** Field homogeneity, Magnetic QA.
**Example in Radiotherapy:** Checked using phantom-based MR uniformity scans.

201. **Zero Momentum Transfer (noun):**
Condition where photon interaction causes no momentum change.
**Related Terms:** Elastic scattering, Quantum mechanics.
**Example in Radiotherapy:** Important in Rayleigh scattering analysis for imaging.

202. **Zero Point Calibration (noun):** Baseline calibration ensuring detector reads zero under non-irradiated conditions.
**Related Terms:** Offset correction, Detector QA.
**Example in Radiotherapy:** Applied to ion chambers before dose verification.

203. **Zero Pressure Ionization (noun):** Ionization chamber measurement condition under standard atmospheric corrections.
**Related Terms:** Environmental correction, Barometric factor.
**Example in Radiotherapy:** Applied in chamber correction factor determination.

204. **Zero Reference Line (noun):** Imaging or planning line used as geometric reference baseline.
**Related Terms:** Coordinate alignment, Treatment geometry.
**Example in Radiotherapy:** Defined on DRR for couch shift verification.

205. **Zero Relative Error (noun):** Condition where measured and planned values are identical.
**Related Terms:** Dosimetric accuracy, QA metrics.
**Example in Radiotherapy:** Observed in recalculated IMRT QA passes.

206. **Zero Spin Relaxation (noun):** Hypothetical state where MR signal decay is absent.
**Related Terms:** T1 relaxation, MR physics.
**Example in Radiotherapy:** Used for simulation modeling in MR-guided systems.

207. **Zero Sum Dose (noun):** Mathematical condition where positive and negative dose deviations cancel out.
**Related Terms:** Gamma index, Dose deviation.
**Example in Radiotherapy:** Observed in composite QA evaluation.

208. **Zero Thermal Drift (noun):** Detector output stability regardless of temperature variation.
**Related Terms:** Detector response, Temperature correction.
**Example in Radiotherapy:** Verified during long beam-on tests.

209. **Zero Velocity Dose Delivery (noun):** Radiation delivered with static gantry or couch motion paused.
**Related Terms:** Step-and-shoot IMRT, Beam gating.
**Example in Radiotherapy:** Used during gated lung treatments.

210. **Zero Voltage Bias (noun):** Detector operated without applied potential to test intrinsic signal.
**Related Terms:** Ion collection efficiency, Leakage current.
**Example in Radiotherapy:** Conducted during diode performance testing.

211. **Zeolite Filter (noun):** Mineral-based filter used for trapping radioactive isotopes.
**Related Terms:** Waste management, Decontamination.
**Example in Radiotherapy:** Applied in exhaust filtration for isotope labs.

212. **Zeptosecond Interaction (noun):** Photon–electron interaction occurring at $10^{-21}$ seconds scale.
**Related Terms:** Quantum radiobiology, Ultrafast physics.
**Example in Radiotherapy:** Studied for understanding high-energy photon interactions.

213. **Zeolite Dosimeter (noun):** Natural mineral dosimeter exhibiting colorimetric radiation response.
**Related Terms:** Passive dosimetry, Solid-state detectors.
**Example in Radiotherapy:** Used in environmental monitoring near cyclotron.

214. **Zenithal Beam Entry (noun):** Beam incident from directly overhead orientation.
**Related Terms:** Vertical beam, Gantry geometry.
**Example in Radiotherapy:** Applied in brain metastasis treatment planning.

215. **Zenithal Collimation (noun):** Collimator configuration optimized for vertical incidence fields.
**Related Terms:** Beam shaping, Field optimization.
**Example in Radiotherapy:** Used in fixed-gantry proton systems.

216. **Zeolite Shield (noun):** Composite shielding using zeolite and lead for radiation attenuation.
**Related Terms:** Radiation protection, Barrier design.
**Example in Radiotherapy:** Tested for lightweight bunker panels.

217. **Zernike Polynomial (noun):** Mathematical function modeling optical aberrations.
**Related Terms:** Image reconstruction, Adaptive optics.
**Example in Radiotherapy:** Applied in CBCT image correction algorithms.

218. **Zeta Radiation Index (noun):** Composite metric integrating dose uniformity and conformity.
**Related Terms:** Conformity index, Homogeneity index.
**Example in Radiotherapy:** Used in plan comparison of VMAT vs IMRT.

219. **Ziegler Range Formula (noun):** Empirical relation predicting proton penetration in matter.
**Related Terms:** Range calculation, Stopping power.
**Example in Radiotherapy:** Used in proton beam range prediction tools.

220. **Zirconium Marker (noun):** Radiopaque fiducial used for image-guided localization.
**Related Terms:** Fiducial tracking, Localization QA.
**Example in Radiotherapy:** Implanted in prostate for daily setup verification.

221. **Zinc Phosphate Glass Dosimeter (noun):** Radiation-sensitive glass measuring absorbed dose via luminescence.
**Related Terms:** Passive dosimetry, Optical readout.
**Example in Radiotherapy:** Used for patient surface dose audit.

222. **Zinc Sulfide Screen (noun):** Scintillation screen emitting light under radiation exposure.
**Related Terms:** Fluoroscopic imaging, Beam alignment.
**Example in Radiotherapy:** Used for light field verification.

223. **Zirconate Ceramic Detector (noun):** High-density dosimetric sensor with radiation stability.
**Related Terms:** Semiconductor detector, Solid-state dosimetry.
**Example in Radiotherapy:** Employed for stereotactic dose verification.

224. **Zone Axis Diffraction (noun):** Electron diffraction pattern along a crystal symmetry direction.
**Related Terms:** Material analysis, Detector design.
**Example in Radiotherapy:** Used for analyzing dosimeter crystal structure.

225. **Zygomatic Field Avoidance (noun):** Planning constraint to reduce dose near zygomatic bone.
**Related Terms:** OAR sparing, 3D planning.
**Example in Radiotherapy:** Applied in head-and-neck IMRT optimization.

226. **Zero-Flux Boundary Condition (noun):** Boundary where no net particle or energy transfer occurs.
**Related Terms:** Monte Carlo simulation, Neutron transport.
**Example in Radiotherapy:** Applied in dose modeling of treatment room shielding.

227. **Zero-Gradient Field (noun):** Magnetic field with uniform strength in all directions.
**Related Terms:** Magnetic homogeneity, MR calibration.
**Example in Radiotherapy:** Used in MR-Linac QA for field uniformity checks.

228. **Zero-Signal Noise Ratio (noun):** Ratio of background signal to actual noise in detectors.
**Related Terms:** SNR, Detector sensitivity.
**Example in Radiotherapy:** Evaluated in EPID imaging for dark current calibration.

229. **Zero-Order Kinetics (noun):** Reaction rate independent of reactant concentration.
**Related Terms:** Radiochemistry, Dose response.
**Example in Radiotherapy:** Observed in saturation of DNA repair enzymes post-irradiation.

230. **Zero-Order Phase Error (noun):** Constant phase deviation affecting MR imaging uniformity.
**Related Terms:** Gradient correction, Image distortion.
**Example in Radiotherapy:** Corrected during MR-based image registration QA.

231. **Zero-Point Field (noun):** Lowest energy state of quantum electromagnetic field.
**Related Terms:** Quantum energy, Vacuum fluctuation.
**Example in Radiotherapy:** Theoretical background for stochastic photon interactions.

232. **Zero-Point Radiation (noun):** Residual electromagnetic radiation in vacuum.
**Related Terms:** Casimir effect, Quantum noise.
**Example in Radiotherapy:** Considered in photon interaction uncertainty studies.

233. **Zero-Time Acquisition (noun):** Instantaneous data capture minimizing motion blur.
**Related Terms:** 4D imaging, Motion correction.
**Example in Radiotherapy:** Used in gated CBCT acquisitions.

234. **Zero-Time Decay (noun):** Time taken for radioactive decay initiation after production.
**Related Terms:** Half-life, Activation analysis.
**Example in Radiotherapy:** Considered in cyclotron isotope transport timing.

235. **Zero-Variance Simulation (noun):** Monte Carlo variance reduction method for deterministic accuracy.
**Related Terms:** Dose modeling, Computational physics.
**Example in Radiotherapy:** Applied in electron beam dose prediction software.

236. **Zeeman Calibration (noun):** Adjustment of MR frequency under known magnetic field splitting.
**Related Terms:** MR physics, Larmor frequency.
**Example in Radiotherapy:** Used for magnetic field uniformity calibration.

237. **Zeolite Catalyst (noun):** Porous aluminosilicate used in radiochemical purification.
**Related Terms:** Isotope separation, Radiopharmacy.
**Example in Radiotherapy:** Used in radionuclide generator column filters.

238. **Zeolite Nanoparticle Shield (noun):** Nano-composite barrier reducing low-energy photon scatter.
**Related Terms:** Shielding material, Nanotechnology.
**Example in Radiotherapy:** Tested for low-weight bunker panel development.

239. **Zenith Correction Factor (noun):** Adjustment for angular dependence of radiation intensity.
**Related Terms:** Angular response, Dosimetry correction.
**Example in Radiotherapy:** Applied for surface dose calibration in TBI.

240. **Zenith Projection Imaging (noun):** Top-down imaging approach for spatial verification.
**Related Terms:** 3D imaging, Surface guidance.
**Example in Radiotherapy:** Used in cranial SRS for head alignment.

241. **Zepto Gray (noun):** Dose unit equal to $10^{-21}$ gray, used in ultralow exposure studies.
**Related Terms:** Microdosimetry, Radiobiological scaling.
**Example in Radiotherapy:** Applied in single-cell nanodosimetry research.

242. **Zeptosecond Pulse (noun):** Ultrashort light pulse enabling attosecond-level interaction studies.
**Related Terms:** Quantum biology, Laser-plasma physics.
**Example in Radiotherapy:** Used in fundamental radiation–matter research.

243. **Zero-Dose Mapping (noun):** Visualization of zero-exposure regions within a plan.
**Related Terms:** Dose cloud, Dose-volume histogram.
**Example in Radiotherapy:** Used to validate shielding efficiency.

244. **Zero-Energy Photon (noun):** Theoretical photon with no measurable energy transfer.
**Related Terms:** Quantum vacuum, Elastic scattering.
**Example in Radiotherapy:** Modeled for low-dose background analysis.

245. **Zero-Friction Couch (noun):** Couch design minimizing resistance for fine motion correction.
**Related Terms:** Robotic couch, Motion precision.
**Example in Radiotherapy:** Used in MR-Linac adaptive treatments.

246. **Zero-Gate Delay (noun):** Minimal latency between respiratory signal and beam gating.
**Related Terms:** Beam gating, Real-time tracking.
**Example in Radiotherapy:** Achieved using optical surface guidance.

247. **Zero-Gap MLC Design (noun):** Leaf design ensuring no leakage between adjacent leaves.
**Related Terms:** MLC transmission, Beam shaping.
**Example in Radiotherapy:** Used in HD120 MLC configurations.

248. **Zero-Hysteresis Magnet (noun):** Magnet showing no lag between magnetization and field strength.
**Related Terms:** MR magnet, Magnetic QA.
**Example in Radiotherapy:** Used for MR-guided system calibration.

249. **Zero-Latency Tracking (noun):** Real-time tumor tracking without delay.
**Related Terms:** Motion management, Adaptive therapy.
**Example in Radiotherapy:** Implemented in MR-Linac systems for gated delivery.

250. **Zero-Leakage Cable (noun):** High-voltage cable preventing any current leakage.
**Related Terms:** Electrical safety, Linac maintenance.
**Example in Radiotherapy:** Inspected annually in power coupling units.

251. **Zero-Margin Planning (noun):** Treatment planning without geometric expansion margins.
**Related Terms:** PTV margin, Adaptive planning.
**Example in Radiotherapy:** Used in daily MR-guided adaptive sessions.

252. **Zero-Motion Imaging (noun):** Technique capturing anatomy in static state.
**Related Terms:** 4DCT, Motion suppression.
**Example in Radiotherapy:** Applied for liver SBRT breath-hold imaging.

253. **Zero-Noise Imaging (noun):** Acquisition achieving optimal signal clarity without artifacts.
**Related Terms:** Image quality, Noise reduction.
**Example in Radiotherapy:** Used in AI-enhanced CBCT reconstructions.

254. **Zero-Offset Algorithm (noun):** Correction method eliminating baseline detector shift.
**Related Terms:** Calibration, Signal processing.
**Example in Radiotherapy:** Integrated in EPID flat-field calibration.

255. **Zero-Phase Planning (noun):** Treatment planning ignoring temporal phase variations.
**Related Terms:** Motion compensation, 4D planning.
**Example in Radiotherapy:** Used in static phantom plan validation.

256. **Zero-Pressure Chamber (noun):** Ionization chamber operated in vacuum for absolute dose.
**Related Terms:** Standard dosimetry, Air-kerma free calibration.
**Example in Radiotherapy:** Used in metrology-grade measurements.

257. **Zero-Reflection Boundary (noun):** Model boundary with no returning radiation wave.
**Related Terms:** Absorbing boundary, Monte Carlo geometry.
**Example in Radiotherapy:** Implemented in photon transport simulations.

258. **Zero-Response Detector (noun):** Detector showing no measurable output under set conditions.
**Related Terms:** Detector fault, QA testing.
**Example in Radiotherapy:** Identified during chamber leakage inspection.

259. **Zero-Temperature Effect (noun):** Theoretical state of no thermal radiation emission.
**Related Terms:** Cryogenic detector, Blackbody radiation.
**Example in Radiotherapy:** Modeled in thermal noise correction studies.

260. **Zero-Time Decorrelation (noun):** Condition where temporal variations in signal are absent.
**Related Terms:** Temporal noise, Signal stability.
**Example in Radiotherapy:** Used in MR-linac temporal imaging QA.

261. **Zirconia Phantom (noun):** High-density phantom simulating bone-equivalent tissue.
**Related Terms:** Phantom QA, Tissue equivalence.
**Example in Radiotherapy:** Used for stereotactic dose verification.

262. **Zirconium Dioxide Detector (noun):** Ceramic detector material resistant to radiation damage.
**Related Terms:** Semiconductor detector, Solid-state dosimetry.
**Example in Radiotherapy:** Used for long-term output stability monitoring.

263. **Zinc Oxide Film Dosimeter (noun):** Nanostructured thin film used for UV and X-ray dose detection.
**Related Terms:** Nanodosimetry, Passive sensors.
**Example in Radiotherapy:** Applied for surface dose mapping.

264. **Zonal Heat Map (noun):** (rare usage) Thermal representation of energy deposition.
**Related Terms:** Energy deposition, Tissue heating.
**Example in Radiotherapy:** Used for thermal modeling of high-dose regions.

265. **Z-Plasty Algorithm (noun):** Optimization technique for adaptive contour reshaping.
**Related Terms:** Auto-segmentation, Deformable registration.
**Example in Radiotherapy:** Used in adaptive recontouring automation.

266. **Z-Transform (noun):** Mathematical operation for discrete signal frequency analysis.
**Related Terms:** Signal processing, Image reconstruction.
**Example in Radiotherapy:** Used in digital radiograph noise filtering.

267. **Z-Valve (noun):** Precision valve used in vacuum beamline systems.
**Related Terms:** Cyclotron hardware, Vacuum control.
**Example in Radiotherapy:** Maintains beamline integrity during isotope transfer.

268. **Z-Vector Correction (noun):** Longitudinal axis correction during 3D image registration.
**Related Terms:** Couch correction, Image fusion.
**Example in Radiotherapy:** Applied for patient alignment verification.

269. **Zenith Detector Array (noun):** Top-mounted detector system for beam uniformity evaluation.
**Related Terms:** 2D array, Flatness QA.
**Example in Radiotherapy:** Zenith array verified uniformity during VMAT commissioning.

270. **Zero Field Output Factor (noun):** Measured output at a vanishingly small field size for model validation.
**Related Terms:** Output factor, Small-field dosimetry.
**Example in Radiotherapy:** Data refined the Monte Carlo scatter correction model.

271. **Zinc Oxide Nanoparticle (noun):** Metal oxide particle investigated as a potential radiosensitizer.
**Related Terms:** Nanomedicine, Radiosensitization.
**Example in Radiotherapy:** ZnO nanoparticles increased DNA damage under 6 MV exposure.

272. **Z-score Normalization (noun):** Statistical scaling method for image intensity standardization.
**Related Terms:** Image preprocessing, Radiomics.
**Example in Radiotherapy:** MR images normalized using Z-score before segmentation training.

273. **Zero Gap Interface (noun):** Design ensuring no space between detector plates or magnets.
**Related Terms:** Geometric precision, Field homogeneity.
**Example in Radiotherapy:** MR-Linac head redesign used zero gap coils for uniform field.

274. **Zone Boundary Dose (noun):** Transition region dose between PTV and OAR.
**Related Terms:** Gradient index, Dose fall-off.
**Example in Radiotherapy:** Boundary dose tightened to meet liver SBRT constraint.

275. **Zeolite-based Phantom (noun):** Solid phantom using zeolite material for density simulation.
**Related Terms:** Phantom material, Dosimetry QA.
**Example in Radiotherapy:** Zeolite phantom tested for proton range verification.

276. **Zoomed MRI Sequence (noun):** Reduced FOV MR technique for localized imaging.
**Related Terms:** MR-Linac imaging, Artifact reduction.
**Example in Radiotherapy:** Zoomed MRI improved prostate contouring accuracy.

277. **Zigzag Beam Modulation (noun):** Beam fluence modulation pattern used for uniform coverage.
**Related Terms:** IMRT fluence, Field shaping.
**Example in Radiotherapy:** Zigzag modulation optimized target homogeneity index.

278. **Zero-Dose Control Region (noun):** Area shielded to receive no measurable dose.
**Related Terms:** Shielding verification, Dose constraint.
**Example in Radiotherapy:** Rectal balloon ensured zero-dose control zone in prostate plan.

279. **Z-Value Imaging (noun):** Quantitative representation of voxel deviation from mean signal.
**Related Terms:** Radiomics feature, Statistical imaging.
**Example in Radiotherapy:** Z-value map assessed edema evolution post-SRS.

280. **Zinc Finger Repair Protein (noun):** DNA-binding protein family involved in radiation-induced repair.
**Related Terms:** DNA repair, Radiobiology.
**Example in Radiotherapy:** Inhibiting zinc finger proteins enhanced radiosensitivity in glioma cells.

281. **Zero Gradient Coil (noun):** MR coil configuration minimizing magnetic gradient distortions.
**Related Terms:** MR-Linac stability, Magnetic homogeneity.
**Example in Radiotherapy:** Coil used to enhance geometric fidelity for adaptive planning.

282. **Zenithal Dose Projection (noun):** Top-down visualization of cumulative dose in 3D volume.
**Related Terms:** Dose visualization, Plan evaluation.
**Example in Radiotherapy:** Zenithal projection improved target coverage review in lung SBRT.

283. **Zipper Artifact (noun):** Line artifact caused by RF interference in MRI images.
**Related Terms:** MR artifact, Image QA.
**Example in Radiotherapy:** Zipper artifact removed after shielding cable repair on MR-Linac.

284. **Zonal Registration Index (noun):** Numeric index quantifying spatial alignment accuracy in zones.
**Related Terms:** Image registration, CBCT matching.
**Example in Radiotherapy:** Index dropped after AI-assisted registration update.

285. **Zero Suppression Mode (noun):** Electronics function eliminating low-level signal noise.
**Related Terms:** Detector readout, Noise reduction.
**Example in Radiotherapy:** Zero suppression improved SRS detector signal clarity.

286. **Zirconium Filter (noun):** High-Z filter element enhancing spectral shaping.
**Related Terms:** Beam hardening, Filtration.
**Example in Radiotherapy:** Zirconium filter applied to flatten kV imaging beam.

287. **Zone-of-Interest Reconstruction (noun):** CBCT technique reconstructing partial anatomy to reduce dose.
**Related Terms:** ROI imaging, Adaptive verification.
**Example in Radiotherapy:** Partial pelvis scan reconstructed via zone-of-interest technique.

288. **Z-axis Collimator (noun):** Collimator controlling longitudinal beam extent.
**Related Terms:** Multi-leaf collimator, Field shaping.
**Example in Radiotherapy:** Z-axis collimator calibrated for 10 cm dynamic field.

289. **Zero Check Protocol (noun):** Routine QA ensuring all meters and chambers read baseline zero.
**Related Terms:** Daily QA, Equipment verification.
**Example in Radiotherapy:** Protocol logged before first patient beam each day.

**290. Z-score Mapping (noun):** Quantitative map of statistical deviations in voxel intensity.
**Related Terms:** Image analytics, Radiomics.
**Example in Radiotherapy:** Z-score mapping aided tumor heterogeneity study.

**291. Zygomatic Dose Constraint (noun):** OAR limit protecting zygomatic bone from excess radiation.
**Related Terms:** Bone tolerance, Head & neck planning.
**Example in Radiotherapy:** Constraint enforced during parotid reirradiation plan.

**292. Z-value Thresholding (noun):** Segmentation rule based on voxel intensity deviation.
**Related Terms:** Image segmentation, Threshold mapping.
**Example in Radiotherapy:** Automated Z-thresholding detected necrotic regions in MR images.

**293. Zero-Gap Multileaf (noun):** MLC design minimizing interleaf radiation leakage.
**Related Terms:** MLC transmission, Leaf design.
**Example in Radiotherapy:** New zero-gap leaves reduced leakage by 25%.

**294. Zenith Beam Pathway (noun):** Superior-inferior beam route aligned along patient's vertical axis.
**Related Terms:** Beam geometry, Entry angle.
**Example in Radiotherapy:** Zenith beam optimized dose fall-off in spine SBRT.

**295. Zirconium Oxide Film (noun):** Film dosimeter using $ZrO_2$ layer for high-energy photon sensitivity.
**Related Terms:** Film dosimetry, Detector materials.
**Example in Radiotherapy:** Used for 6 MV beam film calibration.

**296. Zero-Flux Chamber (noun):** Electrometer configuration ensuring no net current flow.
**Related Terms:** Ion chamber, Current measurement.
**Example in Radiotherapy:** Chamber verified leakage current of <0.1%.

**297. Zonal Beam Symmetry Index (noun):** Quantitative value for lateral dose balance.
**Related Terms:** Beam QA, Symmetry analysis.
**Example in Radiotherapy:** Index confirmed acceptable symmetry in $10\times10$ $cm^2$ field.

**298. Zeta Potential Shift (noun):** Electrokinetic change indicating nanoparticle surface modification post-irradiation.
**Related Terms:** Nanodosimetry, Surface charge.
**Example in Radiotherapy:** Zeta potential shift detected after proton exposure.

**299. Zero-Collision Model (noun):** Simplified transport model assuming no secondary interactions.
**Related Terms:** Monte Carlo approximation, Photon transport.
**Example in Radiotherapy:** Used for fast proton dose estimation in QA software.

**300. Zero-Phase Response Filter (noun):** Digital filter maintaining waveform integrity without phase distortion.
**Related Terms:** Signal processing, Detector calibration.
**Example in Radiotherapy:** Applied in EPID signal correction for accurate portal dosimetry analysis.

**301. Zeeman-Effect Correction (noun):** Adjustment accounting for magnetic field splitting of spectral lines.
**Related Terms:** MR-Linac, Magnetic field calibration.
**Example in Radiotherapy:** Zeeman correction ensured accurate field homogeneity during adaptive MR imaging.

**302. Zinc-Binding Radiosensitizer (noun):** Compound targeting zinc-dependent enzymes to enhance radiation damage.
**Related Terms:** Radiobiology, Molecular therapy.
**Example in Radiotherapy:** Zinc-binding agents improved tumor oxygenation and radiosensitivity in hypoxic models.

303. **Zonal Fourier Transform (noun):** Mathematical tool decomposing spatial dose variations.
**Related Terms:** Image analysis, Dose uniformity.
**Example in Radiotherapy:** Fourier mapping identified periodic leaf pattern in IMRT delivery.

304. **Z-Type Calibration Phantom (noun):** Phantom with stepped density layers for energy verification.
**Related Terms:** QA phantom, Beam quality.
**Example in Radiotherapy:** Used in annual beam energy calibration for proton machine QA.

305. **Z-Pathway Sequencing (noun):** Algorithm determining optimal particle trajectory for dose uniformity.
**Related Terms:** Proton planning, Beam optimization.
**Example in Radiotherapy:** Sequencing improved conformity index in cranial proton treatments.

306. **Zeolite Cavity Dosimeter (noun):** Solid-state dosimeter utilizing microporous zeolite matrix.
**Related Terms:** Solid dosimetry, Detector materials.
**Example in Radiotherapy:** Zeolite dosimeter showed linearity up to 20 Gy in photon beam.

307. **Zeta-Dose Mapping System (noun):** Software tool visualizing electrostatic dose influence in ion beams.
**Related Terms:** Ion beam physics, Dose reconstruction.
**Example in Radiotherapy:** Mapping aided in analyzing stray ion dose near magnetic lenses.

308. **Zenith Correction Grid (noun):** Grid compensating for vertical gantry drift during arc therapy.
**Related Terms:** Mechanical QA, Gantry sag.
**Example in Radiotherapy:** Correction grid applied in high-precision cranial SRS delivery.

309. **Zero-Delay Feedback Circuit (noun):** Electronic control system minimizing latency in beam steering.
**Related Terms:** Beam control, Linac electronics.
**Example in Radiotherapy:** Circuit stabilized magnet current in MR-Linac adaptive workflows.

310. **Zinc-Ion Diffusion Model (noun):** Mathematical representation of ion movement under radiation stress.
**Related Terms:** Radiobiology, Ion kinetics.
**Example in Radiotherapy:** Model predicted diffusion-mediated DNA damage enhancement.

311. **Z-Score-Based Deformable Registration (noun):** Statistical image alignment method using voxel deviation normalization.
**Related Terms:** Deformable registration, CBCT matching.
**Example in Radiotherapy:** Improved liver motion tracking accuracy in adaptive SBRT.

312. **Zeolite Composite Shielding (noun):** Radiation barrier combining zeolite with polymer or metal composites.
**Related Terms:** Shielding design, Material science.
**Example in Radiotherapy:** Used to reduce neutron scatter around proton therapy vault.

313. **Zero-Leak Vacuum Chamber (noun):** Sealed containment ensuring no gas leakage for beamline stability.
**Related Terms:** Accelerator vacuum, Beamline engineering.
**Example in Radiotherapy:** Chamber integrity verified during proton nozzle maintenance.

314. **Z-Plane Adaptive Collimation (noun):** Dynamic control of collimator aperture along patient's longitudinal axis.
**Related Terms:** Collimation, Dynamic shaping.
**Example in Radiotherapy:** Enhanced field adaptation during MR-guided abdominal treatment.

315. **Zeeman-Resolved MR Coil (noun):** Coil optimized for fine magnetic resolution through Zeeman signal differentiation.
**Related Terms:** MR-Linac, Signal fidelity.
**Example in Radiotherapy:** Coil provided high-resolution field mapping for geometry QA.

316. **Zircon-Enhanced Bolus (noun):** Tissue-equivalent bolus containing zircon particles for beam modulation.
**Related Terms:** Bolus design, Surface dose enhancement.
**Example in Radiotherapy:** Used in photon chest wall treatments for improved buildup dose.

317. **Z-Axis Intensity Control Algorithm (noun):** Software function managing longitudinal intensity profiles in scanning beams.
**Related Terms:** Proton therapy, Beam shaping.
**Example in Radiotherapy:** Algorithm refined distal fall-off in spread-out Bragg peak.

318. **Z-Profile Dosimetry (noun):** Depth-dose analysis performed along beam's central longitudinal axis.
**Related Terms:** Depth-dose curve, PDD.
**Example in Radiotherapy:** Used for verifying range precision in proton beams.

319. **Zero-Drift Amplifier (noun):** Amplifier circuit maintaining constant output despite temperature variation.
**Related Terms:** Signal stability, Detector electronics.
**Example in Radiotherapy:** Integrated in electrometer to stabilize low-current readings.

320. **Zeolite-Carbon Composite Filter (noun):** Hybrid filtration element reducing neutron activation and gas byproducts.
**Related Terms:** Air filtration, Radiation safety.
**Example in Radiotherapy:** Used in MR-Linac cooling systems to trap airborne ions.

321. **Zonal Adaptive Masking (noun):** Image processing technique emphasizing clinically relevant regions.
**Related Terms:** Image enhancement, AI segmentation.
**Example in Radiotherapy:** Adaptive masking improved delineation of GTV in rectal MRI.

322. **Zirconium Alloy Marker (noun):** Fiducial marker resistant to corrosion and MR interference.
**Related Terms:** Fiducial tracking, MR compatibility.
**Example in Radiotherapy:** Implanted in prostate for MR-guided localization.

323. **Zero-Current Mode (noun):** Operational mode where circuit bias current is minimized to prevent noise.
**Related Terms:** Low-noise electronics, Detector readout.
**Example in Radiotherapy:** Enabled precise current measurement in micro-chambers.

324. **Zonal Dose Predictor (noun):** AI model forecasting regional dose variations using voxel features.
**Related Terms:** Dose prediction, Machine learning.
**Example in Radiotherapy:** Predictor optimized dose distribution in pelvic VMAT.

325. **Zinc Chelation Therapy (noun):** Adjunctive treatment reducing zinc-mediated tumor repair post-irradiation.
**Related Terms:** Radiomodification, Radiobiology.
**Example in Radiotherapy:** Zinc chelators tested to delay tumor regrowth in xenografts.

326. **Zero-Angle Scatter (noun):** Photon scattering event maintaining incident trajectory.
**Related Terms:** Coherent scatter, Photon transport.
**Example in Radiotherapy:** Zero-angle contribution factored in Monte Carlo simulations.

327. **Zeta-Field Simulation (noun):** Simulated model representing electrostatic field variations.
**Related Terms:** Beam dynamics, Particle transport.
**Example in Radiotherapy:** Simulation used to optimize magnetic lens design.

328. **Zeolite Nanocarrier (noun):** Porous nanoparticle delivering radiosensitizers to tumor microenvironments.
**Related Terms:** Nanomedicine, Drug delivery.
**Example in Radiotherapy:** Enhanced targeted uptake in hypoxic glioma regions.

329. **Zero-Signal Calibration (noun):** Calibration procedure ensuring null detector response at baseline.
**Related Terms:** Detector QA, Calibration.
**Example in Radiotherapy:** Applied before in-vivo diode QA sessions.

330. **Zonal Stability Constant (noun):** Value representing mechanical stability under rotational motion.
**Related Terms:** Gantry QA, Mechanical accuracy.
**Example in Radiotherapy:** Stability constant monitored during annual gantry isocenter check.

331. **Zirconium-Based Detector (noun):** High-sensitivity radiation detector using zirconium thin films.
**Related Terms:** Semiconductor detector, Novel materials.
**Example in Radiotherapy:** Detector validated for ultra-high dose rate FLASH beams.

332. **Zero-Crossing Analysis (noun):** Method detecting signal inflection points for waveform reconstruction.
**Related Terms:** Signal processing, Timing calibration.
**Example in Radiotherapy:** Used for dose synchronization in gated treatments.

333. **Zinc Oxide Dosimeter (noun):** Nano-dosimeter using ZnO for high spatial resolution dose mapping.
**Related Terms:** Nanodosimetry, Fluorescent detectors.
**Example in Radiotherapy:** Demonstrated linear response up to 10 Gy.

334. **Zeolite-Based Immobilizer (noun):** Composite immobilization material providing structural rigidity and radiolucency.
**Related Terms:** Patient setup, Immobilization.
**Example in Radiotherapy:** Used for thoracic immobilization in MR-guided treatments.

335. **Zero-Voltage Drift Control (noun):** Feedback system maintaining stable reference voltage.
**Related Terms:** Detector calibration, Signal accuracy.
**Example in Radiotherapy:** Integrated into electrometer to reduce baseline noise.

336. **Zeta Flux Density (noun):** Measure of localized electrostatic field intensity in beam optics.
**Related Terms:** Field mapping, Beam dynamics.
**Example in Radiotherapy:** Zeta flux patterns analyzed during MR-Linac gradient coil QA.

337. **Zero-Delay Synchronizer (noun):** Timing circuit ensuring no phase lag between trigger and beam delivery.
**Related Terms:** Gating system, Timing control.
**Example in Radiotherapy:** Synchronizer aligned beam pulse with respiratory phase gating.

338. **Zeolite Fiber Shield (noun):** Composite fiber layer reducing neutron scatter in vault walls.
**Related Terms:** Radiation protection, Neutron moderation.
**Example in Radiotherapy:** Installed near gantry rotation path for neutron shielding efficiency.

339. **Zinc-Assisted Radiosensitization (noun):** Enhancement of tumor radiosensitivity via zinc-induced oxidative stress.
**Related Terms:** Radiosensitizer, Radiobiology.
**Example in Radiotherapy:** Zinc-assisted sensitization increased DNA double-strand breaks in glioblastoma cells.

340. **Zonal AI Reconstruction (noun):** Artificial intelligence algorithm reconstructing dose distributions regionally.
**Related Terms:** Deep learning, Dose estimation.
**Example in Radiotherapy:** AI reconstruction improved voxel-based dosimetry accuracy in liver SBRT.

341. **Zirconate Crystal Detector (noun):** Scintillator crystal with high light yield for MV photon beams.
**Related Terms:** Scintillation detector, Dosimetry.
**Example in Radiotherapy:** Used in portal dosimeters for high-resolution imaging.

342. **Zero-Collision Pathway (noun):** Idealized trajectory free of scattering events in transport models.
**Related Terms:** Monte Carlo simulation, Particle transport.
**Example in Radiotherapy:** Applied in fast proton dose computation modules.

343. **Z-score Intensity Normalizer (noun):** Statistical module adjusting image brightness by mean deviation.
**Related Terms:** Image preprocessing, Standardization.
**Example in Radiotherapy:** Used to normalize CT datasets for AI-based segmentation.

344. **Zinc-Ferrite Nanocarrier (noun):** Magnetic nanoparticle enabling radiosensitizer delivery and imaging.
**Related Terms:** Theranostics, Radiobiology.
**Example in Radiotherapy:** Provided targeted MRI visibility in head and neck cancer therapy.

345. **Zero-Flux Magnet Core (noun):** Transformer core ensuring stable inductance with no residual magnetism.
**Related Terms:** Beamline electronics, Magnetic stabilization.
**Example in Radiotherapy:** Maintained current consistency during beam steering calibration.

346. **Z-Gradient Compensation Algorithm (noun):** Computational correction for magnetic field nonuniformity along longitudinal axis.
**Related Terms:** MR-Linac, Gradient mapping.
**Example in Radiotherapy:** Algorithm improved geometric fidelity of adaptive MR images.

347. **Zirconium Dioxide Nanoparticle (noun):** Nano-additive enhancing radiation dose absorption in tumor microenvironments.
**Related Terms:** Radiosensitizer, Nanomedicine.
**Example in Radiotherapy:** Increased oxidative stress under 6 MV photon exposure.

348. **Zenith Tracking System (noun):** Overhead tracking device aligning gantry motion to spatial reference.
**Related Terms:** Motion management, Image guidance.
**Example in Radiotherapy:** Used for auto-positioning during cranial VMAT delivery.

349. **Zero-Noise Amplifier (noun):** Electronic amplifier minimizing signal distortion during data acquisition.
**Related Terms:** Detector electronics, Noise filtering.
**Example in Radiotherapy:** Improved signal-to-noise ratio in ion chamber readout.

350. **Z-score-Based Anomaly Detector (noun):** Algorithm identifying abnormal voxel intensity patterns in QA imaging.
**Related Terms:** Machine learning, Image QA.
**Example in Radiotherapy:** Detected gantry tilt deviations during CBCT QA test.

351. **Zirconate-Ceramic Dosimeter (noun):** Solid-state dosimeter with high radiation hardness and linearity.
**Related Terms:** Ceramic detector, Dosimetry.
**Example in Radiotherapy:** Calibrated for proton dose verification at isocenter.

352. **Zero-Fault Monitoring System (noun):** Integrated QA system continuously verifying operational status.
**Related Terms:** Linac QA, Safety interlock.
**Example in Radiotherapy:** System logged gantry interlock response time during QA.

353. **Zonal Thermal Mapping (noun):** Temperature distribution mapping in equipment under operation.
**Related Terms:** Thermal QA, Equipment stability.
**Example in Radiotherapy:** Used for MR gradient coil heat monitoring.

354. **Zinc Chelate Nanogel (noun):**
Hydrogel structure carrying zinc ions to radiosensitize tumor cells.
**Related Terms:** Drug delivery, Nanomedicine.
**Example in Radiotherapy:** Enhanced oxygenation prior to fractionated treatment.

355. **Zero-Latency Feedback Module (noun):** Real-time correction system minimizing lag between measurement and response.
**Related Terms:** Beam control, Feedback electronics.
**Example in Radiotherapy:** Module synchronized couch motion with respiratory pattern.

356. **Zeolite-Based Radioabsorber (noun):** Material absorbing stray secondary radiation in treatment rooms.
**Related Terms:** Radiation safety, Scattered dose reduction.
**Example in Radiotherapy:** Applied near treatment head to reduce leakage radiation.

357. **Z-Axis Modulated Beam (noun):** Longitudinally intensity-modulated beam improving dose conformity.
**Related Terms:** IMRT, Dose shaping.
**Example in Radiotherapy:** Used in proton spot scanning for uniform target coverage.

358. **Zero-Variance Estimator (noun):** Mathematical approach reducing statistical noise in Monte Carlo dose results.
**Related Terms:** Dose simulation, Statistical analysis.
**Example in Radiotherapy:** Enhanced convergence in GPU-based proton dose modeling.

359. **Zr-Ti Composite Shield (noun):** Zirconium–titanium composite barrier attenuating secondary neutron radiation.
**Related Terms:** Radiation shielding, Structural protection.
**Example in Radiotherapy:** Installed near cyclotron beam exit port for neutron control.

360. **Zero-Error Synchronization Test (noun):** QA procedure ensuring alignment between trigger pulses and beam delivery.
**Related Terms:** Timing QA, Gating accuracy.
**Example in Radiotherapy:** Test verified respiratory gating delay within 5 ms.

361. **Zinc Finger Transcription Inhibitor (noun):** Compound targeting repair proteins to increase radiosensitivity.
**Related Terms:** Molecular radiosensitizer, DNA repair.
**Example in Radiotherapy:** Inhibitor delayed DNA repair in lung carcinoma cells.

362. **Zonal Dose Gradient Curve (noun):** Graphical representation of dose fall-off between target and OAR.
**Related Terms:** Gradient index, Dose fall-off.
**Example in Radiotherapy:** Used for SBRT lung plan evaluation.

363. **Zero-Velocity Beam Gate (noun):** System pausing radiation delivery during zero tumor motion phase.
**Related Terms:** Motion gating, Synchronization.
**Example in Radiotherapy:** Triggered beam hold between respiratory peaks.

364. **Zeolite-Coated Detector (noun):** Detector coated with zeolite film for enhanced sensitivity and shielding.
**Related Terms:** Detector design, Material science.
**Example in Radiotherapy:** Improved dose linearity under low-energy photon exposure.

365. **Zirconium Alloy Collimator (noun):** Collimator material offering corrosion resistance and MR compatibility.
**Related Terms:** Collimator design, MR-Linac integration.
**Example in Radiotherapy:** Used in adaptive MR-guided head treatments.

366. **Z-Coordinate Matrix (noun):** Matrix describing voxel positions along longitudinal imaging axis.
**Related Terms:** Image reconstruction, Coordinate geometry.
**Example in Radiotherapy:** Utilized in deformable registration during adaptive re-planning.

367. **Zero-Field Magnetometer (noun):** Instrument detecting minimal magnetic fluctuations within shielded systems.
**Related Terms:** Field stability, MR QA.
**Example in Radiotherapy:** Monitored MR-Linac field drift during gantry rotation.

368. **Zinc Oxide Nanocomposite Film (noun):** Thin dosimetric film incorporating ZnO nanoparticles for improved response.
**Related Terms:** Film dosimetry, Nanodosimeter.
**Example in Radiotherapy:** Demonstrated uniform response up to 20 Gy.

369. **Z-Plasma Generator (noun):** Ion source producing confined plasma columns for accelerator research.
**Related Terms:** Accelerator physics, Particle source.
**Example in Radiotherapy:** Evaluated for high-efficiency ion beam generation.

370. **Zero-Field Relaxation Time (noun):** Decay constant of magnetization without external magnetic field.
**Related Terms:** MR physics, Relaxation parameter.
**Example in Radiotherapy:** Used to validate MR-Linac T1 calibration.

371. **Zeeman Resonance Detector (noun):** Device measuring frequency shifts in magnetic fields.
**Related Terms:** Magnetic calibration, MR QA.
**Example in Radiotherapy:** Verified homogeneity of 1.5 T MR-Linac magnet.

372. **Zirconium Carbonate Coating (noun):** Protective surface coating reducing scatter on collimator leaves.
**Related Terms:** Surface treatment, Beam shaping.
**Example in Radiotherapy:** Improved transmission uniformity in MLC QA.

**373. Zero-Leak Vacuum Seal (noun):** Ultra-tight sealing mechanism preventing air ingress in beamlines.
**Related Terms:** Vacuum technology, Beam quality.
**Example in Radiotherapy:** Used in proton nozzle maintenance protocols.

**374. Zinc Enzyme Modulator (noun):** Compound regulating zinc-dependent enzymes post-irradiation.
**Related Terms:** Cellular repair, Radiosensitivity.
**Example in Radiotherapy:** Reduced repair efficiency in DNA damage studies.

**375. Z-Factor Correction Model (noun):** Empirical model adjusting detector readings under varied beam conditions.
**Related Terms:** Calibration, Detector response.
**Example in Radiotherapy:** Improved output factor precision during small-field QA.

**376. Z-Map Reconstruction (noun):** Three-dimensional mapping of magnetic susceptibility differences in MRI-guided radiotherapy for dose adaptation.
**Related Terms:** MR-Linac imaging, Susceptibility correction.
**Example in Radiotherapy:** Z-map reconstruction improved soft-tissue visualization during adaptive liver SBRT.

**377. Zero Field Leakage Test (noun):** Verification that no radiation escapes when beam-shaping jaws and MLCs are fully closed.
**Related Terms:** Leakage tolerance, Linac QA.
**Example in Radiotherapy:** Annual QA included a zero field leakage test under IEC standards.

**378. Zero Lag Dose Response (noun):** Immediate detector signal response without delay during dynamic irradiation.
**Related Terms:** Detector sensitivity, Real-time dosimetry.
**Example in Radiotherapy:** EPID testing confirmed near-zero lag during VMAT delivery.

**379. Zero-Point Correction (noun):** Adjustment to baseline detector signal to ensure accurate dose readout.
**Related Terms:** Chamber calibration, Reference setup.
**Example in Radiotherapy:** Zero-point correction applied before ion chamber constancy check.

**380. Zero-Drift Chamber (noun):** Ionization chamber type minimizing charge drift and leakage current.
**Related Terms:** Chamber stability, QA instrumentation.
**Example in Radiotherapy:** Zero-drift design used in precision proton beam calibration.

**381. Zero-Gap MLC Alignment (noun):** Calibration ensuring leaves fully close without radiation leakage at isocenter.
**Related Terms:** Leaf calibration, Transmission QA.
**Example in Radiotherapy:** Verified using film dosimetry and log file analysis.

**382. Zero-Field Background Dose (noun):** Residual environmental radiation dose with beam off condition.
**Related Terms:** Ambient dose, Shielding QA.
**Example in Radiotherapy:** Background dose monitored weekly in treatment bunker.

**383. Zero-Position Gantry Check (noun):** Mechanical validation of gantry returning precisely to 0° reference.
**Related Terms:** Mechanical accuracy, Rotation QA.
**Example in Radiotherapy:** Laser projection verified zero-position stability within ±0.1°.

384. **Zero-Sum Dose Mapping (noun):** Algorithm ensuring total absorbed dose conservation across recalculated adaptive plans.
**Related Terms:** Dose accumulation, Adaptive planning.
**Example in Radiotherapy:** Employed to validate accumulated dose after plan re-optimization.

385. **Zero-Tolerance QA (noun):** Quality assurance protocol allowing no deviation from specified parameters.
**Related Terms:** High precision QA, Error minimization.
**Example in Radiotherapy:** MR-Linac adaptive workflow maintained zero-tolerance for alignment errors.

386. **Zirconium Filter (noun):** Filter material used in diagnostic or therapy imaging to shape X-ray spectrum.
**Related Terms:** Beam filtration, Spectrum hardening.
**Example in Radiotherapy:** Zirconium filter improved contrast in CBCT imaging.

387. **Zirconium Oxide Detector (noun):** Radiation sensor using zirconium oxide for high thermal and mechanical stability.
**Related Terms:** Semiconductor dosimeter, In-vivo detector.
**Example in Radiotherapy:** Evaluated for proton range verification applications.

388. **Zinc Sulfide Screen (noun):** Scintillation material converting radiation energy into visible light.
**Related Terms:** Scintillator, Portal imaging.
**Example in Radiotherapy:** Utilized in early phosphor screen-based portal imagers.

389. **Zone of Electron Equilibrium (noun):** Region where energy deposition equals energy loss, stabilizing dose.
**Related Terms:** Charged particle equilibrium, Depth dose.
**Example in Radiotherapy:** Achieved beyond build-up region in megavoltage photon beams.

390. **Zone of Homogeneity (noun):** Volume within which radiation dose uniformity remains within tolerance.
**Related Terms:** Uniformity index, Dose verification.
**Example in Radiotherapy:** PDD profiles confirmed homogeneity in isocentric region.

391. **Zoom Collimation Mode (noun):** Imaging technique narrowing FOV for enhanced visualization accuracy.
**Related Terms:** kV imaging, Field reduction.
**Example in Radiotherapy:** Used in spine SBRT setup verification.

392. **Zoomed MRI Acquisition (noun):** Reduced field-of-view MRI technique minimizing geometric distortion.
**Related Terms:** MR imaging, Distortion correction.
**Example in Radiotherapy:** Applied in MR-Linac prostate tracking.

393. **Zonal Fusion Algorithm (noun):** Computational model merging dose data from multiple zones for total dose evaluation.
**Related Terms:** Dose summation, Hybrid plan QA.
**Example in Radiotherapy:** Used to blend MR-Linac and photon plan contributions.

394. **Zoned Tissue Segmentation (noun):** Automated algorithm dividing anatomy into functional or density zones.
**Related Terms:** Auto-contouring, AI segmentation.
**Example in Radiotherapy:** Enabled density-based dose adaptation in lung planning.

395. **Z-Spectroscopy (noun):** MRI-based technique analyzing chemical exchange saturation transfer.
**Related Terms:** MR biomarker imaging, Metabolic mapping.
**Example in Radiotherapy:** Explored for tumor hypoxia quantification pre-RT.

396. **Z-Stack Image Fusion (noun):** Integration of sequential image slices into a volumetric dataset.
**Related Terms:** 3D reconstruction, Image registration.
**Example in Radiotherapy:** Used for 3D fiducial tracking verification.

397. **Zonal Plan QA Log (noun):** Documentation of QA performed on each treatment region separately.
**Related Terms:** Plan QA, Record keeping.
**Example in Radiotherapy:** Maintained to track multi-lesion SRS QA reports.

398. **Z-Test Statistical Analysis (noun):** Parametric test for comparing treatment mean values.
**Related Terms:** Statistical validation, Dosimetric comparison.
**Example in Radiotherapy:** Z-test applied to verify plan accuracy between modalities.

399. **Zonal Response Calibration (noun):** Adjustment ensuring consistent detector output across measuring zones.
**Related Terms:** Chamber calibration, Detector mapping.
**Example in Radiotherapy:** Used during EPID calibration routine.

400. **Zylindrical Phantom (noun):** Typographical variant for cylindrical phantom, used for rotational symmetry checks.
**Related Terms:** QA phantom, Dosimetric calibration.
**Example in Radiotherapy:** Cylindrical phantom verified beam concentricity in proton gantry.

401. **Z-Matrix Computational Model (noun):** Mathematical construct representing system variables in radiation simulation.
**Related Terms:** Dose algorithm, Monte Carlo matrix.
**Example in Radiotherapy:** Used in TPS dose kernel derivation.

402. **Zonal Radiation Density Index (noun):** Metric quantifying photon flux per zone volume.
**Related Terms:** Beam intensity, Field mapping.
**Example in Radiotherapy:** Index helped normalize dose in IMRT QA.

403. **Z-Order Mapping (noun):** Spatial indexing for efficient image data organization in treatment planning.
**Related Terms:** Image compression, Data mapping.
**Example in Radiotherapy:** Used for GPU-accelerated dose reconstruction.

404. **Zeta Dose Correction (noun):** Empirical adjustment applied to fine-tune dose discrepancies.
**Related Terms:** Calibration factor, QA correction.
**Example in Radiotherapy:** Implemented in Monte Carlo-based recalculations.

405. **Zenith Gantry Alignment (noun):** Mechanical check ensuring precise vertical positioning of gantry.
**Related Terms:** Gantry calibration, Laser alignment.
**Example in Radiotherapy:** Verified in annual Linac QA.

406. **Zeeman Interaction Mapping (noun):** MRI method mapping magnetic interactions affecting tissue relaxation.
**Related Terms:** MR physics, Paramagnetic effects.
**Example in Radiotherapy:** Used in adaptive MR-guided prostate workflow.

407. **Zeolite Filter (noun):** Material used to absorb airborne radionuclide contaminants in nuclear medicine.
**Related Terms:** Filtration system, Decontamination.
**Example in Radiotherapy:** Installed in isotope handling room exhaust.

408. **Zeotropic Mixture (noun):** Mixture of refrigerants with non-constant boiling composition.
**Related Terms:** Cooling system, Linac engineering.
**Example in Radiotherapy:** Used in cryogenic cooling of MR coils.

409. **Zonal Scatter Evaluation (noun):** Assessment of scattered radiation within subfield areas.
**Related Terms:** Scatter analysis, QA measurement.
**Example in Radiotherapy:** Performed during flatness verification.

410. **Zero-Emission Shield (noun):** Protective barrier designed to eliminate leakage dose from system housing.
**Related Terms:** Shielding, Safety barrier.
**Example in Radiotherapy:** Used in proton nozzle shielding design.

411. **Zeta Potential Dosimeter (noun):** Device measuring electric potential at particle interfaces to assess surface charge response under radiation.
**Related Terms:** Electrostatic detector, Ionization potential.
**Example in Radiotherapy:** Used in nanoparticle-mediated dose enhancement research.

412. **Zero-Angle Beam Entry (noun):** Radiation beam incidence perpendicular to patient surface minimizing geometric distortion.
**Related Terms:** Orthogonal entry, Field alignment.
**Example in Radiotherapy:** Applied in breast tangential field setup to reduce skin folds.

413. **Zenithal Field Dose (noun):** Maximum dose delivered along the central vertical beam axis.
**Related Terms:** Central axis dose, Depth dose.
**Example in Radiotherapy:** Measured during isocentric verification in cranial SRS.

414. **Zonal Calibration Coefficient (noun):** Correction factor applied to dose readings in region-specific calibration.
**Related Terms:** Field uniformity, Detector correction.
**Example in Radiotherapy:** Used to fine-tune lateral profile uniformity.

415. **Zero-Flux Boundary Condition (noun):** Mathematical condition assuming no net particle flow across boundary surface.
**Related Terms:** Transport modeling, Monte Carlo simulation.
**Example in Radiotherapy:** Employed in dose transport equations during TPS verification.

416. **Zeta Radiograph (noun):** High-contrast radiographic image using filtered photon beam to enhance soft-tissue edges.
**Related Terms:** Contrast optimization, Beam filtration.
**Example in Radiotherapy:** Used in phantom imaging for contour validation.

417. **Zinc Oxide Nanoparticle (noun):** Radiation-sensitizing nanoparticle enhancing tumor dose absorption via secondary electron generation.
**Related Terms:** Nanodosimetry, Radiosensitizer.
**Example in Radiotherapy:** Investigated for enhanced cell-killing in proton therapy.

418. **Zeeman Relaxation Effect (noun):** Magnetic field-induced change in relaxation time affecting MR image contrast.
**Related Terms:** MR-Linac physics, Spin relaxation.
**Example in Radiotherapy:** Evaluated for artifact reduction in adaptive MRI-guided plans.

419. **Z-Coordinate Correction Factor (noun):** Adjustment ensuring vertical coordinate consistency between imaging and treatment planes.
**Related Terms:** Coordinate registration, Image alignment.
**Example in Radiotherapy:** Applied during 4D CBCT setup validation.

420. **Zonal Dose Gradient Map (noun):** Graphical representation of dose fall-off within delineated regions.
**Related Terms:** Dose gradient, Hot spot analysis.
**Example in Radiotherapy:** Used in plan evaluation to assess conformity near OARs.

421. **Zero-Crosstalk Imaging (noun):** Image acquisition method reducing interference between dual detectors or coils.
**Related Terms:** MR imaging, Signal isolation.
**Example in Radiotherapy:** Applied in MR-Linac dual-coil calibration.

422. **Zeta-Phase Proton Drift (noun):** Minor energy deviation in proton paths due to magnetic interaction in gantry.
**Related Terms:** Beam transport, Proton optics.
**Example in Radiotherapy:** Corrected in energy layer calibration for uniform Bragg peak.

423. **Zinc Ionization Constant (noun):** Energy threshold for ionization of zinc atoms under radiation exposure.
**Related Terms:** Ionization energy, Atomic interaction.
**Example in Radiotherapy:** Modeled in Monte Carlo dose computation.

424. **Zero-Bias Detector Mode (noun):** Detector configuration without applied potential to measure intrinsic current response.
**Related Terms:** Passive dosimetry, Current leakage.
**Example in Radiotherapy:** Used in thermoluminescent dosimeter calibration.

425. **Zonal Dose Constraint Table (noun):** Structured dataset defining dose tolerances by anatomical zone.
**Related Terms:** Constraint template, Planning objectives.
**Example in Radiotherapy:** Utilized for liver SBRT constraint verification.

426. **Zenithal Imaging Protocol (noun):** Imaging protocol aligned along vertical axis to minimize distortion.
**Related Terms:** Orthogonal imaging, Setup verification.
**Example in Radiotherapy:** Used for cranial and spine radiosurgery.

427. **Z-Score Normalization (noun):** Statistical method standardizing dosimetric datasets for comparison.
**Related Terms:** Data normalization, Statistical QA.
**Example in Radiotherapy:** Applied in comparing plan complexity metrics.

428. **Z-Layer Dose Fusion (noun):** Integration of dose data across depth layers to form composite profile.
**Related Terms:** Dose accumulation, Image fusion.
**Example in Radiotherapy:** Used in adaptive proton therapy dose reconstruction.

429. **Zonal Monte Carlo Grid (noun):** Grid-based structure dividing calculation space for particle transport simulation.
**Related Terms:** Dose grid, Monte Carlo modeling.
**Example in Radiotherapy:** Enhanced computational efficiency in head-and-neck plan recalculations.

430. **Zero-Variance Simulation (noun):** Variance reduction method improving Monte Carlo efficiency without bias.
**Related Terms:** Statistical weighting, Dose computation.
**Example in Radiotherapy:** Used in proton transport models to accelerate computation.

431. **Zygomatic Arc Dose Check (noun):** Verification of dose coverage along zygomatic bone in head plans.
**Related Terms:** Bony anatomy contour, Facial structure QA.
**Example in Radiotherapy:** Checked in orbit-sparing head-and-neck planning.

432. **Z-Axis Gantry Drift (noun):** Vertical mechanical deviation of gantry rotation axis.
**Related Terms:** Mechanical QA, Gantry calibration.
**Example in Radiotherapy:** Monitored quarterly using laser tracking systems.

433. **Zinc-Silicate Scintillator (noun):** Detector material emitting visible light upon radiation exposure.
**Related Terms:** Scintillation, Detector material.
**Example in Radiotherapy:** Used in high-resolution portal imaging panels.

434. **Z-Vector Registration (noun):** Mathematical mapping aligning volumetric imaging coordinates.
**Related Terms:** Image registration, Deformation field.
**Example in Radiotherapy:** Employed during adaptive MR-guided planning.

435. **Z-Direction Dose Spread (noun):** Longitudinal expansion of absorbed dose due to scatter or range uncertainty.
**Related Terms:** Dose falloff, Proton range.
**Example in Radiotherapy:** Monitored in distal falloff analysis.

436. **Zero-Point Field Stability (noun):** Assessment of electromagnetic field baseline over time.
**Related Terms:** Magnet stability, MR calibration.
**Example in Radiotherapy:** Ensures MR-Linac field constancy.

437. **Zonal Density Reconstruction (noun):** Recalculation of voxel density for adaptive dose recalibration.
**Related Terms:** CT density correction, Adaptive planning.
**Example in Radiotherapy:** Updated mid-treatment in adaptive workflows.

438. **Zeolite Ion Trap (noun):** Component capturing charged radionuclides to prevent contamination.
**Related Terms:** Filtration, Shielding safety.
**Example in Radiotherapy:** Installed in isotope handling modules.

439. **Zero-Noise Signal Averaging (noun):** Technique enhancing detector signal-to-noise ratio through repeated sampling.
**Related Terms:** Signal processing, Noise reduction.
**Example in Radiotherapy:** Used in low-dose MR acquisitions.

440. **Z-Layer Proton Reconstruction (noun):** Proton range mapping across discrete energy layers.
**Related Terms:** Range verification, Layered scanning.
**Example in Radiotherapy:** Validated in spot scanning QA.

441. **Zinc-Phosphate Gel Dosimeter (noun):** Polymer gel dosimeter using zinc phosphate as active compound.
**Related Terms:** 3D dosimetry, Gel measurement.
**Example in Radiotherapy:** Tested for small-field IMRT verification.

442. **Zonal Dose Response Function (noun):** Mathematical function linking regional dose with biological effect.
**Related Terms:** Dose-response, Radiobiology.
**Example in Radiotherapy:** Used in tumor control probability modeling.

443. **Z-Dimension Image Scaling (noun):** Vertical dimension scaling correction in reconstructed CT or MR datasets.
**Related Terms:** Geometric calibration, Image correction.
**Example in Radiotherapy:** Ensured consistent voxel geometry in 4DCT.

444. **Z-Plug Collimator (noun):** Collimator insert with adjustable cylindrical apertures.
**Related Terms:** SRS collimation, Field shaping.
**Example in Radiotherapy:** Used in Gamma Knife QA.

445. **Zeta Phase Transition (noun):** Molecular phase change affecting material dosimetric properties.
**Related Terms:** Material physics, Detector calibration.
**Example in Radiotherapy:** Considered in dosimeter temperature correction.

446. **Zero-Error Transfer Function (noun):** Calibration ensuring dose output matches theoretical values.
**Related Terms:** System linearity, Output calibration.
**Example in Radiotherapy:** Verified during beam output QA.

447. **Zonal Tissue Compensation Map (noun):** Map defining compensator thickness by tissue zone.
**Related Terms:** Bolus design, Heterogeneity correction.
**Example in Radiotherapy:** Generated in chest wall tangential planning.

448. **Z-Beam Energy Verification (noun):** Energy validation for beams along vertical axis.
**Related Terms:** Beam QA, Energy constancy.
**Example in Radiotherapy:** Used in proton energy layer testing.

449. **Zinc-Doped Phosphor Plate (noun):** Imaging plate coated with zinc-based phosphor for X-ray capture.
**Related Terms:** CR imaging, Detector plate.
**Example in Radiotherapy:** Used in DRR generation for verification.

450. **Zero-Tolerance Dosimetry (noun):** Dosimetric policy permitting no deviations beyond threshold limits.
**Related Terms:** QA protocol, Error analysis.
**Example in Radiotherapy:** Applied in stereotactic cranial treatments.

451. **Zygomatic Beam Pathway (noun):** Anatomical beam trajectory through the zygomatic arch region during cranial planning.
**Related Terms:** Skull-base planning, Facial contouring.
**Example in Radiotherapy:** Used to avoid optic structures during IMRT for sinonasal tumors.

452. **Zygomatic Bone Shield (noun):** Customized lead or thermoplastic shield protecting the zygomatic area during head-and-neck therapy.
**Related Terms:** Surface shielding, Bolus design.
**Example in Radiotherapy:** Applied for parotid gland irradiation to prevent cheek overdose.

453. **Zeta Adaptive Algorithm (noun):** AI-based optimization algorithm dynamically adjusting dose weights during adaptive therapy.
**Related Terms:** Machine learning, Dose prediction.
**Example in Radiotherapy:** Integrated in MR-Linac adaptive workflows for on-table replanning.

454. **Zero-Beam Deviation Protocol (noun):** remains below tolerance limits.
**Related Terms:** Gantry accuracy, Mechanical QA.
**Example in Radiotherapy:** Verified monthly using Winston-Lutz test data.

455. **Z-Indexed CT Reconstruction (noun):** CT reconstruction method indexing slices along z-axis for 3D modeling accuracy.
**Related Terms:** Image reconstruction, Volumetric imaging.
**Example in Radiotherapy:** Used for deformable image registration in 4DCT datasets.

456. **Zinc-Infused Gel Dosimeter (noun):** Experimental polymer gel infused with zinc for high-resolution 3D dose verification.
**Related Terms:** Gel dosimetry, Polymerization tracking.
**Example in Radiotherapy:** Tested in SBRT QA for micro-dosimetric precision.

457. **Zeta Mapping Interface (noun):** Software tool integrating radiation dose maps with z-coordinate grid alignment.
**Related Terms:** Image fusion, Dose accumulation.
**Example in Radiotherapy:** Used for adaptive MR-guided dose accumulation studies.

458. **Zero-Drift Electrometer (noun):** High-precision dosimetry device minimizing signal drift during current measurement.
**Related Terms:** Electrometer stability, Chamber calibration.
**Example in Radiotherapy:** Used in reference dosimetry for output constancy checks.

459. **Zonal Energy Absorption Factor (noun):** Parameter describing absorbed dose fraction per anatomical region.
**Related Terms:** Absorbed fraction, Dose modeling.
**Example in Radiotherapy:** Implemented in organ-at-risk dose summation algorithms.

460. **Zenithal Radiation Profile (noun):** Beam intensity profile measured along the vertical field axis.
**Related Terms:** Beam symmetry, Flatness measurement.
**Example in Radiotherapy:** Profile confirmed central-axis stability in photon beams.

461. **Z461. Zero-Dose Verification Field (noun):** Non-delivery field used to verify imaging or mechanical alignment without dose output.
**Related Terms:** Setup verification, QA field.
**Example in Radiotherapy:** Used for MR-Linac dry-run alignment testing.

462. **Z-Sequence Energy Modulation (noun):** Sequential adjustment of beam energy layers along depth direction.
**Related Terms:** Energy layering, Proton scanning.
**Example in Radiotherapy:** Optimized for uniform Bragg peak coverage.

463. **Zinc-Doped Fiber Optic Sensor (noun):** Fiber optic dosimeter enhanced with zinc compounds for increased radiation sensitivity.
**Related Terms:** Optical dosimetry, Real-time detection.
**Example in Radiotherapy:** Applied in surface dose measurements.

464. **Zero-Field Leakage Shield (noun):** Barrier minimizing radiation leakage during zero-field conditions.
**Related Terms:** Leakage control, Shielding QA.
**Example in Radiotherapy:** Evaluated in Linac head leakage measurements.

465. **Z-Loop Control Mechanism (noun):** Feedback loop maintaining positional accuracy in automated couch movements.
**Related Terms:** Positioning system, Couch QA.
**Example in Radiotherapy:** Implemented in robotic couch verification routines.

466. **Zenith Dose Evaluation (noun):** Assessment of dose delivered at the highest anatomical point.
**Related Terms:** Peak dose, Dose uniformity.
**Example in Radiotherapy:** Used in total body irradiation dose mapping.

467. **Zero-Error Calibration Model (noun):** Calibration framework ensuring measured and true values align perfectly within uncertainty.
**Related Terms:** Calibration accuracy, QA benchmarking.
**Example in Radiotherapy:** Applied in beam output cross-calibration procedures.

468. **Zeta Radiation Index (noun):** Composite metric integrating dose rate, energy, and exposure time.
**Related Terms:** Dose index, Exposure calculation.
**Example in Radiotherapy:** Used for comparing treatment plan efficiencies.

469. **Zinc Oxide Semiconductor (noun):** Radiation-sensitive semiconductor material for solid-state dosimeters.
**Related Terms:** Semiconductor dosimetry, Detector physics.
**Example in Radiotherapy:** Incorporated in proton range monitoring sensors.

470. **Zonal Histogram Mapping (noun):** Visualization technique for voxel intensity distribution by defined region.
**Related Terms:** DVH analysis, Dose mapping.
**Example in Radiotherapy:** Applied in plan quality evaluation dashboards.

471. **Zero-Latency Imaging (noun):** Real-time image acquisition technique minimizing temporal delay.
**Related Terms:** Real-time guidance, Image registration.
**Example in Radiotherapy:** Used in motion-managed MR-guided therapy.

472. **Zirconium Alloy Collimator (noun):** Collimator component constructed from zirconium for superior radiation resistance.
**Related Terms:** Beam collimation, Material engineering.
**Example in Radiotherapy:** Used in high-dose-rate proton gantries.

473. **Zenith Beam Modeling (noun):** Simulation of radiation beams along the vertical incidence axis.
**Related Terms:** Monte Carlo modeling, Beam geometry.
**Example in Radiotherapy:** Validated for cranial radiosurgery plan QA.

474. **Zero-Offset Imaging Calibration (noun):** Correction ensuring zero baseline bias in image intensity scales.
**Related Terms:** Image correction, Flat-fielding.
**Example in Radiotherapy:** Used in kV imaging systems QA.

475. **Zeta Decay Analysis (noun):** Study of exotic radionuclide decay pathways influencing dose distribution.
**Related Terms:** Nuclear physics, Radioisotope decay.
**Example in Radiotherapy:** Investigated for Yttrium-90 dose modeling accuracy.

476. **Zinc Matrix Detector (noun):** Solid-state detector matrix built with zinc composite layers for high-energy photon detection.
**Related Terms:** Matrix detector, Photon detection.
**Example in Radiotherapy:** Used in novel EPID research.

477. **Zonal Variance Graph (noun):** Plot showing deviation of measured doses within subregions.
**Related Terms:** QA analytics, Plan homogeneity.
**Example in Radiotherapy:** Used for IMRT QA statistical evaluation.

478. **Zero-Deflection Beam Path (noun):** Radiation path unaffected by external forces ensuring direct linear trajectory.
**Related Terms:** Beam geometry, Mechanical alignment.
**Example in Radiotherapy:** Verified during magnetic field QA.

479. **Zenith-Axis Field Scan (noun):** Measurement of dose distribution along vertical central axis.
**Related Terms:** Central axis scan, PDD verification.
**Example in Radiotherapy:** Used in electron beam commissioning.

480. **Zonal Scatter Probability (noun):** Mathematical estimate of photon scattering within specific regions.
**Related Terms:** Scatter model, Dose prediction.
**Example in Radiotherapy:** Applied in Monte Carlo secondary dose corrections.

481. **Zero-Temperature Detector Drift (noun):** Thermal stabilization property reducing detector current drift at constant temperature.
**Related Terms:** Detector stability, Temperature correction.
**Example in Radiotherapy:** Used in reference chamber calibration.

482. **Z-Plasma State (noun):** Ionized state of matter achieved under extreme radiation conditions.
**Related Terms:** Plasma interaction, Particle physics.
**Example in Radiotherapy:** Modeled in high-energy proton physics research.

483. **Zonal Dose Amplification Factor (noun):**
Ratio of local dose enhancement compared to baseline region.
**Related Terms:** Dose ratio, Hotspot analysis.
**Example in Radiotherapy:** Evaluated for nanoparticle-enhanced dosimetry studies.

484. **Zirconium-Doped Scintillator (noun):** Scintillator crystal doped with zirconium to improve light yield.
**Related Terms:** Scintillation detector, Photon conversion.
**Example in Radiotherapy:** Used for EPID panel development.

485. **Zero-Flux Gradient Zone (noun):** Region with no net dose gradient, indicating uniform distribution.
**Related Terms:** Homogeneity zone, Field flatness.
**Example in Radiotherapy:** Verified using planar film dosimetry.

486. **Zeta-Proton Coupling Constant (noun):** Parameter defining interaction strength between protons and magnetic fields.
**Related Terms:** Magnetic focusing, Proton dynamics.
**Example in Radiotherapy:** Applied in proton beamline simulations.

487. **Zero-Signal Drift Chamber (noun):** Ionization chamber designed for negligible baseline signal drift.
**Related Terms:** Electrometer, Stability test.
**Example in Radiotherapy:** Used in daily output constancy QA.

488. **Zonal Histogram Equalization (noun):** Image enhancement process balancing contrast within segmented regions.
**Related Terms:** Image normalization, CT preprocessing.
**Example in Radiotherapy:** Used in auto-contouring AI preprocessing.

489. **Zinc-Carbon Target (noun):** Composite target material for generating diagnostic X-rays.
**Related Terms:** Target assembly, X-ray tube physics.
**Example in Radiotherapy:** Used in imaging subsystem design.

490. **Zenith Calibration Axis (noun):** Vertical alignment axis used as reference during calibration.
**Related Terms:** Coordinate alignment, Gantry QA.
**Example in Radiotherapy:** Verified for zero-angle setup consistency.

491. **Zero-Field Ionization Effect (noun):** Spontaneous ionization of gas molecules in absence of applied field.
**Related Terms:** Ionization chamber physics, Leakage current.
**Example in Radiotherapy:** Monitored during long-term detector tests.

492. **Z-Order Dose Sorting (noun):** Efficient computational sorting of dose matrices in volumetric grids.
**Related Terms:** Data indexing, Algorithm optimization.
**Example in Radiotherapy:** Applied in GPU-based TPS dose calculations.

493. **Zirconium-Based Detector Array (noun):** Detector grid using zirconium materials for high-energy detection.
**Related Terms:** Detector array, Photon measurement.
**Example in Radiotherapy:** Used in experimental high-dose verification systems.

494. **Zeta-Radiation Stability Factor (noun):** Coefficient describing source output stability over time.
**Related Terms:** Output constancy, QA tolerance.
**Example in Radiotherapy:** Used for Linac output trend analysis.

495. **Zinc-Fluoride Scintillator (noun):** Detector crystal producing high-yield light output from radiation.
**Related Terms:** Scintillation physics, Optical conversion.
**Example in Radiotherapy:** Used in secondary electron emission dosimetry.

496. **Zero-Tolerance Geometry QA (noun):** Quality control method ensuring absolute geometric alignment in treatment systems.
**Related Terms:** Isocenter QA, Spatial precision.
**Example in Radiotherapy:** Used in stereotactic frame calibration.

497. **Zonal Radiobiological Index (noun):** Quantitative value expressing biological response within specified tissue zones.
**Related Terms:** BED modeling, Radiobiology.
**Example in Radiotherapy:** Calculated for tumor control probability mapping.

498. **Zero-Dose Reconstruction Algorithm (noun):** Computation reconstructing anatomical setup without delivering radiation dose.
**Related Terms:** Non-irradiating imaging, Dose-free guidance.
**Example in Radiotherapy:** Used in MR-guided planning QA.

499. **Zeta-Gamma Coupling Parameter (noun):** Coefficient describing energy exchange between gamma photons and field particles.
**Related Terms:** Photon interaction, Quantum dosimetry.
**Example in Radiotherapy:** Incorporated in dose distribution modeling.

**500. Zenithal Reference Beamline (noun):**
Primary calibration beamline aligned vertically for reference dosimetry.
**Related Terms:** Reference calibration, Beamline QA.
**Example in Radiotherapy:** Used for absolute dose calibration at national labs.

# Reference


1. Khan FM, Gibbons JP. *The Physics of Radiation Therapy*. 6th ed. Philadelphia: Wolters Kluwer; 2021.
2. Hall EJ, Giaccia AJ. *Radiobiology for the Radiologist*. 7th ed. Philadelphia: Lippincott Williams & Wilkins; 2018.
3. Attix FH. *Introduction to Radiological Physics and Radiation Dosimetry*. New York: Wiley; 1986.
4. Podgorsak EB. *Radiation Physics for Medical Physicists*. Vienna: IAEA Publishing; 2016.
5. Podgorsak EB, editor. *Radiation Oncology Physics: A Handbook for Teachers and Students*. Vienna: IAEA; 2005.
6. DeVita VT Jr, Lawrence TS, Rosenberg SA, editors. *Cancer: Principles and Practice of Oncology*. 11th ed. Philadelphia: Lippincott Williams & Wilkins; 2018.
7. Van Dyk J, editor. *The Modern Technology of Radiation Oncology*. New York: Springer; 1999.
8. Bushong SC. *Radiologic Science for Technologists: Physics, Biology and Protection*. 12th ed. St. Louis: Mosby; 2021.
9. Bushberg JT, Seibert JA, Leidholdt EM, Boone JM. *The Essential Physics of Medical Imaging*. 3rd ed. Philadelphia: Lippincott Williams & Wilkins; 2011.
10. Khan FM. *The Physics of Radiation Therapy Workbook*. Philadelphia: Lippincott Williams & Wilkins; 2016.
11. Knoll GF. *Radiation Detection and Measurement*. 4th ed. Hoboken: Wiley; 2010.
12. International Commission on Radiological Protection (ICRP). *ICRP Publications*. Oxford: Elsevier; [Multiple years].
13. International Atomic Energy Agency (IAEA). *Technical Reports Series (TRS)*. Vienna: IAEA; [Multiple years].
14. NCRP. *Structural Shielding Design and Evaluation for Megavoltage X- and Gamma-Ray Radiotherapy Facilities*. Report No. 151. Bethesda: NCRP; 2005.
15. AAPM Task Group Reports. *American Association of Physicists in Medicine Publications*. Madison: AAPM; [Multiple years].
16. Almond PR, Biggs PJ, Coursey BM, Hanson WF, Huq MS, Nath R, et al. *AAPM TG-51: Dosimetry Protocol for Photon and Electron Beams*. Madison: AAPM; 1999.
17. Klein EE, Hanley J, Bayouth J, Yin FF, Simon W, Dresser S, et al. *AAPM TG-142: Quality Assurance of Medical Accelerators*. Madison: AAPM; 2009.
18. Huq MS, Fraass BA, Dunscombe PB, Glover PM, Ibbott GS, Mechalakos J, et al. *AAPM TG-100: Risk Analysis Methods in Radiation Therapy*. Madison: AAPM; 2016.

**19.** ICRU. *International Commission on Radiation Units and Measurements Reports*. Bethesda: ICRU; [Multiple years].

**20.** Pawlicki T, Jiang SB, Renaud J. Principles of IGRT. In: Palta JR, Mackie TR, editors. *On-Board Imaging and Adaptive Radiation Therapy*. New York: Springer; 2014.

**21.** Palta JR, Mackie TR, editors. *Image-Guided Radiation Therapy in Cancer Treatment*. New York: Springer; 2010.

**22.** Purdy JA. *Intensity Modulated Radiation Therapy: The State of the Art*. Madison: Medical Physics Publishing; 2006.

**23.** Méndez R, Méndez J, editors. *Radiation Oncology: Rationale, Techniques, Outcomes*. Philadelphia: Lippincott Williams & Wilkins; 2017.

**24.** Paganetti H. *The Physics of Proton Therapy*. Bristol: IOP Publishing; 2019.

**25.** Webb S. *The Physics of Radiotherapy: Clinical Dosimetry*. London: Institute of Physics Publishing; 2011.

**26.** Kirby MC. *Radiation Therapy Simulation and Treatment Planning*. [Year not specified].

**27.** Washington CM, Leaver DT. *Principles and Practice of Radiation Therapy*. 4th ed. St. Louis: Mosby; 2016.

**28.** Bentel GC. *Radiation Therapy Planning*. New York: McGraw-Hill; 1996.

**29.** Brahme A, editor. *Comprehensive Textbook of Radiation Oncology*. Boca Raton: CRC Press; 2012.

**30.** Gagel B. *Radiation Therapy: Technology and Techniques*. [Year not specified].

**31.** Mettler FA Jr, Guiberteau MJ. *Essentials of Nuclear Medicine and Molecular Imaging*. 7th ed. Philadelphia: Elsevier; 2018.

**32.** Cherry SR, Sorenson JA, Phelps ME. *Physics in Nuclear Medicine*. 4th ed. Philadelphia: Elsevier; 2012.

**33.** Seeram E. *The Physics of Digital Radiography and Computed Tomography*. 3rd ed. Boca Raton: CRC Press; 2018.

**34.** Mahesh M. *Computed Tomography: Physical Principles, Clinical Applications, and Quality Control*. 4th ed. Philadelphia: Elsevier; 2013.

**35.** Kak AC, Slaney M. *Principles of Computerized Tomographic Imaging*. Philadelphia: SIAM; 2001.

**36.** Spitzer VM. *The Physics of Computed Tomography*. Boca Raton: CRC Press; [Year not specified].

**37.** Liang ZP, Lauterbur PC. *Magnetic Resonance Imaging: Physical Principles and Sequence Design*. New York: Wiley; 2000.

**38.** Stabin MG. *Radiation Protection and Dosimetry: Introduction to Health Physics*. New York: Springer; 2007.

**39.** Turner JE. *Radiological Health Handbook*. Washington, DC: US Department of Energy; 1995.

**40.** Cember H, Johnson TE. *Introduction to Health Physics*. 4th ed. New York: McGraw-Hill; 2009.

**41.** Shleien BN, Slaback LA, Birky BK. *Health Physics: Principles and Practices*. [Year not specified].

**42.** Profio AE. *Radiation Shielding and Dosimetry*. New York: Wiley; 1979.

**43.** Morgan KZ. *Principles of Radiation Protection*. New York: Wiley; 1975.

**44.** Stabin MG. *Radiation Protection and Dosimetry* (Multiple editions). New York: Springer; [Multiple years].

**45.** Mendez TE. *Radiation Oncology: Clinical Practice and Disease Site Management*. [Year not specified].

**46.** Webb S, Nahum AE. *The Physics of Radiation Therapy: Clinical Applications*. Boca Raton: CRC Press; 2002.

**47.** Solberg TD, De Salles AA, editors. *Principles and Practice of Stereotactic Radiosurgery*. New York: Springer; 2015.

**48.** Purdy JA, Kaisersberg I, editors. *Intensity Modulated Radiation Therapy: Practical Essentials*. Madison: Medical Physics Publishing; 2007.

**49.** Wang G. *Practical Essentials of Intensity Modulated Radiation Therapy (IMRT)*. [Year not specified].

**50.** Pawlicki T. *Principles of Image-Guided Radiation Therapy*. [Year not specified].

**51.** Verellen D. *Surface Imaging for Patient Setup and Motion Monitoring*. [Year not specified].

**52.** Palta JR. *On-Board Imaging: Adaptive Radiation Therapy*. [Year not specified].

**53.** Mackie TR. *Tomotherapy and IMRT Techniques*. Madison: Medical Physics Publishing; 2003.

**54.** Solberg TD. *Stereotactic Radiosurgery: Clinical Practice Guide*. [Year not specified].

**55.** Followill DS, Jordan TA. *Quality Assurance in External Beam Radiation Therapy*. [Year not specified].

**56.** Washington CM. *Radiation Therapist Handbook: Practical Techniques*. [Year not specified].

**57.** Smith PJ. *Mould Room Techniques in Radiation Therapy*. [Year not specified].

**58.** Gollnick P. *Basic Radiation Protection Technology*. [Year not specified].

**59.** Slobodan PS. *Applied Dosimetry*. [Year not specified].

**60.** Ahn S. *Clinical Dosimetry: Concepts and Practices*. [Year not specified].

**61.** Darafsheh A. *Radiation Therapy Dosimetry: A Practical Handbook*. Boca Raton: CRC Press; 2020.

**62.** Hall EJ. *Radiobiology Texts and Compendia* (Supplementary Series). [Year not specified].

**63.** Klein M, Mendonca M. *Fundamentals of Radiation Biology*. Boca Raton: CRC Press; 2018.

**64.** International Atomic Energy Agency (IAEA). *Radiation Biology: A Handbook for Teachers and Students*. Vienna: IAEA; 2010.

**65.** Saha GB. *Fundamentals of Nuclear Pharmacy*. 6th ed. New York: Springer; 2010.

**66.** Stabin MG. *Radiation Protection and Dosimetry* (Additional Editions). New York: Springer; [Multiple years].

**67.** Valk PE. *Quality Assurance in Nuclear Medicine*. [Year not specified].

**68.** Ryan DG. *Clinical Nuclear Medicine: A Practical Guide*. [Year not specified].

**69.** Sorenson JA, Phelps ME. *Physics in Nuclear Medicine*. 3rd ed. Philadelphia: W.B. Saunders; 2003.

**70.** Mende TE. *Radiation Oncology: Techniques and Outcomes*. [Year not specified].

**71.** Webb S. *Radiation Therapy Texts on Algorithms and Optimization*. [Year not specified].

**72.** Kirke M. *Radiation Therapy Simulation and Treatment Planning Manuals*. [Year not specified].

**73.** Washington CM, Leaver DT. *Radiation Therapy Practice Manuals*. St. Louis: Mosby; [Year not specified].

**74.** *Mould Room and Immobilization Techniques: Clinical Manual*. [Year not specified].

**75.** QARC. *Quality Assurance Review Center Manuals and Auditing Guidelines*. Providence: QARC; [Multiple years].

**76.** National Research Council. *The Biological Effects of Low-Level Radiation*. Washington, DC: National Academies Press; 1990.

**77.** Jorgensen TJ. *Radiation Exposure: History, Measurement and Risk*. Amherst: Prometheus Books; 2014.

**78.** Rhodes R. *The Making of the Atomic Bomb*. New York: Simon & Schuster; 1986.

**79.** Blume S. *Fallout: The Hiroshima Cover-Up and the Reporter Who Revealed It to the World*. New York: Simon & Schuster; 2020.

**80.** Redniss L. *Radioactive: Marie and Pierre Curie—A Tale of Love and Fallout*. New York: HarperCollins; 2010.

**81.** Fagin D. *Toms River: A Story of Science and Salvation*. New York: Bantam Books; 2013.

**82.** Mole RH. *Radiation and Health*. London: Routledge; 1985.

**83.** Osborn AG. *Radiology Review Manual*. 8th ed. Philadelphia: Wolters Kluwer; 2017.

**84.** Hickey JM. *Review of Nuclear Medicine Technology*. 4th ed. Reston: SNMMI; 2018.

**85.** Seeram E. *Digital Radiography and CT Physics*. Boca Raton: CRC Press; 2019.

**86.** Papp J. *Concise Physics of Medical Imaging*. Oxford: Oxford University Press; 2014.

**87.** Curry TS, Dowdey JE, Murry RC. *Christensen's Physics of Diagnostic Radiology*. 4th ed. Philadelphia: Lippincott Williams & Wilkins; 1990.

**88.** Burch SF. *Physics of Medical Imaging*. [Year not specified].

**89.** Birks JB. *The Theory and Practice of Scintillation Counting*. Oxford: Pergamon Press; 1964.

**90.** Lamarsh JR, Baratta AJ. *Introduction to Nuclear Engineering*. 3rd ed. Upper Saddle River: Prentice Hall; 2001.

**91.** Profio AE. *Radiation Shielding and Dosimetry* (Supplementary Edition). New York: Wiley; 1979.

**92.** Stabin MG. *Radiation Safety in Nuclear Medicine*. Boca Raton: CRC Press; 2020.

**93.** Saha GB. *Radiation Safety and Control*. New York: Springer; 2019.

**94.** Brijlal, Subramanyam NV. *Atomic and Nuclear Physics*. New Delhi: S. Chand Publishing; 2008.

**95.** Krieger H. *Handbook of Radiation Doses*. New York: Springer; 2019.

**96.** Stabin MG. *Radiation Protection and Dosimetry: Textbook Edition*. New York: Springer; 2017.

**97.** Mende TE. *Radiation Oncology: Techniques and Clinical Outcomes*. [Year not specified].

**98.** Washington CM, Leaver DT. *Principles and Practice of Radiation Therapy — Therapist Edition*. St. Louis: Mosby; 2016.

**99.** *The Medical Dosimetrist's Handbook*. [Year not specified].

**100.** Kak AC, Slaney M. *Tomographic Imaging Handbook*. Philadelphia: SIAM; 2001.

**101.** QARC. *Manuals and Auditing Guidelines for Radiotherapy Trials*. Providence: QARC; [Multiple years].

**102.** Gunderson LL, Tepper JE, editors. *Clinical Radiation Oncology*. 4th ed. Philadelphia: Elsevier; 2016.

**103.** Followill DS. *Practical Guide to Quality Assurance in Radiation Oncology* (Updated). Madison: Medical Physics Publishing; [Year not specified].

**104.** International Atomic Energy Agency (IAEA). *Radiation Oncology Physics: Handbook for Teachers and Students*. Vienna: IAEA; 2005.

**105.** Attix FH, Roesch WC, Tochilin M, editors. *Radiation Dosimetry Volumes I–III*. New York: Academic Press; 1968.

**106.** National Research Council. *The Biological Effects of Low-Level Ionizing Radiation*. Washington: National Academies Press; 1990.

**107.** *Fundamentals of Radiation Biology: Lecture Notes*. [Year not specified].

**108.** International Commission on Radiological Protection (ICRP). *ICRP Publication Series: Recommendations and Reports*. Oxford: Elsevier; [Multiple years].

**109.** National Council on Radiation Protection and Measurements (NCRP). *Shielding, Scatter, and Environmental Reports*. Bethesda: NCRP; [Multiple years].

**110.** Washington CM, Leaver DT. *Therapist's Practical Handbook for External Beam Therapy*. St. Louis: Mosby; 2015.

**111.** *Radiation Therapy: Technology and Techniques — Training Manual*. [Year not specified].

**112.** *Practical Essentials of IMRT Planning and Delivery*. [Year not specified].

**113.** *Principles and Practice of Adaptive Radiation Therapy*. [Year not specified].

**114.** *IGRT Clinical Protocols and Implementation Guides*. [Year not specified].

**115.** Verellen D. *Surface Imaging and Motion Management in Radiotherapy: A Clinical Guide*. [Year not specified].

**116.** *Clinical Radiation Oncology: Disease-Site Management Guides*. [Year not specified].

**117.** *Radiation Oncologist's Pocket Guide to Treatment Planning*. [Year not specified].

**118.** *Radiation Therapist's Handbook: Patient Setup & Immobilization*. [Year not specified].

**119.** *Radiation Therapist's Clinical Procedures Manual*. [Year not specified].

**120.** *Radiotherapy Safety and Emergency Procedures Handbook*. [Year not specified].

**121.** *Radiation Dose Management: Principles and Practice*. [Year not specified].

**122.** *Radiation Protection in Diagnostic and Interventional Radiology*. [Year not specified].

**123.** *Radiation Oncology Workflow and Process Maps: A Practical Guide*. [Year not specified].

**124.** *Clinical Imaging for Radiation Therapy: A Practical Guide*. [Year not specified].

**125.** *Radiation Oncology Dosimetry Protocols: National and International*. [Year not specified].

**126.** *Radiation Therapy Machine Operation: Linear Accelerator User Manuals and Service Guides*. Various manufacturers; [Multiple years].

**127.** *Radiation Oncology Nursing and Patient Care: Practical Handbook*. [Year not specified].

**128.** *Clinical Tutorials in Radiotherapy: Case-Based Learning Manual*. [Year not specified].

**129.** *Radiotherapy Physics: Problem Solving and Worked Examples*. [Year not specified].

**130.** *Radiation Therapy Treatment Planning — Algorithms and Commissioning Guide*. [Year not specified].

**131.** *Radiotherapy Equipment QA: Protocols and Checklists*. [Year not specified].

**132.** Radiation *Protection for the Occupational Worker: Guide and Regulations*. Governmental Publications; [Multiple years].

**133.** *Radiation Biology for Clinicians: Core Concepts*. [Year not specified].

**134.** *Radiobiological Modeling in Treatment Planning*. [Year not specified].

**135.** *Clinical Commissioning of Radiotherapy Services: A Practical Guide*. [Year not specified].

**136.** *Dose Calculation Algorithms: Theory and Practice*. [Year not specified].

**137.** *Radiotherapy Contouring Atlases and Organ-at-Risk Guidelines*. Various oncology societies; [Multiple years].

**138.** ESTRO/ASTRO. *Clinical Practice Guidelines and Protocols*. Brussels/Arlington: ESTRO & ASTRO; [Multiple years].

**139.** ESTRO. *RTT Handbook and Educational Materials*. Brussels: ESTRO; [Multiple years].

**140.** ASTRO. *Evidence-Based Guideline Series for Radiation Oncology*. Arlington: ASTRO; [Multiple years].

**141.** IAEA. *Safety Standards Series: Radiation Protection in Radiotherapy*. Vienna: IAEA; [Multiple years].

**142.** World Health Organization (WHO). *Radiotherapy Programme Guidelines and Technical Publications*. Geneva: WHO; [Multiple years].

**143.** European Commission. *Radiation Protection Reports (RP Series)*. Luxembourg: European Commission; [Multiple years].

**144.** *National Radiotherapy Guidelines — Country-Specific Compilations*. Health Ministry Publications; [Multiple years].

**145.** *Clinical Trials QA and Protocol Manuals: Cooperative Group Publications*. Various QA centers; [Multiple years].

**146.** IAEA. *Dosimetry Protocols: TRS-398 and Successor Documents*. Vienna: IAEA; 2000–present.

**147.** *Clinical Radiobiology: Dose Fractionation and Modeling Texts*. [Year not specified].

**148.** *Radiation Therapy in Pacemaker Patients: Clinical Case Collections*. [Year not specified].

**149.** Varian Medical Systems. *HyperArc™ and VMAT Implementation Guides*. Palo Alto: Varian; [Multiple years].

**150.** *Stereotactic Body Radiation Therapy (SBRT) Clinical Practice Manuals*. [Year not specified].

**151.** *Stereotactic Radiosurgery (SRS) Technical and Clinical Guidelines*. [Year not specified].

**152.** *Brachytherapy: Principles and Practice Textbooks*. [Year not specified].

**153.** *Interventional Radiotherapy: Practical Handbooks*. [Year not specified].

**154.** *Proton Therapy: Clinical Protocols and Physics Textbooks*. [Year not specified].

**155.** *Particle Therapy Physics: Theory and Clinical Implementation*. [Year not specified].

**156.** *Radiotherapy in Pediatric Oncology: Guidelines and Handbooks*. [Year not specified].

**157.** GEC-ESTRO. *Brachytherapy Working Group Reports*. Brussels: ESTRO; [Multiple years].

**158.** *Radiotherapy Dosimetry: Practical Checklists for Clinics*. [Year not specified].

**159.** *Radiotherapy Safety Culture: Practical Manuals for Departments*. [Year not specified].

**160.** *Patient Immobilization and Motion Management: Clinical Handbook*. [Year not specified].

**161.** *Radiotherapy Treatment Verification: CBCT and Portal Imaging Guides*. [Year not specified].

**162.** *Manual Matching vs Automatic Matching in CBCT: Clinical Studies Compendium*. [Year not specified].

**163.** *Interobserver Variability in Image Matching: Methods and Recommendations*. [Year not specified].

**164.** *Radiotherapy Workflow Efficiency: Best Practice Guides*. [Year not specified].

**165.** *RTT-Led Workflows and Scope of Practice: International Position Papers*. [Year not specified].

**166.** *Adaptive Radiotherapy: Clinical Implementation and QA Guides*. [Year not specified].

**167.** *Online Adaptive Radiotherapy (oART): Technical and Clinical Publications*. [Year not specified].

**168.** *Radiation Oncology Education: Lecture Series Compendia*. [Year not specified].

**169.** *Training Manuals for Radiation Therapists: Clinical Competency Guides*. [Year not specified].

**170.** *Professional Practice and Ethics in Radiation Therapy: Handbooks*. [Year not specified].

**171.** *Radiation Therapy Documentation and Record Keeping: Administrative Guides*. [Year not specified].

**172.** *Radiation Oncology Commissioning Checklists: National and International Examples*. [Year not specified].

**173.** *Clinical Implementation of New Technologies: Change Management for RTTs and Physicists*. [Year not specified].

**174.** *Radiotherapy Equipment Acceptance Testing: Protocols and Procedures*. Various manufacturers & AAPM; [Multiple years].

**175.** *Radiation Therapist Competency Frameworks: National Standards and Curricula*. [Year not specified].

**176.** *Patient Counselling and Communication in Radiotherapy: Clinical Guides*. [Year not specified].

**177.** *Radiation Therapy Emergency Procedures: How-To Manuals*. [Year not specified].

**178.** *Clinical Audit in Radiotherapy: Methods and Case Studies*. [Year not specified].

**179.** *Radiotherapy Economics and Resource Planning: Health Systems Guides*. [Year not specified].

**180.** *Radiation Oncology Leadership and Teamwork: Practical Texts*. [Year not specified].

**181.** *Imaging Physics for RTTs: Essentials and Practical Tips*. [Year not specified].

**182.** *Radiotherapy Safety Case Studies: Incident Learning System Manuals*. [Year not specified].

**183.** International Bodies (ICRP/IAEA). *Radiation Protection for Patients: Clinical Recommendations*. Vienna/Oxford: IAEA/ICRP; [Multiple years].

**184.** *Radiation Dose Tracking and Registry Implementation Guides*. [Year not specified].

**185.** *Imaging Artefacts in CBCT and CT: Identification and Correction Guides*. [Year not specified].

**186.** *Plan QA and Secondary Check Systems: Practical Handbooks*. [Year not specified].

**187.** *Radiotherapy Outcome Measurement and Follow-Up: Clinical Guides*. [Year not specified].

**188.** *Radiation Oncology Informatics: Data Management and Interoperability Texts*. [Year not specified].

**189.** *Radiotherapy Physics for Clinical Trials: Protocols and QA Guidance*. Cooperative groups; [Multiple years].

**190.** ESTRO/IAEA/ASTRO. *Radiotherapy Education: Curriculum for RTTs and Trainees*. Brussels/Vienna/Arlington; [Multiple years].

**191.** IAEA. *The Role of Medical Physicists in Radiation Oncology: A Practical Handbook*. Vienna: IAEA; 2019.

**192.** *Practical Radiotherapy: A Handbook for Clinicians and Therapists*. [Year not specified].

**193.** *Radiation Oncology Reference Manuals: Disease-Site Specific Protocols*. [Year not specified].

**194.** *Radiation Oncology Peer-Reviewed Text Collections: State-of-the-Art Reviews*. [Year not specified].

**195.** IAEA/WHO. *Radiotherapy Handbook for Low- and Middle-Income Countries*. Vienna/Geneva: IAEA/WHO; [Multiple years].

**196.** *RAD-AIDE Editorial Framework and Reference Guide (Internal Compendium)*. [Internal publication]; [Year not specified].

**197.** *Manufacturer Service Manuals, QA Tools, and Vendor Protocol Compendium for Radiotherapy Equipment*. Varian/Elekta/Accuray; [Multiple years].

**198.** *Clinical Case-Based Problem Solving in Radiotherapy*. [Year not specified].

**199.** *Advanced Radiotherapy Techniques: A Comprehensive Training Manual*. [Year not specified].

**200.** *Radiation Oncology Comprehensive Reference Compendium — Multi-Disciplinary Edition*. [Year not specified].